# Emergency Triage of the Horse

# Emergency Triage of the Horse

*Edited by*

*Rolfe M. Radcliffe*
*Cornell University*
*Ithaca, NY, USA*

*Jamie J. Kopper*
*Iowa State University*
*Ames, IA, USA*

WILEY

Published by John Wiley & Sons, Inc., Hoboken, New Jersey.



***Library of Congress Cataloging-in-Publication Data***

Names: Radcliffe, Rolfe M. editor | Kopper, Jamie J. editor
Title: Emergency triage of the horse / edited by Rolfe M. Radcliffe, Jamie J. Kopper.
Description: Hoboken, New Jersey : Wiley, [2026] | Includes bibliographical references.
Identifiers: LCCN 2025021872 (print) | LCCN 2025021873 (ebook) | ISBN 9781119817642 cloth | ISBN 9781119817659 adobe pdf | ISBN 9781119817666 epub
Subjects: LCSH: Horses–Diseases–Diagnosis | Horses–Diseases–Treatment | Triage (Medicine) | Veterinary medicine
Classification: LCC SF951 .E49 2026 (print) | LCC SF951 (ebook)
LC record available at https://lccn.loc.gov/2025021872
LC ebook record available at https://lccn.loc.gov/2025021873

Cover Design: Wiley
Cover Images: Courtesy of Rolfe M. Radcliffe

Set in 9.5/12.5pt STIXTwoText by Straive, Pondicherry, India

Printed in Singapore
M117617081225

## Dedication

*Rolfe M. Radcliffe*

*For my family – Erin, Mopane, Sawyer, and Haley. Thanks for your understanding when I was away late into the night as an emergency doctor. Without your love and support, my career and this book would not have been possible.*

*Jamie J. Kopper*

*For my family – Jarrod and Addison. Thank you for your support in pursuing a career in unpredictable emergency medicine. To my mentors for instilling in me a love for all things emergency and supporting me in my growth as a clinician, educator and person. I am incredibly grateful to you all.*

# Contents

## About the Editors

*Rolfe M. Radcliffe, DVM, DACVS, DACVECC*

*Associate Clinical Professor of Large Animal Surgery and Emergency Critical Care, College of Veterinary Medicine, Cornell University, Ithaca, NY, USA*

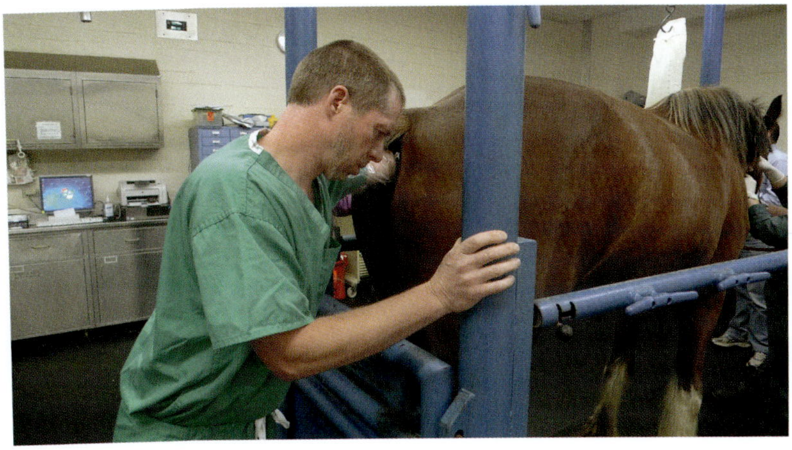

I have an interest and expertise in large animal emergency and critical care medicine and surgery acquired through years of veterinary experience and training. I completed my veterinary school education, and later residency training in Large Animal Surgery under the guidance of Dr. Tracy A. Turner, at the University of Minnesota, College of Veterinary Medicine. In addition, I have several years of both general and referral private practice experience, essential for understanding the challenges and needs of a large animal veterinarian. I have also completed a fellowship in Large Animal Emergency and Critical Care Medicine and Surgery under the mentorship of Dr. Thomas J. Divers at the Cornell University, College of Veterinary Medicine. Since 2005, I have led the Large Animal Emergency and Critical Care service of the Cornell University Large Animal Veterinary Hospital. I also developed and direct a Large Animal Emergency and Critical Care hospital rotation that combines intense clinical training in the field of emergency medicine and surgery together with hands-on clinical case management through our large animal emergency service. A large part of my faculty appointment involves teaching veterinary students and residents in large animal emergency diseases and clinical techniques, as well as contributing toward continuing education programs and collaborative research projects.

*Jamie J. Kopper, DVM, PhD, DACVIM, DACVECC*

*Assistant Professor of Large Animal Internal Medicine and Emergency and Critical Care, College of Veterinary Medicine, Iowa State University, Ames, IA, USA*

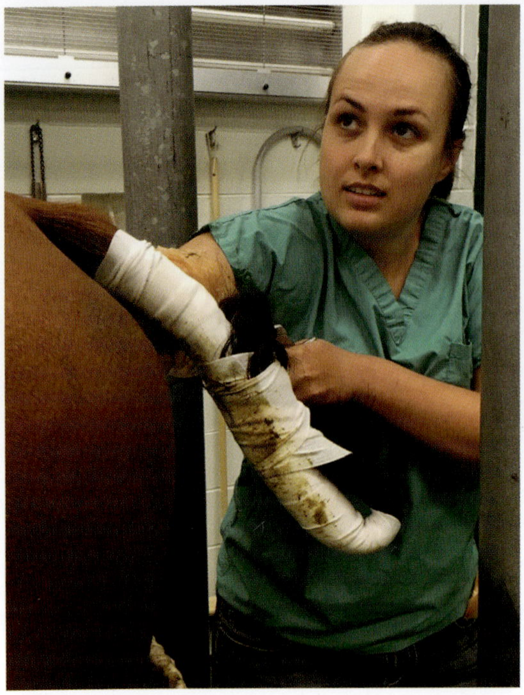

After completing veterinary school at Michigan State University, I subsequently completed an internship at the University of Pennsylvania's New Bolton Center before returning to Michigan State University for residencies in Large Animal Internal Medicine and Emergency and Critical Care. Throughout my training I was fortunate to have mentors who shared their enthusiasm for and love of emergency and critical care medicine and surgery and fostered a similar passion in myself. Since 2017 I have provided critical care services in academic institutions where I have also had the opportunity to share my passion with veterinary students, interns and residents in training. I am a tenure track assistant professor within the Department of Veterinary Clinical Sciences at Iowa State University's College of Veterinary Medicine. Here, I am the service leader for the Equine Internal Medicine service as well as I provide clinical support to the Equine Emergency Service. In addition to providing hands-on training to veterinary students, interns, and residents on the clinical service, I participate in the pre-clinical didactic education of the veterinary students and provide numerous invited continuing education lectures for equine veterinarians at national conferences. Finally, my laboratory focuses on improving survival of horses with gastrointestinal disease, inspired by the cases that we see in the clinic.

## List of Contributors

***Maia R. Aitken***
Department of Clinical Studies - New Bolton Center
University of Pennsylvania School of Veterinary Medicine
Kennett Square, PA
USA

***Mariana Diel de Amorim***
Department of Clinical Sciences
College of Veterinary Medicine
Cornell University
Ithaca, NY
USA

***Karyn Bischoff***
California Animal Health and Food Safety and
Department of Molecular Biosciences
University of California Davis
Davis, CA
USA

***Rebecca Bishop***
Department of Veterinary Clinical Medicine
College of Veterinary Medicine
University of Illinois Urbana-Champaign
Urbana, IL
USA

***Lauren Bookbinder***
Large Animal Clinical Sciences
College of Veterinary Medicine
Michigan State University
East Lansing, MI
USA

***Brandy A. Burgess***
Department of Population Health
College of Veterinary Medicine
University of Georgia
Athens, GA
USA

***Megan Burke***
College of Veterinary Medicine
North Carolina State University
Raleigh, NC
USA

***Soon Hon Cheong***
Department of Clinical Sciences
College of Veterinary Medicine
Cornell University
Ithaca, NY
USA

***Sarah F. Colmer***
Department of Clinical Studies - New Bolton Center
University of Pennsylvania School of Veterinary Medicine
Kennett Square, PA
USA

***Julie Dechant***
Department of Surgical and Radiological Sciences
School of Veterinary Medicine
University of California, Davis
Davis, CA
USA

***Barbara Delvescovo***
Department of Clinical Sciences
College of Veterinary Medicine
Cornell University
Ithaca, NY
USA

***Sally Anne L. DeNotta***
Large Animal Internal Medicine
College of Veterinary Medicine
University of Florida
Gainesville, FL
USA

**Thomas J. Divers**
Department of Clinical Sciences
College of Veterinary Medicine
Cornell University
Ithaca, NY
USA

**Hope F. Douglas**
Department of Clinical Studies - New Bolton Center
University of Pennsylvania School of Veterinary Medicine
Kennett Square, PA
USA

**Norm G. Ducharme**
Department of Clinical Sciences
College of Veterinary Medicine
Cornell University
Ithaca, NY
USA

**Edward T. Earley**
Department of Clinical Sciences
College of Veterinary Medicine
Cornell University
Ithaca, NY
USA

**Rachel Gardner**
BW Furlong and Associates
Oldwick, NJ
USA

**Rebecca (Gimenez) Husted**
Technical Large Animal Emergency Rescue (TLAER)
Macon, GA
USA

**Jenifer R. Gold**
Gold Equine Medical Consulting
Florence, MT
USA

**Erin L. Goodrich**
Animal Health Diagnostic Center
College of Veterinary Medicine
Cornell University
Ithaca, NY
USA

**Eileen S. Hackett**
Department of Clinical Sciences
College of Veterinary Medicine
Cornell University
Ithaca, NY
USA

**Dean A. Hendrickson**
Department of Clinical Sciences
College of Veterinary Medicine and Biomedical Sciences
Colorado State University
Fort Collins, CO
USA

**Klaus Hopster**
Department of Clinical Studies - New Bolton Center
University of Pennsylvania
School of Veterinary Medicine
Kennett Square, PA
USA

**Samuel D. Hurcombe**
Department of Clinical Studies - New Bolton Center
University of Pennsylvania School of Veterinary Medicine
Kennett Square, PA
USA

**Amy L. Johnson**
Department of Clinical Studies - New Bolton Center
University of Pennsylvania School of Veterinary Medicine
Kennett Square, PA
USA

**Kelly Knickelbein**
Department of Clinical Sciences
College of Veterinary Medicine
Cornell University
Ithaca, NY
USA

**Jamie J. Kopper**
Department of Veterinary Clinical Sciences
College of Veterinary Medicine
Iowa State University
Ames, IA
USA

**Laurence Leduc**
Faculté de Medécine Vétérinaire
Département des Sciences Cliniques
Université de Montréal
Saint-Hyacinthe, Quebec
Canada

**Alicia Long**
Department of Clinical Studies - New Bolton Center
University of Pennsylvania School of Veterinary Medicine
Kennett Square, PA
USA

**Elizabeth Williams Louie**
Biomedical and Biological Sciences
College of Veterinary Medicine
Cornell University
Ithaca, NY
USA

**K. Gary Magdesian**
School of Veterinary Medicine, Department of Medicine and Epidemiology
University of California
Davis, CA
USA

**Sue McDonnell**
Department of Clinical Studies - New Bolton Center
University of Pennsylvania School of Veterinary Medicine
Kennett Square, PA
USA

**Rebecca C. McOnie**
Department of Clinical Sciences
College of Veterinary Medicine
Cornell University
Ithaca, NY
USA

**Santiago Mejia**
Cornell Ruffian Equine Specialists (CRES)
College of Veterinary Medicine
Cornell University
Elmont, NY
USA

**Jaime Miller**
Department of Clinical Studies - New Bolton Center
University of Pennsylvania School of Veterinary Medicine
Kennett Square, PA
USA

**Katharyn J. Mitchell**
Department of Clinical Sciences
College of Veterinary Medicine
Cornell University
Ithaca, NY
USA

**Garett Pearson**
Department of Clinical Studies - New Bolton Center
University of Pennsylvania School of Veterinary Medicine
Kennett Square, PA
USA

**John Pigott**
Cornell Ruffian Equine Specialists
Cornell University
Elmont, NY
USA

**Toby L. Pinn-Woodcock**
Animal Health Diagnostic Center
College of Veterinary Medicine
Cornell University
Ithaca, NY
USA

**Brenna R. Pugliese**
North Carolina State University
College of Veterinary Medicine
Raleigh, NC
USA

**Rolfe M. Radcliffe**
Department of Clinical Sciences
College of Veterinary Medicine
Cornell University
Ithaca, NY
USA

**Heidi L. Reesink**
Large Animal Surgery
Department of Clinical Sciences
College of Veterinary Medicine
Cornell University
Ithaca, NY
USA

**Megan Romano**
Department of Veterinary Sciences, Veterinary Diagnostic Laboratory
University of Kentucky
Lexington, KY
USA

**Nicole Scherrer**
Department of Clinical Studies - New Bolton Center
University of Pennsylvania School of Veterinary Medicine
Kennett Square, PA
USA

**Eric L. Schroeder**
Galbreath Equine Center, College of Veterinary Medicine
The Ohio State University
Columbus, OH
USA

***Cristobal Navas de Solis***
Department of Clinical Studies - New Bolton Center
University of Pennsylvania School of Veterinary Medicine
Kennett Square, PA
USA

***Meri Stratton***
Clinical Veterinary Nutritionist and President
All Creatures Veterinary Nutrition Consulting, Inc.
Fairfield, CA
USA

***Joy E. Tomlinson***
Department of Clinical Studies - New Bolton Center
University of Pennsylvania School of Veterinary Medicine
Kennett Square, PA
USA

***Cade Torcivia***
Department of Clinical Studies - New Bolton Center
University of Pennsylvania School of Veterinary Medicine
Kennett Square, PA
USA

***Jarrod Troy***
Department of Veterinary Clinical Sciences
College of Veterinary Medicine
Iowa State University
Ames, IA
USA

***Ashlee E. Watts***
College of Veterinary Medicine and Biomedical Sciences
Texas A&M University
College Station, TX
USA

***Pamela Wilkins***
Departments of Veterinary Clinical Medicine and
Comparative Biosciences
College of Veterinary Medicine
University of Illinois Urbana-Champaign
Urbana, IL
USA

***Alexandra L. Wright***
Department of Clinical Sciences
College of Veterinary Medicine
Cornell University
Ithaca, NY
USA

***Cynthia Xue***
Department of Clinical Sciences
School of Veterinary Medicine
Ross University
Basseterre, St. Kitts
West Indies

# Prologue

Horses are impressive animals that have been domesticated and highly regarded by human civilizations for thousands of years. Horses have changed the lives of people in momentous ways throughout the advancement of human culture and continue to provide important functions for human societies as both working and pleasure animals. Veterinary medicine developed around the health of the horse because of people's dependence on the horse for various tasks from transportation, agriculture, and war time support to shipping, commerce, and sport.

Advances in the human and veterinary medical fields flourished during the last century and continue to develop at a rapid pace. Emergency and critical care medicine and surgery only recently blossomed in veterinary medicine over the last three decades and advances continue in both large and small animals (Mathews 2017). Emergency triage in human medicine is an older field – dating to the 1960s, and its scope and importance continue to evolve (Suter 2012).

Veterinarians often look to human physicians for guidance on emerging ideas and techniques since they often lead the medical field. Similarly, we can look to our human colleagues for advice on emergency triage and learn from their mistakes and experiences.

More than three decades have passed since the publication of "The Ten Commandments of Emergency Medicine" where Wrenn and Slovis provided emergency doctors with guidance on triage of the critically ill human patient (Wrenn and Slovis 1991). Recently, Evans and Slovis updated this editorial, providing a resident's perspective (Evans and Slovis 2020).

The editors are excited to present the first "Ten commandments of Equine Emergency Medicine" as applied to the horse, and based upon the recommendations from Wrenn, Evans, and Slovis.

*Ten commandments of Equine Emergency Medicine*:

1) *Secure the ABCs quickly, carefully, and safely*
2) *Remember fluids, electrolytes, oxygen, and glucose*
3) *Always perform a thorough physical exam*
4) *Assume the worst and prioritize triage over diagnosis*
5) *Stabilize patients first and triage effectively*
6) *Look for the common red flags*
7) *Trust no one, believe nothing (not even yourself)*
8) *Learn from your mistakes*
9) *Do unto others as you would your family (including clients, colleagues, trainers, and referring veterinarians)*
10) *When in doubt, always err on the side of the patient*

## 1. Secure the ABCs Quickly, Carefully, and Safely

The most important aspect of emergency triage is stabilization of the patient's airway, breathing and circulation (Wrenn and Slovis 1991; Evans and Slovis 2020). Specifically, the veterinarian should act to ensure the airway is patent, the patient's ventilation is adequate, and the cardiovascular function is sufficient (Chapter 1 – *How to triage emergency conditions in the horse*). Securing these vital parameters first will allow continued safe evaluation and management of the horse whether medical or surgical treatment is indicated. In human medicine, an ABCDE approach to emergency triage assessment has been described and is considered standard of care (Thim et al. 2012). The letters D and E represent the level of Disability or consciousness and Exposure of the body to look for any problems, respectively. Wrenn and Slovis expanded ABCDE to ABCDEFG, adding F and G; the letter F stands for Fetal viability, an essential part of evaluation for the pregnant female patient. The letter G in humans represents injury from falling off the stretcher and a reminder to always ensure the guard rails are in place. In the horse, the authors propose G stands for danGer. Horses are potentially dangerous animals, and when injured or sick they become more unpredictable and the risk of human injury increases. Veterinarians must prioritize human safety for themselves and all others working near the animal.

*ABCDEFG emergency triage of horses*:

A – secure animal's Airway
B – maintain adequate Breathing
C – ensure sufficient Cardiovascular function
D – evaluate level of consciousness or Disability
E – perform thorough physical Exam
F – assess Fetal viability in pregnant mare
G – prioritize human safety as horses are danGerous

## 2. Remember Fluids, Electrolytes, Oxygen, and Glucose

Emergency fluid resuscitation is the foundation of veterinary emergency critical care, and targeted fluid therapy is invaluable in both primary and referral clinical practice. Fluid therapy with crystalloids and colloids will help stabilize the cardiovascular system and restore tissue and organ oxygenation in states of hypovolemia and shock. Electrolytes are an important step in emergency assessment as many conditions result from or are exasperated by electrolyte abnormalities. Oxygen therapy via face mask, intranasal or intratracheal routes in the critical equine patient is a simple, effective step for stabilizing animals suffering cardiorespiratory problems or other critical illness. The provision of nutritional support via glucose or other treatments should be considered with all emergency cases in horses, especially those that are malnourished, chronically ill, or have not eaten for several days.

## 3. Always Perform a Thorough Physical Exam

Emergency problems in horses may result from disease, injury, or abnormalities with many body systems. A concise, preliminary evaluation will guide emergency triage, and, in many situations, veterinarians must work quickly to stabilize the animal. Following patient stabilization, a more focused clinical exam is indicated to assess the affected body system(s). This exam should be focused yet thorough to avoid missing associated problems, complications, or sequalae. For example, a horse suffering thoracic trauma may initially need the following for emergency stabilization: close or bandage open chest wounds, control hemorrhage if required, remove pleural air, provide intranasal oxygen therapy, administer intravenous fluids, antibiotic, and anti-inflammatory medications. Once stable, a focused examination of the thoracic and abdominal cavities is indicated to determine the extent of injury. This may include palpation of the chest wall for asymmetry or signs of chest wall instability and rib fracture, thoracic and abdominal auscultation and ultrasound, rectal palpation, thoracic and/or abdominal fluid collection, and evaluation of the patient for other extra-thoracic injury.

## 4. Assume the Worst and Prioritize Triage Over Diagnosis

Remember it is the primary goal of the emergency clinician to identify or rule out problems that are life-threatening (Evans and Slovis 2020). We must consider the most serious problems that could be associated with a given clinical sign, even if they are unlikely (Wrenn and Slovis 1991). To do this effectively, veterinarians should work to identify problems that require emergency attention and not focus on obtaining a diagnosis. For example, it is not paramount to know that a horse with colic has colitis versus a large colon volvulus, but rather to make the correct decision for medical or surgical management. Once that decision is made, securing the diagnosis parallels triage, and if the patient's condition deteriorates despite management, re-evaluation of that initial decision is appropriate. Making the correct triage decisions is the foundation of emergency medicine whether human or horse.

## 5. Stabilize Patients First and Triage Effectively

Emergency stabilization of humans, horses, and other animals is the primary responsibility of the emergency clinician; and effective triage skills are essential. Navigating the triage of a critical horse patient requires knowledge, experience, and leadership. *Knowledge*: the clinician must consider the various clinical problems and diseases that may cause various clinical signs; *experience*: nothing replaces experience for stabilizing a sick or injured horse; *leadership*: effective clinicians will be able to manage the situation to secure the safety of themselves and others, and to provide quick decisions for management. Most horses with emergency conditions present with some degree of hypovolemia, and fluid therapy is one foundation of patient stabilization. Other life-saving triage decisions may include blood transfusion for acute hemorrhage, limb stabilization for long bone fractures, tracheostomy for respiratory distress, and fetal manipulation for dystocia.

## 6. Look for the Common Red Flags

Because emergency triage happens quickly with limited medical history and patient information, understanding important signs and problems to look for in patients will help guide effective triage (Wrenn and Slovis 1991). First and foremost, evaluation of a horse's vital signs is indicated: *Heart Rate, Respiratory Rate, Body Temperature, and Blood Pressure*. Effective triage depends upon early recognition of disease, and these vital parameters help detect problems and guide decision making. For example, a horse with a high respiratory rate or labored breathing will receive respiratory support (e.g., intranasal oxygen or tracheostomy) and a focused respiratory exam. Second, an animal's age – especially neonates and older horses – may have unique comorbidities that affect management. For example, foals are more likely to be hypoglycemic or hypotensive secondary to many types of problems including sepsis, colic, respiratory disease, cardiac abnormalities, neurologic disease, or trauma, and this must be addressed during emergency triage and patient stabilization. Third, suspicion should arise whenever an animal re-presents for the same emergency problem as this may signal a failure of initial treatment, misdiagnosis, or secondary complications. Other red flags may also include important information such as acute vs chronic disease, response to therapy, degree of lameness, or severity of pain.

## 7. Trust No One, Believe Nothing (Not Even Yourself)

Emergency triage decisions often occur in the background of incomplete or inaccurate histories, presenting complaints or other medical information (Evans and Slovis 2020). It is the responsibility of the emergency clinician to confirm the patient information and verify the medical history. In addition, it is important to listen carefully to the client concerns and the advice of colleagues to make sure you are following the pertinent path forward. Emergency clinicians should keep an open mind during triage as serious errors may occur when we follow our initial perception and do not consider new evidence or opinions (Wrenn and Slovis 1991). Remember that medical errors may be prevented by not following others blindly, but rather checking and rechecking your own decisions. Strive to follow the evidence and facts based upon scientific discovery rather than abide by tradition and lore. Lastly, never be afraid to ask for help or admit uncertainty when working in emergency medicine.

## 8. Learn from Your Mistakes

Mistakes are an inevitable part of life and human and veterinary medicine are no exception. Expect to make mistakes; however, how you respond to those mistakes is most important. Strive to embrace your mistakes and learn from them (Wrenn and Slovis 1991). Mistakes can be an important path to learning if you take the opportunity to develop and grow. Try not to dwell on your mistakes, instead move on with the knowledge you have gained. How you respond to the mistakes of others is equally important. Do not disparage other people's mistakes, but rather help them through the experience and learn together.

## 9. Do Unto Others as You Would Your Family (Including Families Different from Yours, Colleagues, and Coworkers)

How you treat the owners and families of emergency animal patients is arguably more important than your medical knowledge and triage skills. Working as a veterinarian involves building close relationships, trust, honesty, and empathy with their human owners. We service both animals and humans, and to be an effective clinician we must respect, understand, and help owners, often through the challenging times of an emergency crisis. Such respect and empathy also apply to our coworkers who often support our veterinary mission with little recognition or thanks. As veterinarians we depend heavily on our support staff whether it be our colleagues, secretaries, interns, residents, technicians, or janitorial workers and it behooves us to treat them with our full respect.

## 10. When in Doubt Always Err on the Side of the Patient

Human and veterinary medicine are full of challenges. Both fields are advancing rapidly with large volumes of information and disease conditions to understand and apply (Evans and Slovis 2020). In Veterinary Medicine we do not have the ability to speak with our patients, and a concise, yet thorough, physical exam and history are fundamental aspects of triage. In many situations – especially emergency critical care medicine – we make decisions without a diagnosis or a comprehensive understanding of the problem. When in doubt always think about what is best for the patient. Try to limit how a patient's clinical picture, prognosis, or other factors (such as time, other commitments, and client concerns) may affect patient care. Always advocate for the patient (which may include recommending euthanasia) and work to limit suffering.

The 10 commandments of Equine Emergency Medicine will guide clinicians working in the veterinary medical field. The authors thank Wrenn, Slovis, and Evans for their leadership in the human field, providing the foundation for its application to veterinary medicine. As we reflect on the above commandments, we stress the following when triaging an emergent horse or foal.

1) Secure the breathing and circulation first
2) Perform a thorough yet focused physical exam
3) Prioritize triage over seeking a diagnosis
4) Learn from your own and others' mistakes
5) Always advocate for the patient

Also remember the practice of medicine is part art and part science, and we are helping both people and animals as we practice our trade. The future of human and veterinary medicine is unknown; what lies ahead is likely inspiring, but also challenging. As we face the inevitable advances in medicine, emergency clinicians should not forget the importance of the patient exam and the commandments that were succinctly outlined by Wrenn, Slovis, and Evans for humans, and applied here to the horse.

## References


Evans, C.S. and Slovis, C.M. (2020). Revisiting the ten commandments of emergency medicine: a resident's perspective. *Ann. Emerg. Med.* 77 (3): 367–370.

Mathews, K.A. (2017). Emergency and critical care medicine: an essential component of all specialties and practices. *Front. Vet. Sci.* 4: 165. https://doi.org/10.3389/fvets.2017.00165.

Suter, R.E. (2012, 2012). Emergency medicine in the United States: a systemic review. *World. J. Emerg. Med.* 3 (1): 5–10. https://doi.org/10.5847/wjem.j.1920-8642.2012.01.001.

Thim, T. et al. (2012). Initial assessment and treatment with the airway, breathing, circulation, disability, exposure (ABCDE) approach. *Int. J. Gen. Med.* 5: 117–121.

Wrenn, K. and Slovis, C.M. (1991). The ten commandments of emergency medicine. *Ann. Emerg. Med.* 20 (10): 1146–1147.

# Foreword

I am honored to have been asked to write this foreword to Drs. Radcliffe and Kopper's textbook entitled, *Emergency Triage of the Horse*. I have a long-time interest in equine emergency medicine, beginning with my ambulatory internship at the University of California, Davis where my first written notes were for veterinary students: a hand-typed, 25-page guide (which I still have) on equine emergencies. There have been so many advances in equine emergency medicine and surgery since then! My interest in equine emergencies as a discipline was further stimulated later when my close colleague and friend, Dr. Doug Byars, suggested to Dr. Fairfield Bain and myself that the three of us should complete the training and examination required to be members of the American College of Veterinary Emergency and Critical Care (ACVECC). Doug had attended both human and small animal emergency and critical care meetings and was convinced that much of the knowledge from those conferences could be applied to equine practice. Henceforth, the three of us became the first equine veterinarians to train for and pass the examination to gain entrance into the ACVECC. There are now ACVECC-trained equine veterinarians at many universities and several private practices.

I had the great pleasure of mentoring Dr. Radcliffe during his pursuit of ACVECC certification. Both Dr. Radcliffe, a board-certified equine surgeon, and Dr. Kopper, a board-certified equine internist, are also board-certified in emergency and critical care and have now produced a textbook, *Emergency Triage of the Horse*. This book should complement other outstanding equine textbooks as it uniquely focuses on stabilizing and triaging horses needing emergency care while also offering advice on choosing the most important diagnostic tests for the emergency equine patient. In addition, the book provides other important information often required in the immediate management of the equine emergency, such as biosecurity, anesthesia management, nutritional support, and welfare response, to name a few. The co-editors have recruited an outstanding group of chapter authors who provide pertinent information that will help practitioners triage equine emergencies. Most chapters in the book are organized by clinical signs and body system, making it easy to quickly find the important triage information. I know how much effort is required to author a book like this and applaud Drs. Radcliffe and Kopper for completing this project. Although any monetary reward is modest compared to the work required to edit a quality textbook, Drs. Radcliffe and Kopper's greatest reward for their labors will be practitioners telling them that the textbook has provided valuable information for triaging equine emergencies and improving healthcare for the horse.

*Thomas J. Divers, Professor Emeritus, Cornell University*

# Preface

*Of this I am assured, that he (or she) will be the best practitioner who begins his (or her) life work as a student among patients, learning for himself (or herself) under guidance how to observe, how to think, learning what disease is and how it is to be treated.*

—William Osler

The Natural Method of Teaching the Subject of Medicine, *JAMA* 36:1673–1679, 1901

Learning through experience remains a cornerstone of human and veterinary medical training, and guidance through mentorship and written works are important for such learning.

Several textbooks are available to the veterinarian working with emergency problems of horses.

However, our book is unique. Unique because our book is a manual to use in your daily work – your guide during *triage*. Unique because the authors share their extensive knowledge and experience and answer important questions about the method and art of effective triage. Unique because the authors guide the reader on how to triage emergency problems – "what is the disease and how to treat it." Unique because they mentor the reader on what questions to ask, what things to look for, and what things to monitor – "how to observe." Finally, unique because the authors provide clinical examples to illustrate the principles and thought processes important during triage and how to make challenging decisions – "how to think."

They discuss the important steps in effective triage:

1) How to stabilize patients
2) How to formulate a diagnostic plan
3) How to treat beyond stabilization

They guide the veterinarian on how to proceed under varying circumstances:

1) What can be done at the farm
2) What can be done at the referral hospital
3) How to decide when timing is critical

They offer advice on how to make important decisions:

1) How to decide between medical vs surgical treatment
2) How to manage important complications
3) How to estimate prognosis and decide for euthanasia

This is the first edition of *Emergency Triage of the Horse*. The 2 editors and 54 contributing authors are experts in the field of emergency and critical care medicine and surgery. The book is composed of five parts, including 35 chapters and 6 appendices. The first four parts guide the reader in effective triage:

Part 1 – Emergency Triage Methods and Techniques
Part 2 – Emergency Conditions of the Horse
Part 3 – Specific Problems in Horses and Donkeys
Part 4 – Support of the Emergency Patient

Part 5 provides valuable references important during triage:

Appendix 1 – Reference Values for Adult Horses, Foals and Adult Donkeys
Appendix 2 – Equine Emergency Medications and Fluids
Appendix 3 – Emergency Treatment Protocols
Appendix 4 – Resuscitation Guidelines in the Horse (online)
Appendix 5 – Biosecurity and Isolation Protocols (online)
Appendix 6 – Calculations in Emergency Medicine (online)

The editors and contributing authors hope the *Emergency Triage of the Horse* guides you like a trusted mentor, whether you are a new student, developing resident, or experienced faculty, and whether you happen to be on the phone, at the farm, or in the hospital.

*Rolfe M. Radcliffe*
November 2024 *Jamie J. Kopper*

## Acknowledgments

The editors would like to thank the wonderful team at Wiley, especially Erica Judisch, Judit Anbu Hena Daniel, Vallikannu Narayanan, Susan Engelken and Merryl Le Roux, who were able to efficiently guide us through the challenges of our first book project. A special thank you to Erica, our executive editor, who inspired and encouraged Dr. Radcliffe to pursue this project for so many years. The editors would also like to acknowledge the help of our amazing authors who have shared their noteworthy experiences and worked hard to bring this material to the reader. We are also indebted to our colleagues and mentors who have unselfishly shared their knowledge and inspired a younger generation to follow their lead. A special thank you to Drs. Thomas Divers, Susan Fubini, Norm Ducharme, Alan Nixon and Lisa Fortier who have always been willing to provide advice and guidance for Dr. Radcliffe during his tenure at Cornell University. And to our residents, students and technicians who have been there, by our side, late into the night on our veterinary journey.

## About the Companion Website

This book is accompanied by a companion website:

**www.wiley.com/go/radcliffe/triage**

The website includes:

- Additional content in Chapter 3: Emergency Supplies and Equipment for Triage
- Additional content in Chapter 9: Oral and Maxillofacial Emergencies
- Additional content in Chapter 12: Cardiovascular Emergencies
- Appendix 4 – Resuscitation Guidelines in the Horse
- Appendix 5 – Biosecurity and Isolation Protocols
- Appendix 6 – Calculations in Emergency Medicine

# Part 1

# Emergency Triage Methods and Techniques

# 1

# How to Triage Emergency Conditions in the Horse

*Rolfe M. Radcliffe*[1] *and Jamie J. Kopper*[2]

[1] *Department of Clinical Sciences, College of Veterinary Medicine, Cornell University, Ithaca, NY, USA*
[2] *Department of Veterinary Clinical Sciences, College of Veterinary Medicine, Iowa State University, Ames, IA, USA*

## Introduction

Effective triage of emergency problems is the foundation of veterinary and human critical care medicine (Mathews 2017, Wrenn and Slovis 1991, Evans and Slovis 2020). Astute clinicians must work quickly with limited information to make life-and-death decisions, often under stressful circumstances. Learning how to triage in emergency medicine will help you make these decisions even when the case information is lacking or confusing. Below the editors outline the important triage steps, followed by an example of thoracic injury to illustrate such triage in an emergency patient.

## Emergency Triage Steps

### Step 1: Patient Stabilization

The priority of emergency triage is to ensure patient survival. This will vary with the type and severity of the emergency condition. For example, some problems require immediate attention such as performing a tracheostomy in a horse with respiratory obstruction, while others may be stable and allow for further evaluation. The most important task is to quickly assess the patient to determine the need for emergency intervention (Wrenn and Slovis 1991, Evans and Slovis 2020, Thim et al., 2012) (see Prologue).

a) Secure the patient's airway, breathing, and circulation, and begin immediate life-support measures if needed.
b) Perform a concise, focused exam on the affected body system(s).
c) Treat emergent medical problems, such as shock, fractured limb, pneumothorax, or other problems based upon preliminary exam.
d) Establish venous access and administer the appropriate fluids or other medications.
e) Reassess the patient frequently to determine success of initial stabilization and the need for further emergency support.

### Step 2: Formulating a Diagnostic Plan

Once the animal is stable, additional diagnostic testing is often valuable to help guide further treatment. Remember your goal should be to provide the best outcome for the animal and client, not necessarily to provide the correct diagnosis. Therefore, appropriate triage should focus on patient stabilization and supportive care followed by specific treatments for medical diseases, and early referral for surgical problems.

*Emergency Triage of the Horse*, First Edition. Edited by Rolfe M. Radcliffe and Jamie J. Kopper.

Published 2026 by John Wiley & Sons, Inc.
Companion website: www.wiley.com/go/radcliffe/triage

#### In the Field

When in the field, and lacking diagnostic support, the clinician should follow his or her intuition and make decisions based upon several factors, including physical exam findings and serial patient monitoring, as well as the response to initial stabilization and treatment. Remember to follow the guidelines above, providing immediate patient stabilization before looking for a diagnosis. Let's look at the example of a horse with acute colic. An important guideline for evaluating horses with colic is monitoring the response to sedation or analgesia. Most horses with a surgical problem will have episodes of recurrent pain despite analgesia or other medical treatments. One of the key principles of emergency colic triage is recommending referral for horses non-responsive to or exhibiting recurrent pain despite analgesic administration. Other factors that may also prompt referral are abnormal rectal palpation or ultrasound exams suggestive of a surgical problem, abnormal peritoneal fluid (e.g., serosanguinous), progressive abdominal distention, high heart and respiratory rates, large amounts of gastric reflux, and patient deterioration despite medical management. Remember that several of these same findings (e.g., high HR and RR, reflux, abnormal rectal and ultrasound exams) may also present in horses with medical conditions. However, it is prudent to recommend early referral when a surgical problem is possible and with horses not responding to medical treatment.

#### In the Hospital

With patients in a hospital, specific testing for common sequelae is indicated once the patient is stable. For example, horses presenting with acute colic signs often require immediate stabilization via fluid therapy for hypovolemia and analgesics for pain control. Monitoring the response to such patient stabilization is an important diagnostic step during emergency triage. Horses with acute colic should also receive nasogastric intubation to assess the gastric contents early in your examination; horses with distended small intestine are susceptible to gastric rupture with strangulating small intestinal lesions. Stomach impaction may also be suspected based upon the inability to pass the nasogastric tube completely into the stomach. Once the cardiovascular deficits and pain are addressed, and the stomach has been evaluated for reflux, additional testing is indicated to make the best decision for continued medical vs surgical treatment. Such testing for a horse with colic may include rectal palpation, CBC and chemistry panels, abdominal fluid evaluation, abdominal ultrasound, and abdominal radiography.

### Step 3: Emergency Treatment Guidelines

Following emergency patient stabilization and initial diagnostic testing, specific treatment is often indicated for the clinical problem. Such treatment will vary with the type of emergency and will be based upon the physical exam findings, diagnostic testing, patient monitoring, and response to stabilization. Some horses may receive only supportive treatments and then monitoring pending further diagnostics, while others may require specific medical or surgical treatment.

#### In the Field

Many emergency treatments may be performed in the field, and often these procedures are essential for patient stabilization. A colicky horse with a suspected large colon impaction may receive analgesics, anti-spasmotic drugs, oral cathartics or laxatives, and fluid therapy, while another horse with a nephrosplenic entrapment may also receive phenylephrine followed by exercise as part of the early directed treatment plan. Horses having marked abdominal distention associated with obstructive diseases of the large intestine may benefit from per-cutaneous decompression of the large colon. Exceptions to field emergency treatment include horses that are violently painful, dangerous, or difficult to restrain.

#### In the Hospital

For other horses, hospital referral may be the best option for management. When a horse or foal has a life-threatening injury where advanced treatments or surgery are required, early recommendation for referral is indicated. For example, when a surgical lesion is suspected in a colic horse based upon the presenting clinical signs, physical exam findings, specific testing, and response to analgesic medications or other treatments, referral for surgery should be discussed with the owner. In other cases, the horse may require advanced diagnostic imaging or testing to determine the next step in management. For example, a horse with a laceration into a synovial structure may require both diagnostic and surgical support, unavailable to many clinicians in private equine practice.

## Step 4: Assessment and Monitoring

Frequent physical examination, reassessment, and monitoring is critical for the management of emergency patients. For horses with colic, repeating the physical exam, rectal and ultrasound, abdominal fluid, and essential blood work during triage will improve decision making. Many sequelae are possible with emergency problems and monitoring patients during triage will help direct life-saving treatment. For example, horses with colic may develop endotoxemia, laminitis, post-operative ileus, peritonitis, adhesions, and other problems associated with the primary disease. In addition, the progression of disease often changes following stabilization and frequent assessments will allow timely redirection of therapy.

## Step 5: Decision Making During Triage

### Referral vs Farm Management

The goal of the emergency clinician is to make the best decision for the horse based upon the circumstances. For example, a colic horse with uncontrollable pain, non-responsive to analgesics should be directed for referral directly following patient stabilization if that is even possible. If the client cannot afford referral of the horse, your options are limited on the farm to continued medical management or euthanasia. For horses with medical causes of colic, such as colitis or enteritis, referral may also be indicated for severe disease and where management cannot be accomplished on the farm. For horses with colic, when referral is not possible, humane euthanasia should be recommended for animals with severe, unrelenting pain, non-responsive to analgesics, horses with recurrent pain, and where a surgical lesion is confirmed or highly suspected.

### Medical vs Surgical Treatment

Emergency clinicians often face the decision of whether to pursue medical vs surgical treatment. Further, when surgery is necessary, standing vs general anesthesia is another important consideration. When possible medical or conservative treatment and standing over general anesthesia should be elected to reduce added complications. For horses presenting with colic, many factors will help guide the decision for medical vs surgical treatment. Colic horses with the following should be referred for surgery:

1) Severe, unrelenting pain, non-responsive to analgesics or chronic, recurrent pain.
2) Abnormal rectal exam consistent with a surgical problem.
3) Abnormal ultrasound suggesting a surgical lesion.
4) Abnormal peritoneal fluid (e.g., serosanguinous, elevated total nucleated and red blood cell counts, twice peritoneal compared to systemic L-lactate).
5) Progressive abdominal distention (large intestinal diseases).
6) Progressive deterioration of patient's cardiovascular status or other parameters despite medical management.
7) Lack of borborygmi, high heart rate, large amounts of gastric reflux (not specific for a surgical lesion, but present in many cases).

### Managing Complications

Complications are common in emergency medicine and the presenting problem or sequelae may be life-threatening. When triaging emergent conditions in horses, clinicians should consider what complications are most likely to recognize and address such problems early. For example, horses with colic may develop many sequelae including endotoxemia, ileus, laminitis, peritonitis, adhesions, and recurrent colic among other problems. Complications should be discussed with owners early in case management.

### Estimating Prognosis

Providing an accurate prognosis for horse owners is often challenging during emergency triage because of the limited information available. The response to patient stabilization is valuable for initial estimates until more diagnostic information is known. Serial monitoring will also help guide prognosis and the need for further treatment or surgery. Many retrospective studies or other peer-reviewed literature sources often report a range of survival information that may be helpful to clinicians when discussing prognosis, the decision for various treatment options or euthanasia with clients.

### Decision for Euthanasia

Making the decision to euthanize an animal is one of the most difficult choices facing veterinarians. This decision should be made only after careful consideration of the circumstances, available treatment options, and welfare of the horse. Many different diseases and problems of horses may warrant consideration of euthanasia such as incurable disease, chronic severe pain, severe traumatic injury, inoperable colic, and dangerous behavioral traits. Excellent guidelines for euthanasia of horses and other animals are summarized by the AAEP and AVMA. Remember the veterinarian must always act as an advocate for the horse – whether recommending euthanasia for severe disease or denying it when unjustified.

**Case Example 1.1 Thoracic Trauma**

Patient: *18-year-old Appaloosa gelding*

History: *Impaled on a wooden post several hours prior to presentation. A 10 cm laceration was identified in R axilla at the location of injury. Horse was in respiratory distress with difficulty breathing and marked pain* (Figure 1.1a, b).

Step 1: Patient Stabilization

Provide immediate stabilization steps (Hassel 2007, Laverty et al. 1996, Radcliffe et al. 2009, Sprayberry and Barrett, 2015) (see Chapter 7: wounds, trauma, and other injury):

1) *Bandage or pack thoracic wounds quickly.*
2) *Provide intranasal oxygen.*
3) *Remove pleural air.*
4) *Provide fluids, pain control, anti-inflammatory and antibiotic medications.*

Perform a quick, yet focused patient assessment to evaluate the following:

1) *Respiratory rate, effort and evidence of distress.*
2) *Evaluate mucous membranes for perfusion status.*
3) *Wounds that may penetrate the chest cavity.*
4) *Palpate and examine chest wall for rib fractures, symmetry, and stability.*

(a)

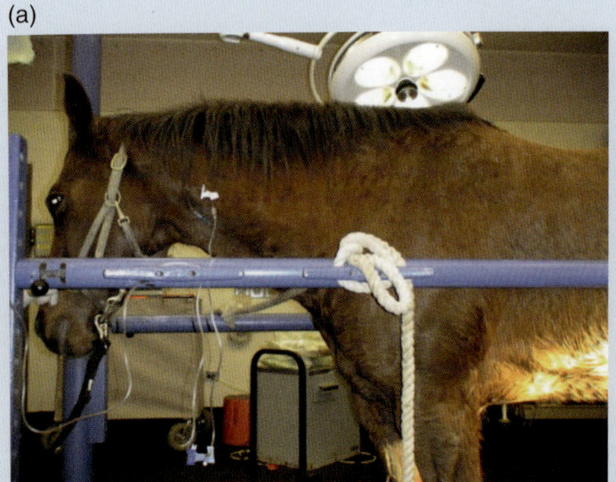

(b)

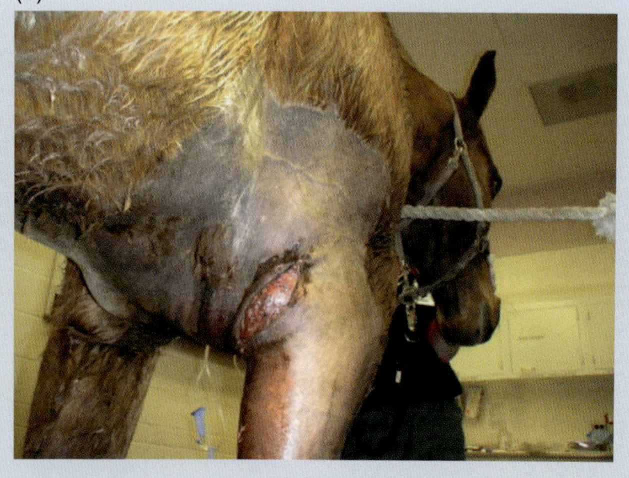

**Figure 1.1** An 18-year-old Appaloosa gelding several hours following impalement on a wooden fence post in the right axillary region (a, b). The horse presented in severe respiratory distress with elevated heart and respiratory rates (84 and 44, respectively), abnormal and absent lungs sounds bilaterally, evidence of thoracic asymmetry, and marked pain during respiration. Immediate stabilization included sealing the chest wound, intranasal oxygen delivery, and removal of pleural air.

- Wounds to the thorax may lead to open or tension pneumothorax. Listening during breathing will help determine if wounds communicate with the chest cavity.
- Sealing and bandaging thoracic wounds early will help limit the progression of pneumothorax. If tension pneumothorax is suspected, open the chest wound or perform thoracocentesis.
- Removal of pleural air may be accomplished via placement of a 4-in. teat cannula or thoracic trocar high in the 12–15 intercostal space (see Chapters 4 and 5: basic and advanced clinical triage procedures).

Step 2: Formulating a Diagnostic Plan

Once the horse is stable, further assess the animal to determine the extent of injury and development of possible sequelae (Hassel 2007, Laverty et al. 1996, Radcliffe et al. 2009, Sprayberry and Barrett, 2015):

1) *Pneumomediastinum and pneumothorax.*
2) *Hemorrhage into the pleural cavity (hemothorax).*
3) *Subcutaneous emphysema.*
4) *Rib fracture and flail chest.*
5) *Diaphragmatic hernia.*
6) *Pleuritis and pleuropneumonia (later following injury).*
7) *Specific thoracic or abdominal injury.*
   - Assessment of the above problems will require astute physical exam skills and serial patient monitoring as many of these problems will develop over time. For example, subcutaneous emphysema may occur following wounds (especially to the axillary or inguinal regions), and dissection of the air beneath the skin and along facial planes may lead to pneumomediastinum or pneumothorax.
   - Involvement of the abdomen should also be considered with blunt or penetrating thoracic injury because the crus of the diaphragm extends cranial to the level of the $6^{th}$ rib in the horse. Ultrasound and radiography are valuable tools to assist with thorough evaluation following thoracic trauma.

Step 3: Emergency Treatment Guidelines

Following initial stabilization and diagnostic evaluation, further specific treatment is indicated (Hassel 2007, Radcliffe et al. 2009).

- Many horses with thoracic injury may require continuous removal of pleural air and or fluid; placement of a thoracic trocar is indicated in such horses. For removal of pleural air and fluid, trocars may be placed into both the dorsal and ventral aspects of the thoracic cavity, respectively (Figure 1.2). Alternatively, an active suction device may be used (e.g., Pleur-evac Chest Drainage System) that will remove fluid and air via one portal.

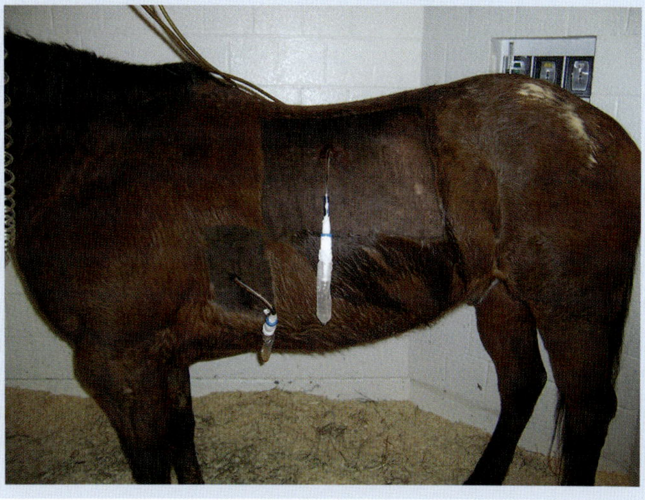

**Figure 1.2** The left hemithorax of the Appaloosa horse with thoracic injury. Chest tube placement was performed for the initial stabilization of this horse and for ongoing removal of pleural air during treatment. The horse had both hemorrhage (hemothorax) and air (pneumothorax) present bilaterally within the pleural cavity. Note the ventral tube placed for fluid removal, and the dorsal one for evacuation of air from left hemithorax of the horse.

- Once the horse is stable, conservative or surgical treatments may also be indicated depending upon the severity of injury. Wounds communicating with the thoracic cavity may require debridement, lavage, and packing with sterile saline-soaked gauze as part of conservative treatment or until more specific therapy may be performed (Figure 1.3).
- As a guideline, horses with superficial trauma, simple rib fractures, and normal ventilatory mechanics will respond to conservative treatment via standing sedation and local analgesia. However, horses having multiple or displaced rib fractures, flail chest, deep penetrating injury, suspected lung laceration, or involvement of the abdominal cavity may require surgery under general anesthesia using positive-pressure ventilation.

Step 4: Assessment and Monitoring

Serial patient monitoring is essential during emergency triage because horses suffering thoracic trauma may develop serious complications even several days or longer following injury.

- Routine assessment should include a physical exam including monitoring of respiratory and heart rates, respiratory effort, dyspnea or distress, and quality of ventilation.
- For example, horses with rib fractures often display severe pain that interferes with a normal ventilatory pattern. Such horses require attention to analgesia, and a multimodal approach using both systemic and local analgesic techniques often proves valuable (Figure 1.4). In addition, rib fractures that are displaced in both foals and adult horses may cause intra-thoracic injury to the lungs, pericardium, heart, and great vessels prompting early surgical intervention.
- Serial monitoring of thoracic trauma patients may also include objective measurements of lung function such as oxygenation measurements and blood gas evaluation.

Step 5: Decision Making During Triage

The emergency clinician faces many difficult decisions while working with thoracic trauma patients (Radcliffe et al. 2009).

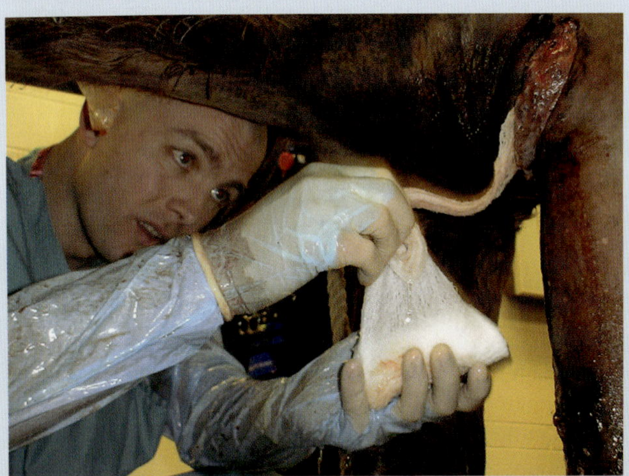

**Figure 1.3** Emergency wound triage for this horse involved debridement, aggressive lavage with sterile saline, and packing the wound with saline-soaked sterile roll gauze until further evaluation and treatment could be performed under general anesthesia. Packing thoracic wounds (especially in the axillary region) is important to prevent subcutaneous emphysema and secondary pneumomediastinum and pneumothorax.

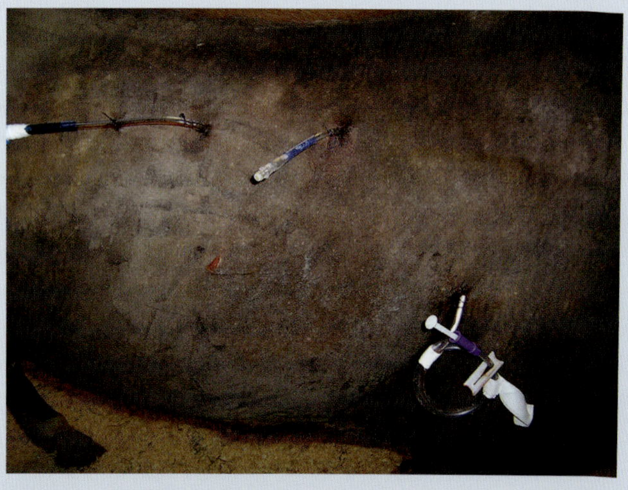

**Figure 1.4** The right hemithorax of the Appaloosa horse with thoracic injury. The horse had multiple displaced rib fractures and secondary flail chest (an unstable section of chest wall) involving its right, cranial thorax. Emergency triage included placement of a chest tube for air removal high in the right caudal thorax, a "soaker catheter" for providing bupivacaine regional analgesia above the fractured ribs in the dorsal cranial thorax, and use of an oxygen line to limit anaerobic bacterial growth in the cranial ventral thorax. The horse was euthanized the following day under general anesthesia after exploration revealed severe injury and contamination of the thoracic cavity.

- Following stabilization, referral is recommended for horses with severe injury where general anesthesia may be required for evaluation and treatment. General anesthesia with positive pressure ventilation ensures sufficient ventilation, enabling thorough exploration of the wound, thoracic and abdominal cavities, control of hemorrhage, repair of lung lacerations and rib fractures, and reconstruction of the wound and chest wall.
- Standing wound repair is possible in many animals with less severe trauma provided the patient remains stable. Some horses may not tolerate an open chest wound during treatment (developing respiratory distress because of progressive pneumothorax), and close monitoring is required during standing procedures.
- Complications (pneumothorax, hemothorax, rib fracture and flail chest, diaphragmatic hernia, pleuritis, pleuropneumonia) are common during the management of thoracic injury in horses, and early recognition and treatment will improve outcomes (Figure 1.5). Pleuritis or pleuropneumonia affects approximately half of all horses suffering thoracic trauma, is challenging to treat, and carries a guarded prognosis for survival (Laverty et al. 1996).
- Other problems sharing a poor prognosis include extra-thoracic injury to the abdominal cavity, musculoskeletal system or other organs, and euthanasia of these animals may be necessary (Laverty et al. 1996). However, most horses without severe injury and complications often respond favorably to management of thoracic injury.

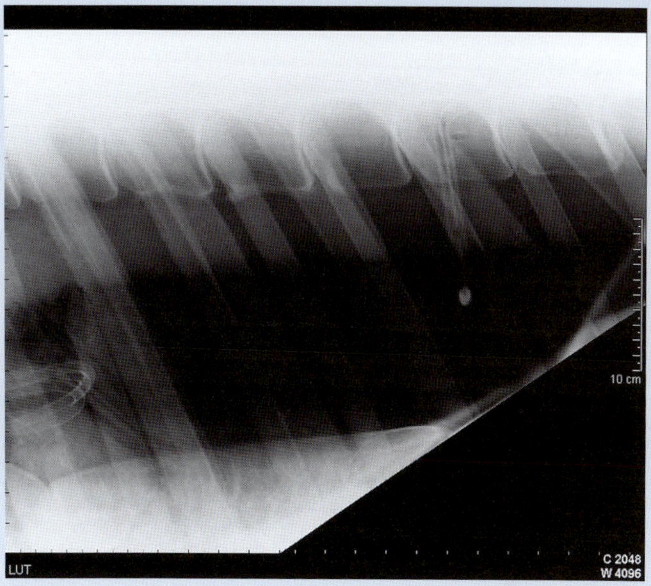


**Figure 1.5** Lateral radiographic view of the dorsal thorax of the Appaloosa horse following thoracic trauma. The horse suffered bilateral pneumothorax following penetrating thoracic injury. Note the displaced rib fracture on the left side of the image, as well as the chest tube for air removal and a "soaker catheter" for regional analgesia in the caudodorsal and craniodorsal thorax, respectively.

## References

Evans, C.S. and Slovis, C.M. (2020). Revisiting the ten commandments of emergency medicine: a resident's perspective. *Ann. Emerg. Med.* 77 (3): 367–370.

Hassel, D.M. (2007). Thoracic trauma in horses. *Vet. Clin. Equine* 23: 67–80.

Laverty, S., Lavoie, J.P., Pascoe, J.R., and Ducharme, N. (1996). Penetrating wounds of the thorax in 15 horses. *Equine. Vet. J.* 28 (3): 220–224.

Mathews, K.A. (2017). Emergency and critical care medicine: an essential component of all specialties and practices. *Front. Vet. Sci.* 4: 165. https://doi.org/10.3389/fvets.2017.00165.

Radcliffe, R.M. et al. (2009). Treating thoracic injuries. *Compend. Contin. Educ. Vet.* 4 (5): 208–223.

Sprayberry, K.A. and Barrett, E.J. (2015). Thoracic trauma in horses. *Vet. Clin. Equine.* 31: 199–219.

Thim, T., Krarup, N.H.V., Grove, E.L. et al. (2012). Initial assessment and treatment with the Airway, Breathing, Circulation, Disability, Exposure (ABCDE) approach. *Int. J. Gen. Med.* 5: 117–121.

Wrenn, K. and Slovis, C.M. (1991). The ten commandments of emergency medicine. *Ann. Emerg. Med.* 20 (10): 1146–1147.

# 2

# Working Safely with Horses During Emergencies: Behavioral Considerations

*Sue McDonnell, Cade Torcivia, and Jaime Miller*

*Department of Clinical Studies - New Bolton Center, University of Pennsylvania School of Veterinary Medicine, Kennett Square, PA, USA*

## Introduction

While any horse can pose threats to safety of health care staff, emergency situations typically offer particular safety challenges. While chemical sedation and/or analgesia is likely the best strategy for human safety and animal welfare, in many emergency situations chemical sedation may be contra-indicated. This chapter addresses key features of equine behavior and management related to safe handling and veterinary care in emergency situations, whether on-farm or in a clinic.

Most of the animated behavior of horses that poses a danger to health care staff, whether during routine or emergency care, is related to fear and/or acute physical discomfort. A recently published open-access scholarly review outlines current welfare and safety concerns regarding routine health and veterinary care procedures (Carroll et al. 2022). In emergency situations, painful and sick horses are especially likely to be fearful. Unfamiliar people and procedures, anxious familiar people, and clinic environments all tend to heighten fear in horses. This can be the case even with the most well-trained and well-experienced horses, but is generally much greater in young, feral, and/or previously unhandled or abused horses. Fear and pain are not always evident to or appreciated by handlers or care staff (Pearson et al. 2021; Rogers and Bell 2022). Moreover, horses have a natural tendency to reflexively show less outward indication of discomfort or fear in novel situations, with perceived threats, and in the presence of caretakers (Torcivia and McDonnell 2020). At various levels, both pain and fear tend to affect sensitivity and reactivity to tactile, auditory, visual, and olfactory stimulation. Some painful and depressed patients may give the impression that they are not likely to react dangerously. Even when recumbent and sedated, most horses can instantaneously arouse to react explosively to what may seem relatively ordinary stimulation. Especially stoic-appearing horses may suddenly express what is called displaced aggression, usually in the form of an out-of-character response, typically a lunging bite toward anything nearby, or sudden strike or kick and squeal. There usually are behavioral warning signs, but they can be quite subtle. Often increased tension of skeletal muscles, with or without subtle escape intention ear movements, head gestures, or limb weight shifting, just moments before an explosive response is the only perceptible indication. So, for most emergency care situations, extra attention to maximizing patient comfort along with attentive monitoring of patient's relative muscle relaxation versus tension can be expected to increase the safety of staff and patient. Aspects to consider include the most suitable staff available for the situation, best environment available for your work and the patient's comfort, and low-stress handling and veterinary procedures suitable for the particular situation and patient condition.

## Staff Considerations

Evolving as an open-plains, grazing prey species, horses are especially perceptive and reflexively responsive to emotional states of other organisms in their environment, both positive ("relaxation, all-clear") and negative ("heads up, alarm"). They are known both anecdotally and recently in scientific research to respond to sensory cues to the emotional states of humans to which they are exposed (Smith et al. 2016; Lanata et al. 2018; Ferretti and Papaleo 2019; Sabiniewicz et al. 2020). Voice tone, body posture,

*Emergency Triage of the Horse*, First Edition. Edited by Rolfe M. Radcliffe and Jamie J. Kopper.

Companion website: www.wiley.com/go/radcliffe/triage

facial expression, and body odors of handlers have all been shown to affect horse behavior. Personnel who work routinely with horses, particularly in emergency situations, usually develop skills at remaining calm, thereby minimizing inadvertently communicating alarm signals to the patient. They tend to speak in a relaxed and soothing voice tone, move about in a normal relaxed fashion, and maintain relaxed body posture and facial expressions. This manner typically serves to reduce the tension and stress not only for the patient, but for everyone present. They also seem more able to remain attentive to the patient's subtle changes in comfort. Inexperienced staff can be encouraged to develop these skills. A recently published open-access discomfort ethogram can be a useful tool for training staff to recognize subtle signs of physical discomfort (Torcivia and McDonnell 2021). Similarly, recognition of pain and emotional discomfort based on facial expression, if not intuitive, can be taught. Training materials can be readily found on-line for the Equine Facial Grimace Scale (Dalla Costa et al. 2014; Dai et al. 2020) and Horse Pain Face (Gleerup and Lindegaard 2016). Training resources for low-stress and low-fear animal handling for veterinary care with specific equine modules are becoming more readily available, both through non-profit and commercial educational organizations (https://www.theveterinarynurse.com/Review/article/let-s-talk-about-stress-equines https://lowstresshandling.com/low-stress-handling/what-is-low-stress-handling/; Fear-Free$^{T}$, fearfreepets.com).

While use of personal safety gear is not required for veterinary care in most jurisdictions, it is becoming more commonly used, especially for work involving a high risk of personal injury. Even when nothing dangerous happens, a helmet, safety vest, and safety shoes can greatly improve relaxed confidence when working around painful horses. See Chapter 34 for recommendations on safety gear for working with down horses, where personal safety gear and training are essential.

## Work Environment Considerations

When working in an on-farm emergency situation, options for location in which to work and control over the environment may be limited. However, to the extent possible, a location selected to balance the comfort of the horse with staff comfort and ability to do good work will maximize safety for all. For patient comfort, desirable features of the veterinary care environment include familiar space, near calm known companions whenever possible, and a relatively quiet, uncluttered space. In the clinical situation, the location, of course, will be unfamiliar to the patient. It is unlikely to have a known companion available. For most anxious patients, any other horse that is comfortable and relaxed in the particular clinical environment is usually somewhat comforting to an otherwise isolated patient. Some clinics have a designated companion horse or pony and safe holding stall in the examination room for this purpose. Even if the clinic is relatively quiet, the sound, visible equipment, and activities will most likely be novel. Examples of common equipment and sounds that can be frightening to patients but are often not noticed by care staff are squeaky wheels on approaching rolling carts, noisy clippers, ring tones on devices, and timer alarms.

When in new environments, patients generally appear less anxious in large open spaces with high ceilings. Non-slip familiar footing also seems to be better than more slippery or unfamiliar footing. While bright lighting can be helpful for examinations, horses often appear more comfortable with lower lighting. Dimmer controls can be a useful addition to emergency receiving areas. Hand-held spot lighting can sometimes be as or more effective at examining wounds and can reduce the need for bright overhead lighting.

## Restraint Considerations

Low-stress, low-fear handling is especially important when restraining horses during emergency procedures. Two important features of low-stress, low-fear restraint of horses include:

a) Maintaining a respectful, non-confrontational, non-reactive manner whenever restraining a patient. Respectful specifically means taking care to monitor the physical and mental state of the patient and the effect of the handler's behavior and the circumstances, modifying the restraint and environment according to the horse's level of comfort. Non-reactive handling includes quietly ignoring, and especially not punishing, any stress-releasing behavior (e.g., head raising, shaking, fidgeting, pawing, stress vocalizations). Reacting to or punishing stress-release behaviors will only increase fear and the associated risk of displaced aggression toward the handler or explosive escape or dangerous defensive aggression. A thoughtful attentive handler can often adjust the restraint and the positioning of the patient to allow and safely abide stress-releasing behaviors.

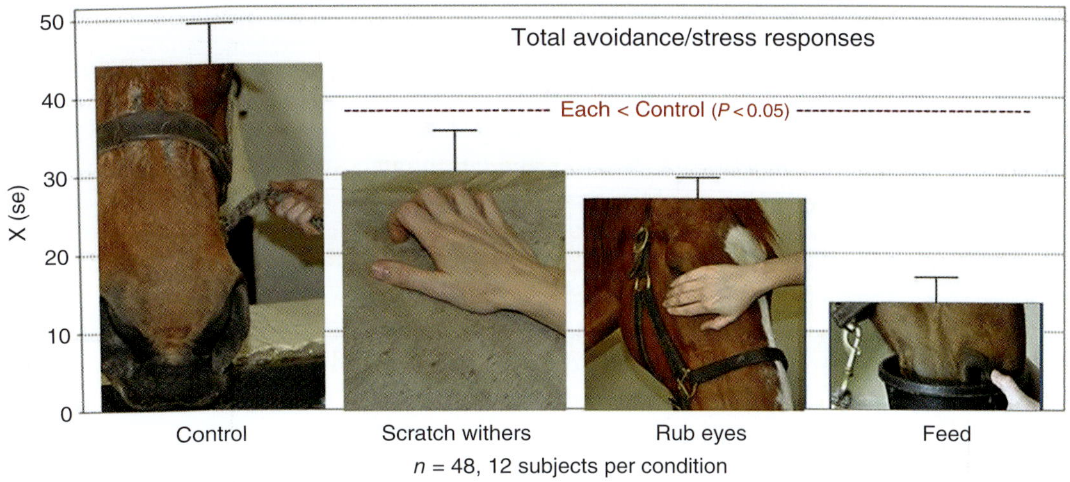


**Figure 2.1** For each of 3 handling interventions and control (12 healthy horses per group) avoidance/stress behavior was compared during a standard health care scenario. Horses were separated from their herd and placed in an examination stock and then exposed for three minutes to a standard aversive auditory stimulus (sheep shear, 85 db at ear level of horse). Interventions by the handler standing near the head included the holding the lead shank loosely while rhythmically scratching at the withers in the manner of mutual grooming, figure-eight rhythmic rubbing of face and eyes, or feeding a highly palatable senior feed. Control involved only holding the lead shank loosely. *Source:* Watson and McDonnell (2018)/Elsevier.

b) Employing soothing positive distraction and reinforcement for tolerating mildly aversive procedures. If the patient is willing to take food and their condition allows, in most instances food is likely the best positive distractor for uncomfortable procedures. As an alternative to feed, the horse can be offered a sweet or salty lick. Commercially made sweet licks for horses are readily available in a variety of flavors, but also can be quickly prepared by applying any syrup or sugary water to a rubber feed bowl. Similarly, a small salt mineral block can be offered. Stressed patients often quickly seem to become fixated on the licking, which appears to relieve stress. When food or a lick is not appropriate, or the patient is uninterested, soothing tactile interaction can also reduce avoidance/stress responses (Watson and McDonnell 2018). Rhythmic scratching at the withers in the manner of mutual grooming or rhythmic rubbing of the face were both found to be effective substitutes for feeding (Watson and McDonnell 2018) (Figure 2.1). Another handling intervention meant to distract horses in these situations is softly scratching, tapping, or knocking the knuckles on the horse's forehead. With these methods, the key is to adjust the rhythm and force of the action with the goal of achieving a soothing positive distraction that relaxes and calms the patient. For an anxious or aggressive handler, it is easy for the rate and intensity of the knocking or tapping to induce greater fear in the patient. With increased fear, horses may become less active due to entering a momentary fear-freeze state. The freeze may give the handler a false impression that they are effectively calming the patient. Typically, a freeze state, if not alleviated, soon leads to an explosive escape or defensive aggressive instantaneous reaction to any additional stimulation. Whether the resulting quiet is fear-related freezing or relaxation can be assessed by monitoring muscle tension and facial expression. Horses vary in their response to these techniques, so when possible, it is worth the time for the handler to evaluate different available techniques to assess which methods and manner appear most soothing and distracting for a particular patient in a particular situation.

## Consideration of Handling Aids

### Examination Stocks

Examination stocks can be quite helpful for safely containing a horse for examination and/or procedures, even for horses that may not have previous experience being restrained in stocks. However, if sufficiently stimulated, a horse can jump out or flip in stocks. Some key features of well-designed examination stocks are quiet, non-slip footing, easy one-hand latches that don't bind with weight, quiet hinges and latches, padding for comfort as well as sound attenuation should the horse kick or hit the stocks, and both a front, back, and side option for entering and exiting. Horses tend to be more comfortable loading in more "open" designs and in an open area.

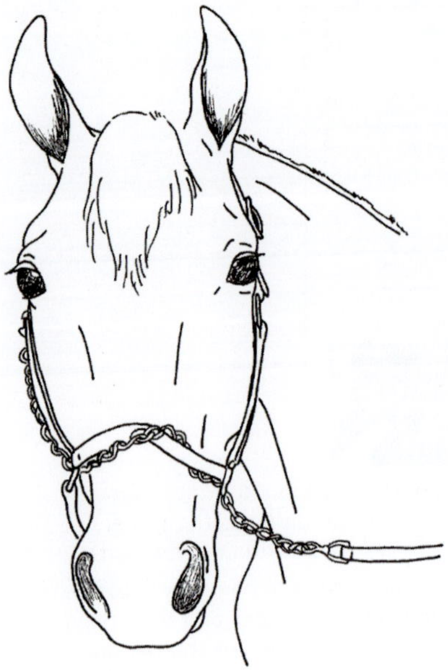

Figure 2.2 Chain over the noseband restraint.

## Chain Over Nose

A chain over the nose can provide more directional control of the head compared to simple attachment of the lead to the lower central ring of the halter. The chain is run through the near-side lower ring of the halter, over the noseband (to protect the delicate tissues of the face), and out through the off-side ring. Various locations of attachment of the chain have different effects (Figure 2.2). If the chain is long enough, attachment to the high off-side ring adds even more effective and smoother directional control of the head than a more rostral attachment. Caution should be taken to keep the halter away from the eye when applying tension to the lead rope. Running the chain under the chin to the ring on the underside of the noseband or to the near-side lower or upper ring can better stabilize a loose-fitting halter from rotating with tension on the lead, but may be more severe and less smooth for directing the head. In lieu of a chain shank, a simple cotton or nylon lead in any of these configurations can be similarly effective.

## Neck Skin Twitch

With one or both hands, grasp and maintain a firm grip on a handful of skin cranial to the shoulder (Figure 2.3). It is often more comfortable to maintain an effective grasp by rolling the fingers into the flesh. Like a nose twitch, full effect may take two to three minutes, and the two-hand grasp and roll are typically often easiest to maintain during that initial wait for the horse to relax.

## Gum Chain

Gum chain restraint involves placement of a chain lead through the side rings of the halter and under the upper lip to be seated at the junction of the gums and upper lip above the incisors (Figure 2.4). When applied gently and held in place with moderate steady tension as illustrated in Figures 2.5, it can effectively calm most horses for moderately aversive procedures. The response is more immediate than for the lip twitch. Of utmost concern for humane use and continued willingness to accept this restraint is that it is not applied in a confrontational or punitive manner, or that it inadvertently inflicts pain. Either outcome can quickly lead to significant specific aversion to subsequent use. In many cases the aversion will generalize to mouth and head shyness. What appears to be most uncomfortable for the horse, and is likely to lead to an aversion of the procedure, is inadvertently scraping the chain over the teeth or gums, or jerking on the chain. This can usually be avoided during placement by carefully

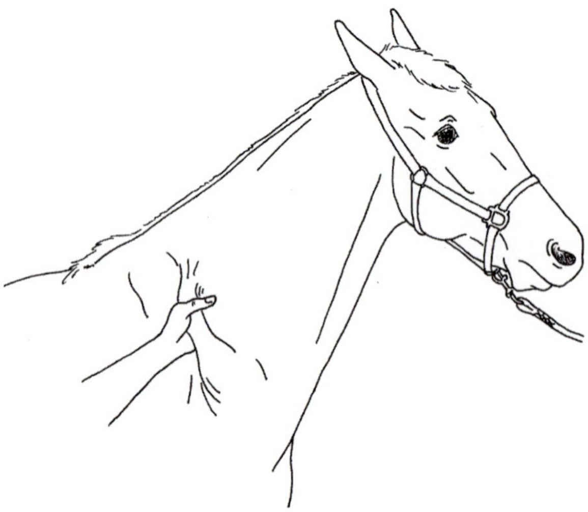

Figure 2.3 One-handed skin grasp restraint.

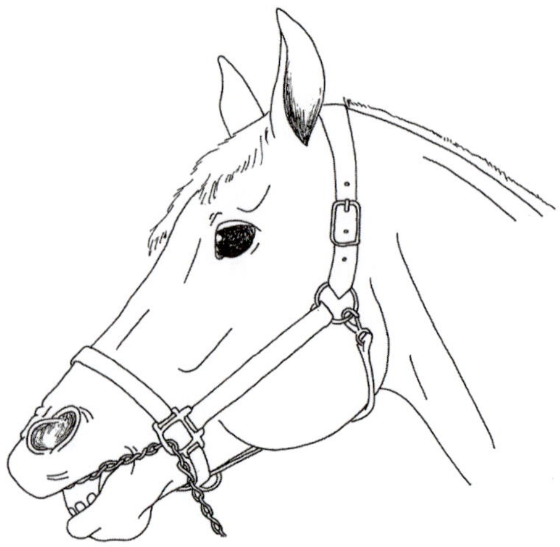

Figure 2.4 Gum chain restraint.

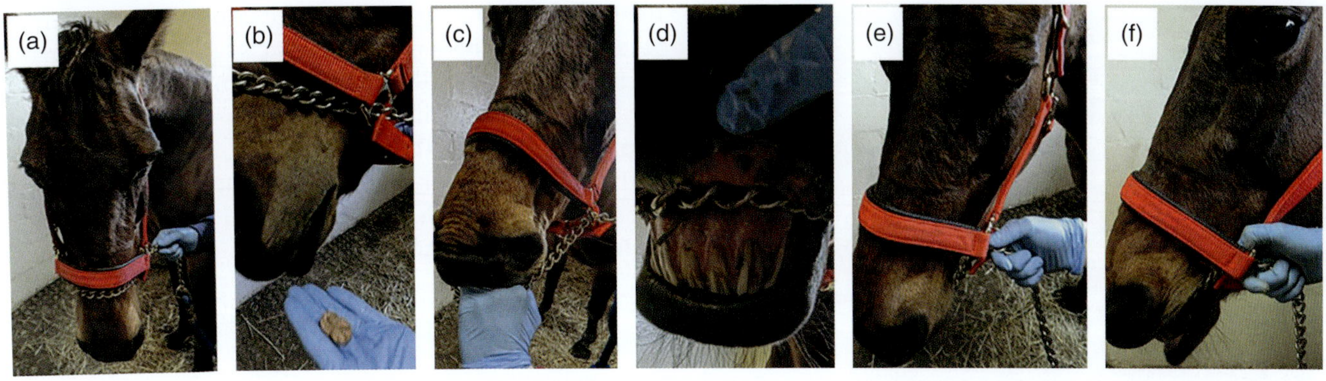


**Figure 2.5** Gentle, respectful application of a gum chain. First, the chain shank is placed through the near-side lower ring on the halter, over the nose and through the off-side ring and clipped to the off-side upper ring (a). The horse is offered a treat if allowed (b). Then, with the chain clasped through the closed hand, the knuckles can be used to gently lift the upper lip (c) as the fingers open to seat the chain at the junction of the gum with the upper lip (d). Once in place, steady tension on the chain is maintained with the hand held close to the near-side ring of the halter. That arm remains relaxed to move with any head movements, so as to avoid jerking on the chain (e). To move the horse, the thumb is reached over the noseband aside the ring to guide the horse by the halter pressure without adding greater pressure on the gums (f).

keeping your fingers between the teeth and gums until the chain is well-seating at the junction of the gums and base of upper lip. Nervous or uninformed handlers may tend to intermittently jerk, sometimes rhythmically, on the chain, in an attempt to focus the horse's attention. In most cases this does not appear helpful to the horse, and often counter-productive by increasing discomfort and fear. Most horses appear far more comfortable with a high-quality soft English brass chain, as is used for handling breeding stallions. Chrome-plated chains on the more common lead shanks have an obviously less tolerable mouth feel. They tend to develop cracks in the plating that more readily lacerate the delicate tissues. A poor-quality chain can be covered with a leather or vinyl sleeve or wrapped with self-adhesive bandage wrap. Also, a half-inch cotton lead is almost as effective as a chain and stays in place better than a chain (Figure 2.6). A hands-free substitute for a gum chain device, known as a Stableizer, is commercially available. The device uses cotton cord that runs from under the lip to over the poll, with a locking pulley system to maintain effective tension. Silastic tubing covers the portion of cord under the lip.

### Lip or Nose Twitch

A lip twitch is a device that tightly squeezes a handful grasp of the upper lip. There are various styles. A traditional loop and pole type twitch is depicted in Figure 2.7. While both rope and chain loops have been used, rope is considered

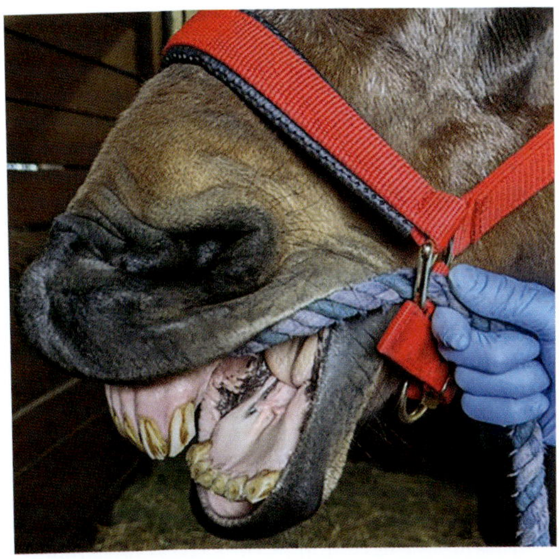

**Figure 2.6** Cotton rope used as a "gum chain" restraint.

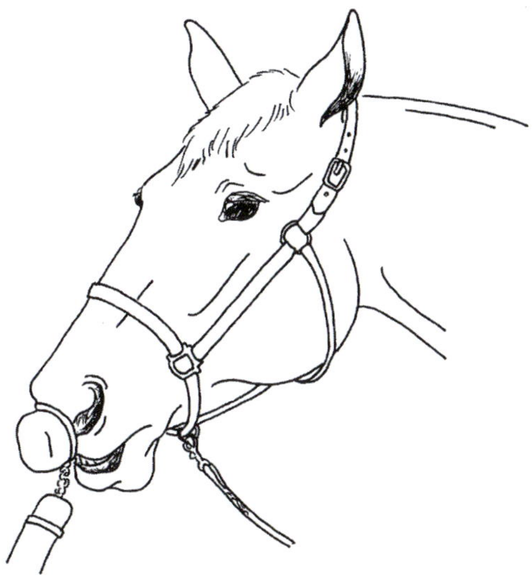

**Figure 2.7** Pole and rope loop twitch restraint.

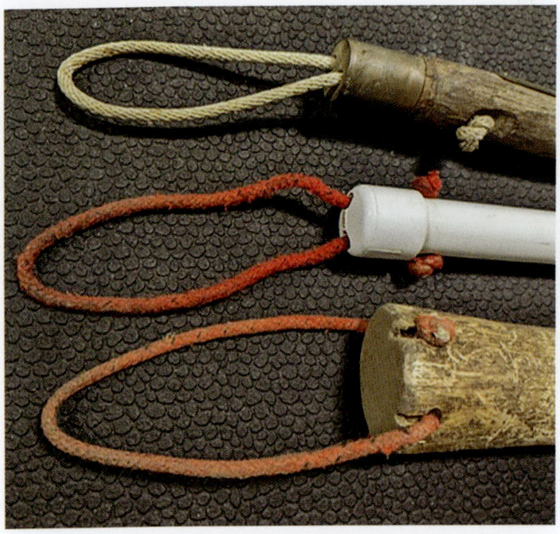

**Figure 2.8** Examples of preferred and non-preferred twitch pole head styles. To avoid pain and injury to teeth, gums, and inner surface of lip, the smooth, rounded plastic head shown in the center is preferred over either the sharp-edged copper collared hickory stick style (top) or the wide axe handle style (bottom).

safer for the horse than a loop of chain. A chain may be preferred by some because it gets a better "bite" and so is less likely to slip off the lip, but it can be more difficult to avoid inflicting excessive pain and/or damaging the delicate tissues of the muzzle. Another potentially painful aspect of the twitch that can lead to aversions is scraping the gums, teeth, or inner lip with the head of the pole. As illustrated in Figure 2.8, a smooth, small, rounded style pole head is preferred, as it is most likely to avoid additional pain or injury.

The twitch is so commonly used for restraint in emergency situations that it is worth listing detailed recommendations for safest and most humane application.

a) Offer a treat just before application.
b) Approach and apply the twitch in a calm, confident, non-confrontational, unhurried manner. Avoid contacting the teeth and gums with the twitch; this can be especially and unnecessarily painful.
c) Maintain appropriate tension–not too tight, not too loose. Maintain control of the pole while allowing the twitch to move with the horse by keeping the holding arm relaxed and flexible. Avoid pulling on the twitch or leading the horse by the twitch, which can be especially uncomfortable.
d) Monitor the horse's response to respect limits of analgesia. Don't proceed with the aversive procedure until signs of analgesia are evident (glassy eye, relaxed drooping lower lip). Aim to stop the aversive procedure and remove the twitch while those signs are still present. This will avoid leaving the horse with a bad memory of the twitch.
e) If the procedure is almost complete, but the patient is becoming restless, remove the twitch before the horse becomes explosively resistant. For most horses, only a few minutes break restores the ability to have another fairly good rise in endorphins when the twitch is re-applied.
f) Upon removal, immediately offer a treat.
g) Just as with chemical sedation, the twitch can be expected to provide the most comfort to the horse when applied before the horse reaches a state of high sympathetic tone. For this reason, it is typically better to use it from the start when the horse is most relaxed.

Figure 2.9 illustrates recommended step-by-step application of the pole and rope loop twitch. A pliers type twitch, often referred to as a humane or "hands-free" twitch, is shown in Figure 2.10. While these can be helpful if working without assistance, the pliers are easily dislodged if the horse is within reach of objects (stocks, wall, foreleg, or chest) against which it instinctively attempts to rub the irritated muzzle.

Figure 2.11 schematically illustrates the concept of various distinct phases of behavioral response associated with a lip twitch, corresponding to pattern of beta endorphin release and depletion. This information is based on results of unpublished work involving continuous serial sampling of venous and intercavernous sinus plasma for assay of beta endorphin during twitch application (McDonnell and Toolan 1991 unpublished). When a twitch is first applied, it provides some additional physical restraint and what appears to be uncomfortable distraction. This has been referred to as the distraction phase. The additional physical restraint and painful distraction will sufficiently control some horses for some procedures; however, some will become more fractious during this stage, fighting the twitch. The third and usually greatest calming benefit of the twitch comes as endorphins are released, evidenced by signs of light sedation. Waiting for the endorphin release will give the patient the greatest benefit. The typical latency to the analgesia phase ranges from three to five minutes after application of the twitch and corresponds to reaching of a plateau in endorphin concentrations.

Development of aversion to the twitch is common. Many clients consider the practice inhumane. Unfortunately, a common misunderstanding is that a twitch should be in place for as little time as possible. So many handlers apply the twitch, then immediately start and rush to complete the aversive procedure, and then remove the twitch as quickly as possible. In that scenario, the twitch may not be in place long enough to reach an effective level of analgesia. All that the horse has

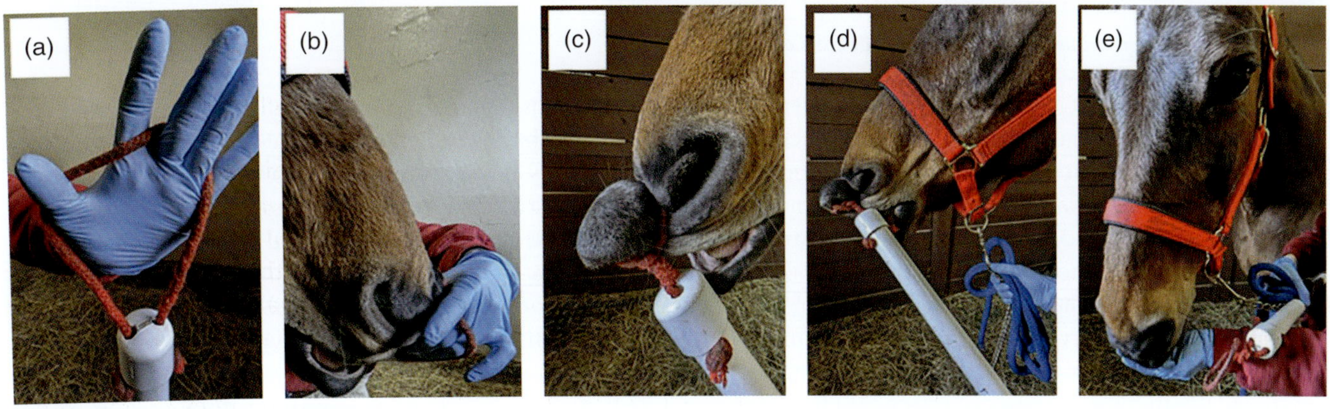


**Figure 2.9** Relaxed, non-confrontational application of a rope twitch. The loop of rope is positioned over the fingers such that it will not slide down to the wrist (a) and then can be more easily slid from the fingers around the grasped handful of upper lip (b). The pole is then calmly rotated to tighten the loop (c). An unrushed rhythmic turn-pause, turn-pause style appears to reassure the horse that it will not continue too tightly. Once tightly in place, care should be taken to not pull or push the horse by the lip. Use the lead shank to direct the horse and remain flexible with the arm holding the twitch handle, moving with any movement of the horse (d). Twitched horses are typically less comfortable walking and more difficult to steer. Immediately after removal, rub the rub the muzzle and offer a treat (e). *Source:* M. Ziad Al-Ani, Robin J.M. Gray.

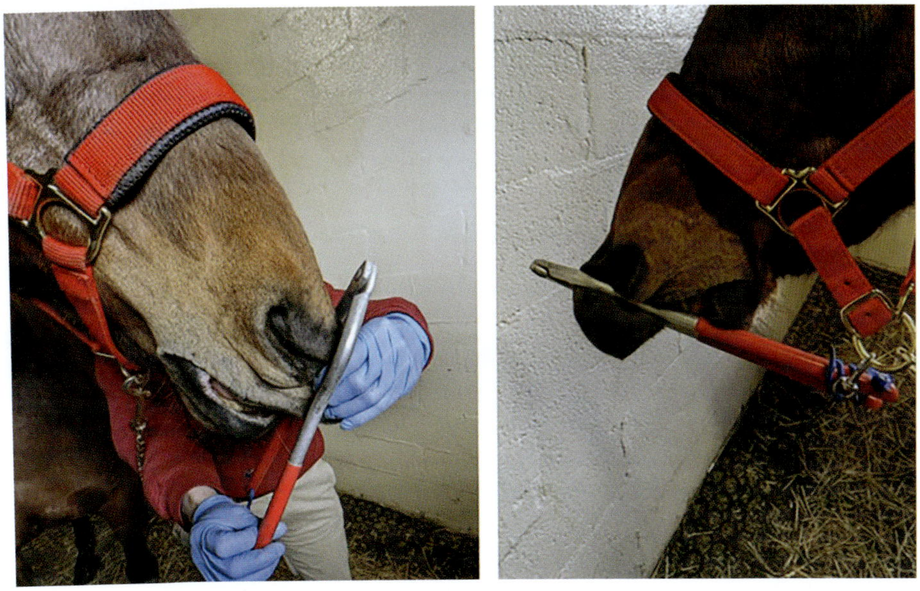

**Figure 2.10** Pliers type twitch, also called "humane twitch." The pliers are clamped over a handful of upper lip and secured with a cord wrapped around the handles and then clipped to the halter.

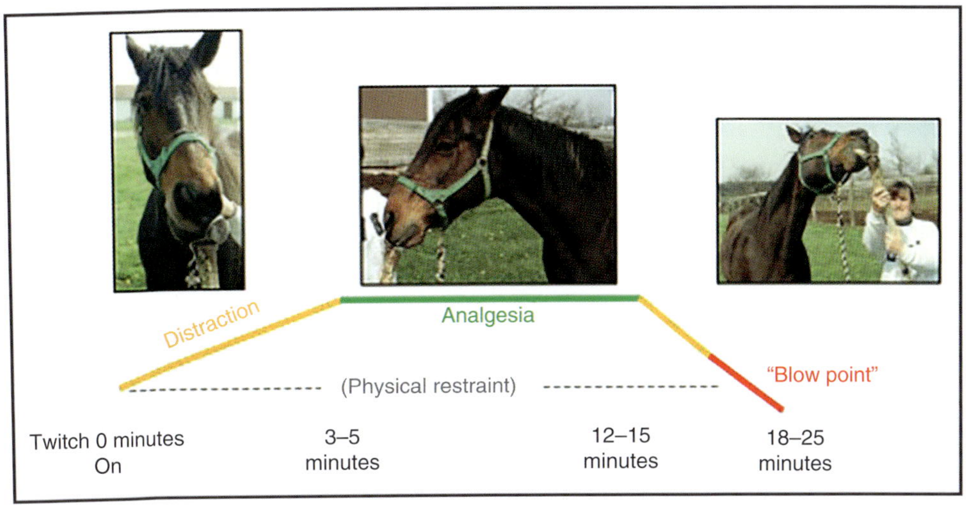


**Figure 2.11** Schematic illustration of phases of endorphin levels and corresponding behavior during twitch application.

experienced, and all that it will be expected to remember about the twitch, is that it was painful, additionally confining, and associated with additional painful procedures. Once analgesia is evident, that phase typically ranges from 12 to 15 minutes after application. At that point, the horse begins to become intermittently more restless for a moment, and then relaxed again. Once that restlessness is noticed, it is recommended to remove the twitch during the next moment of relaxation. If the twitch is not removed and the aversive procedure continued, most horses will become more and more restless, reactive, and eventually agitated to the point of explosively over-running the handler or rearing or bolting to escape the twitch. This has been referred to as the "blow point." It corresponds to circulating endorphin levels dropping below baseline.

It can be helpful to view the twitch like a tranquilizer or pain medication. It takes some time to work and has a duration of effectiveness. Just as with chemical sedation and analgesia, the latency and duration of effect vary among animals and situations. Waiting for the onset of effect, and finishing up while it is still working, or pausing to re-dose, is perhaps the most important concept in humane and effective use. Re-application of the twitch after a few-minutes' rest typically results in another brief rise in endorphin levels and associated relaxation and tolerance of completion of a procedure. One wouldn't think of injecting an analgesic or tranquilizer and trying to immediately begin the aversive procedure, or continuing to finish a procedure when sedation or analgesia had subsided.

Some horses may wiggle the muzzle or otherwise struggle when the twitch is first applied, before effective endorphin release, or during particularly uncomfortable or stimulating moments. If the twitch slips off during a struggle, the behavior that led to escaping the twitch is negatively reinforced ("pressure and release") by successful escape. With negative reinforcement, horses are especially quick to learn escape and then avoidance behavior, often with only one or two successful escapes. Most will naturally repeat the action and escalate the effort with each subsequent attempt. In such cases, persisting by simply repeating attempts often leads to a more confrontational, rough, or rushed approach to application, which just increases the patient's fear and pain. For the current and future welfare of the horse, as well as safety of personnel, it is usually best to give up on the twitch after two successive escapes rather than to persist.

## Veterinary Procedure Considerations

Another general principle of low-stress handling includes taking care to make each procedure as painless as possible. Many of the accepted practices that we expect patients to tolerate, can be made considerably less uncomfortable. Examples include using the finest-gauge needles and catheters that are practical for the job and using topical or injectable numbing agents whenever possible. Modern commercially available skin-numbing products have been shown to be effective for injections for horses within two minutes of application (Torcivia and McDonnell 2022).

Not all horses in emergency situations will have had experience with even the most common veterinary procedures; and, of course, some may have had negative experiences leading to an established aversion. A helpful habit that can reduce the risk of eliciting a potentially dangerous response is to take a moment (literally usually less than a minute) to acclimate the patient to each piece of equipment or instrument that may be novel, and certainly to any potentially uncomfortable procedures. For example, in the case of clipping, before turning on the clipper, first rub the handle soothingly against the shoulder, as if grooming, until the horse relaxes. Then turn the clipper on at a distance in view of the horse, allowing the horse to voluntarily inspect. Next, with the clipper turned on, with your hand around the handle, rub your hand against the shoulder, and then the vibrating handle directly against the shoulder. While maintaining contact, move the clipper toward the area to be clipped. The brief step-by-step acclimation can greatly improve acceptance, especially in clipper-naïve horses. Other common examples are sprays (e.g., disinfectants), examination gloves, radiographic mitt and plate, or nasogastric tube.

## Working with "Wild," Feral, and Previously Unhandled Horses

Horses that have had little previous handling can be especially challenging to work with in emergencies. Whenever possible, sedation is likely the most humane approach. Because of the generally high level of fear, and resulting high sympathetic tone, sedation and general anesthesia are often difficult to effectively gauge. "Wild" horses in domestic care – that is, horses that have been born in free-roaming herds, captured and transitioned to domestic care and training – often retain certain behavioral characteristics of a wild animal. Specifically, their threshold for panic bolting appears lower than for domestically born and managed horses. And once in a state of panic, these individuals appear to exhibit super-strength and athletic ability to jump over or break through fences, gates, walls, or stocks. With blind panic, they have no regard for their own safety. A padded livestock squeeze chute is likely the only safe physical restraint for some of these wild horses now in domestic care. Even when adequately physically contained, veterinary care can be extremely stressful for these animals. Maintaining and recovering these animals from general anesthesia is also challenging for teams not experienced with wild hoof stock species. For these reasons, in emergency situations, particularly thoughtful consideration should be given to whether facilities and staff are adequate to proceed, with both human safety and animal welfare in mind. Low-stress stockmanship methods work well for moving and loading unhaltered wild horses (Hibbard 2022).

## References


Carroll, S.L., Sykes, B.W., and Mills, P.C. (2022). Moving toward fear-free husbandry and veterinary care for horses. *Animals* 2022 (12): 2907.

Dai, F., Leach, M., MacRae, A.M. et al. (2020). Does thirty-minute standardised training improve the inter-observer reliability of the horse grimace scale (HGS)? A case study. *Animals* 10 (5): 781.

Dalla Costa, E., Minero, M., Lebelt, D. et al. (2014). Development of the horse grimace scale (HGS) as a pain assessment tool in horses undergoing routine castration. *PLoS One* 9 (3): e92281.

Ferretti, V. and Papaleo, F. (2019). Understanding others: emotion recognition in humans and other animals. *Genes Brain Behav.* 18 (1): e12544.

Gleerup, K.B. and Lindegaard, C. (2016). Recognition and quantification of pain in horses: a tutorial review. *Equine Vet. Educ.* 28 (1): 47–57.

Hibbard, W. (2022). Stockmanship Journal. https://stockmanshipjournal.com/the-editor/ (accessed January 2022).

Lanata, A.; Nardelli, M.; Valenza, G. et al. (2018). A case for the interspecies transfer of emotions: a preliminary investigation on how humans odors modify reactions of the autonomic nervous system in horses. *Proceedings of the 2018 40th Annual International Conference of the IEEE Engineering in Medicine and Biology Society (EMBC)*, Honolulu, HI, USA (18–21 July 2018). IEEE: Piscataway, NJ, USA, pp. 522–525.

Pearson, G., Waran, N., Reardon, R.J. et al. (2021). A Delphi study to determine expert consensus on the behavioural indicators of stress in horses undergoing veterinary care. *Appl. Anim. Behav. Sci.* 237: 105291.

Rogers, S. and Bell, C. (2022). Perceptions of fear and anxiety in horses as reported in interviews with equine behaviourists. *Animals* 12 (21): 2904.

Sabiniewicz, A., Tarnowska, K., Świątek, R. et al. (2020). Olfactory-based interspecific recognition of human emotions: Horses (Equus ferus caballus) can recognize fear and happiness body odour from humans (Homo sapiens). *Appl. Anim. Behav. Sci.* 230: 105072.

Smith, A.V., Proops, L., Grounds, K. et al. (2016). Horses give functionally relevant responses to human facial expressions of emotion: a response to Schmoll (2016). *Biol. Lett.* 12 (9): 20160549.

Torcivia, C. and McDonnell, S. (2020). In-person caretaker visits disrupt ongoing discomfort behavior in hospitalized equine orthopedic surgical patients. *Animals* 10 (2): 210.

Torcivia, C. and McDonnell, S. (2021). Equine discomfort ethogram. *Animals* 11 (2): 580.

Torcivia, C. and McDonnell, S. (2022). Efficacy of lidocaine topical solution in reducing discomfort reaction of horses to intramuscular vaccination. *Animals* 12 (13): 1659.

Watson, J.C. and McDonnell, S.M. (2018). Effects of three non-confrontational handling techniques on the behavior of horses during a simulated mildly aversive veterinary procedure. *Appl. Anim. Behav. Sci.* 203: 19–23.

# 3

# Emergency Supplies and Equipment for Triage

*Santiago Mejia*[1] *and Elizabeth Williams Louie*[2]

[1] *Cornell Ruffian Equine Specialists (CRES), College of Veterinary Medicine, Cornell University, Elmont, NY, USA*
[2] *Biomedical and Biological Sciences, College of Veterinary Medicine, Cornell University, Ithaca, NY, USA*

## General Equipment List

To provide adequate patient care, it is essential to have a list of equipment to manage primary care emergencies in equine medicine. Many different supplies and equipment are available; however, understanding the market, as well as the local and regional cases, can help you better tailor the equipment needed to provide the best services for your clients.

## General Equipment

| Quantity | Product | Indications |
|---|---|---|
| 1 | Stethoscope | Physical exam |
| 1 | Thermometer | Physical exam |
| 1 | Pen light | Physical exam/eye exam |
| 1 | Ophthalmoscope | Eye exam |
| 1 | Twitch | Physical restraint |
| 1 | Nasogastric tube (assorted sizes) and pump | Colic exam |
| 1–3 | Halters assorted sizes | Physical restraint |
| 1–3 | Lead rope +/− chain | Physical restraint |
| 2 | Surgery pack | Emergency surgery |
| 3–4/each | Assorted suture packs PDS, Vicryl, Prolene, Monocryl | Wound management |
| 2 | Carry Kits | Transport supplies |
| 1 for each | Dispensing bottles (antiseptics) | Antisepsis |
| 1 | Snare OB | Dystocia |
| 1 of each | Flashlight and headlamp | Procedures |
| 1 | Clippers + 3 blades #40 | Hair removal |
| ~ | Dispensing bottles, pill vials, labels, etc. | Dispensing medication |
| 1 | Extension cord | Procedures |
| 1 box | Exam glove | Exams and procedures |
| 3 packs | Gauze 4×4 | Scrubbing, hemostasis, procedures |

(*Continued*)

*Emergency Triage of the Horse*, First Edition. Edited by Rolfe M. Radcliffe and Jamie J. Kopper.

Companion website: www.wiley.com/go/radcliffe/triage

| Quantity | Product | Indications |
|---|---|---|
| 1 box | Sterile Gloves | Surgery and procedures |
| 2 | Lily pads | Frog support |
| 2 gallons | Lubrivet | Rectal exam |
| 2 | Teat cannulas, stainless steel | Abdominocentesis, wound probing, wound flushing |
| 4 | Towels asst. sizes | Different uses |
| 1 | Oral Speculum | Exams |
| 2 | Stallion Catheters | Urinary tract catheterization |
| 4 | Sterile Lube | Wounds, Urogenital |
| 1 box | Syringe 1 mL | Injections |
| 1 box | Syringe 3 mL | Injections |
| 1 box | Syringe 5 mL | Injections |
| 1 box | Syringe 12 mL | Injections |
| 1 box | Syringe 20 | Injections |
| 1 box | Syringe 30–35 mL | Injections |
| 1 box | Syringe 30–35 mL catheter tip | Oral medications |
| 1 box | Syringe 60 mL box | Injections |
| 1 box | Syringe 60 mL box catheter tip | Oral medications |
| 1 box | Hypodermic needle 14 g 1–1.5 in. | Injections |
| 1 box | Hypodermic needle 16 g 1–1.5 in. | Injections |
| 1 box | Hypodermic needle 18 g 1–1.5 in. | Injections |
| 1 box | Hypodermic needle 21 g 1–1.5 in. | Injections |
| 1 box | Hypodermic needle 23 g 1 in. | Injections |
| 1 box | Hypodermic needle 25 g 5/8 in. | Injections |
| 1 gallon | Mineral oil | Colic work-up |
| 2 | Buckets, stainless steel 2 sizes | Assorted procedures |
| 2 | OB chains and handles set | Dystocia |
| 1 bag | OB sleeves | Dystocia/Rectal exams |
| 1 box | Ophtho Q-tips sterile | Ophthalmology procedures |
| 1 box | Ophtho fluorescein strips | Ophthalmology procedures |
| 1 box of each | Scalpel blades #22, 10, 15 | Surgical procedures |
| 2 | Epsom Salts (lbs) | Variety of procedures |
| 3 | Cotton roll 1 lb | Scrubbing |

## Creams, Ointments, and Dressings

| Quantity | Product | Indications |
|---|---|---|
| 3 | Limb Sweat Mixture (Nitrofurazone base + Anti-inflammatory drug such as Dexamethasone or Diclofenac + DMSO) | Limb swellings and cellulitis |
| 1 | Silver sulfadiazine (SSD) | Local antibiotic, burns, wound dressings |
| 2 | Surpass | Local anti-inflammatory |
| 2 | Hydrogel | Wound debridement/dressing |
| 1 | Magna Paste | Poultice |
| 1 | Lidocaine gel | Local anesthetic |
| 1 | A + D Ointment | Burns, skin irritation |
| 2 | Triple antibiotic ointment | Local antibiotic |

## Medication Stock

| Quantity | Product | Indications |
|---|---|---|
| 1 | Acepromazine (10 mg/mL) 50 mL | Tranquilizer |
| 1 | Activated Charcoal Toxiban | Intoxications |
| 1 | Amikacin (250 mg/mL) 4 mL | Antibiotic |
| 2 | Atropine Ointment | Ophthalmic dilate pupil |
| 1 | E-SE 100 mL | Vitamin E and selenium |
| 1 | Buscopan (20 mg/mL) 100 mL | Spasmolytic, abdominal pain analgesic |
| 2 | Carbocaine (20 mg/mL) 100 mL | Local anesthetic |
| 1 | Detomidine (10 mg/mL) 20 mL vial | Sedation (Alpha-2 adrenoceptor agonist) |
| 4 | Detomidine Paste (wear gloves) | Sedation (Alpha-2 adrenoceptor agonist) |
| 1 | Dexamethasone (2 mg/mL) 100 mL | Anti-inflammatory. (corticosteroid) |
| 1 | DMSO Dimethyl sulfoxide 90% | Free radical scavenger |
| 1 | Enrofloxacin (100 mg/mL) 100 mL | Broad-spectrum antibiotic |
| 1 | Excede (200 mg/mL) 100 mL | Broad-spectrum antibiotic |
| 1 | Eye wash | Flush eye, nasolacrimal duct flush |
| 1 | Firocoxib (57 mg tab) 60ct | Non-steroidal anti-inflammatory drug (selective Cox-2 inhibitor) |
| 1 | Flunixin Meglumine (50 mg/mL) 250 mL | Non-steroidal anti-inflammatory drug |
| 6 | Flunixin Paste oral | Non-steroidal anti-inflammatory drug |
| 1 | Furosemide (50 mg/mL) 50 mL | Diuretic |
| 1 | Gentamicin (100 mg/mL) 250 mL | Broad-spectrum antibiotic |
| 1 | Levothyroxine (Thyro-L) | Equine metabolic disease |
| 2 | Lidocaine (2%) 250 mL | Local anesthetic |
| 1 | Methocarbamol (500 mg/tab or 100 mg/mL) | Muscle relaxant |
| >500 | Metronidazole 500 mg tablets | Antibiotic antiparasitic |
| 2 | Naxcel 1 g vials | Broad spectrum antibiotic |
| 2 | Naxcel 4 g vial | Broad-spectrum antibiotic |
| 2 | NeoPolyDex Ointment | Ophthalmic antibiotic and anti-inflammatory |
| 2 | NeoPolyBac Ointment | Ophthalmic antibiotic |
| 1 box | Omeprazole | Proton pump inhibitor |
| 1 | Oxytetracycline (100 mg/mL) 500 mL vial | Broad-spectrum Antibiotic |
| 1 | Oxytocin 100 mL | Stimulate uterine contractions |
| 100 | Phenylbutazone 1-g tablets 100 | Non-steroidal anti-inflammatory drug |
| 1 | Phenylbutazone (250 mg/mL) 100 mL vial | Non-steroidal anti-inflammatory drug (refrigerated) |
| 2 | Phenylephrine HCL (10 mg/mL) 1 mL | Vasoconstrictor |
| 1 | Procaine Penicillin 250 mL vial | Broad-spectrum Antibiotic (refrigerated) |
| 100 | Sucralfate 1 g tablets | Gastro protectant |
| 1 | Tetanus Antitoxin | Vaccine |
| 1 | Tetanus Toxoid | Vaccine |
| 1 | Thiamine 100 mL | Vitamins |
| 5 | Trimethoprim Sulfa 960 mg #100 | Broad-spectrum antibiotic |
| 1 | Trimethoprim Sulfa 960 mg #500 | Broad-spectrum antibiotic |
| 1 | Vitamin B 12 100 mL | Vitamin, weak, anorexic animals |
| 1 | Vitamin B Complex 100 mL | Vitamin, weak, anorexic animals |
| 1 | Vitamin E 250 mL | Vitamin, neuroprotectant |
| 1 | Water Sterile 250 mL | Medication reconstituting |
| 2 | Xylazine (100 mg/mL) 50 mL | Sedation (Alpha-2 adrenoceptor agonist) |

## Emergency Drugs

| Quantity | Product | Indications |
|---|---|---|
| 1 | Atropine 100 mL | Anticholinergic/bradycardia |
| 1 | Doxapram | Respiratory stimulant |
| 1 | Epinephrine 1 : 1,000 | Anaphylaxis, cardiac arrest |

## Catheter Supplies, IV Fluids, and Electrolytes

| Quantity | Product | Indications |
|---|---|---|
| 5 | 0.9% Saline 1 L | Fluid therapy |
| 1 | 5% Dextrose 1 L | Adjunctive therapy |
| 2 | 50% Dextrose 500 mL | Adjunctive therapy |
| 2 | 7.2% Hypertonic saline 1 L | Resuscitation |
| 2 | Calcium Borogluconate 23% 500 mL | Adjunctive therapy |
| 5 | IV Administration set 10 drop/mL | Fluid therapy |
| 3 of each | IV Catheter 14 Ga × 13 cm (5.25 in.)/14 Ga × 9 cm (3.5 in.) | Fluid therapy |
| 3 of each | IV Catheter 16 Ga × 13 cm (5.25 in.)/16 Ga × 9 cm (3.5 in.) | Fluid therapy |
| 5 | IV Injection caps | Fluid therapy |
| 5 | IV T-port extension set | Fluid therapy |
| 2 | IV Blood/Filter Set | Plasma or blood administration |
| 2 | Equine Plasma 1 L bag | Failure Passive Transfer, Endotoxemia |
| 15 | Lactated Ringers 1 L bag | Fluid therapy |
| 4 | Lactated Ringers 5 L bag | Fluid therapy |
| 15 | Plasmalyte 1 L bag | Fluid therapy |
| 4 | Plasmalyte 5 L bag | Fluid therapy |
| 1 | Sodium Bicarbonate 500 mL | Adjunctive therapy |

## Controlled Substances

| Quantity | Product | Indications |
|---|---|---|
| 1 | Butorphanol 10 mg/mL | Opioid, sedation analgesia |
| 2 | Diazepam 5 mg/mL | Muscle relaxant anticonvulsant |
| 2 | Phenobarbital (Fatal Plus) 390 mg/mL Approximately 1 mL/10 lbs body weight | Euthanasia |
| 2 | Ketamine 100 mg/mL | Dissociative, anesthetic, analgesic |
| 2 | Midazolam 5 mg/mL | Muscle relaxant anticonvulsant |

## Bandage and Splints

| | | |
|---|---|---|
| 2 | Poultice Pads (Animalintex) | Foot abscess |
| 12 | Brown Gauze roll 6″ | Bandage |
| 1 | Duct Tape roll | Splint fixation |
| 12 | Elasticon 4″ | Bandage |
| 1 | Kimzey Splint front | Fracture splinting |
| 1 | Kimzey Splint Hind | Fracture splinting |
| 2–3 | PVC assorted sizes | Fracture splinting |
| 1 | Scissors bandage | Bandage removal |
| 3 | SteriRoll each size 14″ | Bandage |
| 3 | SteriRoll each size 16″ | Bandage |
| 12 | Telfa Pads asst. sizes | Wound dressing |
| 12 | VetWrap 4″ roll | Bandage |
| 24 | Gauze Rolls Pack - 4 Inches X 4.1 Yards | Conforming Stretch Bandages |
| 2 of each | White tape 1″, 3″, 4″ | Different procedures |
| | Sheet and Roll Cotton | Bandage |

## Antiseptics

| Quantity | Product | Indications |
|---|---|---|
| 1 | 2% Chlorhexidine Solution gallon | Antiseptic |
| 1 | 4% Chlorhexidine Scrub gallon | Antiseptic |
| 1 | 70% Isopropyl Alcohol | Antiseptic |
| 1 | Povidone Iodine scrub gallon | Antiseptic |
| 1 | Povidone Iodine solution gallon | Antiseptic |

## Podiatry Equipment

| Quantity | Product | Indications |
|---|---|---|
| 1 | Steel Hoof Nipper 14″ | Hoof procedures |
| 1 | Steel Shoe Puller 12″ | Shoe removal |
| 1 | Hoof Rasp | Hoof procedures |
| 2 | Hoof knives | Hoof procedures |
| 1 | Hoof testers | Hoof procedures |
| 1 | Shoe pullers | Hoof procedures |
| 1 | Clinch Cutter | Hoof procedures |

## Intravenous Catheterization

Intravenous (IV) catheter placement is a basic and common skill needed in routine equine clinical practice; this procedure must be learned by students of veterinary medicine prior to going into practice (Hobbs et al. 2021). IV catheters are used for multiple reasons clinically that can include but are not limited to administration of large volumes of fluids, maintenance of continuous fluid therapy, IV medications, parenteral nutrition, blood sampling (Hay 1992; Barakzai and Chandler 2003; N.A. 2014; Schoster 2017; Hobbs et al. 2021).

Many supplies are valuable in preparation for different emergency problems and clinical techniques. Below is list of various items that may prove helpful during emergency triage in the horse.

## Catheter Supplies

An IV catheter should be placed when fluid therapy and/or ongoing IV medication therapy is required (Figure 3.1). The right or left jugular groove is clipped, aseptically prepared, and the catheter is placed using aseptic technique. Reported complications when placing the catheter may include but are not limited to: thrombophlebitis, vein thrombosis, vein damage, accidental intracarotid catheterization, hematoma formation, septic thrombi, cellulitis, and local fibrosis.

*Materials*

1) Sedation (Xylazine/Detomidine hydrochloride and Butorphanol tartrate) (optional for restraint).
2) Twitch or Chain (optional for restraint).
3) Clippers with #40 blade.
4) 4% Chlorhexidine Scrub.
5) 70% Isopropyl Alcohol.
6) 4×4 gauze.
7) Exam Gloves.
8) Sterile Gloves.
9) Lidocaine 2%.
10) 3 mL syringe with 25 g needle.
11) 10 mL syringe with 20 g needle.

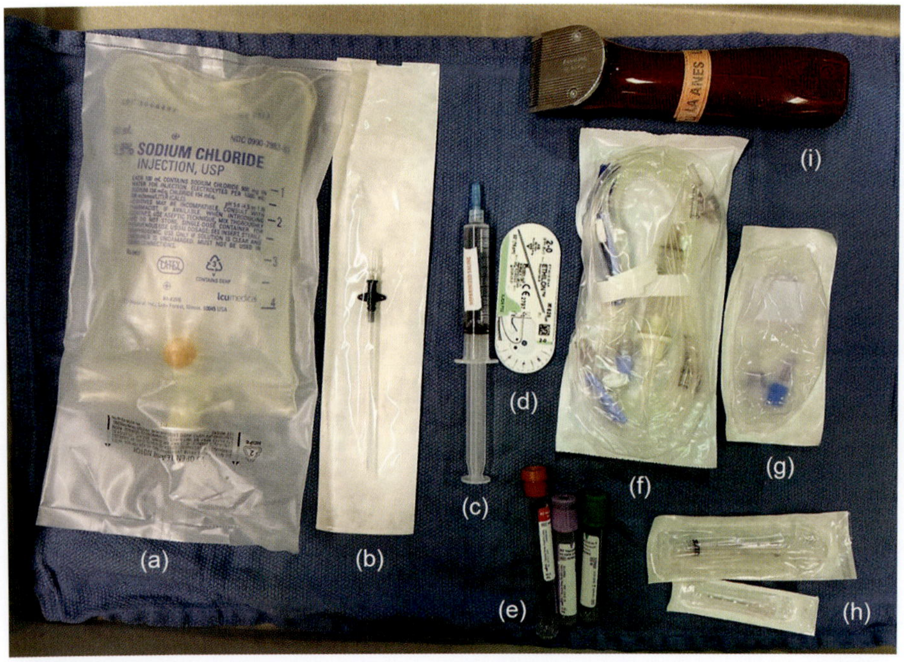


**Figure 3.1** Materials used for IV catheter placement. From left to right (a) Fluids for injection as required (b) Extended Use MILACATH 14 gauge catheter, (c) heparin saline (flush), (d) No. 2-0 ETHILON®, (e) Blood/sample collection tubes, (f) IV infusion set, (g) T-port extension set, (h) 3 mL syringe and 20G 1 in. needle, and (i) cordless clippers.

12) Catheter of choice (Mila Extended Use Catheters – 18–10 g).[1]
13) T-port extension set (B. Braun Medical Inc.).[2]
14) Injection Cap.
15) Suture (2-0 ETHILON® BLACK 1X30″ KS).[3]
16) Adhesive elastic bandage.

*Procedure*

1) Clip the cranial 1/3 of the left or right jugular groove. The authors prefer the left jugular to reduce risk of iatrogenic damage to the right recurrent laryngeal nerve (RLN) specially in horses with disfunction of the left RLN.
2) Aseptically prep the clipped region for five to seven minutes with chlorhexidine scrub, followed by isopropyl alcohol.
3) If desired, local anesthesia (1 mL of 2% lidocaine) can be administered subcutaneously at the intended site of the catheter placement with a 25 g needle.
   a) Local anesthesia should be used for needle-shy patients or neonates.
   b) No more than 1 mL should be used. Placing large blebs can make visualization difficult.
4) A small stab incision in the skin, using a No. 15 scalpel blade, may ease the placement in difficult cases.
5) An appropriate-size catheter (Extended Use catheter required for more than 24 h) should be placed in routine fashion.
6) After placement of the catheter, a previously primed with heparin saline T-port extension set should be attached and flushed again with heparin saline to prevent clot formation.
7) The catheter and extension set are secured with non-absorbable, monofilament suture. The authors prefer on a straight needle.
8) To protect the catheter, apply 4×4 gauze against the catheter and lightly apply an elastic adhesive bandage circumferentially around the neck.

## Medication Administration

There is a diverse range of routes, dosage forms, and delivery systems that have been developed to provide medications. Understanding of pharmaceutics, pharmacokinetics (PK), pharmacodynamics (PD), and therapeutics is a crucial concept to determine the best route and medication formulation. Routes for medication administration can be grouped as parenteral (any non-oral means of administration) and enteral (oral means of administration). There are four basic types of injections used with horses: intravenous (IV), subcutaneous (SQ), intramuscular (IM), and Oral (PO). Other routes of drug administration, including intraarticular administration, pulmonary, rectal, local infiltration, and ocular administration, are useful in equine medicine. The intraarterial, intrathecal, intramedullary, and intraperitoneal routes are used only rarely in equine medicine (Table 3.1).

*IV materials and technique*

- 18–21 gauge needle.
- Assorted syringe sizes 1–60 mL syringes.
- The preferred site for IV drug administration is the right or left jugular vein (authors prefer the proximal 1/3 of the left jugular). However, alternative peripheric vessels that can be used when the jugular veins are thrombosed are cephalic, saphenous, and lateral thoracic veins.
- The vein is held to ease visualization. The needle should be inserted first unattached to a syringe to ensure no accidental intracarotid injections (bright red stream/pulsatile blood flow). An 18-guage needle is the appropriate size for the jugular vein in adult horses; using this needle without a syringe attached will easily inform the clinician if the jugular versus the carotid artery is entered.
- The medication should be injected following manufacturer or other specific drug recommendations.
- The venipuncture site should be compressed for a few seconds after needle removal.
- Common complications of IV administration are adverse reactions, extravasation, intracarotid administration or wrong medication formulation (e.g., procaine penicillin given IV instead of IM).

1 MILA International, Inc. 7984 Tanners Gate Lane Florence, Kentucky USA.
2 B. Braun Medical Inc. Bethlehem, PA USA.
3 Ethicon US, LLC. 2020. 085133-171129.

**Table 3.1** Common routes of drug administration.[a]

| Route | Absorption | Use | Precautions |
|---|---|---|---|
| Intravenous IV | None (directly into the circulation); potentially immediate effects | Emergency use or large volumes; absorption is bypassed | Increased risk of adverse effects; inject solutions slowly<br>Not suitable for most lipid solutions or insoluble substances |
| Subcutaneous SQ | Rapid in aqueous solution; less rapid if deposit formulations | Some less soluble suspensions and implantation of solid pellets or deposit forms | Not suitable for large volumes; irritant substances cause pain and/or necrosis |
| Intramuscular IM | Rapid in aqueous solution; less rapid if deposit formulations | Moderate volumes; lipid vehicles; alternate for venous route | Inadvertent intravenous injection; pain or necrosis at injection site |
| Oral PO | Rate and extent of absorption are highly variable | Maximize compliance (convenient); economical; usually safe | Absorption (bioavailability) may be erratic and incomplete |
| Pulmonary | Rapid; local application for pulmonary disease | Usually for the treatment of pulmonary disease | Absorption (bioavailability) may be erratic and incomplete |

[a] Adapted from Bertone and Horspool (2005).

*IM materials and technique*

- 14–20 gauge needle.
- Assorted syringe sizes 1–60 mL syringes.
- The preferred sites for IM drug administration in the horse are the neck triangle, as well as the pectoral, semimembranosus, semitendinosus or gluteal muscles. The authors prefer the neck and pectoral muscle region for IM injections.
- To administer the IM injection, the needle should be introduced completely, angled perpendicular to the skin.
- Connect the syringe to the needle and aspirate to ensure no blood is obtained. If blood is observed the needle should be redirected or change locations to avoid adverse reactions to the medication.
- When large volumes need to be injected, the volume should be divided into 2 or more sites (no more than 15–20 mL per site) to reduce risk of complications.
- Common complications of IM injections are muscle soreness and pain, abscess formation, or bacterial myonecrosis.

*SQ materials and technique*

- 19–25 gauge needle.
- Assorted syringe sizes 1–10 mL syringes.
- For SQ injections tent the skin and introduce the needle at an angle beneath the skin.
- Prior to medication administration, aspirate the syringe to ensure no blood is obtained. If blood is observed the needle should be redirected or change locations to avoid adverse reactions to the medication.
- Common complications include post injection pain, abscess formation, and hair discoloration.

*PO materials and technique*

- 30–60 mL catheter tip syringe.
- The syringe should be introduced into the side of the mouth (between cheek and molar teeth); next the medication should be delivered slowly but continuously to allow the animal to swallow. Some medications can have a bitter taste and may have horses stop eating; therefore, rinsing the mouth 15–20 minutes after medications can be useful, especially when long-term medications re-prescribed.
- Complications associated with oral medications are uncommon; however, aspiration pneumonia (specially in neonates) or swallowing of foreign bodies (syringes) has been reported.

## Bandaging, Cast, and Splint Supplies

External coaptation can help protect wounds, prevent excessive edema, support the underlying structures, absorb wound exudates, allow application of local therapies (topical medications), reduce dead space, and prevent excessive granulation tissue (Theoret and Schumacher 2017; Canada et al. 2018; Eggleston 2018). Bandages usually are made of three layers (Figure 3.2). The primary or inner/contact layer is one of the most important layers of the bandage since it is in direct contact with the wound; different dressing options are available depending on the wound-healing stage and various applications can be modified, depending on the intended goal. These options can be classified depending on the material (synthetic, semi-synthetic, or biologic), gas and fluid exchange (occlusive, semi-occlusive, or non-occlusive occlusive), or if adherence to the wound bed is desired or not (adherent or non-adherent) (Theoret and Schumacher 2017; Canada et al. 2018; Eggleston 2018). The secondary or intermediate provides absorption and protection to the wound. This layer is usually composed of laminated sheet cotton or cotton roll (Theoret and Schumacher 2017; Canada et al. 2018; Eggleston 2018). The third or outer/external layer is the holding layer of the bandage and is usually accomplished by using an adhesive or cohesive bandaging tape. Splints or casts are typically used to manage lesions or wounds (located in high-motion areas or if compromises supporting structures, such as tendons and ligaments) that require complete or partial immobilization. The type of bandage, cast and/or splint is chosen on the basis of the location and the nature of the injury (Howard et al. 1993; Gomez and Hanson 2005; Moyer et al. 2011a; Theoret and Schumacher 2017; Canada et al. 2018; Eggleston 2018).

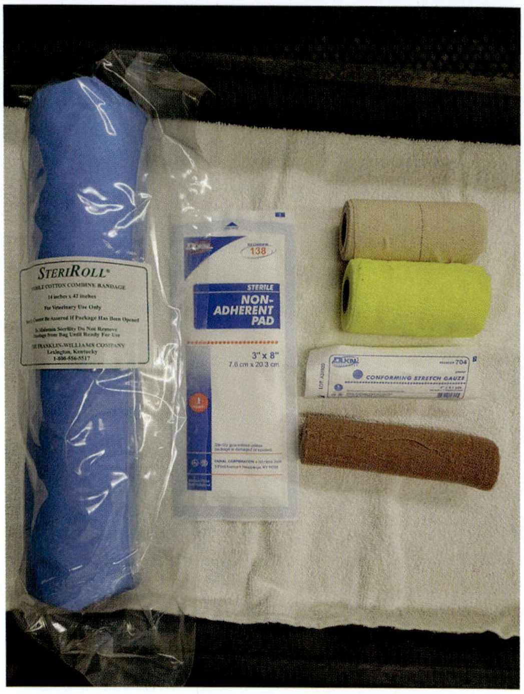


**Figure 3.2** Bandaging supplies for bandage application. From left to right: SteriRoll sterile sheet cotton, non-adherent pad, conforming stretch gauze (white package for attaching non-adherent or other dressing), brown gauze (6-in. for compressing sheet cotton for primary bandage), VetWrap (4-in. for further compressing the bandage), and Elasticon (elastic bandage for covering the top and bottom of the bandage to prevent debris from entering).

*Bandage materials*

1) Inner layer: Desired dressing and sterile comfort stretch gauze roll (e.g., Kling®).[4]
2) Intermediate layer: Sterile or non-sterile combine cotton bandage (e.g., CombiRoll®, RediRoll®, SteriRoll®).[5]
   2.1 The sterile or non-sterile roll can be held in place using a non-stretch brown cling gauze roll to add compression (e.g., Brown cling gauze, JorVet).[6]
3) External layer: Simple tear cohesive bandage (e.g., Vetwrap®, Coban®)[7] and/or adhesive elastic tape to seal the bandage (e.g., Elasticon®, 3M Veterinary Elastic Adhesive Tape®).[7]

*Procedure*

1) Apply the inner layer using aseptic technique. The purpose of this layer is determined by the therapeutic objective. This layer is not used for compression; an elastic material should be used to reduce the risk of strangulation.
2) The intermediate layer keeps the inner layer in place, absorbs the exudate, and acts as padding. This layer can be applied with passive pressure.
3) The outer layer holds the intermediate layer in place and prevents contamination, trauma, and motion. This layer should ideally be breathable but waterproof and adds compression to the bandage.

4 Dynarex Corporation. 10 Glenshaw street, Orangeburg, NY 10962.
5 The Franklin-Williams Company, 116 Venture Court, Suite 12, Lexington, Ky 40511.
6 Jorgensen Laboratories, LLC, 1450 Van Buren Ave, Loveland, Co, 80538.
7 Covertrus North America, 400 Metro Place North, Dublin, Oh, 43017. Or Corporate office, 12 Mount fort Street, Portland, ME 04101.

Tips: In layer circumferential bandage (e.g., limb, abdomen, thorax, neck), each new wrap should overlap the previous one by 50%. The bandage should have even tension throughout the length to prevent uneven pressure that can lead to injuries. A loose bandage or unevenly pressure bandage is more likely to create injuries than an even tension bandage.

- Apply the bandage from distal to proximal.
- Apply even tension through the entire length of the bandage to prevent wrinkles and ridges (pressure points).
- Consider additional padding to narrow areas of the limb to obtain an overall even bandage pressure.
- Make a relief incision to alleviate pressure in areas of concern (e.g., accessory carpal bone, calcaneus tuberosity of tarsus).

## Splints

Splints are commonly made of sturdy, light weight, and readily accessible materials such as polyvinyl chloride (PVC) pipe, wood boards (1 × 3 or 4-in. hardwood), cast material or metal; commercially available splints (e.g., Kimzey®)[8] are also available (Figure 3.3, A and B). Wooden splints of cylindrical shape (e.g., dowels or broom sticks) are contraindicated for splinting in animals as the shape facilitates splint movement along the vertical axis of the limb, compromising stability and causing more damage at the fracture site. Splints are typically used in emergency situations for temporary stabilization of severe bone, joint, or soft-tissue injuries (Box 3.1), and can be used for transportation or in adjunction with selective treatments (intermediary step after removal of a cast and wound healing). However, in most situations, splints should not be used as the only means of fracture treatment.

(a) (b)

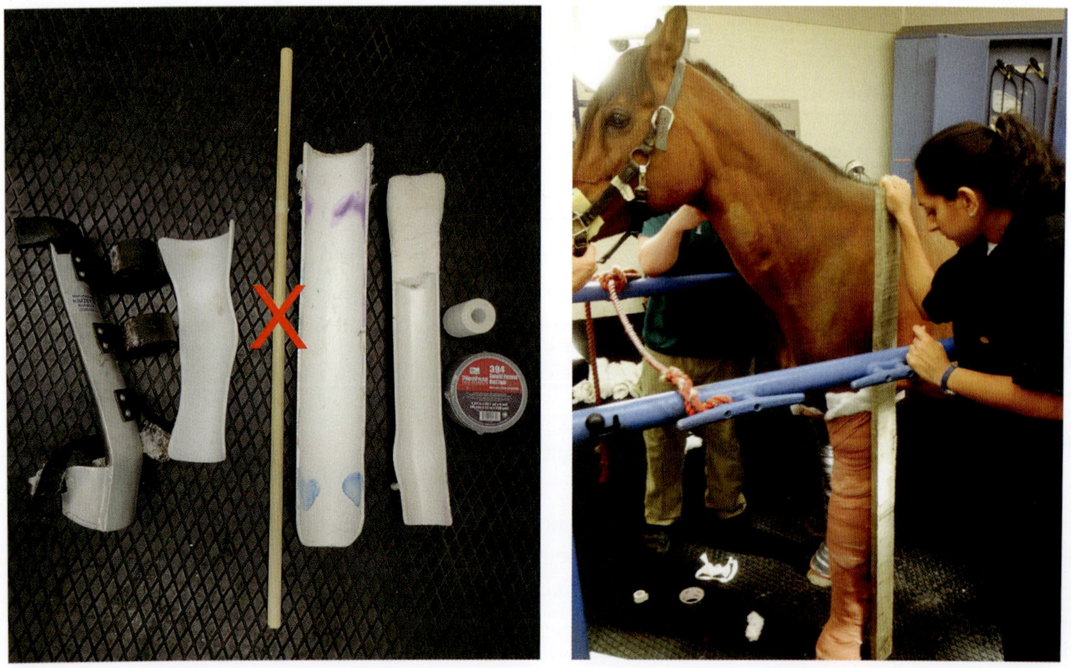

**Figure 3.3** (a) Different splinting materials. From left to right: front-limb Kimzey splint, equine easy splint, wood board, PVC pipe splints, 4″ white tape and duct tape. *Note:* the round wood dowel splint shown (X) is *contraindicated* for limb stabilization as it often rotates under the bandage, ending up over the unstable fracture site and causing further injury. (b) Rather, a hardwood board (ash, oak, hickory, 1 × 3 in. in size) cut to the level of the proximal scapula or greater trochanter is recommended to provide support for mid-limb fractures of the radius or tibia, respectively.

8 Kimzey Welding Works, 164 Kentucky Avenue, Woodland, CA 95695 USA.

**Box 3.1 Principles of splint application for long bone fracture**

1) Apply the splint following the rule of cast application: *stabilize the joint above and below the fracture.*
2) Apply two splints when possible to provide orthogonal stabilization (support along 90° planes); excellent choice for cannon bone and distal tibial or radial fractures.
3) Never end rigid fixation (including splints, casts, bone plates, etc.) in the middle of a long bone; this causes a stress riser effect with possible injury including fracture at the end of the splint or implant.
4) Attach the splint(s) over the entire circumference of the bandage from top to bottom with non-elastic tape (e.g. Duct tape) to increase stability of the bandage/ splint construct.

*Splint materials*

1) Standard bandage materials for appropriate immobilization (for full bandage types and indications, please refer to literature) (Auer 2018).
2) Available splint (examples given above).
3) Non-elastic tape (white tape or duct tape is preferred by the authors).
4) Elastic adhesive tape (e.g., Elasticon®).

*Procedure*

1) Apply a standard Robert Jones bandage.
2) Apply the splint over appropriate anatomic location depending on primary injury/pathology (caudal, dorsal, lateral, or combination of two).
3) Secure splint with non-elastic tape (white tape or duct tape).
4) Elastic adhesive tape (e.g., Elasticon®) to seal top and bottom of the splint bandage. This reduces the bedding and debris that enters the bandage.

Tips: When appropriate padding is placed the splint should be secured tightly against the limb throughout its length to avoid movement of the splint that can act as fulcrum, further damaging the affected structures. Additional bandage materials may be added to the limb or splint to improve contact with the limb.

## Wound Repair Supplies

Basic wound repair supplies include materials to clean and disinfect the wound, repair lacerations, and bandage wounds (Figures 3.4 and 3.5). There are several factors involved with the initial management and repair of a wound. Some of these include the type of wound (e.g., puncture vs. laceration), the location, the degree of trauma, and amount of contamination. Closure of an open, full-thickness wound may be by primary, delayed-primary, or secondary closure techniques. Wounds also may be left to heal by second intention wound healing. The decision on how to treat and manage the wound is often dependent on the intrinsic factors of the wound itself and the clinician's experience (Howard et al. 1993; Gomez and Hanson 2005; Theoret and Schumacher 2017; Auer 2018; Canada et al. 2018; Eggleston 2018).

*Materials*

1) Sedation – often a combination of an alpha 2 agonist and opioid (xylazine/detomidine hydrochloride and butorphanol tartrate).
2) Twitch, chain, or other restraint methods (optional).
3) Clippers with #40 blade.
4) Sterile lubricant.

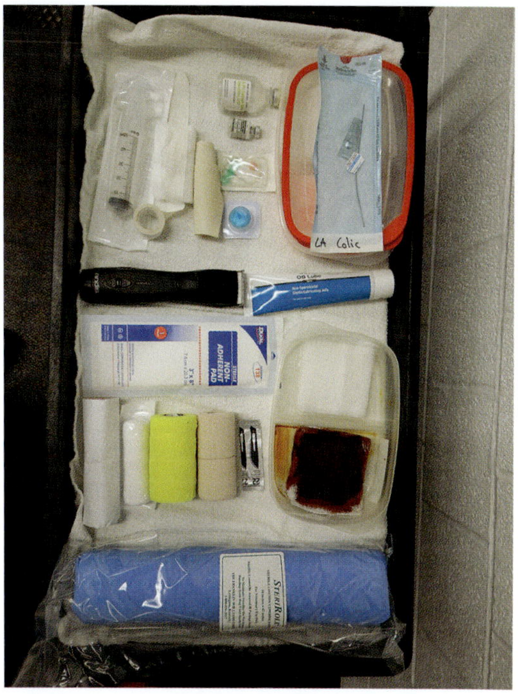


**Figure 3.4** Bandaging, scrubbing, wound probing, and intravenous regional limb perfusion materials for working on patients with wounds or other traumatic injury.

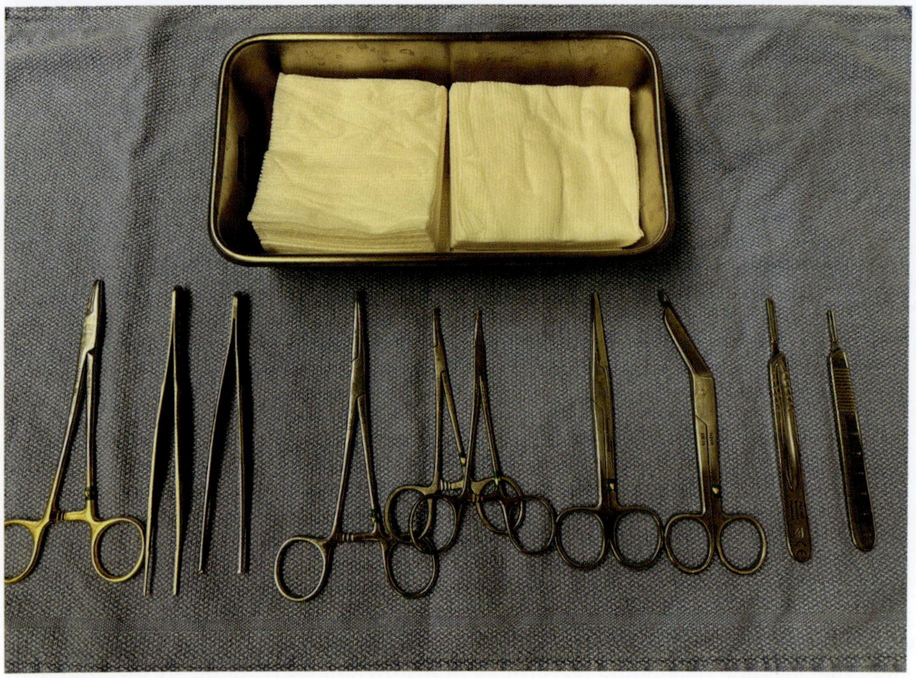

**Figure 3.5** Wound closure basic pack composed of basic instruments: needle drivers, hemostat (crile and mosquito), suture scissors, dissection scissors (Mayo and Metzenbaum), thumb tissue forceps, blade handles (#3 and #4).

5) Scrub Materials.
   5.1 70% Isopropyl Alcohol.[9]
   5.2 Chlorhexidine gluconate scrub (CH) 2–4% (e.g., Pro-Tec® ChlorSeptic 2% with aloe vera).[10]
   5.3 Chlorhexidine gluconate (CH) 2%.[9]
   5.4 Povidone iodine (PI) scrub and solution.[9]
   5.5 0.9% Physiologic Saline Solution.[11]
6) Exam gloves.
7) Sterile gloves.
8) Flexible probe/teat cannula (wound probing).
9) 22–25 gauge needles for local anesthesia.
10) 19–21 gauge needles for injection.
11) 5–35 mL slip tip syringe.
12) IV extension line (optional, for difficult patients).
13) Culture media: Port-a-Cul, blood culture bottles (optional).
14) Wound bandaging materials for the limb:
   14.1 Non-adherent dressing (e.g., Telfa pad® – Curity™ abdominal pad).[12]
   14.2 Sterile comfort stretch gauze roll (e.g., Kling®).[13]
   14.3 Sterile and non-sterile combine cotton bandage (e.g., CombiRoll®, RediRoll®, SteriRoll®).[14] The sterile or non-sterile roll can be held in place using a non-stretch brown cling gauze roll to add compression (e.g., Brown cling gauze, JorVet).[15]
   14.4 Self-adherent bandage (e.g.,Vetwrap®, Coban®).[16]
   14.5 Adhesive elastic tape to seal the bandage (e.g., Elasticon®, 3M Veterinary Elastic Adhesive Tape®).[16]

---

9 Covertrus North America, 400 Metro Place North, Dublin, Oh, 43017. Or Corporate office, 12 Mount fort Street, Portland, ME 04101.
10 Aurora Pharmaceutical, Inc. Northfield, MN 55057.
11 MDMAXX LLC, 1762 Benson Ave, Brooklyn, NY 11214.
12 Covidien LLC, 15 Hampshire Street, Mansfield, MA 02048.
13 Dynarex Corporation. 10 Glenshaw street, Orangeburg, NY 10962.
14 Jorgensen Laboratories, LLC, 1450 Van Buren Ave, Loveland, Co, 80538.
15 The Franklin-Williams Company, 116 Venture Court, Suite 12, Lexington, Ky 40511.
16 Covertrus North America, 400 Metro Place North, Dublin, Oh, 43017. Or Corporate office, 12 Mount fort Street, Portland, ME 04101.

*Procedure*

1) Sedate the patient. Recommended dosages are:
   a) Adult horses: Xylazine 0.3–0.5 mL/kg or Detomidine 0.01 mg/kg IV +/− Butorphanol 0.01–0.02 mg/kg IV for adult horses.
   b) Foals: Midazolam 0.05–0.1 mg/kg or Diazepam 0.1–0.25 mg/kg IV +/− Morphine 0.03–0.06 mg/kg or Butorphanol 0.05–0.1 mg/kg IV.
2) While wearing gloves, apply a generous amount of sterile lubricant over the wound. This helps eliminate debris from entering the wound while clipping.
3) Clip the wound margins. Give yourself enough room to comfortably close the wound when indicated.
4) Perform a rough scrub around the intact skin. Avoid introducing 70% isopropyl alcohol and/or chlorhexidine scrub over the wound bed as it is cytotoxic.
5) The wound itself should be gently and effectively cleaned with 0.9% physiologic saline or a diluted antiseptic solution until all dirt or gross contamination is removed.
   a) CH solution should be diluted 0.05% solution (1 : 40 = 25 mL 2% concentrate diluted with 975 mL sterile isotonic crystalloid solution).
   b) PI 0.1% – 0.2% (10–20 mL/1 L of sterile isotonic crystalloid solution).
6) Change gloves (ideally use sterile gloves) and perform a sterile scrub following the previous guidelines.
7) Using the sterile flexible probe or teat cannula, explore the wound to assess the extent of the wound, and help determine which structures are involved.
8) If surgical closure is indicated, perform local anesthesia (local nerve block or ring block) prior to suturing. Please refer to the literature (Moyer et al. 2011a; Grimm et al. 2015; Auer 2018).
9) Suture the wound using the appropriate suture techniques (appositional vs tension relieving patterns). For better decision making on appropriate closing techniques refer to Chapter 7 or additional literature (Theoret and Schumacher 2017; Auer 2018).
10) Cover the wound with the appropriate bandage material when possible.

## Joint Fluid Collection

Synoviocentesis is a common procedure performed in horses to diagnose or treat joint pathology (Figure 3.6). In horses, joint disease is the most common cause of lameness resulting in morbidity for the patient and loss of income for owners and trainers (Lee et al. 2013). Infectious processes can not only be life threatening, but also reduce future athletic performance secondary to joint pain, fibrosis, and reduced range of motion even if appropriate surgical and/or medical management is performed (Bertone 1999; Morton 2005; N.A. 2011; Grimm et al. 2015; Auer 2018; Baxter 2020).

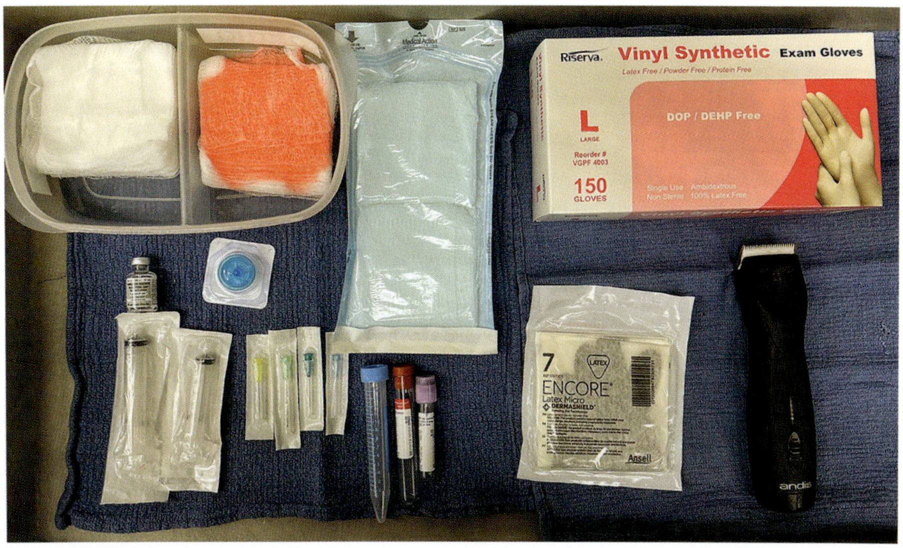


**Figure 3.6** Image shows joint fluid collection materials. Scrubbing materials, assorted syringes and needles, antibiotics (Amikacin), fluid collection tubes (EDTA and plain), exam gloves, sterile gloves, and clippers.

**Table 3.2** Synovial fluid cytology in various clinical conditions.

| Parameter | Normal | Mild synovitis | Osteoarthritis | [a]Septic arthritis | Arthrocentesis |
|---|---|---|---|---|---|
| Total leukocytes (/μ) | 50–500 | 20–250 | ≤1×103 | 20–200×$10^3$ | 1–4×$10^3$ |
| Neutrophils (%) | <10 | <10 | <15 | >90 | 50 |
| Mononuclear cells (%) | >90 | >90 | >85 | <10 | 50 |
| Total protein (g/dL) | 0.8–2.5 | 0.8–3 | 0.8–3.5 | 4.0–8+ | 1.5–2.5 |
| Appearance | Pale yellow, clear | Yellow translucent | Yellow, clear | Yellow-green, turbid | Yellow, clear (in normal circumstances) |
| Viscosity | Hi | Low | Low (variable) | Increased | High |
| Volume | Low | Generally increased | Variable | High | Mildly increased |

[a] Significant elevations in leukocyte counts and total protein concentration occur within the first 12 h in experimentally inoculated joints. Values shown represent those observed at 24 h.
Listed ranges are approximate. Considerable variability exists in published reports.
*Source:* Adapted from Auer, Stick, Kümmerle & Prange.

Iatrogenic septic arthritis has been associated with the experience level of the veterinarian as well as the injection site preparation method, use of sterile gloves, and type of corticosteroid administered (Moyer et al. 2011b; Gillespie et al. 2016; Brunsting et al. 2018; Steel et al. 2013). Other risk factors associated with septic arthritis post-injections include, but are not limited to, clipping the hair at the injection site, use of a single needle for drawing and injecting, and use of dexamethasone (Gillespie et al. 2016). Early recognition and aggressive treatment of synovial sepsis has been associated with a better prognosis for survival and return to athletic function than when treatment is delayed (Morton 2005). Reference ranges for synovial fluid in normal conditions, mild synovitis, osteoarthritis, septic arthritis, and arthrocentesis can be found in Table 3.2.

*Materials*

1) Sedation with a combination of alpha 2-agonist and opioid (xylazine/detomidine hydrochloride and butorphanol tartrate).
2) Twitch (upper lip or ear) or Chain.
3) Clippers with #40 blade.
4) 4% Chlorhexidine Scrub.
5) Isopropyl Alcohol.
6) Exam Gloves.
7) Sterile Gloves.
8) 4×4 Gauze.
9) 18–22 gauge needles.
10) 5–10 mL slip tip syringes.
11) EDTA and Red Top Serum vacutainer tubes.
12) Culture media (port-a-Cul blood culture bottles).
13) Antibiotic of choice (e.g., 125–500 mg Amikacin).

*Procedure*

1) Locate the joint of interest and identify any important landmarks. Please refer to the literature for joint injection guidelines (N.A. 2011; Grimm et al. 2015; Auer 2018; Baxter 2020).
2) Clip the site for needle placement. Clipping may not always be necessary. However, horses with long hair or significant contamination should be clipped to improve sterile preparation of the injection site. Also, injection lower on the limb, especially near the hoof, carries increased risk of contamination.

3) Sedate the patient. Recommended dosages are:
   a) Adult horses: Xylazine 0.3–0.5 mL/kg or Detomidine 0.01 mg/kg IV +/− Butorphanol 0.01–0.02 mg/kg IV for adult horses.
   b) Foals: Midazolam 0.05–0.1 mg/kg or Diazepam 0.1–0.25 mg/kg IV +/− Morphine 0.03–0.06 mg/kg or Butorphanol 0.05–0.1 mg/kg IV.
4) A lip twitch or other method of restraint can be used or added for difficult patients.
5) While wearing exam gloves, the appropriate site should be aseptically prepped for three to five minutes (until no gross contamination is observed) with chlorhexidine scrub followed by isopropyl alcohol.
6) To perform a final sterile prep, place sterile gloves and continue to prep site using sterile gauze with chlorhexidine followed by isopropyl alcohol.
7) For the joint injection, place new sterile gloves and open supplies in the sterile field (glove wrapping) using aseptic technique.
8) If an antibiotic is desired, it should be drawn up with a different needle than the one used for the arthrocentesis.
9) Palpate the injection site with your thumb or index finger (authors recommend only using one finger to locate the injection site as this finger is considered contaminated after palpation).
10) Quickly insert the needle through the skin and into the joint space.
    a) It is very important for the patient to be still at this stage.
    b) Care should be taken to prevent damage to the cartilage and soft-tissue structures as well as to prevent blood contamination to the sample.
11) Synovial fluid frequently appears at the hub of the needle and can run freely.
12) If no fluid is observed, the needle may be rotated or repositioned. An assistant can push the joint capsule from the opposite side as well.
13) Fluid can be collected directly into the appropriate tubes or aspirated with a syringe.
    a) If a syringe is used, the transfer to the tubes or cultures should be quick to avoid the sample from clotting (this is important for the cell count).
    b) Red Top Serum tubes and Port-a-Cul blood culture bottles are designated for culture analysis.
    c) EDTA tubes are designated for cell count and cytology.
14) After you have collected the fluid, you may inject the antibiotic medication and remove the needle.

## References

Auer, J.A. (2018). *Equine Surgery*, 5e. Elsevier.

Barakzai, S. and Chandler, K. (2003). Use of indwelling intravenous catheters in the horse. *In Pract.* 25 (5): 264–271. https://doi.org/10.1136/inpract.25.5.264.

Baxter, G.M. (ed.) (2020). *Adams and Stashak's Lameness in the Horse*. Wiley.

Bertone, A.L. (1999). Update on infectious arthritis in horses. *Equine Vet. Educ.* 11 (3): 143–152. https://doi.org/10.1111/j.2042-3292.1999.tb00936.x.

Bertone, J.J. and Horspool, L.J.I. (ed.) (2005). *Equine clinical pharmacology*, Repr.e. London: W. B. Saunders.

Brunsting, J.Y., Pille, F.J., Oosterlinck, M. et al. (2018). Incidence and risk factors of surgical site infection and septic arthritis after elective arthroscopy in horses. *Vet. Surg.* 47 (1): 52–59. https://doi.org/10.1111/vsu.12699.

Canada, N.C., Beard, W.L., Guyan, M.E., and White, B.J. (2018). Effect of bandaging techniques on sub-bandage pressures in the equine distal limb, carpus, and tarsus. *Vet. Surg.* 47 (5): 640–647. https://doi.org/10.1111/vsu.12914.

Eggleston, R.B. (2018). Equine wound management. *Vet. Clin. N. Am. Equine Pract.* 34 (3): 557–574. https://doi.org/10.1016/j.cveq.2018.07.010.

Gillespie, C.C., Adams, S.B., and Moore, G.E. (2016). Methods and variables associated with the risk of septic arthritis following intra-articular injections in horses: a survey of veterinarians: risk factors for septic arthritis following intra-articular injections in horses. *Vet. Surg.* 45 (8): 1071–1076. https://doi.org/10.1111/vsu.12563.

Gomez, J.H. and Hanson, R.R. (2005). Use of dressings and bandages in equine wound management. *Vet. Clin. N. Am. Equine Pract.* 21 (1): 91–104. https://doi.org/10.1016/j.cveq.2004.11.004.

Grimm, K.A., Lamont, L.A., Tranquilli, W.J. et al. (ed.) (2015). *Veterinary Anesthesia and Analgesia*, 5e. Wiley Blackwell.

Hay, C.W. (1992). Equine intravenous catheterisation. *Equine Vet. Educ.* 4 (6): 319–323. https://doi.org/10.1111/j.2042-3292.1992.tb00976.x.

Hobbs, K.J., Johnson, P.J., Scharf, M.E. et al. (2021). Use of a jugular vein model for the instruction of equine intravenous catheter placement by third-and fourth-year veterinary students. *Equine Vet. Educ.* 33 (5): 249–254. https://doi.org/10.1111/eve.13260.

Howard, R.D., Stashak, T.S., and Baxter, G.M. (1993). Evaluation of occlusive dressings for management of full-thickness excisional wounds on the distal portion of the limbs of horses. *Am. J. Vet. Res.* 54 (12): 2150–2154.

Lee, C.M., Kisiday, J.D., McIlwraith, C.W. et al. (2013). Synoviocytes protect cartilage from the effects of injury in vitro. *BMC Musculoskelet. Disord.* 14 (1): 54. https://doi.org/10.1186/1471-2474-14-54.

Morton, A.J. (2005). Diagnosis and treatment of septic arthritis. *Vet. Clin. N. Am. Equine Pract.* 21 (3): 627–649. https://doi.org/10.1016/j.cveq.2005.08.001.

Moyer, W.W., Schumacher, J.N., Schuhmacher, J. et al. (2011a). *Equine Joint Injection and Regional Anesthesia*. Academic Veterinary Solutions.

Moyer, W., Schumacher, J., Schumacher, J., and Moyer, W. (2011b). *Equine Joint Injection and Regional Anesthesia*, 5e. Academic Veterinary Solutions, LLC.

Orsini, J.A. and Divers, T.J. (ed.) (2014). *Equine Emergencies*. Elsevier. https://doi.org/10.1016/C2010-0-68789-X.

Ross, M.W. and Dyson, S.J. (ed.) (2011). *Diagnosis and Management of Lameness in the Horse*. Elsevier. https://doi.org/10.1016/C2009-0-50774-X.

Schoster, A. (2017). Complications of intravenous catheterization in horses. *Schweizer Archiv für Tierheilkunde* 159 (9): 477–485. https://doi.org/10.17236/sat00126.

Steel, C., Pannirselvam, R., and Anderson, G. (2013). Risk of septic arthritis after intra-articular medication: a study of 16,624 injections in Thoroughbred racehorses. *Aust. Vet. J.* 91 (7): 268–273. https://doi.org/10.1111/avj.12073.

Theoret, C. and Schumacher, J. (ed.) (2017). *Equine Wound Management*, 3e. Wiley.

# 4

# Basic Clinical Triage Procedures

*Barbara Delvescovo*[1], *Rebecca C. McOnie*[1], *Kelly Knickelbein*[1*], *Katharyn J. Mitchell*[1*], *and Nicole Scherrer*[2*]

[1] *Department of Clinical Sciences, College of Veterinary Medicine, Cornell University, Ithaca, NY, USA*
[2] *Department of Clinical Studies - New Bolton Center, University of Pennsylvania School of Veterinary Medicine, Kennett Square, PA, USA*

## Establishing Intravenous Access and Catheter Placement

Intravenous (IV) catheter placement is indicated for the administration of medications and fluid therapy, as well as for the acquisition of blood for serial testing. The primary sites for IV access in the foal and adult horse are the external jugular veins. In the adult horse, the lateral thoracic vessel (superficial thoracic) is also possible, and the only other IV access site that will support large volume fluid therapy. The external jugular veins are large, readily palpable, and usually easily accessed in both the foal and adult horse. However, catheter placement into the external jugular vein in the foal and the lateral thoracic vein of adult horses is more challenging, and an over-the-wire catheter system is highly recommended.

A 14 G, 5.25″ long catheter is commonly placed in the jugular vein of adult horses for fluid and medication administration. If rapid fluid resuscitation is required, a 10 or 12 G catheter is recommended, as the lumen diameter of the catheter can otherwise represent the limiting factor for the rate of fluid administration (Auckburally et al. 2019). A small skin cut down at the site of catheter insertion can improve ease of catheter placement and decrease the likelihood of burring the catheter tip. This is particularly relevant when placing a large (>14 G) catheter, or when working on donkeys. At times, the jugular veins might be inaccessible due to abnormalities such as thrombosis, wounds, or emphysema. Alternatively, the lateral thoracic, cephalic, or saphenous veins can be accessed for IV catheter placement (Barakzai and Chandler 2003). Catheter placement in these locations requires additional catheter protection to avoid dislodgement. Regardless of the site of placement, the catheter should be flushed with heparinized saline four times daily and thoroughly examined at least twice daily. Remove the catheter promptly when it is no longer required to minimize complications.

*Materials* (Figure 4.1)

1) Clippers.
2) Supplies for aseptic skin preparation – antiseptic (chlorhexidine, alcohol), gauze sponges.
3) 2% Lidocaine, 3 mL syringe with a 25 G needle.
4) Intravenous catheter (e.g., 14 G × 5.25″ standard size for adult horses).
5) T-port catheter extension.
6) Injection cap.
7) Heparinized saline flush.
8) 1″ medical tape.
9) Non-absorbable suture on a straight needle.
10) Sterile gloves.
11) Optional: #15 blade, bandage materials (gauze sponges, Elastikon).

*Contributing author

*Emergency Triage of the Horse*, First Edition. Edited by Rolfe M. Radcliffe and Jamie J. Kopper.

Published 2026 by John Wiley & Sons, Inc.
Companion website: www.wiley.com/go/radcliffe/triage

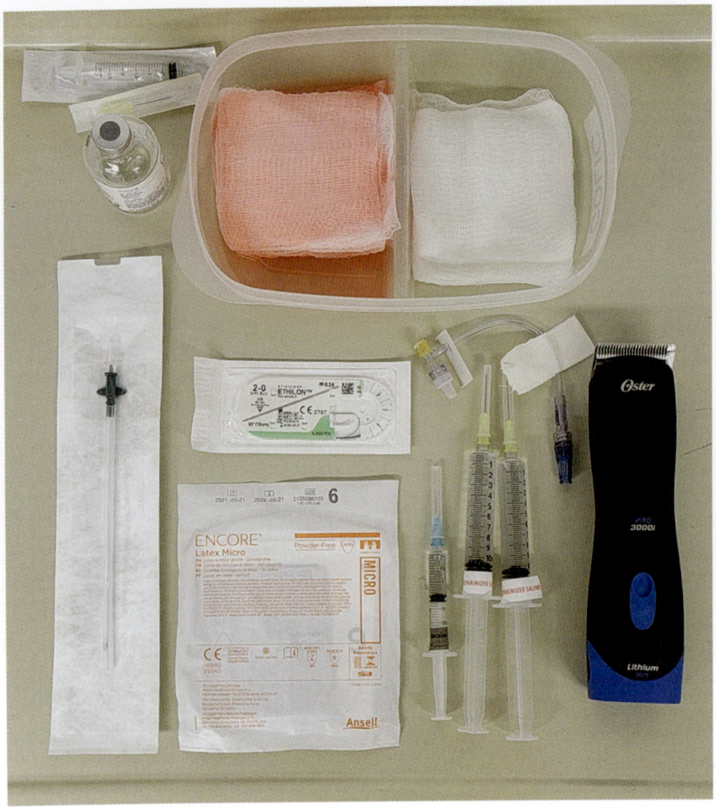


**Figure 4.1** Materials for placement of an intravenous catheter.

*Procedure*

1) Appropriately restrain the patient. Although most horses will tolerate jugular catheter placement with only local anesthesia, some require sedation.
2) Clip a ~3 × 3″ area of hair in the cranial third of the neck over the external jugular vein. The superficial jugular vein and deeper carotid artery are maximally separated in the cranial third of the neck, making this the safest location for catheter placement.
3) Aseptically prepare the clipped site.
4) Deposit a 1″ subcutaneous (SC) line block of lidocaine over the jugular vein to anesthetize the site for catheter placement and securing sutures.
5) Perform final aseptic preparation of the clipped site.
6) Prepare the T-port extension by priming it with heparinized saline and attaching the injection port. Leave the disposable cap on the distal end of the T-port until ready to secure it to the catheter. Apply a small tape butterfly to the extension, near the injection port.
7) Don sterile gloves.
8) Use the #15 scalpel blade to make a ~5 mm skin cut-down at the intended site of catheter placement. If right-handed, use the left hand to pinch up the anesthetized skin and insert the #15 blade in a stab motion through the skin, parallel to the jugular vein with the blade pointing upward. Pinch the #15 blade with the thumb and index finger just below the level of the blade (i.e., "choke up" on the blade) to avoid an inadvertent, excessive depth of penetration.
9) Grasp the sterile catheter. A non-sterile assistant can flush heparinized saline through the catheter. Place a gloved finger over the open hub of the catheter. Use the non-dominant hand to distend the jugular vein. Align the catheter at a 45° angle to the skin, parallel to the length of the jugular vein.
10) Press the catheter firmly through the skin cut-down and into the jugular vein. When a flash of blood is observed, decrease the angle of insertion (i.e., bring the hand toward the horse) and advance the catheter half an inch into the vein.

11) Use your non-dominant hand to stabilize the stylette and use the dominant hand (clean) to advance the catheter off the stylette, into the vessel, positioning the catheter hub at the level of the skin. Remove the stylette. Ensure the catheter continues to bleed back by distending the jugular vein. Immediately secure the T-port extension to the catheter to avoid air embolism.
12) Secure the catheter to the patient's skin with several interrupted sutures. This can include a suture just above the hub of the catheter, suture through the catheter wings, and a suture through the tape butterfly on the T-port extension (Figure 4.2).
13) Flush the catheter with heparinized saline.
14) The catheter can be protected by covering the hub and extension with gauze sponges, and securing these around the neck, limb, or trunk depending on the location of the catheter. The catheter should be secured so the quick release clamp can be easily accessed. Additionally, the bandage should be moved or changed regularly to evaluate the vessel integrity, and to look for signs of infection around the catheter hub.

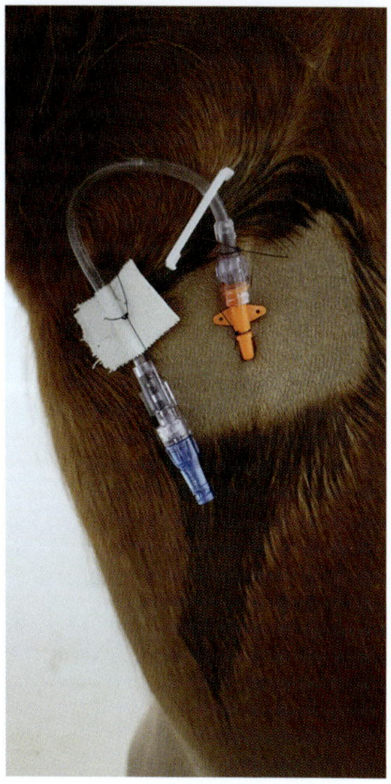

**Figure 4.2** An intravenous catheter placed in the left jugular vein, with the T-port extension and catheter hub appropriately secured to the patient's skin.

*Potential complications*

1) Injury to the carotid artery, noted by blood spurting from the catheter or rapid formation of a large hematoma: Remove the catheter and apply digital pressure with gauze sponges, or secure a large stack of gauze sponges with Elastikon around the neck. A residual hematoma is commonly present (Schoster 2017).
2) Clotting of the catheter during a prolonged attempt at insertion: Flush the catheter with heparinized saline prior to starting the procedure. If a thrombus develops in the catheter, dispose of the catheter and restart.
3) Thrombophlebitis: Inflammation of the catheterized vessel can occur, with or without infection. The diagnosis can be made on clinical examination in many cases and confirmed with ultrasound evaluation of the vessel. The catheter should be removed, and its tip should be cultured. Anti-inflammatory +/− antibiotic therapy should be instituted (Schoster 2017).
4) SC placement of the catheter with difficulty entering the jugular vein or advancing the catheter into the vein: Ensure the catheter and stylette are well seated in the vein prior to advancing the catheter off the stylette. Use of an over-the-wire catheter can ease placement. Ultrasound guidance can be beneficial in hypovolemic foals when catheter placement is extremely difficult. Alternatively, initial fluid resuscitation through a butterfly catheter prior to over-the-needle catheter insertion can improve visualization or palpation of the jugular veins.
5) Venous air embolism: A venous air embolism most commonly occurs when the catheter hub and extension set become detached (often due to the horse rubbing the catheter site). When the horse's head is elevated, an air embolism will result. The effect will depend on the extent of air introduced into the circulatory system, and will range from mild, transient signs to life-threatening consequences. Common signs include abnormal behavior, neurologic symptoms, and cardiac arrhythmias. The horse should be promptly treated symptomatically and closely monitored (Parkinson et al. 2018).
6) Catheter fragmentation: Uncommonly, a catheter will break at the hub and be released into the blood stream. A catheter can also become fragmented or sheared if attempts are made to blindly rethread the catheter over the stylet. If a portion of the catheter is embolized, it often becomes lodged in the pulmonary vasculature; in smaller animals, it can become wedged in the right heart. The location of the catheter embolus should be assessed by ultrasonography and thoracic radiographs. Catheter emboli rarely cause a problem when lodged in pulmonary vasculature; however, removal is likely indicated if the catheter fragment is stuck in the heart (Schoster 2017).

## Fluid Administration Techniques

Fluid administration can be accomplished by numerous methods. The most common and straightforward of these include enteral and IV administration. Selection of the method of fluid administration is dependent on the urgency of fluid resuscitation, the ability to gain vascular access, the patient's tolerance for enteral administration, cost, the type of fluids available, and the disease process(es) affecting the patient (Crabtree and Epstein 2021).

## Intravenous Fluids (IVF)

After IV access and catheter placement have been established, as described earlier in this chapter, a primed fluid line is connected to the IV catheter. IV fluid therapy is the fastest mechanism for expanding the vascular volume and improving the patient's systemic condition in cases of hypovolemic shock.

*Materials*

1) Sterile, isotonic fluids.
2) 1″ medical tape.

*Procedure*

1) Attach a fluid line to the desired fluid bag(s). For adult horses, 5 L fluid bags are recommended and for foals, 1 L fluid bags will likely suffice.
2) Prime the fluid line to remove air.
3) Set the fluid rate. If using a fluid pump for administration to a foal, set a fluid pump with the total volume to be administered and rate for administration.
4) Flush the patient's IV catheter with heparinized saline.
5) Secure the fluid line to the catheter extension.
6) Ensure the extension set and fluid line are patent (all clamps are open). Double check the fluid rate.
7) Create a stress loop for the fluid line by securing it with 1″ medical tape to the patient's halter or a braid in their mane. Avoid creating a large loop through which a foot could get caught.

## Enteral Fluids

Fluid can be administered continuously through a narrow, indwelling nasogastric tube (NGT), or bolused at intervals (often q 2–6h). Isotonic fluids can be administered in combination with mineral oil and/or concentrated electrolyte solutions. The patient must not be "third spacing" fluids into the gastrointestinal tract (e.g., producing gastric reflux) for enteral fluids to be administered. Additionally, the patient must tolerate NGT placement. Enteral fluids are an economic and efficient method of providing fluid resuscitation.

*Materials*

1) Nasogastric tube (NGT).
2) Buckets (2).
3) Stomach pump.
4) Clean, non-sterile isotonic fluids: 4 g KCl (lite salt) + 50 g NaCl (table salt) + 40 g $NaHCO_3$ (baking soda) in 10 L water (Fielding 2018).
5) Optional: fluid carboy or used, clean 5 L fluid bag, used clean fluid line, Christmas tree adapter.

*Procedure*

1) Confirm placement of an NGT in the stomach.
2) Check for gastric reflux by creating a siphon.
3) If there is no gastric reflux, administer 4–6 L fluids as a bolus (for a 450–600 kg horse).
4) For an indwelling NGT: Cover the end of the NGT using a glove finger with a small slit. This will act as a one-way valve to allow the efflux of gastric contents if needed, without allowing gas to enter the NGT. Secure the NGT to the patient's halter using 1″ medical tape. Apply a muzzle if needed to avoid having the patient rub out the NGT. Boluses of fluid can be administered at two to four hours intervals.
5) If a small bore NGT has been placed for continuous infusion of enteral fluids, a hanging carboy (or clean, used 5 L fluid bags) will be required to supply fluids. This set-up does not allow an easy check for gastric reflux. Therefore, it is important that the horse's level of comfort be closely monitored and that the fluid rate be controlled so that the horse does not

receive an overload of fluids. A constant rate infusion of ~1–2 L/h is recommended, depending on the horse's fluid requirements. Assessment for stomach distension should be evaluated ultrasonographically.

6) The horse should not have access to oral fluids or feed when a large bore NGT is in place, since aspiration is possible. Therefore, it is important to ensure that fluid and nutrient requirements are being met by enteral or IV administration.

## Rectal Fluids

Isotonic fluids are administered through an indwelling rectal catheter by continuous gravity drip. They are an inexpensive method of fluid administration and can rehydrate manure in cases of small colon impaction. Defecation or straining can result in displacement of the rectal catheter, making this method of fluid administration less reliable than others. Rectal fluids should not be administered when irritation to the anus or rectum is present, or when a rectal tear is suspected.

*Materials*

1) Fluid carboy or clean, used 5 L fluid bags.
2) Large gauge red rubber catheter or stallion catheter.
3) Christmas tree adapter.
4) Used fluid line.
5) Rectal lubricant.
6) 1″ medical tape.
7) Elastikon.
8) Rectal sleeve.
9) Clean, non-sterile isotonic fluids.

*Procedure*

1) Braid or secure the tail in a rectal sleeve to keep it clean.
2) Fill and hang a fluid carboy or clean, used 5 L fluid bags with isotonic solution.
3) Insert ~12″ of the red rubber or stallion catheter into the horse's rectum. Secure it at the tail base with tabs of medical tape and Elastikon. Do not overtighten circumferentially placed Elastikon or tape around the tail.
4) Attach the Christmas tree adapter to the rectal catheter and connect the fluid line to the adapter.
5) Allow gravity flow of isotonic fluids.
6) Monitor for catheter displacement and irritation at the tail base, anus, and rectum. The patient's manure will be very soft and might become diarrhea.

## Intraosseous Fluids

The administration of intraosseous fluids should be reserved for patients in which IV access cannot be secured and rapid fluid resuscitation is required. This technique is most valuable in compromised foals or miniature donkeys, when vessels can be extremely difficult to access in cases of severe hypovolemia. A temporary intraosseous port can be established by several methods: using an EZIO commercial catheter kit, use of a Jamshidi bone biopsy instrument, or direct insertion of a large gauge needle (14–16 G). Direct insertion of a large gauge needle carries the most risk of breakage and is likely to work only in a neonate (Golenz et al. 1993).

*Materials*

1) Clippers.
2) Aseptic skin scrub.
3) 2% lidocaine, 3 mL with a 25 g needle.
4) #15 scalpel blade.
5) Sterile gloves.
6) EZIO catheter set or Jamshidi bone biopsy instrument and 14 G needles.
7) Bandage supplies: 1″ medical tape, gauze sponges, Elastikon, or Vet Wrap.

*Procedure*

1) Ensure adequate restraint of the patient. If they are a candidate for intraosseous fluid administration, they are likely severely compromised and will be adequately restrained by manual force and local anesthesia.
2) Clip the proximomedial tibia or proximomedial radius.
3) Aseptically prepare the skin in the clipped area.
4) Palpate the medial aspect of the tibia or the radius in the proximal third of the bone. Deposit a focal bleb of lidocaine.
5) Complete aseptic preparation of the skin.
6) Don sterile gloves. Make a ~5 mm stab incision through the skin, and SC tissues down to the bone using a #15 scalpel blade at the site of lidocaine deposition.
7) Establish IO access by:
   a) Using the EZIO drill to insert a commercial catheter into the bone.
   b) Using a 13 g Jamshidi bone biopsy instrument to make a pilot hole, then insert a 14 G needle into the medullary cavity.
   c) Directly inserting a 14 G, 0.5–1″ needle through the cortex of the bone (Golenz et al. 1993).
8) Care must be taken during placement of either catheter or needle to maintain axial alignment and to avoid breaking the tip or creating multiple cortical abrasions.
9) When the medullary cavity has been successfully breached, blood should be present on aspiration. A fluid line can be attached to the catheter or needle. The fluids might require pressure to run at an adequate rate.
10) Secure the needle or catheter using a tape loop. A "donut" with gauze or stockinette secured by vet wrap around the limb can be helpful to stabilize the catheter. Protect this set-up until fluid resuscitation is sufficient or IV access is established.

## Methods of Medication Administration

Medications can be administered by a variety of techniques, depending on the type of medication, indication for treatment, and the horse's temperament (Chapman 2017a, b).

### Oral (PO) Administration

Depending on the consistency of the medication and appetite of the horse, ground or crushed medications can be mixed into a palatable grain for some horses to eat. Alternatively, an oral dosing syringe can be used, in which the medication is softened with warm water to form a paste or dissolved and mixed with a palatable treat such as apple sauce. Tablets can also be effectively hidden in a hollowed-out piece of carrot, apple, or alfalfa cube.

*Procedure*

1) Remove any large chunks of forage from the horse's mouth. Rinse the mouth with water using an oral dosing syringe if it is inevitable that the medication is administered directly after eating.
2) Restrain the horse with a halter and lead rope. Placing a hand over the bridge of the horse's nose can provide additional control over the horse's movements.
3) Slide an oral dosing syringe into the corner of the horse's lips. Administer the medication in aliquots of ~10–20 mL at a time.

### Rectal (PR) Administration

Rectal administration of medications often compromises absorption and requires increases in dosing. It can be accomplished by softening medications into a paste and injecting them into the rectum through a catheter.

*Procedure*

1) Ideally administer the medication after the horse has passed manure.
2) Ensure the horse is appropriately restrained by a handler.
3) Lubricate the tip of a red rubber catheter.

4) Insert the red rubber catheter into the rectum.
5) Inject the medication, followed by a small amount of air to empty the catheter.
6) Remove the catheter from the rectum. Inspect the catheter for blood.

## Intravenous (IV) Administration

IV injection provides a reliable, rapid method of medication administration. Some medications can cause substantial irritation to tissues if the medication extravasates during administration. Therefore, appropriate restraint of the patient, combined with clean needle placement and timely administration limit the likelihood of collateral injury.

*Procedure*

1) Ensure the horse is appropriately restrained.
2) Use the non-dominant hand to hold-off and distend the jugular vein.
3) Place a needle (18–20g, 1–1.5″) into the external jugular vein in the proximal third of the neck.
4) Blood should fill the hub and drip out while the jugular vein is distended.
5) Use the non-dominant hand to steady the needle hub and attach the syringe of medication with the dominant hand.
6) If aspiration confirms the presence of blood and needle placement within the vein, inject the medication. The vein can be distended during aspiration to confirm needle placement.

## Intramuscular (IM) Administration

Intramuscular (IM) injections can be performed in the cervical region, pectorals, and hamstrings. IM injection is variably tolerated by horses, particularly after several injections. Rotate injection sites and limit the total volume of injection at one site to ~15–20 mL. Repeat IM injections can cause significant irritation and discomfort to the horse; however, IM medication formulations might be a more economic option than IV formulations (e.g., PPG vs crystalline penicillin).

*Procedure*

1) Ensure the horse is appropriately restrained.
2) Select the muscle group for injection. If using the cervical region, the appropriate site for injection is within a triangle bordered by the cranial aspect of the scapula, the nuchal ligament, and the dorsal aspect of the cervical vertebrae (Figure 4.3).
3) Place a clean needle (16–20 G) into the muscle to the needle hub. If no blood fills the hub, attach the syringe of medication. Aspirate by pulling back on the plunger to confirm that no blood fills the hub or syringe. Inject ~15–20 mL of medication prior to redirecting the needle or selecting a different site for injection.
4) If blood fills the hub of the needle or is obtained on aspiration with the syringe, the needle should be removed from the muscle. A new needle can be inserted into a different location.

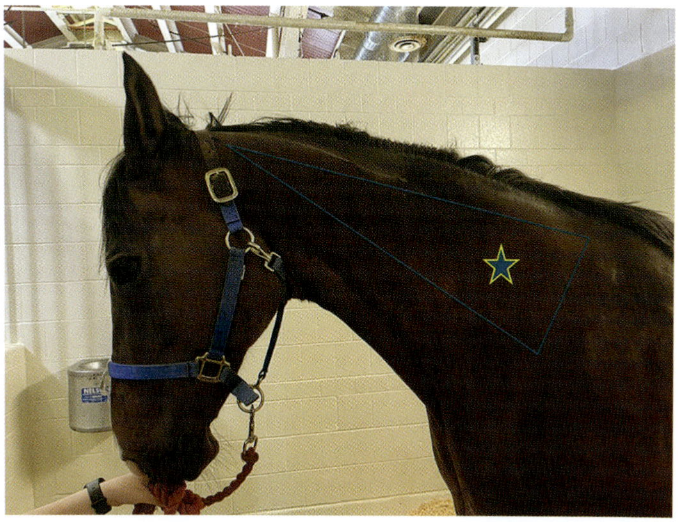

**Figure 4.3** Ideal location for cervical intra-muscular injection indicated by the star. The blue triangle approximates the region of cervical musculature bounded by the nuchal ligament (dorsally), cervical vertebrae (ventrally), and cranial border of the scapula (caudally).

### Subcutaneous (SC) Administration

SC administration of medications in the horse is uncommon. It can be performed in the cervical region or over the pectorals. Due to limited skin mobility, the total volume of SC medication administration should be limited in the horse.

*Procedure*

1) Ensure the horse is appropriately restrained.
2) Elevate skin between the non-dominant thumb and index finger to form a tent.
3) Insert a needle (16–20 G) into the tent of skin so that the tip rests in the SC space. Relax with the non-dominant hand.
4) Use the non-dominant hand to stabilize the needle hub and attach the syringe to the hub.
5) Aspirate by drawing back on the syringe plunger. If no blood fills the hub or syringe, inject the medication.
6) If blood fills the hub of the needle or is obtained on aspiration with the syringe, the needle should be removed. A new needle can be inserted into a different location.

### Transdermal Administration

Transdermal patches are used infrequently in emergency medicine but can be beneficial for amplifying analgesia over a longer term and can be readily secured over the proximomedial antebrachium.

*Procedure*

1) Ensure the horse is appropriately restrained.
2) Clip hair over the proximomedial antebrachium.
3) Wipe the skin with alcohol to remove scurf. Allow the alcohol to dry.
4) Wear exam gloves and remove the backing from the adhesive transdermal patch(es). Apply the adhesive patches to the clean skin on the proximomedial antebrachium.
5) Secure and cover the patches with Elastikon.
6) Use a felt marker to record on the Elastikon the name of the underlying medication, dosage, and date of medication application.

## Nasogastric Intubation

Nasogastric intubation is an important diagnostic and therapeutic procedure. Passing a NGT can be used to confirm the patency of the esophagus or to dislodge a soft food bolus obstructing the esophagus. Its placement in the stomach can also allow the expulsion of gastric reflux that can cause gastric distension. When gastric reflux is not present, nasogastric intubation facilitates the administration of enteral fluids and medications (Londoño 2017a). The NGT diameter should be selected so that it readily passes in the ventral meatus of the nasal passage and enables the clinician to accomplish the goal of the procedure. For example, a large NGT is generally desirable to enable siphoning of thick or large volumes of gastric fluid, whereas a smaller diameter NGT might be sufficient when the primary goal is electrolyte fluid administration. If the horse is producing a large volume of gastric reflux and is being trailered to a referral center, the NGT should be secured indwelling to decrease the patient's risk of gastric rupture.

*Materials* (Figure 4.4)

1) NGT.
2) Sterile lubricant or lidocaine gel.
3) Optional: 20 mL, 2% lidocaine if no lidocaine gel available.
4) Buckets (2; ideally with measurement increments) – one empty, one with lukewarm water.
5) Fluid pump.

*Procedure*

1) Appropriately restrain the patient. Depending on the horse's temperament and systemic condition, this might include sedation and/or use of a twitch.
2) Administer lidocaine lubricant to the floor of the nasal passage. Alternatively, administer ~20 mL of lidocaine topically to the nasal passage as a splash block. Apply a small amount of lubricant to the end of the NGT.
3) Standing beside the horse and facing the same direction, place your dominant hand (closest to the horse) over the bridge of the horse's nose. Use your thumb to dilate the nares as well as elevate the false nostril. Your non-dominant hand

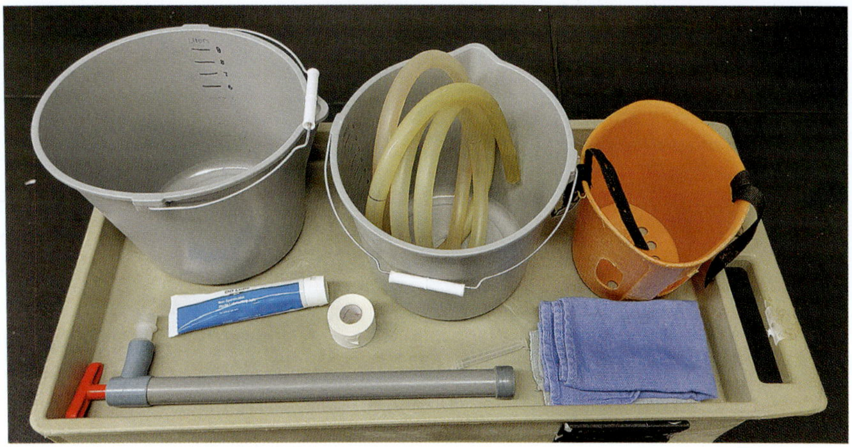

**Figure 4.4** Materials for nasogastric intubation *Source:* M. Ziad Al-Ani, Robin J.M. Gray.

should advance the NGT into the ventral meatus of the nasal passage. Your dominant thumb can direct the tube ventrally and medially.

4) Advance the tube carefully through the pharynx until slight resistance is met. (If you meet firm resistance, you are most likely hitting the ethmoids.) Advance the tube with careful, gentle pressure. A swallow should be felt against the tube, at which point the tube can be more rapidly advanced. Alternatively, you can place the external end of the NGT in your mouth as it is advanced. When gentle pressure is met in the pharynx, you can blow through the tube, which often stimulates a swallow. Poll flexion also increases the likelihood of the horse swallowing the NGT. As the tube is advanced down the esophagus, there should no longer be resistance meeting the end of the tube, but there is an increase in friction when advancing the tube. Negative pressure should be detected if the tube is in the clinician's mouth. Other methods of confirming placement of the stomach tube within the esophagus are outlined in Box 4.1.
5) Once the tube is passed into the esophagus, it should be visualized and palpated in the cervical region to confirm appropriate placement.
6) Move the tube down the esophagus, into the stomach in swift, firm strokes. A mild increase in resistance can again be felt as the NGT is passed through the cardia. Stomach gas is often readily detected from the NGT once the stomach is reached. Tube placement in the stomach can also be confirmed by spontaneous reflux or by blowing air into the tube while a clinician auscults the stomach to confirm the presence of gurgling gas sounds.
7) Evaluate the stomach contents and volume. If there is no spontaneous reflux, create a siphon by pumping ~0.5–1 L of warm water into the stomach. The NGT often needs careful repositioning for the siphon to be effective. Repeat several times if abnormal stomach contents are obtained.
8) Enteral fluids can be administered to a maximum recommended volume of ~6–8 L for a 500 kg horse. Release the NGT attachment from the stomach pump and elevate the tube (to the level of the horse's ears), so that any inadvertently pressurized fluid can be released from the stomach. If there is no return of fluid, kink the NGT and remove it from the stomach by pulling in gentle, long arcing strokes.

**Box 4.1 Methods of confirming NGT placement into the esophagus and stomach**

1) Moderate resistance to passage of the NGT occurs when entering the esophagus compared to little to no resistance when entering the trachea.
2) Direct palpation of the NGT is possible in the lower left aspect of the neck region high in the jugular groove just proximal to the shoulder.
3) Negative pressure obtained while clinician is aspirating on the tube while it is in the esophagus.
4) Visualization and palpation of the NGT in the esophagus while passing the NGT.
5) Return of stomach contents (fluid or gas). NGTs might have a chronic odor from use – do not confuse this with the release of stomach gas.
6) Auscultation of the stomach while gas is injected through the tube. Gurgling noises should be audible during auscultation of the stomach.
7) When the NGT is intra-tracheal, there is free flow of air in and out of the tube when the clinician blows or aspirates. Upon manipulation of the trachea, a rattle can sometimes be detected (Dechant 2021).

*Potential complications* (Londoño 2017a; Dechant 2021)

1) Mal positioning of the tube (i.e., tracheal intubation).
2) Laryngeal, esophageal injury.
3) Injury to personnel if horse is inadequately restrained.
4) Nasopharyngeal trauma, rhinitis (particularly in cases of indwelling NGT).
5) Aspiration pneumonia following administration of fluid or feed through a mal-positioned NGT.
6) Epistaxis due to trauma of the mucosa, nasal turbinates, or ethmoid turbinates is usually self-limiting unless an underlying coagulopathy is present or trauma is extensive. To decrease the likelihood of epistaxis, restrain the horse adequately, lubricate the NGT, and pass the NGT carefully in the ventral meatus. If bleeding starts, place a small towel over the horse's nose so that if the horse coughs, the trajectory of the blood is limited in the environment. Topical phenylephrine can be useful to slow the hemorrhage. Slight elevation of the horse's head to wither height might prevent worsening or persistence of bleeding. If the blood loss becomes severe, packing of the nasal passage, fluid therapy or blood transfusion, in addition to medications such as aminocaproic acid, might be appropriate.

## Sedation Techniques in Horses

Sedation can provide analgesia, a calming effect and restraint in emergent scenarios. These effects are important for keeping the patient, personnel, and clinician(s) safe. Multimodal use of sedation medications can be particularly effective at establishing the depth and duration of desired sedation (Michou and Leece 2012). For short procedures requiring limited analgesia, Xylazine or Detomidine are often adequate. However, a commonly used combination of medications for a moderate duration (~30–45 minutes) of sedation and analgesia is Detomidine and Butorphanol. This combination can be modified to decrease the duration of effect by substituting Xylazine for Detomidine or Romifidine, or to increase the duration and potency of analgesia by substituting Morphine for Butorphanol. Xylazine is not recommended for use in pregnant mares during their last trimester of gestation (Michou and Leece 2012). Acepromazine might increase the depth of sedation achieved, with no additional analgesia, when administered with an α2-adrenoreceptor agonist +/− opioid. It should not be used in hypovolemic or endotoxemic patients, as its vasodilatory effect can compromise systemic compensation for hypotension (Michou and Leece 2012). Benzodiazepines (diazepam, midazolam) can provide sedation in neonatal or sick foals. Since they do not have an analgesic effect, benzodiazepines are commonly paired with an opioid.

Dosing of sedation in adult horses is notoriously variable. Experienced clinicians commonly estimate doses based on their assessment of the horse's temperament, level of pain, size, and condition, as well as the desired effect of the sedation, the clinician's comfort with the medications, and the type of medication selected. The horse's systemic condition should be considered, and the dosing minimized to decrease the risk of adverse effects in compromised patients. Reversal agents for α2-adrenoreceptor agonists and opioids are available but are costly and uncommonly required for horses.

Oral, sublingual, IM, and IV routes can be used for administration of sedatives. IV access might be difficult if a horse is excited or painful, although it provides the fastest onset of action. IM administration of medication can sufficiently alter the patient's behavior to allow further administration of sedatives IV. Horses intolerant of needles can be administered sedatives orally or sublingually to make the patient pliable for the intended procedure, or to facilitate injection of additional sedation. Efficacy of the sedatives is improved by administration prior to stimulation; however, this is nearly impossible in most emergent scenarios (Michou and Leece 2012). Adjunct use of locoregional analgesia and securing a quiet environment might decrease sedation dosing requirements.

Ataxia is anticipated following administration of sedatives. If relocation is required, horses should only be walked. The sedated horse can be steadied by the handler placing a hand on the halter and, if needed, an additional spotter to provide tail support. Often, horses exhibit stertorous respiration due to low head position and nasopharyngeal collapse. To limit nasal edema formation during prolonged periods of sedation, the head should be rested on a stand at wither-height. Bradycardia and second-degree atrioventricular block often accompany α2-adrenoreceptor agonist administration; they are transient and uncommonly affect oxygenation or perfusion. Decreased gastrointestinal motility results from administration of α2-adrenoreceptor agonists and opioids. Following extended periods of sedation, care should be taken to monitor the patient's manure output and gradually refeed them. The excitement that sometimes accompanies opioid administration can be curtailed by concurrent administration of an α2-adrenoreceptor agonist or acepromazine (Michou and Leece 2012).

## Electrocardiogram

The electrocardiogram (ECG) is used to diagnose abnormal cardiac rhythms. Physiologic arrhythmias such as sinus arrhythmias, first and second atrio-ventricular degree block are commonly detected in horses and typically of little clinical relevance, provided they disappear with increasing heart rate (e.g., stress or exercise). Investigation of the specific abnormal rhythms and cardiovascular consequences is a fundamental step to establish the need for treatment. Although arrhythmias can be commonly recognized in horses, most don't require immediate anti-arrhythmic treatment; however, some arrhythmias can be life threatening and need emergency treatment (see Chapter 12).

In emergency settings, the ECG evaluation becomes particularly useful in cases of unexplained tachycardia or bradyarrhythmia, in cases of unexplained weakness or collapse, and in general as a tool to define any auscultated abnormal rhythm to determine clinical importance.

In the emergency setting, a modified base-apex lead recording is sufficient to accurately diagnose most rhythm abnormalities (Figure 4.5a–d) (Box 4.2).

*Materials*

1) Electrodes (clip-on or self-adhesive gel patch).
2) Electrical cables and recording device.
3) Display and recording system.

Emergency, short-duration ECG recordings in field settings can be obtained with hand-held devices (Box 4.3). These devices provide diagnostic quality traces and can display and record on cell phones and tablets and therefore be very helpful for real-time interpretation and prompt sharing of acquired data (Kraus et al. 2019). Longer-term recordings with telemetric systems can be useful to continuously monitor the rhythm and evaluate response to treatment.

## Abdominocentesis

Abdominocentesis is an important aspect of the colic work-up, and a useful diagnostic tool when evaluating communication of wounds or masses with the abdomen. Evaluation of peritoneal fluid parameters and cytology can confirm colic etiology, including strangulating intestinal lesions, infectious peritonitis, and a ruptured gastrointestinal viscus. Aseptically collected fluid can be submitted for culture and sensitivity. Abdominocentesis can be readily performed in the field with a well-behaved horse, an experienced handler, and an assistant. It is normal to obtain peritoneal fluid that is pale, straw-colored, and transparent.

*Materials* (Figure 4.7)

1) Clippers.
2) Supplies for aseptic skin preparation (chlorhexidine, alcohol, gauze sponges).
3) 2% lidocaine, 3 mL syringe with 25 G needle.
4) Purple, green, and red top tubes +/− culturette with transport media.
5) Microscope slides.
6) Sterile gloves.
7) Method 1: #15 scalpel blade, teat cannula or bitch catheter, sterile gauze.
8) Method 2: spinal needle (18g, 3″).

*Procedure* (Figure 4.8a–d)

1) Ensure appropriate restraint of the patient. The procedure can be safely performed in many horses with light sedation and local anesthesia. If available, stocks can facilitate restraint.
2) Identify a cranioventral site for abdominocentesis based on the presence of an ultrasonographically identified fluid pocket or predetermined landmarks. A standard location for abdominocentesis with a teat cannula is 1–4″ to the right of midline, one hand's breadth caudal to the pectoral convergence on the ventral trunk. This site commonly corresponds to the junction of the cranial third and caudal two-thirds of the abdomen. Abdominocentesis with an 18-gauge, 1.5-in. needle can be performed on midline (through the linea alba) at the same craniocaudal location (Walton and Southwood 2013; Radcliffe et al. 2022).

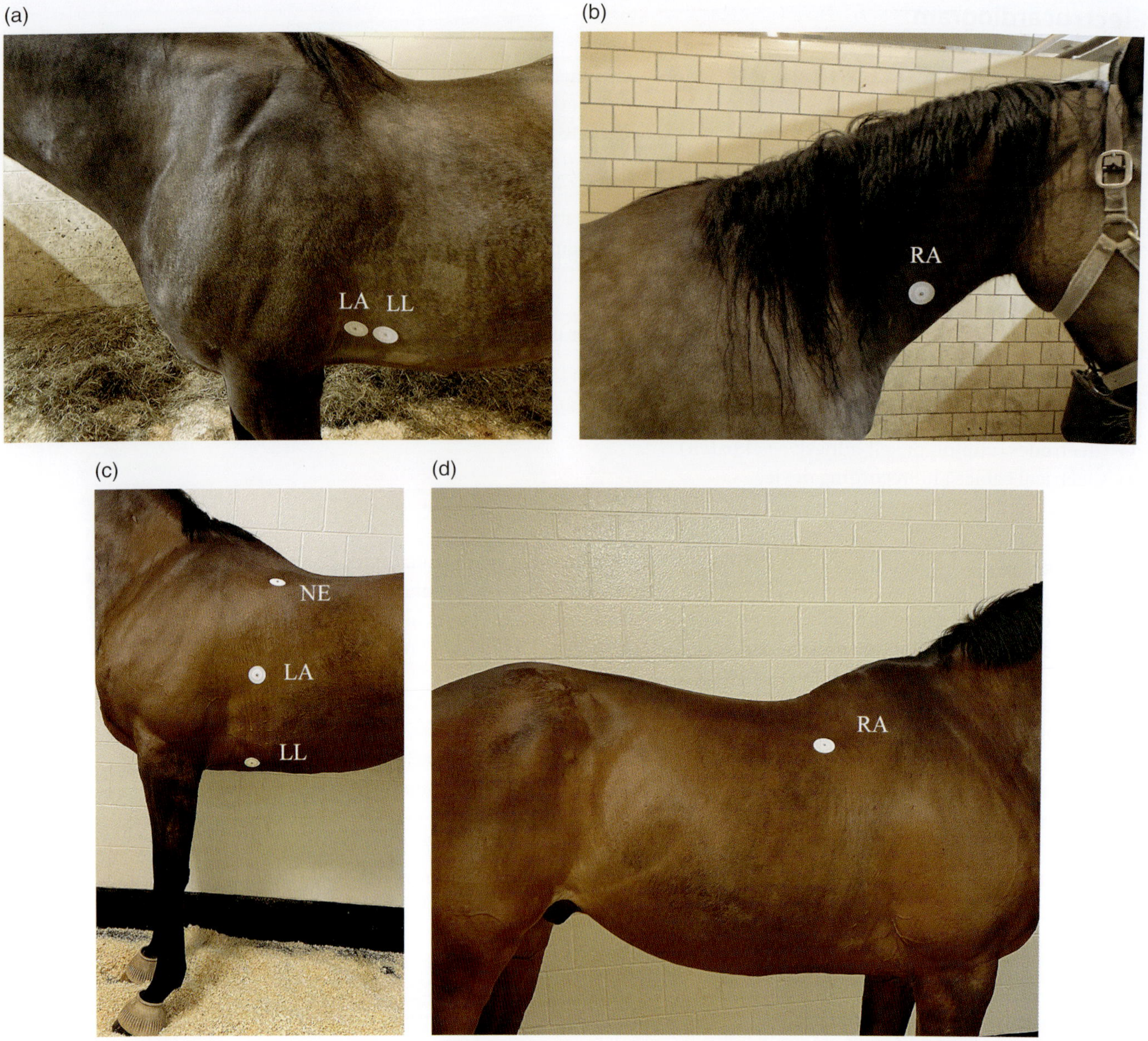


**Figure 4.5** (a,b) One of several methods to record a modified base-apex electrocardiogram (ECG) in a resting horse. The left arm (LA) electrode and the left leg (LL) electrode are placed over the base of the heart on the left side (Figure 4.5a), while the right arm (RA) electrode is placed on the right neck in the jugular furrow (Figure 4.5b). In this configuration both Lead I (RA-LA) and Lead II (RA-LL) will provide the largest negative QRS complex morphology, while Lead III (LA-LL) will only have a small amplitude QRS-T complex. Paper speed is typically set at 25 or 50 mm/s. (c, d) A three-lead modified base-apex can also be obtained and is particularly useful for telemetric or longer-term recordings. Place the LA electrode on the left, at the intersection of the base of the heart and point of the shoulder, and the LL electrode on the left, at the level of the elbow, below the LA electrode (Figure 4.5c). Place the RA electrode on the right 15 cm below the level of the withers, behind the shoulder (Figure 4.5d). Finally, place the neutral electrode (NE) somewhere between LA and RA (in this horse on the left above the LA). In this configuration Lead I (RA-LA) will highlight the atrial electrical activity, magnifying P waves, Lead II (RA-LL) will produce the typical ECG trace visualized with a modified base-apex configuration (negative S wave morphology), and Lead III (LA-LL) will produce an alternative QRS morphology that can be useful when identifying ventricular ectopy. Paper speed is typically set at 25 or 50 mm/s. *Source:* M. Ziad Al-Ani, Robin J.M. Gray.

**Box 4.2 Procedure for setting up a modified base-apex lead useful for emergency cardiac rhythm evaluation and longer term monitoring with ECG recorders (e.g., Televet 2[1] telemetric ECG)**

1) Dry the coat if damp or wet in the pre-established areas where the electrodes will be placed for a modified base apex recording (Figure 4.5a–d).
2) Clip small patches on designed areas for electrodes placement if long coat is present (e.g., winter coat, cushingoid horse).
3) Apply the self-adhesive gel patches. A small quantity of electrode gel or a drop of saline can also be added to the self-adhesive gel patch electrodes to improve contact. Do not apply gel or saline to the horse directly as this might prevent the patches from sticking well.
4) Connect the electrodes to the ECG cables and the recording device ensuring that batteries are charged.
5) If the intention is to leave the ECG in place for a prolonged time (e.g., exercise test or hours-long monitoring), it is advisable to cover the patches with self-adhesive foam to secure the position of the electrodes.
6) Commercially available surcingle or a sticky elastic bandage can be used to cover the electrodes and the cables.

**Box 4.3 Procedure for short-duration ECG with hand-held devices (e.g., Alivecor,[2] Figure 4.6)**

1) Ensure you have downloaded the specific app on your device.
2) There is usually no need for clipping.
3) Apply water, alcohol, or gel in contact with the skin at the site where the apex beat can be felt, slightly lower than the left atrium level.
4) Apply the device at this level.
5) Observe and record the trace on your device. Optimize signal by repositioning device if P-QRS-T complexes are not diagnostic.

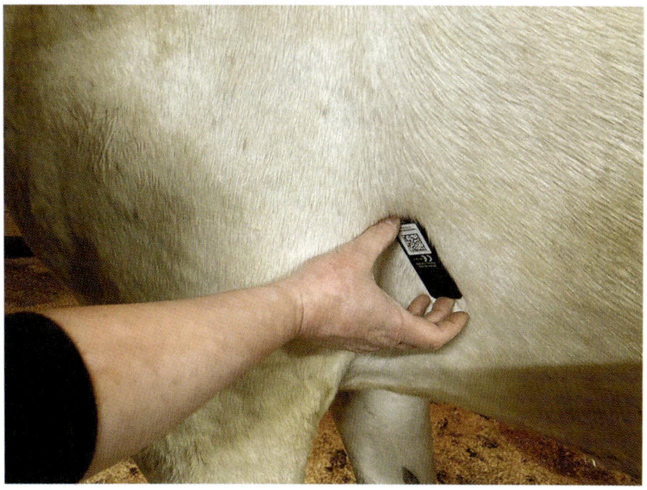

**Figure 4.6** Placement of a hand-held ECG recording device. The electrodes are placed against the damp skin, where the apex beat can be palpated, with the device on a 45° angle, with the top electrode angled toward the head. If the QRS complex is small and difficult to visualize then you can have the leg pulled forward or push the device further under the triceps or slide up the chest a few centimeters for better contact over the base of the heart. *Source:* M. Ziad Al-Ani, Robin J.M. Gray.

1 Televet 2, Heusenstamm, Germany.
2 Alivecor, Inc, Woodside, CA 94062.

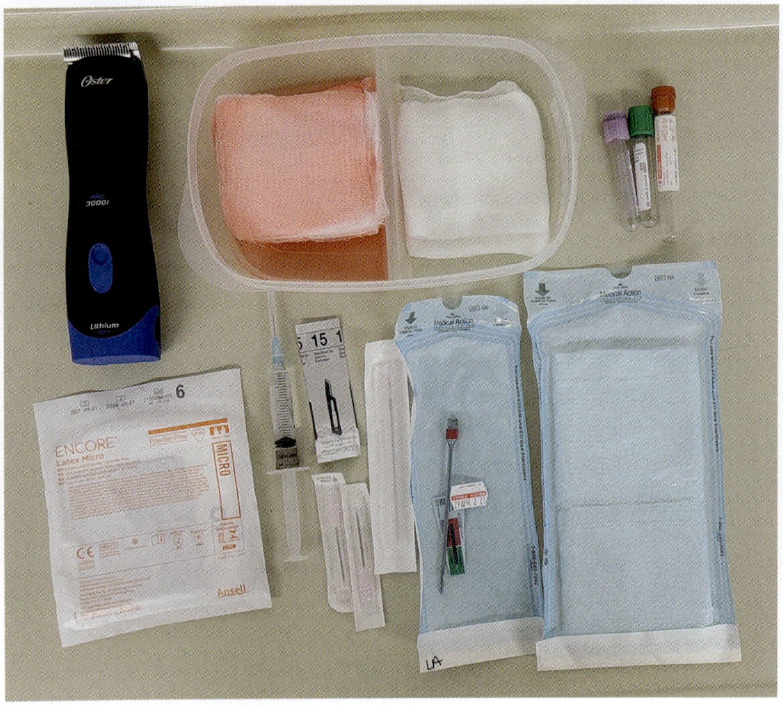


**Figure 4.7** Materials for abdominocentesis.

3) Clip a ~3 × 3″ area at the site of intended abdominocentesis.
4) Aseptically prepare the skin in the clipped area.
5) Deposit local anesthetic in a nodule subcutaneously, then place the needle through this bleb to infiltrate the rectus muscle layer. This step is optional if using method 2 (needle aspirate).
6) Complete the aseptic skin preparation over the clipped area.
7) Don sterile gloves.
8) Method 1: Make a ~5 mm stab incision through the skin and external rectus sheath with a #15 blade (Figure 4.8a). Thread a 3.75-in. teat cannula[3] through the center of a gauze sponge so that blood contamination of the sample is avoided. Choke up on the teat cannula with your dominant hand and use your non-dominant hand to create a friction bridge while advancing the cannula perpendicular into the abdomen (Figure 4.8b,c). There will be two small releases of pressure ("pops") as the cannula moves through the internal rectus sheath and the peritoneum into the abdomen (Radcliffe et al. 2022).
9) Method 2: Insert the 18-gauge, 1.5-in. needle through skin and advance it half the working length of the needle (¾″). Advance the needle slowly (2–3 mm at a time) checking for fluid or movement. Independent movement of the needle (often in a circular motion) may indicate needle contact with viscera. When such movement is detected, the needle should be withdrawn slightly as further advancement will yield enterocentesis. Continue slowly advancing the needle until fluid is obtained (Figure 4.8d), movement is detected, or the base of the needle reaches the abdominal wall. The use of an 18-gauge, 3.5 in. spinal needle may also be performed; however, without ultrasound guidance inadvertent enterocentesis is likely (Radcliffe et al. 2022).
10) Fluid should be spontaneously retrieved from the abdomen. If this is not the case, gentle repositioning of the teat cannula can be attempted. Alternatively, the horse can be stepped forward or backward a half or full step. If no fluid is retrieved, the abdomen should be re-evaluated by ultrasound for an appropriate location to perform abdominocentesis, or the horse might require fluid resuscitation to have a significant volume of abdominal fluid.
11) An assistant should be positioned on the opposite side of the horse (if safe to do so) with tubes for fluid collection.
12) Remove the needle or cannula from the abdomen. Hold digital pressure over the site for a couple of minutes if bleeding is faster than a slow drip.
13) Evaluate the clinicopathologic parameters of the collected fluid (nucleated cell count, total solids, lactate, cytology). Make at least one slide for cytology.

3 JorVet, Jorgensen Labs, Loveland, CO.

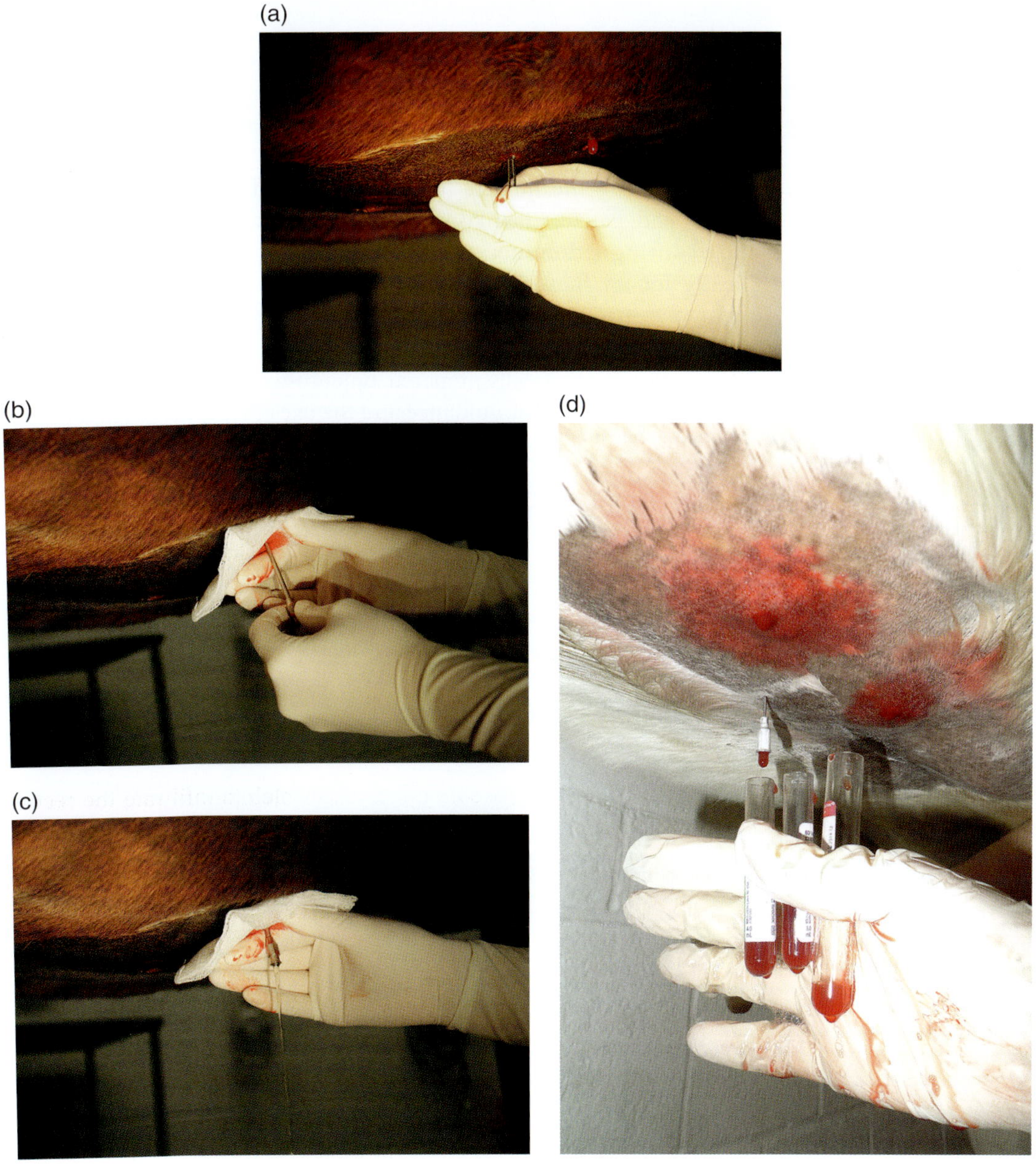


**Figure 4.8** (a–c) Abdominocentesis procedure for placing a 3.75-in. teat cannula. After clipping and sterile preparation of the abdomen, a #15 blade is advanced through the skin and external sheath of the rectus abdominus muscle (a). Next, a 3.75-in. udder infusion cannula (JorVet, Jorgensen Labs, Loveland, CO) is inserted perpendicular to the abdominal wall at a 30° outward angle from vertical (b). The cannula is inserted through the skin and external sheath of the rectus muscle. Continue advancing slowly and two "pops" should be felt as the cannula penetrates the internal sheath of the rectus muscle and peritoneal lining. The teat cannula is usually within 1 in. of the abdominal wall when the peritoneal lining is reached (c). A firm thrust through the peritoneal membrane is recommended to avoid "tenting" of the membrane away from the retro-peritoneal tissues. Note the normal gross appearance of light yellow, clear abdominal fluid in this horse. (d) Abdominocentesis procedure using an 18-gauge, 1.5-in. needle. After clipping and sterile preparation of the abdomen, an 18-gauge, 1.5-in. needle is inserted on midline to a depth of approximately ¾ of inch. Advance the needle slowly (2–3 mm at a time) checking for fluid or movement. Independent movement of the needle (often in a circular motion) may indicate needle contact with viscera. When such movement is detected, the needle should be withdrawn slightly as further advancement will yield enterocentesis. Continue slowly advancing the needle until fluid is obtained (a), movement is detected, or the base of the needle reaches the abdominal wall. Note the bloody peritoneal fluid in this horse. Peritoneal fluid evaluation revealed an elevated RBC count, normal nucleated cell count and normal L-lactate levels. The horse was non-painful and recovered with medical management. *Source:* Radcliffe et al. (2022) / with permission of John Wiley & Sons.

*Potential complications*

1) Enterocentesis occurs most commonly when the needle or teat cannula penetrates a heavy colon (e.g., sand-filled or dehydrated impaction). Brown-green, malodorous fluid with feed particulate is generally obtained. The needle or teat cannula should be removed. The rate of significant complication is low. Systemic antimicrobial treatment can be considered (Walton and Southwood 2013).
2) Hemorrhage can occur uncommonly when vasculature in the muscle layer is punctured. This bleeding can be treated with a pressure bandage (e.g., non-adherent pad, gauze, Elastikon) around the horse's trunk. Hemorrhagic fluid can be obtained when the spleen is punctured during abdominocentesis. The bleeding is usually self-limiting; the horse can be monitored ultrasonographically for an increase in hemorrhagic abdominal fluid (Radcliffe et al. 2022).
3) Omental herniation occurs most commonly in foals when abdominocentesis is performed using a teat cannula. If omental herniation occurs, the foal should be sedated, the site aseptically prepared, omentum returned to the abdomen, and a staple or interrupted suture placed in the skin. Ultrasonographic guidance and the use of a needle for abdominocentesis are recommended when evaluating foals (Walton and Southwood 2013).

## Synoviocentesis

Synoviocentesis is performed to evaluate joints, tendon sheaths, or bursas for infection or inflammation (Figure 4.9a–d). The approach used for synoviocentesis will depend on the quality of overlying soft tissues, the presence of wounds, and the temperament of the horse. The ideal site for synoviocentesis should allow for synovial fluid collection without injury to collateral structures (e.g., cartilage), while avoiding contaminated tissues (such as skin wounds, areas of septic cellulitis, or abscessation). Appropriate restraint with sedation and locoregional anesthesia can facilitate synoviocentesis (Auer et al. 2018).

*Materials*

1) Optional: clippers, mepivacaine for locoregional anesthesia (at the discretion of the clinician).
2) Supplies for aseptic skin preparation (chlorhexidine, alcohol, gauze sponges).
3) Needles, 18–21G.
4) Syringes, 3–10 mL.
5) Red and purple top tubes +/− culturette with transport media.
6) Microscope slides.
7) Sterile gloves.
8) Sterile gauze, Elastikon.

*Procedure* (Figure 4.9a–d)

1) Secure a space with limited environmental contamination (e.g., clean exam room or barn aisle with no blowing dust).
2) Ensure appropriate restraint of the patient. This can include sedation, locoregional anesthesia, and/or use of a twitch.
3) If working with a wound or laceration in the horse, select a location for synoviocentesis-based digital and/or sterile probe examination of the wound (Figure 4.9a) and ultrasonographic or radiographic exams.
4) Rough aseptic skin preparation of the site for synoviocentesis.
5) Sterile aseptic skin preparation of the site for synoviocentesis.
6) If required, an assistant can help to position the limb appropriately (e.g., in flexion).
7) Select an appropriately sized needle (18–21g, 1–1.5″), depending on the joint to be sampled. Use the largest needle that can be introduced without injury to increase the chance of an adequate synovial fluid collection.
8) Assertively place the needle in the landmarked location into the synovial structure (Figure 4.9b). Synovial fluid is retrieved spontaneously from many joints on successful penetration of the synovium (Figure 4.9c). The needle sometimes requires redirection until the tip is free, and there is no synovium obstructing the tip. Stabilize the hub of the needle with your non-dominant hand and attach a syringe with your dominant hand. Aspirate to withdraw synovial fluid. If fluid is not readily retrieved, loosen the attachment between the needle and syringe. Decreasing the pressure of aspiration can allow the efflux of synovial fluid from the joint. Carefully moving the limb through its range of motion can facilitate fluid retrieval but increases the risk of cartilage injury or needle breakage. As a last resort, a small volume of sterile saline can be injected to aid in collecting diluted synovial fluid.

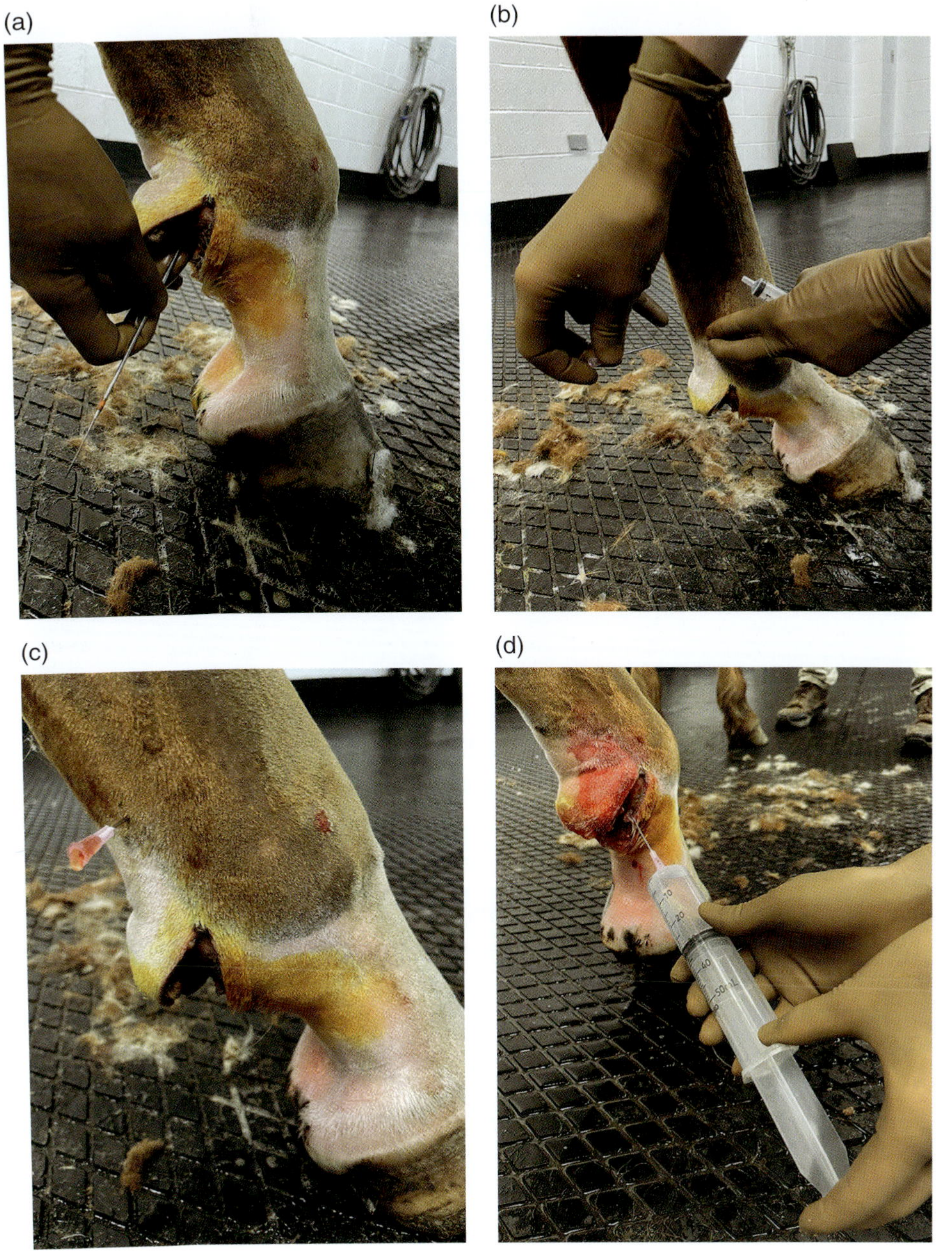


**Figure 4.9** (a–d) Synoviocentesis procedure: A horse presented with a severe laceration of the plantar region of the RH fetlock joint. Following clipping and sterile preparation of the region, a sterile probe was placed into the wound to determine the direction and depth of penetration (a). Ultrasonographic and radiographic guidance will help determine what structures may be involved. Distention of nearby synovial structures may be used to confirm communication with the wound. Because of confirmed communication with the digital flexor tendon sheath, synoviocentesis was performed using a 20-gauge, 1.5 in. needle above the wound (b, c). Note lavage of the wound with sterile, isotonic fluids using a 50 mL syringe and an 18-gauge, 1.5-in. needle. Further treatment to explore and lavage the tendon sheath was performed under general anesthesia.

9) Save the fluid in your choice of purple top tube (cytology, nucleated cell count [NCC], total solids [TS]), red top tube, or culturette. Make at least one slide for cytology. The clinicopathologic parameters of the synovial fluid analysis will need to be interpreted in light of saline dilution if this technique was implemented.
10) Wound lavage is indicated and may be performed both standing (Figure 4.9d) and recumbent. General anesthesia is recommended for most cases where synovial involvement requires aggressive lavage and exploration of the synovial compartment.
11) Place a light wrap over the sampled joint with sterile gauze and Elastikon.
12) Administer a systemic ant-inflammatory medication of choice.

## Thoracocentesis

Thoracocentesis or thoracentesis or pleural tap is a procedure that aims to remove fluid or air from the pleural space. This procedure is indicated when pleural effusion is suspected upon chest auscultation, and it is then identified on ultrasound or radiographic examination. This procedure is indicated in conditions such as pleuropneumonia, pleural abscesses, neoplastic effusion, hemothorax, or pyothorax. The procedure can provide samples for diagnostic purposes and/or provide therapeutic drainage of the effusion. Placement of chest tubes for continuous or repeated drainage of effusion or air is also achievable with a similar procedure, and it is described in more detail in Chapter 5.

*Materials*

1) Clippers.
2) Sterile scrub material.
3) Local anesthetic, 2–4 mL of 2% Lidocaine.
4) 1 × 25 G 5/8″ needle for local block.
5) 1 mL × 2 mL syringe for local block.
6) Sterile gloves.
7) Sterile scalpel blade (#15) - Optional if not using a blunt instrument.
8) Sterile blunt teat cannula or 12–14 G IV catheter (blunt instruments are preferred as less likely to penetrate and injure the lung parenchyma).
9) Three-way tap (stopcock).
10) 1 mL × 10 mL or 5 mL syringe for collection.
11) Material for collection: EDTA vacutainer tubes, plain vacutainer tubes, aerobic/anaerobic culture media.
12) Sedation (use of sedatives will vary based on patient's attitude and cardio-vascular stability): A combination of Detomidine IV 0.01 mg/kg and Butorphanol IV at 0.01 mg/kg is recommended if the patient is stable.
13) Ultrasound.

*Procedure*

1) Identify the site. Ultrasound guidance is recommended for the selection of the thoracocentesis's site. When ultrasonography is not available, careful auscultation can be helpful to determine the site. Often an eligible site is located ventrally between the 6th and 8th intercostal spaces at about 10 cm dorsal to the olecranon. Precise placement is fundamental to avoid puncturing cardiac structures.
2) Clip and aseptically prepare the site chosen.
3) Infiltrate local 2–3 mL of local anesthetic in the SC tissue and intercostal muscle, trying to instill some close to the pleural surface. Care should be taken when choosing the site of the local infiltration, avoid the caudal aspect of the ribs as intercostal vessels and nerve run on the caudal aspect of each rib and should be strategically avoided. Care should also be taken to avoid the lateral thoracic vein.
4) Perform a final aseptic preparation.
5) Make a stab incision through the skin and fascia taking care of incising cranial to the caudal rib of the chosen intercostal space. The incision can be extended into the intercostal muscle to facilitate the cannula insertion. If using a catheter there might not be the need for a stab incision.
6) Attach the three-way tap at the end of the sterile cannula or catheter. Alternatively, a sterile syringe can be attached to prevent air influx in the pleural cavity and subsequent pneumothorax.
7) Pass the cannula or catheter through the stab incision or where the local was instilled until a loss of resistance is experienced.
8) Open the three-way tap.
9) Pleural fluid might flow freely at this point, or you might need to gently aspirate with a syringe to obtain it. If fluid is expected but not flowing, the cannula can be gently twisted or slightly advanced. Do not advance the cannula if not much fluid is expected due to the high risk of lung puncture.
10) Close to three-way tap.
11) Remove the cannula at the end of the procedure.
12) There is usually no need to suture the skin.

*Potential complications*

1) Pneumothorax, if there is inadvertent air influx in the pleural cavity.
2) Hemothorax, if a large vessel is accidentally punctured.
3) Accidental cardiac puncture. Not placing the canula too cranial and ventral and ultrasound guidance to elect the puncture site, can help prevent this complication.

## Tracheal Wash and Bronchoalveolar Lavage

These procedures are indicated in horses with lower airway disease and as part of investigation of exercise intolerance/poor performance. Tracheal wash (TW) is indicated for evaluation of pathologies that might be infectious, focally extensive, or affecting larger airways (i.e., bacterial bronchopneumonia, pulmonary hemorrhage). Bronchoalveolar lavage (BAL) is used to investigate diffused lower airways diseases such as Equine Asthma. BAL might miss pathologies that are not diffuse and, if performed via blind technique, is not suitable to obtain samples for reliable culture.

### Tracheal Wash

TW may be performed via a trans-tracheal or endoscopic approach. The trans-tracheal procedure bypasses the upper airways representing the best method to retrieve a sample for bacterial culture. Note that samples obtained through the biopsy channel of the endoscope, without the use of a guarded endoscopic aspiration catheter[4]are not suitable for culture as there will be contamination from the upper airways. The endoscopic technique has the advantage of direct visualization of the area to sample.

*Materials: trans-tracheal technique*

1) Sedation. A combination of Detomidine IV 0.01 mg/kg and Butorphanol IV at 0.01 mg/kg is recommended if the patient is stable. Butorphanol can help suppress cough during the procedure.
2) Clippers.
3) Material for scrub.
4) Sterile gloves.
5) #15 scalpel blade.
6) 25 G 5/8′ needle for local block.
7) 2 mL syringe for local block.
8) 2 mL local anesthetic (i.e., lidocaine 2%) for skin block.
9) 20–50 mL of sterile 0.9% saline solution.
10) 20–50 mL syringe.
11) 12–14 G 3″ catheter or 12 G 1″ needle *.
12) 5 F polyethylene tubing or a 5 F dog urinary catheter.
13) Commercially available kits for trans-TW are an alternative to 11 and 12.[4]
14) EDTA tube for cytology, slides, aerobic and anaerobic media for culture.
15) Antibiotic for SC infiltration.

* Note: catheters might be too soft and bend within the tracheal rings; needles are preferred

*Procedure: trans-tracheal technique*

1) Ensure the animal is well sedated and restrained with the head elevated and the neck extended.
2) The site for the procedure is localized on midline of the mid-cervical region, proximal to the fusion of the sternocephalic muscles.
3) Clip and aseptically prepare the site (approximately 3 cm × 3 cm).

4 Large Animal Transtracheal Wash kit/TTL Mila International, Inc., Florence KY.

4) Palpate between the tracheal rings and instill 2 mL of local anesthetic in skin and SC tissue.
5) Perform a final aseptic preparation.
6) Perform a small stab incision along the midline between the tracheal rings where the needle is going to be inserted. This can help to avoid excessive skin drag when inserting the needle.
7) Stabilize the trachea between your index finger and your thumb using one hand.
8) Palpate the trachea and identify the tracheal rings, then insert the needle with the other hand entering between the tracheal rings until the needle is about 1–2 cm seeded in the lumen of trachea. Aim the needle bevel downward. If using a catheter, remove the stylet once seeded in the tracheal lumen.
9) Advance the sterile tubing provided in the kit or the urinary dog catheter through the needle/catheter, stabilizing the latter with one hand and passing the tubing with the other.
10) Once the tubing is few centimeters within the tracheal lumen, start injecting 30–50 mL of sterile saline (20 mL for a foal), then advance the tubing toward the thoracic inlet.
11) Immediately pull back with the syringe in order to retrieve the saline injected.
12) Move the sampling tube proximo-distally to retrieve as much volume possible, ideally 10–20 mL.
13) If retrieval of the sample is unsuccessful, inject an additional saline solution, using the same amount used the first time and try to retrieve again.
14) Withdraw the tubing first through the needle/catheter until it is completely out, then withdraw the needle/catheter. This avoids skin contamination from the tubing. However, if while withdrawing the tubing there is resistance, stop and withdraw the needle/catheter first until the sharp end is outside the skin and visible. This will prevent cutting off the tubing in the airways.
15) You can instill local antibiotics (e.g., 3 mL procaine penicillin) subcutaneously at the site of puncture.
16) Place a few mL of the sample in EDTA tube for cytology and prepare few fresh smears on glass slides, place some sample in culture media for aerobic and anaerobic cultures.

*Materials: endoscopic technique*

1) Sedation. A combination of Detomidine IV 0.01 mg/kg and Butorphanol IV at 0.01 mg/kg is recommended if the patient is stable. Butorphanol can help suppress cough during the procedure.
2) Endoscope with light source.
3) Guarded TW/aspiration catheter.[5]
4) 30 mL of sterile 0.9% saline solution.
5) 30 mL syringe.
6) EDTA tube for cytology, aerobic and anaerobic media for culture.

*Procedure: endoscopic technique*

1) Ensure the endoscope is clean and flushed to reduce contamination.
2) Advance the scope through the larynx, in the tracheal lumen.
3) Once the proximal/mid-trachea or once a pool of mucus/secretions is reached, pass the guarded tubing in the biopsy channel.
4) Most commercially available kits are designed so that the sterile tubing is protected by a guarded line to avoid contamination from the scope that was just advanced through the upper airways. Once the area of sampling is reached, advance the sterile tubing through the guarded line and aspirate the sample in a sterile syringe. If there is no visible fluid, inject 20–30 mL of sterile saline in the trachea and pull back with the syringe in order to retrieve the saline injected. The advantage of this technique is the direct visualization of the sample in the airways.
5) Place a few mL of the sample in EDTA tube for cytology and prepare fresh smears, place some sample in culture media for aerobic and anaerobic cultures.

*Potential complications* (predominantly associated with the trans-tracheal technique):

1) SC emphysema at the injection site. This is usually mild and does not cause a problem; however, if severe, it can result in pneumomediastinum. Horses in respiratory distress are more likely to develop severe pneumomediastinum.
2) Tubing laceration and loss in the airways. Usually this gets coughed up in the larynx within minutes.

5 Tracheal wash/Aspiration catheters Mila International, Inc., Florence KY.

3) SC abscessation or cellulitis at the site of injection of the transtracheal technique.
4) Chondritis of the tracheal rings due to damage of the rings' cartilage during the transtracheal technique. This can lead to local tracheal stenosis if severe.

## Bronchoalveolar Lavage (BAL)

BAL can be performed via endoscope or blindly via BAL tube. The advantage of the endoscopic technique is the direct visualization of the airways and the possibility of directing the scope in a specific lung and focal areas.

*Materials*

1) Sedation. A combination of Detomidine IV 0.01 mg/kg and Butorphanol IV at 0.01 mg/kg is recommended if the patient is stable. Butorphanol can help suppress cough during the procedure.
2) 20 mL syringe with local anesthetic (2% Lidocaine).
3) 4 mL × 60 mL syringes with sterile 0.9% saline solution.
4) EDTA tube for cytology, and plain tube or container.
5) 5 mL syringe.
6) BAL silicone tube[6] for the blind technique.
7) Endoscope, at least 2 m long, with light source for the endoscopic technique.

*Procedure: blind technique*

1) Sedate and restrain the horse appropriately. The head will need to be extended to facilitate the tube passage in the trachea.
2) Pass the BAL catheter in the ventral nasal meatus until it reaches the trachea. No resistance should be felt in the trachea. You can confirm the tracheal placement by holding the proximal trachea between your index finger and your thumb and gently shake it latero-laterally, this will allow to feel the tube moving against the tracheal wall.
3) When in the trachea, gradually instill the local anesthetic solution while advancing the tube distally until the tube gets lodged in the bronchial tree.
4) Inflate with air the tube balloon cuff once the tube is well lodged as distally as possible.
5) Instill the 4 mL × 60 mL syringes of saline and then gently retrieve the infused fluid immediately. You might not retrieve more than 50–60% of the instilled volume. The fluid obtained should be foamy, indicating the presence of surfactant.
6) Deflate the tube cuff and pull out the BAL tube.
7) The sample obtained can be pooled. Submit for analysis immediately. If submission is going to be delayed place a few mL of the sample in the EDTA tube to better preserve the cell morphology.

*Procedure: endoscopic technique*

1) Sedate and restrain the horse appropriately.
2) Pass the endoscope into the trachea and start instilling the local anesthetic gradually while passing it distally.
3) Stop when lodged into the distal bronchial tree and use the biopsy channel to instill the sterile saline solution and retrieve it immediately.
4) Pool the sample obtained and submit for analysis immediately. If submission is going to be delayed place a few mL of the sample in the EDTA tube to better preserve the cell morphology.

*Potential complications*

1) Focal or locally extensive pneumonia is a rare complication. Temperature and attitude should be monitored for a few days after the procedure.
2) Hemorrhage is also a rare complication, and it happens more likely after severe cough or in the presence of severely remodeled lung parenchyma. Fatal hemorrhage after the procedure has been reported in one case.

6 Large Animal Broncho-alveolar Lavage catheter Mila International, Inc., Florence KY.

## Diagnostics for Ophthalmology

This subchapter will describe some of the basic ophthalmic diagnostics in the context of ophthalmic emergencies. Chapter 16 will discuss in detail how to recognize and triage specific ocular emergencies.

Accurate assessment of ocular emergencies is fundamental to establish appropriate and aggressive intervention to attempt to preserve vision. The first step in ocular emergencies is to obtain a thorough history regarding the time and nature of the disease and treatments already received. A complete physical exam of the patient should follow. Many systemic diseases have ocular manifestations, and ocular disease can have systemic consequences. The goals of the initial assessment are to establish severity of the disease, visual deficits, and prognosis. The unaffected eye should always be fully examined as owners might not recognize previous impaired vision that could contribute to the presenting disease. Ideally, the ophthalmic exam should be carried out in an area that can be darkened. Basic instruments and supplies needed for basic diagnostics are outlined below.

### General Ophthalmic Exam

*Materials*

1) Bright, focal light source (otoscope or Finoff transilluminator with a strong light source or a penlight, avoid LED lights).
2) Direct ophthalmoscope.
3) Slit lamp biomicroscope - Optional.
4) Indirect lens.
5) Camera (cell phone or other).

*Procedure*

1) Evaluate facial and orbital symmetry.
2) Complete cranial nerve evaluation, focusing on the palpebral reflexes, dazzle reflexes, menace responses, and direct and consensual pupillary light reflexes (PLR).
3) Examine carefully the eyelids, conjunctiva, sclera, nictitating membrane, cornea, anterior chamber, iris, pupil and lens using a bright focal light source or, ideally, a direct ophthalmoscope.
4) The use of a slit lamp is ideal for evaluation of the anterior segment as it provides magnification and versatile illumination.
5) Evaluate the fundus using a focal light source and indirect lens or a direct ophthalmoscope. Pupillary dilation is achieved using a mydriatic agent (1% tropicamide 0.2 mL/eye is preferred over atropine for diagnostic purposes due to fast onset and short duration), allowing for full evaluation of the fundus. Indirect ophthalmoscopy is indicated especially when cloudy media is present (e.g., hyphema).
6) Take pictures of lesions for documentation/monitoring purposes and/or to consult an ophthalmologist if required.

### Schirmer Tear Test

Start with a Schirmer tear test (STT) if the eye is possibly dry (e.g., in cases of facial paralysis, corneal disease, suspected keratoconjunctivitis sicca). Perform STT before any staining or other topical medication. Do not perform this test in fragile eyes including those with deep corneal ulcers or lacerations or that have ruptured.

*Materials*

1) Schirmer tear test strips.

*Procedure*

1) Fold the strip 90° at the notch while the strip is still contained within the plastic wrap.
2) Place the bent part gently under the lower eyelid margin. You can close the lids with your hand to ensure the strip remains in place.
3) Wait one minute.
4) Remove the strip and read how far the moisture has migrated along the strip. Normal values: >15 mm/min.

## Fluorescein/Rose Bengal Staining

Fluorescein stain adheres to the hydrophilic corneal stroma and therefore is useful to identify corneal ulcers in which the epithelium is missing. It is indicated in every painful eye, eyes with a trauma history, and eyes with chronic corneal disease. A cobalt blue filter highlights fluorescein uptake and is included on most direct ophthalmoscopes. Fluorescein staining can be also helpful in determining patency of the nasolacrimal duct. This can be achieved by verifying that fluorescein appears at each nostril within about 20 minutes from corneal application.

Rose Bengal staining is used to detect devitalized corneal and conjunctival epithelial cells. This stain is useful in cases of suspected viral or fungal infection, for detection of qualitative tear film deficiency, or to assess the extent of some conjunctival neoplasms like squamous cell carcinoma. This stain can also help detect the presence of very small foreign bodies. The procedure is similar to that described for fluorescein staining. However, interpretation is strictly related to time and concentration: ensure to interpret the results immediately after application (no later than one to two minutes) and keep in mind that an excessive concentration can stain healthy epithelial cells.

*Materials*

1) Fluorescein strips[7] or Rose Bengal strips.[8]
2) 3 mL syringe.
3) 1–2 mL of sterile saline solution.
4) 25 G needle.
5) Direct ophthalmoscope or slit lamp or other light source.

*Procedure*

1) Place the stain-containing part of the strip (tear off the white part and discard) in an empty 3 mL syringe by removing then replacing the plunger.
2) Attach the needle to the syringe and draw up 1–2 mL sterile saline, then break the needle off at the hub.
3) Gently spray the solution on the cornea.
4) Gently close the eye lid two to three times to ensure the solution distributes well onto the cornea.
5) Assess for uptake using a light source (preferably with a cobalt blue filter).

## Corneal Culture and Cytologic Examination

Many corneal lesions in horses are associated with bacterial or fungal infections; therefore, obtaining samples for cytology and culture and sensitivity is important to inform the diagnosis and guide treatment.

Cytology should be carried out with any ulcer that appears infected (cellular infiltrate, stromal loss) and in any case of prolonged ulcerative keratitis. Retrieval of a cytological sample should not be attempted if the cornea is perforated or if a descemetocele is present. Topical anesthetic (proparacaine or tetracaine) should be applied to the ocular surface prior to the collection of samples for cytology and culture. Topical anesthetic solutions should not negatively affect culture positivity rates and aid in the collection of diagnostic samples by preventing contamination from the conjunctiva or eyelids in blepharospastic patients.

*Materials*

1) Topical anesthetic (proparacaine 0.5%, tetracaine 0.5%).
2) Sterile scalpel blade (use the non-cutting side) or cytology brush or Kimura spatula.
3) Culture swabs.
4) Cotton swabs to use after cytological scraping.
5) Glass slides.
6) Aerobic and anaerobic culture media.
7) Diff-Quik stain +/− Gram stain.

7 Wyeth Ayerst Laboratories, Rouses Point, NY 12979.
8 Amcon laboratories, St Louis, MO 63123.

*Procedure: cytology*

1) Sedate and restrain the horse properly.
2) Apply 0.1–0.2 mL of topical anesthetic.
3) Remove excessive debris if needed before collecting the sample. This will increase the chances of obtaining a diagnostic sample.
4) Scrape the corneal lesion with the non-cutting end of the blade held at a 45 degree angle or brush/spatula.
5) Place the sample collected on the glass slide.
6) After scraping, the excessive epithelium can be cleared with the use of a dry cotton swab.
7) Slides can then be stained, after they dry, and be evaluated for the presence of inflammatory cells, bacteria, and fungi. The slides can be submitted to a clinical pathologist for further evaluation. If fungal hyphae are identified or the clinical disease could be consistent with fungal infection, fungal culture and anti-fungal treatment are recommended.

*Procedure: culture*

1) Confirm the eye is NOT ruptured and there is no descemetocele.
2) Gently roll the swab on the lesion, avoiding touching the conjunctiva or eyelids.
3) Place the swab in culture media.

## Tonometry

Intraocular Pressure (IOP) measurement is indicated when there is suspicion for or a previous diagnosis of glaucoma or uveitis as well as in cases with corneal edema, historical trauma, unexplained painful or red eyes, and lens luxation. Do not perform tonometry in eyes with deep corneal ulcers or lacerations, descemetoceles, or in ruptured globes.

Both eyes should be evaluated, and a difference of less than 5 mmHg between the eyes is considered consistent with normal variation. Two measurements per eye should always be taken since repeatability plays a major role in accurate interpretation of the results.

*Materials*

1) Topical anesthetic (proparacaine 0.5%, tetracaine 0.5%).
2) Tono-Pen[9] (and tip covers) or TonoVet (and probes).[10]
3) Sedation and/or auriculopalpebral perineural anesthesia might be needed for some horses. Note that sedation decreases IOP or can increase the IOP if the head position lowers, always maintain the head in neutral or slightly elevated position.

*Procedure*

1) Sedate and perform an auriculopalpebral nerve block, if needed.
2) Apply topical anesthetic if using a TonoPen.
3) Open the eyelids using your index finger and thumb, stabilize the lids against the orbit and not the globe as this will falsely elevate the measurement.
4) Keep the instrument perpendicular to the corneal surface and obtain the readings.
5) Obtain IOP readings in the most central area of the cornea or the most normal area of the cornea.
6) Read the instructions and understand how to use your tonometer prior to use – comfort with your instrument is critical to obtaining an accurate measurement.

## Ultrasound

Ocular ultrasonography is a safe and simple procedure that can provide important information about the structural integrity of the globe despite the presence of severe eyelid, corneal or lens pathology that prevents a direct view into the eye. Ultrasonography is indicated when a complete ocular exam is not possible due to the presence of pathologies that impede visualization of deeper structures. Ultrasonography can aid in establishing treatment plan and prognosis for many diseases

9 Medtronic Solan, Jacksonville, FL, USA.
10 Icare, Helsinki, Finland.

involving the globe, the periorbital tissues, and the retrobulbar structures (e.g., retinal detachments, lens abnormalities, and retrobulbar masses). Care should be taken when performing an ultrasound if there is risk of globe rupture.

Some training is needed to confidently identify abnormalities and distinguish them from artifacts. For more details about image acquisition and abnormalities, see Slack J. "Emergency Ocular Examinations" in "Equine Emergencies treatment and procedures" (Slack 2014).

*Materials*

1) Ultrasound – 5–14 MHz probe. Rectal probes can provide reasonable images of the globe.
2) Coupling agent safe for use around the eye (Optixcare, other corneal lubricant).

*Procedure*

1) Sedation and/or auriculopalpebral nerve block, if needed.
2) Apply the coupling agent.
3) Place the probe on the lid and begin acquiring images.

Additional diagnostic procedures include skull radiography or computed tomography in cases of facial trauma involving the orbit.

## Rectal Examination

Rectal examination is a core diagnostic for evaluating horses with signs of colic, reproductive tract disease or other problem involving the abdominal cavity (Figure 4.10) (Box 4.4). Abnormalities are uncommonly detected within the rectum (e.g., tear, obstipation), and it is used as a sleeve through which organs can be palpated to assess positioning, distension, and consistency. A safe environment should be established, where the horse's ability to swing the hind quarters is limited and, ideally, where a protective barrier is present between the horse's hind limbs and the clinician. A set of metal stocks is desirable for this procedure. Alternatively, a stack of hay bales can be piled between the horse and clinician (Londoño 2017b).

*Materials*

1) Sedation.
2) 2% lidocaine, 60 mL in slip tip syringe.
3) Plastic pipette or red rubber catheter.
4) Rectal sleeve.

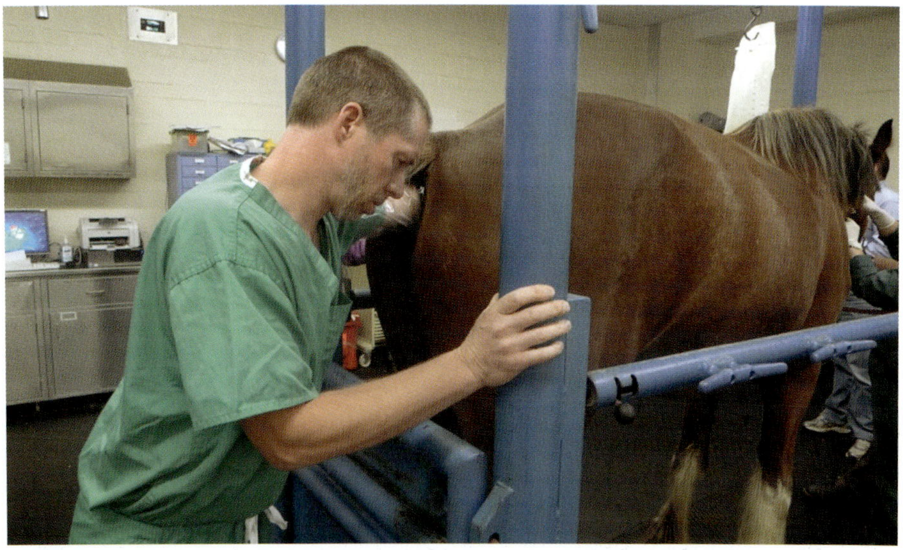

**Figure 4.10** Rectal examination in the horse. Appropriate preparation for a rectal exam may include the use of sedation, restraint, intra-rectal Lidocaine, or other drugs. When performing a rectal exam in the horse for the evaluation of colic, the clinician should attempt to answer three questions: (i) is the exam normal or abnormal? (ii) is the problem involving the small or large intestine or another organ? and (iii) what differentials correspond to the exam findings?

**Box 4.4 Questions to answer during rectal exam**

The clinician should attempt to answer three questions during the rectal exam:

1) Is the exam normal or abnormal?
2) Does the abnormality involve the small or large intestine or another organ?
3) What list of differentials is consistent with the rectal exam findings?

5) OB lubricant.
6) Optional: further chemical restraint – butylscopolamine (Luo et al. 2006), caudal epidural.
7) Optional: brown gauze and 1″ tape for tail wrap.

*Procedure* (Figure 4.10)

1) Establish appropriate restraint of the patient to facilitate clinician safety. If desired, wrap the horse's tail and secure it forward by looping brown gauze around the neck and between the fore limbs. Do not tie the tail to stocks.
2) Don a rectal sleeve and apply copious lubricant to the hand and arm.
3) Enter the rectum with fingers in a cone shape. Dilate the anus gradually with a couple of fingers if it is not possible to enter with the entire hand. Gently maneuver fingers to cup fecal balls and sweep them out of the rectum. Empty the rectum of manure.
   Note: Do not force against peristaltic contractions.
4) Introduce a pipette or red rubber catheter into the rectum with the tip protected and clasped in a hand. Inject 60 mL lidocaine into the rectum through a pipette or red rubber catheter.
5) Develop a consistent method for evaluation of the caudal abdomen by rectal exam (Luo et al. 2006).
   a) Orient yourself by palpating the aorta along dorsal midline. It can be followed caudally to its bifurcation of iliac arteries. The pulses should be readily identified and equal.
   b) Palpate the caudal pole of the left kidney. Palpate the clear trough (nephrosplenic space) formed by the nephrosplenic ligament and head of the spleen.
   c) Palpate the head of the spleen and follow the margin of the spleen caudoventrally.
   d) Evaluate the caudal abdomen for intestinal contents – palpate ventrally for fecal balls within the small colon, distended loops of small intestine (not normally palpable, but often mid-caudal abdomen when present), and the pelvic flexure (smooth, soft viscus in the left caudal abdomen).
   e) Palpate the body and horns of the uterus and follow the uterus to each ovary. The uterus is usually palpable by curling a hand over the pelvic brim.
   f) Palpate the bladder. Confirm its identity by following the left and right lateral ligaments. It might not be easily palpable if empty.
   g) Each of the inguinal rings can be palpated in the lateral, caudoventral abdomen.
   h) Identify the cupula and medial band of the cecum in the right, caudal abdomen
6) Remove hand from the rectum. Evaluate the sleeve for the presence of blood, which can indicate mucosal irritation or rectal tearing. If blood is present, further evaluation of the horse and communication with the owner is immediately warranted.
7) Clean up lubricant and manure from the horse's perineum.

## Field Necropsy

A field necropsy can be performed to obtain a definitive diagnosis, either on gross examination or by histopathology, to educate the clinician or client, to provide legal documentation, and/or to support the decision for euthanasia (Ness and Bain 2009). A timely, systematic approach to field necropsy, with appropriate case selection, is most likely to result in an accurate diagnosis. Referral to a pathologist is recommended when an insurance provider requests a necropsy, medical decision making is questioned by the owner or a third party, or when the field clinician's familiarity with necropsy or the complex nature of the suspected disease is low (Frank et al. 2015). Contraindications for field necropsy include the suspicion of neurologic disease and reportable, zoonotic diseases such as anthrax, equine encephalitides, and rabies (Ness and Bain 2009).

Location selection for field necropsy is important to ensure isolation from other animals (including scavengers), easy disposal of the cadaver, and adequate disinfection after necropsy (Ness and Bain 2009). The number of assistants should be minimized to avoid accidents and minimize biosecurity risks. Necropsy should be undertaken as soon as possible after death to avoid loss of tissue integrity and artifact associated with autolysis, as well as rigor mortis. A focused field necropsy for tissue evaluation and collection can be adequate when a single organ is of concern; however, examination should be performed in a consistent, thorough manner. At a minimum, grossly abnormal tissue should be sampled; a fresh and formalin-fixed sample of each lesion should be collected for submission to the lab (Frank et al. 2015). Follow lab recommendations for tissue handling and shipping.

*Materials*

1) Personal protective equipment (PPE): gloves, plastic sleeves, boot covers, coveralls or disposable suit, protective eye wear.
2) Containers for sampling: culture media, cassettes and formalin for histopathology, blood tubes, whirl-pacs or similar sealable storage bags.
3) Identification tags or markers.
4) Camera.
5) Knife.
6) Sharpening steel.
7) Disposable surgical blades.
8) Rib cutters, hack saw.
9) S-curve needle.
10) Umbilical tape.

*Procedure* (Ness and Bain 2009; Frank et al. 2015)

1) Move the cadaver to the selected, appropriate location as described above.
2) Don PPE.
3) Evaluate the body for overall condition and evidence of injury. An assistant can help to collect photographic documentation of the necropsy and/or keep notes during the procedure.
4) Position the cadaver in left lateral recumbency.
5) Using a scalpel blade, make a skin incision from the xiphoid to the tuber coxa, following the paracostal arch. Make a second, transverse incision from the xiphoid toward the base of the wither (caudal to the triceps).
6) Paying attention to avoid entering the abdominal and thoracic organs, use a knife to transect the remaining tissue along the path of the skin incision.
7) Gas should flow into the abdomen upon puncturing the peritoneum.
8) Reflect dorsally the musculature overlaying the ribcage.
9) Separate the diaphragm from its attachment on the right side of the ribcage. Gas should flow into the thorax upon puncturing the diaphragm and pleura.
10) Using rib cutters or a hack saw, transect the exposed ribs at their dorsal and ventral extents.
11) Fold the ribcage cranially, maintaining its cranial muscular attachment.
12) If the thorax is the point of focus for the field necropsy, reflection of the right fore limb is recommended at this stage for thorough evaluation of the lungs, pleura, mediastinum, and heart with related vasculature. The limb can be reflected by elevating it and incising the axillary soft tissues. The thoracic organs are accessible for removal alongside the pluck (tongue, larynx, trachea, esophagus). Skin and soft-tissue transection abaxial and parallel to the pluck will facilitate its removal.
13) Examination of the abdominal cavity begins with evaluation of organ positioning *in situ*. Exteriorize the large colon from the abdomen to facilitate examination of the remaining abdominal organs. Examine the stomach, small intestine, cecum, and small colon. Improved access for exteriorizing and examining intestine can be accomplished by transection of the mesentery.
14) Additional organs for examination include the liver and spleen. Access to the retroperitoneal (kidneys and adrenal glands) and urogenital organs can be optimized by reflection of the right hind limb by incising the inguinal soft tissues and dislocating the coxofemoral joint.
15) Collection of the brain is achieved for neurologic disease testing (e.g., rabies) by first reflecting the skin and muscle from the frontal and caudal aspects of the skull. Three bone cuts (forming a triangle) are recommended to

elevate the cranium and expose the brain. Make a transverse bone incision connecting the supraorbital fossae. Extend the incision from each supraorbital fossa to the foramen magnum. Digitally elevate and remove the brain. Wear appropriate PPE if neurologic, zoonotic infectious disease (such as rabies, equine encephalitides) is suspected. Referral for necropsy in cases of suspected neurologic, zoonotic infectious disease is strongly recommended.

16) Limb harvest for careful dissection is recommended to evaluate focal musculoskeletal injury.
17) Replace exteriorized organs in the abdomen or thorax. Replace the ribcage and muscular skin flap. Use umbilical tape on an S-curve needle to close the body wall and skin in a single layer.

## Isolation and Biosecurity

Emergency consultations can represent a potential risk for the spread of contagious and/or zoonotic diseases. This can be the case for patients admitted to facilities such as equine hospitals and cases seen by practitioners attending emergency calls in the field. Most equine practices have biosecurity programs involving isolation protocols, disinfection protocols, and surveillance testing to limit the risk of transmission of infectious diseases. This subchapter will focus on the field approach to biosecurity and isolation protocols in the context of emergency situations for the equine practitioner. Please see Chapter 17 for additional information regarding infectious disease and biosecurity.

### Identification of Patients at Risk

Patients affected by any stressful events such as illness and/or discomfort are more likely to acquire infectious agents. For this reason, it is important to recognize that the emergency patient might be at increased risk of carrying and spreading infectious diseases. Identification of higher-risk patients becomes important so that preventive measures can be implemented during the emergency exam to limit the exposure to personnel and other animals. A thorough investigation regarding other horses on the premises and type of premises is always warranted and might start over the phone, even before the patient is examined.

Examples of patients at increased risk of developing infectious and contagious diseases are:

- Horses with a recent history of travel. It is important to have knowledge of the geographical areas travelled with the specific endemic diseases as they might differ from the area of origin.
- Horses with recent exposure to new horses: horses that travel to horse shows, barns that hosted horse shows, recent contact with new arrivals, horses in layout facilities with a lot of in and out traffic.
- Horses on premises where there are multiple sick horses.
- Horses that are already receiving antibiotic treatment (risk for *C. difficile* or *Salmonella spp.* colitis).
- Horses presented for bite wounds of other animals including wildlife.
- Horses with fever of unknown origin.
- Horses with respiratory signs such as nasal discharge, cough, enlarged mandibular lymph nodes.
- Horses that have been in contact with animals infected with transmissible diseases.
- Horses presenting acute neurologic disease with or without concurrent fever and without evidence of trauma or other cause.
- Horses presenting with diarrhea.
- Mares presented for abortion.

### Emergent Patient Handling

Helpful guidelines to decrease the likelihood of disseminating infectious disease spread by fomites:

- Always wear disposable gloves when handling any patient.
- Hands should be washed between patients using water and soap as hand hygiene can assist in the prevention of disease transmission.
- Clean equipment of organic matter scrubbing with soap and water then rinse and disinfect the equipment between horses. Thermometers should be cleaned of organic debris and disinfected between horses.
- Examine high-risk patients or patients known to be infectious last.

- Wear PPE and implement isolation protocols on the farm for the cases described below*.
- Ensure your clothes and footwear are clean before entering your vehicle to leave the premises.
- Ensure your equipment is cleaned and disinfected before leaving the premises and attending to other calls.

### Isolation/Quarantine

*It is advised to place the following patients in isolation/quarantine:

- Horses with enterocolitis, or with colic and fever with or without diarrhea.
- Horses with small colon impactions as they have higher incidence of *Salmonella spp*. shedding.
- Horses with obvious diarrhea.
- Fever of unknown origin.
- Horse with respiratory signs such as nasal discharge, and coughing.
- Multiple horses with limb or ventral body wall edema in multiple horses.
- Horses that present oral or coronary band vesicular or ulcerative lesions.
- Horses with acute neurologic symptoms with or without fever and with no clear evidence of trauma. This is particularly important if other horses on the same premises or that have been in close contact are showing upper respiratory signs/abortions (suspected EHV-1 infection). It might be wise to place the entire farm might need to be placed in isolation when EHV-1 is suspected until test results are finalized.
- Horses where multi-drug-resistant (MDR) bacteria have been isolated from draining wounds or surgical sites.

### Isolation in Field Settings

Achieving complete isolation with appropriate barriers can be challenging in the field.

- Ideally, isolate the patient in a separate facility (e.g., physically separate barn). If this is not possible, place the patient as far away as possible from other animals (e.g., at the end of the barn).
- Place footbaths with disinfectant outside the stall of the isolated horse and advise personnel to dip their feet when entering and exiting the stall. You can place an additional footbath at the entrance of the affected barn. Ensure that shoe wear is clean before using footbath as many disinfectants do not work when there is organic material present.
- Ensure the personnel are trained to wear disposable full gowns or coveralls to wear when accessing the isolated stall. Train personnel in how to properly apply and remove the gown or coverall without getting contaminated. Waterproof coveralls are recommended when dealing with diarrhea.
- Consider using separate utensils to clean the stall – shovel, wheel barrow, etc.
- Disposable face covers (masks) and hair covers are required for diseases that can be transmitted via aerosol or via nasal secretions (e.g., EHV-1, Strangles).
- No dogs or other pets should be allowed to get in any sort of contact with the affected animal to avoid them becoming fomites.

Note: The attending veterinarian should work together with owners and barn personnel to outline isolation protocols based on the specific situation presented.

The state or federal animal health official will oversee restrictions on at-risk animals in the event of a reportable disease.

More details on how to isolate patients on the farm can be found at: https://equinediseasecc.org/biosecurity/isolation-quarantine

## References

Auckburally, A., Petruccione, I., and Voss, S. (2019). Providing fluid therapy to equine colic patients. Part 1. *In Pract.* 41: 445–454. https://doi.org/10.1136/inpl6035.

Barakzai, S. and Chandler, K. (2003). Use of indwelling intravenous catheters in the horse. *In Pract.* 25: 264–271. https://doi.org/10.1136/inpract.25.5.264.

Chapman, A. (2017a). Injection techniques. In: *Manual of Clinical Procedures in the Horse*, 1ste (ed. L.R.R. Costa and M.R. Paradis), 72–87. John Wiley & Sons https://doi.org/10.1002/9781118939956.ch6.

Chapman, A. (2017b). Other routes of medication administration. In: *Manual of Clinical Procedures in the Horse*, 1ste (ed. L.R.R. Costa and M.R. Paradis), 88–94. John Wiley & Sons https://doi.org/10.1002/9781118939956.ch7.

Crabtree, N.E. and Epstein, K.L. (2021). Current concepts in fluid therapy in horses. *Front. Vet. Sci.* 29 (8): 648774. https://doi.org/10.3389/fvets.2021.648774. PMID: 33855057; PMCID: PMC8039297.

Dechant, J.E. (2021). Complications of nasogastric intubation. In: *Complications in Equine Surgery*, 1ste (ed. L.M. Rubio-Martinez and D.A. Hendrickson), 29–35. John Wiley & Sons https://doi.org/10.1002/9781118939956.ch7.

Fielding, L. (2018). Practical fluid therapy and treatment modalities for field conditions for horses and foals with gastrointestinal problems. *Equine Pract.* 34: 155–168. https://doi.org/10.1016/j.cveq.2017.11.013.

Frank, C., Madden, D.J., and Duncan, C. (2015). Field necropsy of the horse. *Vet. Clin. North Am. Equine Pract.* 31 (2): 233–245. https://doi.org/10.1016/j.cveq.2015.04.002. Epub 2015 May 26. PMID: 26021522.

Golenz, M.R., Carlson, G.P., Madigan, J.E., and Craychee, T. (1993). Preliminary report: the development of an intraosseous infusion technique for neonatal foals. *J. Vet. Intern. Med.* 7: 377–382. https://doi.org/10.1111/j.1939-1676.1993.tb01034.x.

Kraus, M.S., Rishniw, M., Divers, T.J. et al. (2019). Utility and accuracy of a smartphone-based electrocardiogram device as compared to a standard base-apex electrocardiogram in the horse. *Res. Vet. Sci.* 125: 141–147.

Londoño, A.S. (2017a). Nasogastric intubation. In: *Manual of Clinical Procedures in the Horse*, 1ste (ed. L.R.R. Costa and M.R. Paradis), 172–176. John Wiley & Sons https://doi.org/10.1002/9781118939956.ch14.

Londoño, A.S. (2017b). Rectal examination. In: *Manual of Clinical Procedures in the Horse*, 1ste (ed. L.R.R. Costa and M.R. Paradis), 182–189. John Wiley & Sons https://doi.org/10.1002/9781118939956.ch7.

Luo, T., Bertone, J.J., Greene, H.M., and Wickler, S.J. (2006). A comparison of N-butylscopolammonium and lidocaine for control of rectal pressure in horses. *Vet. Ther.* 7 (3): 243–248. PMID: 17039447.

Michou, J. and Leece, E. (2012). Sedation and analgesia in the standing horse 1. Drugs used for sedation and systemic analgesia. *In Pract.* 34: 524–531. https://doi.org/10.1136/inp.e6423.

Ness, S.L. and Bain, F.T. (2009). How to perform an equine field necropsy. *AAEP Proceedings* 55: 313–316.

Parkinson, N.J., McKenzie, H.C., Barton, M.H. et al. (2018). Catheter-associated venous air embolism in hospitalized horses: 32 cases. *J. Vet. Intern. Med.* 32 (2): 805–814. https://doi.org/10.1111/jvim.15057. Epub 2018 Feb 20. PMID: 29460300; PMCID: PMC5866986.

Radcliffe, R.M., Hill, J.A., Liu, S.Y. et al. (2022). Abdominocentesis techniques in horses. *J. Vet. Emerg. Crit. Care* 32: 72–80. https://doi.org/10.1111/vec.13118.

Schoster, A. (2017). Complications of intravenous catheterization in horses. *Schweiz. Arch. Tierheilkd.* 159 (9): 477–485. https://doi.org/10.17236/sat00126.

Schumacher, J. and Schramme, M. (2019). Diagnostic and regional surgical anesthesia of the limbs and axial skeleton. In: *Equine Surgery*, 5the (ed. J.A. Auer and J.A. Stick), 1220–1243. MO: Saunders Elsevier.

Slack, J. (2014). Imaging techniques and indications for the emergency patient. In: *Equine Emergencies: Treatment and Procedures*, 4e (ed. J.A. Orsini and T.J. Divers), 97–102. St Louis: Elsevier Saunders.

Walton, R.M. and Southwood, L.L. (2013). *Abdominocentesis and Peritoneal Fluid Analysis.* Practical Guide to Equine Colic https://doi.org/10.1002/9781118704783.ch10.

# 5

# Advanced Clinical Triage Procedures

*Barbara Delvescovo[1], Brenna R. Pugliese[2], Klaus Hopster[3]*, Kelly Knickelbein[1]*, and Nicole Scherrer[3]**

[1] Department of Clinical Sciences, College of Veterinary Medicine, Cornell University, Ithaca, NY, USA
[2] North Carolina State University, College of Veterinary Medicine, Raleigh, NC, USA
[3] Department of Clinical Studies - New Bolton Center, University of Pennsylvania School of Veterinary Medicine, Kennett Square, PA, USA

## Regional Perfusion Techniques

Regional limb perfusion (RLP) may be used to deliver antimicrobials to infected tissues at high concentrations. Compared to systemic administration, RLP provides increased levels of antimicrobials to infections of the limb, reducing side effects and medication costs. Two techniques of RLP are described in horses based upon the delivery method – intravenous (IV-RLP) and intraosseous (IO-RLP). Intravenous RLP is most applied, especially for the treatment of septic synovial structures, infected wounds, complicated hoof abscesses, and osteomyelitis (Figure 5.1a–c). Intraosseous RLP is an alternative for severe bone or joint infections, especially when venous access is not possible (e.g., with severe cellulitis), or when longer treatment times are required. The procedure can be performed in the field or the hospital under appropriate sedation with the use of a manually applied hemostatic tourniquet (Esmarch or Pneumatic) to occlude blood flow. The drug is then delivered to the region of interest through a local vein (IV-RLP) or into the medullary cavity of a long bone (IO-RLP) to achieve a high antimicrobial concentration. The concentration-dependent aminoglycoside antibiotics, such as Amikacin and Gentamicin, are most employed.

*Materials*

1) Recommended intravenous sedation: detomidine hydrochloride (0.005–0.01 mg/kg IV) and butorphanol tartrate (0.005–0.01 mg/kg IV); re-dose as needed throughout procedure.
2) Clippers.
3) Aseptic preparation supplies.
4) Sterile gloves.
5) Esmarch or pneumatic tourniquet (narrow rubber tourniquets are ineffective).
6) 21–25 g × ¾-in. butterfly needles (Winged Infusion Set[1]).
7) Sterile NaCl, 50 mL.
8) Amikacin sulfate 1–2 g (adult horse dose).
9) Two gauze pads folded and prepared with 1-in. white tape roll started on their edge.

*Additional materials for IO-RLP*

1) 4.5 mm cannulated screw.
2) 3.2 mm drill bit and 4.5 mm tap.
3) 3.2 mm drill guide and tissue protector.
4) 3.2 mm screwdriver.

*Contributors

1 Winged Infusion Set, Terumo Medical Corporation, Somerset, NJ.

*Emergency Triage of the Horse*, First Edition. Edited by Rolfe M. Radcliffe and Jamie J. Kopper.
 Published 2026 by John Wiley & Sons, Inc.
Companion website: www.wiley.com/go/radcliffe/triage

(a) (b) (c)

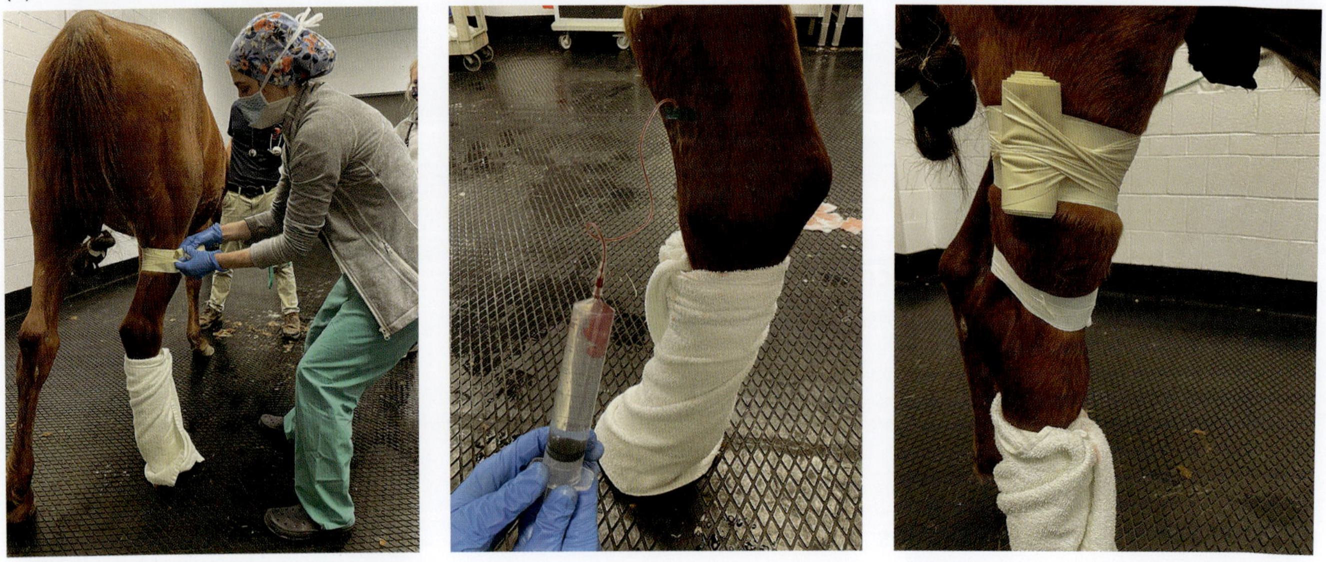

**Figure 5.1** (a–c) Intravenous regional limb perfusion (RLP) procedure in a horse for the treatment of a septic fetlock joint. Place an Esmarch tourniquet above treatment region and proximal to vein, wrap tightly, and secure (a). Introduce a butterfly needle (21–25 gauge, Winged Infusion Set) into the vein in a proximal-to-distal orientation, seating the length of the needle to the hub. Allow venous blood to flow back into the extension set to confirm placement; do not aspirate as to prevent collapse, venous laceration, and/or hematoma (b). Slowly inject 50 mL perfusate over three to five minutes. As the needle is removed, place folded gauze pads onto injection site and wrap limb tightly with white tape to secure bandage in place (c). Remove the tourniquet and temporary bandage after 20–30 minutes.

5) Air or electric drill.
6) Extension set.
7) Lidocaine, 2%, 3–10 mL.
8) #3 scalpel handle and #15 blade.

*IV-RLP procedure* (Figure 5.1a–c)

1) Prepare a 50 mL syringe containing 1–2 g amikacin, diluted to 50 mL with sterile NaCl. Use a smaller dose (500 mg) and volume (25 mL) for foals. Attach a butterfly needle and prime the extension line. *Note: Remember to subtract the RLP dose from the daily systemic amount of an aminoglycoside to prevent overdose and possible acute renal injury especially in foals.*
2) Sedate the patient. The horse should be minimally responsive to external stimuli to tolerate the tourniquet. Foals should be restrained in recumbency.
3) Aseptically prepare skin overlying superficial vein.
   a) For treatment of the distal limb below the fetlock, consider the medial or lateral palmar/plantar digital vein at level of the proximal sesamoid bones.
   b) For the mid-distal forelimb (metacarpus, carpus) consider the cephalic vein at the level of, or just distal to, the chestnut.
   c) For the mid-distal hindlimb (metatarsus, tarsus) consider the saphenous vein as it is coursing medially over the tibia.
4) Place Esmarch tourniquet above treatment region and proximal to vein, wrap tightly and secure (Figure 5.1a). Perform last sterile preparation if needed. A second tourniquet placed distal to the lesion may also be used to further isolate the region if needed; this may be valuable for more proximal limb injuries.
5) Introduce a butterfly needle (21–25 gauge, Winged Infusion Set[1]) into vein in a proximal-to-distal orientation, seating the length of the needle to the hub.
6) Allow venous blood to flow back into the extension set to confirm placement; do not aspirate as to prevent collapse, venous laceration, and/or hematoma (Figure 5.1b).
7) Slowly inject 50 mL perfusate over three to five minutes. Intermittently release the plunger on the syringe to watch blood flow back and confirm continued correct placement (blood will appear dilute over time). Monitor vein to ensure it is not "blown" or leaking into surrounding tissue.

8) As needle is removed, place folded gauze pads onto injection site and wrap limb tightly with white tape to secure bandage in place (Figure 5.1c).
9) Remove tourniquet and temporary bandage after 20–30 minutes (Kilcoyne et al. 2018; Gustafsson et al. 2020; Kilcoyne et al. 2021).

*IO-RLP procedure*

1) Follow the steps above for the RLP technique with the following exceptions.
2) Place the cannulated screw under sterile conditions.
3) When placing a 4.5 mm cannulated screw, use a small amount of lidocaine at the site of screw placement.
4) Use a #15 blade to make an incision down to the bone (commonly the third metacarpal or metatarsal bone).
5) Make a unicortical hole in the bone with the 3.2 mm drill bit using a drill guide or tissue protector.
6) Tap the hole with a 4.5 mm tap.
7) Place the screw with the 3.2 mm screwdriver at a length to allow the end of the screw to penetrate into the medullary cavity.
8) Some horses may become painful following the increased intraosseus pressure of IO-RLP. Inject 3–10 mL of lidocaine into the medullary cavity prior to the antibiotic infusate to prevent this problem.
9) Following IO-RLP, make sure the luer lock connection to the cannulated screw is well protected under a sterile, heavy bandage.

## Fracture Stabilization Methods

In the equine limb, prompt fracture stabilization is critical to improving the chance of a successful fixation after referral (Box 5.1). Therefore, external coaptation is used to immobilize the limb in the emergency setting, with the goal of stabilizing the joint above and below the fracture. The equine limb lacks stabilizing musculature in the distal limb, and further, the upper-limb musculature is mostly confined to the lateral aspect. Very proximal limb fractures such as the humerus and femur cannot be adequately stabilized; however, immobilization of fractures between the coronary band and olecranon or stifle can and should be immobilized for transport. Immobilization helps prevent the development of open fractures, further fracture displacement or propagation, or stretching of and trauma to the local vasculature and nerve supply, complications which decrease patient outcomes and prognosis for survival. Few supplies are needed to provide adequate stabilization in the field; only bandage materials and various splints are required. Splints may include PVC splints (4–8-in. diameter), wooden boards (1-in. thick by 3 or 4-in. wide), or the Kimzey splint. Splints should be sufficiently strong and wide enough to span the width of the limb, but never heavy or cumbersome, such that the horse is still able to walk and balance itself during transport. Do not use a wooden broom handle or dowel in place of a PVC or wooden splint as the round shape will allow splint migration under the bandage. The round splint will migrate to the fracture site causing further trauma and injury.

*Materials*

1) Non-adherent wound dressing and roll gauze (if wound present).
2) 8–10 rolls of roll cotton.
3) 6-in. brown gauze.
4) Vet wrap and Elastikon, 4-in.
5) PVC or wooden splints of appropriate length.
6) Duct tape.
7) Sedation and analgesia (Xylazine and butorphanol).
8) Clippers, betadine and saline, gauze, and saline flush (for wound cleaning if indicated).

**Box 5.1 Principles of fracture immobilization**

1) Stabilize the joint above and below the fracture.
2) Provide orthogonal (90°) stabilization when possible.
3) Never end rigid fixation (splint, cast, bone plate, etc.) in the middle of a long bone.
4) Rigid fixation should not end near the fracture site.

*Procedure – placing a lower-limb splint (below the carpus or tarsus for fractures of P1, P2, or stable distal cannon bone fractures).*

1) Examine the limb for skin wound (i.e., open fracture). Clip and clean wound if indicated.
2) Apply non-adherent wound dressing and secure with roll gauze if needed.
3) Place a modified Robert Jones bandage.
   a) Have an assistant hold the limb, at or above the level of the carpus or tarsus, such that the horse is non-weightbearing and the toe is pointed.
   b) Apply three to six thin layers of roll or sheet cotton from hoof to carpus or tarsus, being sure to provide good coverage over the coronary band.
   c) Applying significant pressure, secure cotton with 6-in. brown gauze to secure and tighten the bandage. Apply Vet Wrap at full stretch to further strengthen and tighten the bandage. Do not apply brown gauze or vet wrap onto skin; leave 1–2 in. at the top of the bandage. Elastikon may be applied to seal the top of the bandage.
   d) For fractures of P1, P2, or the distal cannon bone in the front limb, apply a PVC or wooden splint to the dorsal surface.
   e) The splints should extend from the ground to the level of the distal carpus or tarsus
   f) Ensure the toe is pointed (fetlock and pastern straight) for stabilization of forelimb fractures of the phalangeal region.
   g) For the hindlimb, apply splint to the plantar surface of the limb with the fetlock in flexion and the solar surface in line with the cannon bone. A flat wooden board works best for this application as it helps align and stabilize the hoof, and pastern and cannon bones.
   h) If medial or lateral instability is appreciated and enough room is present, apply a second lateral splint at 90° to the first.
   i) Secure splint(s) over bandage using duct tape. The entire surface of the splint and bandage should be covered with tape.

*Alternative: commercial splint application (Leg-Saver by Kimzey for phalangeal fractures)*

1) Only consider in cases without medial-lateral instability and for injuries distal to the fetlock. Do not use in unstable fractures.
2) Place a basic, well-padded standing wrap to the distal limb. Ensure that it ends above the most proximal portion of the splint bones and covers the coronary band.
3) Pick up the limb and slide the hoof all the way into the toe of the splint. While holding the knee in flexion (it is helpful to face the horse's head and rest the toe on your knee), begin closing the distal Velcro straps to secure the splint. Once held in place, you may set the toe on the ground. The horse will then step further into the toe.
4) Tighten the Velcro straps while placing pressure on the dorsal splint. It is critical that the straps are tight, and the splint is well-secured to the limb to provide adequate fracture stabilization.
5) You may have to repeat tightening after the horse walks to achieve sufficient stability.
6) White tape may be applied over the Velcro straps to provide additional security and to prevent loosening of the splint.
7) Horses walk very well with the Kimzey splint; this splint may also be used for recovery from general anesthesia in horses suffering fractures or other injury to the phalangeal region.

*Procedure – placing an upper-limb splint (to the level of the elbow or stifle for fractures of the metacarpus or metatarsus and olecranon fractures of the ulna)*

1) Place a modified Robert Jones bandage, as described for the lower limb, extending from hoof across the carpus or tarsus, extending as proximal as possible (i.e., to the olecranon or stifle).
2) For front-limb fractures of the cannon bone, place a palmar and lateral PVC or wooden splint, extending from the ground to the elbow. Tape the splints to the bandage separately to maximize strength of the bandage and splint support.
3) Olecranon fractures are an exception to the rules of fracture immobilization. Horses with these fractures present with a dropped elbow and inability to extend the forelimb. The goal is not to stabilize the fracture since the radius (and not the ulna) is the weight bearing bone of the proximal forelimb, but rather to allow use of the limb. For these fractures, place a splint from the ground to the level of the elbow on the caudal aspect of the limb to lock the carpus in extension. This allows the horse to ambulate, decreasing anxiety and allowing appropriate transport.

4) For the hind-limb fractures of the cannon bone, secure a lateral splint from the ground to the stifle crossing over the tarsus. A second PVC or metal splint can also be modified to follow the shape of the front or back of the hindlimb to provide orthogonal stabilization.
5) Where the splint does not contact the body well (e.g., lower limb) you may have to pad with additional gauze stacks or roll cotton. The authors suggest padding the PVC or wood directly with gauze or cotton and covering with tape.
   a) Note: Humeral and femur fractures should not be splinted, as the splint may act as a fulcrum and cause further displacement.

*Procedure – placing an upper-limb splint (to the level of the scapula or hip for fractures of the radius and tibia, respectively)*

1) Place a modified Robert Jones bandage, as described for the upper limb, extending from hoof across the carpus or tarsus, extending as proximal as possible (i.e., to the olecranon or stifle).
2) For middle-to-proximal radial fractures, place a lateral wooden splint (hardwood, 1-in. thick by 3–4-in. wide), extending from the ground to the top of the scapula region.
3) For distal radial fractures, placing second splint from the ground to the level of the elbow will provide additional strength via orthogonal stabilization.
4) For tibial fractures, place only a lateral splint from the ground to the region of the greater trochanter of the proximal femur.
5) Where the splint does not contact the body well (for example at the olecranon, or at the hip) you may have to add additional gauze stacks or roll cotton to provide full contact with the limb and splint. The authors suggest padding the PVC or wood directly with gauze or cotton and covering with tape.
   a) Note: humeral and femur fractures should not be splinted, as the splint may act as a fulcrum and cause further displacement and injury.

## Cast Application Techniques

Casts are commonly applied to stabilize the distal limb in cases of bone or soft-tissue injury, as well as for lacerations requiring immobilization for healing. Lightweight fiberglass casting tape is commercially available in a variety of widths and is durable and easy to apply. The horse should be appropriately restrained, sufficiently sedated, and the limb should be clean and dry prior to cast application. The limb must be held in an anatomically correct orientation and positioned in flexion, extension, or weightbearing position depending on the intended function of the cast. In the adult horse, casts are uncommonly applied to the limb in the field due to challenges of placement, compliance, personnel availability, and the fact that most fractures will require hospitalization and internal fixation.

*Casting materials*

1) Warm water in small bucket.
2) Exam gloves.
3) Stockinette – cut to twice as long as required cast plus several extra centimeters of length. Roll from each end toward the middle; one end should be rolled inward, and one end should be rolled outward.
4) Cast padding.
5) Adhesive casting felt.
6) Fiberglass cast tape.
7) Obstetrical wires and fluid line (for wire placement during cast application to allow cast removal without a cast cutter).
8) Methyl methacrylate.
9) 2-in. white tape.
10) Elastikon adhesive bandage.
11) Standing wrap, brown gauze, vet wrap if applying a bandage cast.
12) Non-adherent wound dressing and roll gauze (if wound present).
13) Two wooden blocks.
14) Hoof stand with cradle.

*Procedure – applying a hoof cast* (Fitzgerald et al. 2006)

1) Remove shoe if present, trim to remove excessive frog and sole.
2) Dress and bandage wounds with non-adherent dressing and roll gauze, being sure to be sparing and keeping this layer thin. Secure with a thin layer of Elastikon if needed for additional protection.
3) Cut stockinette to length: approximately twice as long as the distance from toe just above the fetlock. Roll as described above.
4) Apply the outward rolled half to the hoof and pastern. Twist at the toe, then roll the inward rolled half up the leg.
5) Cut a piece of adhesive casting felt to the circumference of the pastern and approximately 5 cm wide. Apply around pastern such that it fits snugly and has no overlap of ends.
6) Place obstetrical wires, encased within a fluid line, on the medial and lateral aspects of the foot and secure to the surface of the stockinette proximally and distally using 2–3 in. strips of 2 in. white tape. The ends should protrude from the top and bottom of the cast and the fluid line such that handles may be attached and used to saw off the cast at the time of removal.
7) Sedate horse. For the forelimb, rest the cannon bone on the cradle of a hoof stand such that the fetlock and digit hang in a weightbearing position. Alternatively, an assistant can hold the limb in this position.
8) For the hindlimb, rest foot on edge of wooden block. Position the foot so as much of the foot is hanging off the back of the block as possible; the bottom of the foot should remain parallel to the ground so that the hoof–pastern axis is in the neutral position. Position contralateral on a block of similar height.
9) Submerge the first roll of fiberglass cast material in warm water for 10–20 seconds, then gently squeeze out excess water so that the material is not dripping wet. About three rolls of material will be needed for the average adult horse. Start with 2–3 in. wide cast material to allow smooth application around the foot and pastern, then increase size to 3–4 in.
10) Apply the first roll of cast material to the hoof and pastern with moderate tension. There should be 50% overlap between passes, and the material should overlap the felt around the pastern by 50% such that there is no sharp edge contacting the skin of the horse.
11) After the first 1–2 passes of cast material, you may fold down the top edge of the stockinette to create a finished edge (cut holes to pass the obstetrical wire through), then continue with casting.
12) For the hindlimb, once only the toe is remaining, an assistant holds the limb off of the board, extending it cranially. This position aids in maintaining extension of the fetlock and digit.
13) Cover the toe and bottom of the foot using a figure 8 pattern around the heels and place the foot back onto the board for the casting material to set.
14) Once hardened, apply methyl methacrylate to the sole of the cast. When prepared methyl methacrylate should be a thick paste consistency, such that it can be scooped onto the bottom of the hoof to shape and cure. In the author's experience, it works well to mix this in a urine cup, and scoop onto the open surface of the foil cast material packaging. You can then apply the entire piece of foil to the bottom of the foot and let the material set, leaving the foil in place. This contains the methyl methacrylate, and lets you gently press and distribute it until flat and covering the entire sole and toe.
15) Coil the obstetrical wires and secure to the top and bottom of the cast using white tape.
16) Finally, to give the horse traction, apply Elastikon to the sole of the cast.
17) Seal the top edge of the cast to the horse's pastern by wrapping with Elastikon to prevent debris from falling side. Change this layer every 24 h to inspect for cast sores.

*Procedure – applying a half- or full-limb cast*

1) Ensure limb is clean and dry.
2) Cut stockinette and prepare as described above and apply to limb by rolling the outward rolled half up the limb, twisting at the toe, then rolling the inward half up the leg.
3) Place circumferential strips of felt adhesive at anatomic prominences and also at the top of the cast. For example, the author recommends placing felt around the base of the proximal sesamoid bones, the coronary band, and accessory carpal bone.
4) Apply a thin layer of cast padding, achieving 50% overlap with each pass. Two total passes should be sufficient to pad the limb.

5) Place fluid line-sheathed obstetrical wires medially and laterally and secure with 2–3 in. strips of white tape, such that enough length remains proximally and distally to use for future removal of the cast.
6) An assistant must hold the limb in a weightbearing position such that no significant varus or valgus is resulting. Wire placed through the toe of the hoof can help to hold the distal segment in extension but requires additional equipment.
7) After submerging in warm water for 10–20 seconds and wringing out excess water, apply from proximal to distal, spirally down the leg and overlapping each pass by 50%. The cast material should be applied under moderate tension such that it is slightly stretched, and results in no wrinkles or folds.
8) Continue spiraling up and down the limb until 4–8 total passes are achieved. After the first 1–2 passes, you may fold down the stockinette and incorporate into the cast to create a finished edge. You will have to cut holes in the stockinette to pass the obstetrical wires through.
9) The heel may require bulking, which is easily achieved by removing the core of a roll of cast material and flattening the whole roll; place this at the heel and cover with several additional layers of cast material.
10) Other areas which may need additional reinforcement include the toe and over the joints. The foot can be additionally reinforced using methyl methacrylate as described previously.
11) Coil wires proximally and distally and secure with white tape. Cover weight bearing surface and seal top of cast with Elastikon.

## Emergency Tracheostomy

Emergency tracheostomy is indicated in the case of acute or chronic, upper airway obstruction (UAO). Depending on timing of intervention, the procedure may be performed in the standing (Figure 5.2a, b) or in the down horse. Tracheostomy is the creation of an airway which bypasses obstruction of the nasal passages, larynx, or proximal trachea. Once the surgical approach is made, a temporary tracheostomy tube can be placed and secured. If a permanent tracheostomy is likely to be needed (e.g., chronic upper respiratory diseases such as neoplasia of upper airways) temporary tracheostomy should be placed in the middle neck instead of the proximal third (see ideal location in procedure description). This location will not preclude the subsequent creation of a permanent tracheostomy. Note that due to the nature of UAO some patients will not

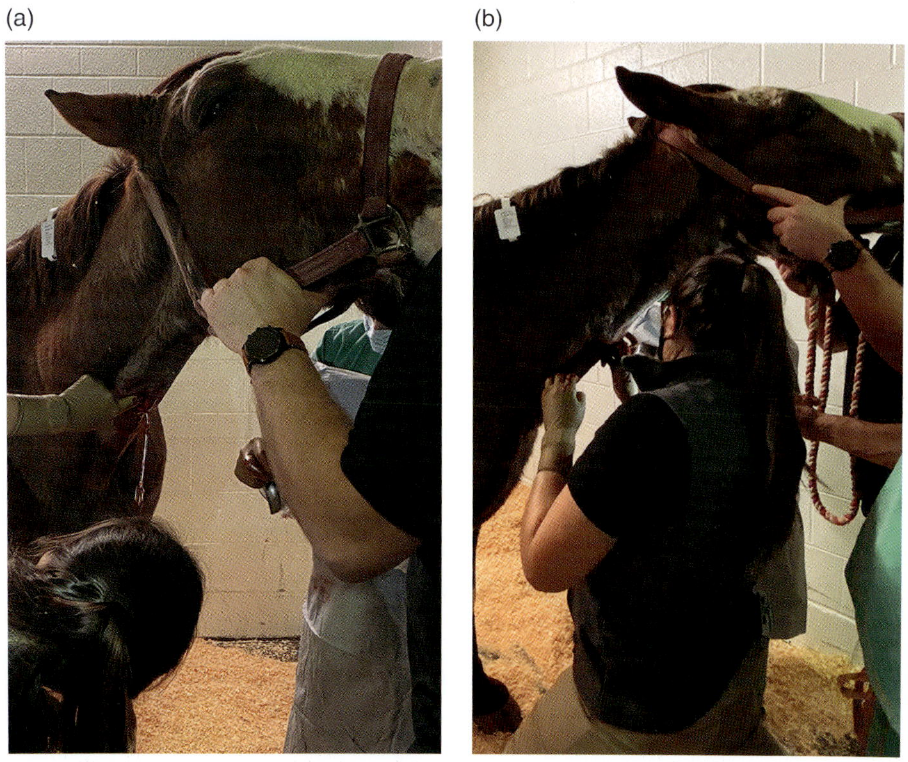

**Figure 5.2** (a, b) Emergency tracheostomy is indicated in the case of acute or chronic, upper airway obstruction (UAO), and may be performed in the standing or recumbent horse. Identify the trachea and make a 7–10 cm incision starting at the junction between the proximal and middle third of the neck and extending caudally. Use blunt finger dissection or Mayo scissors to separate the muscle bellies of the sternothyroideus, retracting them laterally on either side to visualize the tracheal rings (a). Palpate the annular ligament between two tracheal rings in the center of the incision. Make a full-thickness, transverse incision through the annular ligament and into the tracheal mucosa no longer than 1/3 of the tracheal circumference. Insert self-retaining metal tracheostomy tube (b). Alternatively, if using a cuffed silicone tube, hemostats can be useful to grasp the end of the tube and guide it into the tracheal lumen.

require sedation, and in others, sedation will further compromise respiratory function. The horse should be sedated if (i) indicated to maintain human safety and/or (ii) sedation is necessary to provide intervention. Under life-threatening circumstances clipping, aseptic preparation, and local anesthesia may be forgone to expedite creation of an airway. Safety of the animal handlers and veterinarians are important in emergent cases. A horse in severe respiratory distress that is dangerous may be allowed to collapse prior to creating a tracheostomy. If a tracheostomy tube is not available the handle of a plastic gallon jug, a trimmed 50 mL syringe case, nasogastric tube, or garden hose can be used as alternatives.

*Materials*

1) Clippers.
2) Aseptic preparation supplies.
3) Sterile gloves.
4) 2% lidocaine or mepivacaine, 10 mL syringe, 19–23 g × 1-in. Needle.
5) #10 scalpel blade, on handle (disposable recommended).
6) Variety of tracheostomy tubes in range of approximate, appropriate sizes (metal self-retaining[2] or cuffed silicone[3]).
7) If using cuffed silicone tube: large hemostats, size 2-0 nonabsorbable suture on a straight needle, and umbilical tape.

*Procedure* (Figure 5.2a, b)

1) Landmarks: the trachea is readily palpable in the upper ventral neck. Identify the junction between the proximal and middle third of the neck – the incision begins at this junction and extends caudally. The tracheal rings are palpated on midline.
2) If circumstances allow, aseptically prepare the surgical site.
3) When time allows, subcutaneously inject 5–10 mL of 2% local anesthetic on ventral midline overlying the trachea to create a 5–10 cm bleb.
4) Using a #10 scalpel blade, make an approximately 7–10 cm proximal-to-distal full-thickness skin incision.
5) Bluntly finger-dissect the subcutaneous tissues between the muscle bellies of the sternothyroideus, retracting them laterally on either side (Figure 5.2a). If available, Mayo scissors can be used bluntly to achieve this separation and visualization of the tracheal rings.
6) Palpate the annular ligament between two tracheal rings in the center of the incision. Using the #10 blade, make a full-thickness, transverse incision through the annular ligament and into the tracheal mucosa. The incision should be parallel to the tracheal rings and be no longer than 1/3 of the tracheal circumference.
7) Insert self-retaining metal tracheostomy tube[2] (Figure 5.2b). Alternatively, if using a cuffed silicone tube,[3] hemostats can be useful to grasp the end of the tube and guide it into the tracheal lumen. The silicone tube will require suturing into place, which is facilitated by using nonabsorbable suture on a straight needle. Umbilical tape can additionally be used to create a loop around the horse's neck which is tied to either side of the tube for added security.
8) Place hand over tracheostomy lumen to confirm adequate airflow.
9) Tracheostomy tube maintenance and complications:
   Because secretions may build up surrounding and within the tracheostomy tube, it is essential to monitor and clean the tracheostomy site and tube daily during use in any animal. Failure to do so may lead to obstruction of the airway. Other complications of tracheostomy tube use include local infection and subcutaneous emphysema.

## Chest Tube Placement

Chest tube placement is indicated in conditions such as pleuropneumonia, pleural abscesses, neoplastic effusion, pyothorax or hemothorax for sampling, release of pleural effusion, collection of blood for autotransfusion, instillation of medication, or lavage of the pleural cavity. The procedure can be easily performed with the horse standing under sedation. Chest tube placement may be required in the ventral or dorsal thorax depending upon the disease and removal of fluid or air from the thorax, respectively (Figure 5.3a–c). The chest tubes can be left in place for repeated drainage or medication administration. Note that both sides may need to be drained separately as most horses with pleural disease will have an intact, complete mediastinum.

---

2 Two-part metal tracheostomy tube – Pape's model; 22 mm internal diameter (Jorgensen laboratories, Inc., Loveland, Colorado).
3 Silicone Equine Tracheostomy Tube, 15 mm internal diameter (Jorgensen laboratories, Inc., Loveland, Colorado).

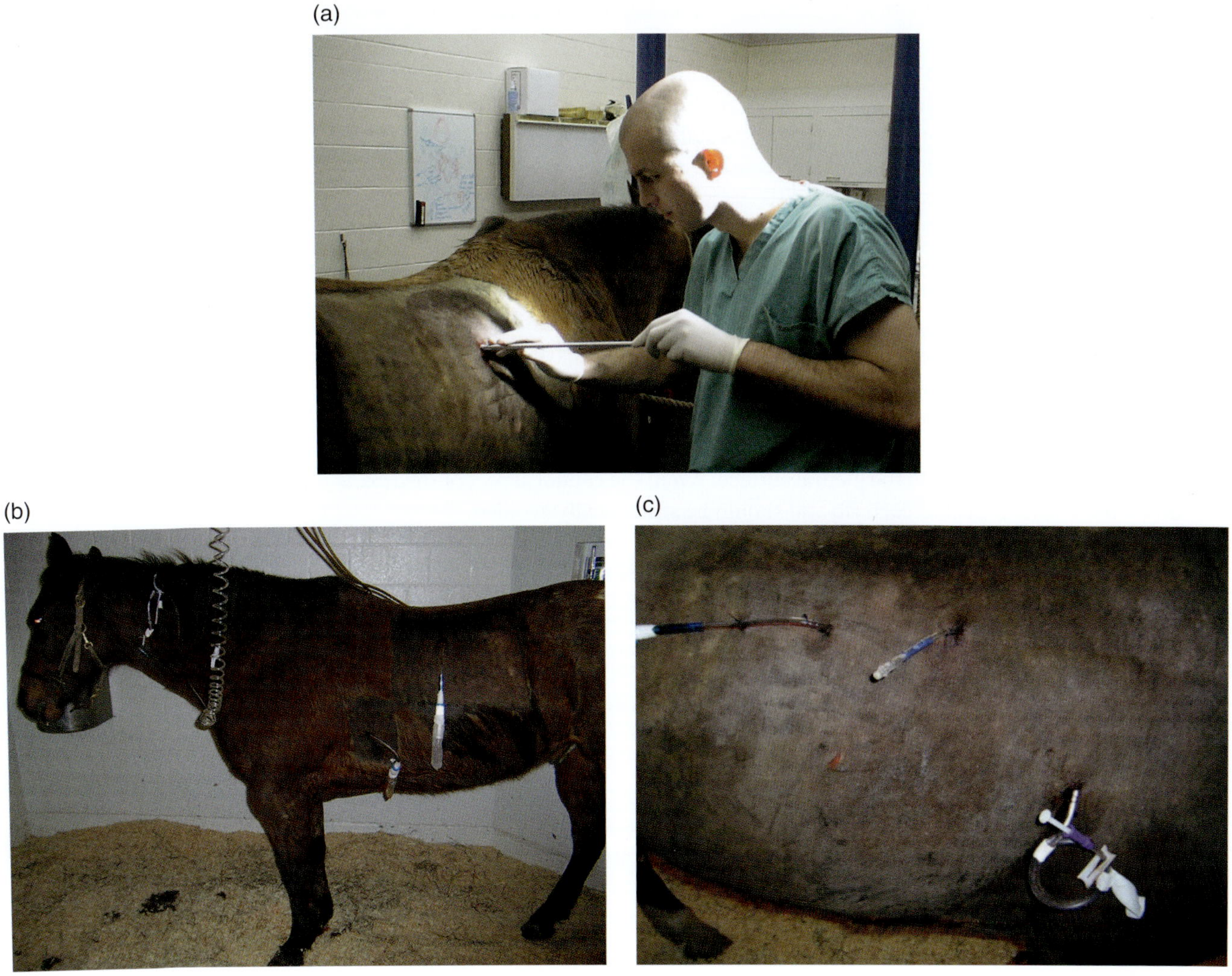

**Figure 5.3** (a–c) Placement of a chest tube to relieve pneumothorax in a horse with penetrating axillary thoracic injury, bilateral pneumothorax, and respiratory distress. Identify the site caudo-dorsally between the 13th and 15th intercostal spaces. After sterile preparation, make a stab incision through the skin and fascia along the cranial border of the caudal rib in the selected rib space. Hold the chest tube firmly and pass it through the stab incision, pushing the tube through the tissues until you penetrate the pleural membrane, and a loss of resistance is felt (a). Air may be removed via a 60 mL syringe and three-way stopcock or a suction pump (not to exceed 20 mmHg), and a Heimlich valve may be placed. (b) The left hemithorax of a horse where the dorsal tube is for removal of air and the ventral tube for removal of pleural fluid. (c) The right hemithorax of the same horse showing placement of a chest tube in the dorsocaudal thorax, a "soaker" catheter for delivery of bupivacaine analgesia in the craniodorsal thorax above multiple, adjacent rib fractures, and an oxygen line for infiltration of oxygen into severely injured tissues at the site of trauma to prevent anaerobic infection.

*Materials*

1) Clippers.
2) Sterile scrub.
3) Local anesthetic (e.g., Lidocaine 2% 5–10 mL).
4) 1 × 21 G 1.5′-in. needle for local block.
5) 1 × 5 mL syringe for local block.
6) Sterile gloves.
7) Sterile scalpel blade (#15).
8) Sterile indwelling trocar catheter (chest tube) 20–24 F.
9) Sterile clamp.

10) One-way valve if leaving the tube in place (e.g., Heimlich one-way valve[4] or a condom).
11) Non-absorbable 0 or 1 suture.
12) Sampling equipment: EDTA vacutainer tubes, plain vacutainer tubes, aerobic/anaerobic culture media, slides.
13) Sedation (use of sedatives and options may vary based on patient's attitude and cardiovascular stability). Detomidine IV 0.01 mg/kg is recommended if the patient is stable.
14) Ultrasound for guidance of chest tube placement.

*Procedure*

1) Identify the site for fluid removal from the lower thoracic cavity. For chest tube placement in the dorsal thorax (indicated for removal of air following pneumothorax), please see the end of this chapter. Ultrasound guidance is recommended. When ultrasonography is not available, careful auscultation can be helpful to determine the site. A suitable site is often located between the 6th and 8th intercostal spaces at about 10 cm dorsal to the olecranon. Precise placement is fundamental to avoid the cardiac structures and to avoid the lateral thoracic vein.
2) Clip and aseptically prepare the site chosen.
3) Infiltrate 5–10 mL of local anesthetic in the subcutaneous tissue and intercostal muscle at the cranial aspect of the rib, trying to instill some close to the pleural surface. Avoid the caudal aspect of the ribs as the intercostal vessels and nerve run on the caudal aspect of each rib and should be strategically avoided.
4) Perform a final aseptic preparation.
5) Make an approximately 0.5–0.8 cm stab incision through the skin and fascia close to the cranial border of the caudal rib of the chosen intercostal space. The incision can be extended into the intercostal muscle to facilitate the chest tube insertion.
6) Hold the chest tube firmly and pass it through the stab incision. In order not to push the tube in excessively, restrain it firmly using one hand to hold it against the body while the other hand at the bottom of the tube applies steady pressure. When in contact with the pleura some resistance will be felt, push the tube through it gently until loss of resistance is felt. You can apply gentle rotation to the tube while putting pressure to facilitate insertion through the thoracic wall tissues.
7) Once in the pleural cavity, pass the chest tube over the stylet and remove the stylet. Pleural fluid should start to flow out. Clamp the chest tube if fluid is not coming out constantly to prevent air influx in the pleural cavity and subsequent pneumothorax.
8) If the tube is staying in place, secure the tube to the skin using a purse string suture followed by a finger-trap pattern.
9) If the tube is staying in place, apply a one-way valve at the end of it, such as the Heimlich valves[4]. Alternatively, a sterile condom (with a small cut at the end) can be taped to the tube and can act as a one-way valve. If no one-way valve is applied, leave the tube clamped when not in use to avoid possible air entry into the thoracic cavity and subsequent pneumothorax.
10) The tube can stay in for several weeks if well secured in place. Daily flushing with sterile balanced solutions may help prevent occlusion from debris and fibrin, maintaining patency.
11) Once removed, the skin can be sutured with absorbable or non-absorbable 0 suture using a single cruciate or two simple interrupted sutures.

*Possible complications*

1) Pneumothorax, if there is inadvertent air influx into the pleural cavity.
2) Hemothorax, if a large vessel is accidentally punctured.
3) Cardiac puncture during chest tube placement. Use of ultrasound guidance during tube placement will help prevent this complication.
4) Cellulitis around the tube-skin insertion site.

## Pericardiocentesis

Indications: Sampling and/or release of pericardial fluid accumulation. It should be performed only when enough pericardial effusion is visualized; otherwise, the risk of cardiac puncture is substantial. This procedure is indicated in cases of pericarditis,

4 Heimlich chest drainage valve (Advanced Anesthesia Specialists, LLC, Prescott Arizona).

neoplastic effusion, transudate or blood causing tamponade. It is performed under ultrasonographic guidance. Pericardiocentesis can provide samples for diagnostic purposes (cytology and culture) and/or provide therapeutic drainage of the effusion.

*Materials*

1) Clippers.
2) Sterile scrub material.
3) Local anesthetic, 5–10 mL of 2% Lidocaine.
4) 1 × 21 G 1.5-in. needle for local block.
5) 1 × 5 mL syringe for local block.
6) IV catheter.
7) Sterile surgical gloves.
8) Sterile scalpel blade (#11).
9) Sterile indwelling thoracic catheter (chest tube) 28–32 F if the effusion is substantial, 12–24 F is the volume of the effusion is small or 10–14 G 5.25-in. intravenous catheter.
10) Three-way tap (stopcock) if using the intravenous catheter or sterile clamp if using the chest tube.
11) 30–60 mL syringe.
12) Ultrasound with sterile probe cover and sterile gel.
13) ECG monitoring for real-time monitoring.
14) 0 or 1 non-absorbable suture.
15) Collection equipment: EDTA vacutainer tubes, plain vacutainer tubes, aerobic/anaerobic culture media.
16) Sedation (use of sedatives may vary based on patient's attitude and cardiovascular stability). A combination of Detomidine IV at 0.01 mg/kg and Butorphanol IV at 0.01 mg/kg is recommended if the patient is stable.
17) Emergency anti-arrhythmic drugs.

*Procedure*

1) Place ECG and ensure to have a diagnostic trace to be able to monitor heart rhythm during procedure as arrhythmias could be induced.
2) Place an IV catheter in case emergency anti-arrhythmic drugs are needed during the procedure.
3) Consider administering IV fluids if cardiac tamponade is present to help improve cardiac output during the procedure.
4) Elect the site for puncture via echocardiographic guidance. In most cases, a suitable site is found at the 5th left intercostal space, in the area included between the lateral thoracic vein and a line level with the point of the shoulder.
5) Clip and aseptically prepare the area elected.
6) Infiltrate local 5–10 mL of local anesthetic in the subcutaneous tissue and intercostal muscle. Avoid the caudal aspect of the ribs as intercostal vessels and nerve run on the caudal aspect of each rib.
7) Perform a final aseptic preparation.
8) Make an approximately 0.5–0.8 cm stab incision through the skin and fascia taking care of incising cranial to the caudal rib of the chosen intercostal space.
9) Pass the chest tube or the catheter through the stab incision. Perform the puncture echo guided to avoid injury to the myocardium.
10) Once in contact with the pericardial surface the tube or catheter will be noticed to move in conjunction with the heart beats. Advance slowly and carefully until fluid starts flowing out. When using an indwelling chest tube, in order not to push in excessively, restrain the tube firmly using one hand to hold it against the body while the other hand at the bottom of the tube applies steady pressure. You can apply gentle rotation to the tube while putting pressure to facilitate insertion through the pericardium.
11) If using a catheter, connect it to the three-way stopcock and keep it closed until you are in the pericardial cavity.
12) Once in the pericardial cavity, fluid should flow out spontaneously. If not flowing immediately, after ensuring the positioning using the ultrasound, use the sterile syringe to apply gentle suction.
13) Monitor the ECG trace during the procedure. Occasional arrhythmias induced by the advancement of the tube/catheter are possible. Stop the advancement if frequent arrhythmias are detected during placement. Repositioning of the tube sometimes will ameliorate the arrhythmias.
14) If arrhythmias do not resolve with withdrawing or repositioning of the tube, specific treatments may be needed (see Chapter 12).
15) Check final placement of the tube via echocardiography.

16) The tube can then be left clamped after drainage and sutured in place using a purse string and a finger-trap pattern. It is recommended not to remove all the fluid from the pericardial cavity as this might cause friction of the pericardium.
17) Lavage of the pericardial cavity after drainage can be achieved infusing 1–2 L of warm sterile 0.9% saline solution. Antibiotics might be added in the lavage in cases of septic pericarditis (10,000–20,000 Sodium penicillin/L or 1 g of Gentamicin/L). Intra-pericardial tissue plasminogen activator (tPA) could be also valuable to reduce fibrin production (Jesty 2014).
18) Remove the tube when the fluid does not re-accumulate.

*Possible complications*

1) Pneumopericardium if there is inadvertent air influx in the cavity.
2) Trauma to the coronary arteries or cardiac puncture during placement. This is best avoided with the use of ultrasound guidance during placement.
3) Onset of sustained arrhythmias that require intervention.
4) Cellulitis around the tube skin insertion.

## Preparation for Field Anesthesia in the Emergent Horse

Short-term field anesthesia is a valuable tool in emergency situations with multiple purposes: immobilize the patient reducing risks for the personnel, reduce risk of further injury for the patient itself, enable immediate treatments to be administered, stabilize life-threatening conditions, move the animal safely from a precarious or dangerous environment to a safer area, and gain time to formulate a rescue plan.

General anesthesia's risks are substantially increased in compromised patients, especially in field settings where there is no access to hospital facilities and personnel. Therefore, stabilization prior to induction can be key in decreasing morbidity and mortality associated with the anesthetic event.

This subchapter is meant to be a quick guide on stabilization of the emergent patient for field induction and anesthesia (Figure 5.4); please refer to Chapter 30 of this book, *Anesthesia in emergency medicine,* for details on field induction and anesthesia.

### Pre-anesthetic Stabilization

1) Perform a complete physical exam. Realistically, in an emergency, you might be able to perform part of a physical exam. Focus on the cardiovascular and respiratory system. Salient steps are:
   - Evaluate respiratory rate and effort; if the horse is in respiratory distress evaluate if lung sounds are present and if airways are patent. Prepare for tracheostomy or pneumothorax/pleural fluid relief if needed.
   - Evaluate heart rate, mucous membrane color and moisture, capillary refill time (CRT), temperature
   - jugular refill, peripheral pulses, jugular refill to detect signs of hypovolemia.
2) Place an IV catheter and start fluid resuscitation. You can place a catheter of larger diameter (10 or 12 gauge) in hypovolemic/severely dehydrated horses; the placement of two catheters is also helpful. This will greatly facilitate faster fluid resuscitation.
3) If the heart rate is >60 bpm and the gastrointestinal system cannot be ruled out as cause of the emergency and/or there are signs of colic pass a nasogastric tube to release possible gastric distention.
4) Evaluate abdominal distention and consider percutaneous trocarization if distention is life threatening.
5) Check for signs of external or internal hemorrhage.
6) Evaluate the musculoskeletal system to establish the need to stabilize fractures.
7) The patient might need sedation. Refer to Chapter 4, *Basic clinical triage procedures,* for sedation of the emergent horse.

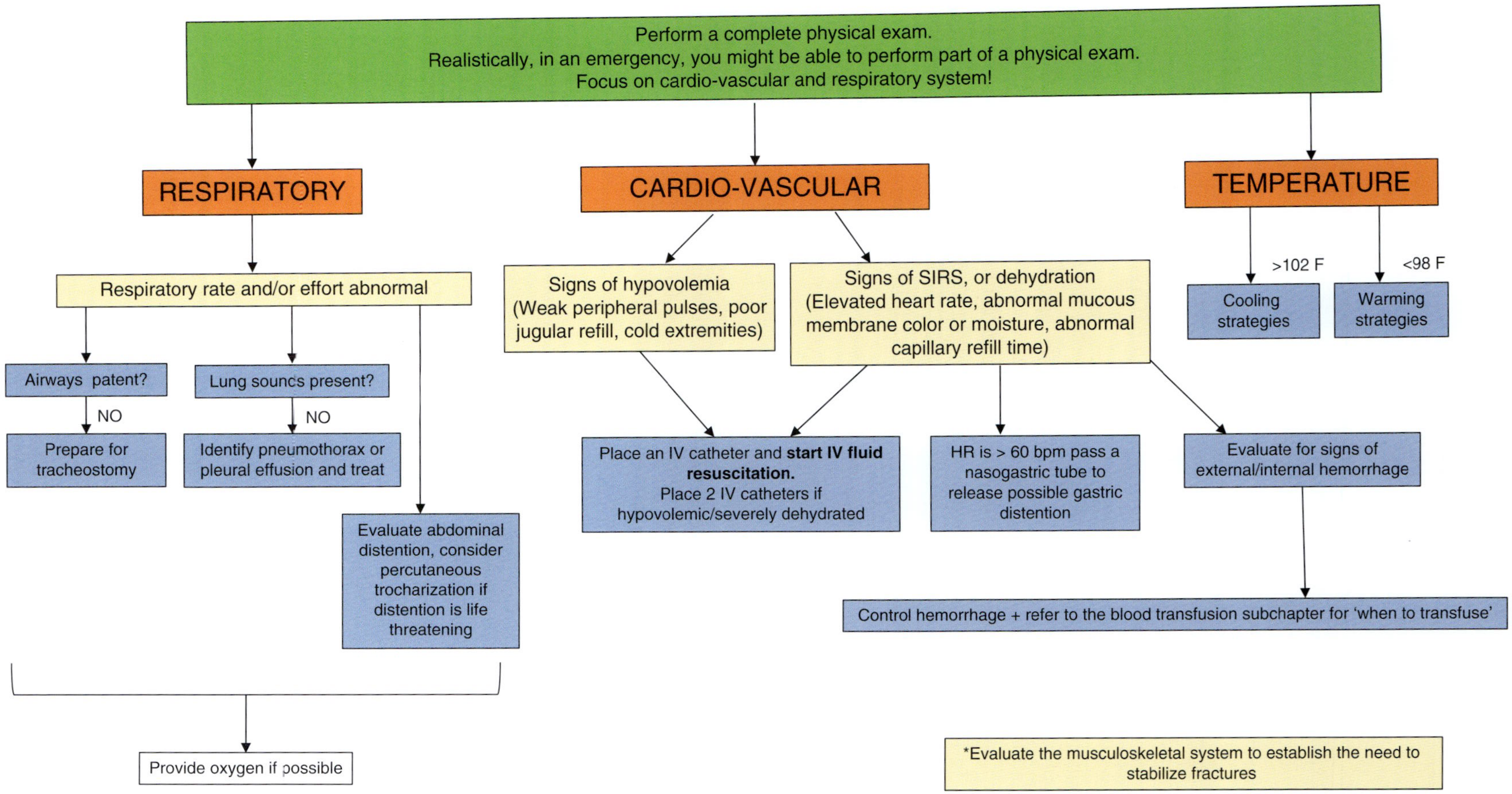


**Figure 5.4** Pre-anesthetic flow chart for the stabilization of the horse prior to field anesthesia. Many emergency problems may require short-term anesthesia for the management of life-threatening conditions or to remove a horse from a dangerous situation. Stabilization prior to anesthesia is a critical first step.

*The goal of pre-anesthetic stabilization is to get the patient in the best condition possible before the anesthetic event. This will depend on cooperation, personnel, equipment, and time availability.*

## Fluid Therapy

- Hypertonic saline (7.2% sodium chloride): A 4 mL/kg bolus should be administered in all cases of hypovolemia for its intravascular volume expanding properties. This is not considered a replacement of balanced solution. Administration should be followed by isotonic crystalloids. Monitoring of electrolytes warranted with prolonged use. Do not administer hypertonic saline if there is uncontrolled hemorrhage or in cases of pre-existing hypernatremia.
- Isotonic crystalloids (PlasmaLyte, Lactated Ringer's, Hartmann solution): Start with 10–20 mL/kg bolus in cases of hypovolemia/dehydration (which is 20–25% of the total shock bolus for adult horses of 80–90 mL/kg), re-assess clinical parameters and administer additional boluses until indices of perfusion (heart rate, CRT, extremities temperature, pulse quality) have improved (Crabtree and Epstein 2021). Isotonic crystalloids are safe to give to replace volume as their electrolyte's concentration approaches the physiological values.

  After resuscitation and loss replacement maintenance rate can be set at 60 mL/kg/day in adult horses.
- If possible, run point-of-care bloodwork including PCV/TS, lactate, electrolytes profile, and renal values to monitor effects of fluid resuscitation and establish the best fluid therapy plan.
- Care should be taken when treating horses in cardiac failure with large volume resuscitation as they might be euvolemic or even hypervolemic. Patients in renal failure might also be easily volume overloaded; therefore, the ability to produce urine and signs of volume overload should be closely monitored.
- Please refer to Chapter 28 for specific recommendations on fluid therapy in the emergent horse.

## Analgesia

Treating pain as soon as possible is part of stabilization of a patient in order to reduce distress and help reach better plains of anesthesia (Matthews and Carroll 2007). Many clinical parameters can be reliably monitored to establish pain levels and duration. Tachycardia, tachypnea, lameness, sweating, colic behavior, unwillingness to move, restlessness, inappetence, abnormal posture, immediate reaction to palpation of a specific area are all signs of pain. Multimodal or balanced analgesia is often required to treat pain consequent to inflammation or tissue injury (Matthews and Carroll 2007). The purpose of balanced analgesia is to target different site of neuronal conduits and involves using drugs of different classes often together with local anesthetics and regional blocks.

Non-steroidal anti-inflammatory drugs (NSAIDs) are a common class of analgesics used as first line for mild-to-moderate pain. They are indicated in inflammatory pain. Use NSAIDs when renal function is appropriate and after fluid resuscitation. Opioids are indicated in moderate-to-severe pain. Morphine and Butorphanol are commonly used drugs and are often used in combination with alpha-2 agonists for sedative purposes too. As part of balanced analgesia, lidocaine and other local anesthetics are commonly used in severe localized pain in conjunction with systemic analgesics. Some anesthetics at subanesthetic dose (i.e., Ketamine) can be also added for moderate-to-severe pain. Table 5.1 reports common dosages and uses of the above-mentioned medications.

## Oxygen Therapy

If possible, providing intra-nasal oxygen therapy can be beneficial in any horse in distress. Oxygen can be provided holding a mask or tubing in front of patent nostrils or suturing oxygen delivering tubing in the nostrils. Flow by oxygen therapy has been proven to be effective when high flow rates of 15 L/min or higher are used in adult horses. Intratracheal oxygen administration is also possible and will provide improved oxygen delivery.

## Transfusion

Refer to Chapter 28, where a summary of blood transfusion is provided. The indications and clinical procedure of blood collection and transfusion in the horse are described later in this chapter.

**Table 5.1** Analgesic medications in the horse.

| Drug | Dose/frequency | Route of administration | Common uses |
|---|---|---|---|
| Detomidine | 0.05–0.02 mg/kg q1–2 h | IV or IM | Abdominal pain |
| Xylazine | 0.2–1 mg/kg | IV or IM | Abdominal pain |
| Flunixin meglumine | 1.1 mg/kg | IV or PO | Abdominal pain |
| Phenylbutazone | 2.2–4.4 mg/kg | IV or PO | Musculoskeletal pain |
| Morphine | 0.1–0.2 mg/kg q4–6 h | IV or IM | Moderate to severe pain |
| Butorphanol | 0.01–0.04 IV or 0.04–0.2 IM q2–4 h | IV or IM | Low analgesic effect at the lower doses |
| Tramadol | 9–10 mg/kg q3–6 h | PO | |
| Ketamine | 1–2 mg/kg IM q1 h or 0.4–0.8 mg/kg/h, IV in CRI | IM or CRI IV | For severe acute or chronic pain and somatic pain |
| Gabapentin | 20–40 mg/kg | PO | Neuropathic and chronic pain |
| Lidocaine | 1.3 mg/kg as bolus Followed by 3 mg/kg/h in CRI | IV | Abdominal pain or musculoskeletal pain in conjunction with other analgesics |

### Positioning and Padding

If the horse is down, provide padding to the pressure points (hips, elbows, etc.) and protection to the limbs with bandages, and to the eyes with eye lube, especially when moving the horse.

## Cecal or Colonic Trocarization

This technique can be performed to release moderate-to-severe cecal or colonic tympany. Often this procedure is used when surgical intervention is not an option, when the bowel distention is life-threatening and decompression cannot wait referral, or to improve patient ventilation and perfusion prior to the induction of general anesthesia.

*Materials*

1) Clippers.
2) Sterile scrub material.
3) Local anesthetic, 3–5 mL of 2% Lidocaine.
4) 1 × 25 G 5/8-in. needle for local block.
5) 1 × 5 mL syringe for local block.
6) Sterile gloves.
7) 14 or 16 G IV catheter.
8) 30-in. extension set.
9) Plain container with small amount of water.
10) Suction pump (optional).
11) Ultrasound.
12) 3 mL syringe with 2 mL of procaine penicillin.
13) Sedation.

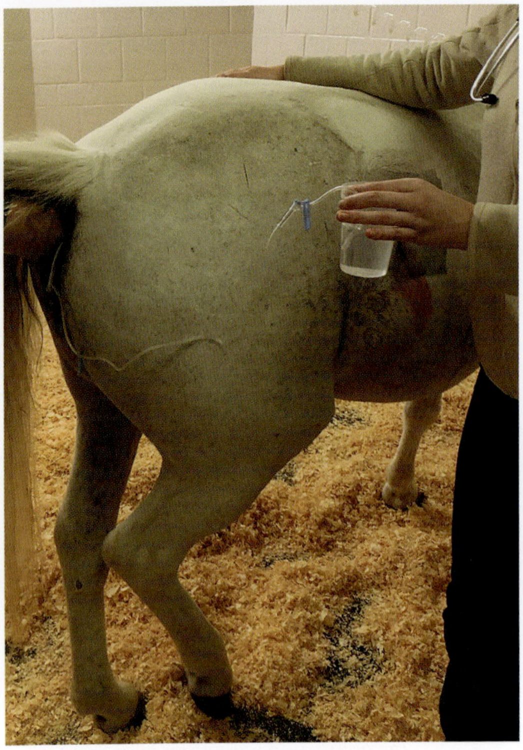

**Figure 5.5** Colonic trocarization via the rectum in a horse with a large intestinal displacement. Note it is important to hold and guard the IV catheter within your hand while entering the rectum to avoid rectal laceration or puncture. Transcutaneous trocarization is employed more often and avoids the additional complication of rectal injury.

*Transcutaneous procedure*

1) Sedate or restrain the patient.
2) Detect the area of gas distention in the paralumbar fossa ultrasound guided. If ultrasound is not available rectal palpation and auscultation can help identify the correct area to trocarize. A "ping" can often be heard in the right paralumbar fossa when gas distention is present. Ultrasound guidance is recommended when trocarizing the colon on the left side due to the close presence of vital structures like kidney and spleen.
3) Clip and scrub the area elected.
4) Instill 2–3 mL of local anesthetic in skin, subcutaneous muscle, and underlying muscles.
5) Perform a final aseptic preparation.
6) Insert the catheter through the layers until losing resistance and gas should start flowing out. The catheter should be kept perpendicular to the skin during insertion. Remove or withdraw the stylet once into the lumen of the cecum/colon.
7) Attach the sterile extension to the catheter end and put the end of the extension in the plain container with water. Colonic or cecal gas decompression is confirmed when bubbles are seen erupting in the water cup.
8) A suction pump can be used to release gas distention faster.
9) Remove the catheter once the gas is no longer retrievable. While withdrawing the catheter inject 2–3 mL of Procaine Penicillin or 3 mL of Gentamicin.

*Transrectal procedure* (Figure 5.5)

The transrectal trocharization technique is suitable in patients that have severe colonic gas distention easily palpable transrectally (Figure 5.5).

1) Sedate or restrain the patient.
2) Administer Buscopan 0.1–0.3 mg/kg IV to facilitate the rectal exam and procedure.
3) Clean rectum from feces.
4) Instill 30 mL of Lidocaine intrarectally.
5) Connect the IV catheter to the extension and place the end of the extension in the plain container with water.
6) Hold and guard the IV catheter within your hand while entering the rectum. Care should be taken to avoid rectal laceration or puncture.
7) Place the catheter against the distended colon and penetrate through it perpendicularly.
8) Air should start flow once you enter the lumen of the distended viscera.
9) A suction pump can be used for faster gas release.
10) Remove the catheter attached to the extension all together once gas no longer flows. Guard carefully the tip of the catheter with your hand while exiting the rectum.
11) The horse should be placed on systemic antibiotics.

*Possible complications*

1) Septic or aseptic peritonitis. The risk is higher with intra-rectal technique or repeated trocarizations. Peritonitis can present focally and low grade or more diffuse.
2) Focal cellulitis or abscess at the catheter insertion.
3) Abscess or injury on the cecal/colonic wall or abdominal wall.
4) Rectal injury with the transrectal technique.

## Caudal Epidural Anesthesia

Caudal epidural injection provides regional anesthesia and analgesia to the tail and perineal area. Several types of medications may be placed into the epidural space depending upon the desired affect; Table 5.2 lists the commonly used drugs for caudal epidural anesthesia in the horse. Caudal epidural anesthesia allows for surgery and interventions of the urogenital tract (dystocia, rectal prolapse, uterine prolapse, surgery of the rectum, vagina, or bladder, urethra). Using higher volumes more cranial analgesia (i.e., hindlimbs) can be achieved; however, caution should be taken when using higher volumes of local anesthetics. The caudal epidural space is accessible caudal to the sacrum, with no risk of dural puncture or acquisition of CSF at this location. If the patient is going to require repeated drug administration, a caudal epidural catheter may be inserted.

*Materials*

1) Clippers.
2) Sterile scrub material.
3) Local anesthetic, 2–3 mL of 2% Lidocaine.
4) 1 × 25 G 5/8-in. needle for local block.
5) 1 × 5 mL syringe for local block.
6) Sterile gloves.
7) 18 G 1.5-in. injection needle, 18 G Spinal needle or 18 G Tuohy epidural needle.
8) 10 mL syringe.
9) Sterile drugs, ideally preservative free, to be injected.
10) Sedation.
11) Stocks for restraint if available.

*Procedure*

1) Sedate and restrain the patient. Ensure the horse is standing squarely. The clinician should stand on one side of the horse's hind end rather than directly behind the horse to allow for safe injection.
2) Identify the site for injection located between coccygeal vertebra 1 and 2 (Co1-Co2). Move the tail up and down while feeling on midline for the first palpable depression caudal to the sacrum. This depression created by the last immovable spinous process and the first movable spinous process that normally correspond to Co1 and Co2, respectively. This location is usually approximately 1–3 in. cranially to the beginning of tail hairs.
3) Clip and aseptically prepare the site.
4) Infiltrate approximately 2 mL of lidocaine in the skin and direct some local anesthetic deep to the insertion site to block the approach more fully. Local anesthetic may not be required when horses are sedated.

**Table 5.2** Epidural medications in the horse.

| Drug | Dose | Duration | Onset |
|---|---|---|---|
| **Detomidine 10 mg/mL** | **0.03–0.06 mg/kg** | **2–3 h** | **5–15 minutes** |
| Lidocaine 20 mg/mL | 0.2–0.35 mg/kg | 45–60 minutes | 6–10 minutes |
| Mepivacaine 20 mg/mL | 0.2–0.25 mg/kg | 45–60 minutes | 6–10 minutes |
| Ketamine 100 mg/mL | 0.5–2 mg/kg | 30–75 minutes | 5–10 minutes |
| Morphine PF 25 mg/mL | 0.1 mg/kg | Lasts up to 18 h | 1–5 h |
| Xylazine 100 mg/mL | 0.17–0.35 mg/kg | 165–210 minutes | 10–30 minutes |
| Xylazine + MORPHINE | X: 0.17 mg/kg M: 0.1 mg/kg | >12 h | 30–60 minutes |
| Xylazine + LIDOCAINE | X: 0.17 mg/kg L: 0.22 mg/kg | 5.5 h | 5–15 minutes |
| Detomidine + Morphine | D: 0.01–0.03 mg/kg M:0.1 mg/kg | 20–24 h | 20–30 minutes |
| Tramadol | 1 mg/kg | 8–12 h | 30 minutes |

*Source:* Adapted from Robinson and Natalini (2002) and Driessen (2014).

5) Prepare the sterile syringe with the drug/drugs to be administered.
6) Insert the injection, spinal or Tuohy needle on midline over the palpated space. The bevel of the needle should be pointed cranially. Angle the needle perpendicular to the slope of the rump at this location. This angle may need to be adjusted depending on the conformation of each individual, generally tilting the needle hub in a caudal direction.
7) Start advancing the needle maintaining the same angle and direction, the depth of insertion varies depending on individual anatomy, presence of subcutaneous fat, and angle of insertion. Continue to advance the needle until confirmation of epidural placement.
8) Different methods can be used to verify placement of needle tip in epidural space.
   Method 1: Hanging drop technique: Insert the needle ¾-in. into the skin and other soft tissues. If using the spinal or Tuohy needle, remove the stylet. Next fill the hub of the needle with the epidural medication or sterile saline. Advance slowly through the remaining soft tissues until the needle passes through the interarcuate ligament and a loss if resistance is perceived. At this location, the drop is quickly lost (negative atmospheric pressure), confirming entrance into the epidural space. Alternatively, attempt to push a small volume of injectate while there is an air bubble within the syringe. If the air bubble compresses, this indicates proper needle placement.
   Method 2: Advance the needle until slight resistance is felt at the level of the interarcuate ligament; advance just beyond the resistance and attach a loss of resistance syringe. This syringe filled with air allows confirmation of epidural placement. This special syringe has a low-resistance plunger seal that allows confirmation of a low-pressure space. Use a very small volume and quick injection technique to confirm presence in the epidural space. If the air in the syringe compresses, and the plunger does not return to its original location, then the needle is properly placed in the epidural space.
9) For either of these methods, if the needle is advanced too far, the floor of the vertebral canal might be reached. Before injecting drugs always aspirate to make sure the venous sinus is not involuntarily punctured.
10) Connect the syringe and start injecting drugs slowly, if the needle is in the space, no resistance should occur; instead, if resistance is noted while injecting, the needle is not in the correct position and will need to be replaced. You can also use the air bubble technique reported above to ensure proper placement.
11) Even standard doses of local anesthetics placed into the epidural space can sporadically cause ataxia and recumbency in horses without a specific obvious cause. Caution must be taken with high volumes; >8–10 mL can cause cranial spread and paralysis of the lumbosacral nerves to the hind legs (Robinson and Natalini 2002).

## Subpalpebral Lavage System Placement

A subpalpebral lavage (SPL) system is a catheter system used to facilitate delivery of ophthalmic solutions to the ocular surface. Kits are commercially available from MILA and can be placed in the field using sedation and local anesthesia. Indications include the treatment of corneal ulcers or lacerations, severe uveitis, or any case in which eye medications are necessary and the horse's behavior prevents administration. An SPL allows the caretaker to deliver topical treatments to a painful eye without manipulating the eyelids or extensive handling of the horse's head; this reduces further trauma to the globe and risk of rupture. The system may be maintained for several weeks or months in cases necessitating prolonged therapy. Placement in either the superior or inferior eyelid is appropriate, though placement in the inferior eyelid results in less risk of a footplate ulcer due to protection from the third eyelid and a tendency for the footplate to stay in place in the lower conjunctival fornix due to gravity (Figure 5.6a, b).

*Materials*

1) SPL kit.
2) Sterile gloves.
3) 0.2% povidone iodine solution and gauze.
4) 0.5% proparacaine or tetracaine ophthalmic solution.
5) 2% lidocaine or mepivacaine, 3 mL syringes, 25 g × 5/8-in. needles.
6) Detomidine hydrochloride (0.02–0.04 mg/kg IV).
7) Roll of 1-in. white tape.
8) 20 g × 1–1.25-in. catheter.
9) Injection cap.
10) Wooden tongue depressor.
11) Nonabsorbable suture, size 2-0, straight needle.

(a) (b)

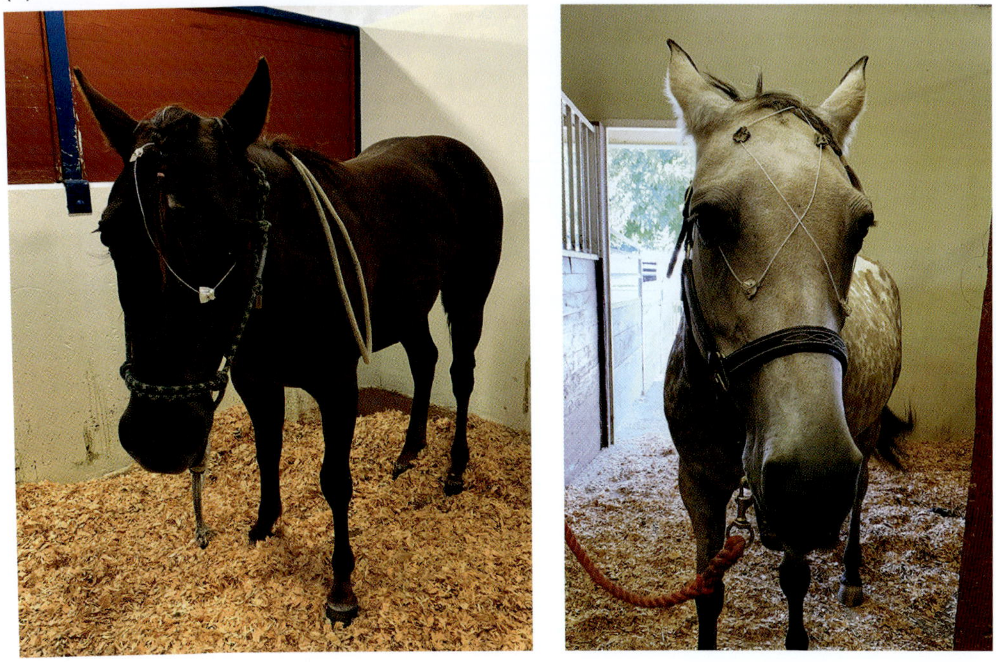

**Figure 5.6** (a) Unilateral and (b) bilateral lower lid SPL placement. Note that placement in either the superior or inferior eyelid is appropriate, though placement in the inferior eyelid results in less risk of a footplate ulcer due to protection from the third eyelid and a tendency for the footplate to stay in place in the lower conjunctival fornix due to gravity.

*Procedure*

1) Braid the forelock and mane.
2) Sedate the horse and restrain with the head rested on an elevated surface (e.g., stacked hay or shavings bales).
3) Prepare the ocular surface and eyelids with dilute povidone iodine solution; palpate the auriculopalpebral nerve as it crosses the zygomatic arch and prepare this site. If placing the SPL in the upper lid, also prepare the skin overlying the supraorbital foramen by placing a thumb below the dorsal orbital rim and middle finger in the supraorbital fossa – the foramen is palpated as a depression with the index finger, midway between the thumb and middle finger, above the medial canthus. Also prepare the skin at the site at which the SPL will be placed through the eyelid.
4) Using 1–2 mL of 2% lidocaine or mepivacaine at each site, deposit local anesthetic subcutaneously over the auriculopalpebral nerve, the supraorbital foramen, and lid placement site using a 25 g needle.
5) Apply topical anesthetic onto the corneal surface via a syringe and 25 g needle with the needle broken off from the hub.
6) Wearing sterile gloves, insert a finger into the deepest recession of the conjunctival fornix (upper or lower lid). If the horse is reactive, give the local block more time to take effect, consider additional sedation, or place a twitch.
7) Using the index finger of your dominant hand as a guard between the trocar and the globe, guide the trocar to pass through the conjunctival fornix to exit the eyelid skin adjacent to the orbital rim *(central if upper lid, nasal if lower lid)*.
8) Push the trocar tip through the eyelid until it exits the skin, then pull the trocar and tubing through the lid until the footplate of the SPL rests in the conjunctival fornix.
9) Check placement of the footplate with your finger before securing the line. Care should be taken to make ensure the oblique angle of the footplate matches the slant of the eyelid margin.
10) Using white tape, create two to three tape butterflies to secure the line to the skin of the face (see photos). A simple interrupted suture using 2-0 nonabsorbable material should be placed through each butterfly wing, taking care not to suture through or encircle the SPL tube. An alternative to sutures is placing a small amount of anesthetic at each site and using the SPL trocar to place the SPL tubing under the skin in the same locations (Figure 5.7a, b).
11) Use the trocar to thread the length of the tubing through the forelock braid, then through the braids in the mane. It should extend nearly to the withers.

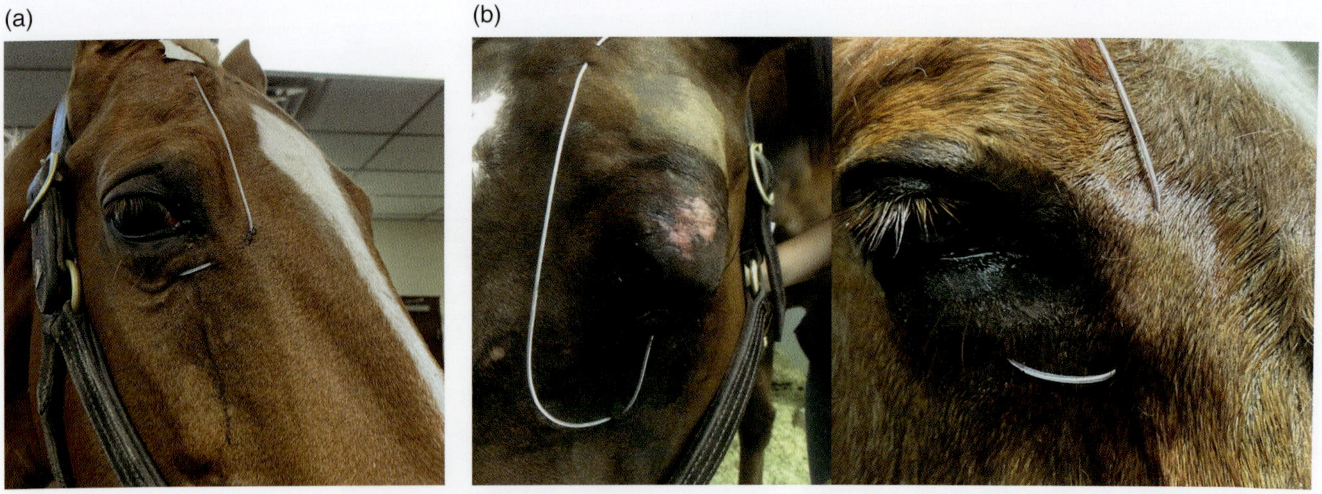

**Figure 5.7** (a) This is an example of a correct placement of a lower eyelid SPL with the SPL tubing placed under the skin near the eye and in the forehead. (b) In the image on the left, this bite is too small, and the image on the right is the correct placement.

12) If excessively long, cut the end of the tubing and thread a 20 g × 1.5-in. catheter into its lumen (retract the tip of the stylet inside the catheter to avoid puncturing the tubing). Once firmly inserted to the hub, remove the stylet and attach an injection cap.
13) Cover a wooden tongue depressor with white tape and secure the injection port and adjacent tubing to the tongue depressor with tape, then tape it to the last mane braid, leaving only the injection cap visible (Dwyer 2013).

## Blood Collection and Transfusion

*Indications*

- Decreased packed cell volume (PCV) <12% over one to two days indicates the need for a transfusion.
- Abnormally elevated lactate values greater than 4 mmol/L after crystalloid fluid resuscitation.
- PCV of <20% in acute bleeding (first 12 h). However, this is not always reliable (see below).
- In acute bleeding, the need for a blood transfusion is not always dictated by a decreased PCV because the value may be falsely increased due to splenic contraction. In these cases, the need for a transfusion is based on evidence of severe bleeding or hemolysis, elevated lactate values, tachycardia, pale mucous membrane, signs of hypoperfusion and hypotension (weak pulses, cold extremities, and generalized weakness).
- A low but stable PCV (12–20%) might not require a transfusion if lactate and clinical parameters are stable.
- Whole blood provides red cells, as well as proteins and fresh clotting factors, and might be helpful in an actively bleeding horse. The amount of blood to safely collect and transfuse will depend upon the size of the recipient and donor horses, respectively, as well as the extent of blood loss (Box 5.2).

**Box 5.2 How much blood to take from donor**

- It is safe to collect up to 20% of the total blood volume of the donor. In an adult horse 8–10% of the body mass in kg is the total blood volume (40–50 L/500 kg), and the blood volume that can be safely collected ranges from 8 to 10 L.

*How much blood to transfuse*

- The amount of blood needed for a blood transfusion can be calculated with the formula:

$$\text{Amount of blood (L)} = \frac{\text{Desired PCV} - \text{PCV recipient}}{\text{PCV of donor}} \times (0.08 \times \text{Body weight in kg of recipient})$$

*Ideal donor characteristics*

- Ideally the donor should be cross matched to the recipient.
- If cross match is not possible, the ideal donor should be a gelding of >400 kg in body weight that has never received a transfusion and has not donated blood in the previous three to four weeks. The donor should be Aa, Qa negative. If blood type is unknown draft breeds and cold blood breeds are usually preferred as they are more likely to be Aa and Qa negative. The donor PCV should ideally be >35% and he should be clinically healthy and up to date on vaccinations. Ideally, the donor should be previously tested and negative for transmissible hepaciviruses and other infectious diseases (EIA).

*Materials for collection and administration*

1) Clippers.
2) Sedation.
3) Sterile scrub material.
4) Sterile surgical gloves.
5) 10–14 G IV catheter.
6) 2-0 non-absorbable sutures.
7) Blood collection set - Collection bag (3–4 L for adults) with connected collection tubes, anticoagulant (some collection bags will already have anti-coagulant).
8) Blood filtration fluid administration set.

*Collection procedure*

1) Clip and sterilely prepare the mid 1/3 of the left jugular vein for catheter placement of the donor.
2) Place a 10–12 G IV catheter "upstream" (with the catheter tip directed toward the head) in the jugular vein. This will facilitate blood flow in the collection bag.
3) Add the anticoagulant in the collection bag if not already included. Sodium citrate and acid-citrate-dextrose (ACD) are the most common. Use 1 : 9 ratio for ACD (ACD:blood). Otherwise add 1 mL of sodium citrate for each 7 mL of blood intended to collect.
4) Connect the collection bag to the secured catheter and let the blood flow and fill the bag to the volume desired.
5) Gently mix the bag while the blood is flowing in to ensure the anticoagulant gets mixed homogeneously.
6) If collecting the maximum amount from the donor, give a fluid bolus of 20 mL/kg after collection.

*Administration procedure*

1) Place an IV catheter in the recipient.
2) Acquire heart rate, respiratory rate, and rectal temperature of the recipient before starting the transfusion to have baseline values.
3) Attach the blood collection bag to the filter.
4) Rate of administration: Start with 1 mL/kg for the first 30 minutes, monitor vital signs every 5 minutes for about 15–20 minutes to detect any sign of a transfusion reaction. If no reactions are noted, increase the rate to 10–20 mL/kg/h and continuing monitoring vital signs closely.
5) Change the filter every 3–4 L of blood.

## Autotransfusion

Consider autotransfusion if the patient has accumulated blood in a body cavity (hemoabdomen, hemothorax), and there is no evidence of neoplasia or sepsis. Collect blood from the cavity aseptically (using a teat cannula or a chest tube) and transfer it in a collection bag pre-filled with anticoagulant (Figure 5.8). Use approximately 1/3 the normal amount of

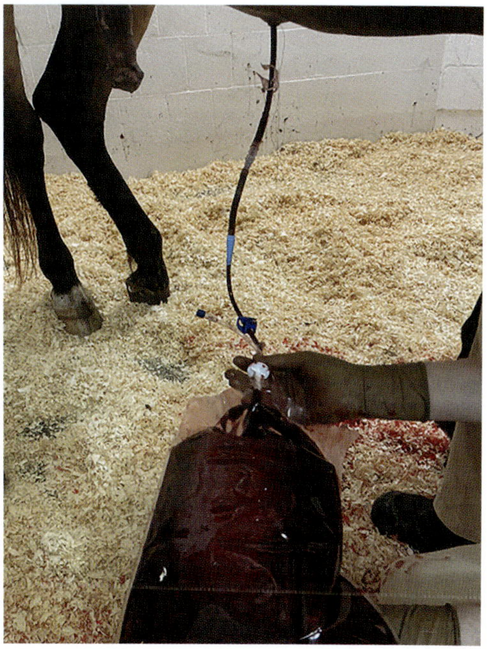

**Figure 5.8** Collection of blood from a horse with hemoabdomen to perform an autotransfusion. Autotransfusion may be considered for horses with blood in a body cavity (hemoabdomen, hemothorax), and there is no evidence of neoplasia or sepsis. Collect blood from the cavity aseptically (using a teat cannula or a chest tube) and transfer it in a collection bag pre-filled with anticoagulant. Note, use approximately 1/3 the normal amount of anticoagulant (ACD or citrate-phosphate-dextrose [CPD] or sodium citrate), or 1 unit heparin per mL of blood.

anticoagulant (ACD or citrate-phosphate-dextrose [CPD] or sodium citrate). Alternatively, use 1 unit heparin per mL of blood. Filters should be changed every 2 L during autotransfusion administration (Divers 2014).

### Possible Complications

Signs of transfusion reaction: Tachycardia, sweating, increased in baseline temperature, tachypnea, respiratory distress, urticaria, restlessness, edema, colic signs, fasciculations.

Stop or slow down the transfusion if reaction signs are noticed. Corticosteroids or diphenhydramine administration might be needed if reaction signs are moderate. Treat with IV fluids and epinephrine in case of severe anaphylactic reaction.

## Fasciotomy

Fasciotomy is indicated in cases of compartment syndrome, which may occur in cases of acute swelling (due to muscular trauma, snake, or insect bite). Hemorrhage or edema can cause a marked elevation in pressure within the fascial compartment, leading to ischemia, pain, and lameness if associated with the limbs. In the proximal limbs, consider fasciotomy if conservative management (i.e., compressive bandaging, systemic NSAID administration, topical NSAID application, cold water hydrotherapy) yields inadequate improvement. Compartment syndrome may also affect the head; fasciotomy should be considered if upper airway obstruction is imminent, or if prehension of food/water is limited by swelling.

*Materials*

1) Clippers.
2) Aseptic preparation supplies.
3) Sterile gloves.
4) 2% lidocaine or mepivacaine, 10 mL syringe, 19–23 g × 1-in. Needle.
5) #10 scalpel blade and handle.

*Procedure*

1) Palpate for most fluctuant areas and those near vital structures necessitating acute reduction in swelling. In the limbs, the affected area may be very firm, sensitive to palpation, or cold to the touch (Sullins et al. 1987).
2) Aseptically prepare site(s).
3) Perform line block(s) with 2% local anesthetic and sedate the patient as needed.
4) Using a #10 scalpel blade, make full-thickness skin incisions ranging from stab incisions to longer incisions of 5–15 cm in length.
   a) In the proximal limbs (i.e., antebrachial compartment syndrome), create an 8–15 cm proximal-to-distal incision over the affected area, extending through the skin, subcutaneous tissues, and the fascia of the affected muscle. A 3–4 cm facial release should be noted and there should be no fascial tension remaining (Sullins et al. 1987).
5) Leave all incisions open for drainage and to heal by second intention.
6) Consider placement of a Penrose drain through the distal aspect of proximal limb fasciotomies to promote continued drainage.
7) Where possible, apply a supportive bandage to reduce dead space.
8) Institute systemic antimicrobial therapy and apply petroleum jelly or vitamin A and D ointment ventral to draining incisions to prevent skin scalding.

## Relief of Pneumothorax

Pneumothorax results when there is presence of air between the lungs and the chest wall causing collapse of the lung. Evacuation of the air from the chest cavity is needed to reinflate the lungs and re-establish negative intrathoracic pressure (e.g., open pneumothorax), and to provide release of increased intra-thoracic pressure (e.g., tension pneumothorax) that leads to cardiopulmonary collapse and severe hypoxia (Figure 5.9a, b). Diagnosis can be achieved via auscultation and percussion of the chest wall; however, ultrasonography and radiography are more specific and reliable methods to identify pneumothorax and other abnormalities (rib fractures, fluid accumulation, or foreign bodies) (see Chapter 11). When the pneumothorax is unilateral, the patient is relatively stable, while bilateral pneumothorax

(a) (b)

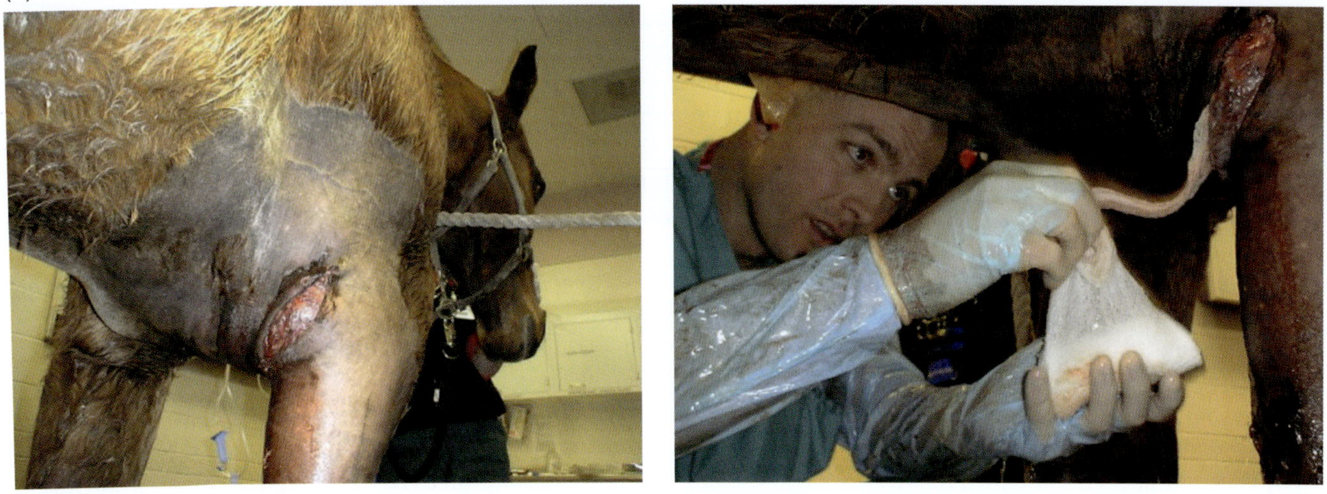

**Figure 5.9** (a, b) Packing of the axillary wound in the same horse from Figure 5.3 following removal of air from the thorax. The horse landed on a wooden post while jumping a fence, suffering severe thoracic trauma, bilateral pneumothorax, multiple rib fractures, and flail chest. The horse improved markedly following emergency stabilization; however, euthanasia was elected – following surgical exploration under general anesthesia – because of extensive disruption of the chest wall and gross contamination of the thoracic cavity.

can cause severe and progressive respiratory distress. When inflammatory diseases are present (e.g., pleuropneumonia) the pneumothorax is more likely to be unilateral due to the presence of a complete mediastinum. In addition to removal of air from the thorax, it is important to bandage or pack chest or axillary wounds (Figure 5.9a, b) to prevent progressive pneumothorax.

*Materials*

1) Clippers.
2) Sterile scrub material.
3) Local anesthetic, 5–10 mL of 2% Lidocaine.
4) 1 × 21 G 1.5-in. needle for local block.
5) 1 × 5 mL syringe for local block.
6) Sterile gloves.
7) Sterile scalpel blade (#15).
8) Sterile trocar catheter (chest tube) 20–28 F. A 4-in. teat cannula or a 14–16 G IV catheter are valid alternatives for immediate air release but are not suitable for repeated evacuations.
9) One-way valve if leaving the tube in place (e.g., Heimlich one-way valve[5] or a condom).
10) Non-absorbable 0 or 1 suture.
11) Sedation (use of sedatives and options may vary based on patient's attitude and cardiovascular stability). Detomidine IV 0.01 mg/kg is recommended if the patient is stable.
12) Ultrasound to guide placement.
13) Suction pump or 60 mL Luer tip syringe for suction.

*Procedure* (Figure 5.3a–c)

1) Identify the site. Ultrasonographic or radiographic guidance is recommended. Usually, the suitable site is located caudo-dorsally between the 13th and 15th intercostal spaces.
2) Clip and aseptically prepare the area elected.
3) Infiltrate local anesthetic in the subcutaneous tissue and intercostal muscle, trying to instill some close to the pleural surface. Avoid the caudal aspect of the ribs as intercostal vessels and nerve run on the caudal aspect of each rib.
4) Perform a final aseptic preparation.

5 Heimlich chest drainage valve (Advanced Anesthesia Specialists, LLC, Prescott Arizona).

5) Make an approximately 0.5–0.8 cm stab incision through the skin and fascia along the cranial border of the caudal rib. The incision can be extended into the intercostal muscle to facilitate the chest tube insertion. If using an IV catheter there is no need for a stab incision.
6) If using a chest tube, hold it firmly and pass it through the stab incision. Push the tube through it gently until loss of resistance is felt when entering the pleura. Restrain the tube firmly using one hand to hold it against the body while the other hand at the bottom of the tube applies steady pressure. You can apply gentle rotation to the tube while putting pressure to facilitate insertion through tissues (similar to a chest tube for fluid drainage).
7) If using an IV catheter or a cannula connect a three-way stopcock before insertion. When using a catheter remove the stylet once in the pleural space, advancing the catheter.
8) Once in the pleural cavity, air may not enter the chest cavity with an open pneumothorax; however, if pressurized air escapes, this indicates the presence of a more severe tension pneumothorax. Connect the suction pump (an adaptor might be needed) or the 60 mL syringe to the tube or the catheter and start suctioning air. If using a suction pump do not exceed – 20 mmHg of pressure to avoid re-expansion pulmonary edema.
9) If the indwelling tube is staying in place, secure the tube to the skin using a purse string suture followed by a finger-trap pattern.
10) It is recommended to apply a one-way valve at the end of the indwelling tube. Heimlich valves[5] or, alternatively, a condom (with a small cut at the end) can be taped to the tube and can act as a one-way valve. If no one-way valve is applied, leave the tube clamped when not in use.
11) Once removed the skin can be sutured with absorbable or non-absorbable 0 suture using a single cruciate or two simple interrupted sutures.
12) Protect the tube by covering it with a sticky elastic bandage (Elastikon[6]).

*Possible complications*

1) Progressive pneumothorax with inadvertent air influx in the pleural cavity through the tube.
2) Hemothorax if a large vessel is accidentally punctured.
3) Lung puncture during placement if aggressive and careless during insertion or if the site is not elected accurately.
4) Cellulitis around the tube skin insertion.

## References


Crabtree, N.E. and Epstein, K.L. (2021). Current concepts in fluid therapy. *Horses. Front. Vet. Sci.* 8: 29.

Divers, T.J. (2014). Liver failure, anemia, and blood transfusion. In: *Equine Emergencies: Treatment and Procedure*, 4e (ed. J.A. Orsini and T.J. Divers), 269–288. St Louis: Elsevier Saunders.

Driessen, B. (2014). Pain management. In: *Equine Emergencies: Treatment and Procedure*, 4e (ed. J.A. Orsini and T.J. Divers), 749–763. St Louis: Elsevier Saunders.

Dwyer, A.E. (2013). How to insert and manage a subpalpebral lavage system. *AAEP Proceedings* 59: 164–173.

Fitzgerald, B.W., Honnas, C.M., Plummer, A.E., and Eastman, T.G. (2006). How to apply a hindlimb phalangeal cast in the standing patient and minimize complications. *AAEP Proceedings* 52: 631–635.

Gustafsson, K. et al. (2020). Time to peak concentration of amikacin in the antebrachiocarpal joint following cephalic intravenous regional limb perfusion in standing horses. *Vet. Comp. Orthop. Traumatol.* 33 (5): 327–332.

Jesty, S.A. (2014). Cardiovascular system. In: *Equine Emergencies: Treatment and Procedure*, 4e (ed. J.A. Orsini and T.J. Divers), 124–156. St Louis: Elsevier Saunders.

Kilcoyne, I., Nieto, J.E., Knych, H.K., and Dechant, J.E. (2018). Time required to achieve maximum concentration of amikacin in synovial fluid of the distal interphalangeal joint after intravenous regional limb perfusion in horses. *Am. J. Vet. Res.* 79 (3): 282–286.

Kilcoyne, I., Nieto, J.E., Galuppo, L.D., and Dechant, J.E. (2021). Time required to achieve maximum amikacin concentration in the synovial fluid of the tarsocrural joint following administration of the drug by intravenous regional limb perfusion in horses. *Am. J. Vet. Res.* 82 (2): 99–104.

Matthews, N.S. and Carroll, G.L. (2007). Review of equine analgesics and pain management. *AAEP Proceedings* 53: 240–244.

Robinson, E.P. and Natalini, C.C. (2002). Epidural anesthesia and analgesia in horses. *Vet. Clin. N. Am. Equine Pract.* 18 (1): 61–82.

Sullins, K.E., Heath, R.B., Turner, A.S., and Stashak, T.S. (1987). Possible antebrachial flexor compartment syndrome as a cause of lameness in two horses. *Equine Vet. J.* 19 (2): 147–150.


6 Elasticon (Johnson and Johnson, New Brunswick, NJ, USA).

# 6

# Emergency Diagnostic Assessment During Triage

*Toby L. Pinn-Woodcock*[1]*, John Pigott*[2]*, and Sally Anne L. DeNotta*[3]

[1] *Animal Health Diagnostic Center, College of Veterinary Medicine, Cornell University, Ithaca, NY, USA*
[2] *Cornell Ruffian Equine Specialists, Cornell University, Elmont, NY, USA*
[3] *Large Animal Internal Medicine, College of Veterinary Medicine, University of Florida, Gainesville, FL, USA*

## Diagnostic Testing

### Point-of-Care Testing

Point-of-care testing (POCT) refers to diagnostic analysis that can be performed close to the patient, where care is being provided (Slovis et al. 2020). POCT assays range from dip-stick indicators to handheld devices that can be used in both equine ambulatory practice and hospital-based settings. POCT tools offer rapid diagnostic results during emergency triage to facilitate timely patient management decisions. POCT assays are available for the assessment of blood glucose, blood gas analysis, L-lactate, serum amyloid A (SAA), immunoglobulin G, cardiac troponin I, biochemical analysis, hematology, and select pathogen screening. Practitioners should bear in mind that some POCT devices can be climate or temperature sensitive, thereby limiting their use in certain settings. Whenever possible, select POCT devices that have been validated for use in equine patients but take into consideration that the accuracy, precision, sensitivity, and specificity of these assays may vary from laboratory diagnostic options. Due to the constantly evolving field of POCT technology, clinicians are encouraged to perform market research prior to investing in POCT systems for their practice.

### Laboratory Diagnostic Considerations During Emergency Triage

The specimens required for a diagnostic work-up will depend on the nature of the emergency being triaged. Use of the correct collection container and appropriate specimen handling will influence sample quality and its suitability for laboratory testing. Specimen collection for infectious disease diagnostics may be required during emergency triage (Table 6.1). Infectious disease considerations can vary regionally and seasonally. Appropriate test selection will aid in making a definitive diagnosis, guiding treatment, and determining what biosecurity protocols are warranted. Due to the variation in test catalogs and submission requirements among diagnostic laboratories, consultation with your laboratory prior to submission is encouraged to help shape the diagnostic work-up.

### How to Interpret and Implement Culture and Susceptibility Results

Antimicrobial therapy will often be a component of stabilization in the critically ill patient following triage. Appropriate interpretation and implementation of antimicrobial susceptibility results will contribute to a favorable patient outcome (Gajic et al. 2022). Employ the following principles during antimicrobial selection (Box 6.1) (adapted from Craig Altier, DVM, PhD, Cornell University):

*Emergency Triage of the Horse*, First Edition. Edited by Rolfe M. Radcliffe and Jamie J. Kopper.

Companion website: www.wiley.com/go/radcliffe/triage

**Table 6.1** Laboratory diagnostics for equine infectious disease investigations.

| Sample collection for infectious disease diagnostics | | |
|---|---|---|
| **Test performed** | **Specimen(s)** | **Sample handling** |
| **Equine abortion** | | |
| Aerobic culture | Submit 3 fresh tissue samples for individual culture: placenta, lung, and stomach contents | Labeled and individually packaged in sterile leak-proof container, refrigerate, ship overnight in insulated container with ice packs |
| Equine arteritis virus (EAV) SN | Maternal serum (separated) in red top tube | Refrigerate or freeze, ship overnight in insulated container with ice packs |
| Equine arteritis virus FA or PCR | Fresh tissue: placenta, liver, lung, kidney | Labeled and individually packaged in sterile leak-proof container, refrigerate, ship overnight in insulated container with ice packs |
| Equine herpesvirus 1 FA or PCR | Fresh tissue: lung (preferred), placenta (use only if lung not available) | Labeled and individually packaged in sterile leak-proof container, refrigerate, ship overnight in insulated container with ice packs |
| Equine herpesvirus -1 SN | Maternal serum (separated) in red top tube | Refrigerate or freeze, ship overnight in insulated container with ice packs |
| Equine Hherpesvirus-4 SN | Maternal serum (separated) in red top tube | Refrigerate or freeze, ship overnight in insulated container with ice packs |
| Equine influenza virus (EIV) HAI | Maternal serum (separated) in red top tube | Refrigerate or freeze, ship overnight in insulated container with ice packs |
| Histopathology | Formalin-fixed tissues: placenta, liver, lung, brain, adrenal, heart, thymus, small intestine, kidney, and fetal skin | Fixed tissues can be co-mingled in one formalin jar with tissue:formalin ratio of 1 : 10 |
| Leptospira MAT, 5 standard serovars | Maternal serum (separated) in red top tube | Refrigerate or freeze, ship overnight in insulated container with ice packs |
| Leptospirosis PCR | Submit 2 fresh tissue samples: placenta and kidney preferred; stomach contents acceptable | Labeled and individually packaged in sterile leak-proof container, refrigerate, ship overnight in insulated container with ice packs |
| Selenium | Maternal EDTA whole blood in purple top tube | Refrigerate, ship overnight insulated container with ice packs |
| **Equine diarrhea** | | |
| Anaerobic culture | Fecal swab in anaerobic transport media | Maintain at room temperature, ship overnight |
| Clostridium difficile PCR – A and B genes | Feces in sterile leak-proof container | Refrigerated and less than 24 h old or frozen |
| Clostridium difficile toxins (A/B) ELISA | Feces in sterile leak-proof container | Refrigerated and less than 24 h old or frozen |
| Clostridium perfringens PCR – alpha toxin and beta toxin | Feces in sterile leak-proof container | Refrigerated and less than 24 h old or frozen |
| Coronavirus PCR, Beta | Feces in sterile leak-proof container | Refrigerate, ship overnight in insulated container with ice packs |
| Fecal floatation | Feces in sterile leak-proof container | Refrigerate (do not freeze), ship overnight in insulated container with ice packs |
| Lawsonia intracellularis (consider in foals from three months to one year of age) | Feces in sterile leak-proof container | Refrigerate, ship overnight in insulated container with ice packs |
| Potomac horse fever (*Neorickettsia risticii*) IFA | Separated serum in red top tube | Refrigerate, ship overnight in insulated container with ice packs |

**Table 6.1** (Continued)

| Test performed | Specimen(s) | Sample handling |
|---|---|---|
| **Sample collection for infectious disease diagnostics** | | |
| Potomac horse fever (*Neorickettsia risticii*) PCR | EDTA whole blood in purple top tube or feces in sterile leak-proof container (sample type may vary by laboratory) | Refrigerate, ship overnight in insulated container with ice packs |
| Rotavirus types A and B PCR | Feces in sterile leak-proof container | Refrigerate, ship overnight in insulated container with ice packs |
| Salmonella culture and antimicrobial susceptibility | Feces in sterile leak-proof container or aerobic transport media | Refrigerate, ship overnight in insulated container with ice packs |
| Sand recovery analysis | Feces in leak-proof container | Refrigerate, ship overnight in insulated container with ice packs |
| **Equine neurologic disease**[a] | | |
| Aerobic culture and antimicrobial susceptibility | CSF sample taken using sterile technique and placed in aerobic blood culture media (preferred) or sterile red top tube | Refrigerate, ship overnight in insulated container with ice packs |
| Anaplasma phagocytophilum PCR[b] | EDTA whole blood in purple top tube | Refrigerate, ship overnight in insulated container with ice packs |
| *Borrelia burgdorferi* PCR | CSF in red top tube | Refrigerate, ship overnight in insulated container with ice packs |
| Cerebrospinal fluid cytology | CSF in EDTA purple top tube and two to three air-dried, unstained slides | Refrigerate CSF and ship overnight in insulated container with ice packs; separate slides from icepack during shipping to prevent condensation |
| Eastern equine encephalitis virus IgM ELISA | Separated serum (preferred) or CSF in red top tube | Refrigerate, ship overnight in insulated container with ice packs |
| Eastern equine encephalitis virus PCR | EDTA whole blood | Refrigerate, ship overnight in insulated container with ice packs |
| Equine herpesvirus-1 PCR | Nasal swab in red top tube with 0.5 mL sterile saline to keep moist and EDTA whole blood in purple top tube | Refrigerate, ship overnight in insulated container with ice packs |
| Equine Lyme multiplex ELISA | Separated serum and CSF in red top tubes | Refrigerate, ship overnight in insulated container with ice packs |
| Equine protozoal myeloencephalitis serum: CSF ratio | Separated serum and CSF in red top tubes | Refrigerate, ship overnight in insulated container with ice packs |
| Fungal culture and susceptibility | CSF sample taken using sterile technique and placed in aerobic blood culture media (preferred) or sterile red top tube | Refrigerate, ship overnight in insulated container with ice packs |
| Rabies virus direct fluorescent antibody test | Whole head or fresh cross section of brain, including caudal cerebrum, cerebellum and brainstem | Refrigerate, ship overnight in insulated container with ice packs |
| Selenium | EDTA whole blood in purple top tube | Refrigerate, ship overnight in insulated container with ice packs |
| Vitamin E | Separated serum | Refrigerate, protect from light, ship overnight in insulated container with ice packs |
| West Nile virus IgG/IgM capture ELISA | Separated serum (preferred) or CSF in red top tube | Refrigerate, ship overnight in insulated container with ice packs |

(*Continued*)

**Table 6.1** (Continued)

| Test performed | Specimen(s) | Sample handling |
|---|---|---|
| **Sample collection for infectious disease diagnostics** | | |
| **Equine respiratory disease** | | |
| Aerobic culture and antimicrobial susceptibility | Tracheal wash fluid in red top tube or swab of fluid in aerobic transport media | Refrigerate, ship overnight in insulated container with ice packs |
| Anaerobic culture | Tracheal wash fluid in red top tube or swab of fluid in anaerobic transport media | Maintain at room temperature, ship overnight in insulated container |
| Equine adenovirus 1 PCR | Nasal swab in red top tube with 0.5 mL saline to keep moist or nasopharyngeal wash in sterile leak-proof container. | Refrigerate, ship overnight in insulated container with ice packs |
| Equine arteritis virus PCR | Nasal swab in red top tube with 0.5 mL saline to keep moist or nasopharyngeal wash in sterile leak-proof container. | Refrigerate, ship overnight in insulated container with ice packs |
| Equine herpesvirus-1 PCR | Nasal swab in red top tube with 0.5 mL saline to keep moist or nasopharyngeal wash in sterile leak-proof container. | Refrigerate, ship overnight in insulated container with ice packs |
| Equine herpesvirus-4 PCR | Nasal swab in red top tube with 0.5 mL saline to keep moist or nasopharyngeal wash in sterile leak-proof container. | Refrigerate, ship overnight in insulated container with ice packs |
| Equine herpesvirus-5 PCR | Bronchoalveolar lavage fluid in red top tube | Refrigerate, ship overnight in insulated container with ice packs |
| Equine influenza virus PCR | Nasal swab in red top tube with 0.5 mL saline to keep moist or nasopharyngeal wash in sterile leak-proof container. | Refrigerate, ship overnight in insulated container with ice packs |
| Equine rhinitis virus A and B PCR | Nasal swab in red top tube with 0.5 mL saline to keep moist or nasopharyngeal wash in sterile leak-proof container. | Refrigerate, ship overnight in insulated container with ice packs |
| Fungal culture and susceptibility | Tracheal wash fluid in red top tube or swab of fluid in aerobic transport media | Refrigerate, ship overnight in insulated container with ice packs |
| Rhodococcus equi PCR | Tracheal wash fluid in red top tube | Refrigerate, ship overnight in insulated container with ice packs |
| Strep equi subsp. equi culture | Discharge from abscess, nasal swab or nasopharyngeal wash in aerobic transport media | Refrigerate, ship overnight in insulated container with ice packs |
| Strep equi subsp. equi PCR | Discharge from abscess, nasal swab in red top tube with 0.5 mL saline to keep moist or nasopharyngeal wash in red top tube. | Refrigerate, ship overnight in insulated container with ice packs |
| Tracheal wash cytology | Tracheal wash fluid in EDTA purple top tube with two to three unstained air-dried slides | Refrigerate, ship overnight in insulated container with ice packs; separate slides from icepack during shipping to prevent condensation |

[a] Adapted from Cornell Animal Health Diagnostic Center.
[b] Horses with *Anaplasma phagocytophilum* infection may present with ataxia, although more often this clinical sign is not observed and instead horses more commonly present with fever, lethargy, distal limb vasculitis, and jaundice.

**Box 6.1 Antibiotic selection guidelines**

1) Understand the antimicrobial susceptibility interpretation categories:
   - Susceptible (S): Efficacy and pharmacodynamic information indicate that antibiotics in the susceptible category may be clinically effective.
   - Intermediate (I): The concentration of antibiotic needed to prevent the growth of the bacterial strain is equal to the antibiotic concentration that can be achieved in the body. Antibiotics in this category may be clinically effective if administered appropriately, but stringent compliance to the proper dosing regimen is essential. Consider this class only if no appropriate susceptible antibiotic is available.
   - Resistant (R): Avoid the use of any antibiotic in this category.
   - No interpretation (NI): Pharmacokinetic and efficacy studies are required to generate data indicating whether in vitro susceptibility results can be translated into successful clinical outcomes. When data do not exist for a specific combination of bacteria, antibiotic, and animal species, then a result of "No Interpretation" is given. If no suitable antibiotic is available in either the "Susceptible" or "Intermediate" category, then clinicians should contact the laboratory for more information about this group.
2) Do not base antimicrobial selection on the minimum inhibitory concentration (MIC): The MIC provides no useful means to compare among *Susceptible* antibiotics and should not have bearing on antimicrobial selection. The MIC is a measure of how much antibiotic is needed to prevent the growth of a bacterial isolate in *vitro* but does not consider whether this concentration of antibiotic is achievable in every species. Antibiotics vary greatly in their achievable animal concentrations.
3) Consider the site of infection: Choose an antibiotic that reaches the site of infection in high concentration. Susceptibility interpretations are based upon predicted *serum* concentrations. These concentrations will be similar in most soft tissues but in some anatomical locations the achievable concentrations may be substantially lower (e.g., CSF and bone) or higher (e.g., urine) than in serum.
4) Practice good antibiotic stewardship: Choosing a "first-line" antibiotic, if available, helps to prevent resistance to more modern antibiotics and thus preserves their efficacy.

## How to Collect and Prepare Specimens for Cytology

1) *Sample collection*

*Fluid specimens and effusions*

- Aseptically collect body cavity fluids into an ethylenediaminetetraacetic acid (EDTA) anticoagulant purple top tube for cytology evaluation. The EDTA anticoagulant is required to preserve cell features, prevent clot formation, and inhibit bacterial proliferation prior to cytologic evaluation. A fluid specimen should also concurrently be collected into a sterile non-additive tube (red top or white top tube) with a portion placed in bacterial transport media (aerobic and anaerobic media) for potential ancillary testing such as bacterial/fungal culture or biochemical analysis.
- Make smears from well-mixed fluid immediately following fluid collection to prevent artifacts that may skew interpretation, such as erythrophagia or phagocytosis of bacteria by macrophages. Clinical pathologists will often compare the smears provided by the practitioner to those made in the laboratory to aid their interpretation.

*Solid lesion cytology*
*Collection techniques*

- Aspiration Cytology – fine needle aspirate (FNA)
  1) Use a 21–22 gauge needle and 5–12 mL syringe.
  2) Aseptically prepare the aspiration site, then upon insertion of the needle apply gentle suction to remove cells.
  3) Redirect the needle and repeat aspiration several times before exiting the site.
  4) When finished, remove the needle from the syringe. Fill the syringe with air, reconnect to the needle, then gently use air to expel the contents of the needle onto the slide, with needle bevel facing the slide. Repeat this action several times to create several slides for evaluation.
  5) Gently make contact (squash) smears with these slides and promptly air-dry (see instructions below).

- Exfoliative Cytology
  - *Impression smears* are used to evaluate exudative skin lesions and fresh biopsy specimens prior to formalin fixation. They may only detect surface contamination in certain instances and may not be representative of the lesion.
    1) Using a freshly cut surface, first blot the tissue with gauze to remove excess fluid/blood.
    2) Next, gently touch/roll the cut surface onto several clean slides, making several impressions per slide. Submit multiple slides for evaluation.
  - *Tissue Scrapings* are used for biopsies that will not exfoliate using an impression smear or lesions that cannot be aspirated. Gently create contact smears from tissue scrapings and include the "spreader" slide for evaluation as well.
    1) Using the edge of a scalpel blade angled perpendicular to the cut surface of tissue, gently scrape off cells.
    2) Wipe the cells that have accumulated on the scalpel blade onto a glass slide, then make a contact (squash) smear for cytologic evaluation.

2) *Slide Preparation of effusions/fluids*
   - Smears can be made either from fluids that have not been concentrated (direct smears) or those that have been concentrated by centrifugation. Only centrifuge a portion of your fluid sample, in case other ancillary diagnostic testing is indicated on the non-centrifuged fluid. Reference values for joint, peritoneal, pleural, and cerebral spinal fluid in adult horses are listed in Table 6.2.
   - Smear types and applications:
     - Video Tutorials of cytology slide preparation are available through eClinPath (Cornell University 2016) on-line (credit Tracy Stokol): https://eclinpath.com/cytology/procedure-videos/
     - Helpful hints:
       - Prepare smears from well-mixed fluid.
       - A hair dryer can be used to quickly air-dry slides.
   - Wedge smear: For assessment of peripheral blood or centrifuged and high cellularity fluids of low viscosity. If centrifugation is performed, take an aliquot of fluid for this purpose, preserving the rest for other diagnostics or laboratory cytologic evaluation. Centrifuge on low speed to preserve cell integrity, then remove most of the supernatant and resuspend the pellet in approximately 0.25 mL of the remaining fluid. Use this suspension to create the wedge smear.
   - Contact (squash) smear: Indicated for aspirates, tissue scrapings, or viscous fluids (synovial fluid, tracheal wash, mucous) which don't spread well with the wedge smear. Excessive pressure during contact smear preparation can damage cells.
   - Line smears: Indicated for concentrating low cellularity fluids that are transparent to only slightly turbid, such as body cavity effusions, CSF, and urine. Line smears are especially useful when a centrifuge is not available to concentrate a pellet in a fluid of low cellularity.
3) *Cytology specimen evaluation*
   - Fluid analysis can be performed in-house with the appropriate hemocytometer equipment or referred to a clinical pathology laboratory. Total protein can be measured in-house using a refractometer. Note that total protein can be falsely elevated when a small volume of fluid is placed in a large EDTA tube.
   - If sending samples to a diagnostic laboratory for evaluation by a clinical pathologist, include two to three unstained air-dried slides from solid lesions and effusions/fluids. Ship slides in secure, break-proof slide-holders. Effusion and fluid samples for cytology should be immediately placed in EDTA purple top tubes upon collection and shipped next-day, refrigerated with ice-packs. Use Styrofoam or other packing material to insulate slides from ice-packs in the same shipping container to prevent slide condensation.

**Table 6.2** Reference values for joint fluid, peritoneal/pleural fluid, and cerebral spinal fluid (CSF) in adult horses.

| | Gross appearance | Nucleated cell count (cells/uL) | Red blood cell count | Protein |
|---|---|---|---|---|
| Joint fluid | Translucent, colorless to light yellow, high viscosity | <1000 | None-few | <2.5 g/dL |
| Peritoneal and Pleural Fluid | Translucent to slightly turbid, colorless to straw-colored | <5000 | None-few | <2.5 g/dL |
| CSF | Clear, colorless | 0–5 | None-few | 60–120 mg/dL |

**Box 6.2 Interpreting fluid cytology specimens**

*Distinguishing hemorrhage from blood contamination*

- Observe the fluid as it first begins to flow from the body cavity upon collection to determine if it starts to clear and becomes red or vice versa, as this would suggest blood contamination rather than hemorrhage.
- Most hemorrhagic effusions do not clot when placed in a red top tube because they defibrinate rapidly.
- The presence of platelets indicates blood contamination or peracute hemorrhage.

*Use inflammatory cell populations to understand the timeline and disease process*

- Majority neutrophils (>85–90%) suggests acute inflammation.
- Majority small cell lymphocytes with some reactive lymphocytes indicates chronic inflammation.
- Macrophage dominance (histiocytic inflammation) with or without vacuolization or phagocytic activity suggests chronic inflammation potentially secondary to the presence of a persistent antigenic stimulation.
- Eosinophilic inflammation indicates a response to parasitic or allergic stimulus.
- Mixed inflammation consisting of lymphocytes, macrophages, and few neutrophils indicates a chronic process.

- Diff-Quik is appropriate when evaluating cytology smears in-house. Ensure stain reagents are fresh without precipitates to prevent under-staining and artifact, respectively. Be advised that some mast cells will not stain with Diff-Quik and can be mistaken for other round cells or macrophages.

4) *Helpful hints for fluid cytology interpretation* (Box 6.2)

## Emergency Imaging

### Radiography Techniques

Radiographs are a common component to many emergency evaluations, particularly in situations warranting further evaluation of acute-onset lameness, suspected fractures, to better assess wounds for any bone or joint involvement, and to characterize penetrating foreign bodies relative to deeper structures. Radiographic techniques are specific to the x-ray generator and digital radiography system being used. Further, different anatomic regions will require specific techniques to help optimize image quality. Companies provide radiographic technique charts for their systems, to give practitioners a starting point to achieve the best image quality with their units. They are typically generated for an average-sized adult horse, so adjustments will be needed for foals, miniature, and draft horses. As an example, MinXray has a TR90+ system with recommendations for several body parts including the foot (lateral projection kV 74, time 0.08 seconds), fetlock and carpus (kV 78, time 0.08 seconds), and stifle (lateral projection kV 80, time 0.16 seconds, caudal-cranial projection kV 90, time 0.24 seconds) at a distance of 26 in. from the generator source to the plate. Appropriate personal protective equipment such as lead aprons and thyroid shields should be utilized for all people in the room or area while taking radiographs, including lead gloves for the holder of the plate.

#### General Considerations

If the horse is standing, the limbs should be as square as possible, with even weight bearing on all four feet to optimize positioning. In an emergency situation, particularly with pronounced lameness, radiographs are taken with the horse in whichever position they are comfortable in, which may include minimal weight bearing on the limb. In general, if the radiograph is too dark (overexposed), time can be decreased by 1/4-1/2x. If the radiograph is too light (underexposed), time can be increased by 2-4x (MinXray, Equine Technique Chart).

#### Foot Considerations

Standing the horse on wooden blocks is useful for taking radiographs of P2 and P3, to elevate the foot off the ground, away from the margin of the plate. A tunnel can be utilized to obtain radiographs of the solar margin of P3 and the navicular bone. Playdough can be utilized to lightly pack the sulci of the frog to decrease gas artifact on the radiograph. If an open-heel shoe is on with no pad, 60° DP radiographs of the P3 margin can still be taken with oblique projections to see the palmar/plantar processes of P3 and the navicular bone margins. If a full pad or bar shoe is on the foot, remove the shoe for the clearest radiographs of the region.

### Penetrating Injuries

With cases of penetrating injuries, contrast or metallic probes can be inserted into the wounds to help determine depth, potential involvement of nearby synovial and soft-tissue structures and bone.

## Endoscopy Examination

Endoscopic examination on an emergency basis may be utilized to evaluate the source of epistaxis or nasal discharge, the cause of a respiratory noise or difficulty breathing, or the integrity of the esophagus or trachea after trauma. Endoscopy may also be utilized for further evaluation of the cause of esophageal obstruction. Common endoscopes for equine use come in a 1 or 3 m length, with 1 m scopes used more commonly on an emergency basis in the field. Videoendoscopes in the ambulatory setting are becoming more common, with the ability to take pictures and video. Alternatively, fiberoptic endoscopes are available with direct visualization through the eye piece.

### General Considerations

If accurate assessment of laryngeal function is important, an unsedated endoscopic evaluation should be performed if possible. After, sedation can be administered to complete the rest of the exam if necessary. With someone holding the horse and utilizing a twitch if appropriate, the scope is passed in the ventral meatus of the nasal passage. This can be performed by the same person operating the endoscope, or by your assistant if available. If there is no water channel on the scope, any mucus or blood that is present on the end of the scope can be gently rubbed off against the mucosa of the pharynx to enhance visibility. To enter the guttural pouches, an endoscopic probe is inserted through the biopsy channel of the scope into the guttural pouch openings. The scope can then be gently rotated to enter the pouch. If no biopsy channel is present, a bent insemination pipette or chambers catheter can be placed through the opposite nostril to facilitate opening the entrance to the pouch.

### Examination and Triage

With cases of epistaxis or nasal discharge, evaluation of both nasal passages, pharynx, larynx, trachea, esophagus, and guttural pouches should be performed. Blood coming from the guttural pouch opening can be observed with mycosis, trauma, or infection (Figure 6.1). For respiratory noise or difficulty breathing, examine both nasal passages, pharynx, larynx, trachea, and guttural pouches. If there is prominent laryngeal or pharyngeal swelling, the stress of the exam can sometimes exacerbate the degree of respiratory obstruction. If significant upper airway obstruction is observed (Figure 6.2), a temporary tracheostomy should be considered to secure an airway prior to further investigation (see Chapter 5, *Advanced Clinical Triage Procedures*).

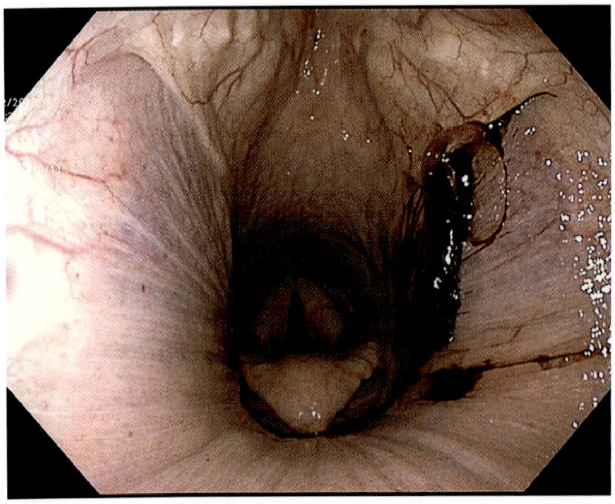

**Figure 6.1** Endoscopic image of the pharynx in a horse with epistaxis. Coagulated blood is observed coming from the left guttural pouch opening. The case was diagnosed with guttural pouch mycosis causing hemorrhage from the internal carotid artery.

## Ultrasound Examination

### Abdominal Ultrasonography

"Transabdominal ultrasonography is a rapid, non-invasive diagnostic technique invaluable to emergency triage of the equine patient. The emergence of affordable, high-quality portable devices has made this diagnostic modality readily accessible to both the hospital and field clinician. The ability to assess the appearance, location, and contents of internal organs provides clinicians with critical information to determine a diagnosis, recommend surgical or medical management, and later, monitor response to treatment. While the acute abdomens represent the most common indications for ultrasound examination, the modality has broad application including assessment of soft-tissue swellings and injury sites, fracture identification, jugular vein assessment, and facilitation of ultrasound-guided diagnostic procedures.

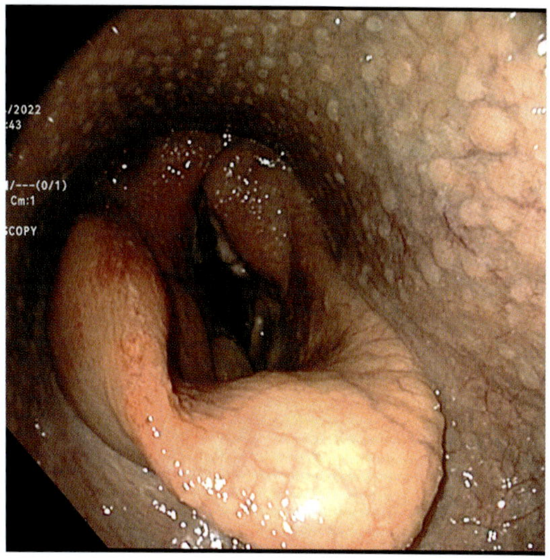

**Figure 6.2** Endoscopic image of the larynx in a horse with a moderate upper respiratory noise at rest. Severe swelling is observed along the right aryepiglottic fold and laryngeal wall with bilateral arytenoid chondritis present. Severe narrowing of the rima glottidis is also observed and a temporary tracheostomy was immediately performed.

### General Considerations

A low-frequency (2–8 MHz), curvilinear transducer works well for imaging the equine abdomen. Higher-frequency probes have the advantage of better image resolution and quality, but often lack the penetration required for a complete abdominal exam. Higher-frequency probes may be utilized for foal examination. Isopropyl alcohol is used as an acoustic coupling agent. Long coated horses may require clipping and application of a coupling gel to achieve adequate image quality.

*Sonographic evaluation of the normal equine abdomen*

- The ultrasound examination should be performed much like a physical examination; methodically and thoroughly. Exact technique is not as important as developing one's own systematic approach that is performed in repeatable fashion on every patient. The author's preference is to start with the left cranial abdomen in order to quickly identify horses with gastric reflux that require immediate intervention. Approximate sonographic viewing locations of abdominal organs are provided in Figure 6.3.
- Starting near the elbow at the cranial-most aspect of the left abdomen, consecutive dorsal-to-ventral sweeps are made while moving caudally over the abdomen one intercostal space at a time, ending in the paralumbar fossa. This is followed by several cranial-to-caudal passes over the ventralmost aspect of the abdomen, starting at the xyphoid and ending in the inguinal region. The process is repeated on the right side of the abdomen.
- In the left cranial abdomen, the liver is visible adjacent to the cranial edge of the spleen. The echogenicities of the two organs can be compared from this view. Moving caudally brings the stomach into view in the 9th–12th ICS, characterized by its large semi-circular gas echo and location medial to the spleen. The splenic vein can often be seen adjacent to the stomach wall. In contrast to normal intestinal wall thickness (which should be less than 4 mm), stomach wall frequently measures up to 8 mm and can have a double-layer or "halo" appearance.
- The spleen is visible over most of the left abdomen, positioned between the body wall and large colon. Large colon is characterized by its hyperechoic gas-to-wall interface and sacculated (ventral colon) or smooth (dorsal colon) appearance.
- Large colon wall thickness should not exceed 4 mm and is often too thin to easily measure in normal horses. Small colon is also sacculated and may be observed deep to the spleen.
- The left kidney and nephrosplenic space are visible in the dorsal left flank, medial to the caudal spleen at a depth of approximately 15–25 cm.
- Small intestine can be imaged in the left inguinal region; generally appearing as variable layers of motile structures with or without luminal fluid. Round and/or amotile loops of small intestine are an abnormal finding. The ventral abdomen is useful for evaluating large colon wall thickness and locating a suitable site for abdominocentesis.
- Moving to the right abdomen, again starting cranially near the elbow, colon wall is imaged just caudal to the diaphragm. Moving caudally reveals the liver in the 8–15th ICS and the adjacent right dorsal colon. The duodenum is visible between the medial surface of liver and the right dorsal colon and can be traced caudally as it courses along the body wall before turning medially just ventral to the caudal pole of the right kidney. It is usually collapsed, and peristaltic waves can be easily observed during real time scanning.
- In geriatric horses, hepatic atrophy may make imaging the liver difficult. The right kidney is located superficially and dorsally between the 15th and 17th ICS.
- The cecum encompasses most of the right paralumbar fossa and can be followed ventrally and cranially to its apex on the abdominal floor. Unlike the large colon, cecal blood supply courses both medially and laterally, the latter of which can be visualized against the body wall in the ventral right paralumbar fossa. When imaged transversely, these vessels appear

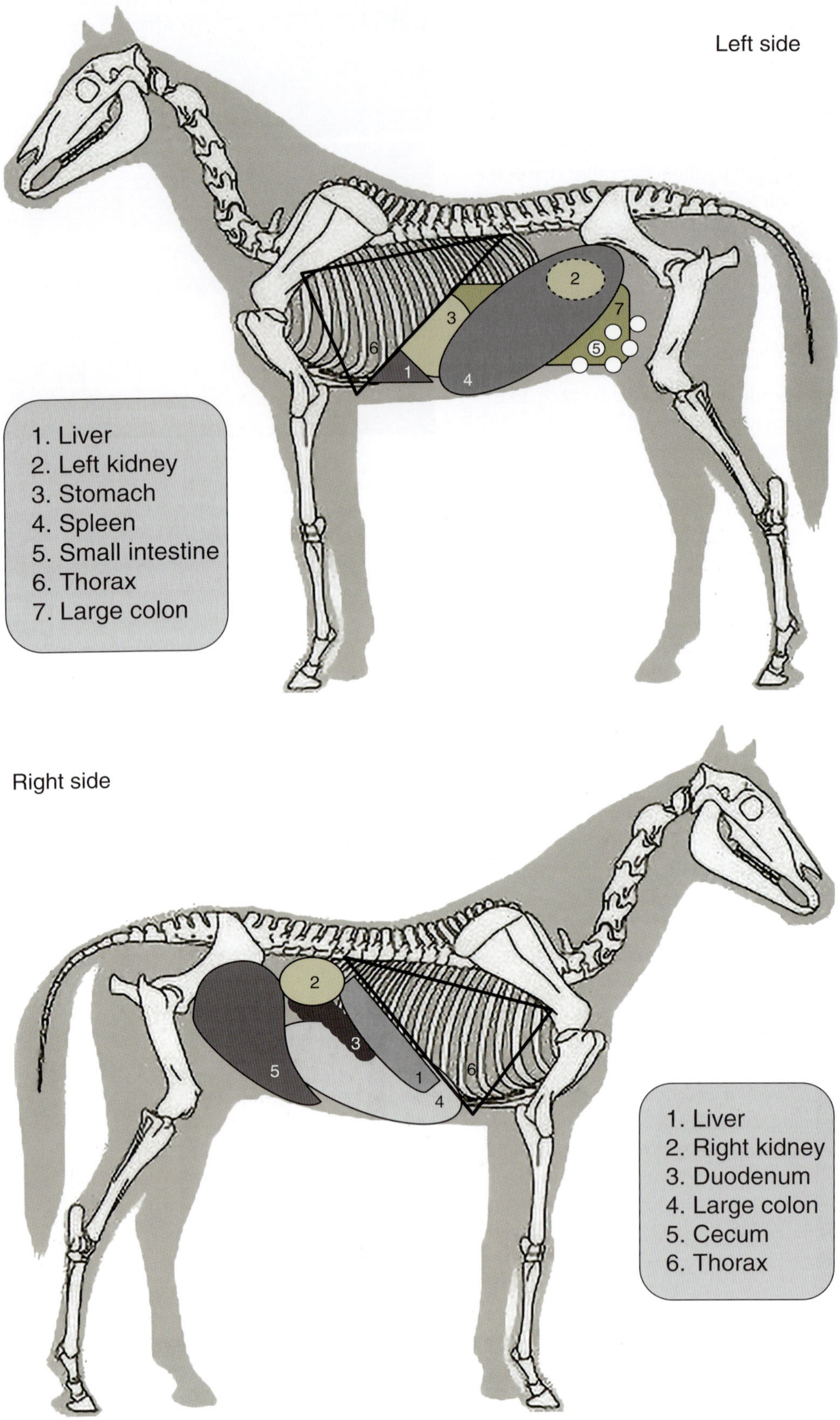


**Figure 6.3** Approximate sonographic viewing locations of abdominal organs in the horse.

**Box 6.3 The FLASH sonographic viewing locations are as follows**

Left:
- Ventral abdomen
- Gastric window
- Spleno-renal window
- Left middle third of the abdomen

Right:
- Duodenal window
- Right middle third of abdomen
- Cranial ventral thorax

as small hypoechoic circular structures adjacent to the cecal wall. Intestinal peristalsis and wall thickness, and peritoneal fluid volume and character, are assessed throughout the examination."

*Source: DeNotta, SL. Proceedings, Vermont Veterinary Medical Association Winter CE Conference, Burlington, VT. February* (2016).

A rapid FLASH abdominal ultrasound technique described by (Busoni et al. 2011) assesses the equine abdomen in specific regions and may be utilized to facilitate rapid assessment of emergency patients (Box 6.3).

## Sonographic Evaluation of the Equine Acute Abdomen

### "Gastric Disorders

A gastric echo spanning more than four intercostal spaces that contains large volumes of hypoechoic "swirling" fluid is an immediate indication for passage of a nasogastric tube. This is a common finding with proximal small intestinal obstructive lesions and/or small intestinal ileus. Gastric impactions can be difficult to diagnose sonographically but can appear as an enlarged gastric echo containing hyperechoic material casting a sharp acoustic shadow.

### Small Intestinal Disorders

Distended, fluid-filled loops of small intestine can be observed with strangulating or obstructive lesions, anterior enteritis, and ileus (Figure 6.4). Decreased peristalsis and sedimentation of ingesta within the ventral lumen may also be noted. Sections of strangulated small intestine often have thickened walls (>5 mm) and minimal peristaltic activity. Increased peristalsis is sometimes observed with anterior enteritis. Distended loops of small intestine in the cranial left abdomen can occur with epiploic foramen entrapments, sometimes obscuring visualization of the normal stomach–spleen interface.

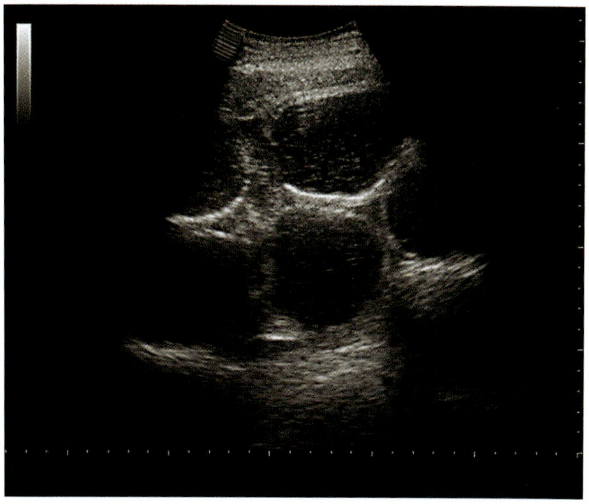

Figure 6.4 Image obtained from the ventral abdomen of a horse with a strangulating lipoma. Note the loops of distended small intestine observed throughout the viewing field.

### Colonic Disorders

Nephrosplenic entrapments are diagnosed sonographically by inability to visualize the left kidney due a large gas-filled viscus in the caudodorsal left abdomen (Figure 6.5). The spleen will be pushed ventrally, and its dorsal edge can often be observed displacing medially off the body wall where it meets the offending large intestine. Colonic mesenteric vessels observed coursing laterally along the right side of the abdomen is suggestive of a right dorsal displacement and/or 180° large colon volvulus (Figure 6.6) (Ness et al. 2012). Thickened large colon wall is frequently observed in the ventral abdomen with volvulus of the large colon.

Impending diarrhea is often visible as variably echogenic swirling ingesta in the cecum and/or large colon that may be accompanied by increased wall thickness (>5 mm) in cases of colitis (Pease et al. 2004). Right dorsal colitis is characterized by thickened and edematous right dorsal colon (often > 15 mm), imaged in the right 10th–14th ICS, adjacent to the liver.

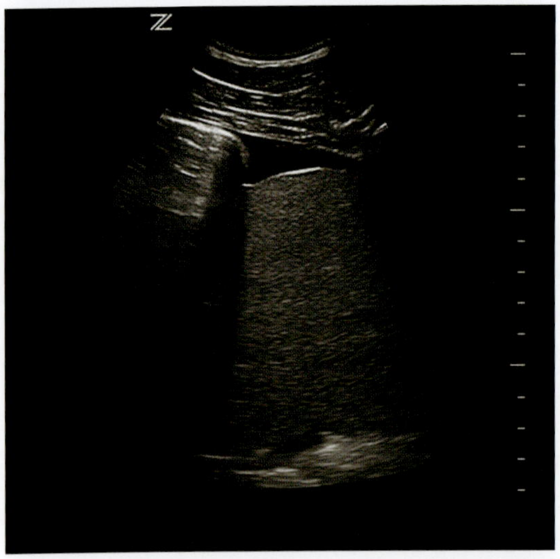

**Figure 6.5** Image obtained from the left caudodorsal abdomen of a horse with nephrosplenic entrapment. Note that the spleen (right) is being displaced off the body wall by a gas-filled viscus (left), likely the large colon. Left kidney is not visible due to acoustic shadowing by the entrapped section of bowel.

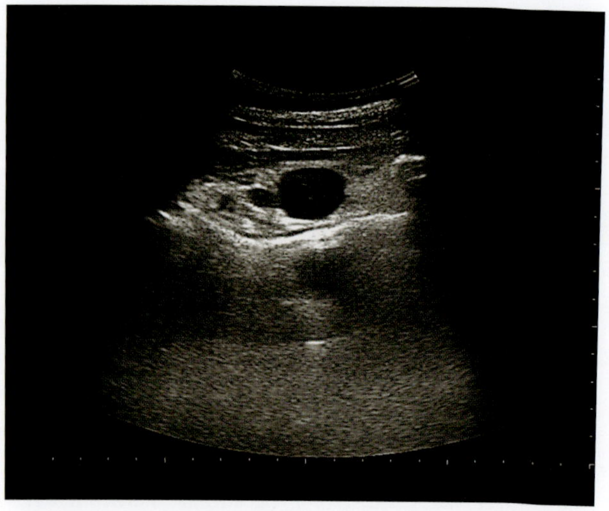

**Figure 6.6** Image obtained from the right mid abdomen of a horse presenting for colic. The presence of colonic vessels (black circular structures in center of image) suggests a right dorsal displacement or 180° volvulus of the large colon. A right dorsal colon displacement was identified at surgery.

## Thoracic Ultrasonography

Indications for thoracic ultrasound include evaluation of horses and foals with signs of respiratory disease, fever of unknown origin, exercise intolerance, abnormal thoracic auscultation, inappetence, weight loss, thoracic and abdominal trauma, some types of colic and unexplained hematological abnormalities.

### General Considerations

A medium–high frequency (6–10 MHz), curvilinear or straight transducer works well for imaging the equine thorax. Traditional rectal probes work very well for foal exams, but generally lack the depth capability to image an adult thorax. Isopropyl alcohol is used as an acoustic coupling agent. Long coated horses may require clipping and application of a coupling gel to achieve adequate image quality."

*Source: DeNotta, SL. Proceedings, Vermont Veterinary Medical Association Winter CE Conference, Burlington, VT. February* (2016).

*Thoracic ultrasound examination*

- Alcohol is applied to the chest wall one section at a time and immediately imaged with consecutive dorsal-to-ventral sweeps of the probe, advancing in a cranial-to-caudal direction one intercostal space at a time. Advancing the probe slowly allows assessment of both inspiratory and expiratory phases. Both sides of the thorax should be evaluated, as well as the right cranial lung lobe, which can be imaged through the right triceps musculature.
- The normal equine lung surface should appear smooth and hyperechoic (white) with a back-and-forth sliding motion (Figure 6.7). Vertical hyperechoic streaks "comet tails" (Figure 6.8), pleural surface irregularities, and/or fluid accumulation between the pleural surface and body wall (Figure 6.9) are all suggestive of pulmonary disease. The ability to image past the pleural surface into the lung parenchyma is also abnormal and may be observed in conditions causing lung consolidation, atelectasis, fibrosis, and/or abscessation.
- It is important to recognize that because ultrasound waves cannot travel through air, it is only possible to evaluate the surface of the lungs, and thus, lesions below the surface, e.g., lung abscesses, may be missed.

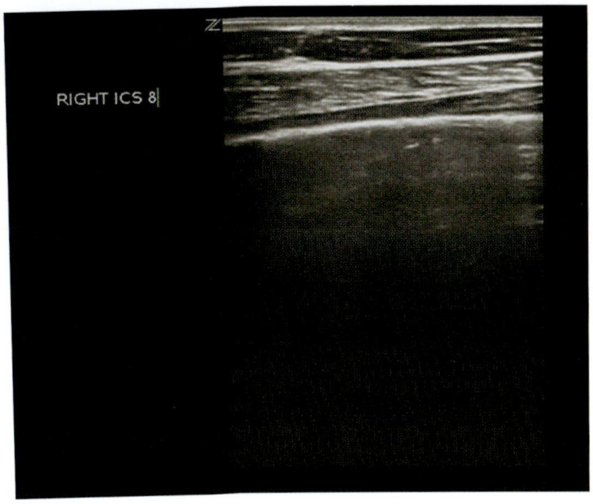


**Figure 6.7** Normal thoracic ultrasound demonstrating a smooth, hyperechoic (white) pleural surface.

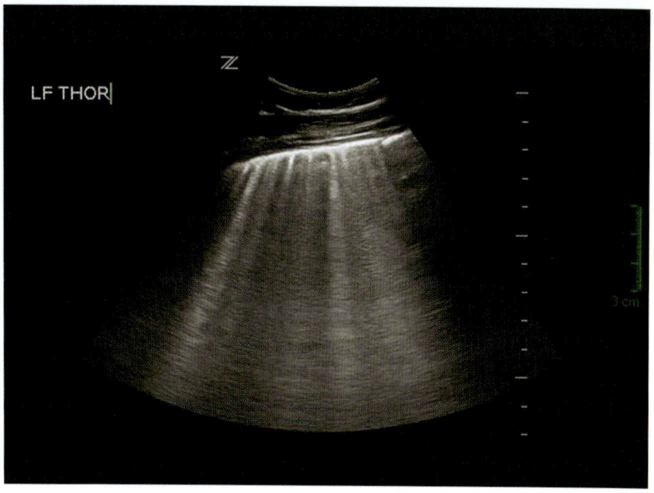


**Figure 6.8** Vertical "comet tails" in a horse with pneumonia.

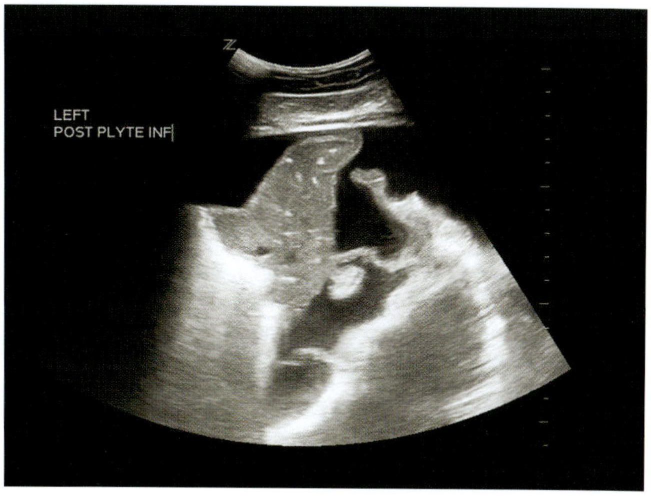


**Figure 6.9** Consolidated lung lobe tip surrounded by pleural fluid in a horse with pleuropneumonia.

## References

Busoni, V., De Busscher, V., Lopez, D. et al. (2011 Apr). Evaluation of a protocol for fast localised abdominal sonography of horses (FLASH) admitted for colic. *Vet. J.* 188 (1): 77–82. https://doi.org/10.1016/j.tvjl.2010.02.017. Epub 2010 Mar 26. PMID: 20347357.

Cornell University (2025). eClinPath.com. https://eclinpath.com/cytology/ (accessed May 2025).

DeNotta, S.L. (February 2016). Abdominal and thoracic ultrasound of the horse. *Proceedings, Vermont Veterinary Medical Association Winter CE Conference,* Burlington, VT.

Gajic, I., Kabic, J., Kekic, D. et al. (2022). Antimicribial susceptibility testing: a comprehensive review of currently used methods. *Antibiotics* 11 (427): https://doi.org/10.3390/antibiotics11040427.

Ness, S.L., Bain, F.T., Zantingh, A.J. et al. (2012). Ultrasonographic visualization of colonic mesenteric vasculature as an indicator of large colon right dorsal displacement or 180° volvulus (or both) in horses. *Can. Vet. J.* 53 (4): 378–382. PMID: 23024382; PMCID: PMC3299504.

Pease, A.P., Scrivani, P.V., Erb, H.N., and Cook, V.L. (2004). Accuracy of increased large-intestine wall thickness during ultrasonography for diagnosing large-colon torsion in 42 horses. *Vet. Radiol. Ultrasound* 45: 220–224.

Slovis, N.M., Browne, N., and Bozorgmanesh, R. (2020). Point-of-care diagnostics in equine practice. *Vet. Clin. N. Am. Equine Pract.* 36 (1): p161–p171. https://doi.org/10.1016/j.cveq.2019.12.007.

# Part 2

# Emergency Conditions of the Horse

# 7

# Wounds, Trauma, and Other Injury

*Rolfe M. Radcliffe[1], Heidi L. Reesink[2], and Dean A. Hendrickson[3]*

[1] *Department of Clinical Sciences, College of Veterinary Medicine, Cornell University, Ithaca, NY, USA*
[2] *Large Animal Surgery, Department of Clinical Sciences, College of Veterinary Medicine, Cornell University, Ithaca, NY, USA*
[3] *Department of Clinical Sciences, College of Veterinary Medicine and Biomedical Sciences, Colorado State University, Fort Collins, CO, USA*

## Introduction

Veterinarians are mindful of the high incidence of wounds and other trauma in horses. Injury is common because of their curious nature and tendency toward a flight response, as well as their large size and associated high forces and energy during trauma. Because horses suffer many different types of injury throughout their bodies – and healing, return to function, and complications vary depending upon body location – they require individual wound management decisions (Gaughan 2018). Patient stabilization is the first requirement of wound triage, followed by evaluation; cleaning, debridement, and lavage; wound closure and support. Wound management often involves a strategic combination of both medical and surgical interventions (Hendrix and Baxter 2005). Complications are common and frequent reevaluation is necessary to guide healing and improve prognosis and outcome. Traumatic wounds in horses are frequently challenging and euthanasia may be an option; however, with appropriate management outcomes are often favorable (Hendrix and Baxter 2005).

## Emergency Wound Triage

Patient stabilization is the foundation of emergency triage and is summarized in Boxes 7.1 and 7.2.

## Emergency Wound Evaluation and Management

### Wound Examination

It is imperative that veterinarians prevent iatrogenic contamination of wounds with proper hand hygiene and other techniques.

Hand Hygiene

1) When contaminated – **wash hands** with gentle, **neutral pH, non-medicated soap**.
2) When hands are clean – use an alcohol-based sanitizer having **>60% ethyl alcohol**.
3) Use products that contain **hand conditioners** to maintain skin health and integrity.

*Emergency Triage of the Horse*, First Edition. Edited by Rolfe M. Radcliffe and Jamie J. Kopper.
 Published 2026 by John Wiley & Sons, Inc.
Companion website: www.wiley.com/go/radcliffe/triage

**Box 7.1 Patient Stabilization**

**Systemic Considerations**

STEP 1 – Examine animal from a distance and make sure it is in a safe location. Perform a quick physical exam to assess the systemic stability of the patient.

Evaluate first **ABC – airway, breathing, circulation**. If airway, breathing, or circulation is abnormal, stabilize first.

**Airway**: First make sure the airway is patent; place an endotracheal tube via the oral or nasal cavity if necessary to secure the airway; perform a tracheostomy if an airway cannot be secured.

**Breathing**: Restore ventilation and provide intra-nasal or tracheal oxygen at 10–15 L/min for an adult horse (5 L/min for a foal).

**Circulation**: Assess shock and begin fluid therapy (shock dose: 20–80 mL/kg IV isotonic crystalloids over several hours or 1–2 L of hypertonic saline followed by crystalloid fluids).

If these are normal, proceed with routine physical exam followed by attending to the specific injury. If the wound requires immediate attention, triage wound care (below) before general PE.

STEP 2 – If the horse is stable, sedate or restrain horse for hands-on palpation and evaluation of the wound or injury if necessary. If horse is in shock or requires emergency fluid resuscitation, place catheter and begin fluids.

**Box 7.2 Patient Stabilization**

**Wound Factors**

STEP 3 – Immediate wound triage

A) **Stop hemorrhage by direct pressure, ligature, or hemostat**: If that is not possible, apply a pressure bandage while stabilizing the horse and gathering your supplies.

B) **Provide structural support**: Bandaging and/or splinting may be indicated for tendon, ligament, or bone injury prior to movement and referral. If the wound is associated with a long-bone fracture, follow both wound triage and emergency fracture stabilization guidelines.

C) **Examine the wound to determine what structures are involved**: Visually examine and palpate the affected area noting damage to soft tissues especially muscles, ligaments and tendons, nerves and blood vessels, injury to bone and periosteum, evidence of synovial cavity involvement (e.g., joint effusion, synovial fluid drainage, lameness).

D) Prepare the wound with isotonic crystalloid fluid lavage, clipping, and disinfection prior to deeper wound evaluation. **Use palpation, ultrasound, and radiographs to guide complete evaluation** of the affected structures.

E) Make a plan for management… **Referral should be considered for injuries requiring specialist care:** wounds involving joints, tendon sheaths and bursae, tendon and ligament injury, damage to bones or periosteum, hoof wall and coronary band, extensive degloving injury, injury to the cranium and sinuses, wounds into the abdomen or thorax, and other complicated problems.

F) **Wounds into the abdomen or thoracic cavity require immediate patient stabilization** and often referral depending upon severity (below).

G) Lacerations lacking significant contamination, swelling, or drainage and without communication of synovial structures, the abdomen or thorax may be **closed primarily** following routine cleaning, debridement and lavage.

H) Lacerations with marked contamination, swelling, or drainage may benefit from **delayed closure** techniques.

I) **Antibiotics, anti-inflammatory drugs, and tetanus toxoid** (when tetanus vaccination status is unknown or exceeding six months) should be considered for most wounds and other penetrating injuries in the horse.

A thorough examination of the wound is imperative to help determine appropriate management steps (Gaughan 2018). Follow these steps below:

1) ***Take a history***... ask questions including: is your horse stable, how much hemorrhage, degree of lameness, where is the wound located, how old is the wound, how did it happen, have you given any treatments, current on vaccinations including tetanus?
2) ***Watch horse walk***... with severe lameness (Grades 4–5/5) keep horse still and quiet. Access limb for evidence of fracture, soft-tissue support injury, or communication with synovial structure. Care should be taken to avoid exercising the horse when bone fracture is suspected. Remember horses with open synovial compartment wounds may not be severely lame as compared to horses with a closed septic injury.
3) ***Note wound location*** of distal limb, trunk, head, and neck. Wounds of the distal limb are often complicated because of lack of overlying tissue, involvement of vital structures, high degree of movement, increased contamination, increased tension and wound retraction, and tendency toward exuberant granulation tissue formation (Gaughan 2018). Wounds of the trunk (including axillary and inguinal regions) may involve the abdomen and/or thorax.
4) ***Note wound type*** such as a flap, degloving injury, puncture wound, abrasion, or contusion and if the wound is acute or chronic. Also note if the wound is associated with blunt or penetrating trauma as this will affect both wound characteristics and tissues possibly involved.
5) ***Sedate horse and consider local anesthesia*** for wound evaluation. A combination of systemic sedative and analgesic drugs together with local nerve and/or ring blocks above the wound are often necessary for standing wound repair. General anesthesia may be indicated for dangerous horses or those with severe injury where wound exploration, cleaning, and management may be improved. Consider GA and referral for horses suffering synovial cavity disruption, bone or soft-tissue injury, penetration of the abdomen or thorax, presence of foreign material, and other injury where standing management may be challenging (Gaughan 2018).
6) ***Perform a careful visual examination*** of the wound. Think about the size and location of the wound, type and depth of injury, degree of contamination, what tissues are involved (e.g., skin, muscle, bone, tendon, ligament, synovial structure), evidence of foreign bodies, and possible complications. Also note the degree of swelling, drainage, and other signs of infection.
7) ***Palpate and manipulate the limb*** to determine what structures may be involved. Try to understand what vital structures may be compromised – vascular, neurologic, structural (bone, tendon, ligament), and synovial (joint, tendon sheath, bursa). Manipulation of the injured limb through passive range of motion will give additional information about the type and depth of injury, structures involved, and help you plan further diagnostics. Imaging is recommended prior to limb manipulation in cases of bone, tendon, ligament and synovial involvement to avoid further structural injury and air accumulation beneath the skin (Gaughan 2018).

## Diagnostic Techniques

### Wound Palpation

After wound cleansing and lavage, manual palpation with sterile gloves will help determine the specific tissues affected as well as depth and extent of injury. Use your fingers or a sterile metal probe to determine the depth and direction of injury and to examine what tissues are involved from deepest to most superficial. Look carefully for evidence of tissue trauma, degree of contamination, presence of foreign material, and signs of inflammation or infection. Digital palpation may also be combined with passive range of motion to help elucidate the full extent of injury.

### Ultrasound

Ultrasound is a valuable tool for understanding both bone and soft-tissue injury during wound evaluation. Use ultrasound to look for damage to soft-tissue structures, especially synovial cavities, tendons and ligaments, and for bone injury. Synovial involvement should be suspected with enlarged synovial cavities and or changes in normal fluid acoustic appearance from anechoic to hyperechoic. The full extent of tendon and ligament injury may be possible via ultrasound, although this is more difficult with increasing tissue injury. Bone fracture should be suspected where the bone surface is irregular or has a step in the acoustic outline.

#### Radiographs

Radiographic assessment is important to rule out bone injury with most limb wounds and other injury where the skeleton may be involved. Radiographs may also help identify foreign material following trauma and confirm synovial involvement using sterile metal probes or when intra-articular gas is identified. Common problems that may be missed without survey radiographs include non-displaced fractures, osteochondral fragmentation, sequestrum formation, as well as the presence of foreign bodies and other debris.

#### Injection Techniques

Survey radiographs are best performed prior to injecting solutions near wounds as image artifacts may occur. Various injection techniques are often necessary for complete wound evaluation, especially for suspected synovial cavity involvement, puncture wounds, and foreign bodies (Gaughan 2018). Isotonic crystalloid solutions, vital stains, and radiographic dyes are most commonly used. For suspected synovial involvement, inject isotonic, crystalloid solutions into the questioned synovial cavity away from the wound using aseptic technique. Maximal distention of the compartment is often required, and fluid will leak or squirt from the wound confirming communication. Radiographic dyes (e.g., iohexol) may also be injected into a synovial cavity – use radiographic guidance to determine if leakage occurs outside of the structure. Vital stains are useful to help determine the depth of a wound and presence of foreign material. Avoid injecting solutions directly into a wound when communication with a synovial cavity or other body cavity is suspected as this may force bacteria and debris deeper into the tissues and further contaminate the structure.

### Wound Cleaning and Lavage

Infection is the most important problem leading to delayed wound healing. The most common bacteria of traumatic horse wounds include *Staphylococcus aureus*, *Streptococcus pyogenes*, Gram-negative aerobic enteric bacteria, and anaerobes (Adam and Southwood 2006; Brumbaugh 2005). The wound-healing steps of *inflammation*, *debridement*, *repair*, *and remodeling* are negatively affected by prolonged inflammation, swelling, and drainage. Wound cleaning, lavage, and debridement are the foundation of appropriate wound care (Frees 2018) (Figure 7.1a and b) (Box 7.3).

### Wound Debridement

Debridement of traumatic wounds is an essential step of treatment that removes organic or foreign material, damaged and necrotic tissues, as well as bacteria and other pathogens. Debridement is also essential for the treatment of non-healing wounds (Maher and Kuebelbeck 2018). Several types of debridement are possible including direct lavage, surgical and biosurgical methods, use of a laser, as well as enzymatic or chemical debridement. Mechanical methods of debridement such as lavage, surgical excision, and wet-to-dry bandages are most commonly used in acute wound management.

#### Debridement

1) Use **saline-soaked gauze or soft sponge** to remove organic and foreign material, blood, and other debris.
2) Lavage wound as directed above…
3) **Surgical excision** of damaged and contaminated tissue is indicated with a **sharp #10 or #15 scalpel blade**.
4) With **large flap wounds, do not remove any devitalized skin**; instead, lavage and sharply remove or scrape the underlying dermis with a sharp scalpel blade.
5) **Sharp excision of the margins of a flap is indicated** and will freshen the edges and remove organic material and bacteria prior to closure.
6) **Bandage debridement** is effective for damaged tissue that may not be surgically removed.
7) Prepare a **wet-to-dry bandage** by placing saline-soaked gauze over the wound followed by a Robert Jones bandage; removal at 12–24 h debrides the wound of necrotic material and other wound debris.
8) Wound debridement is also necessary during delayed wound closure techniques.

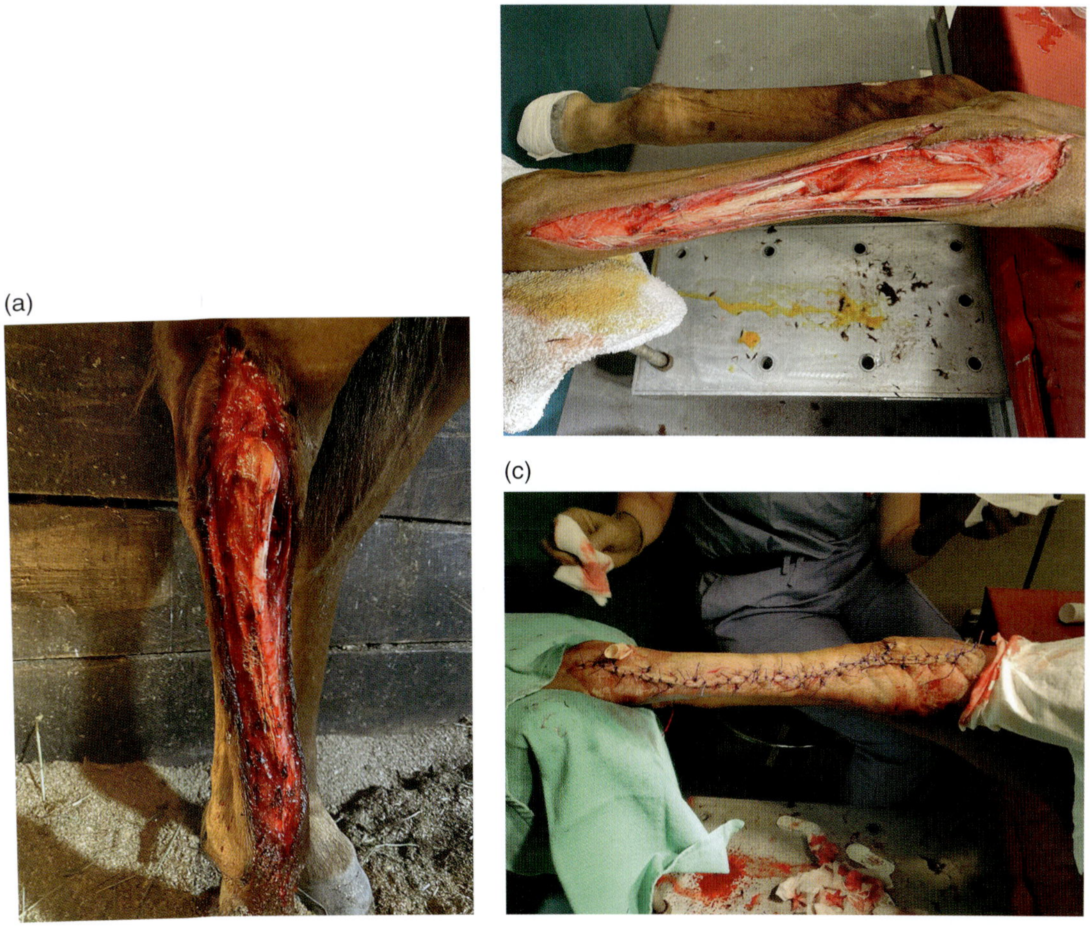

**Figure 7.1** A long 40 cm laceration extending from the proximal aspect of the tarsocural joint across the dorsal aspect of the right hind metatarsus to the level of the fetlock joint (a). Although the wound is recent, significant contamination is still present in the wound. After wound lavage and debridement (b). Following primary closure using a combination of vertical mattress and simple interrupted suture patterns (c). Note the presence of a passive (Penrose) drain placed across the length of the wound to provide distal drainage.

### Box 7.3 Wound Cleaning

1) Place a **temporary bandage** to control hemorrhage, for brushing hair and debris from horse and when triaging other emergent problems.
2) **Lavage the wound** if necessary to remove severe contamination, debris, blood.
3) Place a **sterile, water-based lubricating jelly** into the wound to prevent further wound contamination.
4) **Clip hair** surrounding the wound starting at the wound and moving outward.
5) **Clean wound carefully** with saline-soaked gauze or sponge side of surgical scrub brush… mechanical scrubbing is for intact skin only.
6) **Povidone iodine and chlorohexidine antiseptic solutions** and isopropyl alcohol are limited to surrounding **intact skin only** as they are cytotoxic (Frees 2018).
7) Use **dilute antiseptic solutions** for heavily contaminated wounds (Leise 2018):
   0.1% Povidone iodine (10 mL 10% PI solution per liter of lavage fluid)
   0.05% Chlorohexidine (25 mL 2% CH solution per liter of lavage fluid)

*Wound Lavage*

1) **Lavage wounds with sterile isotonic fluids** such as normal saline or LRS (Leise 2018). Saline can be made by adding salt to boiled tap water (2 teaspoons/L).
2) Lavage at an oblique angle using a pressure of 8–15 psi.
3) Use a **35 mL syringe and an 18–19 Ga needle** to deliver 10–15 psi.
4) Antibiotics in wound lavage remain controversial and may contribute to bacterial resistance.

## Wound Management Decisions

Wound healing in horses is affected by many variables including wound size and location, age of wound, type of injury, level of contamination, amount of tension, presence of foreign bodies, among many other factors (Kamus and Theoret 2018). Clients should be advised about realistic outcomes and the often-extended healing times, as well as possible complications and the importance of frequent monitoring (Caston 2012). The most functional and cosmetic result of wound management is accomplished with primary or delayed-primary wound closure (Doughty and Sparks 2016, Myers 2004b [Wound healing], Kamus and Theoret 2018). The decision between management techniques is dependent on the amount of tissue loss and the degree of contamination or infection. Wounds with minimal tissue loss should be closed whenever possible. Contaminated and infected wounds with minimal tissue loss should be debrided and closed when necrotic tissue and bacterial loads have been removed. Wounds can be closed at any time during the wound-healing process. Wounds with excessive tissue loss will be managed by second-intention healing. When treating wounds with second-intention healing, skin-grafting techniques should be discussed with the client (Maher and Kuebelbeck 2018).

1) Primary closure: The wound, with minimal tissue loss and contamination, is debrided and sutured. If there is tension on the wound edges, a tension-relieving pattern (Near–Far–Far–Near or Vertical Mattress) is used along with tissue apposition sutures (simple interrupted, cruciate, simple continuous) to improve healing (Figure 7.1c).
2) Delayed-primary closure: The wound, with minimal tissue loss and moderate contamination, is debrided and covered with a debridement dressing until the contamination is minimized. It is then closed as described above for primary closure. Debridement of the wound bed as well as systemic and local antibiotic therapy are important steps in preparation of delayed closure techniques. (Figure 7.2a and b)
3) Second-intention healing: When the wound has too much tissue loss to close primarily or as a delayed-primary closure, it is treated with wound dressings as described in the next section. Degloving injuries to the lower limb are an example where second-intention healing is required (Figure 7.3a–c). Skin-grafting techniques should be considered during second-intention healing and for other large or non-healing wounds (Maher and Kuebelbeck 2018).

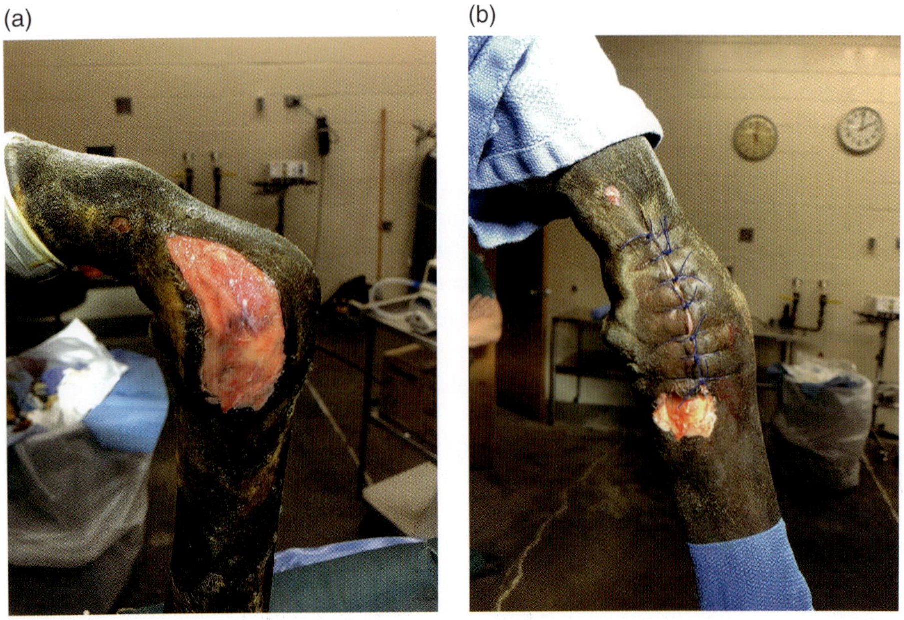


**Figure 7.2** Photos showing delayed-primary closure of a wound that was three days old. Wound following cleaning and lavage, but prior to debridement (a), and after closure (b). Note that the proximal aspect of the wound had too much tissue loss for complete closure.

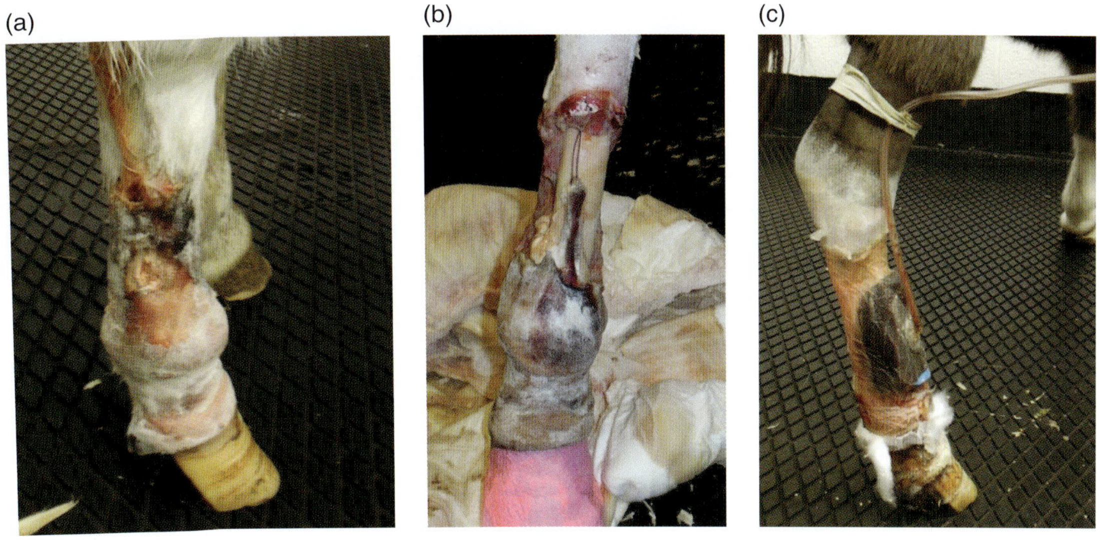


**Figure 7.3** Severe degloving injury on the dorsal metatarsus of a miniature mule mare. (a) Shortly after the time of trauma. (b) Approximately five days following injury. Significant tissue sloughing occurred over the first week despite conservative tissue debridement. (c) Wound management included application of negative pressure wound therapy. See Case Example 7.1 at the end of this chapter for additional details.

## Wound Dressings

Wound dressings maintain a moist environment, allow for gas exchange, protect the wound from infection, allow removal of exudate, and promote epithelialization. Wound healing occurs in various stages – Inflammation, Debridement, Repair, and Remodeling. Wound dressings should be appropriate for the stage of wound healing. In general, wound healing can be broken into several types of wounds that occur over these four stages: Infected or Necrotic Wounds, Dry Wounds, Granulating and Contracting Wounds, and Epithelializing Wounds. If the appropriate dressings are not used for the stage of wound healing the wound-healing process will be delayed. Wounds should always be kept moist. Moist wound healing has been shown to decrease the time of wound healing by approximately 50% (Winter 1962, 1963). For example, the application of manuka honey to open wounds may decrease wound retraction and speed healing of lower-limb wounds in horses compared to untreated wounds (Dart et al. 2015). Dressings can either provide moisture to the wound, maintain moisture at the wound, or remove moisture at the wound. Figure 7.4 illustrates relative moisture control at the wound site. Dressings with red bars remove moisture, dressings with no color simply keep the same amount of moisture at the wound side, and dressings in green add moisture to the wound. The size of the bar indicates relative moisture control. Dressings are also described by their occlusiveness. Completely occlusive dressings hold all exudate in where non-occlusive dressings allow exudate to move relatively freely through the dressing. There are many levels of occlusiveness in dressings. It is important to choose the right level of moisture control to provide the best environment for wound healing (Myers 2004a [Dressing Selection and Bandaging]). Regenerative therapies (e.g., platelet-rich plasma,

**Figure 7.4** Image showing how dressing types impact moisture management. Red bars indicate dressings that remove moisture. Green bars indicate dressings that provide moisture.

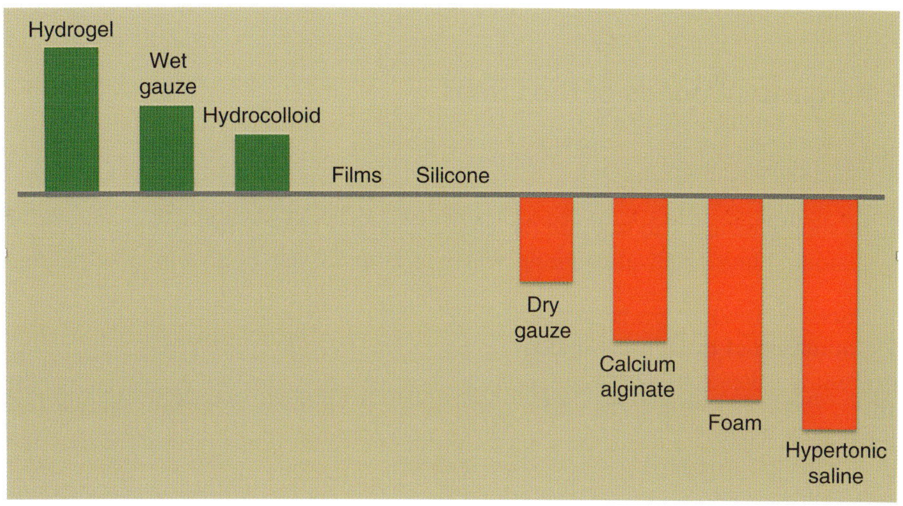

amniotic membrane and mesenchymal stem cells) may be incorporated into wound-healing repair and may function as scaffolds, cells, and/or bioactive factors (Dahlgren 2018).

1) Infected or necrotic wounds: In this stage of wound healing, debridement dressings should be combined with the wound debridement techniques previously described. Examples of debridement dressings include hypertonic saline, antimicrobial dressings, honey, and negative pressure devices.
2) Dry wounds: In this stage of wound healing, a moistening dressing should be used. Examples of moistening dressings include wet-to-wet dressings and hydrogels.
3) Granulating and contracting wounds: In this stage of wound healing, a dressing that encourages healthy granulation tissue and wound contraction should be used. Examples of granulation and wound contraction dressings include calcium alginate dressings and amnion.
4) Epithelializing wounds: In this stage of wound healing a dressing that encourages epithelialization should be used. Examples include semi-occlusive foam dressings.

### Bandages, Splints, Casts

Bandages act to protect the wound, absorb blood, exudate, bacteria and necrotic material, prevent contamination, minimize swelling, stabilize the limb, and decrease motion (Eggleston 2018a [Bandages]). Bandages are made up of different layers. The primary dressing is the layer that is directly adjacent to the wound. Those dressings are covered in the previous section. The next layer is often a compression layer with roll cotton, combine cotton, or reusable quilts. The next layer is typically roll gauze. Wide gauze is better than narrow gauze for distributing pressure. The last layer is another compression material such as VetWrap. It is common to use some type of elastic bandage at the top and bottom of the bandage to keep debris from getting inside the bandage. Finally, consider immobilizing wounds with casts and splints in areas of high motion to improve wound healing (Eggleston 2018a [Bandages]).

1) Select the appropriate primary dressing and cover with either gauze or elastic bandage without applying any pressure.
2) Apply an appropriate compression layer (roll cotton, sheet cotton, combine cotton, etc.)
3) Apply wide width (at least 4-in. [10 cm], preferably 6-in. [15 cm]) gauze with pressure, leaving the proximal 1 cm and distal 1 cm of the cotton open. Overlap the gauze by 50% when wrapping to evenly distribute pressure.
4) Apply a compression layer such as VetWrap to provide additional compression.
5) Apply some type of elastic bandage such as Elastikon to cover the top and bottom of the bandage.
6) *Apply immobilization layer:*
   a) Various types of immobilization are possible: fiberglass casts, cast or splint bandages, or other immobilization devices such as the Kimsey splint.
   b) Fiberglass cast: apply multiple layers of fiberglass cast material (6–8 layers for half-limb casts; 10–14 for full-limb casts).
   c) Cast bandage: apply fiberglass casting material directly over a Robert Jones or other bandage.
   d) Splint bandage: affix with 2-in. (5 cm) wide white tape or Duct tape.
   e) Kimsey Leg Saver Splint: apply directly to lower limb over Robert Jones bandage.

## Emergency Wounds of the Limbs

When triaging limb wounds, it is important to evaluate the horse's ability to bear weight on the limb(s). When a major fracture, collateral ligament rupture, or luxation has been sustained, the alignment of the limb may be grossly abnormal, and steps should be taken to stabilize the limb and relieve anxiety prior to performing more diagnostics, such as radiographic evaluation. Limb stabilization for referral is an essential step in fracture management and is discussed in Chapters 5 and 8.

### Examination of the Limb Wounds

A thorough examination of the wound is imperative to help determine appropriate management steps (Box 7.4). Follow these steps below:

## Box 7.4 Limb Wound Evaluation

1) **Assess for gross malalignment or instability of the limb**: If present, restrain the horse (mechanical ± chemical restraint), apply a bandage and/or temporary coaptation, and obtain radiographic images to assess the nature of the injury prior to contacting an equine referral center (see Chapters 5 and 8).
2) **Watch the horse walk**: If severe lameness (Grade 4–5/5) is present in the absence of gross malalignment or limb instability, the horse should not be walked more than a few steps.
3) **Examine and palpate the wound**: Palpate the limb for evidence of fracture, soft-tissue support injury, or communication with a synovial structure. If the wound is deep or open, clipping the hair (with a #10 blade) and scrubbing the wound with 0.1% povidone iodine or 0.05% chlorhexidine and sterile, isotonic saline may be performed in the standing, sedated horse. Wound evaluation and palpation may be more appropriate in lateral recumbency in young foals (<2–3 months of age).
4) **Achieve hemostasis**: If a major vessel has been lacerated or there is significant hemorrhage, it may be appropriate to place a hemostat or a ligature on the vessel (2–0 absorbable suture). If this is not possible, a pressure bandage can be applied prior to imaging.
5) **Perform diagnostic imaging**: Once the wound has been localized to a specific region or region(s), imaging is appropriate. Radiography is commonly performed prior to ultrasonography, but the order of diagnostic imaging may be dependent upon the nature of the injury and the equipment available.
   a) **Radiography**: A complete radiographic series of 2–4 views, including orthogonal projections, is indicated for many limb wounds. Radiographs can reveal the presence of hairline fractures, bone trauma, osteochondral fragmentation, bone sequestrae, some foreign bodies (e.g., metallic), and occasionally synovial sepsis, if gas is present (Figure 7.5a and b). Note: while radiographs can be used to confirm a diagnosis of synovial sepsis, they should never be used to rule out synovial sepsis since radiographs are not sensitive for early synovial sepsis diagnosis.
   b) **Ultrasound**: Ultrasound is more sensitive for the diagnosis of synovial sepsis and detection of most foreign bodies compared to radiographs; however, false negatives occur, especially in the acute period. Ultrasonographic

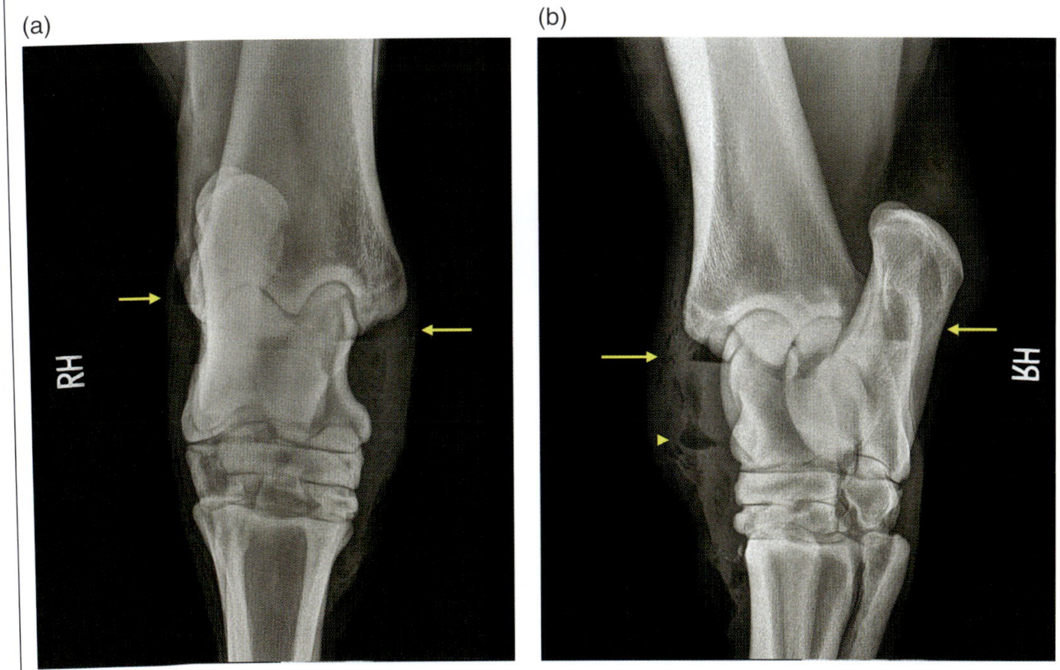


**Figure 7.5** (a) Dorsoplantar (DP) and (b) dorsolateral-plantaromedial oblique (DLPMO) radiographic projections from a horse sustaining a wound (arrowhead) to the dorsomedial aspect of the right tarsus. The wound communicated with the tarsocrural (or tibiotarsal) joint as evidenced by the gas opacities at the proximal aspect of the joint (arrows), with several small loculated gas opacities within the subcutaneous tissues dorsomedially.

signs of synovial sepsis include synovial effusion, synovial thickening, increased synovial fluid echogenicity, and hyperechogenic spots and fibrinous loculations (Beccati et al. 2015). US can also detect superficial bone trauma/fragmentation and can be useful for differentiating cellulitis from synovial joint sepsis or for locating small effusions for synoviocentesis.

6) **Make a management plan**: Referral should be considered for injuries requiring specialist care, including wounds involving bones, joints, tendon sheaths, and bursae; major tendon and ligament injury or soft-tissue support disruption; and extensive degloving injury or other complicated problems. If referral is not an option, some injuries can still be effectively treated in a field scenario, as described below.

## Wounds Involving Bone

While major fractures inducing gross limb malalignment are readily apparent, certain fractures or bone trauma may be difficult to detect. If the potential for bone trauma is suspected, it is important to perform a thorough radiographic evaluation prior to anesthetizing a horse due to the potential for fracture propagation during recovery from anesthesia. Even with a thorough radiographic evaluation, some hairline fractures or small cortical bone defects (Figure 7.6a–d) can be missed; therefore, if there is potential for bone trauma, it is preferable to repair wounds and lacerations in the standing, sedated horse. Direct damage to bone or its periosteum may also result in subsequent bone sequestration and a non-healing wound (Eggleston 2018b [Special Challenges]). Radiographs may not reveal the presence of the abnormal bone and surrounding lysis until up to 21 days following healing.

If the nature of the injury or patient temperament precludes standing treatment and repair, such as with extensive tendon/ligament lacerations or synovial structure involvement, but a hairline fracture or cortical bone defect is present, then precautions should be taken prior to recovery, such as coaptation of the limb with a fiberglass cast or other coaptation device. Referral is advisable in these scenarios as fracture propagation is possible, even with appropriate coaptation.

If radiographic, ultrasonographic, or physical examination reveals that a wound involves a non-destabilizing bone injury, follow these steps below:

1) ***Perform diagnostic imaging***: Once the wound has been localized to a specific region or region(s), imaging should be performed. Radiography is commonly performed prior to ultrasonography, but the order of diagnostic imaging may be dependent upon the nature of the injury and the equipment available.
2) ***Consider referral***: Cases with intra-articular bone or osteochondral fragmentation should be referred to a specialist for arthroscopic treatment, including either fragment removal or fixation. A pressure bandage, such as a Robert Jones

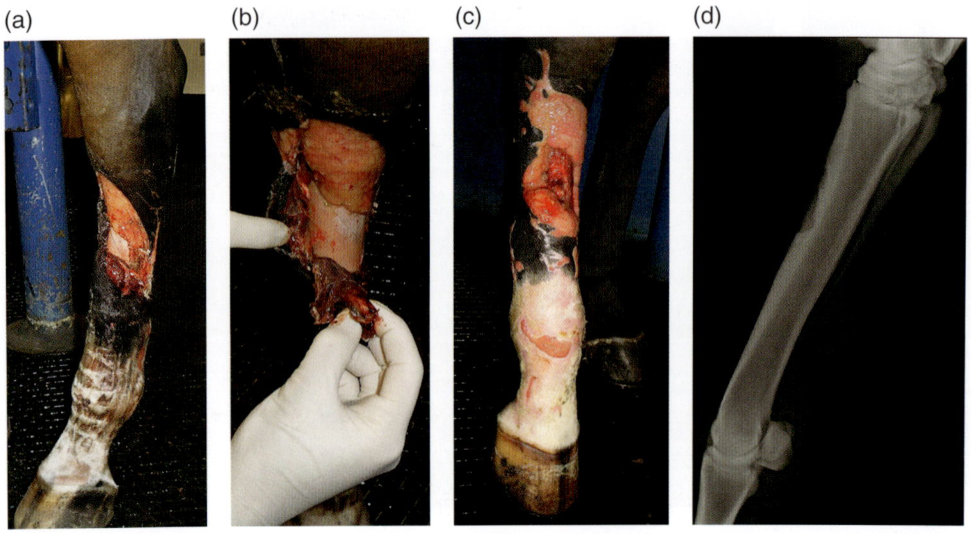

**Figure 7.6** Photos demonstrating a hindlimb laceration with a linear cortical bone defect in the third metatarsal due to fencing wire (a, b). A focal area of discoloration where the bone has been denuded of periosteum (b). Purulent drainage from the dorsal metatarsal bone three weeks post-injury correlated with increased lameness (c). Radiographs three weeks post-injury revealed extensive lysis and bone necrosis at the site of the bone devoid of periosteum (d).

bandage, is generally appropriate for stabilization of joints distal to the carpus/tarsus. If a hairline fracture is detected, a distal limb fiberglass cast may be more appropriate for coaptation. Consult your equine referral specialist to determine the specific recommendations for coaptation and shipping.

3) If referral is not an option, consultation with a specialist may still help guide on-farm treatment.
   a) **For hairline fractures or cortical defects**, the following steps may reduce the likelihood of fracture propagation:
      i) ***Stall confinement ± cross-tying***: Stall confinement to reduce ambulation may enable certain, minimally displaced hairline fractures to heal. Healing may sometimes be possible even with more extensive non-displaced fractures in a horse with a quiet temperament; however, conservative management is associated with an increased likelihood of complications, such as osteoarthritis in cases involving the joint or support limb laminitis. In horses that have already been trained to cross-tie, tying may reduce episodes of lying down, thereby reducing the likelihood for fracture propagation when rising. Straight stalls may be a viable option for the early healing period in horses accustomed to this type of stabling.
      ii) ***Placing a bandage cast*** may be another option for horses with incomplete or hairline fractures managed via stall confinement and/or cross-tying. Casting material may be applied over a Robert Jones bandage to provide additional support during healing. Bandage cast application should follow the same principles of regular cast application, stabilizing the joint above and below the fracture.

## Wounds Involving Synovial Structures

When sepsis affects a closed synovial structure, such as a joint, tendon sheath, or bursa, the horse may be severely lame or unwilling to bear weight on the limb (grades 4–5/5 AAEP lameness). However, in acute injuries, synovial contamination with an actively draining synovial structure may not result in severe lameness until the structure seals, sometimes days or weeks later. The synovial structure will typically be distended, warm, and painful to palpation (Ludwig and van Harreveld 2018). While foals with synovial sepsis are commonly febrile, in many cases, adult horses are not febrile. Subcutaneous edema and/or cellulitis may also accompany the septic synovial structure and may confound diagnosis of synovial sepsis.

If physical examination and survey diagnostic imaging reveal that a wound may involve a synovial structure, follow these steps below:

1) ***Perform additional diagnostic imaging***: Survey radiographs and ultrasonography can be used to screen for synovial sepsis as describe above. Ultrasonographic signs of synovial sepsis include synovial effusion, synovial thickening, increased synovial fluid echogenicity, and hyperechogenic spots and fibrinous loculations (Beccati et al. 2015). Ultrasound is generally more sensitive for the diagnosis of synovial sepsis than radiographs.
   a) ***Ultrasound to differentiate cellulitis from synovial sepsis***: If a horse presents with severe lameness (Grades 4–5/5) and a warm, painful limb with subcutaneous, pitting edema, differential diagnoses may include cellulitis, joint sepsis, or the combination of both. Acute distal limb edema is discussed in Chapter 8, but occasionally, cellulitis is diagnosed in the presence of questionable joint sepsis. There may be concern about performing more invasive diagnostics, such as synoviocentesis and joint distention, for fear of tracking subcutaneous infection into a sterile joint. In such cases, it may be appropriate to begin cellulitis treatment with broad-spectrum antimicrobial therapy and compression bandaging of the distal limb prior to ultrasonographic re-assessment in 24 h. If the lameness and clinical signs have not improved in 24 h and concern for joint sepsis remains, synoviocentesis should be performed.
   b) ***Radiography with a sterile probe***: The presence of gas in a synovial structure following a laceration or puncture wound suggests that the structure may have been inoculated with microorganisms. In the absence of gas but where synovial contamination with a wound or puncture is suspected, probing the wound with a sterile object, such as a malleable probe or teat canula, and obtaining orthogonal radiographic views may be able to confirm penetration of a synovial cavity. It is important to be cautious not to advance the probe too deep to induce joint penetration.
   c) ***Radiography following a "street nail injury"***: When a horse sustains a "street nail injury" after stepping on a nail, screw, or other sharp, metallic object, radiographs should be obtained with the penetrating object in place to evaluate the anatomical location of the object, as long as this can be performed without requiring the horse to ambulate further. It is important to obtain orthogonal views (e.g., dorso-palmar/plantar and lateromedial most commonly); however, non-weightbearing views are appropriate as they do not risk further penetration into deeper structures. Once diagnostic quality radiographs are obtained, the penetrating object should be removed to avoid further injury,

especially prior to shipping to a referral center. If radiographs with the object in place cannot be acquired prior to transport, use a permanent marker to circle the entrance location on the sole of the foot and save the object to be included with the horse for referral.

d) ***Radiography with contrast material***: Sterile radio-opaque contrast material, such as 240 mg/mL iohexol, can be injected aseptically into a synovial structure to assess for leakage, but this should always follow synoviocentesis. While ultrasound is now more commonly used to assess synovial wound communication, contrast material can still be effective when ultrasound is not readily available and when the wound is small or has sealed. In the case of a "street nail injury," if the penetrating object was removed by the owner or is no longer present, contrast material can be injected into the digital flexor tendon sheath, the distal interphalangeal joint, and/or the navicular bursa to assess for solar leakage (Schumacher and Stashak 2017). Contrast material has some advantages over ultrasound for "street nail injuries" since ultrasound cannot easily penetrate the hoof capsule or sole.

2) ***Perform synoviocentesis and distend synovial structure:***

a) ***Synoviocentesis and distension***: Ultrasound can be used to select an appropriate site for synoviocentesis, which should be as distant from the wound as possible in an area with intact skin and absent cellulitis. The skin should be aseptically prepared, and sterile materials should be prepared in advance for synovial fluid collection (18–22 Ga, 1–1.5 in. needles and 3- to 6-mL syringes for most distal limb sites) and distension (0.9% sodium chloride or other isotonic crystalloid and syringes appropriate for the synovial structure). Longer needles and/or larger syringes are required for more proximal limb sites, such as the elbow, shoulder, stifle and hip, in addition to the navicular bursa (Moyer et al. 2011). Synovial fluid should be collected into a syringe or directly into EDTA (purple top) and serum (red top) tubes for synovial fluid analysis. Following synoviocentesis, the structure should be distended with an appropriate volume of isotonic fluid, typically 2–4 times the normal volume of the joint. A sterile extension set may be helpful for distending the synovial structure as the increased pressure can be painful, resulting in movement or kicking (Figure 7.7a and b). Perineural anesthesia and/or a subcutaneous ring block may also facilitate this procedure.

b) ***Synovial fluid analysis*** is typically performed on fluid obtained in EDTA tubes and includes a nucleated cell count (NCC), total protein (TP), and differential cell analysis and typically requires a minimum of approximately 0.5 mL (Table 7.1. Synovial Fluid Analysis for Sepsis Diagnosis) (Steel 2008) (Box 7.5). If limited volume is available, a smear can be prepared and stained with a Wright or Wright–Giemsa stain for a differential analysis. Additional synovial fluid can be transferred to an appropriate medium for bacterial culture, including aerobic/anaerobic blood culture vials, Port-A-Culs, or other culture vials or culturettes. Blood culture vials yield the highest positive culture rates for synovial samples (Dumoulin et al. 2010; Pearson et al. 2023).

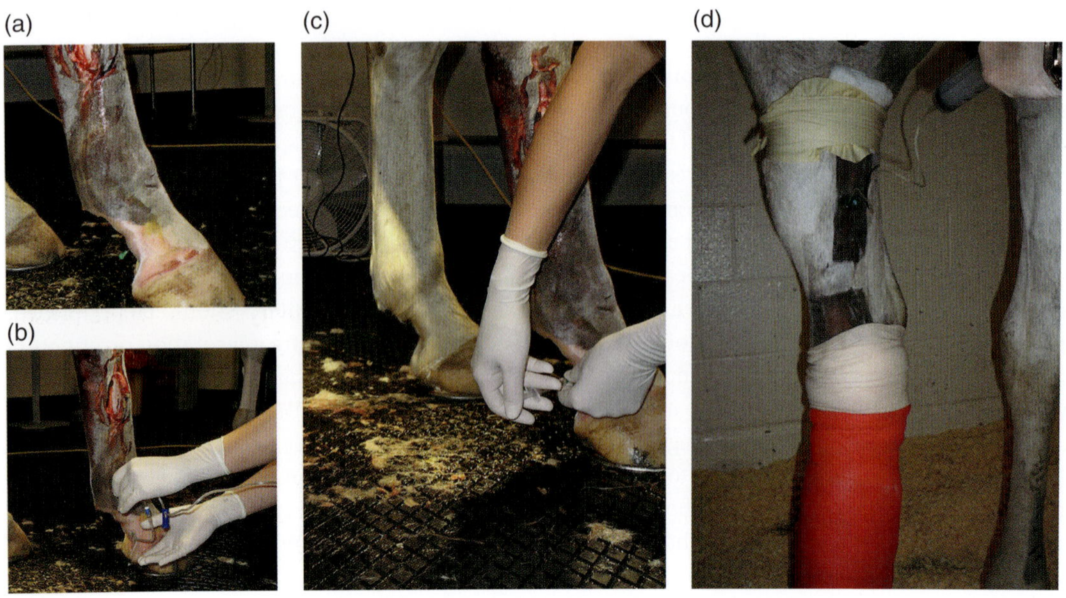

**Figure 7.7** Photos demonstrating a hindlimb laceration with exposed bone and possible synovial structure involvement. A 21 Ga needle was placed in the plantar pouch of the digital flexor tendon sheath for synoviocentesis (a), synovial distension (b), and intra-synovial infusion of amikacin (c). Synovial fluid analysis was within normal limits, and distension yielded positive pressure, so the wound was sutured, and IVRLP was performed following bandaging (d).

**Table 7.1** Synovial fluid analysis for sepsis diagnosis.

| Parameter | Non-septic | Inflammatory or possible early septic | Septic |
|---|---|---|---|
| Color | Clear to pale yellow | Variable but not turbid | Turbid, floccular, variable in color |
| Viscosity | Viscous (2–5 cm mucin string) | Reduced | Reduced |
| Total protein (TP) | <1.5 g/dL | 1.5–2.5 g/dL | >2.5 g/dL |
| Nucleated cell count (NCC) | <2,000 cells/μL | 10–20,000 cells/μL | >30,000 cells/μL |
| Neutrophil % of NCC | <10% of NCC | 20–80% | ≥90% (often degenerate neutrophils) |

**Box 7.5 Synovial Fluid Analysis**

Table 7.1provides cutoff values to help clinicians discriminate between septic and non-septic synovitis, but it is critical to interpret these results in the context of clinical examination and lameness findings. When NCCs and TP are high, septic arthritis is relatively easy to diagnose. However, early infection is difficult to diagnose as parameters may not meet these thresholds in the first 12–24 h post-injury (Ludwig and van Harreveld 2018; Steel 2008). While synovial fluid analysis and cytology can help assist with the diagnosis of sepsis, it alone is insufficient to provide a definitive diagnosis.

Efforts continue to develop improved diagnostics for the detection of early synovial sepsis, including evaluation of synovial fluid enzymes and confirmation with bacterial culture and/or 16S ribosomal DNA PCR (16s rDNA).

3) ***Consider referral***: Cases with suspected synovial structure involvement should ideally be referred to a specialist for arthroscopic, tenosocopic, or bursoscopic debridement and medical therapy.
4) If referral is not an option, successful on-farm treatment may be performed, especially if sepsis is diagnosed acutely, contamination is minimal, and the joint is superficial or readily accessible for needle lavage.
   a) ***Synovial structure lavage***: Lavage of the affected synovial structure is the mainstay of synovial joint or structure involvement when arthro-, teno-, or bursoscopic treatment is not possible (Ludwig and van Harreveld 2018). Sedation and perineural anesthesia facilitate lavage of distal limb structures. IV anesthesia can be used for foals or intractable horses once other bone trauma has been ruled out with radiographs and/or ultrasonography. Multiple, large gauge (18–14 Ga) needles are placed for ingress and egress of fluids in as many compartments as possible (i.e., dorsal and palmar/plantar, lateral and medial, proximal and distal), as appropriate for the synovial structure (Figure 7.8a–c). Sterile, isotonic fluids should be lavaged through the structure using either a hand-held pressure bag or directly via syringe. Aim for larger volumes (3 to 5-L) for fetlock, carpal, and tarsal joints and digital flexor tendon sheaths, with a minimum of 1-L for smaller joints (Ludwig and van Harreveld 2018). Lavage may need to be repeated more than once.
   b) ***Locoregional antimicrobial therapy***: Locoregional antimicrobial therapy should be emphasized in addition to systemic antimicrobials (Brumbaugh 2005; Hanson 2018). Enterobacteriaceae spp. are commonly cultured from joint infections resulting from penetrating wounds (Richardson and Stewart 2019); however, *Staphylococcus aureus*, *Pseudomonas* spp., and other staphylococci spp. are also commonly identified in cases of synovial sepsis (Ludwig and van Harreveld 2018). Antimicrobial choices should be guided by culture & sensitivity results, where possible (Adam and Southwood 2006).
      i) ***Direct injection***: intra-articular or intra-synovial injection can be performed immediately post-lavage (Figure 7.7c). Care should be used to choose an antimicrobial that is appropriate for the source of infection, compatible with the synovial environment, and with consideration of antimicrobial stewardship principles to minimize development of antimicrobial resistance (Brumbaugh 2005; Hanson 2018; Pearson et al. 2023; Pezzanite et al. 2022).
      ii) ***Intravenous regional limb perfusion (IVRLP)*** achieves high local concentrations in synovial structures while minimizing adverse systemic effects such as nephrotoxicity. IVRLP is performed in the sedated horse, commonly after IV detomidine ± butorphanol sedation, and placement of a tourniquet (pneumatic or wide elastic Esmarch-type bandage) proximal to the injection site. Injection of the antimicrobial diluted in an appropriate volume of saline or isotonic solution is made with the tourniquet remaining in place for a duration of 15–20 mins (Figure 7.7d) (Biasutti et al. 2021; Kelmer 2016). Use approximately 30–50 mL for foals or distal to the carpus/tarsus in adult horses and 60–100 mL for sites proximal to the carpus/tarsus.

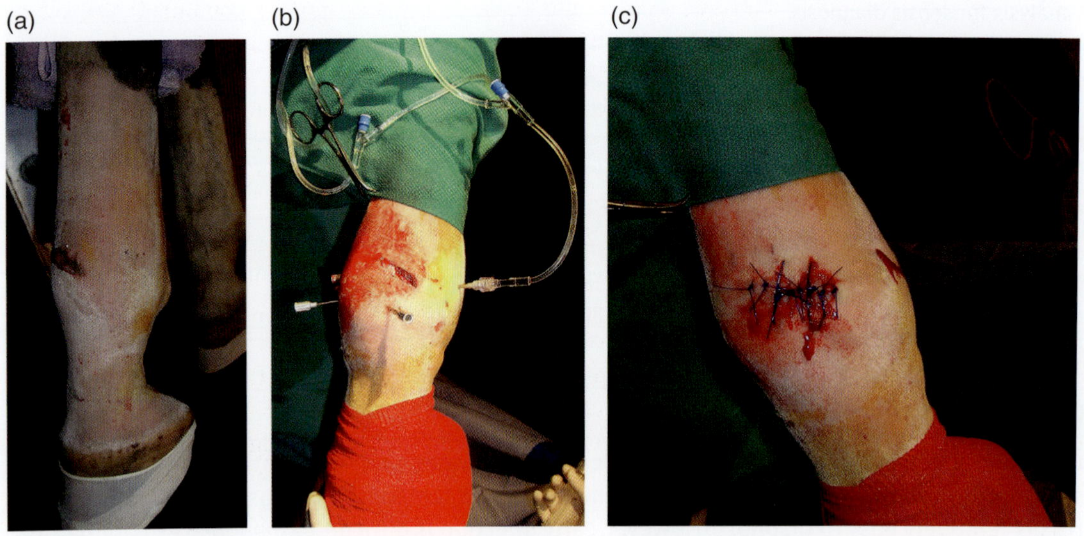


Figure 7.8 (a) Small wound communicating with the dorsal aspect of the fetlock joint. (b) Needle lavage with 14–16Ga needles in the dorsomedial, dorsolateral, plantaromedial, and plantarolateral pouches of the fetlock joint performed under general anesthesia. (c) Sutured wound prior to bandage application for recovery.

c) ***Systemic antimicrobial therapy***: Broad-spectrum antimicrobial therapy may be instituted; however, locoregional delivery should be prioritized. Common systemic antimicrobial combinations include a beta-lactam or cephalosporin combined with an aminoglycoside, such as gentamicin or amikacin. If possible, synovial fluid should be obtained for bacterial culture and sensitivity testing prior to instituting empirical therapy, and antimicrobial choice should be guided by culture and sensitivity results, once available.

d) ***Analgesia and pain management***: Synovial sepsis can induce severe lameness, leaving horses at risk for complications such as support limb laminitis (Ludwig and van Harreveld 2018). Analgesia is commonly provided by systemic non-steroidal anti-inflammatories, such as phenylbutazone or flunixin meglumine, which may provide sufficient pain relief in combination with compression bandaging. Additional analgesia can be provided by perineural anesthesia with bupivacaine or bupivacaine liposome injectable solution. If pain is severe and recalcitrant, caudal epidural anesthesia may be required for hindlimb synovial sepsis, or other analgesic techniques such as systemic ketamine may be attempted. Referral or euthanasia may be appropriate when pain is uncontrollable.

e) ***Bandaging***: Compression bandaging protects synovial structures and deeper tissues from contamination and infection, while counterpressure provides pain relief and decreases edema. Open distal limb synovial structures should be bandaged with a sterile, non-adherent dressing and gauze, followed by sterile roll cotton or a combine bandage, brown gauze, elastic bandage, and sealed with elastic bandage tape at the top and bottom. Proximal limb wounds communicating with synovial structures are more difficult to bandage, but similar principles of applying sterile non-adherent dressings secured with a tie-over or stent bandage may be appropriate for proximal limb structures.

## Wounds Involving Tendons and Ligaments

Due to the minimal soft-tissue coverage, distal limb lacerations commonly affect multiple soft-tissue structures, including tendons and ligaments. The long and lateral digital extensor tendons are commonly involved in hindlimb wounds or degloving injuries, and the common and lateral digital extensor tendons can be involved in forelimb wounds. Fortunately, extensor tendon wounds will often heal with minimal long-term effects on musculoskeletal function, even with significant loss of extensor tendon tissue (Caston 2012). Wounds involving the flexor tendon bundle or suspensory apparatus result in more significant functional impairments with a poorer prognosis for recovery and even survival.

If physical examination and survey diagnostic imaging reveal tendon and/or ligament involvement, follow the steps below:

1) ***Determine the need for limb immobilization:***
   a) **Suspensory apparatus disruption**: Wounds that disrupt the suspensory apparatus (i.e., the suspensory ligament, proximal sesamoid bones, or distal sesamoidean ligaments) result in complete loss of the fetlock support apparatus and the inability to bear weight on the limb. For wounds that cause complete suspensory apparatus disruption,

immediate stabilization of the limb with a Kimzey splint, monkey splint, or cast coaptation combined with a 2×4 splint to align the metacarpus/–tarsus and digits is essential to prevent further trauma, including neurovascular disruption, thrombosis, or other irreversible trauma (Dahlgren 2017).

b) **Collateral ligament rupture**: Complete rupture of collateral ligaments can induce limb instability and, in some cases, limb malalignment. Lameness is usually severe to non-weightbearing. If the limb is grossly malaligned or the horse is unable to bear weight and medial–lateral instability is detected on palpation, coaptation should be applied as described in Chapters 5 and 8 as appropriate for the location of instability.

c) **Flexor tendon injury**: Most wounds involving the flexor tendons will affect superficial structures first, progressively involving deeper structures. Complete transection of the superficial digital flexor tendon results in partial loss of fetlock support and fetlock hyperextension, but weightbearing is still possible. Complete transection of the deep digital flexor tendon causes pathognomonic dorsiflexion of the pedal bone and hoof. Complete transection of both the superficial and deep digital flexor tendons causes more severe fetlock hyperextension and dorsiflexion of the pedal bone and hoof. Horses with complete transection of either flexor tendon, but especially the combination of both, will benefit from bandaging and coaptation support. The combination of a heel wedge and coaptation that aligns the bony column as described in Chapters 5 and 8 will improve comfort and protect the injured structures during the healing process.

d) **Extensor tendon injury**: Complete transection of the extensor tendon bundle, especially in the hindlimb, can acutely interfere with the protraction phase of the stride (Schumacher and Stashak 2017). Application of a dorsal or palmar/plantar splint with a Robert Jones bandage to return the limb to normal alignment will restore the ability to protract the limb, relieve anxiety, and promote ambulation.

2) ***Determine if a synovial structure is involved***: If palpation of the limb or diagnostic imaging confirms that a synovial structure is involved in addition to the tendon/ligament injury, referral for specialist care is recommended. If synovial sepsis is questionable, then synoviocentesis and distension of the synovial structure should be performed as described above in *Wounds Involving Synovial Structures.*

3) ***Consider referral***: Even if a synovial structure is not involved, referral for specialist care should be considered for extensive wounds involving complete or partial transection of one or more flexor tendons.

4) ***If referral is not an option***, successful on-farm treatment may be performed, especially for wounds involving extensor tendons or partial rupture of flexor tendons outside of synovial structures. If flexor tendon involvement is documented, owners should be forewarned about the potential for performance limitation due to fibrotic scar tissue, contracture, adhesion formation, or repeated injury post-healing. If complete suspensory apparatus disruption is present and referral is not an option, euthanasia should be considered.

   a) **Wound management**: General principles of wound cleaning and debridement apply as described in *Emergency Wound Evaluation and Management.* For extensor tendon lacerations, it is critical to sharply debride any necrotic, avascular, or heavily contaminated tendon tissue with a scalpel blade (#10 or #22). Follow principles of wound lavage as described above. When minimal tissue loss is present, the extensor tendon can be sutured with monofilament absorbable suture (0 to 2–0) using an interrupted pattern, such as a horizontal mattress pattern or 3-loop-pulley (Dahlgren 2017). However, suturing of extensor tendons is often not necessary, especially when significant tissue is missing (Figure 7.9a–d). Extensor tendon tissue will typically heal adequately via fibrosis with just apposition of the superficial tissues and bandaging and splinting to return the limb to normal alignment.

   b) **Tendon and ligament suture patterns**: Referral for specialist care is generally recommended when a flexor tendon is completely transected. If referral is not an option, the transected tendon or ligament is not within a synovial structure, and the edges of the tendon are healthy and can be apposed with minimal tension, the following suture patterns can be used to appose the tissue with monofilament, absorbable suture. Suture materials that maintain their strength for longer periods of time, such as polydioxanone, are recommended for suturing tendon due to the longer tissue-healing times of tendon and ligament tissue.

      i) **Locking loop, double-locking loop, and three-loop pulley patterns.**
      ii) **Krackow, continuous cruciate, and far–near–near–far patterns.**
      iii) **Bunnell–Mayer and Mason–Allen patterns.**

## Wound Management and Closure Techniques

General principles of wound closure timing and techniques also apply to limb wounds. While primary closure of acute, non-grossly contaminated limb wounds is preferred where possible, delayed-primary closure may be appropriate when contamination is extensive and/or presentation is delayed, leading to extensive edema and retraction of

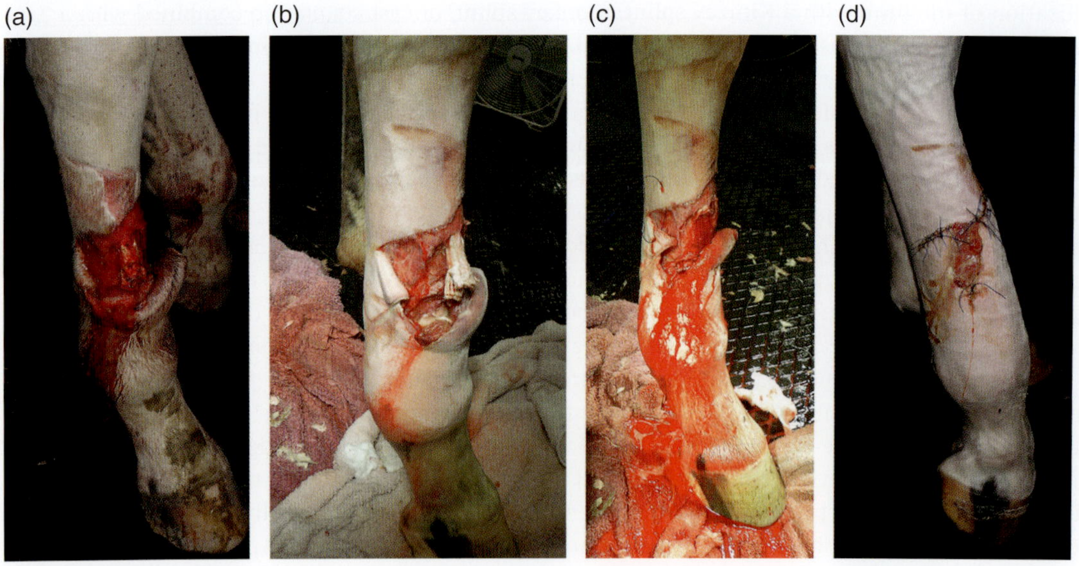


**Figure 7.9** Distal limb wound with transection of the combined long and lateral digital extensor tendons (a). Wound post-clipping and scrubbing (b) and following scalpel debridement and transection of debris-contaminated extensor tendons as the wound is beginning to be sutured (c). One-week post-injury, revealing apposition of the repaired skin edges with a small area that is beginning to granulate (d).

the wound edges. In degloving wounds or wounds with extensive skin loss due to the laceration or skin necrosis, second-intention healing may be required, with the potential for repeated debridement and subsequent skin-grafting techniques.

General principles of wound cleaning, debridement, and closure apply as described in the previous sections, *Emergency Wound Evaluation and Management* and *Wound Management Decisions*. The location of distal limb wounds with high tension, high motion, and limited vascular and soft-tissue coverage amplify the importance of skin preservation and tension-relieving suture techniques. Primary or delayed-primary closure techniques are recommended, when possible, to avoid complications such as excessive granulation tissue formation and chronic inflammation and infection that will delay wound healing. In addition, because of the high-motion areas over distal limb joints, immobilization may be required for some distal limb wounds. Because horses are prone to cast complications, fiberglass coaptation may be used in some cases, especially for heel bulb and hoof wounds, whereas splints and bi-valved splint bandages may be preferred for the metacarpal/–tarsal and antebrachial/crus locations.

Wound management techniques that may assist with distal limb wounds include:

1) ***Tension-relieving suture patterns:***
   a) ***Near–far–far–near.***
   b) ***Near–near–far–far.***
   c) ***Vertical mattress.***
   d) ***Horizontal mattress.***
   e) ***Cruciate suture.***
   f) ***Stents:*** *Any of the above tension-relieving suture patterns can be combined with stents to distribute pressure across the wound margins. Commercially available stents or polypropylene or red-rubber tubing can be cut to size.*
2) **Stent bandages**: "Tie-over" bandages can be used to reduce tension on suture lines and are more applicable for wounds proximal to the carpus/tarsus, especially wounds including the elbow and stifle and more proximal. For these bandages, monofilament, non-absorbable suture can be used to create "loops" on either edge of the wound, several cm away from the wound edge. A sterile towel or dressing can be applied over the wound, and sterile umbilical tape can be tied in a "shoelace" pattern to relieve tension directly on the sutured wound edges.
3) **Tension-relieving incisions**: Multiple, short (~0.5–1 cm), staggered, full-thickness, vertical skin incisions may enable closure of distal limb wounds under significant tension.

4) **Immobilization**: Fiberglass casts, cast bandages, splint bandages, and other commercially available immobilization devices may be used to provide temporary immobilization to allow wounds over distal limb joints to heal and are described in more detail in *Wound Management Decisions* in this chapter and Chapter 5.
5) **Negative pressure wound therapy (NPWT)**: Negative pressure wound therapy (NPWT) is thought to enhance wound healing in both humans and animals and involves the intermittent or continuous application of sub-atmospheric pressure (approximately 125 mmHg) to a wound (Cantatore et al. 2023; Launois et al. 2021). The advantages are reported to include increase of local blood flow, decrease in wound edema, removal of exudate, improved granulation tissue formation, reduced numbers of bacteria in the wound as well as signaling of angiogenesis and stimulation of anti-inflammatory cytokines (Launois et al. 2021).

## Complications of Limb Wounds

Complications of limb wounds are numerous (Hanson 2009). Fortunately, many complications can be managed with additional treatment and wound debridement and management, although some complications may be life-threatening.

Potential complications of limb wounds include:

1) Wound dehiscence.
   a) High motion, high tension areas (e.g., distal limb joints).
   b) Infection.
2) Wound infection.
3) Exuberant granulation tissue (proud flesh).
4) Chronic, non-healing wounds.
5) Sequestrum/sequestrae formation: avascular necrosis of bone, common after cortical bone is denuded of periosteum, especially in hindlimb degloving injuries (Figure 7.6).
6) Osteonecrosis, osteitis, and osteomyelitis.
7) Antimicrobial resistance and/or multi-drug resistance.
8) Contralateral or support limb laminitis.
9) Fracture propagation due to bone trauma, cortical defects, or hairline fractures.
10) Neoplastic transformation (rare).

## Prognosis and Outcome

The prognosis for limb wounds is dependent upon several factors, including bone and synovial structure involvement, tendon and ligament involvement, the degree of contamination, the presence of and antimicrobial resistance profiles of microorganisms, and the duration of time prior to medical treatment. Rapid, aggressive treatment of wounds, especially those involving synovial structures, improve the prognosis.

### Bone

Small osteochondral fragment with minimal articular involvement = better prognosis, can be removed arthroscopically
Large articular fragments, comminution, or displacement = worse prognosis
Non-articular sequestration or avascular necrosis = better prognosis than articular

### Synovial Structure

Multi-joint or multi-structure involvement = worse prognosis
Established infection of synovial structure carries a worse prognosis than acute involvement or communication
Foals = worse prognosis, often due to multiple joints or other comorbidities

### Tendon/Ligament

Multiple structure involvement = worse prognosis
Complete transection of a tendon or ligament carries a worse prognosis compared to partial transection injury
Flexor tendon involvement = much worse prognosis than extensor tendon involvement

## Hoof Trauma

### Wound Examination

The foot is complex with many anatomic structures involved including: hoof wall, third phalanx, navicular bone, deep digital flexor tendon, multiple ligaments, navicular bursa, digital tendon sheath, nerves, and vessels (Redding and O'Grady 2012). The proximal interphalangeal or pastern joint is also located approximately 2cmm above the coronary band and injury to the hoof or heel bulb region may also involve this synovial cavity. Consequently, all structures must be assessed to determine their involvement in the wound. Radiographs should be procured at the minimum. Ultrasound, CT, and MRI should also be considered. To identify possible synovial involvement, pressurization with isotonic saline or polyionic replacement fluid should be performed (Figure 7.10b). In cases of synovial involvement, synovial lavage and regional limb perfusion are the most effective methods to reduce infection risk.

### Types of Hoof Injury

Hoof injuries can take many forms. The most common is the heel bulb laceration (Figure 7.10a–c). Heel bulb lacerations can be relatively superficial or include multiple other structures such as nerves, vessels, tendons, ligaments, navicular bursa, or tendon sheath. Other injuries include penetrating injuries to the bottom of the foot (e.g., nails) and lacerations/avulsions of the hoof wall (Burba 2013; Céleste and Szöke 2005; Stashak 2002) (see Chapter 8).

### Lacerations Involving the Coronary Band

Lacerations of the coronary band should be sutured primarily whenever possible. Wounds having significant swelling, drainage, or infection benefit from delayed-primary closure in combination with wound debridement. In cases where too

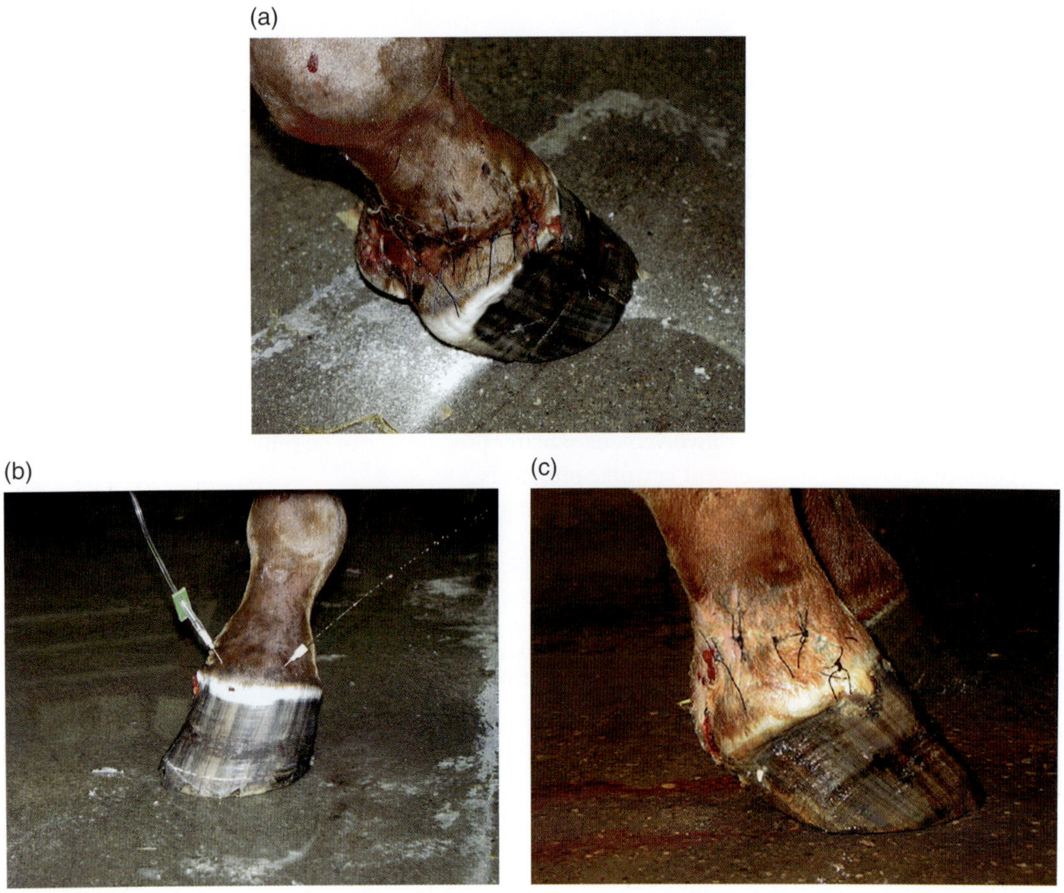

**Figure 7.10** Photos of a heel bulb laceration in a horse. Laceration (a) and joint lavage (b) 24 h after closure. Another image of the healed wound three weeks after closure immediately after foot cast removal (c).

much tissue has been lost, second-intention healing will be required. Occasionally it is difficult to determine the integrity of the coronary band. In some instances, the coronary band appears damaged when it is not and in others it appears healthy when it is damaged. In some horses, it can take up to four weeks to fully determine the impact on the coronary band. Consequently, the coronary band should be preserved whenever possible. Clients should always be warned that hoof cracks or abnormal hoof growth may be a recurrent problem when there is damage to the coronary band.

## Hoof Repair Techniques

Primary or delayed-primary closure of heel bulb lacerations should be attempted whenever possible. Sharp debridement along with debridement dressings will help to prepare the laceration for closure. Medical maggots can be used in cases of deep infection (Burba 2013). A foot cast should be placed to reduce movement and increase the likelihood of successful wound closure and healing (Stewart et al. 2009) (Figure 7.11a and b). Hoof wall avulsions can be treated with primary or delayed-primary closure of the skin component and wire "lacing" of the hoof wall component (Figure 7.12a–e). In this figure there are two cases: the first horse had a primary soft-tissue component that was sutured using tension-relieving sutures. The involved hoof wall was drilled with a 12-Ga needle and Size 2 nylon was placed through the holes and the hoof wall stabilized (Figure 7.12a). Figure 7.12b was taken after three weeks in a foot or slipper cast. In the second horse, the soft tissues were normal, but the hoof wall had been avulsed. The distal section of avulsed hoof wall was resected, and the remaining wall was sutured after drilling with a 12-Ga needle using Size 2 nylon (Figure 7.12c). The foot was placed in a foot/slipper cast (Figure 7.12d) for two weeks. The hoof wall healed back in place and the foot continued to grow normally (Figure 7.12e). The author has had better success with suturing the skin component and removal of the affected hoof wall to allow it to grow back over time. A bar shoe can be placed on the foot with adequate frog support until the hoof wall grows back toward the ground surface (Figure 7.13a–c).

## Complications of Hoof Injury

The most serious complication of hoof injury involves septic synovial structures (Redding and O'Grady 2012). It is imperative to identify synovial structure involvement early in the traumatic period. Painful neuromas can occur when the digital nerve has been severed. Coffin bone osteomyelitis can occur with penetrating injuries. Some lacerations cause enough trauma to the coronary band that normal hoof growth cannot be achieved, and a hoof crack is always present.

## Prognosis and Outcome

The prognosis for heel bulb lacerations without synovial, ligament, or tendon involvement is generally good. Scar tissue formation at the laceration site can lead to eventual lameness. Painful neuromas can also occur and should be discussed with clients at the time of presentation. Synovial, tendon, and/or ligament involvement will decrease the prognosis.

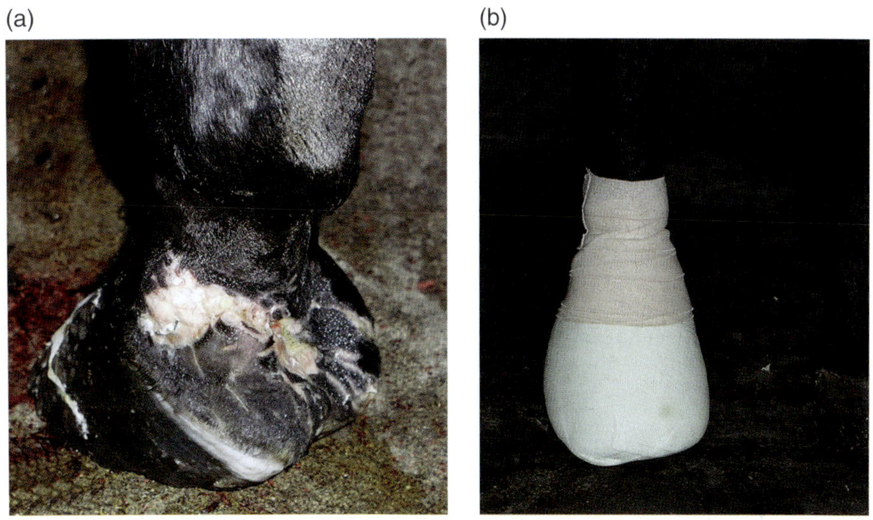

**Figure 7.11** Photos of a heel bulb laceration in a horse following initial repair and early healing prior to (a) and after placement (b) of a foot or slipper cast.

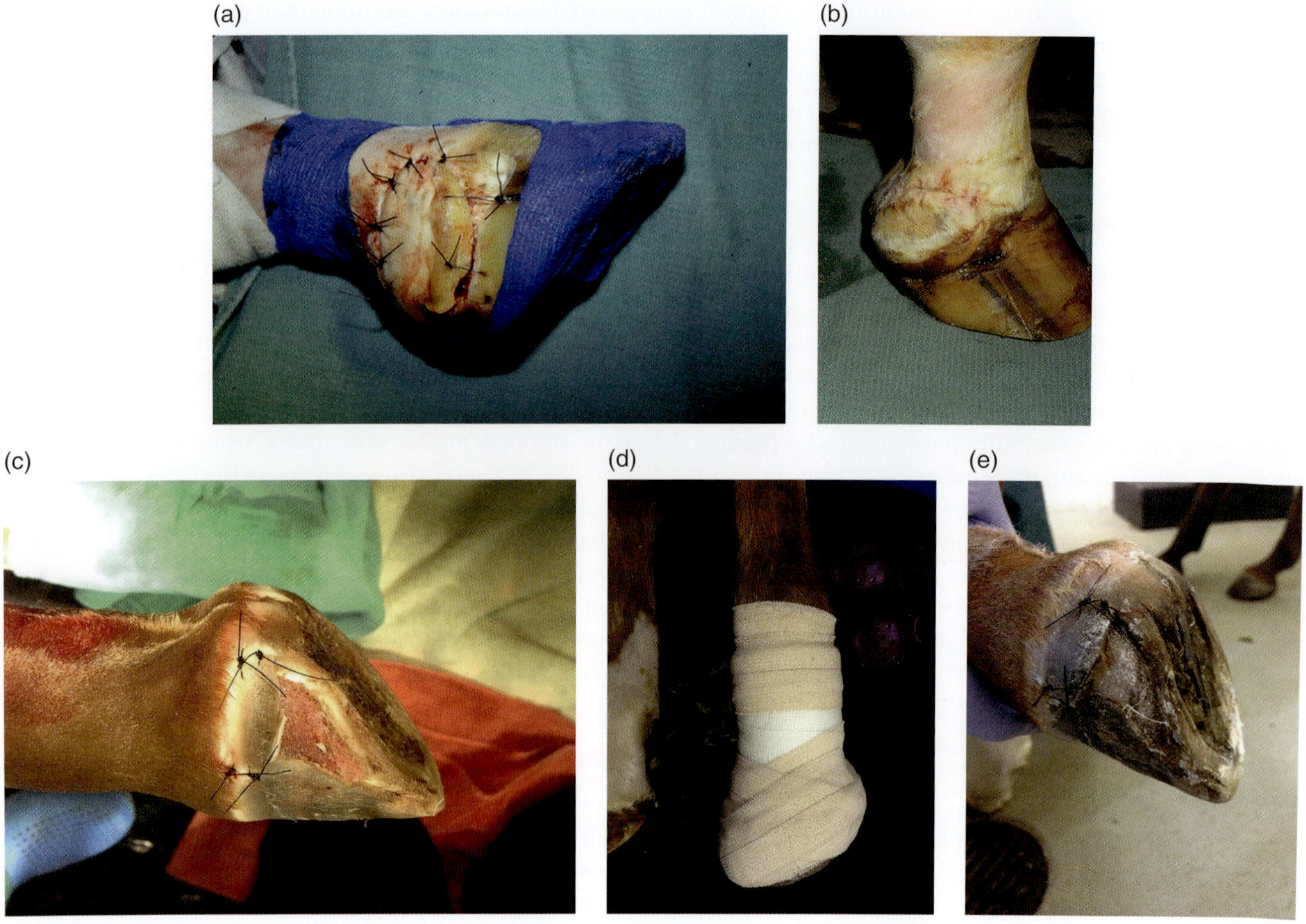


**Figure 7.12** Photos of two horses after heel/hoof laceration repair: Case 1: At time of surgical repair (a), and three weeks after surgical repair at the time of hoof/slipper cast removal (b). Case 2: After surgical repair and removal of the distal hoof wall (c), after hoof/slipper cast application (d), and two weeks following surgical repair, immediately after hoof/slipper cast removal (e).

## Emergency Wounds of the Body and Head

### Wound Management and Closure Techniques

Wounds of the body and head are managed as described above. Wounds of the body generally heal faster than limb wounds and are more amenable to primary or delayed-primary closure as there is often less contamination and tissue loss (Barber 2005; Gaughan 2018). Wounds of the head often heal well because of an excellent blood supply to the head region, and even chronic or contaminated wounds may be candidates for primary wound closure. Wound debridement of head wounds should be performed cautiously, preserving as much tissue and skin as possible to facilitate accurate reconstruction as well as normal function and appearance (Barber 2005). Depending on the wound area, tension-relieving techniques should be considered such as tension-relieving suture patterns (Horizontal Mattress, Vertical Mattress, Near–Far–Far–Near) as well as stents or buttons. Stents or buttons can only be used for the mattress patterns. The horizontal mattress pattern should be reserved for areas of low tension as when used for high tension closure, it will interrupt blood supply to the wound margins. It is important to assess all the deeper layers to investigate penetration into the thorax, abdomen, or skull. Radiographs are valuable when dealing with head wounds. Bone fragments that are unattached and without blood supply should be removed to reduce the possibility of sequestrum formation. Incomplete displaced skull fractures may often be elevated back into position, while complete fractures may require stabilization with orthopedic wire or suture. Wounds that involve the sinuses should be closed in at least 2 layers to reduce the likelihood of wound dehiscence secondary to airflow from the sinus. In addition, trauma to the lips, tongue, and eyelids often requires special repair techniques to achieve appropriate closure (Barber 2005).

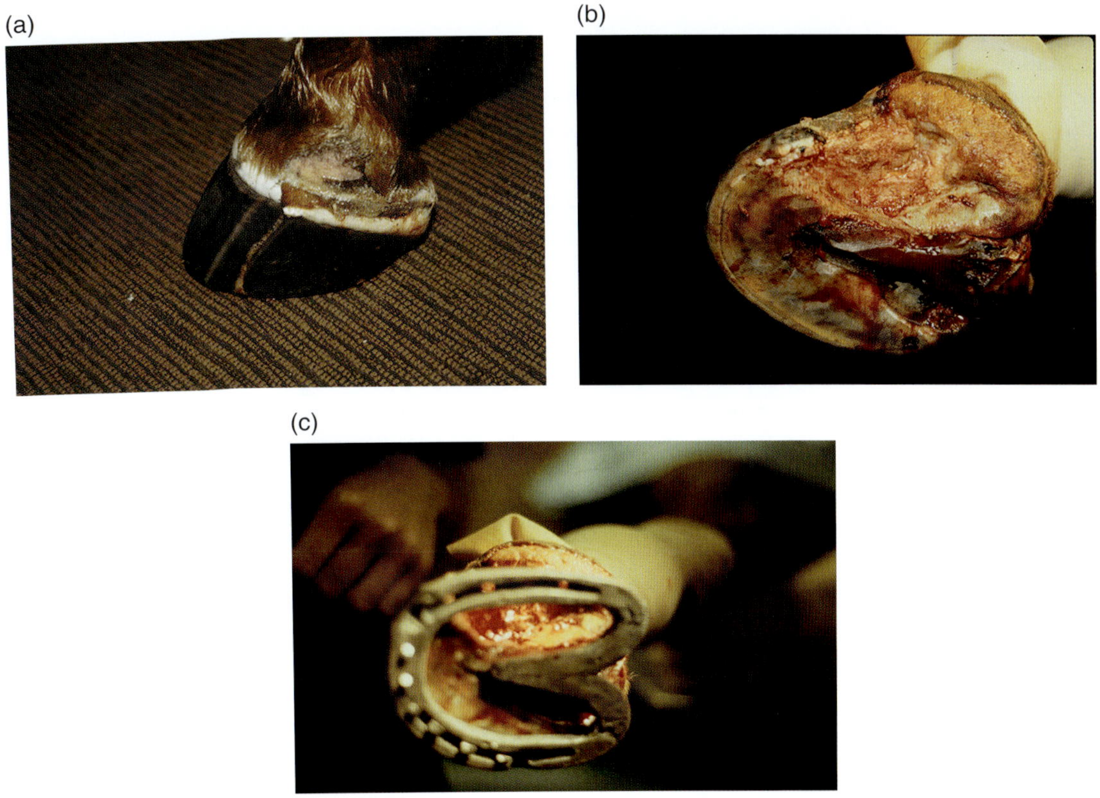

Figure 7.13 Photos of horse with a large hoof wall avulsion. Horse at presentation showing hoof wall avulsion injury (a), foot after removal of the avulsed hoof wall (b), and bar shoe with frog support prior to bandage application (c).

## Bandaging Techniques for the Body and Head

Bandages are not usually necessary for wounds of the body. However, if required, stent or "tie-over" bandages are most appropriate for wounds of the body. The head is a challenging area to bandage. There are many ways to maintain a head bandage, but due to the "conical" shape of the head, the bandages often slip toward the nose or displace over the eyes. As for other wounds, an appropriate primary dressing should be selected. This should be covered with gauze (preferably antimicrobial gauze to reduce bacterial penetration). The author has found that placing a strip of elastic bandage from the rostral aspect of the facial crest on one side, then around the poll behind the ears, and to the rostral aspect of the facial crest on the other side that is incorporated into the bandage will help to keep the bandage from slipping. Cast material can be used to provide a protective "helmet" when there are facial bone fractures.

## Complications of Body and Head Wounds

The most common complication of head and body wounds is dehiscence secondary to movement and/or infection. Consequently, it is important to make sure the bacterial numbers in the wound are low enough for closure. It may mean that 24–48 h of debridement dressings along with sharp debridement should be performed prior to closure. Large wounds of the body and head benefit from drain placement to provide ventral drainage and avoid seroma formation, infection and/or dehiscence. Another complication of head wounds is fistula formation with the sinuses or nasal cavity. Appropriate wound debridement and multi-layer closure will help to reduce the chance of fistula development as well as wound dehiscence. Sinus lavage is often indicated in cases of trauma with sinus involvement. Injuries involving the orbital rim may be associated with abnormal eye movements, corneal ulceration, or uveitis. Since the head has an excellent vascular supply, hemorrhage may be serious and require compression or other steps to control bleeding. Importantly, horses with head wounds should also be evaluated for traumatic brain injury and appropriate triage performed (see Chapter 15) (MacKay 2004).

### Prognosis and Outcome

Compared to the lower limb of the horse, the supporting tissues and blood supply are excellent in the body and head region. Wounds that are managed appropriately generally heal well leading to a good prognosis and outcome. Sinus and nasal fistulas can be quite challenging to treat, and prevention is recommended if possible. Traumatic brain injury will decrease the prognosis and increase the costs of managing head trauma in horses.

## Abdominal Injury

Abdominal injury is common in horses and may be serious especially with penetration of the abdominal cavity (Hanson 2009). Many injuries occur when horses strike an object when running or jumping. When penetration does occur, the prognosis is guarded depending upon the extent of injury and structures affected (Murray 2012). Initial triage of abdominal injury should focus on patient stabilization, followed by close evaluation of the wound and abdominal cavity.

### Patient Stabilization

#### Systemic Considerations

*STEP 1 – Perform a quick physical exam to assess the systemic stability of the patient…* *see Box 7.1.*

### Penetrating Abdominal Injury

#### Wound Factors

*STEP 2 – Immediate wound triage*

A) ***Evaluate the wound*** *considering* ***location, depth, and evidence of communication*** *of the abdominal and thoracic cavities. Communication may be confirmed with direct wound palpation, abdominocentesis, abdominal ultrasound or rectal palpation. With horses having evisceration of intestine or omentum, it is imperative that wounds are closed quickly or covered to prevent further injury.*

B) ***When the wound does not involve the abdominal cavity****: follow the steps above to lavage, debride, and close the wound. Placement of a Penrose drain to facilitate drainage may be indicated. An abdominal bandage may be useful to provide support during wound healing.*

C) ***Wounds with suspected peritoneal communication but no evisceration*** *should be closed using suture or towel clamps or packed with sterile saline-soaked gauze and protected with a full abdominal bandage. A stent bandage may also be used to prevent loss of intestines or omentum.*

D) ***When a small amount of intestine has penetrated and is exposed****: first try to lavage and replace the intestine back into the abdomen or under the skin, temporarily close the wound and then bandage and administer antibiotics prior to referral. This may be performed via standing sedation. A clean bed sheet or garbage bag may be used to support the intestines during lavage and replacement.*

E) ***When larger amounts of intestine are exposed and referral is close and possible****: lavage the intestines, then wrap a large bed sheet around the abdomen to support the intestines and prevent further injury and contamination. Wrap the sheet close to the abdomen and place Elastikon around the edges to seal the bandage. Begin antibiotics and refer the horse for abdominal exploration, lavage and assessment of intestinal or other organ injury.*

F) ***If referral is not an option****: lay the horse down under* ***short-acting chemical anesthesia****. Clip hair and disinfect around the wound, and then lavage intestines judiciously with large volumes of sterile saline or tap water if necessary.* ***Replace intestines back into abdomen*** *and close the abdominal wall defect. Place a Penrose drain under the skin to facilitate drainage. Continue medical management.*

G) ***Euthanasia is indicated for horses where abdominal penetration results in intestinal perforation and contamination or other severe abdominal or extra-abdominal injury****.*

H) ***Complications*** *of penetrating abdominal injury* ***include intestinal perforation, other abdominal organ injury, peritonitis, abscess or adhesion formation, and diaphragmatic and body wall herniation****.*

### Blunt Abdominal Trauma

#### Wound Factors

*STEP 2 – Immediate wound triage*

A) ***Evaluate the wound*** *considering* ***location, depth, and possible injury to underlying structures such as ribs, spleen, or other internal organs.*** *Communication with the abdominal and thoracic cavities is also possible but less likely compared to penetrating injury.*
B) ***Palpate the wound*** *to understand its size and depth and possible communication.*
C) ***Ultrasound the wound region*** *to determine if underlying structures are involved.* ***Evaluate the spleen with left abdominal wall trauma****, and the* ***cecum, large colon, and liver with right-sided trauma****. Rectal palpation may help determine additional abdominal injury.*
D) ***Collect abdominal fluid*** *to rule out: 1) hemoabdomen secondary to splenic or other organ hemorrhage or 2) evidence of intestinal injury.*
E) ***Consider a blood transfusion for hemoabdomen*** *if the horse has clinical evidence of shock (high heart rate, pale or white mucous membranes, poor pulse pressure, cold extremities) in acute hemorrhage*
F) *Blunt and penetrating abdominal or thoracic injury may result in* ***injury to structures outside of these cavities such as skeletal or other organ injury*** *that carries a poor prognosis for survival.*
G) ***Complications*** *of blunt abdominal trauma include* ***severe hemorrhage, splenic or intestinal injury, wound dehiscence, and diaphragmatic and body wall herniation****.*

## Thoracic Injury

Thoracic trauma in horses may be life-threatening depending upon involvement of the thoracic cavity and degree of respiratory tract compromise. Respiratory distress and shock are common consequences of trauma. Injury may occur when horses are fighting, suffer a fall, strike an object while running or jumping, or during other trauma such as vehicular accidents (Sprayberry and Barrett 2015). Many types of trauma may involve the thorax including blunt or penetrating injury, pectoral and axillary lacerations, rib fracture and flail chest, lung lacerations and contusions as well as vessel injury (Hassel 2007). Complications are common and include subcutaneous emphysema, pneumothorax, pneumomediastinum, hemothorax, diaphragmatic hernia, and pleuritis (Hanson 2009). When penetration does occur, the prognosis is usually favorable with appropriate management. Initial triage of thoracic injury should focus on patient stabilization, followed by close evaluation of the wound and thoracic and abdominal cavities (Radcliffe et al. 2009).

### Patient Stabilization

#### Systemic Considerations

*STEP 1 – Perform a quick physical exam to assess the systemic stability of the patient… see Box 7.1. Emergency management should include provision a patent airway, adequate ventilation and shock treatments.*

*In horses with thoracic trauma,* ***assess the horse for the following emergency problems****: airway obstruction, respiratory distress (associated with open or tension pneumothorax and flail chest), massive hemothorax, hemorrhagic shock, and abdominal injury.* ***Examination of thoracic injury includes****: physical exam, thoracic auscultation, wound evaluation, chest wall palpation, diagnostic thoracocentesis, ultrasound and radiographic exams, and blood gas analysis.* ***Observe the horse breathing from above*** *to appreciate thoracic wall asymmetry, rib deformity, concavity, and abnormal or paradoxic respiratory movement.*

### Penetrating Thoracic Injury

#### Wound Factors

*STEP 2 – Immediate wound triage*

A) *Examine wound quickly to assess the movement of air…* ***if air is moving into the thorax but not out during respiration, open wound immediately****. This will convert the pneumothorax from tension to open, helping to stabilize the horse. Movement of air during thoracic injury may also be appreciated via emergency thoracocentesis.* ***Pneumothorax may be open, closed, or tension*** *and is suspected when there are clinical signs of respiratory distress (tachypnea, dyspnea, nostril* *flaring, cyanotic mucous membranes, and restlessness).* ***A tension pneumothorax is most dangerous*** *and characterized by progressive respiratory effort and distress, hypoxemia, and hypotension.*

B) ***Close or bandage chest wounds immediately*** *to prevent worsening pneumothorax.* ***Close the wound with suture or pack with sterile gauze*** *and close with towel clamps. A* ***sterile airtight bandage*** *may also be placed using petrolatum dressings, kitchen plastic wrap or an Ioban drape to create an airtight seal of the thorax. Bandaging is contraindicated with flail chest as it decreases ventilation and exacerbates pulmonary injury.*

C) ***Provide intranasal or intratracheal oxygen supplementation and fluid resuscitation.*** *Oxygen delivery is indicated for horses with signs of respiratory distress or shock: tachypnea, dyspnea, tachycardia, abnormal mucous membrane color, poor pulse pressure. Provide 15 L/min oxygen supplementation in the adult horse and 5–10 L/min in smaller horses and foals. Also, provide emergency fluid resuscitation as directed by the degree of hypovolemia.*

D) ***Remove pleural air to improve alveolar ventilation*** *and further stabilize the horse. Place a 4-in. teat cannula, 14-Ga catheter or thoracostomy tube (24–36 French) high in the 12–15th intercostal space.* ***Make a stab incision and guide the cannula or chest tube directly in front of the rib*** *to avoid the intercostal blood vessels. Connect the teat cannula or catheter to an extension set with a 3-way stopcock and use a 60 mL syringe or suction device to evacuate the thorax. Following thoracic air removal, a* ***Heimlich valve*** *may be connected to the chest tube to allow continuous exiting flow.*

E) ***Examine the chest wall for stability***... *palpate the chest wall and wound for evidence of rib fractures, thoracic penetration, and presence of foreign bodies. If the chest wall moves opposite normal respiratory movements (paradoxyl motion), flail chest is present.* ***Flail chest is difficult to stabilize*** *without surgical repair under general anesthesia, and* ***referral is recommended*** *following patient stabilization.*

F) ***Wounds of the axillary, pectoral, or inguinal regions may result in severe subcutaneous emphysema.*** *Pneumomediastinum and subsequent pneumothorax may develop days later, and continued monitoring is indicated. Suture or pack wounds with saline-soaked sterile gauze and secure to the horse with a stent bandage. Limit movement of the horse with stall rest and cross tying.*

G) ***Severe pain is associated with rib fracture*** *and pleural trauma...* ***multimodal analgesia is indicated; treat with local or regional nerve blocks and systemic analgesics*** *to improve abnormal ventilation.*

H) *Penetrating injury to the thorax may damage the heart, lungs, and great vessels in addition to the chest wall, and varying degrees of hemothorax are possible.* ***Immediate triage of acute thoracic hemorrhage includes stopping hemorrhage, crystalloid fluid therapy, and whole blood transfusion. Aminocaproic acid*** *(10–20 mg/kg) may help stabilize clot formation in horses where severe hemorrhage cannot be controlled.*

I) *Thoracic injury may also involve the abdominal cavity...* ***horses having deep penetrating injury and trauma caudal to the 6th rib may suffer abdominal involvement.*** *Diaphragmatic hernias are also possible with abdominal or thoracic trauma. A complete exam of the abdomen includes wound exploration, ultrasound exam, abdominocentesis, and rectal palpation.*

J) *Referral for thoracic injury will depend upon the severity of injury and associated complications as well the need for general anesthesia.* ***Horses with smaller chest wounds, simple rib fractures without chest wall instability, modest amounts of hemothorax or pneumothorax, and trauma without deep penetration or contamination usually respond well to conservative management*** **via** ***standing techniques.***

K) ***Horses with more severe injury may require general anesthesia and surgical treatment.*** *General anesthesia under positive-pressure ventilation permits improved access to the thoracic and abdominal cavities for exploration and lavage, control of hemorrhage, removal of foreign bodies, closure of lung lacerations, repair of rib fractures, wound reconstruction, and stabilization of flail chest.*

L) *The prognosis for penetrating thoracic trauma will depend upon the severity of injury and associated complications.* ***Many sequelae of thoracic injury include****: hemothorax, pneumothorax, pneumomediastinum, subcutaneous emphysema, pleuritis, diaphragmatic hernia, rib fracture and flail chest, as well as damage to the heart, lungs, and blood vessels (*Radcliffe et al. 2009*).*

## Blunt Thoracic Trauma

### Wound Factors

*STEP 2 – Immediate wound triage*

A) ***Perform a thorough physical exam looking for evidence of blunt trauma:*** *deformation or asymmetry of the chest wall, rib fractures including flail chest, hemothorax, pneumothorax, crepitus in the region of the neck or chest, abdominal trauma, respiratory distress, and shock.*

B) ***Rib fracture or flail chest in combination with hemothorax and pulmonary contusions*** *are likely complications of blunt thoracic trauma in adult horses. The most common injuries during human blunt thoracic trauma include fractures of the thoracic cage, lung contusions and tears, myocardial contusions, aortic rupture, and tracheal damage (*Hassel 2007*).*

C) ***Provide intranasal or intratracheal oxygen supplementation and fluid resuscitation.*** *Oxygen delivery is indicated for horses with signs of respiratory distress or shock: tachypnea, dyspnea, tachycardia, abnormal mucous membrane color, poor pulse pressure. Provide 15 L/min oxygen supplementation in the adult horse and 5–10 L/min in smaller horses and foals. Also, provide emergency fluid resuscitation as directed by the degree of hypovolemia.*

D) ***Treatment of blunt thoracic injury*** *will depend upon the degree of trauma and respiratory compromise and the development of secondary complications.* ***Follow the recommendations listed above for Penetrating Thoracic Trauma*** *for the management of pneumothorax, hemothorax, rib fractures and flail chest, severe pain as well as the secondary abdominal injury and recommendations for conservative* versus *surgical management (*Radcliffe et al. 2009*).*

## Necrotizing Skin Problems

Several types of injury in horses may lead to necrosis and sloughing of affected tissues depending upon the type and extent of injury. Thermal injury to the body affects the skin and underlying tissues to various depths (1st through 4th degree burn injury – see Chapter 22), while extremely cold temperatures may decrease blood flow and lead to tissue damage of the extremities. Venomous bites from snakes and other animals release toxins and other substances that lead to tissue injury, cardiorespiratory failure, and other organ injury. Gas gangrene produces necrotizing cellulitis or myositis secondary to infection from several *Clostridium* species of bacteria (Uzal et al. 2022).

### Thermal Injury

Thermal burn injury is most commonly associated with barn fires, and a four-level classification system has been described based upon the depth of injury (see Chapter 22).

### Frostbite Injury

Extreme cold temperatures may lead to tissue damage when fluid within cells crystallizes injuring cell contents and membranes (Sheridan et al. 2022). Decreased blood flow to tissues may predispose to such injury. The extremities and areas of previous injury having abnormal blood flow are most affected. In addition, diseases such as viral or bacterial infections or ingestion of mycotoxins may lead to secondary vasoconstriction and increased risk of frostbite injury. Older horses, animals with poor nutrition, and those with pre-existing diseases are also predisposed to frostbite. Finally, having a smaller body size, miniature horses and donkeys are more susceptible to cold injury.

Similar to thermal tissue damage, a four-level classification scheme has been reported for human frostbite injury that may be translated to the horse (Sheridan et al. 2022). Although there is substantial overlap, levels 1 and 2 are considered superficial injury and 3 and 4 deep frostbite. Treatment is directed at slow rewarming, anti-inflammatory, thrombolytic and analgesic medications, removal of necrotic tissue as well as topic wound management (Sheridan et al. 2022).

### Patient Stabilization

#### Systemic Considerations

*STEP 1 – Perform a quick physical exam to assess the systemic stability of the patient... see Box 7.1.*

#### Wound Factors

*STEP 2 – Immediate wound triage*

A) ***Carefully assess the extremities and other areas of suspect frostbite damage****: The tips of the ears, the feet and coronary band region, and in males the penis and prepuce should be evaluated.*

B) ***Frostbite will present as areas of hard tissue that may appear pale in color:*** *Later signs of inflammation may include redness, swelling, and black or scaly skin. Tissue necrosis and drainage may also occur as tissues slough and infection develops.*
C) ***Bring the horse into a warm stall or barn:*** *Try to slowly warm the affected tissue. A towel soaked in warm water (40 °C or 104 °F) will work well. Do not use a hair drier or other device that may further damage the tissue.*

#### Treatment of Frostbite

*STEP 3 – Frostbite wound management*

A) ***Topical and/or systemic anti-inflammatory medications and antimicrobials:*** *May be indicated to help control the inflammation and secondary bacterial infection, respectively.*
B) ***Thrombolytic medications:*** *May help reestablish blood flow in early cases.*
C) ***Analgesia:*** *Is also important to control the pain associated with tissue necrosis.*
D) ***Surgical debridement of affected tissue:*** *May be required to help remove damaged or necrotic tissue during healing.*
E) ***Preventing frostbite should include the following:*** *Maintain proper shelter, especially from severe cold, wind, and wet conditions; blanket horses that are at risk or not acclimated to cold weather; provide adequate nutrition, including increased feed or high fat supplements during extreme cold; ensure a constant heated water source throughout winter months.*

## Venomous Bites

Venomous bites may occur from various animals including reptiles, insects, and spiders.

## Snake Bite Envenomation

Snake bite envenomation commonly affects horses in specific regions of the world and because of possible severe complications including death, they should be considered emergencies (Landolt 2007). A large number of horses suffering suspected elapid snake envenomation in Australia (Bamford et al. 2018) and *Daboia palaestinae* envenomation from the Eastern Mediterranean region (Tirosh-Levy et al. 2019), had a favorable outcome following specific antivenom treatment. Rattlesnakes belong to the pit viper family (Crotalidae) and are the most common snake involved in horse envenomation in the United States. Rattlesnake envenomation usually leads to marked swelling around the bite injury, tissue necrosis, and coagulopathy (Gilliam et al. 2012). The most dangerous acute effects of rattlesnake bites in horses include airway obstruction and hemolytic anemia (Landolt 2007), although cardiac abnormalities are common and may also be life-threatening (Gilliam et al. 2012). Most fatalities result from subsequent problems including cardiac injury, laminitis, myopathy, and other organ failure.

## Patient Stabilization

#### Systemic Considerations

*STEP 1 – Perform a quick physical exam to assess the systemic stability of the patient… see Box 7.1.*

#### Wound Factors

*STEP 2 – Immediate wound triage*

A) ***Carefully assess the snake bite region:*** *Because most bites occur on the face in horses, severe swelling of the muzzle and nares may obstruct the nasal passage and require immediate airway support (*Landolt 2007*). Intranasal oxygen therapy may also be indicated.*
B) ***Avoid manipulation of the bite wound:*** *Do not incise over the fang marks, perform a fasciotomy, or place tourniquets, ligatures, or compression bandages that may worsen tissue injury.*

#### Treatment of Snake Bites

*STEP 3 – Snake bite management*

A) ***Fluid therapy*** *is indicated for horses showing systemic problems such as cardiovascular collapse, organ failure, hemolysis, cardiac arrythmias, and colic.*

B) ***Antivenom treatment is indicated for most horses,*** *except those having localized swelling, normal vital parameters, and blood work. Two antivenoms are available in the United States to treat Crotalidae snakebites (*Landolt 2007*):*
   1) *Antivenin (Crotalidae) Polyvalent (equine; ACP, Fort Dodge Animal Health, Fort Dodge, IA).*
   2) *Crotalidae polyvalent immune Fab (ovine; CroFab, FabAV, Protherics, Nashville, TN).*

C) ***Antibiotics, anti-inflammatory medications, and tetanus antitoxin are indicated*** *in horses to prevent secondary infection and help reduce the pain, swelling, and inflammation associated with snake bite envenomation (*Landolt 2007*). Non-steroidal anti-inflammatory drugs (NSAIDs) are commonly prescribed, while corticosteroids remain controversial and are usually reserved for allergic reactions.*

## Gas Gangrene

Gas gangrene of horses is a sporadic disease most commonly caused by *Clostridium perfringens Type A*, although several other clostridial species have been identified (Uzal et al. 2022). The contamination of various wounds with clostridial bacteria following trauma, parturition, vaccination, or other injections is responsible for inciting the disease. Gas gangrene most often develops in horses following intramuscular injections when contamination of the site with clostridial spores or vegetative bacteria occurs (Uzal et al. 2022). Subsequent spore germination or vegetative bacterial proliferation develops in areas of trauma, and toxin production follows leading to the classical clinical signs of bacteremia, toxemia, and myonecrosis.

## Patient Stabilization

### Systemic Considerations

*STEP 1 – Perform a quick physical exam to assess the systemic stability of the patient… see Box 7.1.*

### Wound Factors

*STEP 2 – Immediate wound triage*

A) ***Aggressive antibiotic treatment*** is important to help prevent severe disease and improve prognosis for survival.
B) ***Wound debridement*** and exposure of the bacteria to oxygen are essential treatments.
C) **Supportive care** including fluid therapy is indicated.

### Treatment of Gas Gangrene

*STEP 3 – Gangrene management*

A) ***The most important step in limiting the severity of disease is surgical debridement and opening of the wound*** *(Figures 7.1 and 7.2): Wound debridement allows for removal of necrotic tissue and limits spread of the infection. Opening the wound will also help reduce the anaerobic bacterial load by providing oxygen to the tissues and provide for drainage.*
B) ***Perform an ultrasound evaluation of the affected region*** *prior to surgical wound debridement to help determine the extent of infection and guide incision placement (Figure 7.1). Ultrasound may also be used to monitor the response to treatment and the need for further surgery.*
C) ***Place large penrose drains*** *to help improve ventral drainage following surgical wound exposure. Such drains may be tied across adjacent wound incisions (Figure 7.2).*
D) ***Place oxygen lines into the wound*** *to help limit continued anaerobic bacterial growth (Figure 7.2).*
E) ***Daily wound lavage*** *with cold water hydrotherapy or dilute iodine solution may be used to help improve drainage and promote healing.*
F) ***Broad-spectrum antibiotics*** *are indicated until culture and sensitivity testing are available. Antibiotics should be continued until the wounds are healing and appear healthy, and the evidence of infection (CBC, fibrinogen, SAA) returns to normal.*
G) ***Fluid therapy*** *may be continued as necessary depending upon the severity of infection and secondary complications.*

# Gunshot Injury

Gunshot wounds in horses are not a common problem in equine practice, but when such injury does occur, it may be life-threatening depending upon the organs and tissues involved. A variety of injuries are possible, and the degree of damage and prognosis is related to the kinetic injury and type of projectile, as well as the characteristics of the tissues encountered (Munsterman and Hanson 2014).

Initial triage of gunshot injury should focus on patient stabilization, followed by close evaluation of the wounds and other tissue or organ injury.

## Patient Stabilization

### Systemic Considerations

*STEP 1 – Perform a quick yet thorough physical exam to assess the systemic stability of the patient. Remember that airway, breathing, and cardiovascular problems and support are the priority for immediate triage in trauma patients... see Box 7.1.*

## Gunshot Wound Injury

### Wound Factors

*STEP 2 – Immediate wound triage*

A) ***Perform a thorough physical exam looking for evidence of bullet wounds:*** *Bullet entry wounds in horses often present as a circular wound with distinct, clean margins. Exit wounds are often less circumscribed and larger depending upon the impact energy, type of projectile, and tissues involved.*

B) ***Gunshot wounds may be penetrating, non-penetrating, or perforating depending upon the depth of injury:*** *Non-penetrating injury affect skin and subcutaneous tissues while penetrating gunshot trauma passed deeper into the body; perforating injury is usually most damaging passing completely through the body.*

C) ***The impact energy and injury from a gunshot wound is directly related to the muzzle velocity and design of the bullet:*** *Low-, medium-, and high-velocity weapons create different levels of tissue damage, and different bullet types affect the deformation of the projectile and subsequent wound severity when traveling through tissue (*Munsterman and Hanson 2014*).*

### Injury Classification

***Treatment of Gunshot Wounds*** *STEP 3 – Gunshot wound management*

A) ***The severity and prognosis of gunshot injury is directly related to the tissues and organs involved*** *(*Munsterman and Hanson 2014*): Involvement of vital structures including the heart, lungs, and vessels of the thorax, viscera, and other organs within the abdomen, the head and neck, the central nervous system as well as bone and joints may be life-threatening with a greater likelihood of serious complications compared to other organs such as skin, muscle, and other soft tissues.*

B) ***Bone injury varies depending upon the energy of the bullet and the type of bone:*** *High-energy projectiles cause increased fracture comminution and bone damage compared to lower-velocity injury. Cortical bone injury is usually associated with varying degrees of fracture, while cancellous bone may have perforation or fragmentation.*

C) ***Gunshot wound injury should be assumed to be contaminated and not sterile:*** *Bacteria will be introduced into bullet wounds from the skin and other tissues during penetrating and perforating injury. The risk of infection increases greatly when contaminated structures such as the gastrointestinal tract or airways are involved.*

D) ***Surgical debridement of bullet entrance and exit wounds as well as other tissue damage may be indicated depending upon the tissues involved:*** *When planning surgical debridement of injured tissues, remember damage may extend beyond the bullet tract because of surrounding injury from pressure waves or necrosis.*

E) ***Broad-spectrum antibiotic coverage directed at both aerobic and anaerobic bacteria is indicated with gunshot injury:*** *Because of the high likelihood of bacterial contamination such treatment is especially important when damage occurs to the gastrointestinal or respiratory tracts.*

**Case Example 7.1 Traumatic Limb Wound**

*Patient: Threeyear-old miniature mule mare*

*History: Right hindlimb trauma secondary to limb entrapment between the stall door and frame (Figure 7.14a–f). After struggling to free herself, the mare managed to extract its leg from the door. The limb was bleeding, and the mule was reluctant to walk.*

*Step 1: Patient Stabilization*

Provide immediate stabilization steps (see Chapter 7: wounds, trauma and other injury):

1) *Stop or control hemorrhage with a pressure bandage, hemostat, or suture ligature.*
2) *Examine the wound for extent and depth of injury* via *palpation, sterile probe, and/or limb manipulation.*
3) *Provide structural support if needed for bone or soft-tissue injury.*
4) *Provide pain control, anti-inflammatory, and antibiotic medications.*

Perform a quick, yet focused patient assessment to evaluate the following:

*Assess the wound for communication with synovial structures.*
*Examine the pastern and foot for presence of adequate blood supply.*
*Evaluate the cannon bone and flexor tendons for damage* via *radiography and ultrasound.*

- Severe wounds to the limb may damage blood supply distal to the injury. Assessment via physical exam, ultrasound, venography, and/or thermography may be valuable.
- Traumatic wounds to the cannon bone may cause damage to the periosteum or the bone itself. Radiographs may not be conclusive for sequestration formation or non-displaced fracture for several (3–4) weeks.

*Step 2: Formulating a Diagnostic Plan*

Once the horse is stable, further assess the animal to determine a management plan:

1) *Determine the best choice for wound closure: your three options include primary wound closure, delayed closure, or second-intention healing.*
   a) ***Primary closure*** *– for wounds that are fresh without infection, marked swelling, or drainage.*
   b) ***Delayed closure*** *– for wounds that are infected, swollen, have significant drainage, or tissue damage.*
   c) ***Second-intention healing*** *– for wounds that have large amounts of tissue loss that prohibit primary or delayed closure techniques (Figure 7.14a–f).*
2) *Ultrasound and radiographs are indicated to assess the bone and soft tissues of the injured limb. Ultrasound may help determine synovial communication, injury to tendons and ligaments, presence of foreign bodies, and bone damage. Radiographs are indicated to assess for bone fracture or cortical injury, foreign material in the wound, presence of gas in tissues or synovial structures, and degree of tissue swelling.*
   - For wounds located near synovial structures (joints, tendon sheaths, or bursa) distend the synovial cavity with sterile saline to see if fluid leaks from the wound. Alternatively, contrast may be placed into the synovial cavity to see if leakage occurs outside of the joint, sheath, or bursa. Do not inject contrast or fluid into the wound to determine communication as this will force bacteria and debris into a breached synovial cavity.

*Step 3: Emergency Treatment Guidelines*

Following initial stabilization and diagnostic evaluation, further specific treatment is indicated.

- For wounds with significant loss of tissue as in this case, second-intention healing is required. Initial treatment is directed toward wound cleaning, disinfection, and lavage. Use of dilute iodine (0.1%) and chlorohexidine (0.05%) solutions is safe and effective for open wounds. Never use concentrated disinfectants or alcohol in an open wound as these are cytotoxic.
- Wound debridement is required to remove necrotic and contaminated tissue while salvaging as much tissue as possible. Surgical tissue debridement was performed cautiously in this case to remove devitalized tissue early in wound management.

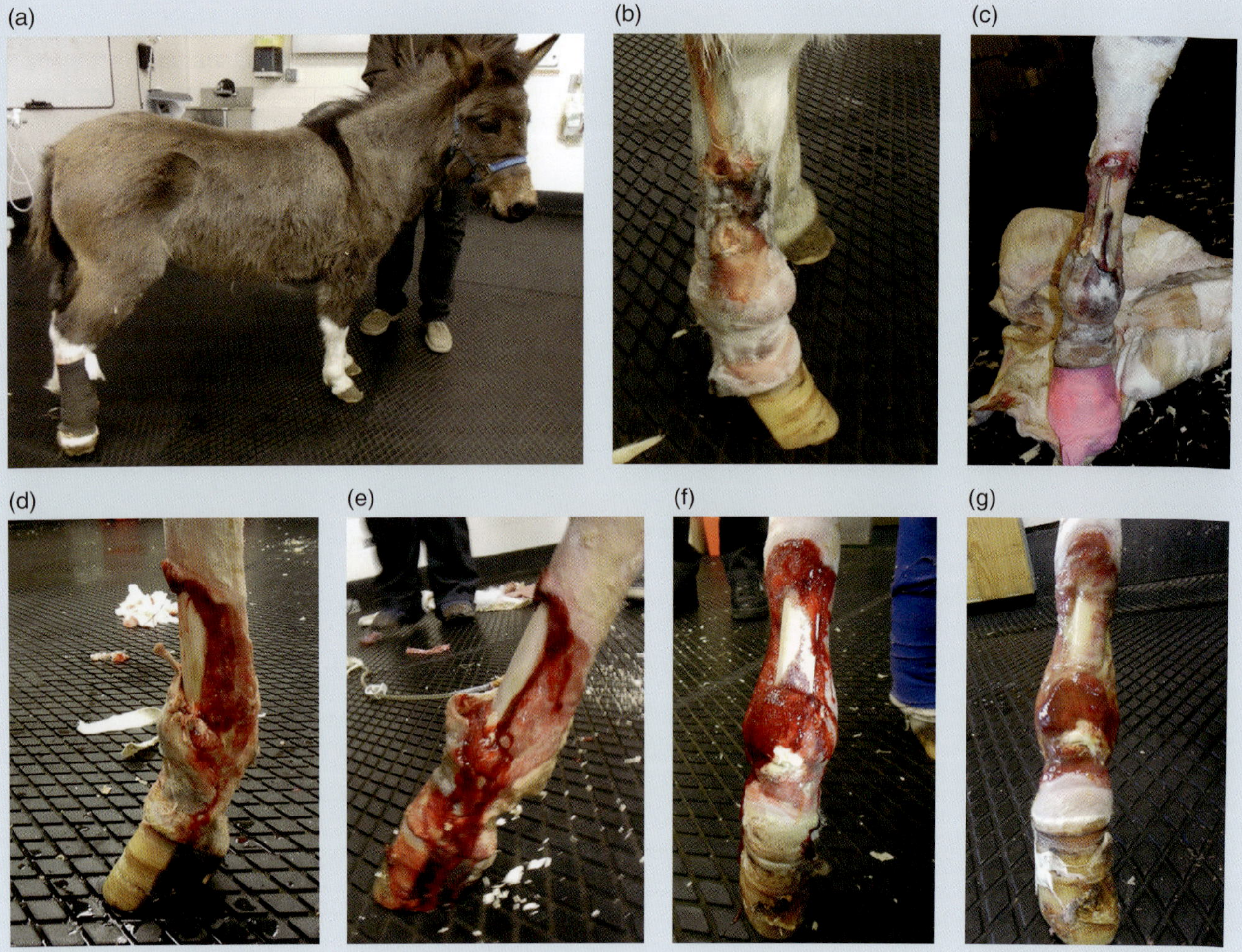


**Figure 7.14** Three-year-old miniature mule mare three hours following RH limb entrapment in a stall door (a and b). Significant tissue injury occurred and the blood supply below the wound was decreased. Communication with synovial structures was not suspected because the injury was located above the fetlock joint on the dorsal aspect of the metatarsus (b). Careful wound debridement and second-intention wound-healing steps were followed and healing progressed well (c–g).

- Bandaging is essential for wounds healing via second intention. Initial bandaging should address the need for tissue debridement followed by techniques to enhance granulation tissue formation and epithelialization. For example, wounds with devitalized tissue benefit from debridement dressings such as wet-to-dry bandages, hypertonic saline, or honey.
- Wound dressings are valuable for wounds healing by second intention. Such dressings should correspond to the stage of wound healing to provide the most benefit and avoid delays in healing. For example, wound dressings may help facilitate tissue debridement, stimulate granulation tissue formation, promote wound contracture, enhance epithelialization, and moisten dry wounds.
- Negative pressure wound therapy (NPWT) is an excellent technique for challenging wounds such as those requiring second-intention management (Figure 7.15a–c). NPWT accelerates wound debridement, reduces edema, decreases bacteria loads, stimulates wound contraction, and increases blood flow and cell proliferation.

*Step 4: Assessment and Monitoring*

Serial wound monitoring is essential during emergency wound management to make important decisions that will decrease wound-healing time and improve outcomes.

- During second-intention healing, careful monitoring will allow appropriate dressing application to correspond with the stage of wound healing.
- To allow epithelial cell migration, wounds that develop exuberant granulation tissue require sharp transection to remove the granulation tissue to at or just below the level of the surrounding skin (Figure 7.16a and b).

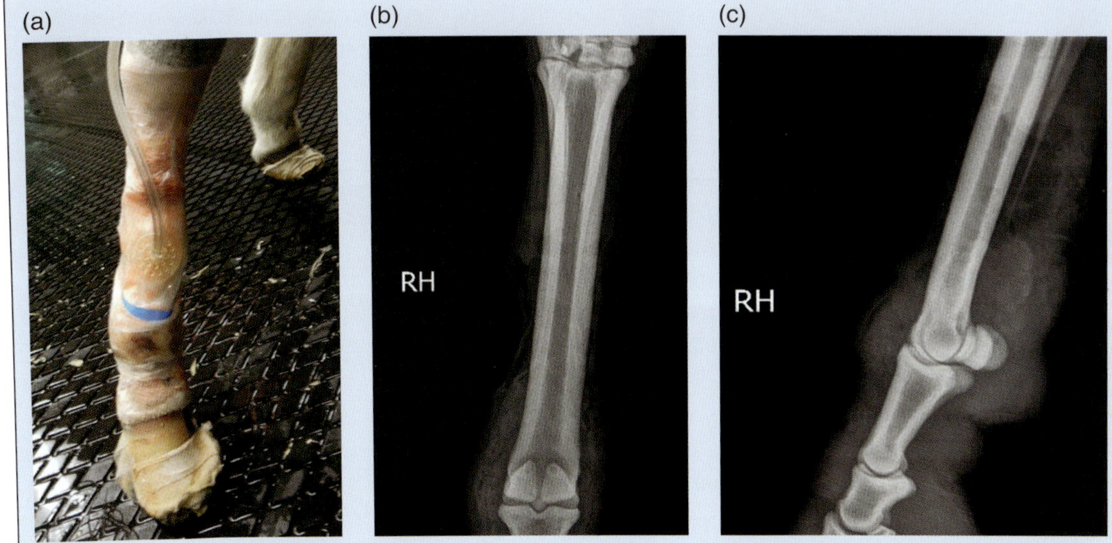


**Figure 7.15** Negative pressure wound therapy was used in this case to help stimulate granulation formation to cover the exposed cannon bone (a). AP and LM Radiographs of the wound region did not reveal bone injury but confirmed severe tissue loss (b and c). Although not a complication in this case, sequestrum formation is common following such cannon bone wounds as the periosteum is easily damaged, leading to avascular bone, drainage and infection.

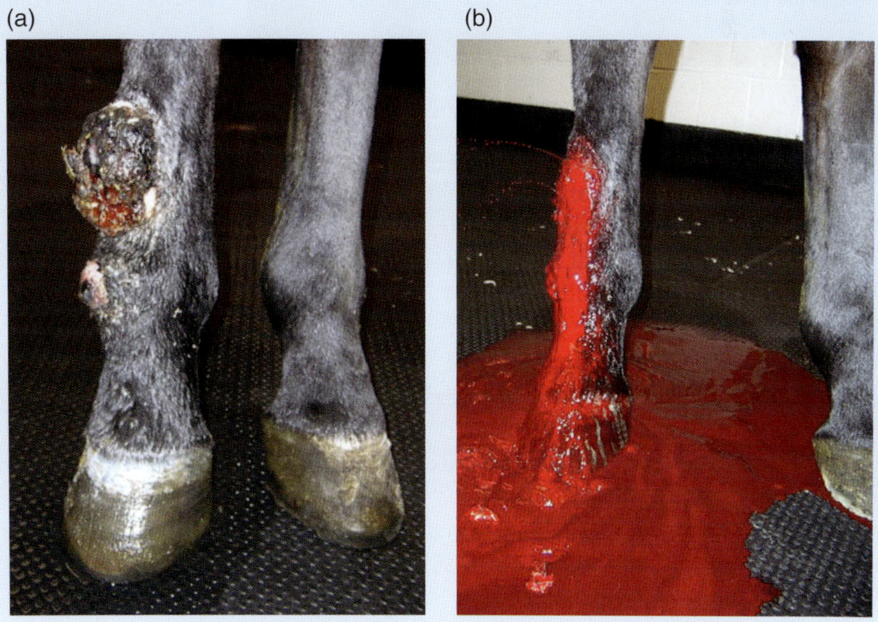


**Figure 7.16** A different horse with a chronic non-healing wound (a). Note the exuberant granulation tissue protruding extensively out beyond the normal limb contour. Such excessive granulation tissue results from chronic irritation, inflammation, and trauma secondary to poor wound management. Sharp transection (b) is the treatment of choice followed by pressure bandage application over a non-adherent dressing to promote epithelialization.

- Skin-grafting techniques may also be valuable to help speed wound healing especially during second-intention healing where large granulation tissue beds occur such as following degloving injuries.

*Step 5: Decision Making During Triage*

The emergency clinician faces many difficult decisions when working with limb wounds in horses.

- Following stabilization, referral is recommended for horses with severe injury involving bone fracture, ligament or tendon damage, or penetration of synovial structures.
- Many factors affect the decision for wound closure including wound type, size and location, degree of contamination, amount of tissue loss and swelling, blood supply, presence of infection or foreign body, communication with synovial structures, degree of wound tension, and local wound-healing properties.

- Complications (wound dehiscence, infection, exuberant granulation tissue, sequestrum formation, non-healing wounds and lameness) are common during wound management in horses, and early recognition and treatment of these problems will improve outcomes (Figure 7.17a and b).

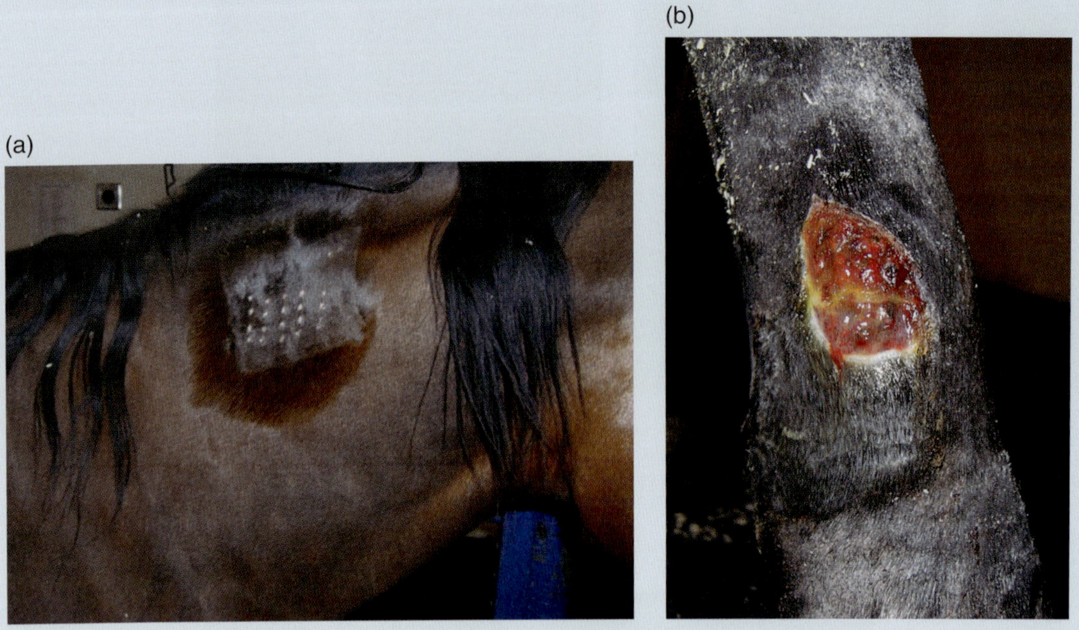

**Figure 7.17** Pinch skin grafting in a horse with a chronic non-healing limb wound (a and b). Horses having large amounts of tissue loss and second-intention healing may benefit from skin-grafting techniques to accelerate epithelialization, reduce healing time, and limit scar formation and other complications. Beneath the mane on the neck and along the ventral abdomen are common sites for donor skin collection (a). The recipient site should have a healthy bed of granulation tissue prior to grafting. Pinch or punch skin grafting places small islands of epithelial tissue into the granulation tissue bed across the wound (b).

## References


Adam, E.N. and Southwood, L.L. (2006). Surgical and traumatic wound infections, cellulitis, and myositis in horses. *Vet. Clin. N. Am. Equine Pract.* 22: 335–361.

Bamford, N.J., Sprinkle, S.B., Cudmore, L.A. et al. (2018). Elapid snake envenomation in horses: 52 cases (2006–2016). *Equine Vet. J.* 50: 196–201.

Barber, S.M. (2005). Management of neck and head injuries. *Vet. Clin. N. Am. Equine Pract.* 21: 191–215.

Beccati, F., Gialletti, R., Passamonti, F. et al. (2015). Ultrasonographic findings in 38 horses with septic arthritis/tenosynovitis. *Vet. Radiol. Ultrasound* 56: 68–76.

Biasutti, S.A., Cox, E., Jeffcott, L.B., and Dart, A.J. (2021). A review of regional limb perfusion for distal limb infections in the horse. *Equine Vet. Educ.* 33: 263–277.

Brumbaugh, G.W. (2005). Use of antimicrobials in wound management. *Vet. Clin. N. Am. Equine Pract.* 21: 63–75.

Burba, D.J. (2013). Traumatic foot injuries in horses: surgical management. *Compend. Contin. Educ. Vet.* 35 (1): E5.

Cantatore, F., Pagliara, E., Marcatili, M., and Bertuglia, A. (2023). Negative-pressure wound therapy (NPWT) in horses: a scoping review. *Vet. Sci.* 10 (8): 507.

Caston, S.S. (2012). Wound care in horses. *Vet. Clin. N. Am. Equine Pract.* 28: 83–100.

Céleste, C.J. and Szöke, M.O. (2005). Management of equine hoof injuries. *Vet. Clin. North Am. Equine Pract.* 21: 167–190.

Dahlgren, L.A. (2017). Tendon and paratenon lacerations. In: *Equine Wound Management* (ed. C. Theoret and J. Schumacher), 403–421. Wiley.

Dahlgren, L.A. (2018). Regenerative medicine therapies for equine wound management. *Vet. Clin. N. Am. Equine Pract.* 34: 605–620.

Dart, A.J., Bischofberger, A.S., Dart, C.M., and Jeffcott, L.B. (2015). A review of research into second intention equine wound healing using Manuka honey: current recommendations and future applications. *Equine Vet. Educ.* 27: 658–664.

Doughty, D.B. and Sparks, B. (2016). Chapter 4. Wound-healing physiology and factors that affect the repair process. In: *Acute and Chronic Wounds: Current Management Concepts*, 5e (ed. R.A. Bryant and D.P. Nix), 63–81. St. Louis, MO: Elsevier.

Dumoulin, M., Pille, F., van den Abeele, A.M. et al. (2010). Use of blood culture medium enrichment for synovial fluid culture in horses: a comparison of different culture methods. *Equine Vet. J.* 42: 541–546.

Eggleston, R.B. (2018a). Equine wound management: bandages, casts and external support. *Vet. Clin. N. Am. Equine Pract.* 34: 557–574.

Eggleston, R.B. (2018b). Wound management: wounds with special challenges. *Vet. Clin. N. Am. Equine Pract.* 34: 511–538.

Frees, K.E. (2018). Equine practice on wound management. *Vet. Clin. N. Am. Equine Pract.* 34: 473–484.

Gaughan, E.M. (2018). Diagnostic approaches to understanding equine limb wounds. *Vet. Clin. N. Am. Equine Pract.* 34: 461–471.

Gilliam, L.L., Holbrook, T.C., Ownby, C.L. et al. (2012). Cardiotoxicity, inflammation, and immune response after rattlesnake envenomation in the horse. *J. Vet. Intern. Med.* 26: 1457–1463.

Hanson, R.R. (2009). Complications of equine wound management and dermatologic surgery. *Vet. Clin. N. Am. Equine Pract.* 24: 663–696.

Hanson, R.R. (2018). Medical therapy in equine wound management. *Vet. Clin. N. Am. Equine Pract.* 34: 591–603.

Hassel, D.M. (2007). Thoracic trauma in horses. *Vet. Clin. N. Am. Equine Pract.* 23: 67–80.

Hendrix, S.M. and Baxter, G.M. (2005). Management of complicated wounds. *Vet. Clin. N. Am. Equine Pract.* 21: 217–230.

Kamus, L. and Theoret, C. (2018). Choosing the best approach to wound management and closure. *Vet. Clin. N. Am. Equine Pract.* 34: 499–509.

Kelmer, G. (2016). Regional limb perfusion in horses. *Vet. Rec.* 178: 581–584.

Landolt, G.A. (2007). Management of equine poisoning and envenomation. *Vet. Clin. N. Am. Equine Pract.* 23: 31–47.

Launois, T. et al. (2021). Use of negative pressure wound therapy in the treatment of limb wounds: a case series of 42 horses. *J. Equine Vet. Sci.* 106: 103725.

Leise, B.S. (2018). Topical wound medications. *Vet. Clin. N. Am. Equine Pract.* 34: 485–498.

Ludwig, E.K. and van Harreveld, P.D. (2018). Equine wounds over synovial structures. *Vet. Clin. North Am. Equine Pract.* 34: 575–590.

MacKay, R.J. (2004). Brain injury after head trauma: pathophysiology, diagnosis, and treatment. *Vet. Clin. N. Am. Equine Pract.* 20: 199–216.

Maher, M. and Kuebelbeck, L. (2018). Nonhealing wounds of the equine limb. *Vet. Clin. N. Am. Equine Pract.* 34: 539–555.

Moyer, W., Schumacher, J., and Schumacher, J. (2011). *Equine Joint Injection and Regional Anesthesia*. Academic Veterinary Solutions, LLC.

Munsterman, A.S. and Hanson, R.R. (2014). Trauma and wound management. *Vet. Clin. N. Am. Equine Pract.* 30: 453–466.

Murray, S.J. (2012). How to manage penetrating wounds in the field. *Proceedings of the 58th Annual Convention of the American Association of Equine Practitioners*, Anaheim, California, USA (228–230 December 1–5).

Myers, B.A. (2004a). Dressing selection and bandaging. In: *Wound Management Principles and Practice* (ed. B.A. Myers), 116–151. Upper Saddle River, NJ: Prentice Hall.

Myers, B.A. (2004b). Wound healing. In: *Wound Management Principles and Practice* (ed. B.A. Myers), 9–21. Upper Saddle River, NJ: Prentice Hall.

Pearson, G.B., Papa, B., Mosaddegh, A. et al. (2023). Equine synovial sepsis laboratory submissions yield a low rate of positive bacterial culture and a high prevalence of antimicrobial resistance. *Am. J. Vet. Res.* 84.

Pezzanite, L.M., Hendrickson, D.A., Dow, S. et al. (2022). Intra-articular administration of antibiotics in horses: justifications, risks, reconsideration of use and outcomes. *Equine Vet. J.* 54: 24–38.

Radcliffe, R.M., Ducharme, N.G., Divers, T.J., and Gleed, R.D. (2009). Treating thoracic injuries. *Compend. Contin. Educ. Vet.* 4 (5): 208–223.

Redding, W.R. and O'Grady, S.E. (2012). Septic diseases associated with the hoof complex. *Vet. Clin. N. Am. Equine Pract.* 28: 423–440.

Richardson, D.W. and Stewart, S. (2019). Synovial and osseous infection. In: *Equine Surgery* (ed. J.A. Auer, J.A. Stick, J.M. Kummerle, and T. Prange), 1458–1470. Elsevier.

Schumacher, J. and Stashak, T.S. (2017). Management of wounds of the distal extremities. In: *Equine Wound Management* (ed. C. Theoret and J. Schumacher), 312–251. Wiley.

Sheridan, R.L., Goverman, J.M., and Walker, T.G. (2022). Diagnosis and treatment of frostbite. *N. Engl. J. Med.* 386: 2213–2220.

Sprayberry, K.A. and Barrett, E.J. (2015). Thoracic trauma in horses. *Vet. Clin. N. Am. Equine Pract.* 31: 199–219.

Stashak, T.S. (2002). Lameness part 1: the foot. In: *Adams Lameness in Horses*, 5e (ed. T.S. Stashak), 725–733. Philadelphia, PA: Lippincott Williams & Wilkins.

Steel, C.M. (2008). Equine synovial fluid analysis. *Vet. Clin. North Am. Equine Pract.* 24: 437–454.

Stewart, A.A., Ketzner, K.M., Byron, C.R., Stewart, M.C. (2009). Equine distal limb wounds managed with phalangeal casts: 50 cases. *Proceedings of the 55th Annual Convention of the American Association of Equine Practitioners*, Las Vegas, Nevada, USA (239–240 December 5–9).

Tirosh-Levy, S., Solomovich-Manor, R., Comte, J. et al. (2019). Daboia (Vipera) palaestinae envenomation in 123 horses: treatment and efficacy of antivenom administration. *Toxins* 11: 168.

Uzal, F.A., Navarro, M.A., Asin, J., and Henderson, E.E. (2022). Clostridial diseases of horses: a review. *Vaccine* 10: 318.

Winter, G. (1962). Formation of the scab and the rate of epithelialization of superficial wounds in the skin of the young domestic pig. *Nature* 193: 293–294.

Winter, G. (1963). Effect of air exposure and occlusion on experimental human skin wounds. *Nature* 197: 91–92.

# 8

# Musculoskeletal Injury

*Ashlee E. Watts*

*College of Veterinary Medicine and Biomedical Sciences, Texas A&M University, College Station, TX, USA*

## Acute Severe Lameness – The Phone Conversation

"The sun should never set on an acute, severe lameness."

The horse with acute, severe lameness should be seen as soon as reasonably possible, but what does this mean? Does it mean the veterinarian should drop everything, reschedule the next appointment, turn the truck around, and head to the farm? Or does it mean the veterinarian should add an appointment at the end of the day?

During the initial contact, the veterinarian gathers information to develop a differential diagnosis ranking – is this likely to be an unstable fracture or luxation that requires the soonest possible attention or is this likely to a be a sub-solar foot abscess that needs to be seen as it fits in the day's schedule? The answer can be surprisingly difficult to ascertain and the experience of the person with the horse has a dramatic influence on the clarity of the answer. Asking the right questions to get the clearest picture is an art and highlights the importance of skills in communication in veterinary medicine. Questions that should be asked are in outlined in Box 8.1. When these questions lead to suspicion of unstable fracture or luxation, synovial sepsis, or there are signs of systemic compromise, the horse should be seen as soon as reasonably possible; otherwise, the veterinarian should balance the needs of other clients and the day's schedule with when the horse will be seen that day.

## Acute, Severe Lameness – The Physical Examination

Prior to homing in on the affected limb, the veterinarian should perform a quick physical examination to assess the systemic state of the horse. Shock due to severe pain should be expected with some conditions such as displaced long bone fractures and severe cases of acute laminitis. Shock and even death due to blood loss can occur with displaced fractures of the pelvis or femur. Shock due to sepsis can occur with severe cellulitis. Systemic derangements should be treated accordingly and considered when making medication decisions.

When the horse is extremely agitated, difficult to handle, unsafe, or further injury is possible due to behavior, judicious sedation may be indicated prior to examination of the limb. When selecting the sedative and dose, the veterinarian should keep in mind that some localizing signs such as pain on palpation or manipulation can be muted by sedation and excessive ataxia could lead to further injury.

Evaluation of the limb should begin with static palpation to assess for heat, synovial swelling, edematous swelling, pain on palpation, abnormal orientation of the limb, abnormal moisture on the limb, wounds, or increased digital pulses. After the static exam, the limb should be picked up and range of motion and pain response should be assessed. If fracture is suspected, the veterinarian should take care to slowly test range of motion as the pain response can be dramatic and explosive (Box 8.2). Following the range of motion exam, the foot should be inspected, including hoof tester evaluation. Again, if a sub-solar foot abscess is suspected, the hoof testers should be applied with care before adding the normal amount of hoof tester pressure as a painful response can be dramatic and explosive.

*Emergency Triage of the Horse*, First Edition. Edited by Rolfe M. Radcliffe and Jamie J. Kopper.

Companion website: www.wiley.com/go/radcliffe/triage

**Box 8.1 Questions to ask during the initial contact for an acute, severe lameness**

- When standing is the foot fully on the ground or is the horse holding it in the air?
- If the foot is on the ground, does the horse stand square or is the limb pointed (forelimb) or cocked (hindlimb)?
- Does the limb hang or swing abnormally, is the limb bending in an unusual location, or is the limb pointing in the wrong direction?
- Is the limb conformation abnormal?
- Is there swelling? If so, where is it and how would you characterize it (e.g., firm, soft, fluctuant, pitting, warm, painful)?
- Is there fever?
- Are there signs of shock such as elevated respiratory rate, profuse sweating, or extreme agitation or distress?
- Is there a history of recent joint injection(s)?
- Is there a wound or draining tract?
- Is there drainage or unusual moisture on the limb?
- Is there a foreign body (e.g., nail in the foot)?
- Is there obvious or known trauma: e.g., the stall boards are broken, the fence is broken, a strange horse is also in the paddock, the horse got loose, a loud crack was heard immediately prior to lameness, etc.?
- Is there a recent history of mild–moderate lameness in the affected limb prior to this acute, severe lameness?

**Box 8.2 The physical examination**

Pain on palpation, range of motion, or hoof tester response, can induce an explosive and violent reaction when examining a horse with acute, severe lameness. Care should be taken to slowly introduce the test whether it is digital pressure, joint flexion, or hoof testers, to avoid injury to the examiner or handler.

## Acute Severe Lameness – The Ambulation Examination

If the horse is waving the limb in the air or there is severe systemic compromise, the ambulation examination should be skipped. If the horse does not have systemic derangements and no obvious limb problems, an ambulation examination can be performed and should be performed if diagnostic anesthesia is needed. Most emergency lameness results in lameness that is visible at a walk, and therefore examination of the trot may not be required. It is useful to observe the horse turning in both directions, particularly for forelimb lameness. Common interpretations during the ambulation exam are summarized in Box 8.3.

**Box 8.3 Common interpretations for the character of lameness**

- Lameness that is exacerbated on the outside of the turn is often a medial problem (e.g., sub-solar abscess at the medial toe quarter).
- A processional type of gait of the forelimbs, where the forelimb is not advanced farther cranial than the contralateral limb, often indicates a proximal problem such as the shoulder.
- In severe hindlimb lameness the haunches will often be displaced with the painful hindlimb more under the horse (e.g., right hindlimb lameness would result in the haunches displaced to the left). Displacement of the haunches can result in a crab-walking type of gait (also known as sidewinder) where the haunches seem disunited from the forelimbs. Crab-walking can also occur with neurological disorders but when due to lameness, it is simply the horse's effort to unload on the affected limb (Aleman et al. 2020).
- Unwillingness to move may indicate severe bilateral (or quadrilateral) lameness (e.g., laminitis, bilateral hindlimb degenerative suspensory desmopathy).
- Unwillingness to move may indicate a movement disorder (e.g., Shivers, Stringhalt).
- Unwillingness to move followed by hyperflexion of a hindlimb may indicate upward fixation of the patella.
- Lameness with a dropped elbow indicates radial nerve paralysis or fracture of the humerus, olecranon, or proximal radius and ulna.

## Acute Severe Lameness – Diagnostic Anesthesia

While diagnostic anesthesia is the mainstay of routine lameness evaluation, it is generally reserved for blocking out the foot during emergent conditions, and continued blocking up the limb is rarely indicated. Diagnostic anesthesia of the foot can confirm that the foot is in fact the cause of lameness when a foot abscess is suspected, or sometimes perineural anesthesia of the foot is required to allow therapeutic interventions.

### Stepwise Blocking of the Foot

- When blocking out the foot for a suspected foot abscess, anesthetizing one side first (medial for example, if the lameness is worse on the outside of a turn) may help in localizing the problem and directing therapeutic measures, particularly when there are no other localizing signs such as a positive hoof tester response.

Prior to diagnostic anesthesia of the foot, the veterinarian should always consider the possibility of fracture of the proximal and middle phalanx as non-displaced phalangeal fractures can progress to complete and displaced fractures after the limb is desensitized with a nerve block. Horses with non-displaced P1 fractures will have a recent history of mild-to-moderate lameness in that limb, fetlock effusion, and a strong withdrawal response to distal limb manipulation and flexion. Radiographically, a peri-articular radioluceny may be seen on the dorsoplantar/palmar (DP) projections and/or a dorsal periosteal proliferation on the lateromedial (LM) projection; however, lack of radiographic abnormalities does not rule out non-displaced fracture (Brünisholz et al. 2015; Ellis et al. 1987). If P1 or P2 fracture is suspected, diagnostic anesthesia should not be performed (Box 8.4).

## Acute, Severe Lameness – Diagnostic Imaging

When there are localizing signs (e.g., swelling, pain, heat, response to local anesthesia) to help identify the region of the problem, diagnostic imaging of the affected area can be performed, which may include radiographs and/or ultrasound.

## Specific Conditions

### Foot Injuries – Sub-solar Foot Abscess

By far, the most common cause of acute, severe lameness is a sub-solar foot abscess. Fortunately, these injuries will usually be resolved on the farm without the need for referral or advanced diagnostics and have a good prognosis. This does not mean that sub-solar abscesses are to be taken lightly – they can be difficult to resolve and can result in prolonged lameness, and other complications such as systemic sepsis, hematogenous infections, and severe local cellulitis – but most of the time sub-solar foot abscesses are self-limiting (Box 8.5).

**Box 8.4 Diagnostic anesthesia should not be performed when first or second phalangeal fracture is suspected**

- Non-displaced P1 or P2 fracture will often have a history of recent development of a moderate lameness in the same limb.
- Non-displaced P1 or P2 fracture will often have a history of recent development of fetlock effusion in the same limb.
- Non-displaced P1 or P2 fracture will have a strong withdrawal response to distal limb manipulation and joint flexion.

**Box 8.5 Foot abscess case progression indicates the need for repeat examination**

- It is important to keep in mind that when a diagnosis of sub-solar foot abscess has been made, if there is not normal case progression with abscess drainage and lameness improvement over the following 1–3 days, additional diagnostics should be performed. If a reason for lack of progression is not identified, referral should be considered.

Foot abscess usually results in lameness that is seen at a walk and is sometimes non-weight bearing. There is usually increased heat in the hoof wall or coronary band, increased digital pulse pressure, and a withdrawal response to hoof testers. There may also be foul-smelling drainage at the coronary band or along the white line of the foot. Sometimes there will be substantial edematous swelling of the limb proximal to the foot or marked effusion of the distal interphalangeal joint (Carmalt 2009). However, the absence of these localizing signs does not preclude the diagnosis of foot abscess; sometimes, there will be the complete absence of localizing signs including hoof tester response.

If foot abscess is still suspected because there is severe lameness and no other abnormal findings of the limb, the foot should be blocked to confirm the suspicion and to rule out a proximal limb problem. For foot abscesses, a palmar digital or an abaxial nerve block can be used to desensitize the foot but may not alleviate foot pain in all cases (Moyer 1989). The veterinarian should keep in mind that a palmar digital block may desensitize much of the pastern as well and neither block should be performed if a pastern fracture is suspected (Box 8.4). When it is not clear which side of the foot is the problem, stepwise blocking of the medial side and then the lateral side, for example, can help to localize the problem.

Diagnostic imaging with radiographs is sometimes utilized to assess for causes of abscessation such as keratoma, foreign body, or sequestrum of the third phalanx. The radiographic study should include a horizontal DP, horizontal LM, and DP60. When keratoma is suspected, the horizontal LM should be obliqued to highlight the area of P3 bone resorption that is evident on the DP60, which will show a double edge of P3 the full distal to proximal extent of the keratoma. Gas lucency in the sub-solar space of a horizontal LM or horizontal DP foot radiograph confirms the diagnosis of sub-solar abscess and can also guide the location for ideal drainage at the white line. Keep in mind that the absence of gas or other radiographic abnormalities does not rule out sub-solar abscess.

When a foot abscess is suspected and there is not already a draining tract, the shoe should be removed (when present) and the area of the white line should be evaluated (Figure 8.1a–e). Take care when removing the shoe as a normally compliant horse can become fractious from the torque of shoe removal with pull-offs. The use of crease pullers to pull each nail individually alleviates this concern. In general, there is no added value in abscess drainage by removing the wall or sole tissue, and this should be avoided (Box 8.6). Evaluation of the white line should commence in the region where there was sensitivity to the hoof testers or heat (Figure 8.1a). When there is no indication of region, the dead and exfoliating hoof tissue should be removed from the entire periphery of the white line with the hoof knife. This will allow the area of abscessation to become apparent as a small dark line, or crack-like appearance, in the fresher, waxy foot (Figure 8.1b). This small dark line can be followed with the hoof knife, and repeated hoof testing if needed, until exudate of the abscess is encountered (Figure 8.1c–e). If hemorrhage is encountered prior to exudate paring at that location should stop as this indicates debridement of sensitive tissue beyond the sub-solar space. Whether foul-smelling exudate or hemorrhage is encountered, the foot should be prepared to enhance drainage (e.g., soak boot). When examining the white line, keep in mind that some abscesses will not drain at the bottom of the foot, rather they will drain at the coronary band. The horseman's term for a sub-solar abscess draining at the coronary band is gravel (Figure 8.2a, b). It will result in separation of the coronary band, sometimes from the heel almost to the toe quarter. While it appears alarming, this separation will grow out with only a small horizontal defect in the hoof wall and no long-term consequence.

Following examination of the foot, the foot should be maintained in a way to enhance drainage of the abscess, which is accomplished by making the hoof tissue as wet and soft as possible. A soaking bandage with wet, soapy cotton secured with tape will suffice, but commercially available poultice pads and boots can also be used. The bandage should be changed as needed to maintain the integrity of the bandage and the continued moisture against the foot. The wet bandage should be changed to a dry bandage when the lameness at a walk is resolved, and there is no longer abscess exudate present in the bandage. The main benefit of the dry bandage is more accurate assessment for continued subsolar drainage. Replacement of the shoe and resumption of normal housing and activity can commence when there is no longer drainage or lameness.

Until the abscess is resolved, the horse should be kept confined and anti-inflammatory medications can be administered as needed. Antibiotics are rarely indicated, except in the rare case with proximal cellulitis. The horse's recent tetanus history should be confirmed or a booster administered.

**Box 8.6 Foot abscess hoof debridement should occur at the white line only**

- Debridement of the sole of the hoof should be avoided as this can result in prolapse of the overlying soft tissues of the foot – a painful problem in and of itself – that is frustratingly slow to resolve. Fortunately, there is rarely a need to debride the sole for a sub-solar abscess as the abscess from the sub-solar space will drain at the white line at the periphery of the foot or along the bar, and this is a much safer place to allow drainage.

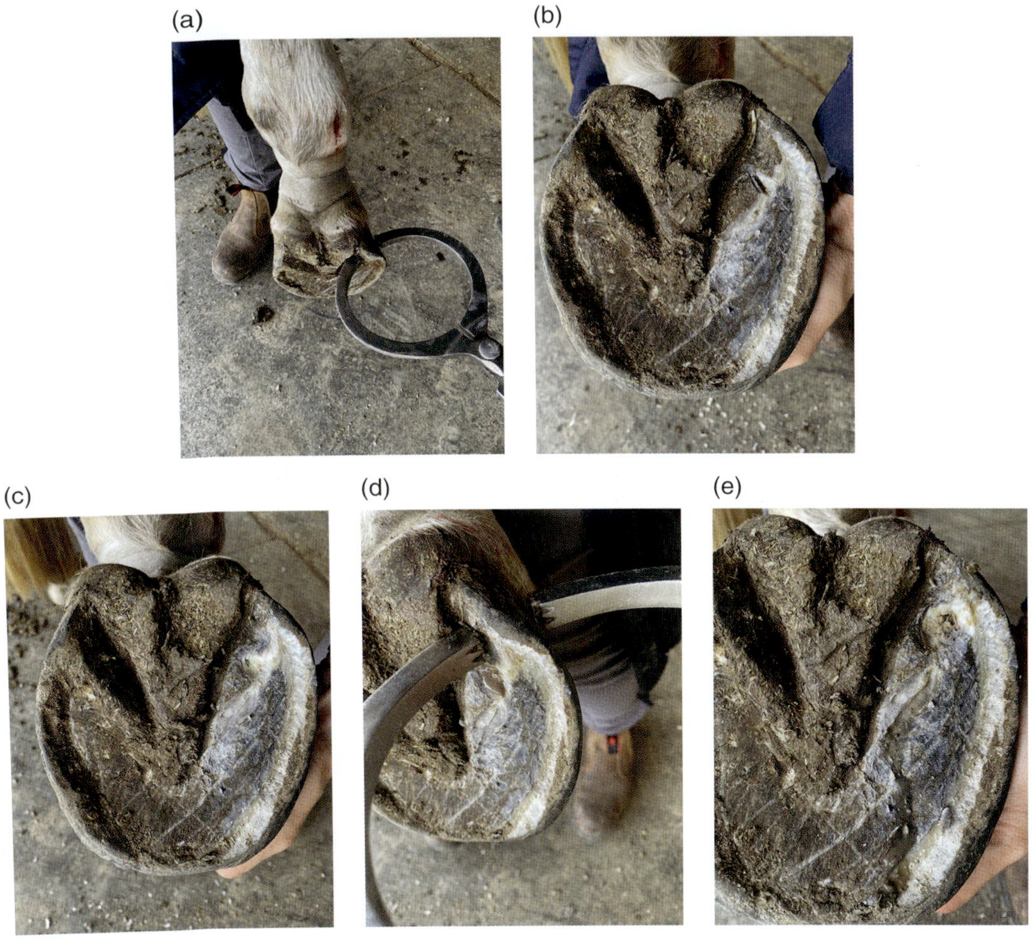

**Figure 8.1** A 9-year-old QH mare was evaluated for acute lameness that was visible at a walk. There were increased digital pulses on the affected limb, and a strong response to hoof testers applied to the lateral bar and the lateral heel. The mare was extremely difficult to manipulate and examine, presumably due to pain. (a) After an abaxial nerve block the lameness was resolved and the mare became quiet and cooperative for manipulation, hoof testing, and paring of the foot. (b) The white line along the lateral heel, heel quarter, and bar was pared until a dark line was visualized along the white line of the lateral bar. (c, d) This tract was followed until exudate could be expressed with pressure from the hoof testers. (e) The final appearance of the foot prior to applying a wet foot bandage. The lameness was improved the following day and drainage resolved quickly. The mare resumed ridden work one week later.

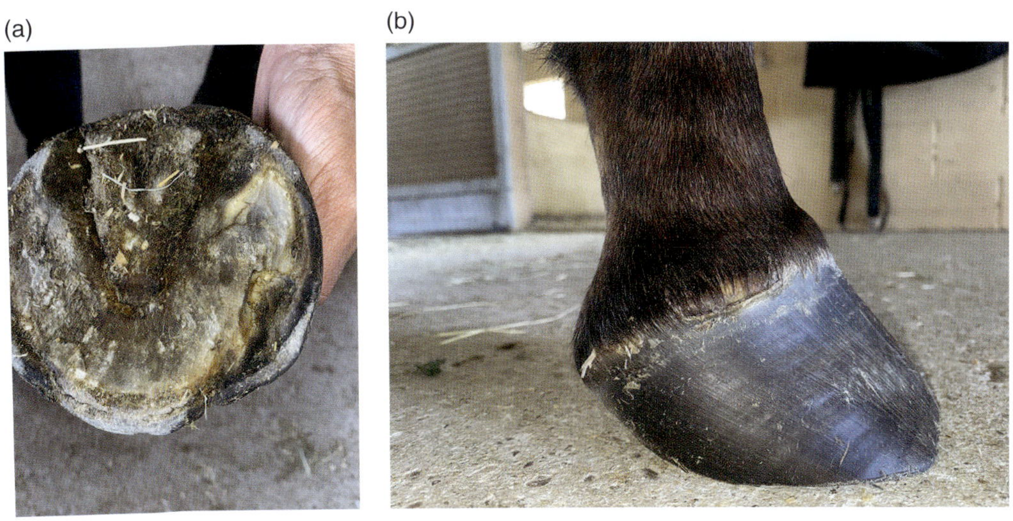

**Figure 8.2** An 8-month-old warmblood colt was presented for an acute, severe lameness at a walk. There was heat palpable in the medial hoof wall, increased digital pulses, and a withdrawal response to hoof testers applied along the medial toe quarter. (a) The white line was pared and a dark crack was followed until exudate drained. The foot was maintained in a soaking foot bandage. The lameness and hoof tester response improved dramatically but did not resolve, so the soaking foot bandage and stall confinement was continued. (b) Ten days after the original presentation pain was present on palpation of the coronary band at the medial toe quarter; the next day malodorous exudate was identified at coronary band separation at that location. The soaking bandage was continued until the lameness and drainage resolved five days later. The long-term outcome was excellent.

**Box 8.7 Gravel management**

- When a sub-solar abscess gravels, or drains at the coronary band (Figure 8.2b), the duration of treatment is often protracted and clinical improvement and worsening can be episodic (Cole et al. 2019). Unlike a sub-solar abscess that is draining at the white line of the foot, recurrent lameness and recurrent drainage over the course of days or even a few weeks should be expected.

The prognosis for most sub-solar foot abscesses is excellent, and most cases will be resolved in 5–10 days. Occasionally, the duration will be much longer, and this is especially true for abscesses that drain at the coronary band rather than the white line (Cole et al. 2019) (Box 8.7). If the lameness has not improved in three days, additional diagnostics, which may be only re-application of hoof testers and paring with a hoof knife, should be pursued. If the reason for lack of improvement is not identified or cannot be addressed, referral should be considered. When the abscess will not resolve or is recurrent, a foreign body, keratoma, or sequestrum of the third phalanx should be suspected and additional diagnostics, or referral, should be pursued.

## Foot Injuries – Penetrating Foreign Body

Penetration of the sole of the foot by nails, metal rods, mesquite thorns, or other objects can be benign or life-threatening (Figures 8.3–8.6). The difference in prognosis is dictated by the structures encountered. When the foreign body has entered one or all three synovial structures within the foot (navicular bursa, coffin joint, and digital flexor tendon

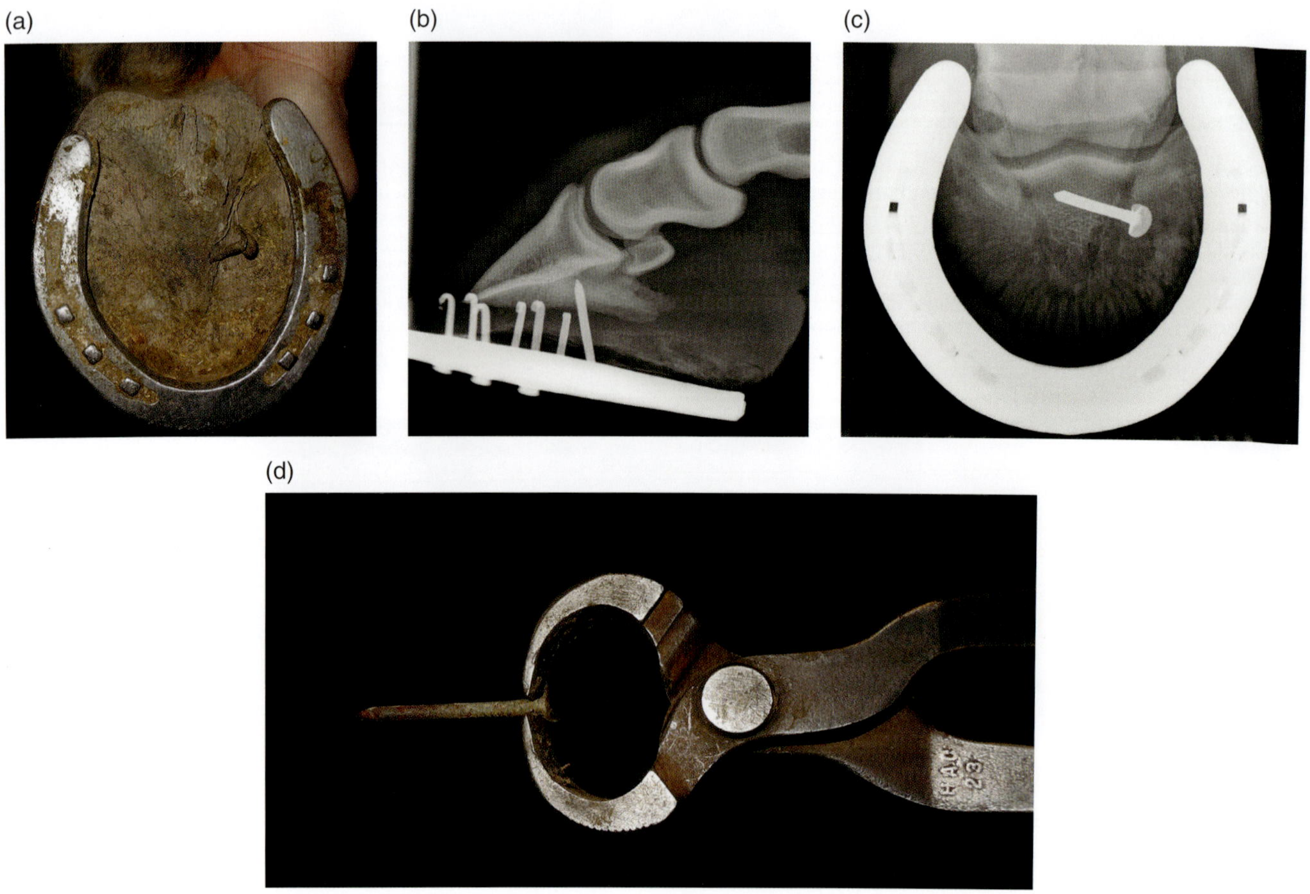

**Figure 8.3** A middle-aged warmblood gelding was presented for acute, severe lameness. (a) A nail was found in the cranial third of the frog. (b, c) Orthogonal radiographs confirmed that the nail had not penetrated a synovial structure. (d) The nail was removed and the foot was treated with a soaking boot, similar to a foot abscess, and the horse was administered an oral antibiotic. The injury healed without complication.

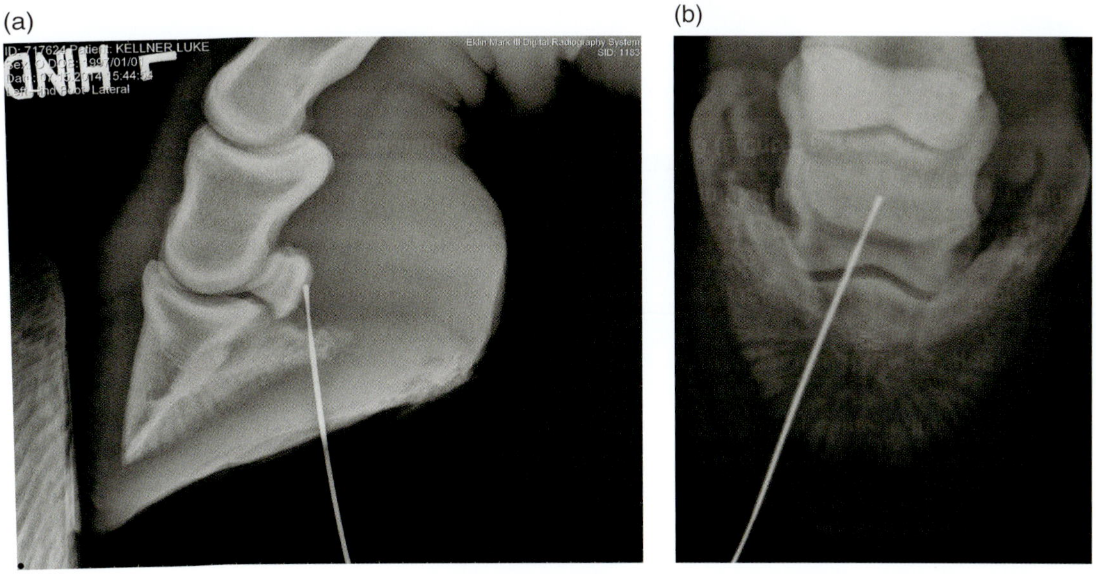


**Figure 8.4** A 4-year-old Quarter Horse mare was presented for severe lameness of several days' duration after a nail had been removed from the foot. Prior to presentation the nail had been removed from the central third of the frog and the nail tract had been pared on the farm. (a, b) A probe was used to explore the tract and radiographic imaging demonstrated communication with the navicular bursa. The horse was euthanized due to a grave prognosis.

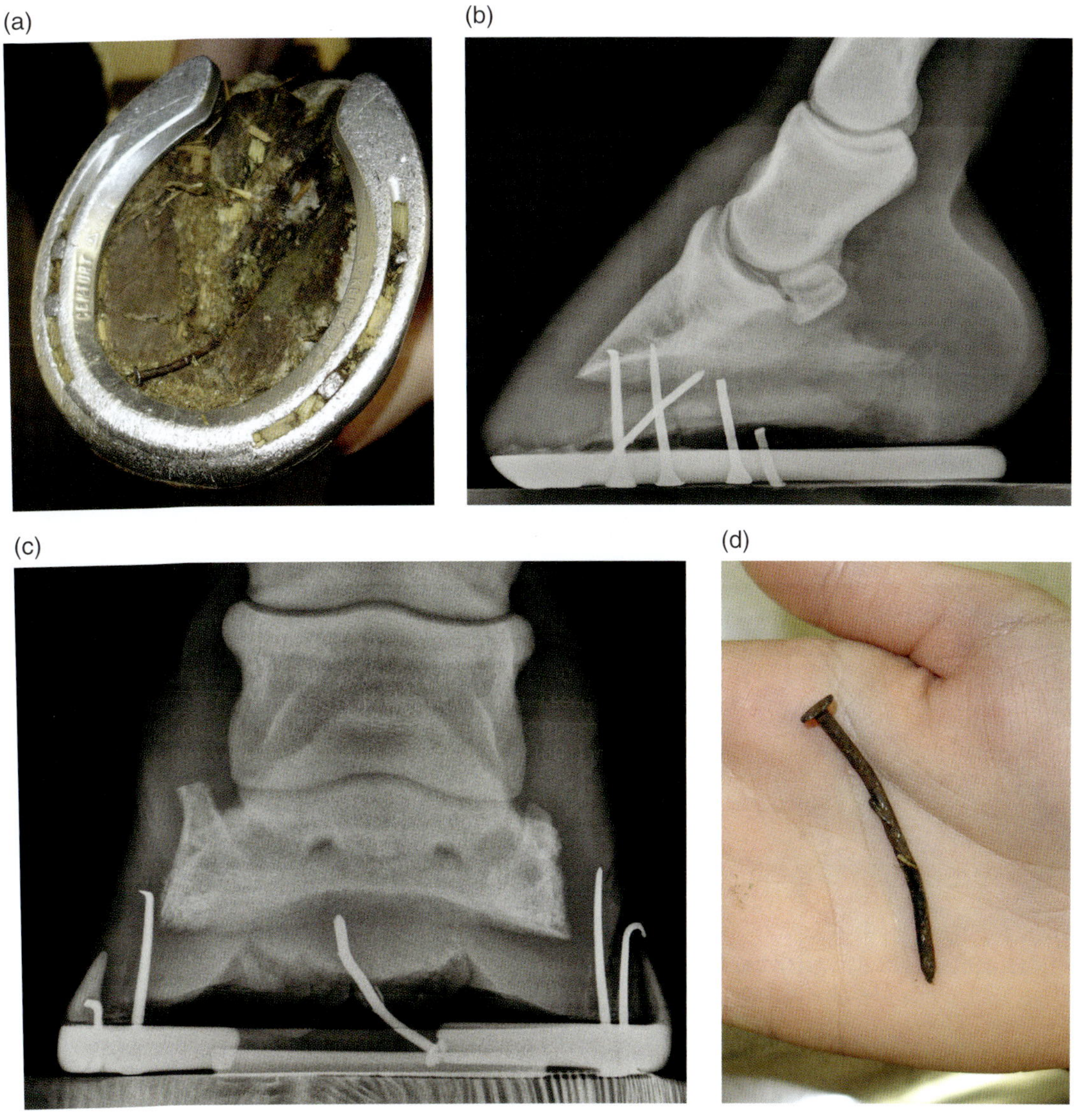


**Figure 8.5** A 9-year-old warmblood gelding was presented for a recent-onset moderate lameness. (a) A nail was found in the foot. (b, c) Orthogonal radiographs confirmed lack of synovial involvement. (d) The nail was removed and the foot was maintained in a soak-type boot overnight. When there was no lameness the following day, soaking was discontinued. The injury healed without incident.

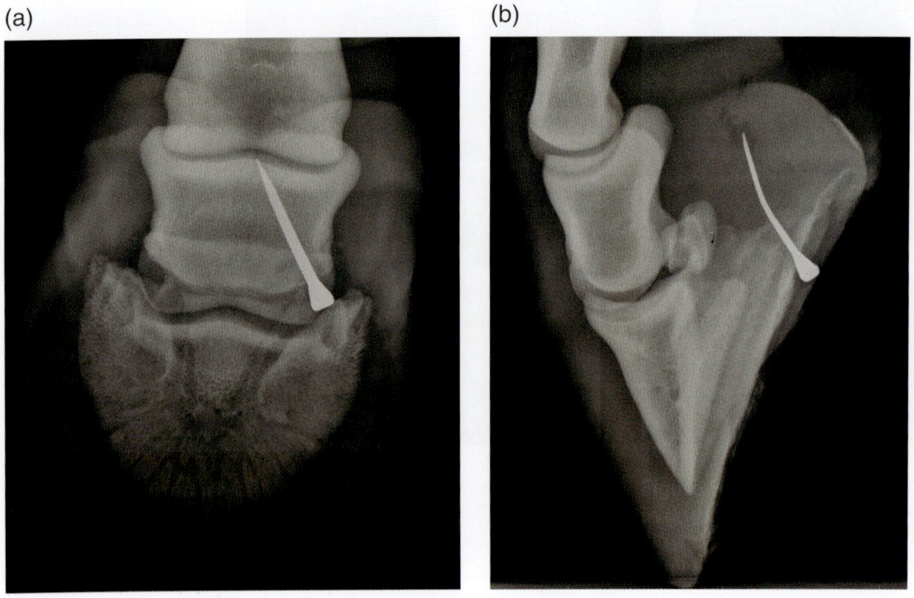


**Figure 8.6** A 4-year-old Quarter Horse gelding was presented for acute, severe lameness. A nail was found in the caudal third of the frog. (a,b) Orthogonal radiographs confirmed that the nail had not penetrated a synovial structure. The foot was maintained in a soak boot similar to a foot abscess for one week, regional limb perfusion with amikacin was performed daily for three days, and the injury healed without complications.

sheath) the situation is dire and requires immediate referral for aggressive medical and surgical care. Rapid referral for thorough lavage and local therapy is the most effective way to optimize prognosis. As a general guide, foreign body penetration of the middle third of the frog or its sulci should increase concern for synovial involvement. When the foreign body has contacted the subsolar space, the distal phalanx, or the digital cushion, the therapy is much simpler; the tract should be treated to facilitate drainage by paring of the tract and maintenance of a soak boot like a foot abscess.

Given the dramatic difference in therapeutic course of action and prognosis, determining the path of the foreign body is of the utmost importance. When the foreign body has been removed, it can be surprisingly difficult to ascertain its path, even on a high field magnetic resonance imaging (MRI). Therefore, when the foreign body is metallic, it should be left in place and orthogonal radiographs used to assess the likelihood of synovial involvement. If the object is not radiopaque or has been removed, synoviocentesis should be performed to check for synovial involvement by collection of synovial fluid and by distention of the synovial structure with sterile fluid to confirm integrity of the synovial capsule. Keep in mind that it is nearly impossible to collect synovial fluid from a navicular bursa and a synovial wash with sterile fluid is often the only way to collect samples for culture and cytology. Alternatively, radioopaque dye can be injected into the synovial structure(s) to document leakage via the tract radiographically. As compared to other synovial spaces, distention of synovial structures within the foot with fluid or radioopaque dye can result in a false negative when the entry wound to the synovial structure was small; therefore, a sample for synovial cytology is especially useful.

The veterinarian can assess synovial involvement on the farm or refer for these diagnostics. If it will be done on the farm, the foot should be desensitized with an abaxial block to facilitate needle placement. The navicular bursa should be assessed prior to the coffin joint or digital flexor tendon sheath as distention of either of these structures can make it difficult to enter the navicular bursa. When synovial involvement (or lack thereof) is not clear, the horse should be referred for additional diagnostics.

## Foot Injuries – Hoof Wall Avulsion

Lacerations of the hoof and coronary band are covered elsewhere in Chapter 7. Hoof wall avulsions can be due to overreach injury at the heel bulb or entrapment of the foot, often at the lateral heel quarter. Like a sub-solar abscess that has graveled, simple hoof wall avulsions rarely need intensive care and can be treated at the farm. Usually, a light bandage with or without topical antibiotics for a few days is sufficient. Severe avulsions may need a bar shoe or foot cast followed by a bar shoe to optimize healing (Figure 8.7a–c). For most injuries without a significant loss of tissue, the area of avulsion will grow out with normal hoof growth as a horizontal crack, similar to that after a gravel (Box 8.7).

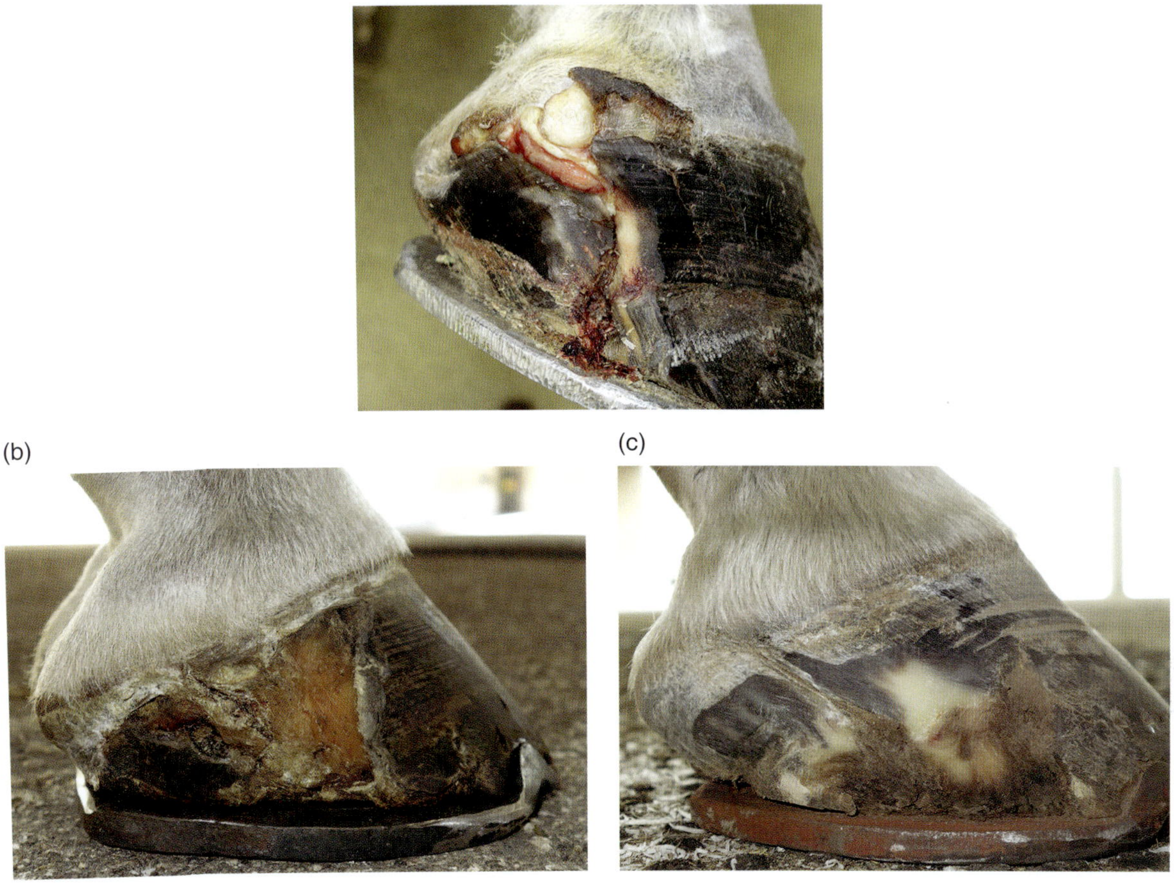

(a) (b) (c)

**Figure 8.7** (a) A middle-aged warmblood gelding was presented for a severe, chronic hoof wall avulsion of three weeks duration. It had been treated with topical antibiotics and a bandage. There was a moderate lameness at a trot and pain on palpation along the adjacent coronary band. (b) The detached hoof wall was debrided and the foot was maintained in a foot cast for one month, followed by application of a heart-bar shoe. (c) Three months after presentation, the horse was sound and had resumed ridden work. The long-term outcome was good with a small vertical line at the lateral heel quarter.

## Synovial Sepsis

Synovial sepsis secondary to a wound is covered in Chapter 7.

Synovial sepsis can also occur in the absence of wounds. Synovial sepsis (other than an extensor tendon sheath) is always a life-threatening condition and should be referred or admitted to a hospital for advanced medical and surgical care immediately. When referral is not an option, joint lavage and antibiotic therapy can be performed on the farm, but referral to a surgical facility should always be suggested.

Synovial sepsis can be iatrogenic following intra-synovial medication administration and development of an acute, severe lameness after synovial medication administration is always an emergency. Post-injection sepsis usually takes several days to a few weeks to become apparent as the administered treatment delays the inflammatory response (Krause et al. 2022). Development of severe lameness at 6–12 h post-injection is rarely sepsis and is most likely joint flare (Box 8.8).

### Box 8.8 Post-injection joint flare

- Post-injection joint flares are self-limiting and with phenylbutazone and rest, the lameness should resolve rapidly. When synoviocentesis is performed during joint flare, the cytology will reveal severe inflammation with proportions of neutrophils ranging from 30% to 80% but will not reach the neutrophil proportion of joint sepsis (90% + neutrophils).

Synovial sepsis can occur by hematogenous inoculation. This is common in foals but also occurs in adult horses (Byrne et al. 2020). It appears that the digital flexor tendon sheath and fetlock joints of the adult horse are a common site for hematogenous infection. Given the rarity of hematogenous synovial infection in adult horses, diagnostics for joint sepsis are often delayed and the horse is unfortunately treated for cellulitis or soft-tissue injury rather than joint sepsis. Given the gravity of synovial sepsis, anytime there is marked synovial swelling and severe lameness, synovial sepsis should be considered and appropriate diagnostics like ultrasound and synoviocentesis should be considered. In chronic, closed joint infections there will be abnormalities on radiographs as well with irregular new bone formation at the joint margins.

In hematogenous synovial sepsis, there will be marked synovial effusion and lameness and sometimes also extension of the infection into peri-synovial cellulitis. Cellulitis occurs in these cases because it is often missed for the dire emergency that they are, either by the people managing the horse at the farm or by the attending veterinarian, or both. An easy diagnostic to help define sepsis versus non-septic synovial inflammation is ultrasound. In sepsis, the fluid will appear flocculent rather than anechoic, which should alert the veterinarian to the need for synoviocentesis. When synoviocentesis reveals abnormal fluid, the horse should be referred immediately. Prognosis for synovial sepsis depends on the duration of infection and the pathogenicity and antimicrobial sensitivity of the infecting agent, but it has been this author's experience that apparently hematogenous synovial infections in the adult horse are often easier to resolve than synovial infections by direct inoculation (e.g., wound, iatrogenic) even when chronic.

## Fractures and Luxations

Fractures and luxations can fall into the no-big-deal category or can be irreparable, requiring euthanasia, and everything in between. The bone(s) and/or joint(s) that are involved dictate the prognosis. For example, a displaced femur fracture in a full-sized adult horse is irreparable with current techniques. Whereas a minimally displaced sagittal first phalanx fracture is easily repaired with lag screws. A list of reparable fractures is not included in this text as the list is ever-expanding with advancement of surgical techniques and equipment. Additionally, the feasibility of repair is dictated by the equipment and expertise that is available at accessible referral facilities (Box 8.9).

Joint luxation is similar – some joint luxations are easily treated on the farm and others cannot be repaired and everything in between. Therefore, the best course of action is to diagnose the luxation, stabilize the horse, and speak to a surgeon about the feasibility of repair.

- A complete metacarpo(tarso)phalangeal luxation (Figure 8.8) may be stabilized for referral or treated on the farm. This luxation is a dire emergency for stabilization to prevent further injury to the limb, especially the surrounding skin, but is relatively easy to treat by closed reduction and a cast, which can be done on the farm. Depending on the degree of damage to the soft tissues and to the tissues of the joint itself, this treatment has a good prognosis (Yovich et al. 1987). When fracture is present along with luxation (i.e., fracture-luxation), the prognosis for recovery is decreased as joint injury is likely; referral for possible surgical options should be performed.
- Luxations of the proximal interphalangeal joint, carpal joints, femoropatellar joint and distal tarsal joints are treatable in most cases but only by advanced surgical care.
- Luxations of the distal interphalangeal joint, tarsocrural joint, and femorotibial joint may not be possible to repair.
- Luxations of the coxofemoral joint and shoulder joint can be treatable with advanced surgical care in ponies and foals but not in full-sized adult horses.

Good-quality orthogonal radiographs are the mainstay of diagnosis and are particularly important if the owner is considering repair. However, some fractures are difficult to document radiographically in full-sized adult horses such as fractures of the spine, pelvis, and femur. Alternative diagnostics like rectal palpation can be useful for identification of some pelvic fractures. Manipulation of the limb while listening for bone-on-bone crepitation over the region of interest

**Box 8.9 Which fractures are fixable and which are not?**

- When faced with a fracture, the best course of action for the veterinarian is to call the surgeon to whom the horse would be referred to for repair for advice. Many times, this call should be made at the time of diagnosis, not the next day. This is because some fractures that are fixable should be transported to the referral facility immediately, and others can be scheduled almost like an elective surgery.

with a stethoscope can be useful for fractures of the humerus, femur, and pelvis. Ultrasound can also be useful to document these proximal fractures. Similarly, some proximal luxations cannot be radiographed well in the field. For coxofemoral luxation, which is nearly impossible to radiograph in the field in anything other than a small pony or miniature horse, the physical examination findings are diagnostic (Figure 8.9).

Stabilization of the fracture or luxation that includes or is distal to the elbow or stifle is of paramount importance when the owner will pursue repair. The main goal is to prevent additional injury; whether the fracture is open or closed and the health of the soft tissues is often a main determining factor in fracture repair success or failure. The secondary goal is to allow the horse to use the limb to some degree, which can reduce the horse's anxiety level. Again, the surgeon that is being referred to is an excellent resource for how the limb and horse should be managed prior to and during transport. Key points in limb splinting are summarized in Box 8.10.

*How to apply a bandage and splint for fracture stabilization:*

- Mild-to-moderate sedation may be necessary for splint application and trailer loading with horses with long bone fractures. Try to avoid heavy sedation so that the animal is not ataxic or near to falling down. In most cases, it is best to apply the bandage and splint prior to trailer loading.
- The bandage under a splint should be well padded and stiff.
- Multiple, thin layers of cotton secured with alternating layers of brown gauze are far more stable than a single, thick layer of cotton with a single, thick layer of brown gauze.
- The bandage should be thick enough to make the limb round with a uniform thickness from top to bottom but not so thick that the splint is too far from the limb. Increasing the distance between the splint and the central axis of the limb increases the stress on the splint material and the chance for splint breakage.
- It is almost impossible to apply a well-padded bandage that is too tight in an adult horse. The end product should be difficult to indent with finger pressure and should make a distinct thumping sound when flicked with the index finger. However, it is possible to overly tighten a well-padded bandage in the foal, and special effort should be made to get even, firm compression that remains indentable with pressure from the finger.
- Except in cases where the splint will extend past the elbow, stifle, or the plantar calcaneus, the bandage should be longer than the splint.
- Splint materials should be strong and light weight and should be appropriate for patient size. For example, a 2×4 in. piece of wood is too large to splint a newborn foal but is appropriate to splint a distal metacarpal fracture in a full-sized horse. A 1×3 or 1×4 in. hardwood board (ash, oak, hickory) is preferred for foals and adult horses, and is commonly available at most farms.

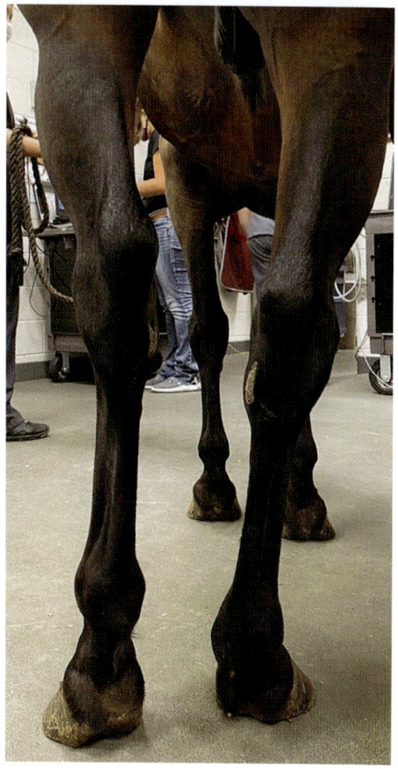

**Figure 8.8** A middle-aged large pony was presented for acute, severe lameness and a left coxofemoral luxation was diagnosed by physical examination and confirmed radiographically. When standing square, the left hindlimb was externally rotated and the point of the left hock was substantially higher than the corresponding right hock.

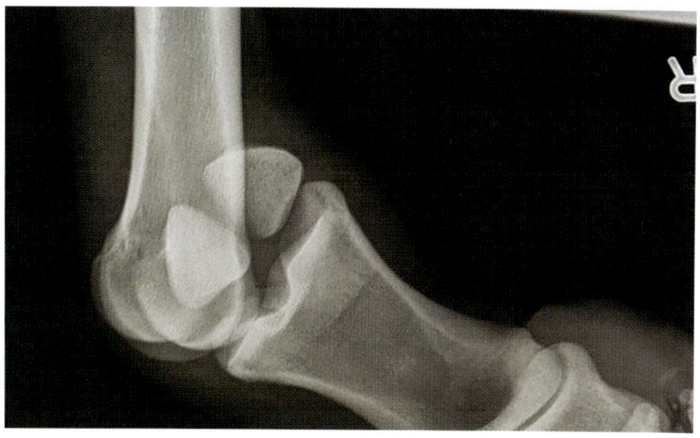


**Figure 8.9** A complete metacarpo(tarso)phalangeal luxation in a horse. Immediate stabilization of the joint is essential to prevent further injury to the soft tissues and bones of the limb. However, treatment by closed reduction and cast immobilization often provides a favorable outcome.

**Box 8.10 Principles of emergency fracture stabilization**

- Multiple forces are acting on the limb during weight bearing and ambulation. These forces include bending, torsion, and compression. Bending and torsional forces are most likely to cause worsened displacement and injury to the overlying skin. Compression forces can also be problematic with highly comminuted or unstable fractures, but rarely results in injury to the soft-tissue envelope.
  1) Attempt to stabilize the limb following the rule of cast application: stabilize the joint above and below the fracture. In some cases this will not be possible or desirable.
  2) Never end rigid fixation in the middle of a long bone (e.g., a full-limb cast should always approach the elbow or stifle joints and not end in the middle of the radius or tibia).
  3) If possible, place splints at 90 degrees to provide orthogonal stabilization. Unfortunately, this often only possible with metacarpal/tarsal bone fracture. Below this level there is no need for two splints, and above this level, the attachment of the limb to the body interferes with splint placement at 90°.
  4) Never end a splint near the fracture site as this will result in further trauma, displacement, and injury; even a splint ending near the fracture may cause added stress concentration at the site of injury.

- The rule of stabilizing at least the joint above and below the fracture does not always apply in the horse. This is because of the additional stabilization provided by the long cannon bone in all four limbs and the additional length of the calcaneus in the hindlimbs. Avoidance of fixing the carpus or tarsus when splinting greatly eases bandage and splint construction and is more tolerable for the horse as well, provided appropriate stabilization is achieved.
- Non-elastic tape, such as duct tape, should be used to secure the splints.
- Some horses will react violently to limb bandages and splint, especially of the hindlimbs. Take care when applying bandages and splints and warn handlers of the possibility of an explosive reaction, which often occurs when the horse first attempts to flex the now rigid limb.

*Fracture examples:*

- Fracture of the first or second phalanx or the distal metacarpus(tarsus) should be stabilized with a dorsal (forelimb) or plantar (hindlimb) splint to the level of the carpus or hock, respectively. This splint will stabilize the fetlock joint and minimize further movement at the fracture site. Raising the heel with some type of wedge will improve biomechanical stability. By aligning the bones of the distal limb, the bending forces acting on the pastern below the fetlock are converted to compression, which is less detrimental than bending and torsion. A Kimsey splint has been designed for this application and is superior to splinting techniques, as it stabilizes the fetlock and pastern joints and aligns the pastern with the cannon bone.
- Fracture of the tibia or radius should receive a single lateral splint from the ground up to the level of the scapula (radius fracture) or greater trochanter (tibia fracture). A palmar splint is recommended in the forelimb if the fracture is in the distal region of the radius but not a proximal fracture as a palmar splint would end too near the fracture site. In the hindlimb a plantar splint may be possible, but would require substantial contouring of the splint material.
- Fracture of the olecranon of the elbow is an exception to the principles of fracture stabilization listed above because the olecranon is not a weight-bearing bone of the forelimb (the radius provides this function). Horses with olecranon fractures have a dropped elbow and inability to advance or extend the limb because the triceps muscle function of limb extension is disrupted. With diseases that affect this bone–muscle–tendon unit (olecranon fracture, radial nerve paralysis, and humeral fracture), limb extension is impaired. When the elbow is dropped due to olecranon fracture or radial nerve paralysis horses respond favorably to maintaining the limb in extension by applying a full-limb bandage and caudal/palmar splint from the fetlock (or ground) to the elbow. Even though this breaks the rules of fracture stabilization outlined above, it enables limb extension and return to near normal weight-bearing.

Another point of advice: when trailering horses with long bone fractures, remember "crack in the back." Face the horse forward in the trailer with hindlimb fractures and backward with fractures of the forelimb. This places the fractured limb in the rear of the trailer away from the increased forces of breaking presented to the limbs in the front of the trailer. Acceleration forces do affect the limbs in the back of the trailer, but these forces tend to be lower and more easily controlled than breaking forces.

## Cellulitis

Cellulitis is a common cause of acute, severe lameness and in most cases can be treated on the farm with a good prognosis. Hindlimbs appear to be affected more commonly than forelimbs, and this may be due to the differences in the lymphatic system of the hindlimb of the horse. Cellulitis is almost always secondary to infection or to a break in the skin somewhere on the limb. When there is not skin injury there is usually a local infection such as a subsolar foot abscess. Cellulitis can be focal to the nidus of infection or can be widespread, affecting the entire limb. A common scenario would be a case with pastern dermatitis (i.e., scratches) that develops secondary cellulitis. The hallmark signs of cellulitis are limb swelling with pitting edema, lameness, and fever as well as abscessation, weeping skin, and necrotic skin in protracted cases. Swelling can be dramatic and is often described as a stove–pipe–limb. Elevations of serum amyloid A, neutrophilia, hyperfibrinogenemia, and hyperproteinemia are expected in all but the mildest cases.

The mainstay of treatment is counter-pressure and anti-inflammatory medications. Counter-pressure is achieved through compression bandaging and cold, compression devices. Anti-inflammatory medications are often administered topically and systemically. For example, a horse might receive a course of 4.4 mg/kg phenylbutazone twice daily, one or two daily doses of 0.04 mg/kg dexamethasone IV, and daily topical diclofenac or DMSO/furacin. Systemic antibiotics are indicated when the condition is severe or has not responded to local therapy. Unless culture and sensitivity are available, antibiotics should be broad spectrum as staphylococci and coliforms are common in cellulitis. Referral or admittance to a hospital is only required in the most severe cases and sometimes is sought for convenience given the labor-intensive bandage management.

Complications of cellulitis include impaired lymphatics leading to recurrent cellulitis or chronic lymphangitis. Chronic lymphangitis is common in draft horses and less common in non-draft breeds. Another complication of cellulitis is subcutaneous abscess formation, which requires surgical drainage under local anesthesia.

## Tendon/Ligament Injury – Complete Rupture

Complete tendon/ligament laceration or rupture on the back of the limb (e.g., flexor tendons, suspensory ligament) can be a life-threatening injury and often requires referral for aggressive surgical or medical care. When the injury can heal, it is almost always career ending. In stark contrast, complete laceration on the front of the limb (extensor tendons and ligaments) is almost without long-term consequence, comparatively. The main difference is that structures at the back of the limb are required to support the weight of the horse and prevent limb hyperextension. With loss of the tendons/ligaments on the front of the limb there is no loss of ability to support the horse's weight and thus it is not a life-threatening condition, it is rarely career-ending, and it often can be managed on the farm.

The presenting clinical signs of limb hyperextension will help localize the specific tendon involvement. For example, complete disruption of the superficial digital flexor tendon leads to partial loss of fetlock support and fetlock hyperextension, yet weightbearing is still possible. Complete disruption of the deep digital flexor tendon (DDFT) causes dorsiflexion of the pedal bone and hoof, yet weightbearing is still possible. Complete disruption of both the superficial and deep digital flexor tendons causes more severe fetlock hyperextension and dorsiflexion of the pedal bone and hoof. Disruption of the suspensory apparatus (i.e., the suspensory ligament, proximal sesamoid bones, or distal sesamoidean ligaments) results in complete loss of the fetlock support apparatus and the inability to bear weight on the limb.

The location of flexor tendon disruption on the limb also dictates prognosis. For example, complete loss of the deep digital flexor tendon at the level of the navicular bone or the insertion on P3 is a dire injury and almost always results in euthanasia; whereas complete loss of the superficial or the DDFT along the mid-metacarpus or even within the pastern will be performance limiting long term, but with appropriate care the horse can survive.

Complete loss of the flexor tendons (superficial or deep) can be managed on the farm or referred depending on the circumstances, but many can be appropriately cared for on the farm. Primary surgical repair with suture of the flexor tendons does not appear to improve prognosis and most horses are managed with strict rest and orthotic devices, such as a dynamic fetlock support shoe (Whitfield-Cargile et al. 2009, 2011) or a limb cast. Another important consideration in complete flexor tendon loss is the involvement of a synovial structure. When the injury is due to a wound, it is often within a tendon sheath, which greatly complicates treatment and worsens the prognosis – these horses should be stabilized and referred immediately to address synovial sepsis.

Complete loss of the suspensory apparatus is always life-threatening and requires aggressive surgical care for a fetlock arthrodesis for the horse to survive. When euthanasia is not elected, these horses should be stabilized and splinted as soon as possible and referred. The bandaging and splint should be applied similar to fracture or luxation at the distal metacarpal(tarsal) level.

Complete loss of the common calcaneal tendon is always life-threatening, and while differing methods of repair have been attempted, they are rarely successful. When euthanasia is not elected, these horses should be stabilized and splinted as soon as possible and referred immediately.

A caveat to the gravity of flexor tendon rupture is the not uncommon injury in the aged horse of complete rupture of the forelimb superficial digital flexor tendon. This appears to be a spontaneous injury at the musculotendinous junction and with adequate rest, will heal. There will be lameness, local swelling, and a palpable absence of the superficial digital flexor tendon (SDFT). On ultrasound examination, the tendon fibers of the SDFT distal to the rupture will be wavy from lack of tension. Orthotic devices and special shoes are not required. Often these horses have an over-at-the-knee conformation after this injury has healed, but they will be pasture sound.

## Tendon Injury Without Complete Rupture

Tendon injury can also be partial, either as a "core lesion" or as a surface tear. These injuries are exercise related, with core injuries being a condition of cumulative sports-related injury and surface tears as a one-time event, often referred to as a misstep injury or accident. Surface tears are almost always within a synovial structure such as the digital flexor tendon sheath or navicular bursa. Core injuries can be within the region of a synovial structure or not; either way it does not involve synovial fluid in most cases.

The clinical signs will depend on the structure injured and the location of the injury. For example, a surface tear of the DDFT at the level of the navicular bone will have lameness alone whereas a surface tear of the DDFT within the digital flexor tendon sheath will have lameness, synovial effusion, and pain on digital palpation. A core lesion of the SDFT or DDFT, whether it is within the digital flexor tendon sheath or mid-metacarpal(tarsal), will have palpable tendon swelling, peri-tendinous swelling, and pain on digital palpation. These injuries rarely result in acute, severe lameness that can be seen at a walk, but there will be consistent lameness at a trot and an increase in lameness in response to distal limb flexion.

Initially, both core lesions and surface tears are difficult to visualize on ultrasound and can be missed. With time, core lesions become easily visualized on ultrasound evaluation. Therefore, if bowed tendon is suspected, the horse should be re-examined 7–10 days later when the core lesion will be more clear ultrasonographically. In contrast, surface tears usually remain difficult to visualize on ultrasound evaluations and often require diagnostic tenoscopy, (Smith and Wright 2006) MRI, (Dyson et al. 2003) or radiographic contrast evaluation (Fiske-Jackson et al. 2013).

Surface and core tendon injuries do not require immediate referral and a plan for treatment including whether the horse will be referred can be made in the days and weeks that follow. In the meantime, the horse should be rested and treated with anti-inflammatory medications and local therapy including compression and ice.

Degenerative suspensory desmopathy is a condition that can affect older horse, especially large breed broodmares, and younger horses with a breed-associated increased risk for the disease. The onset of the disease is usually insidious, taking months or years to progress to the point of severe lameness. However, in some cases there will be an apparent acute onset of severe lameness characterized by unwillingness to move or to rise from recumbency and clear signs of pain and distress. These horses are usually managed on the farm; referral is utilized for surgical options, such as fetlock arthrodesis. The decision for euthanasia is often complicated by the episodic nature of lameness associated with degenerative suspensory desmitis. When the horse has major disruptions to normal patterns of recumbency (either stops laying down or is laying down excessively), refuses to move, or cannot maintain adequate body weight despite adequate nutrition, euthanasia is usually indicated.

Most tendon and ligament injuries have a good prognosis and will heal with appropriate rest and careful return to exercise; however, surface tears within a synovial structure are unlikely to heal without surgical debridement. Again, the decision of when to refer for advanced diagnostics and therapeutics can be made in the days and weeks following injury.

## Muscle Injury

The most common muscle injury is rupture or partial rupture of the inner thigh or hamstring muscles including the semitendinosus, semimembranosus, biceps femoris muscles and, occasionally, the gracilis muscles. These injuries often occur after a known event such as pulling back while tied or during athletic use. Western performance events seem to have a higher incidence of these injuries, probably due to the hard stops and turns at speed. Clinical signs will be lameness, local

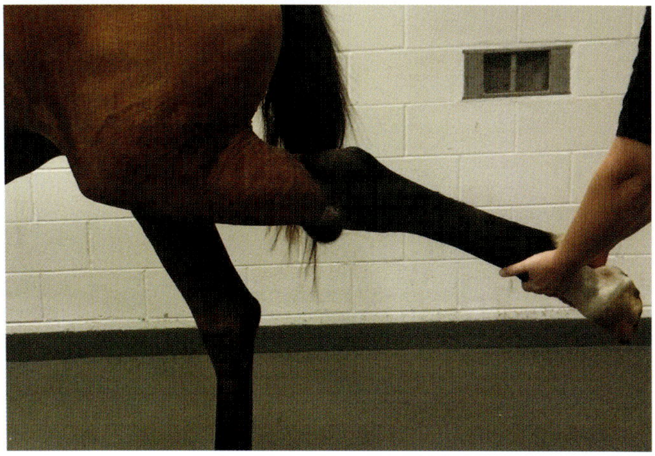

**Figure 8.10** A middle-aged Quarter Horse was presented for acute, severe lameness. The horse would place nearly full weight on the limb during the stance phase, but the limb appeared unstable during the flight phase. Extension of the hock concurrent with flexion of the stifle was possible and led to a diagnosis of peroneus tertius rupture. The horse was treated with stall confinement for six weeks, stall confinement with hand grazing for six weeks, and small paddock confinement for six weeks, and the injury healed without incident.

and severe swelling, dependent swelling in the limb distal to the injury, and pain on manipulation/palpation. The lameness will often be characterized as a shortened stride length or displacement of the haunches as opposed to reduced weight bearing. Ultrasound evaluation will reveal hematoma, edema, and disruption of the muscles involved. These cases do not require immediate referral and should be treated with rest, local therapy (cold therapy), and anti-inflammatory medication. The muscle injury will heal but can result in fibrotic myopathy, which can affect athletic performance.

A less common muscle injury is rupture of the peroneus tertius muscle (Figure 8.10). This injury usually occurs when the limb becomes entrapped behind the horse but sometimes appears to be spontaneous. This injury to the stay apparatus will allow the hock to extend when the stifle is flexed. It will result in lameness at a walk and an odd appearance to the gait, as the hock will remain extended throughout the flight phase of each step. These injuries do not require referral or advanced care. They should be strictly rested, usually for about six weeks, followed by 6–12 weeks of a graduated, controlled exercise program.

## Acute Laminitis

Laminitis can affect a single foot, both front feet, or all four feet. It can be a life-threatening problem with severe lameness and/or persistent recumbency, or it can be a mild lameness of little long-term consequence. It can be due to metabolic disease, systemic illness, severe contralateral lameness, or trauma to the foot. It can result in radiographically apparent displacement of the third phalanx within the hoof capsule or it can remain radiographically silent, without displacement of the third phalanx.

In the most common scenario, there is bilateral forelimb lameness and in acute cases, there will be increased hoof wall temperature, increased digital pulse pressure, and variable withdrawal reaction to hoof testers. The main differential for bilateral forelimb lameness is heel pain due to navicular syndrome, but this is rarely an acute change. Another differential for bilateral forelimb lameness is road founder or sole pain, usually seen in cases where the shoes have recently been removed, the feet recently trimmed, or after the horse has been housed or exercised on harder ground than it is accustomed to. These horses will improve with supportive care and time. If the problem is recurrent, changes to the foot management practices should be considered.

When laminitis is considered a likely diagnosis, radiographic examination is usually performed to include a horizontal beam lateral to medial and horizontal beam dorsal to palmar radiograph to assess for rotational or sinking displacement of the distal phalanx within the hoof capsule. Rotational displacement can be diagnosed as the dorsal edge of the third phalanx lose parallel alignment with the dorsal hoof wall. Sinking laminitis without rotation can be diagnosed using the ratio of the hoof wall thickness obtained at the junction of the middle and distal third of dorsal P3 to the palmar length of P3. Taken with the clinical picture, ratios greater than 0.3 or asymmetrical ratios (e.g., a ratio of 0.25 in one forelimb and a ratio of 0.29 in the contralateral forelimb) should raise concern for sinking laminitis. Alternatively, increase ratios could indicate thickening due to severe inflammation prior to rotational displacement. If it is the first occurrence of laminitis, displacement may not be present at the first exam and repeat imaging 5–7 days later will show displacement of the distal phalanx. Chronic laminitis begins with displacement of the pedal bone within the hoof capsule. Realignment of the hoof and pedal bone and providing support are important principles of managing chronic laminitis in horses.

Management of the foot will depend on clinician preference but usually includes adding frog support, heel elevation, and/or reducing breakover with commercially available boots, pads, or shoes. Other means of foot support include deeply bedded stalls or access to a deep sand area. Submersion of the foot in ice water is also commonly used to mitigate pain and inflammation.

Management of the horse will depend upon the etiology. In metabolic cases or pasture associated cases, the diet should be changed to reduce non-structural carbohydrates and to induce weight loss. Discontinuing access to fresh pasture grass with its high sugar content or limiting grazing to early morning only, and soaking hay for 30 minutes prior to feeding to remove water-soluble carbohydrates should be considered. In cases where Cushing's disease is suspected, testing should be performed and treatment with pergolide should be considered.

Cases with acute laminitis are usually managed on the farm. Immediate referral should be considered when there is systemic illness; otherwise, referral can be sought in the days and weeks that follow the initial diagnosis in cases that are not responding appropriately to routine laminitis management. Working together with a qualified farrier is essential for handling many lameness problems referable to the foot, including laminitis.

## Conclusion

Musculoskeletal injury is a frequent reason for presentation to the equine emergency clinician. Some musculoskeletal injury is devastating and there is no option but euthanasia, other musculoskeletal injury is of minimal consequence and needs diagnostics only, and some musculoskeletal injury is life-threatening, but with appropriate care will heal. Most importantly, the prognosis is optimized with early and skillful emergency triage.

### Case Example 8.1 Fracture of the Radius

Patient: A 21-year-old Thoroughbred gelding used for pleasure riding was presented for an acute, severe right forelimb lameness.
History: Two days prior to presentation the owner noted a small abrasion on the medial right forearm from a presumed kick injury, but no lameness was observed. The day of presentation the owner observed sudden-onset severe right forelimb lameness after the horse rose from recumbency in the stall.

*Emergency triage steps:*

*Step 1: Patient Stabilization:*

- The horse should be restrained and kept calm.
- If a handler will not be available for continuous restraint with a halter and a lead rope, the horse should be kept tied up to prevent the horse from laying down.
- Use of an orthotic device on the foot of the support limb should be considered to help prevent support limb laminitis.

Patient findings: The owner reported non-weight bearing lameness with swelling of the forearm and signs of severe distress including sweating and increased respiratory rate. The owner was instructed to stay with the horse until veterinary arrival.

*Step 2: Formulating a diagnostic plan:*

- A brief physical examination should be performed to assess the systemic state of the horse.
- The limb examination should include inspection of the abrasion on the forearm and the surrounding tissues.
- Radiographic examination of the radius should include at least cranial-caudal and lateral-medial projections with consideration to the addition of cranial to caudal oblique projections.

Patient findings: The physical examination was unremarkable other than tachycardia (54 bpm), tachypnea (40 bpm), diffuse sweating, and mild increase in rectal temperature (101°F). There was a severe right forelimb lameness and mild, firm swelling that did not pit, and was painful on deep palpation centered around the healing abrasion on the medial forearm. Radiographs of the forearm revealed an incomplete radial fracture.

*Step 3: Emergency treatment guidelines:*

- When radial fracture is suspected but a fissure line is not observed radiographically, radiographs should be repeated in 10 days (Derungs et al. 2001).
- Referral for surgical treatment by internal fixation is rarely advised due to the inability to fully assess the fracture configuration resulting in a high risk for failure of the repair postoperatively.
- Propagation of the fracture line(s) to complete, displaced fracture can occur with the increased load and torsional forces of the horse getting up from laying down.
- Cross-tying a horse with a suspected or confirmed non-displaced radial fracture can be used to discourage laying down. However, horses can still lay down when they are tied.
- The only way to prevent the horses from laying down, is the use of a sling support system. The sling not only prevents the horse from lying down but allows horse movement in the stall and many horses will support their weight with the sling during periods of rest.
- Referral to a hospital for maintenance in a sling support system to prevent the horse from laying down while the fracture heals should be considered.
- Most conservatively managed incomplete radial and tibial fractures are maintained in a sling support system for 4-10 weeks, depending on the rate of apparent healing (Fürst et al. 2008).
- Splinting or casting the fracture is rarely performed for long-term management due to the likelihood of the split or cast ending at or close to the level of the fracture.
- A stiff, full-limb compression bandage with a lateral splint from the level of the ground to the wither should be considered for transport.

Patient findings: Given the increased risk of progression to a displaced fracture during rising from recumbency, the horse was tied in the stall to prevent laying down and maintained on phenylbutazone and SoftRide boots on both front feet. The horse stood square and appeared to be comfortable.

*Step 4: Assessment and monitoring:*

- A common complication is support-limb laminitis.
- Comfort level should be monitored daily, and analgesics administered as needed.
- Orthotic devices designed to prevent support-limb laminitis or deep, supportive footing should be used.
- Local wound care and bandaging may be needed at the site of the kick injury.
- Systemic antibiotics may be needed when there is cellulitis associated with the kick injury.
- Horses will initially be visibly sore on the limb while tied, progressing to visible soreness while shifting or turning in the stall, and finally to lack of lameness development after hand walking exercise.
- Serial radiographic examination is used to monitor fracture healing. An important finding that demonstrates developing fracture stability is presence of periosteal and endosteal callus that is initially irregular and becomes smoothly marginated and cortical-like density. The fracture margins themselves will become more apparent (wider and more radiolucent) in the first weeks and eventually develop less crisp margins, less width, and less radiolucency before filling in completely, which will take several months.

Patient findings: Four weeks later, the horse was found lying down in the stall despite being tied and was unwilling to rise. With verbal and physical stimulation, the horse rose from recumbency but was immediately non-weight bearing on the right forelimb. Repeat radiographs revealed additional fracture lines and irregular periosteal new bone formation, but the radial cortices appeared to remain intact, and the fracture was not displaced (Figure 8.11a, b).

The horse was transported to a referral facility to be maintained in an Anderson sling (Figure 8.12). The purpose of the sling was to prevent recumbency and allow the horse to support his body weight by leaning against the sling. During the first week of hospitalization, the horse would frequently rest the right forelimb on its toe and paw with the right forelimb. During the second week of hospitalization, resting and pawing of the right forelimb was less frequent, but the horse appeared to be sore on the right forelimb when moving around in the stall. In the third week, the horse appeared to be comfortable on the right forelimb most of the time. During the fourth week (eight weeks from the original kick injury), the Anderson sling was removed for five-minute daily hand walks. At the end of the walks, mild right forelimb lameness was noted, which steadily improved to no observable lameness when walking over the following two weeks.

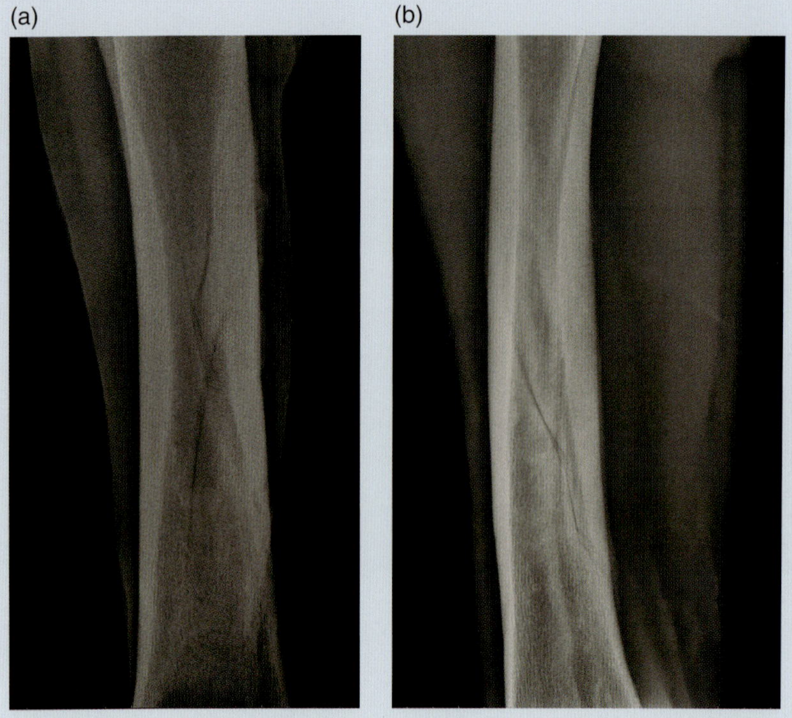

**Figure 8.11** (a) Cranial-caudal and (b) lateral-medial radiographs four weeks after the initial kick injury to the medial forearm. There is an incomplete, comminuted radial fracture with irregular periosteal new bone.

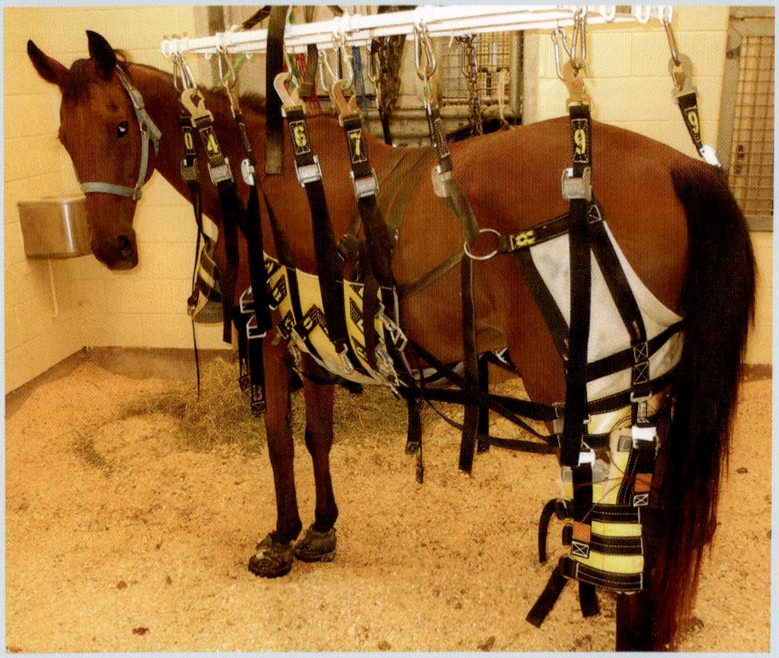

**Figure 8.12** A 21-year-old Thoroughbred gelding was maintained in an Anderson sling to prevent fracture propagation associated with rising from recumbency.

In the sixth week of hospitalization (ten weeks from the original kick injury), the fracture lines remained radiographically visible with smooth, cortical-like periosteal and endosteal new bone (Figure 8.13a, b). The Anderson sling was removed, and the horse was observed to roll several times, rising normally without subsequent right forelimb lameness. The horse was discharged with instructions for an escalating controlled exercise program over the following three months prior to resumption of pasture turnout with others and unrestricted ridden work.

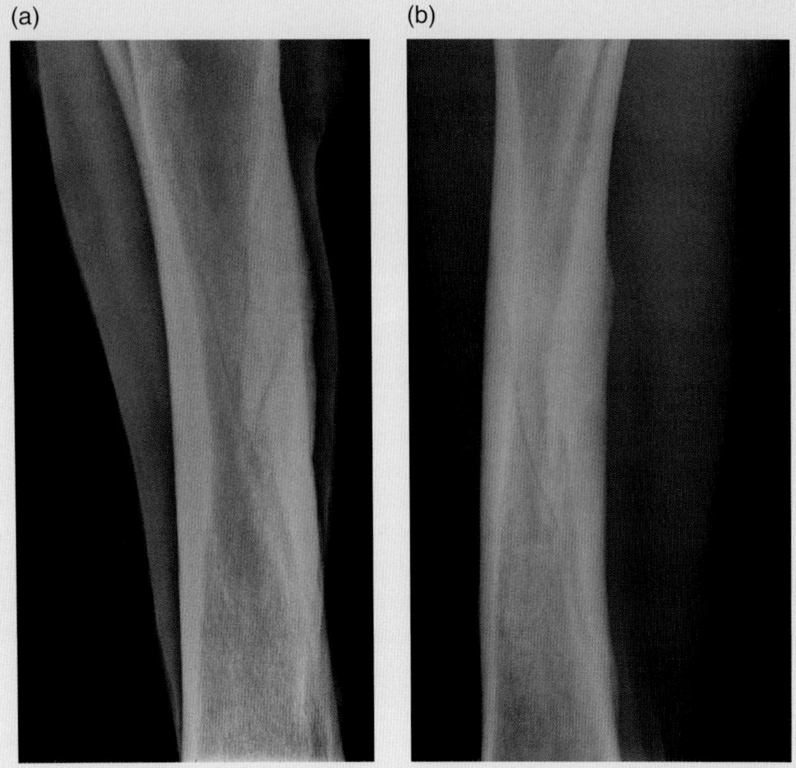


**Figure 8.13** (a) Cranial-caudal and (b) lateral-medial radiographs 10 weeks after the initial kick injury to the medial forearm. There is an incomplete, comminuted radial fracture with smoothly marginated and cortical-like periosteal and endosteal new bone.

*Step 5: Decision making during triage:*

*Decision for referral:*

- Incomplete radial or tibial fracture in the horse is nearly always associated with a kick injury to the medial forearm (crus).
- The fracture may progress to an unstable fracture in the weeks following injury, which usually occurs while the horse is rising from recumbency.
- Owners who would like to minimize the risk of fracture progression to a complete fracture should be referred for in hospital sling support to prevent the horse from laying down.
- If sling support is not available, cross-tying can be utilized to reduce laying down behavior, but cross-tying will not prevent the horse from laying down.

*Medical* vs *surgical treatment:*

- Surgical treatment is not recommended due to difficulty in fully assessing fracture configuration.

*Managing complications:*

- Support limb laminitis is prevented by careful analgesia, orthotic devices on the foot with or without deep bedding, and use of the sling to support the horses body weight.

*Estimating prognosis:*

- With prevention of laying down during the 4–10 weeks after injury, (Fürst et al. 2008) most horses have a good prognosis for survival and resumption of athletic activities.

*Decision for euthanasia:*

- Radial and tibial fractures that progress to a complete fracture are rarely fixable and euthanasia is usually indicated.

## References


Aleman, M., Berryhill, E., Woolard, K. et al. (2020). Sidewinder gait in horses. *J. Vet. Intern. Med.* 34: 2122–2131.

Brünisholz, H.P., Hagen, R., Fürst, A.E., and Kuemmerle, J.M. (2015). Radiographic and computed tomographic configuration of incomplete proximal fractures of the proximal phalanx in horses not used for racing. *Vet. Surg.* 44: 809–815.

Byrne, C.A., Lumsden, J.M., Lang, H.M., and O'Sullivan, C.B. (2020). Synovial sepsis of unknown origin in the adult Thoroughbred racehorse. *Equine Vet. J.* 52: 91–97.

Carmalt, J.L. (2009). What is your diagnosis? *J. Am. Vet. Med. Assoc.* 235: 377–378.

Cole, S.D., Stefanovski, D., Towl, S., and Boyle, A.G. (2019). Factors associated with prolonged treatment days, increased veterinary visits and complications in horses with subsolar abscesses. *Vet. Rec.* 184: 251–251.

Derungs, S., Fuerst, A., Haas, C. et al. (2001). Fissure fractures of the radius and tibia in 23 horses: a retrospective study. *Equine Vet. Educ.* 13: 313–318.

Dyson, S., Murray, R., Schramme, M., and Branch, M. (2003). Lameness in 46 horses associated with deep digital flexor tendonitis in the digit: diagnosis confirmed with magnetic resonance imaging. *Equine Vet. J.* 35: 681–690.

Ellis, D., Simpson, D., Greenwood, R.E., and Crowhurst, J.S. (1987). Observations and management of fractures of the proximal phalanx in young Thoroughbreds. *Equine Vet. J.* 19: 43–49.

Fiske-Jackson, A.R., Barker, W.H.J., Eliashar, E. et al. (2013). The use of intrathecal analgesia and contrast radiography as preoperative diagnostic methods for digital flexor tendon sheath pathology. *Equine Vet. J.* 45: 36–40.

Fürst, A.E., Keller, R., Kummer, M.R. et al. (2008). Evaluation of a new full-body animal rescue and transportation sling in horses: 181 horses (1998–2006): retrospective study. *J. Vet. Emerg. Crit. Care* 18: 619–625.

Krause, D.M., Pezzanite, L.M., Griffenhagen, G.M., and Hendrickson, D.A. (2022). Comparison of equine synovial sepsis rate following intrasynovial injection in ambulatory versus hospital settings. *Equine Vet. J.* 54: 523.

Moyer, W. (1989). Clinical examination of the equine foot. *Vet. Clin. N. Am. Equine Pract.* 5: 29–46.

Smith, M.R.W. and Wright, I.M. (2006). Noninfected tenosynovitis of the digital flexor tendon sheath: a retrospective analysis of 76 cases. *Equine Vet. J.* 38: 134–141.

Whitfield-Cargile, C., Dabareiner, R.M., and Sustaire, D. (2009). How to use a fetlock support brace to manage lacerations of equine flexor tendons. *Medicine.* 394–398. http://aaep.org.

Whitfield-Cargile, C., Dabareiner, R.M., and Sustaire, D. (2011). Use of a fetlock support brace to manage lacerations of equine flexor tendons. *Equine Vet. Educ.* 23: 46–52.

Yovich, J.V., Turner, A.S., Stashak, T.S., and McIlwraith, C.W. (1987). Luxation of the metacarpophalangeal and metatarsophalangeal joints in horses. *Equine Vet. J.* 19: 295–298.

# 9

# Oral and Maxillofacial Emergencies

*Alexandra L. Wright and Edward T. Earley*

*Department of Clinical Sciences, College of Veterinary Medicine, Cornell University, Ithaca, NY, USA*

## Introduction

A complete examination of the oral cavity, skull, and head is indicated for oral emergency in the horse and may include intraoral and extraoral examination, nasal endoscopy, radiographic and computed tomography (CT). Many types of oral and maxillofacial problems may present to the equine veterinarian, including dental, skull, and lingual trauma, as well as other diseases. Box 9.1 summarizes important principles outlined in the chapter.

## Oral and Maxillofacial Examination

A complete summary of *oral and maxillofacial examination* including extraoral (visual and palpation), oral (mirror and endoscopic), nasal endoscopic and radiographic examinations of the head and oral cavity is provided in the online book supplement. Here the authors outline specific examination equipment and methods, radiographic positioning and technique, and endoscopy principles. They also share additional illustrations to guide the clinician through diagnostic examination of the oral cavity and maxillofacial region of the horse (AVDC 2023; Baratt 2013, 2020; Claffey and Ducharme 2020; Dixon et al. 2014; Earley et al. 2020a; Earley and Reiswig 2020c; Easley 2020; Galloway and Easley 2013; Griffin and Vogt 2022; Henry and Bishop 2020; Henry et al. 2022; Menzies 2013; True and Dotzel 2020).

## Case Management

### Dental Trauma

#### Dental Fracture – Classification and Assessment

Dental fractures are classified based on location and extent of the fracture margins. In the horse, the incisors, premolars (excluding the first premolar-wolf tooth), and molars have a hypsodont tooth form which has a short clinical crown, long reserve crown, and short roots. The clinical crown is the portion of the tooth that is visible within the oral cavity. It extends from the margin of the gingival attachment to the occlusal surface. The reserve crown is the most robust and longest portion of the tooth. It extends from the attached gingiva apically to the roots. In the area between the alveolar bone margin and the soft-tissue gingival attachment, additional peripheral cementum is laid down around the tooth. This gives the tooth additional strength as it erupts above the gingiva margin and becomes the clinical crown. The apical aspect of the reserve crown forms short roots at about ~5–6 years post eruption of the tooth. The formation of the roots marks a set length (and time) of reserve crown available for eruption into a functional clinical crown. The incisors have a single root, the mandibular premolars and molars have two roots (mesial and distal), and the maxillary premolars and molar have three roots (palatal, mesial buccal, and distal buccal). The vascular, nerve, and vital cellular supply (collectively termed pulp) to the tooth extends from the roots

*Emergency Triage of the Horse*, First Edition. Edited by Rolfe M. Radcliffe and Jamie J. Kopper.

Companion website: www.wiley.com/go/radcliffe/triage

**Box 9.1 Oral and maxillofacial key points**

- Open-mouth radiographs with a speculum are preferred unless a skull fracture is suspected.
- The oral endoscope gives a high-resolution, detailed image allowing for subtle details not discernable with an intraoral mirror.
- Nasal endoscopic techniques may be used to evaluate conchal bullae and sinus disease.
- A radiographic examination utilizing a bisecting angle technique allows for images that are proportional to the actual anatomy.
- Dental fractures are described as involving the clinical crown, reserve crown, and/or root(s). Additionally, the fracture margin is delineated to determine if the internal pulp of the tooth is involved.
- Not all fractured teeth require extraction. If there is reserve crown with good attachment, oral and radiographic monitoring may be indicated prior to determining if extraction is warranted.
- Equine Odontoclastic Tooth Resorption and Hypercementosis (EOTRH) is a progressive resorptive disease affecting both dentition and surrounding bone.
- Not all skull fractures require fixation. Unilateral rostral fractures may heal with conservative management.
- When a skull fracture (maxilla or mandible) involves the bony alveolus around a tooth, it is usually best to leave the tooth in place initially for stabilization. However, typically (~6–10 weeks post fracture) the tooth will require extraction to allow for complete healing.
- Lingual trauma or foreign body should be considered with horses exhibiting marked tongue swelling, dysphagia, and hypersalivation.

(root canal) into a common pulp chamber and coronally into a vital network of pulp horns. The pulp horns extend through each cusp formation (multiple cusps merged to form the premolars and molars) to a variable distance below the occlusal surface (~3–15 mm) (White and Dixon 2010). Sub-occlusal secondary (irregular) dentin and peripheral secondary dentin (regular) within the pulp horn form the darkly stained occlusal dentin which covers and protects the sensitive pulp tissue of the tooth.

Fractures are assessed based on the depth of the fracture margin and if a pulp horn has been involved. If the fracture extends to the gingival margin it is referred to as a *clinical crown* fracture. If the fracture extends past the gingival attachment, it is a *reserve crown* fracture; however, based on terminology consistent with other species, it is often termed collectively as root and reserve crown and called a *crown–root* fracture. For clarity and specificity, in this chapter the fracture location will be described based on the anatomy involved 1) clinical crown, 2) reserve crown, and 3) root(s). If a pulp horn is involved the fracture is additionally described as a *complicated* fracture. The term complicated arises because of the possibility of internal disease extension through the pulp horn network within the tooth from pulp exposure or insult. An uncomplicated fracture refers to a fracture margin that does not extend into a pulp horn (only involves the dental hard tissues: enamel, dentin, and/or cementum).

#### Anterior Dentition – Incisor and Canine Teeth

Incisor and canine trauma often involve self-inflicted injuries that may not be witnessed or noticed for hours to days. Examples of trauma include incisive bone fracture, tooth luxation or avulsion, alveolar bone fracture, and tooth fracture (Earley and Rawlinson 2013). Both oral and radiographic examinations are indicated to assess the nature and extent of the injury. Local infusion of anesthetic (lidocaine or mepivacaine) should be utilized when cleaning, debriding, and treating the site of injury. Regional anesthesia may be achieved via the inferior alveolar, mental, maxillary, or infraorbital nerve (Campoy and Sedgewick 2020). (*See supplemental material online for nerve block details.*)

*Tooth luxation* refers to different levels of attachment loss (periodontal ligaments and bone) while the tooth remains within the alveolus. Luxation types in order from least to more severe have been described as 1) Concussion, 2) Subluxation, 3) Extrusive, 4) Lateral, and 5) Intrusive (Gracis 2012). A case example of a horse tooth luxation is presented in Box 9.2. If the periodontal ligaments are unharmed and mostly intact, the tooth may be treated with light-to-moderate splinting. Alveolar bone is often compromised and/or fractured. The blood supply to the apex of the tooth may be compromised with the initial trauma. This may lead to "loss of vitality" (non-vital) and potentially endodontic infection/disease. Mildly luxated teeth may be repositioned and splinted with composite material. The splint may need some wire reinforcement. Tooth attachment, bone healing, and splint integrity should be monitored weekly with radiographic monitoring at ~4-, 6-, 8- and 10-weeks post splint application. If secondary endodontic disease develops, root canal therapy or extraction may be indicated.

**Box 9.2 Tooth luxation case example: periodontal splinting (Figures 9.1–9.8)**

- A 7-month-old Thoroughbred colt presents with acute trauma of the incisive bone involving the deciduous incisors.
- Initial oral examination reveals that the right and left maxillary deciduous first incisors (501 and 601) have severe lateral luxation. The left maxillary deciduous second incisor (602) is missing. The right maxillary deciduous second incisor is fully erupted and appears normal. It is also noted that the right and left maxillary deciduous third incisors are just erupting and appear normal (Figures 9.1 and 9.2).
- The site is gently debrided and lavaged (saline) with careful attention to the location of the developing permanent teeth just lingual to the deciduous counterparts.
- The gingival defects and lacerations are closed with a 3–0 absorbable monofilament suture[1] (Figure 9.3).
- With the young unerupted developing permanent dentition present, the erupted luxated deciduous dentition is preserved using an oral splint.
- A wire-reinforced composite splint is created using 22-gauge cerclage wire. The wire is buried submucosal using 18-gauge needles (Figure 9.4).
- The wire is gently tightened using an orthodontic wire tensioner.[2]
- The clinical crowns of the deciduous incisors are etched with phosphoric acid,[3] rinsed, and gently air dried (Figure 9.5).
- An unfilled resin[4] is placed along the exposed surfaces of the clinical crowns and light cured.[5]
- A chemically curing bis-acrylic composite[6] is applied to the labial surface of the teeth and over the wire to protect the soft tissues and strengthen the splint (Figure 9.6).

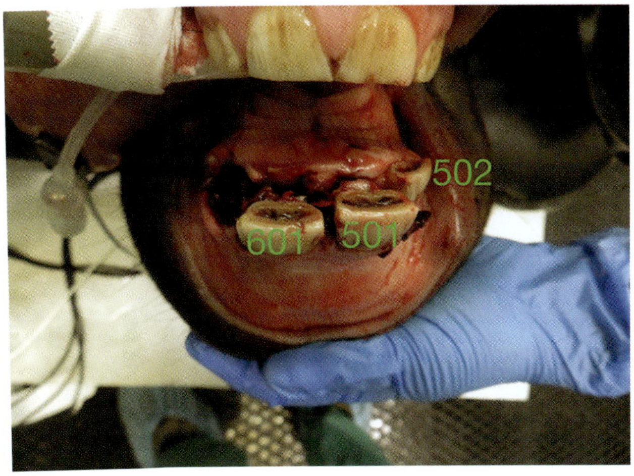


**Figure 9.1** 7-month-old foal with acute trauma of incisive bone. The foal is in dorsal recumbency under general anesthesia. There is severe lateral luxation of both central deciduous incisors (501 and 601). The right maxillary second (middle) deciduous incisor (502) is fully erupted and appears normal. The left maxillary second deciduous incisor (601) is missing.

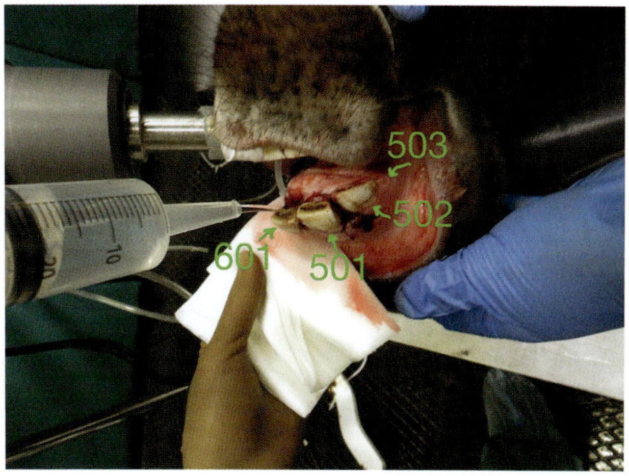


**Figure 9.2** 7-month-old foal with acute trauma of incisive bone in dorsal recumbency. Gentle saline lavage with careful attention not to disturb the dental buds of the developing permanent teeth. The permanent teeth usually emerge just lingual to their deciduous predecessors. The right maxillary third deciduous incisor (503) is normal and actively erupting.

1 Monocryl (poliglecaprone 25) suture, Ethicon Johnson and Johnson Surgical Technologies, Somerville, NJ, 08876.
2 Orthodontic pliers, 3M™ Unitek™ Prestige Series Hand Instruments, Maplewood, MN, 55144.
3 37% Phosphoric Acid etch gel, Benco Dental, Pittson, PA, 18640.
4 Prime&Bond NT, Nano-Technology Dental Adhesive, Dentsply Sirona, Milford, DE, 19963
5 Soleil™ Curing Light, Benco Dental, Pittson, PA, 18640.
6 Protemp™ Plus, 3M ESPE Dental Products, St. Paul, MN, 55144–1000.

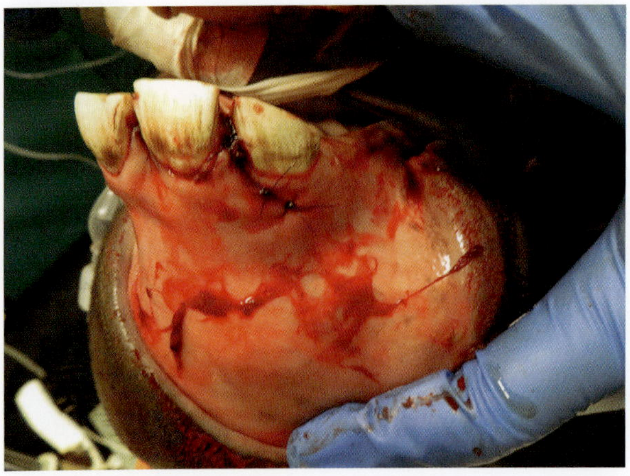

**Figure 9.3** 7-month-old foal with acute trauma of incisive bone in dorsal recumbency. The gingival defects/lacerations are closed with simple interrupted sutures.

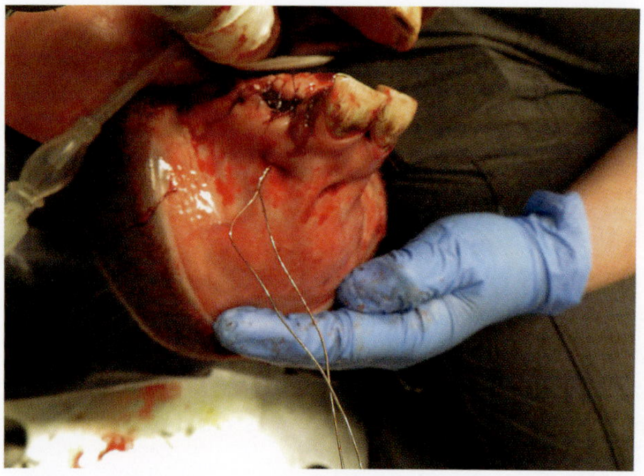

**Figure 9.4** 7-month-old foal with acute trauma of incisive bone in dorsal recumbency. The gingival and mucosal defects are closed with monofilament absorbable suture.[1] 22-gauge stainless steel wire is placed submucosal as an initial cerclage reinforcement for the luxated 501 and 601.

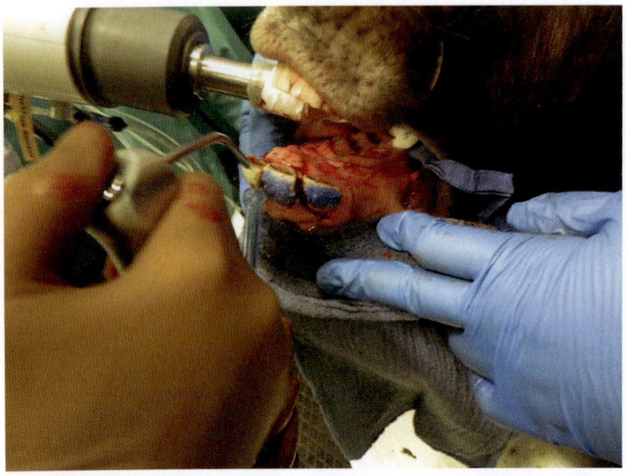

**Figure 9.5** 7-month-old foal with acute trauma of incisive bone in dorsal recumbency. The buccal and palatal surfaces of the incisor clinical crowns are prepared for bonding and splint application by etching with phosphoric acids.

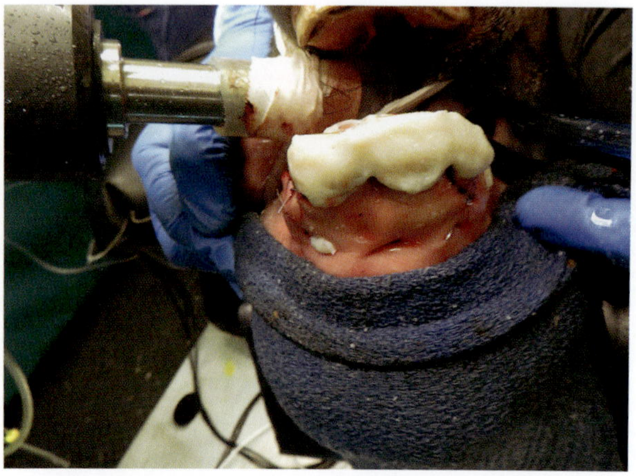

**Figure 9.6** 7-month-old foal with acute trauma of incisive bone in dorsal recumbency. An intraoral splint is created with a bis-acrylic composite.[6]

- An intraoral radiograph is taken following completion of the composite/wire splint (Figure 9.7). Note the irregular/malformation of 601 (red arrows) and the widened periodontal ligament along the mesial aspect of 501 (green arrows).
- At six weeks post splint application, bone and dental healing is evaluated with intraoral radiographs. At that time the oral splint is removed with standing sedation. 501 has no attachment and 601 has very poor attachment (green arrows) (Figure 9.8).

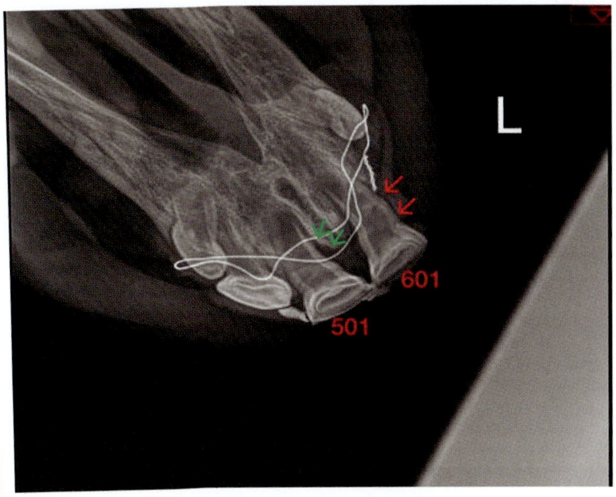


**Figure 9.7** 7-month-old foal with acute trauma of incisive bone. Intraoral radiograph of the completed intraoral splint. Note the irregular/malformation of 601 (red arrows) and the widened periodontal ligament along the mesial aspect of 501 (green arrows).

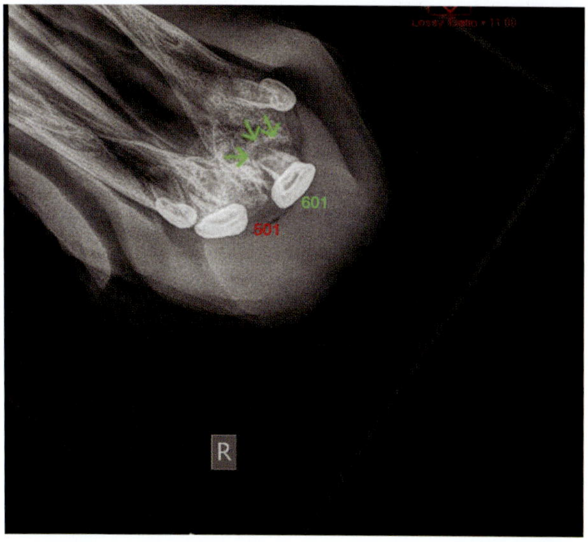


**Figure 9.8** At six weeks post splint application, bone and dental healing is evaluated with intraoral radiographs. At that time the oral splint is removed with standing sedation. 501 has no attachment and 601 has very poor attachment (green arrows) Extraction was indicated.

*Tooth avulsion* refers to complete tooth removal from the alveolus. It often involves more extensive periodontal ligament damage and/or bone fracture. It is likely that the blood supply to the tooth will be compromised. A case example of tooth avulsion in a horse is summarized in Box 9.3. An attempt to repair an avulsed tooth requires replacement into the alveolus and robust splinting with wire-reinforced composite. If avulsion involves deciduous dentition, gentle replacement and splint application may be considered to allow for some type of deciduous dental healing while the underlying permanent tooth continues to develop. If there is extensive bone and soft-tissue damage along with severe contamination it may be better to gently lavage the wound and remove the compromised deciduous components while trying to preserve the underlying developing permanent dental bud(s). A flap may be developed with the remaining soft tissue by creating a release incision and elevating attached periosteum. The mucosal flap can be positioned to protect developing adult teeth and closed using a 2–0 or 3–0 absorbable monofilament suture.[1]

#### Posterior Dentition – Premolar and Molar Teeth (Cheekteeth)

In addition to tooth fractures as described above, disease may extend to the soft tissue (periodontal ligament) and bony attachment (lamina dura) of the tooth within the alveolus. If the soft tissue and bone attachment loss exceeds ~50%, the long-term prognosis for the tooth is poor. Disease extension may develop beyond the alveolus and extend to an overlying sinus, nasal bullae, neighboring tooth, or fistulate through bone. Dental radiography and computed tomography are very helpful when assessing disease attachment loss and disease extension. In the equine patient, not all dental fractures will require extraction. With the reserve crown capability and the robust cellular nature of the pulp, many tooth fractures can internally wall off internal pulp infections (with secondary regular and irregular dentin) and allow time for reserve crown replacement. (Dacre et al. 2007; Dixon et al. 2007, 2021; Earley and Rawlinson 2013; Pollaris et al. 2021) Endoscopic and radiographic monitoring are indicated to assess attachment and tooth vitality.

### Equine Odontoclastic Tooth Resorption and Hypercementosis (EOTRH)

EOTRH is a progressive resorptive disease affecting both dentition and surrounding bone. It is a multifactorial syndrome (Earley et al. 2017; Limone 2020; Smedley et al. 2015; Staszyk et al. 2008) that was first described in 2004 (Klugh 2004) and is currently common among the general horse population. The disease has been diagnosed in horses of all breeds, usually older than 12 years, and affecting all teeth but most commonly incisors and canines. To date, little is known about the etiology of the disease even though it occurs widespread across the world. Because this disease tends to be under-diagnosed in

**Box 9.3 Tooth avulsion case example: deciduous tooth extraction, nonvital bone removal, and preservation of developing adult dentition with a mucogingival flap (Figures 9.9–9.13)**

- A 4-year-old Morgan gelding presents with a chronic fracture of the rostral right mandible.
- Initial oral examination reveals avulsion of the right mandibular permanent second incisor (402) and the right mandibular deciduous third incisor (803). Also noted is exposure and lateral luxation of the right mandibular developing permanent third incisor (403) (Figure 9.9).
- An intraoral radiograph confirms avulsion of 402 and 803 along with lateral luxation of the unerupted 403 (Figure 9.10).
- Due to the chronicity, local infection, and nonvital teeth, all three teeth (402, 803, and 403) are extracted along with the fractured devitalized bone (Figure 9.11).
- The surgical site is gently lavaged and debrided. A double-release advancing mucoperiosteal flap is created to close the remaining defect using a 2–0 monofilament absorbable suture[1] (Figure 9.12).
- The fractured rostral right mandible and close association of the three teeth is reconstructed post extraction (Figure 9.13).

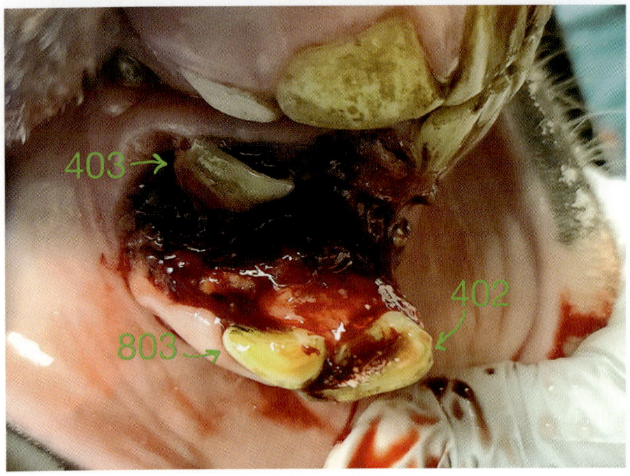


**Figure 9.9** 4-year-old Morgan gelding with a chronic fracture of the rostral right mandible. Avulsion of 402 and 803 and exposure of the developing 403.

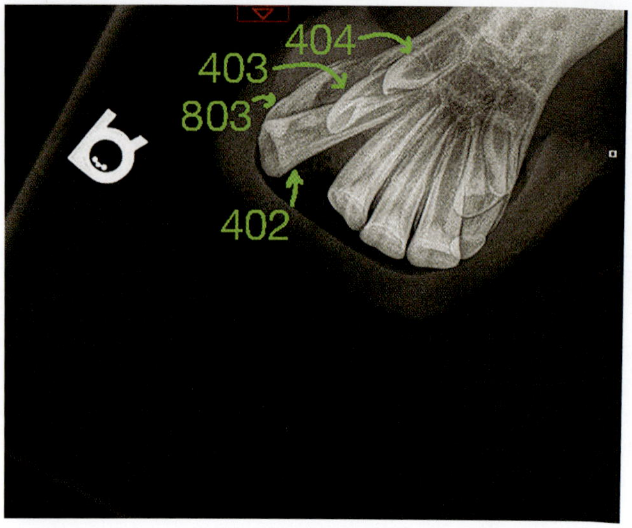


**Figure 9.10** 4-year-old Morgan gelding with a chronic fracture of the rostral right mandible. Intraoral radiograph showing the avulsed 402 and 803.

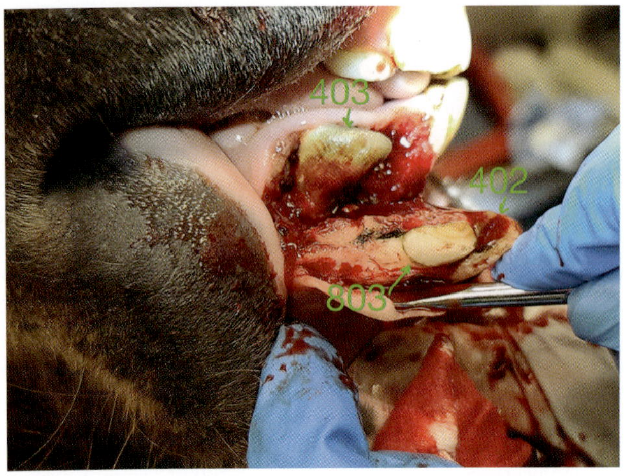


**Figure 9.11** 4-year-old Morgan gelding. Following gentle saline lavage and debridement, the developing 403 appears necrotic and non-vital. Due to the chronic nature of the fracture and guarded prognosis, extraction of all three teeth was performed.

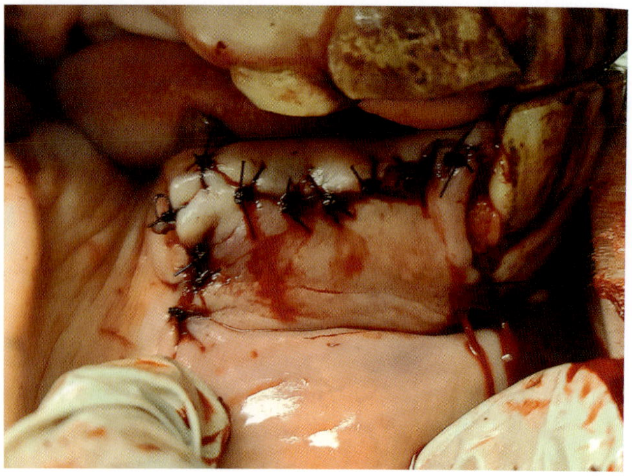

**Figure 9.12** 4-year-old Morgan gelding. A double-release advancing mucoperiosteal flap is created to close the extraction site(s).

**Figure 9.13** 4-year-old Morgan gelding. Note the position and close association of the developing 403 just lingual to 803.

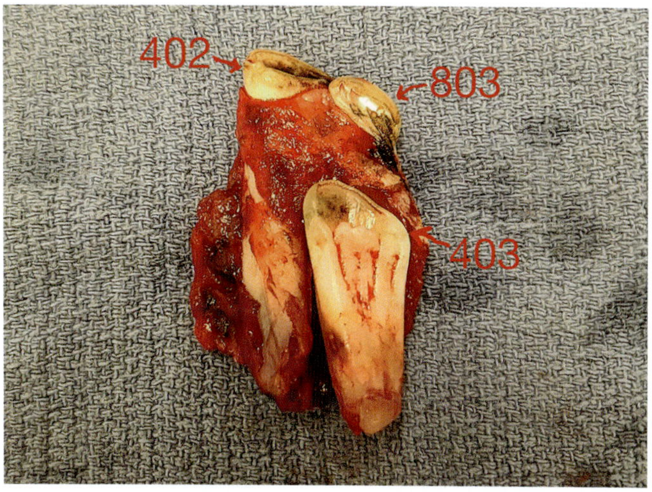


the general horse population (Henry et al. 2017; Rehrl et al. 2018, 2022), cases often present late with significant clinical signs, morbidity, and advanced radiographic changes. No treatments have been effective in slowing the progression of the tooth resorption or hypercementosis. Due to the painfulness of the disease, extraction of all affected rostral dentition (incisors and canines) is typically recommended (Limone 2020).

Pathological incisor fractures are often seen in horses with EOTRH. The integrity of the tooth is compromised with the disease process which may lead to fracture. (Earley and Rawlinson 2013) Extraction of the fractured tooth is indicated to treat the acute pain of the injury. Local and/or regional anesthesia, sulcular incision, and elevation of the tooth ± fragments is indicated. Post-operative radiographs are necessary to ensure complete removal of the tooth fragments. This site can be left to heal by second intention with simple extraction, or a release flap may be utilized to cover the extraction site (Earley and Galloway 2020b). If additional teeth are severely affected with resorptive disease, more extractions may be indicated later as a scheduled, non-urgent procedure. A case example of EOTRH in a horse is presented in Box 9.4.

*EOTRH summary:*

- Clinical signs: Sensitivity to oral speculum use despite sedation, gross changes including gingival recession, gingival bulging, draining tracts, and fractured incisors. Due to the chronic inflammatory process, disease progression may lead to weight loss and occasionally inappetence.
- Radiographic changes: Resorption of the tooth starting at the periodontal ligament space, some teeth will additionally have reactive abnormal cementum that has been termed "hypercementosis." Periapical bone loss can occur due to resorption and expansion of cementum. Radiographs are indicated for diagnosis and monitoring progression of the disease.
- Since EOTRH is a slow progressive disease, extraction is typically not an urgent, emergency surgery. The systemic and oral health should be considered before dental procedures are performed. Tooth floating/grinding may increase dental pain and aggravate/accelerate the disease process. Complete incisor extraction will reduce the occlusal space between the maxillary and mandibular cheek teeth. The reduced space will increase occlusal forces which may be painful with severely affected premolars and molars. Surgical extraction techniques are typically indicated since resorptive teeth tend to fragment and ankylosis to bone is common. Referral to a veterinary dentist for evaluation and possible extraction(s) is recommended (Earley and Galloway 2020b).

  *Practice Tip: If speculum sensitivity is noted during an evaluation of an older horse, intraoral incisor and canine radiographs are indicated to diagnose, stage, and manage the resorptive disease.*

### Skull Fracture

Skull fractures commonly involve the rostral mandible(s) and rostral maxilla (incisive bone). Occasionally, caudal mandible fractures may occur that involve the horizontal or vertical ramus. Caudal maxillae fractures may present due to local blunt trauma from either self-infliction or kick wounds from pasture mates. Mandible and maxillae injuries should be initially evaluated conservatively. Soft-tissue swelling may be noted along the medial or lateral aspects of the ventral border of the mandible or on the dorsal aspect of the long axis of the face. Initial extraoral examination should include palpation

**Box 9.4 EOTRH case example: Incisor fracture (Figures 9.14–9.20)**

- Root fracture of the left maxillary third incisor (203). The tooth has been severely compromised due to the resorptive disease (Figures 9.14 and 9.15).
- The treatment plan is to surgically extract the tooth and root.
- A mucoperiosteal flap is created. Buccal alveolar bone is removed using a high-speed surgical drill[7] (with saline irrigation) and a 5 mm oval carbide bur.[8]
- With the reserve crown and root exposed, the tooth and root are extracted with gentle luxation and elevation (Figures 9.16–9.18).[9]
- A post extraction intraoral radiograph confirms complete extraction of the tooth (Figure 9.19).
- The mucogingival flap (Figure 9.20) is closed using a 3–0 monofilament absorbable suture.[1]
- Once the extraction site is healed, a treatment plan is developed for the remaining teeth severely affected with resorptive disease.

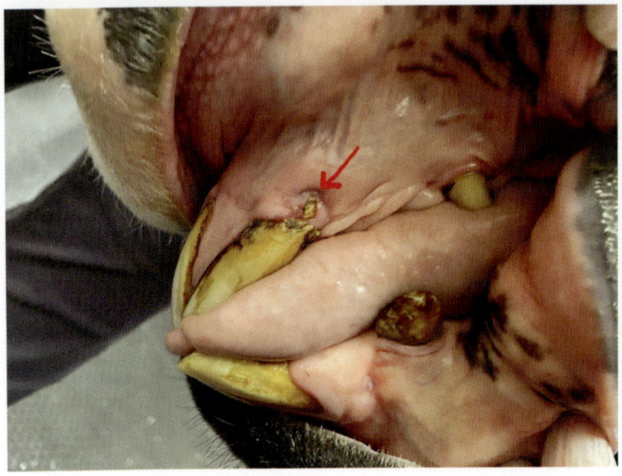

**Figure 9.14** Root fracture of the left maxillary third incisor (203) due to EOTRH (Equine odontoclastic tooth resorption and hypercementosis). Severe resorptive disease of 203 with gingival recession and exposure of the root (red arrow).

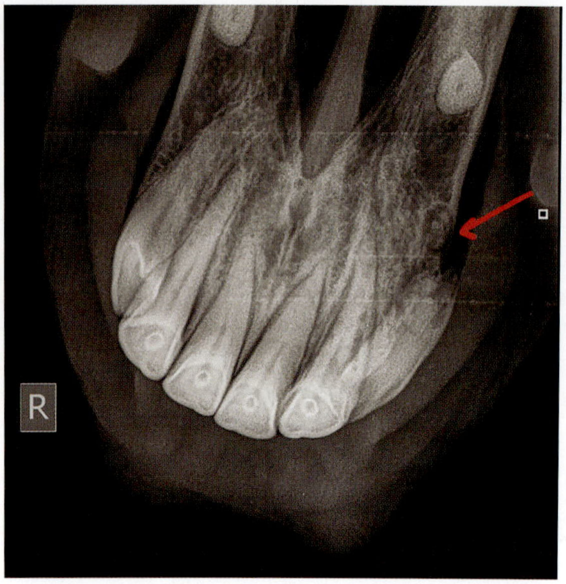


**Figure 9.15** Root fracture of the left maxillary third incisor (203) due to EOTRH. Intraoral radiograph of the maxillary incisors. A pathological root fracture of 203 is evident (red arrow).

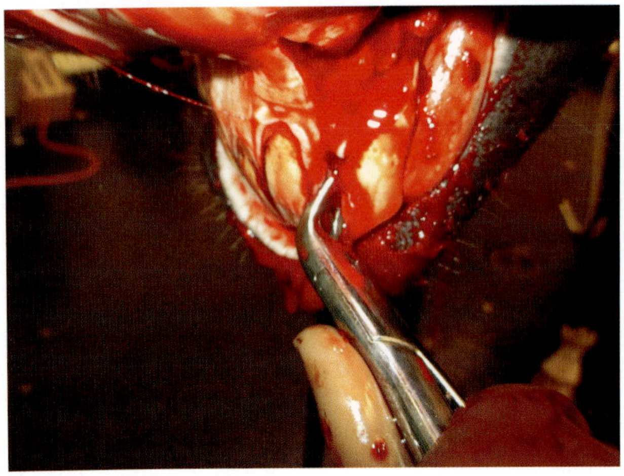

**Figure 9.16** Root fracture of the left maxillary third incisor (203) due to EOTRH. Small right angled cowhorn forceps are used for initial luxation prior to elevation and extraction.

---

7 Hall 5058–5001 Surgairtome 2 Pneumatic Surgical Handpiece, ConMed Linvatec, Largo, FL, 33773–4908.

8 Oval Bur-Medium, ConMed Corporation, Utica, NY, 13502–5994.

9 Atraumair #23 Cowhorn Forceps. Hu-Friedy Manufacturing, Co., LLC, Chicago, IL, 60618–5935.

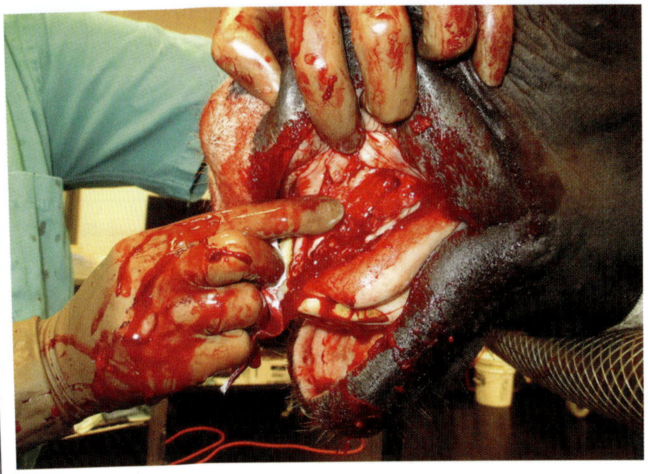

**Figure 9.17** Root fracture of the left maxillary third incisor (203) due to EOTRH. The single-release envelope flap is raised to show complete extraction of 203 and the fractured root.

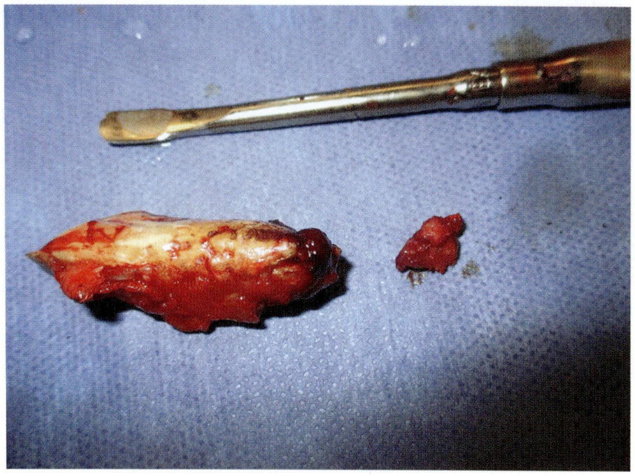

**Figure 9.18** Root fracture of the left maxillary third incisor (203) due to EOTRH. Extracted 203 and root tip.

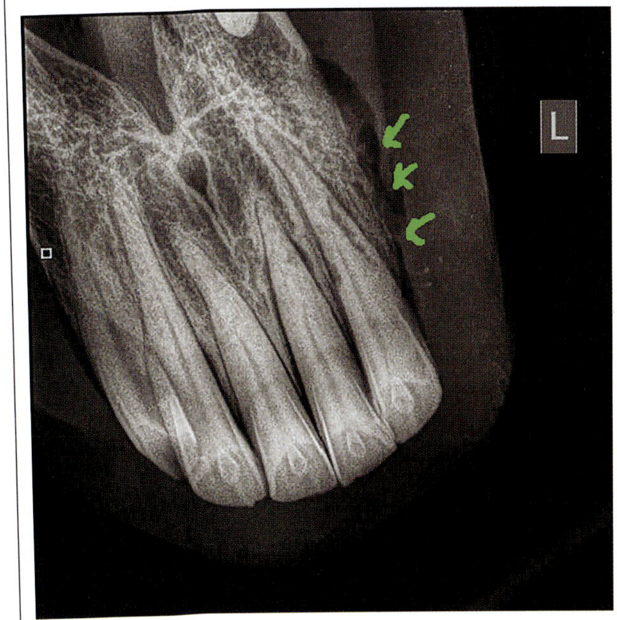


**Figure 9.19** Root fracture of the left maxillary third incisor (203) due to EOTRH. Post extraction intraoral radiograph confirms complete extraction of 203 and the fractured root (green arrows).

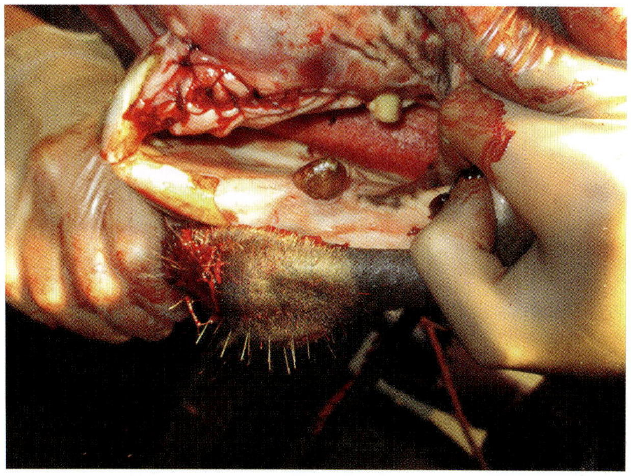

**Figure 9.20** Root fracture of the left maxillary third incisor (203) due to EOTRH. The extraction site is closed with the mucogingival flap and simple interrupted absorbable sutures.[1]

for swelling, asymmetry, crepitus, and skin abrasion/laceration. The initial radiographic examination is performed with the mouth closed utilizing the same extraoral techniques as described for open-mouth techniques in the *radiographic examination* section above. If the fracture is unilateral, intraoral radiographic and oral examination techniques may be utilized with caution. Overextension of the dental speculum may cause further damage to the fracture site and should be avoided. An adequate plane of sedation is necessary to prevent chewing behavior that also may displace the fracture when the speculum is in place. Figure 9.21 is an extraoral radiograph demonstrating a rostral maxillae fracture involving the nasal and palatal processes of the incisive bone. Figure 9.22 is an intraoral radiograph showing a fracture involving the left rostral mandible. Figure 9.23 is a 3-dimensional reconstruction of a computed tomography (CT) examination showing a severe caudal mandible fracture involving the horizontal ramus.

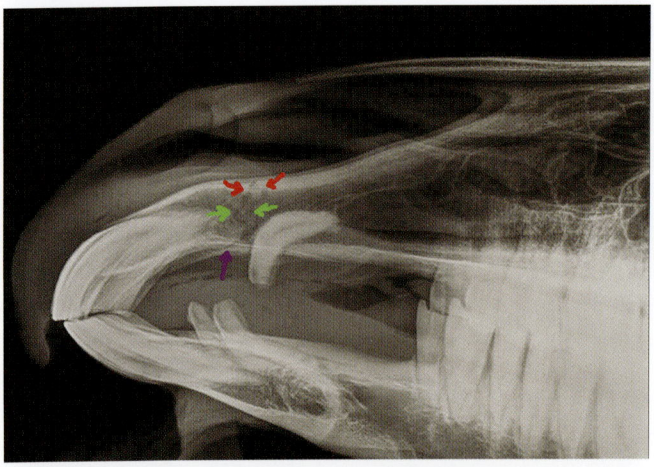

Figure 9.21 Extra oral radiograph of a bilateral rostral maxillae fracture. Several bones are fractured including the nasal process of the incisor bone (red arrows), the rostral maxilla (green arrows) and the palatal process of the incisor bone (purple arrow).

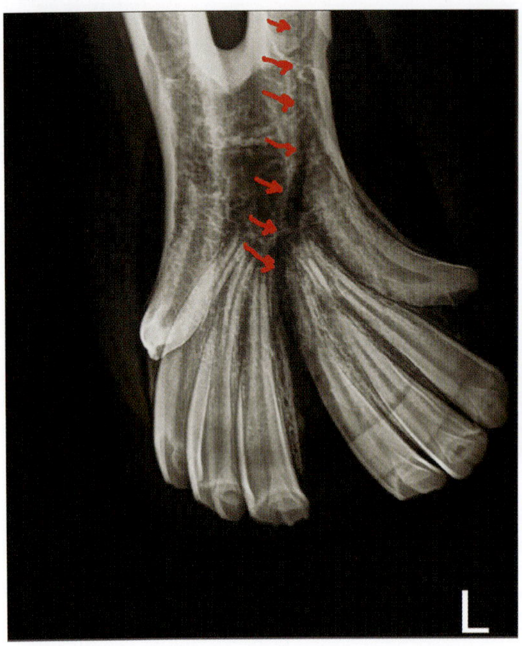


Figure 9.22 Intraoral radiograph of a left rostral mandible fracture. The fracture extends from the interproximal bone between the central mandibular incisors (301 and 401) and caudal past the apical aspect of the left mandibular canine (red arrows).

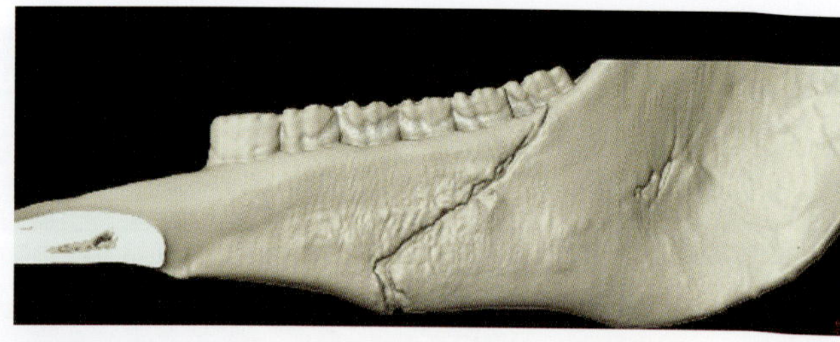

Figure 9.23 Reconstructed 3-dimensional CT examination. Severe caudal mandible fracture of the horizontal ramus.

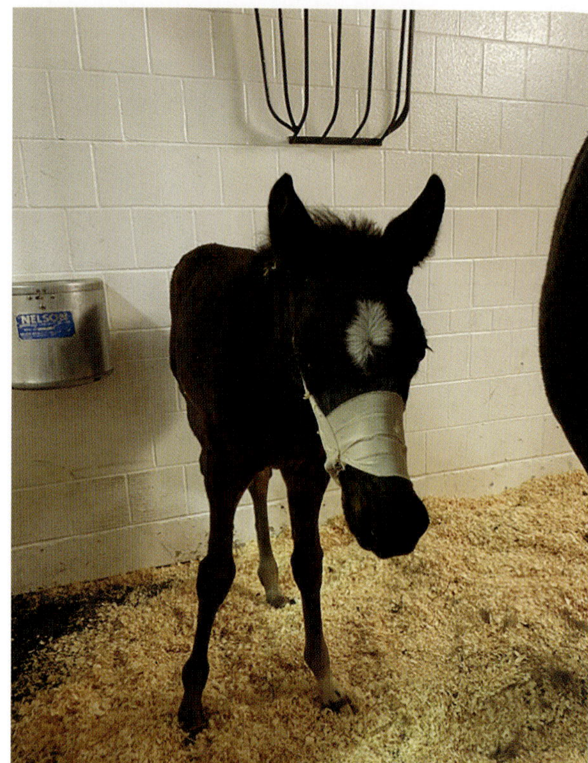


Figure 9.24 A supportive muzzle will not restrict skull growth and give some support for fracture healing.

Following complete examination and diagnostic imaging, discussion for referral and fracture repair is recommended. Fracture stabilization for trailering can be achieved with muzzle therapy (Figure 9.24) and a loose tie in the trailer to avoid excessive pressure on the face. Muzzle therapy is useful in other species that are young, rapid growing animals. The muzzle does not restrict growth while also providing some support of the fragments (Snyder 2019). A wide slightly stretched adhesive bandage[10] may be used to create a muzzle that is somewhat loose to allow for drinking and mastication. Alternatively,

10 Elastikon Elastic Tape, 3"X2.5 yards, Johnson & Johnson Consumer Companies, Inc., Skillman, NJ, 08558–9418.

a snug-fitting halter may also be used as a supportive "muzzle." One to two fingers should comfortably fit between the halter and the face. The muzzle should be changed every ~3–5 days to keep it clean, dry, and allow for continual adjustment with young growing animals. If referral is not an option, there are clinical case reports of successful healing with conservative management with unilateral fractures not involving dental structures (Jansson 2016). Soft feed, adequate pain management, muzzle therapy, and restricted activity is necessary throughout the healing period. Serial radiographic examinations of the fracture site are recommended to monitor healing. Typically, skull fractures should heal within ~6–8 weeks; however, with conservative muzzle therapy the healing time could extend to ~10–12 weeks. Complications such as chronic draining tracts, bone sequestrum, or secondary dental disease could develop during the healing process. A case example of a skull fracture in a foal is summarized in Box 9.5.

**Box 9.5 Skull fracture case example: Maxillofacial trauma with bilateral incisive bone fracture and bilateral mandible fracture (Figures 9.25–9.28)**

- 3-month-old Thoroughbred filly with a history of head trauma.
- 3-dimensional reconstruction from a computed tomographic (CT) study shows the four fractures present involving the right and left nasal processes of the incisive bones and the right and left rostral mandible (Figures 9.25 and 9.26).
- Fracture stabilization of the right and left mandible fractures utilizing cerclage wire of the rostral mandibles and a wire-reinforced composite interdental splint which incorporated the rostral mandibles and deciduous incisors extending bilaterally to the distal aspect of each mandibular deciduous second premolar (706 and 806) (Figure 9.27).

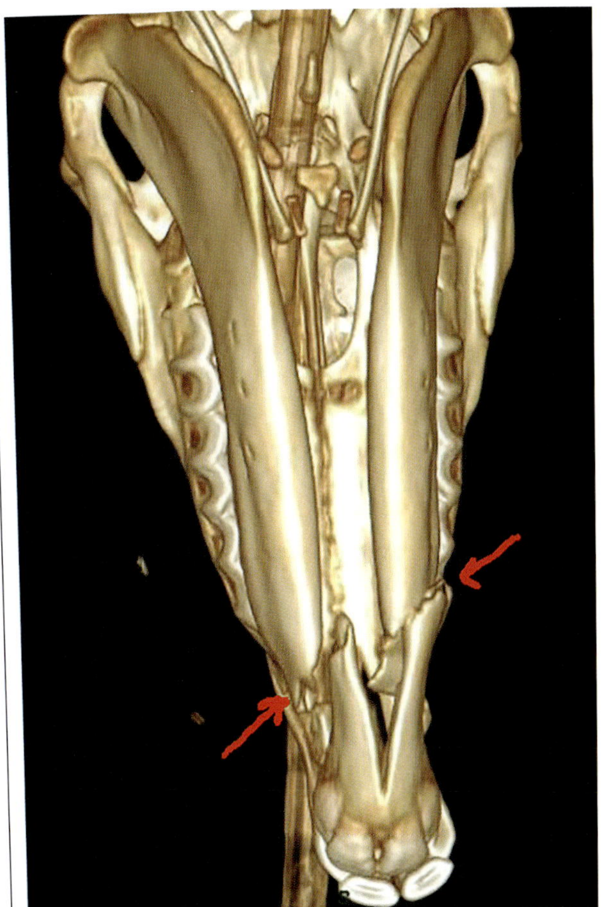

**Figure 9.25** 3-dimensional CT reconstruction shows a bilateral rostral mandible fracture (red arrows).

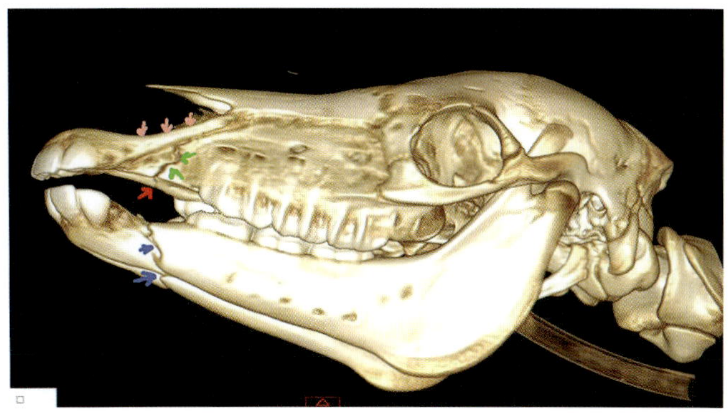

**Figure 9.26** 3-dimensional CT reconstruction. Right rostral maxillary fracture (green arrows) with involvement of the palatine process of the incisor bone (red arrow). The right nasal process of the incisive bone is normal (pink arrows). Both rostral mandibles are fractured (blue arrows).

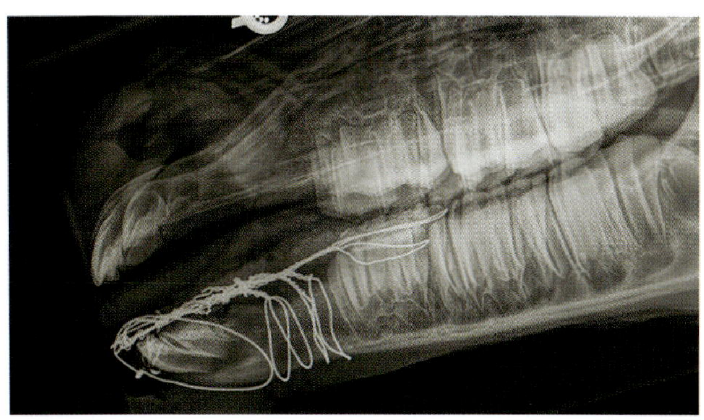

**Figure 9.27** Fracture stabilization of both mandibles using a combination of wiring and composite splint.[6]

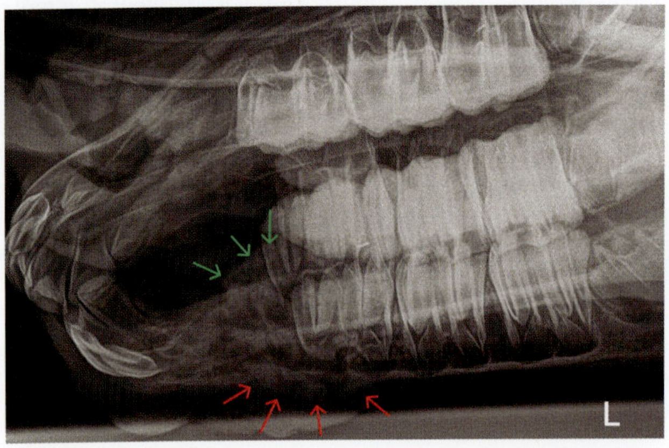


**Figure 9.28** 6-week post operative radiograph following removal of the splint and wires. Bony callous outlined dorsally by green arrows and ventrally by red arrows.

- Fracture stabilization of the incisive bone fractures was managed conservatively utilizing a tape muzzle (Figure 9.24).
- The wire-reinforced composite splint and mandible cerclage wires were removed under general anesthesia at five weeks post-fracture repair.
- Extraoral post-operative radiograph examination at six weeks shows healing with a bony callous present. The filly was nursing and gaining weight (Figure 9.28).
- Muzzle therapy was continued for two more months with frequent monitoring to allow for muzzle adjustment as the foal continued to grow.

If dental and/or alveolar fractures are present, careful monitoring and treatment planning is indicated. With dental fractures, the loose dental fragments can be removed immediately. When reserve crown and/or root tip fragments are involved, it is best to wait approximately 6–10 weeks to give the fracture time to partially heal. (Earley 2014) An embedded cheek tooth (even fractured) will give support for the initial healing of the fracture. Once a bony callous has developed the fractured tooth is extracted to allow for complete healing of the fracture.

## Lingual Trauma

Trauma to the tongue should be a considered differential when a case is presented with dysphagia, hypersalivation, quidding, or oral hemorrhage. (Divers 2014; Geet and Ramzan 2011). A complete oral examination should be performed once external trauma/fracture of the mandible or maxilla is ruled out with an extraoral and radiographic examination. With the intraoral lingual examination, both the dorsal and ventral aspects of the tongue should be evaluated. When examining the ventral aspect, it is important to evaluate the closely associated frenulum and sublingual salivary duct(s). Additional imaging (ultrasound and radiographic) may be indicated when differentiating between laceration, local trauma, foreign-body penetration, and lingual mass. Sedation and local anesthesia are typically indicated for evaluation and treatment of lingual pathology. Additionally, personal protection such as gloves and face mask should be utilized during the examination process since rabies could be a considered rule out with similar presenting clinical signs.

Lacerations of the tongue can be biting injuries, iatrogenic trauma from instruments used during dental procedures, chewing lesions, wounds that occur when a horse bites their tongue during exercise, displaced fractured teeth, or unknown trauma when out in pasture. Acute laceration and tongue trauma may be treated with local debridement and repair using a monofilament absorbable suture.[1] Supportive treatment with pain medication, antibiotics, and soft feed may aid in healing. For more chronic lesions, second-intention healing is indicated (Figure 9.29). The lingual site may benefit with additional supportive care utilizing a local treatment of a sucralfate slurry to coat the lesion(s) (Vaillant and Samimi 2016). A case example of lingual trauma in a horse is presented in Box 9.6.

Tongue foreign-body penetration may involve plant material, wood, or wire. A lingual foreign body will present similar to a laceration with the chief complaint being difficult eating, excessive drooling, quidding, and depression. Additional rule outs would include vasculitis and neoplasia. The site should be cleaned, debrided, and explored for foreign material. Biopsy of the site may be helpful if foreign material is not obvious, and there is suspicion of neoplasia (Figures 9.30 and 9.31). Ultrasound and radiographs of the tongue can be beneficial for a metallic foreign body or localization of the foreign material (Figures 9.32 and 9.33).

Figure 9.29 Second-intention healing of a lingual laceration approximately seven days post injury.

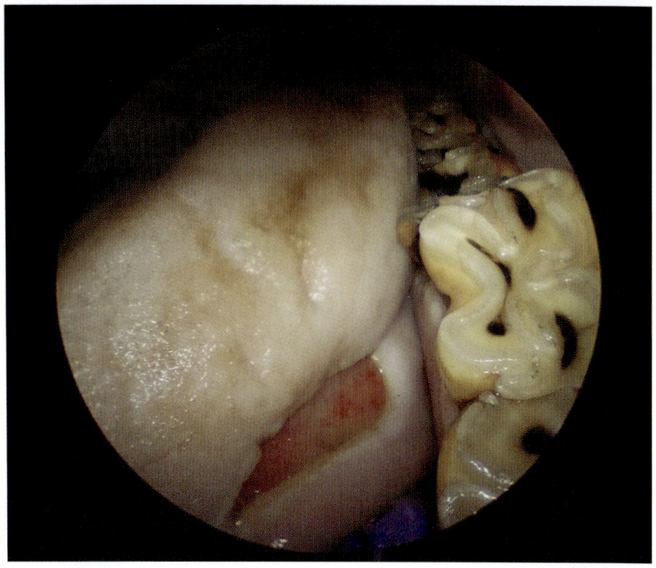

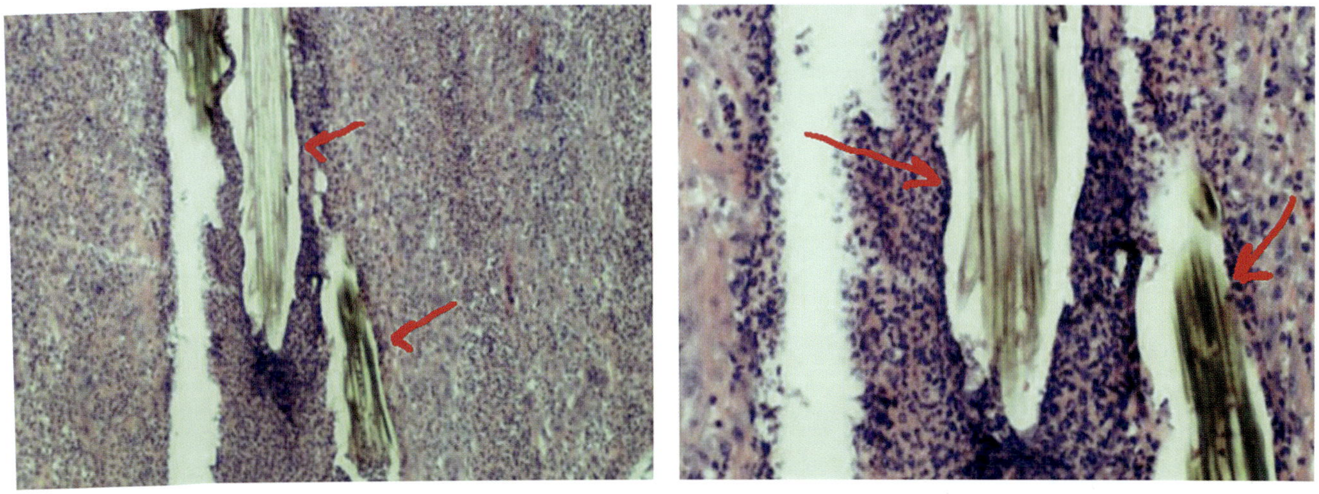

Figure 9.30 Histopathology showing foreign-body material (reported plant material) embedded in a lingual tissue (red arrows). *Source:* Courtesy of Rhinebeck Equine, LLP.

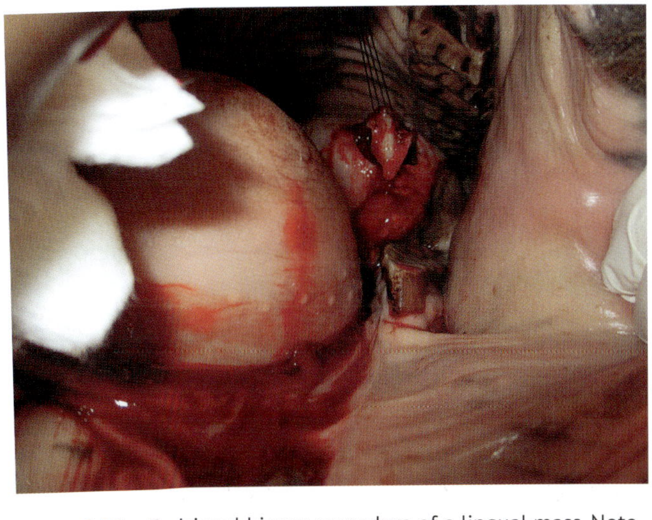

Figure 9.31 Excisional biopsy procedure of a lingual mass. Note the preplaced sutures.

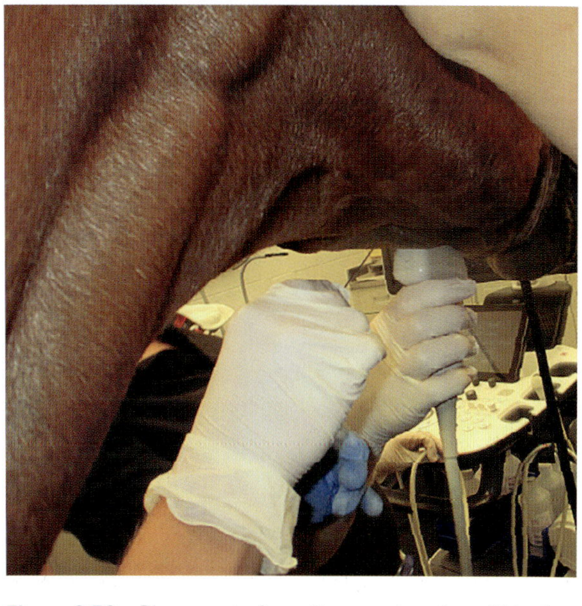

Figure 9.32 Placement of an ultrasound probe within the intermandibular space for evaluation of the tongue.

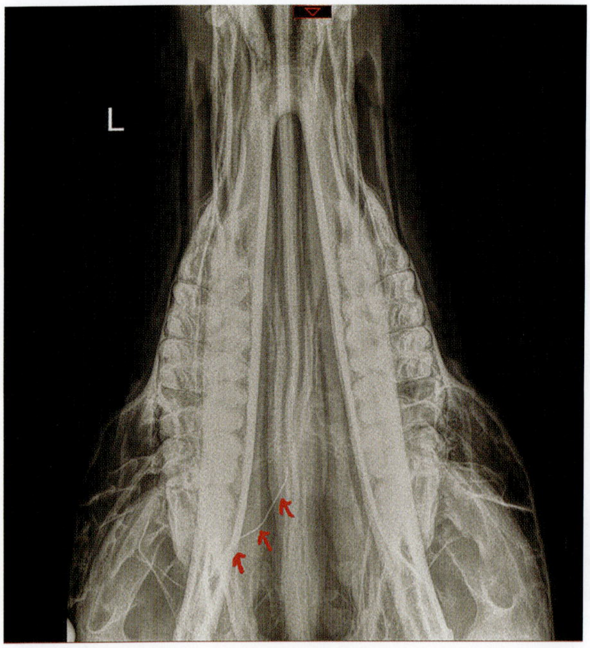


**Figure 9.33** Dorsal ventral radiograph showing a needle embedded in the caudal aspect of the tongue (red arrows). The needle was removed manually after being isolated by palpation of the tongue with an oral speculum in place.

**Box 9.6 Lingual trauma case example: Severe laceration of the tongue (Figures 9.34 and 9.35)**

- 16-year-old Quarter horse mare with a history of tongue trauma that occurred during riding while using a bit.
- Oral exam revealed a severe laceration involving approximately 90% of the dorso-ventral thickness of the tongue, located 1 cm rostral to the frenulum (Figure 9.34).
- The horse was prepared for standing surgery via stock restraint and detomidine sedation and morphine analgesia. Pre-operative antibiotics and anti-inflammatory medications were administered.

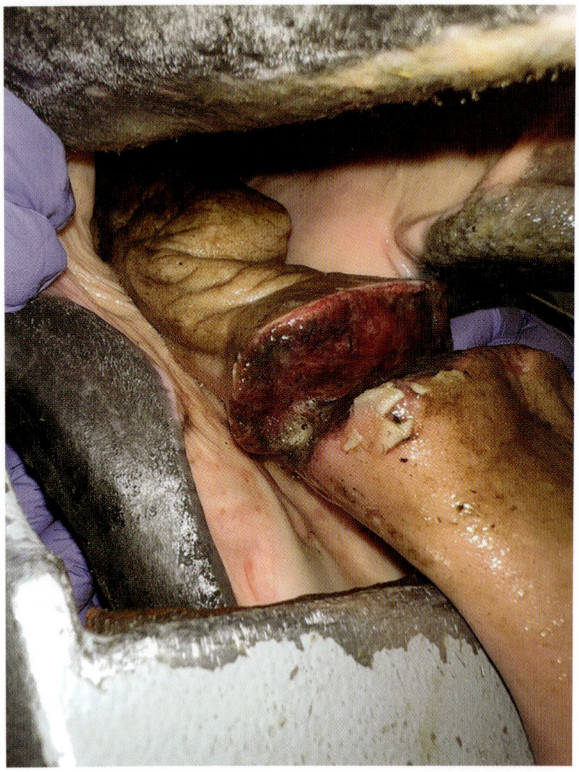

**Figure 9.34** Severe tongue laceration following suspected injury from a bit. The laceration, located 1 cm rostral to the frenulum, involved approximately 90% of the dorso-ventral tongue thickness. *Source:* Courtesy of Dr. Brenna Pugliese.

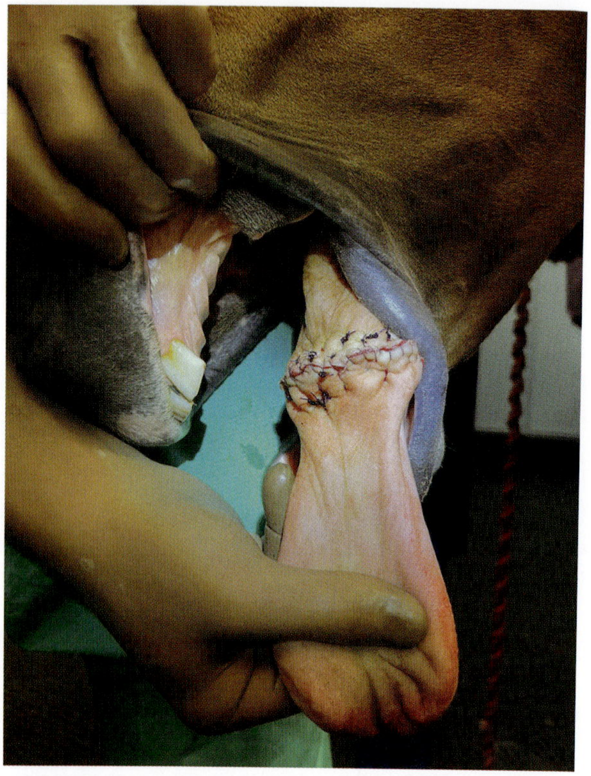

**Figure 9.35** Completed repair of severe tongue laceration. A 3-layer closure of the laceration was performed via a combination of vertical mattress, simple interrupted, and continuous absorbable sutures. *Source:* Courtesy of Dr. Brenna Pugliese.

- The lingual laceration was lavaged, locally anesthetized, and debrided. A 3-layer closure of the laceration was performed via a combination of vertical mattress, simple interrupted and continuous absorbable sutures (Figure 9.35). Layer 1: Vertical mattress sutures pre-placed using 1 Monocryl and held with mosquito forceps until tied after layer 2. Layer 2: Simple interrupted "walking" sutures using 0-monofilament absorbable placed deep to superficial to oppose muscle and eliminate dead space. Layer 3: Simple continuous closure using 2/0 Monocryl. Simple interrupted stitches could also be used for this final layer to close the lingual epithelium.
- Post-operative care included immediate access to water, gradual return to feeding via senior feed mash for several days followed by soaked hay pellets for several months.
- The lingual laceration healed without complications and the mare returned to previous riding performance.

## Conclusion

When evaluating a horse for oral and maxillofacial trauma, the examination process is the most important component in understanding the extent of pathology and developing a treatment plan. Modalities for examination include extraoral evaluation, endoscopy (intraoral and nasal), ultrasound, radiographic (intraoral and extraoral), and occasionally computed tomography. Pathology noted with head trauma involves dental, skull (maxilla and mandible), and lingual. *Dental trauma* will range from mild displacement (luxation) to complete alveolar exfoliation (avulsion). If there is associated tooth fracture, the extent and location of the fracture margin(s) should be identified. *Skull fractures* that are rostral and unilateral may be treated conservatively (diet management and/or a soft fabric muzzle). More severe skull fractures that are caudal and/or bilateral may require some type of oral wiring/splint stabilization or even surgical fixation with bone plate(s) and cortical screws. *Oral soft-tissue and lingual trauma* may be challenging to diagnose. Careful palpation along the dorsal and ventral surface of the tongue, endoscopic examination of the caudal oral cavity, external sublingual ultrasound and dorsal–ventral radiographs are helpful when trying to determine the etiology of lingual pathology. Occasionally, an excisional soft-tissue biopsy of the tongue or associated soft-tissue attachment(s) may be indicated.

## References


AVDC (2023). AVDC nomenclature. http://AVDC.org – American Veterinary Dental College. https://avdc.org/avdc-nomenclature (accessed 16 March 2024).

Baratt, R.M. (2013). Advances in equine dental radiology. In: *Advances in Equine Dentistry, Veterinary Clinics Equine Practice* (ed. J. Easley), 367–395. Philadelphia: Elsevier.

Baratt, R.M. (2020). Dental radiography and radiographic signs of equine dental disease. In: *Equine Dentistry and Oral Surgery, Veterinary Clinics Equine Practice* (ed. E.T. Earley, R.M. Baratt, and S.S. Galloway), 445–476. Philadelphia: Elsevier.

Campoy, L. and Sedgewick, S.R. (2020). Standing sedation and locoregional analgesia in equine dentistry. In: *Equine Dentistry and Oral Surgery, Veterinary Clinics Equine Practice* (ed. E.T. Earley, R.M. Baratt, and S.S. Galloway), 477–499. Philadelphia: Elsevier.

Claffey, E.F. and Ducharme, N.G. (2020). Equine nasal endoscopy: treating bullae disease and sinus disease. In: *Equine Dentistry and Oral Surgery, Veterinary Clinics Equine Practice* (ed. E.T. Earley, R.M. Baratt, and S.S. Galloway), 659–669. Philadelphia: Elsevier.

Dacre, I., Kempson, S., and Dixon, P.M. (2007). Equine idiopathic cheek teeth fractures. Part 1: pathological studies on 35 fractured cheek teeth. *Equine Vet. J.* 39 (4): 310–318.

Divers, T.J. (2014). Acute salivation ptyalism. In: *Equine Emergencies Treatment and Procedures Fourth Edition* (ed. J.A. Orsini and T.J. Divers), 176–177. St. Louis: Elsevier Saunders.

Dixon, P.M., Barakzai, S.Z., Collins, N.M. et al. (2007). Equine idiopathic cheek teeth fractures: part 3: a hospital-based survey of 68 referred horses (1999–2005). *Equine Vet. J.* 39 (4): 327–332.

Dixon, P.M., Froydenlund, T., Luiti, T. et al. (2014). Empyema of the nasal Conchal bulla as a cause of chronic unilateral nasal discharge in the horse: 10 cases (2013-2014). *Equine Vet. J.* 445–449.

Dixon, P.M., Kennedy, R., and Reardon, R.J.M. (2021). Equine idiopathic and infundibular caries related cheek teeth fractures: a long-term study of 486 fractured teeth in 300 horses. *Front Vet. Sci.* 8: 646870.

Earley, E.T. (2014). Dental radiography ambulatory techniques. In: *Equine Emergencies Treatment and Procedures Fourth Edition* (ed. J.A. Orsini and T.J. Divers), 164–175. St. Louis: Elsevier Saunders.

Earley, E.T., Baratt, R.M., and Galloway, S.S. (2020a). Preface: snapshot of equine dentistry: past, present and future. In: *Equine Dentistry and oral surgery, Veterinary Clinics Equine Practice* (ed. E.T. Earley, R.M. Baratt, and S.S. Galloway), xi–xiii. Philadelphia: Elsevier.

Earley, E.T. and Galloway, S.S. (2020b). Equine standing surgical extraction techniques. In: *Equine Dentistry and oral surgery, Veterinary Clinics Equine Practice* (ed. E.T. Earley, R.M. Baratt, and S.S. Galloway), 575–612. Philadelphia: Elsevier.

Earley, E.T. and Rawlinson, J.R. (2013). A new understanding of oral dental disorders of the equine incisor and canine teeth. In: *Advances in Equine Dentistry, Veterinary Clinics Equine Practice* (ed. J. Easley), 273–300. Philadelphia: Elsevier.

Earley, E.T., Rawlinson, J.R., Baratt, R.M. et al. (2017). Hematologic, biochemical, and endocrine parameters in horses with tooth resorption and hypercementosis. *J. Vet. Dent.* 34 (3): 155–160.

Earley, E.T. and Reiswig, J.D. (2020c). Equine dental floating – crown odontoplasty. In: *Equine Dentistry and oral surgery, Veterinary Clinics Equine Practice* (ed. E.T. Earley, R.M. Baratt, and S.S. Galloway), 501–526. Philadelphia: Elsevier.

Easley, J. (2020). A brief history of equine dental practice. In: *Equine Dentistry and Oral Surgery, Veterinary Clinics Equine Practice* (ed. E.T. Earley, R.M. Baratt, and S.S. Galloway), 425–432. Philadelphia: Elsevier.

Galloway, S.G. and Easley, J. (2013). Incorporating oral photography and endoscopy into the equine dental examination. In: *Advances in Equine Dentistry, Veterinary Clinics Equine Practice* (ed. J. Easley), 345–366. Philadelphia: Elsevier.

Geet, T. and Ramzan, P.H.L. (2011). Chapter 9: head and dental trauma. In: *Equine Dentistry Third Edition* (ed. J. Easley, P.M. Dixon, and J. Schumacher), 115–127. Philadelphia: Saunders Elsevier.

Gracis, M. (2012). Chapter 22: management of periodontal trauma. In: *Oral Maxillofacial Surgery in Dogs and Cats* (ed. V. FJM and M.J. Lommer), 201–203. London: Saunders Elsevier.

Griffin, C. and Vogt, C. (2022). Chapter 24: equine dental equipment, materials and instrumentation. In: *Equine Dentistry and Maxillofacial Surgery* (ed. J. Easley, P. Dixon, and N. du Toit), 453–459. Cambridge, Scholars Publishing.

Henry, T. and Bishop, I. (2020). Adjunct extraction techniques in equine dentistry. In: *Equine Dentistry and Oral Surgery, Veterinary Clinics Equine Practice* (ed. E.T. Earley, R.M. Baratt, and S.S. Galloway), 565–574. Philadelphia: Elsevier.

Henry, T., Stoll, M., and Rice, M. (2022). Chapter 28: equine exodontia. In: *Equine Dentistry and Maxillofacial Surgery* (ed. J. Easley, P. Dixon, and N. du Toit), 534–541. Cambridge: Scholars Publishing.

Henry, T.J., Puchalski, S.M., Arzi, B. et al. (2017). Radiographic evaluation in clinical practice of the types and stage of incisor tooth resorption and hypercementosis in horses. *Equine Vet. J.* 49 (4): 486–492.

Jansson, N. (2016). Conservative management of unilateral fractures of the mandibular rami in horses. *Vet. Surg.* 45 (8): 1063–1065.

Klugh, D. (2004). Incisor and canine periodontal disease. In: *Proceedings of the 18th Annual Veterinary Dental Forum*. Fort Worth, TX: Lexington: American Association of Equine Practitioners.

Limone, L.E. (2020). Update on equine odontoclastic tooth resorption and hypercementosis. In: *Equine Dentistry and Oral Surgery, Veterinary Clinics Equine Practice* (ed. E.T. Earley, R.M. Baratt, and S.S. Galloway), 671–689. Philadelphia: Elsevier.

Menzies, R. (2013). Oral examination and charting: setting the basis for evidence-based medicine in the oral examination of equids. In: *Advances in Equine Dentistry, Veterinary Clinics Equine Practice* (ed. J. Easley), 325–343. Philadelphia: Elsevier.

Pollaris, E., Broeckx, B.J.G., Rajasekharan, S. et al. (2021). Fracture resistance of equine cheek teeth with and without occlusal fissures: a standardized ex vivo model. *Front Vet. Sci.* 8: 699940.

Rehrl, S., Schroder, W., Muller, C. et al. (2018). Radiological prevalence of equine odontoclastic tooth resorption and hypercementosis. *Equine Vet. J.* 50 (4): 481–487.

Rehrl, S., Schulte, W., Staszyk, C. et al. (2022). Equine odontoclastic tooth resorption and hypercementosis: investigating individual incisor disease patterns using radiological classification. *Equine Vet. J.* 55 (3): 419–425.

Smedley, R.C., Earley, E.T., Galloway, S.S. et al. (2015). Equine odontoclastic tooth resorption and hypercementosis: histopathologic features. *Vet. Pathol.* 52: 903–909.

Snyder, C.J. (2019). Maxillofacial fracture repair using noninvasive techniques. In: *Oral and Maxillofacial Surgery in Dogs and Cats*, 2e (ed. V. FJM, M.J. Lommer, and B. Arzi), 307. St. Louis: Elsevier.

Staszyk, C., Bienert, A., Kreutzer, R. et al. (2008). Equine odontoclastic tooth resorption and hypercementosis. *Vet. J.* 178: 372–379.

True, C.K. and Dotzel, A.R. (2020). Equine oral endoscopy. In: *Equine Dentistry and Oral Surgery, Veterinary Clinics Equine Practice* (ed. E.T. Earley, R.M. Baratt, and S.S. Galloway), 433–443. Philadelphia: Elsevier.

Vaillant, L. and Samimi, M. (2016). Aphthous ulcers and oral ulcerations. *Presse Med.* 45 (2): 215–226.

White, C. and Dixon, P.M. (2010). A study of the thickness of cheek teeth subocclusal secondary dentine in horses of different ages. *Equine Vet. J.* 42 (2): 119–123.

# 10

# Diseases of the Abdomen

*Megan Burke*[1], *Julie Dechant*[2], *and Alicia Long*[3]

[1] *College of Veterinary Medicine, North Carolina State University, Raleigh, NC, USA*
[2] *Department of Surgical and Radiological Sciences, School of Veterinary Medicine, University of California, Davis, Davis, CA, USA*
[3] *Department of Clinical Studies - New Bolton Center, University of Pennsylvania School of Veterinary Medicine, Kennett Square, PA, USA*

## Evaluation of the Horse with Colic

### Goals

The goals of the colic examination are to try to identify the cause of colic, and to determine whether the horse should be managed on the farm, or referred for further evaluation and treatment. For veterinarians working in a referral hospital, an additional goal is to determine if the horse should be managed medically or if surgery should be recommended. When evaluating a horse for colic, it may help to keep three questions in mind as summarized in Box 10.1.

### History

Depending on the severity of pain, it may be necessary to triage a horse with colic before obtaining a complete history. However, the importance of a thorough history cannot be overstated. Pertinent history questions may include, but are not limited to:

- Previous history of colic, including previous colic surgery.
- Duration and severity of colic signs
  - Identify when the horse was last noted to be normal.
- Fecal output and consistency.
- Medications administered prior to arrival
  - Route given (IV, IM, oral).
  - Response to medications.
- Are any other horses affected?
- Current diet, including any recent changes
  - Changes in appetite or water intake noted before onset of colic signs.
- Current use of the horse, and any recent changes in frequency or intensity of exercise.
- Vaccination and deworming history.
- History of recent travel.
- Reproductive status.
- Dental care regimen.
- Cribbing behavior.
- Concurrent or pre-existing diseases.

*Emergency Triage of the Horse*, First Edition. Edited by Rolfe M. Radcliffe and Jamie J. Kopper.

Companion website: www.wiley.com/go/radcliffe/triage

**Box 10.1 Three main questions to consider when evaluating a horse for colic**

1) Where in the gastrointestinal (GI) tract is the lesion located? Or is it potentially a non-GI cause of colic?
2) Can the problem be managed in the field, or does it require referral?
3) Can the problem be managed medically, or does it require surgery?

## Physical Examination

A thorough physical examination should be performed on any horse being evaluated for colic. Special attention should be paid to the degree of discomfort, gastrointestinal sounds (increased, normal, decreased, absent), and perfusion parameters, which reflect cardiovascular and volume status.

## Diagnostic Procedures

If it can be done safely, all horses evaluated for colic should have a nasogastric tube passed, and abdominal palpation per rectum should also be attempted. Things that might preclude palpation include horse size, temperament, and availability of a competent handler. In most circumstances, safety for horse, handler, and veterinarian can be improved by use of sedation (+/− placement of a twitch) prior to performing these procedures. For an adult horse, xylazine, 0.2–0.6 mg/kg (100–300 mg) +/− butorphanol, 0.004–0.01 mg/kg (2–5 mg) can be administered IV. Detomidine, 0.004–0.01 mg/kg (2–5 mg) is also an appropriate choice. However, detomidine is a very potent analgesic and can mask surgical pain for up to 60 minutes, which may complicate evaluation of the severity of colic signs.

Detailed instructions on nasogastric intubation, and abdominal palpation per rectum are covered elsewhere in this text (Part 1, Chapter 4). Briefly, normal horses should produce <2 L of nasogastric reflux. The presence of nasogastric reflux is consistent with either a functional or mechanical obstruction of the small intestine. Nasogastric reflux and/or abnormal findings on abdominal palpation per rectum may increase the suspicion for a more critical lesion that may benefit from referral.

Targeted sonographic evaluation of the abdomen using a 5–10 mHz curvilinear probe has been described and can be performed by practitioners of varying skill levels from new graduates to specialists (Busoni et al. 2011; LeJeune and Whitcomb 2014). This evaluation should take <10 minutes and does not provide complete evaluation of the abdomen. The goal is to target areas with the highest likelihood of providing information that can be used to guide treatment recommendations.

- Ability to perform hematologic analysis will depend on whether the horse is being evaluated in a field or hospital setting. However, the availability and affordability of hand-held "stall side" analyzers for L-lactate and serum amyloid A (SAA), have increased the "real-time" information available to veterinarians. Both tests can be run on whole blood, or peritoneal fluid. L-Lactate is an indirect measure of tissue perfusion, while SAA is a major acute phase protein in horses and increases with an inflammatory insult. In healthy horses, blood and abdominal fluid lactate concentrations should be <1.0 mmol/L, while SAA concentrations should be <15 μg/mL (Bowlby et al. 2021). Increases in either marker indicate either increased severity or increased duration of disease. These diagnostic tests are summarized in Box 10.2.

## Decision for Referral or Surgery

Ultimately, field practitioners must decide if a horse with colic can be managed on the farm, or if it should be referred to a surgical facility. Veterinarians working in referral centers must decide whether horses can be managed medically, or if surgery is indicated. Figures 10.1 and 10.2, adapted from Gardner et al. (2019) show examples of decision trees that can assist in these cases.

**Box 10.2 Diagnostic procedures during a colic workup**

- Nasogastric intubation.
- Abdominal palpation per rectum.
- +/− Targeted sonographic evaluation of the abdomen.
- +/− Hematologic evaluation of blood and peritoneal fluid.

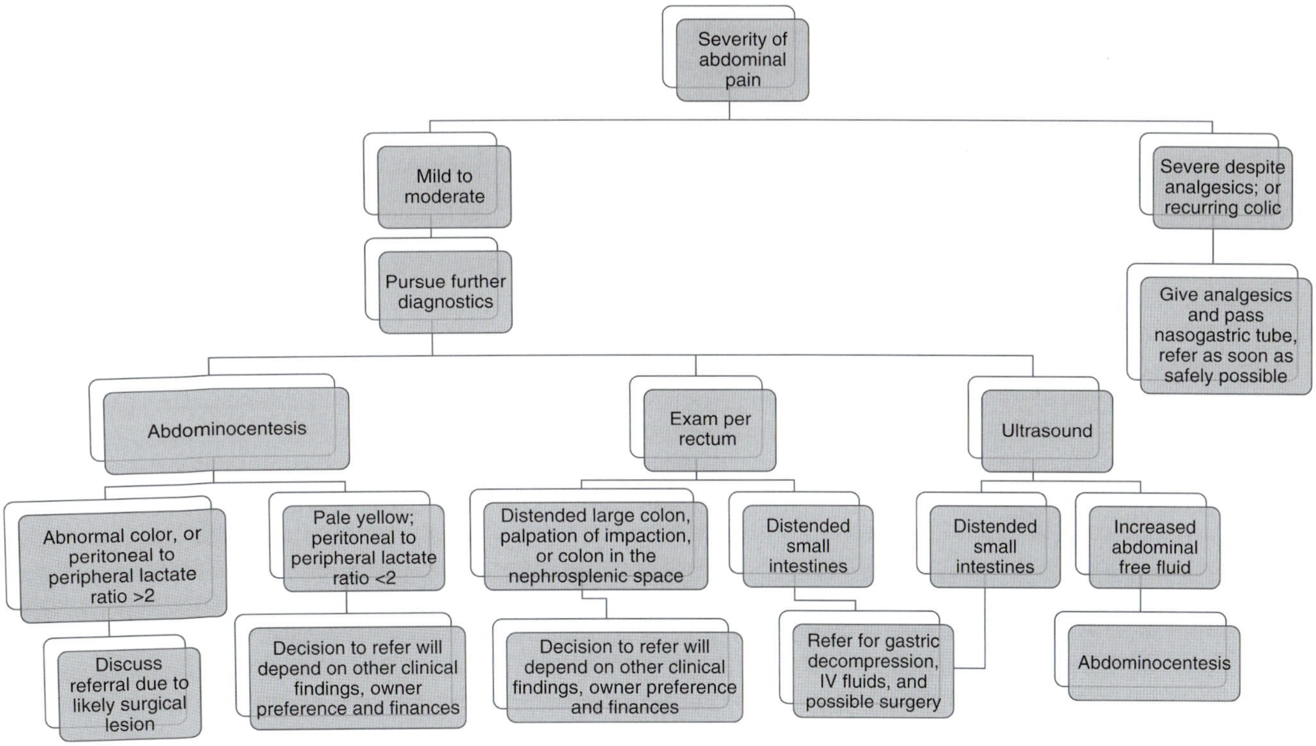


**Figure 10.1** Decision tree for field practitioners evaluating horses for colic.

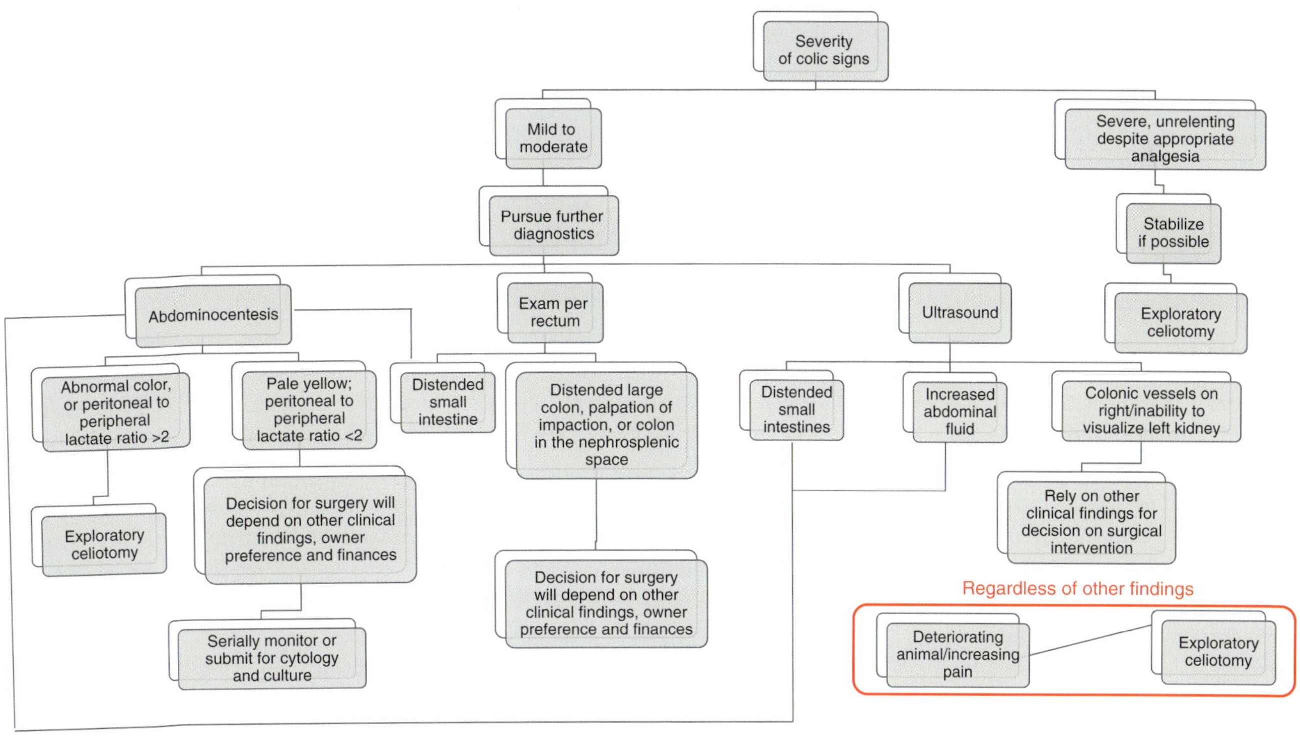


**Figure 10.2** Decision tree for surgical intervention in horses with colic admitted to a tertiary referral center.

## Lesions by Anatomic Location

### Esophageal Obstruction

#### Clinical Signs

Classic clinical signs associated with esophageal obstruction are nasal discharge containing feed and saliva, coughing, frequent swallowing, and ptyalism. Less common clinical signs include extension of head and neck, colic, or obtundation.

#### Triage Over the Phone

Initial phone contact with owner may elucidate a presumptive diagnosis of esophageal obstruction, especially with experienced owners, or if the classic signs of esophageal obstruction are evident after eating. Owners should be instructed to remove feed and water. If signs have been present for less than 15–20 minutes, the owner can be instructed to monitor horse for another 15–20 minutes for resolution; however, if signs have been prolonged, do not resolve spontaneously, or if the horse (or owner) appears distressed, immediate veterinary attention should be provided.

#### Triage at the Farm

***History*** It is important to manage the current presentation, but also to identify risk factors that may predispose to recurrence or warrant further investigation. The signalment, duration of clinical signs, diet, and recent medical history, including past episodes of esophageal obstruction, recent nasogastric intubation, or cervical trauma.

***Examination*** Complete physical examination is performed with particular attention to temperature, heart rate, respiratory rate, mucous membrane color and refill, jugular fill, and cervical palpation. Thoracic and trachea auscultation and rebreathing exam should be performed to assess baseline signs of feed aspiration. The veterinarian should be mindful of the presence of other neurological deficits that might be indicative of other causes of dysphagia.

#### Emergency Triage Steps

***Patient Stabilization*** Signs of cardiovascular compromise or moderate-to-severe dehydration must be addressed with IV fluid therapy prior to treatment. Signs of respiratory distress should be managed with intranasal oxygen, and if upper respiratory tract obstruction is present (which is rare), tracheotomy.

***How to Formulate a Diagnostic Plan*** Initial assessment includes passage of a nasogastric tube to confirm diagnosis and attempt to resolve the obstruction. An oral examination should be performed while the horse is sedated to rule out dental abnormalities. The horse should be given prophylactic antibiotics to prevent aspiration pneumonia. Although not essential for easily resolved, acute esophageal obstruction, Complete Blood Count/CBC (systemic inflammation), esophagoscopy (esophageal injury), and thoracic ultrasound (pneumonia) can be done. If the episode is prolonged, not easily resolved, recurrent, or complicated (recent nasogastric intubation, other neurological signs, respiratory distress, cervical swelling), then CBC and serum biochemistry, endoscopy (esophagus, upper airway, trachea), radiographs (cervical and/or thoracic +/− contrast), ultrasound (thoracic +/− cervical), and other diagnostic tests are indicated.

***Emergency Treatment Guidelines Beyond Stabilization*** If horse appears clinically stable, it can be moderately to heavily sedated with alpha-2 agonists (+/− butorphanol) and a nasogastric tube placed to the level of the obstruction. If the horse's head can be maintained near the ground, lavage of the obstruction via the tube to achieve resolution of the obstruction can be attempted for 15–30 minutes. Administration of oxytocin (0.11–0.22 IU/kg IV) may be useful to help resolve esophageal obstructions (Chiavaccini and Hassel 2010). If the obstruction cannot be resolved within that timeframe, it is advisable to perform esophagoscopy to identify the cause of the obstruction.

#### What Can Be Done at the Farm

Initial assessment and efforts to resolve the obstruction can be easily performed on the farm. The availability of portable, digital endoscopy, ultrasound, and radiographs does allow some of these more advanced assessments in the field; however, cases that are in need of these diagnostic tests often require more supportive care and intensive treatment and are best referred to a referral hospital.

**Box 10.3 Indications for referral in horses with esophageal obstruction**

- Chronic (>18 hours), recurrent, or unresolved esophageal obstruction.
- Ingestion of foreign objects not amenable to lavage.
- Foals (<1 years old).
- Friesian horses.
- Tachypnea.
- Hyperproteinemia (>7.0 g/dL).

### What Can Be Done at the Referral Hospital

Referral hospitals can provide the same care as in the field, with more ready access to blood analyzers, all endoscopic modalities (including 3 m endoscopes), imaging modalities, and hospitalization for IV fluid therapy, antimicrobial treatment, and nutritional management.

### Advice on How to Decide Between Options When Referral Is Time-Critical

If the horse is in respiratory distress, tachypneic, or appears systemically compromised (fever, cervical swelling, dehydrated, tachycardic), referral is indicated for stabilization prior to treatment. If signs of upper airway obstruction are present, tracheotomy should be performed prior to transport (note that this would be an uncommon presentation).

### Important Decisions During Management

***Decision for Hospital Referral vs Farm Management (Box 10.3)*** Acute, easily resolved, first-time occurrences of esophageal obstruction can be managed on the farm. Chronic, recurrent, unresolved, or complicated esophageal obstruction should be referred. Known ingestion of a foreign object not amenable to lavage warrants referral. Esophageal obstruction in foals (<1 year old) or Friesian horses warrants consideration of referral due to the potential for congenital strictures or megaesophagus, respectively (Broekman and Kuiper 2002; Chiavaccini and Hassel 2010). Respiratory rate >22 breaths/min, TP >7.0 g/dL, and chronic duration (>18 hours) are associated with complications and warrant referral (Fiege et al. 2000; Chiavaccini and Hassel 2010).

***Decision for Medical vs Surgical Treatment*** Lavage under general anesthesia is indicated if repeated attempts at standing lavage are unsuccessful or the horse is refractory to sedation and handling. Surgical treatment is indicated with foreign body obstructions, non-resolvable impaction, obstructions causing esophageal perforations, and selected morphologic abnormalities (vascular ring anomalies, severe stricture, esophageal masses or cysts, pulsion diverticulum).

***How to Manage Important Complications*** Intravenous fluid therapy and electrolyte correction are indicated for chronic obstruction or dehydration. Antimicrobial therapy is indicated for aspiration pneumonia. Sucralfate and low-residue soft feeds or mashes are indicated for acute management of esophageal erosions and mucosal injury. Esophageal strictures can be managed with low bulk pellet mash feeding or various directed treatments if conservative management is unsuccessful (bougienage, balloon dilation, surgery).

***Estimating Prognosis*** Prognosis for simple esophageal obstructions, even those complicated by aspiration pneumonia, tends to be very good (>85% survival) (Fiege et al. 2000; Chiavaccini and Hassel 2010). Esophageal obstructions associated with stricture, diverticula, or megaesophagus have an overall poorer prognosis due to likelihood of recurrent obstruction and difficulties in management.

***Decision for Euthanasia*** Horses with chronic, unresolved obstruction or severe systemic compromise without a referral option should be euthanized in the field. Horses with evidence of esophageal perforation have a poor prognosis, and euthanasia is indicated if owner is not financially committed or willing to refer. Horses with recurrent esophageal obstructions due to stricture, diverticula, or megaesophagus are often eventually euthanized due to owner frustration and expense of ongoing treatment.

## Stomach

Horses with gastric lesions can present with a variety of symptoms including acute colic, chronic intermittent colic, weight loss, and bruxism (grinding teeth). Gastric lesions requiring emergency management are relatively rare.

### Equine Gastric Ulcer Syndrome (EGUS)

Equine Gastric Ulcer Syndrome (EGUS) is a blanket term encompassing ulcers of either the squamous or glandular portion of the stomach (Sykes et al. 2015). The prevalence of EGUS increases with the intensity of training, reaching 90% or greater in racehorses and high-level sport horses. However, rates of EGUS in pleasure horses and broodmares on pasture are reported to be as high as 59 and 70%, respectively (LeJeune et al. 2009). Additionally, the use of nonsteroidal anti-inflammatory drugs (NSAIDs) can result in gastric ulceration.

***Pathophysiology*** The squamous portion of the stomach lacks defenses to protect against exposure to acid. Both hydrochloric acid produced in the glandular portion of stomach and volatile fatty acids (VFAs) in grain can cause squamous mucosal damage (ESGD) (Figure 10.3). The glandular portion of the stomach is the site of hydrochloric acid production. Normally, this region has multiple protective mechanisms to prevent mucosal damage. Therefore, glandular ulceration (EGGD) is thought to be due to reduced function of these normal protective mechanisms.

The role of NSAIDs in EGUS is controversial. Experimental studies evaluating rates of EGUS in horses receiving clinical and supra-clinical doses of NSAIDs have shown mixed results. Additionally, the rates of EGUS in the equine population are far higher than the number of animals likely receiving NSAIDs. Therefore, NSAID use may play a role in the development of ulcers in individual animals, but is unlikely to explain the high rates of EGUS at the population level (Sykes et al. 2015).

***Clinical Signs*** Clinical signs of EGUS can be vague but often include chronic intermittent colic, colic after eating, poor appetite, weight loss, bruxism, behavioral changes, and poor performance. EGUS is rarely associated with acute, severe colic signs.

***Diagnosis*** Gastroscopy is the only way to reliably diagnose EGUS. Horses should be fasted for 12–18 hours prior to performing gastroscopy. Treatment for squamous ulcers differs from that for glandular ulcers. Treatment without confirming the presence and location of ulcers via gastroscopy may be unrewarding. It is critical to evaluate the entire stomach as well as the pylorus and proximal duodenum.

A standardized grading system has been validated for ESGD and is summarized in Figure 10.3 (Sykes et al. 2015). Although several grading systems for glandular disease have been proposed, there is currently no validated grading system for EGGD.

***Treatment*** Acid suppression is the cornerstone of treatment for all forms of EGUS. Both proton pump inhibitors and $H_2$ blockers have been used to treat EGUS. Several studies have shown proton pump inhibitors to be more effective in naturally occurring disease (Sykes et al. 2015). Omeprazole is therefore considered the drug of choice for treatment of EGUS. It is important to ensure that a buffered or coated formulation is used; otherwise, omeprazole will be inactivated in the acidic environment of the stomach. Recent studies (Varley et al. 2019) have shown a poor response of EGGD to omeprazole therapy alone. The addition of misoprostol (a prostaglandin $E_1$ analog) to standard omeprazole therapy appears to significantly improve healing and resolution when compared to omeprazole and sucralfate, or omeprazole therapy alone. This is likely due to the role of reduced mucosal defenses in the pathophysiology of EGGD. Treatment recommendations are summarized in Boxes 10.4 and 10.5.

Oral omeprazole therapy alone has shown limited efficacy for EGGD and is no longer recommended as a monotherapy for glandular disease. Omeprazole (as described previously) in combination with Sucralfate: 20 mg/kg PO, q6 for four weeks may be effective for some horses with EGGD.

Regardless of the location of ulceration, repeat gastroscopy is recommended prior to discontinuing treatment.

***Prognosis*** EGUS treated with 28 days of omeprazole: 70–80% (Sykes et al. 2015)

EGGD treated with 28 days of misoprostol: Resolution – 72%; Improvement – 98% compared to 28 days of omeprazole plus sucralfate: Resolution – 20%; Improvement – 65% (Varley et al. 2019).

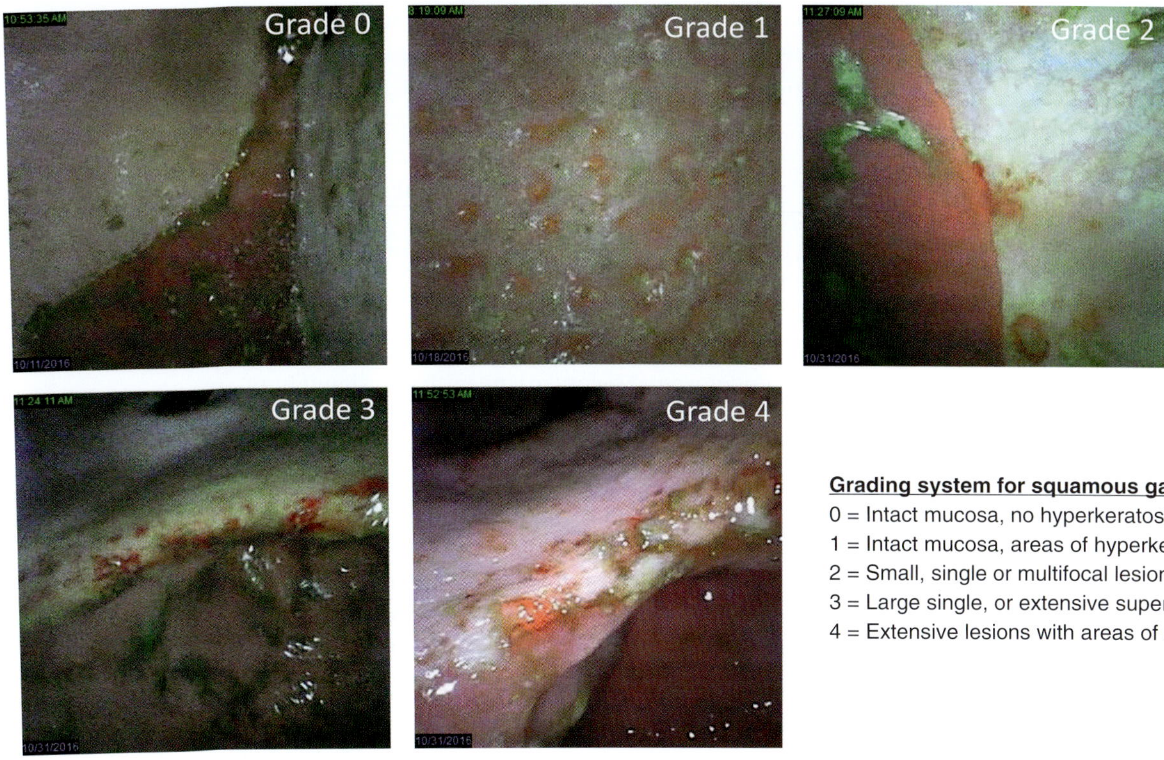


**Grading system for squamous gastric disease**
0 = Intact mucosa, no hyperkeratosis
1 = Intact mucosa, areas of hyperkeratosis
2 = Small, single or multifocal lesions
3 = Large single, or extensive superficial lesions
4 = Extensive lesions with areas of deep ulceration

**Figure 10.3** Grading of squamous gastric ulcers. *Source:* Courtesy of Dr. Kate Hepworth-Warren.

**Box 10.4 Recommended protocol for treatment of ESGD**

Omeprazole buffered formulation (GastroGard®): 4 mg/kg PO, q24 for three to four weeks; OR
Omeprazole enteric granules (Gastrozol): 1 mg/kg PO, q24 for three to four weeks; OR
Famotidine 2–3 mg/kg PO, q12 for three weeks

**Box 10.5 Recommended protocol for treatment of EGGD**

Misoprostol: 2–5 mcg/kg PO, q12 for four weeks PLUS
Omeprazole buffered formulation (GastroGard): 4 mg/kg PO, q24 for four weeks; OR
Omeprazole enteric granules (Gastrozol): 1 mg/kg PO, q24 for four weeks

### Gastric Impaction

Gastric impactions are a relatively rare cause of colic, representing less than 1% of all colic cases admitted to a tertiary referral center in 1 study (Winfield and Dechant 2015). Gastric impactions can be primary or secondary to another abdominal lesion.

***Pathophysiology*** Primary gastric impactions occur when dried ingesta accumulates in the stomach. They can be caused by the feed material itself (e.g., poor quality hay, inadequately soaked beet pulp), inadequate dental care, abnormal gastric motility, abnormal thickening of the muscular layers of the gastric wall, or increased amounts of fibrotic tissue within the wall (Southwood and Wilkins 2015). Masses within the wall of the stomach, or pyloric stenosis can also cause gastric impactions. Horses with gastric impaction are at increased risk of gastric rupture compared to the general colic population (Winfield and Dechant 2015).

***Clinical Signs*** Colic signs may be acute or chronic (days to weeks) and range from mild to severe. Some horses also show signs of weight loss and lethargy.

***Diagnosis*** Gastric impaction can be diagnosed endoscopically, sonographically, at exploratory laparotomy or at necropsy. Endoscopic findings consistent with gastric impaction include a visible impaction on gastroscopy that remains after fasting for 24 hours. Sonographic findings consistent with impaction include a severely enlarged stomach extending beyond left intercostal space (ICS) 15 and often beyond ICS 18. Additionally, the gastric wall may appear thickened on ultrasound.

***Treatment*** Medical treatment of gastric impactions involves passage of a nasogastric tube and repeated lavage with warm water. Passing a large bore tube reduces the incidence of feed material clogging the tube. There are case reports in the literature regarding the use of Diet Coke to assist in the breakup of gastric impactions secondary to persimmon bezoars (Banse et al. 2011). It is the author's experience that Diet Coke is also effective for resolving gastric feed impactions. A single dose of dioctyl sodium sulfosuccinate (DSS), an anionic surfactant, may be used to increase penetration of water into the impaction. Published doses range from 10 to 50 g/kg. DSS should be used cautiously as exceeding the recommended dose can be fatal due to severe osmotic diarrhea and endotoxemia secondary to epithelial sloughing.

Surgical management of gastric impactions in adult horses is limited by the location and accessibility of the equine stomach. Gastrotomy is difficult and the risk of abdominal contamination is high. Successful surgical resolution by hydrating the impaction either using a needle inserted through the gastric wall or using an indwelling nasogastric tube, followed by manual manipulation through the celiotomy incision has been described (Bird et al. 2012).

***Prognosis*** Prognosis is dependent on the underlying cause of the impaction. The prognosis for horses with an acute impaction caused by poor quality hay, or ingestion of expandable feeds appears to be favorable with a low risk of re-impaction. Horses with chronic impactions due to masses or an underlying gastric motility disorder appear to have a poorer prognosis, and an increased risk of recurrence (Bird et al. 2012). Horses with primary gastric impactions are at risk of gastric rupture, regardless of initiating cause. A recent study evaluated horses with primary gastric rupture. In that study 20 of the 23 horses where the cause of rupture was identified at necropsy had primary gastric impactions (Winfield and Dechant 2015).

#### Gastric Rupture

***Pathophysiology*** Gastric rupture can be primary or secondary to a colic lesion distal to the stomach. Primary gastric rupture can be idiopathic, or the result of either a gastric impaction (common) or a perforating gastric ulcer or penetrating foreign body (rare) (Winfield and Dechant 2015). The cause of gastric rupture may be unknown in 20–60% of cases (Todhunter et al. 1986; Kiper et al. 1990; Winfield and Dechant 2015).

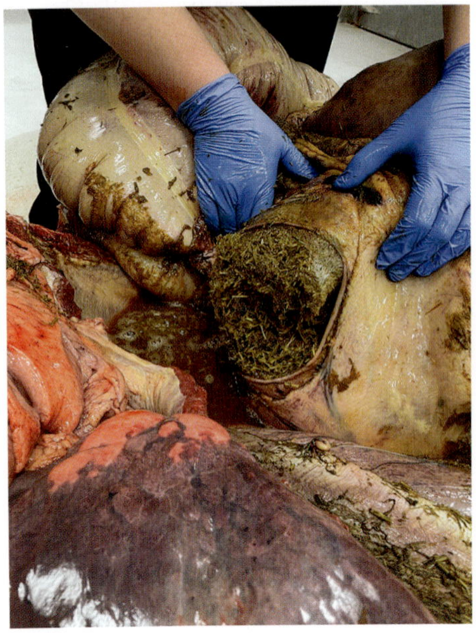

**Figure 10.4** Gastric rupture.

***Clinical Signs*** Horses with gastric rupture secondary to a more aboral lesion are often described as becoming acutely more "comfortable," followed quickly by developing signs of shock (tachycardia, tachypnea, dull demeanor, prolonged jugular fill, abnormal mucous membranes). Horses with gastric rupture are also often reluctant to move. For horses with idiopathic primary gastric rupture there may be no history of colic, and these horses may present initially with clinical signs of shock.

***Diagnostics*** Hematologic changes consistent with gastric rupture include hyperlactatemia, hemoconcentration, and leukopenia. Sonographic evaluation of the abdomen may reveal a large volume of hyperechoic, swirling peritoneal fluid, or free gas within the peritoneum. Abdominocentesis that yields brown, malodorous fluid combined with clinical signs consistent with gastric rupture is highly suggestive. However, unless cytologic analysis confirms the presence of intracellular bacteria, enterocentesis cannot be ruled out. Therefore, definitive diagnosis is made either at surgery, via cytologic analysis of peritoneal fluid, or at necropsy (Figure 10.4).

***Treatment/Prognosis*** Due to the degree of contamination that occurs with gastric rupture, prognosis is grave to hopeless and euthanasia should be pursued.

## Small Intestine

### Obstructive Lesions

#### Duodenitis Proximal Jejunitis

Duodenitis Proximal Jejunitis (DPJ), also referred to as anterior enteritis, is an inflammatory disease which accounts for approximately 3–22% of small intestinal colics (Stewart et al. 2020). Several studies have indicated that there may be geographic differences in prevalence and severity of DPJ, with cases being less frequent and less severe in the western United States. Differentiating DPJ from a small intestinal strangulating obstruction (SISO) can be challenging based on clinical signs.

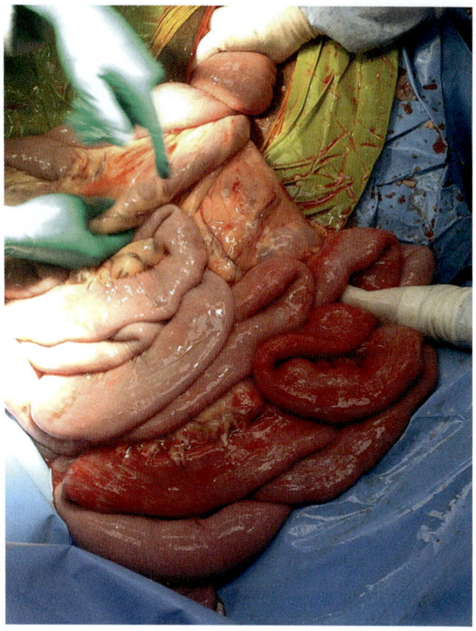

**Figure 10.5** Duodenitis proximal jejunitis.

***Pathophysiology*** Although not fully elucidated, DPJ is thought to be an inflammatory process primary in the duodenum and proximal jejunum which results in initial hypermotility, followed by ileus (Arroyo et al. 2018). This inflammation leads to petechial or ecchymotic hemorrhage on the serosal surface of affected segments (Figure 10.5). Ileus leads to accumulation of electrolyte-rich fluid in the intestinal lumen. Edema in the mucosa and submucosa and sloughing of the villus epithelium increase the absorption of bacteria and bacterial toxins into the blood. Several retrospective studies and one experimental study have suggested a role for *Clostridiodes difficile* toxin A in the pathophysiology of DPJ (Arroyo et al. 2017). However, not all horses with DPJ culture *C. difficile* from feces or GI content; therefore, the pathogenesis is likely multifactorial.

***Clinical Signs*** Mild-to-moderate colic combined with large volumes of nasogastric reflux are the hallmark signs of DPJ. In contrast to most horses with SISO, horses with DPJ will often become markedly more comfortable after gastric decompression. Other clinical signs of DPJ include dull mentation, fever (30%), and tachycardia (85%). Although these clinical signs can be suggestive of DPJ, SISO cannot be ruled out based on clinical signs alone.

***Diagnostics*** Clinical signs, especially response to gastric decompression, are commonly used in the field to distinguish DPJ from other causes of small intestinal colic. Sonographic evaluation often reveals distended small intestine and an enlarged stomach. Abdominocentesis can help to differentiate DPJ from SISO. Peritoneal fluid from horses with DPJ is usually yellow (vs. serosanguinous) and often has an elevated total protein. Definitive diagnosis can only be made at surgery or necropsy and is based on the gross and histologic appearance of the duodenum and proximal jejunum.

***Treatment*** Gastric decompression and IV fluids to replace volume and electrolyte deficits are the cornerstones of treatment for DPJ. For horses with fever or other signs of endotoxemia, icing the feet to prevent laminitis, as well as anti-endotoxic treatments including flunixin meglumine (1.1 mg/kg, q12) and polymyxin B (4,000–6,000 units/kg, IV q8) can be considered. Antimicrobial use is controversial, as a definitive causality between *C. difficile* and DPJ has not been confirmed.

Several studies have compared outcomes between horses managed medically vs those managed surgically (Underwood et al. 2010). Results suggest that surgical intervention does not improve outcomes in horses with DPJ, but that horses managed surgically do not have a worse prognosis than horses managed medically. The current recommendation is that surgical treatment of DPJ be reserved for cases where SISO cannot be ruled out, or in horses where reflux persists despite medical treatment.

#### Ileal Impaction

Luminal obstructions of the small intestine are generally rare, with obstructions in the ileum being most common. Ileal impactions have a prevalence of 0.5–10.8%, and the prevalence varies by geographic location (Fleming and Mueller 2011). Ileal impactions are associated with feeding of Coastal Bermuda grass hay, tapeworm (*Anoplocephala perfoliata*) infestation, or poor-quality hay, and/or dental care.

***Pathophysiology*** Coastal Bermuda hay is the predominant feed type in much of the Southeastern United States, where ileal impactions are common. The high lignin content of this hay decreases digestibility and predisposes to intraluminal impaction. Spasmodic contraction of the ileum combined with dehydration of the feed mass results in exacerbation of the impaction. Less commonly, ileal impactions can be caused by ileal hypertrophy, which may or may not be associated with feeding Coastal Bermuda hay.

***Clinical Signs*** Horses with ileal impactions often display moderate-to-severe pain due to a combination of muscular spasm of the ileum around the impaction, and progressive distension of small intestine proximal to the obstruction. Tachycardia is variable and was reported in 57% of cases in 1 study (Fleming and Mueller 2011). Nasogastric reflux may be present, especially in the later stages of the disease.

***Diagnostics*** In approximately 30% of cases, abdominal palpation per rectum may reveal the impacted ileum in the right dorsal abdomen at approximately the 1 o'clock position. Occasionally, the impaction can be traced laterally to the medial aspect of the cecum (Hanson 2015). Later in the course of disease, generalized small intestinal distension may preclude palpation of the ileum.

Abdominocentesis can be used to try to differentiate ileal impaction (or other small intestinal obstruction) from SISOs. Horses with ileal impactions usually have clear, straw-colored fluid with an elevated lactate.

***Treatment*** In one study evaluating 245 horses with ileal impaction, 54% were successfully treated medically while 46% required surgical correction. Variables that increased the risk of surgery were production of nasogastric reflux and failure to respond to analgesic administration (Fleming and Mueller 2011).

The mainstays of medical therapy are IV fluids and analgesic administration. IV fluids should be given at two to three times maintenance (120–180 mL/kg/day, or 2.5–4 L/h) to promote movement of fluid from the vascular space into the lumen of the ileum to hydrate the impaction. In horses requiring surgery the impaction can be broken down manually and milked into the cecum. Intraluminal injection of polyionic fluids with or without 1% carboxymethylcellulose ("Belly Jelly"), 2% lidocaine, or dioctyl sodium succinate (DSS) have all been described to hydrate the impaction and facilitate manual breakdown (Little and Blikslager 2002; Fleming and Mueller 2011; Hanson 2015). For impactions that fail to resolve with external manipulation, an enterotomy can be performed oral to the impaction and a combination of intraluminal hydration using a hose, and extraluminal massage can facilitate resolution.

***Prognosis*** The prognosis for horses with ileal impactions is good, with >90% of horses treated medically or surgically surviving to hospital discharge (Fleming and Mueller 2011).

## Strangulating Lesions

Small intestinal lesions are found in 32–59% of all horses undergoing exploratory laparotomy for colic (Bergren et al. 2015). There are many potential causes of a SISO, with strangulating lipomas (30%) and epiploic foramen entrapments (10%) being the most common. SISOs require surgical intervention and prognosis is improved by early referral. For the field practitioner, early recognition of horses that may have a SISO is more important than identifying the specific lesion type. This section will focus on general characteristics of SISO. Details for specific lesion types are outlined in Table 10.1, although this is not an exhaustive list.

Only 25–30% of the adult equine abdomen can be felt on rectal or visualized sonographically. Therefore, even with the additional diagnostic capabilities available in referral centers, an exact diagnosis is often not known when the decision for surgery is made (Gardner et al. 2019).

### Clinical Signs

Horses with SISO initially show signs of moderate-to-severe pain. This generally corresponds to the period after strangulation but before devitalization of the bowel. Once the bowel becomes non-viable the severity of colic signs may decrease while signs of shock may become evident. Nasogastric reflux is variably present in horses with SISO and depends on the location of the strangulating lesion (oral or aboral), and the duration of strangulation. Unlike horses with DPJ, colic signs in horses with SISO are not relieved by gastric decompression.

### Diagnostics

Distended loops of small intestine are palpable in approximately 50% of horses with SISO (Pye et al. 2019). Severely gas distended small intestine may feel like bicycle tires or balloon animals on palpation. However, less severely distended

**Table 10.1** Common causes of small intestinal strangulating lesions in adult horses.

| Lesion | Signalment | Pertinent history | Prevalence | Diagnostic findings | Survival to discharge for surgically treated horses |
|---|---|---|---|---|---|
| Strangulating lipoma | Ponies, Arabians, Saddlebreds, age >15 years | | 13% of surgical colics; 30–43% of SI colics | US: 2 populations of SI. One (affected) dilated with thick walls, one (unaffected) normal | 60–80%<br>Garcia-Seco (2005), Mair and Smith (2005), Southwood and Wilkins (2015) and Pye et al. (2019) |
| Epiploic foramen entrapment | TBs and large horses overrepresented | History of cribbing or wind sucking | 5% of surgical colics; 10–19% of SI colics | US: Dilated SI cranially on R side by the liver | 50–74%<br>Englebert et al. (1993), vanBergen (2016, 2021) and Southwood and Wilkins (2015) |
| Segmental volvulus | | Recent gastroscopy | 7.8% of SI colics | | 67%<br>Stephen et al. (2004) |
| Entrapment through a mesenteric rent | | | 0.75 – 3.0% of surgical colics; 13.6% of SI colics | | 38–68%<br>Gayle et al. (2000), Mair and Smith (2005), Kilcoyne et al. (2016) and Pye et al. (2019) |
| Intussusception | Young horses overrepresented, but can occur at any age | | 1.2% of SI colics | Intussusception visible on US in 54% of cases | 64%<br>Haddad et al. (2022) and Pye et al. (2019) |

Key: SI, small intestine; US, ultrasound.

loops, or those distended with fluid rather than gas may be more subtle, and more challenging to palpate. Sonographic evaluation of the abdomen should be performed if equipment is available. The best ultrasound window for identifying distended small intestine is inguinal, on both the right and the left sides. Fluid distended small intestine will sink to the ventral regions of the abdomen, and there are no other abdominal structures located in the inguinal area to block visibility.

Abdominocentesis can provide valuable information for differentiating strangulating and non-strangulating small intestinal obstructions. Serosanguinous fluid (Figure 10.6) consistent with a strangulating lesion has been shown to have a high sensitivity (92%) for the need for surgery (Southwood and Wilkins 2015; Coronado and Beatty 2021). An elevated peritoneal fluid lactate is also strongly associated with the need for surgery. A peritoneal to whole blood lactate ratio of 2 : 1 or higher is strongly associated with the need for surgery, while a peritoneal lactate concentration >16 mmol/L is strongly correlated with non-survival (Radcliffe et al. 2022). Detailed instructions on how to perform abdominocentesis are provided elsewhere (Part 1, Chapter 4). Indications of a SISO based on peritoneal fluid analysis are summarized in Box 10.6.

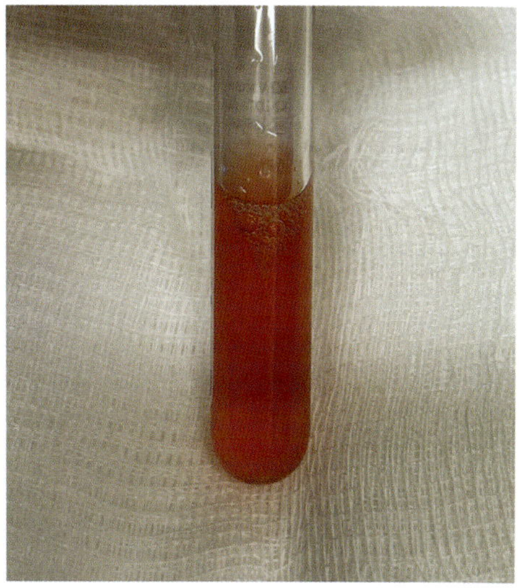

**Figure 10.6** Serosanguinous peritoneal fluid.

**Box 10.6 Peritoneal fluid abnormalities consistent with SISO**

- Serosanguinous color.
- Elevated peritoneal fluid lactate.
  - >16 mmol/L correlated with non-survival.
  - Peritoneal fluid: blood lactate ratio of 2 : 1 or higher associated with the need for surgery.

### Treatment

Regardless of the specific cause, SISO requires surgical intervention or euthanasia if surgery is not an option. Abdominocentesis can be a valuable tool (and visual aid) for field practitioners, when trying to help owners make decisions in horses with suspected SISO without the option for referral to a surgical center.

### Prognosis

Advances in the care of the critically ill equine patient have resulted in improved survival rates for horses with SISO (Garcia-Seco 2005). Recent studies (Mair and Smith 2005; Stewart et al. 2014; Espinosa et al. 2017) reported short-term survival rate for horses undergoing surgery for SISO between 74–80%. Preoperative variables that are consistently associated with non-survival in horses with SISO include increased heart rate, PCV, peripheral and peritoneal lactate, and an increased peritoneal-to-peripheral lactate ratio (Garcia-Seco et al. 2005; Stewart et al. 2014; Espinosa et al. 2017). Increases in these variables are associated with both the severity and duration of colic which underscores the importance of early recognition and referral.

The need for resection and anastomosis is consistently associated with reduced survival in horses with SISO (Garcia-Seco 2005; Mair and Smith 2005; Espinosa et al. 2017). For horses requiring resection, most studies show that jejunocecostomy has decreased short- and long-term survival, compared to jejunojejunostomy or jejunoileostomy (Garcia-Seco 2005; Mair and Smith 2005; Espinosa et al. 2017). Complication rates are high after surgery for SISO. The most common complication is postoperative ileus (POI), which occurs in 18–60% of horses, and has been shown to significantly decrease survival to discharge compared to horses that do not develop POI (Mair and Smith 2005; Stewart et al. 2014; Kilcoyne et al. 2016; Hellstrom et al. 2021). Postoperative colic, endotoxemia, and incisional complications are also common and have a negative effect on survival. Horses that require a second celiotomy have a significantly decreased survival rate compared with horses requiring only a single celiotomy.

## Cecum

The cecum is the primary site of hind gut fermentation in the horse, responsible for the breakdown of cellulose in the diet.

### Cecal Tympany

Cecal tympany is common in horses with colic, and although it can be the primary problem, it is usually secondary to a more aboral obstruction. Horses with cecal tympany often have external abdominal distension, particularly noticeable in the right paralumbar fossa. Auscultation and percussion in this area will often elicit a ping (gas/fluid interface), although it is rarely as obvious or resonant as those encountered in ruminants. Severe tympany results in increased intraabdominal pressure which causes pain, abdominal hypertension, and increased respiratory effort. Cecal trocharization is useful to decrease pain, improve venous return, and improve movement of the diaphragm. Trocharization has been described both percutaneously through the right flank and transrectally (Scotti et al. 2012; Schoster et al. 2019). The transrectal approach requires a specialized canula which is not commonly available to field practitioners. The transcutaneous approach can be performed in the field in the standing sedated horse with a 14 g over the stylet catheter, local anesthetic, sterile gloves, an extension set, and a cup to hold water (Figure 10.7). This procedure is described in further detail in Chapter 5.

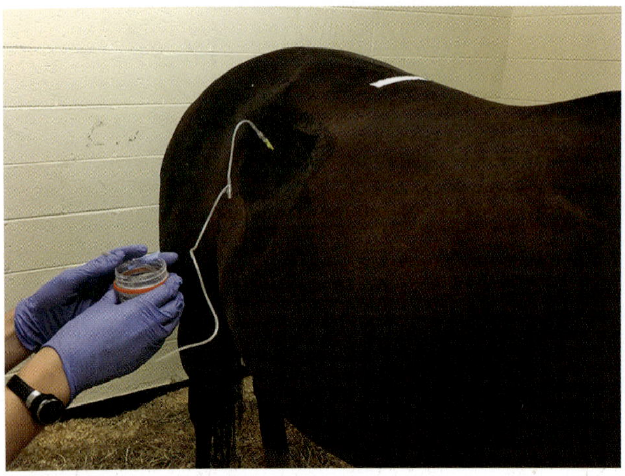

Figure 10.7 Cecal trocharization.

### Cecal Impaction

Cecal impaction is the most common primary disease of the cecum, and represents 4.1–5.0% of colics admitted to referral hospital, and 40–50% of all cecal disease (Plummer et al. 2007; Aitken et al. 2014). Two distinct types of cecal impaction have been described: primary (Type 1) impactions consisting of dehydrated feed material, and secondary (Type 2) impactions which have a more fluid content and are thought to be secondary to changes in cecal motility (Plummer 2009; Aitken et al. 2014). It has been hypothesized that cecal impactions may be more common in horses undergoing stall rest or receiving NSAIDs due to non-gastrointestinal injury, although this association has not been confirmed.

#### Clinical Signs

Horses with cecal impaction generally demonstrate mild-to-moderate signs of pain, although horses with type 2 disease can be severely painful (Plummer et al. 2007). Horses with cecal impactions initially respond favorably to analgesic therapy, which may delay recognition of the problem. Horses with cecal impactions often have a decreased appetite and reduced manure production.

#### Diagnostics

Abdominal palpation per rectum is the best way to diagnose a cecal impaction. Differentiating a cecal impaction from a large colon impaction is critical because many horses with cecal impaction will require surgery, while large colon impactions often respond to medical management. The cecum is located in the right ventral quadrant of the abdomen and can be difficult to definitively identify on palpation when it is normal. In horses with cecal impaction, a large viscus can be appreciated filling the right dorsal and ventral quadrants of the abdomen. The easiest way to identify the impacted structure as the cecum is to attempt to sweep the hand dorsally and laterally around the structure. The cecum has dorsal body wall attachments which prevent or limit the ability to continue to move the hand dorsolaterally. If the impacted structure is the large colon, movement of the hand will not be impeded because the colon does not have attachments to the body wall in this location.

#### Treatment/Prognosis

Both medical and surgical therapy have been described. Before medical management is pursued, owners should be advised of the high risk of fatal cecal perforation, which occurs in 25–30% of cases. Medical management consisting of analgesia, and enteral fluid therapy has a reported success rate of 61–81% (Plummer et al. 2007; Aitken et al. 2014). Horses with mild colic signs of short duration, and who have small-to-moderately sized impactions on abdominal palpation are the best candidates for medical management. Horses with a long duration of colic, more severe signs of pain, and large impactions on abdominal palpation are at a higher risk of cecal rupture, and more likely to require surgery. Survival to discharge after surgery is reported to be between 82 and 95%. Surgical treatment options include typhlotomy and evacuation of the cecal contents, or typhlotomy combined with cecal bypass. In one study, the overall re-impaction rate after surgery was 22%, and was significantly higher if the initial impaction was a type 2 with liquid-ingesta (36%), vs a type 1 with dry ingesta (11%) (Aitken et al. 2014).

### Ileocecal, Cecocecal, and Cecocolic Intussusception

Intussusceptions occur when one segment of intestine invaginates into another segment. Altered motility in one segment due to inflammation, or obstruction can result in intussusceptions if adjacent segments continue to move normally, resulting in telescoping of one segment over the other (Bell and Textor 2010). The inner segment is the intussusceptum, while the outer segment is the intussuscepiens. Intussusceptions are most common in horses between 1 and 3 years of age, but they can occur at any age (Southwood and Wilkins 2015). Intussusceptions are also thought to be associated with *Anoplocephala perforliata*, although causality has not been proven (Bell and Textor 2010).

#### Clinical Signs

Colic signs associated with intussusceptions are varied and can range from severe, acute abdominal discomfort to mild, intermittent colic sometimes with accompanying weight loss. Severe pain occurs when the intussusceptum is tightly trapped within the intussuscepiens resulting in compromised blood flow. Conversely, in cases where colic is mild and intermittent, the intussusceptum may slide in and out of the intussuscepiens.

#### Diagnostics

In a recent retrospective, 54% of cases of intussusception were diagnosed using abdominal palpation per rectum, abdominal ultrasound, or both (Bell and Textor 2010). Ileocecal intussusceptions may be palpable on rectal as a tubular mass. They

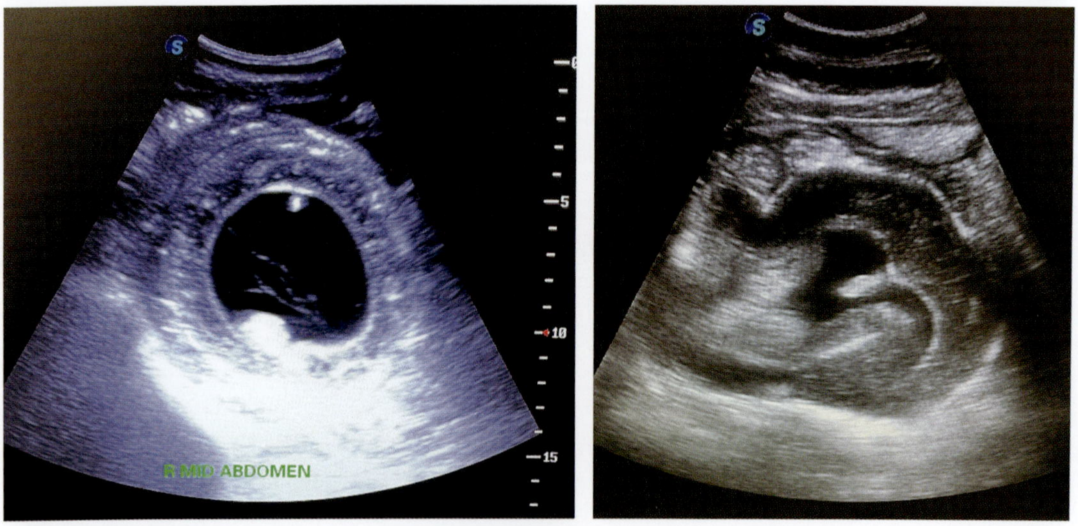


**Figure 10.8** Ultrasonographic images of an intussusception.

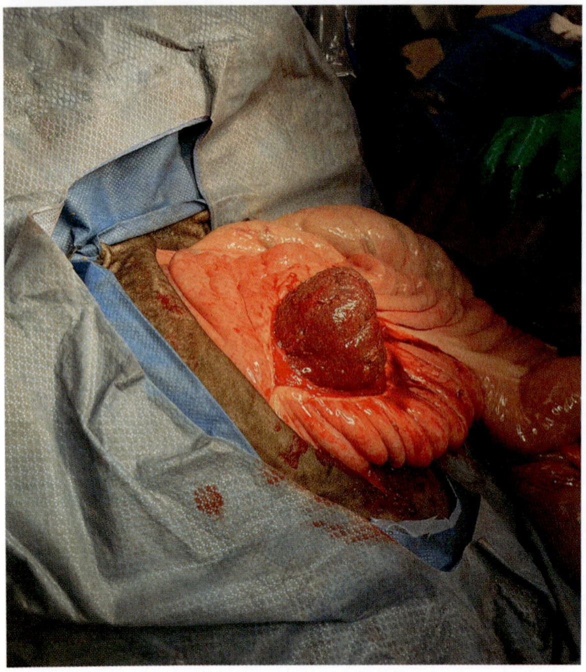

**Figure 10.9** Cecocolic intussusception.

are less likely to be visible on ultrasound because the ileum is located medial to the cecum. Horses with cecocecal or cecocolic intussusceptions may have a firm mass palpable within the cecum or colon on the right side. Additionally, a "target lesion" can be seen on sonographic evaluation of the abdomen on the right side (Figure 10.8).

Due to sequestration of the compromised segment of bowel within the intussuscepiens, peritoneal fluid may not always reflect the severity of damage to the entrapped bowel. However, abdominal fluid analysis was found to be abnormal in 63% of ileocecal, 67% of cecocecal, and 81% of cecocolic intussusceptions.

#### Treatment

Intussusceptions result in compromise of the intussusceptum and therefore require surgical treatment. Ileocecal intussusceptions can be very difficult to reduce and often involve only a short segment of invaginated ileum. Even if reduction is possible, the risk of contamination is high due to the friable nature of the intussusceptum. It is currently recommended to perform an incomplete ileocecostomy without reducing the intussuceptum. Cecocecal intussusceptions can often be manually reduced, and the compromised apical tissue removed by typhlectomy. Cecocolic intussusceptions involve invagination of the cecum through the cecocolic valve. Manual reduction is usually unrewarding. Creating a colotomy and performing an amputation of the invaginated cecum within the lumen of the colon may facilitate eventual reduction of the intussusception (Figure 10.9). Techniques have been described using suture, umbilical tape, or poly amide tie wraps (zip ties) to ligate cecum prior to amputation (Martin et al. 1999; Bell and Textor 2010; de Bont 2018). There is a high risk of contamination with this procedure. A recent paper (Lores and Ortenburger 2008) described a technique for complete cecal bypass and ileocolotomy in three horses where the cecocolic intussuception could not be reduced.

#### Prognosis

In one study, survival to discharge for horses allowed to recovery from surgery for ileocecal and cecocecal intussusceptions was 81 and 75%, respectively. In that same study, survival for horses with cecocolic intussusceptions was lower at 44% (Bell and Textor 2010).

## Large Colon

### Obstructive Lesions

#### Large Colon Impaction

***Feed Impaction*** Large colon impactions are the second most common cause of colic in the horse, representing approximately 15% of cases (Hanson and Schumacher 2021b). Although most large colon impactions are successfully treated in the field, in one study they still made up 13% of colic cases admitted to a referral hospital (Plummer 2009). Impactions are most common at the pelvic flexure (70%) and at the junction of the right dorsal and transverse colons (10%). This is due to changes in luminal diameter that occur in these locations (Plummer 2009). Changes in management including feed change, housing change, or increased/decreased exercise may predispose horses to developing large colon impaction. In one study 54% of horses had a change in management that occurred within two weeks of a diagnosis of a large colon impaction (Plummer 2009). Additionally, large colon impactions have a seasonal distribution, with the highest occurrence during fall and winter (Hanson and Schumacher 2021b).

***Sand Impaction*** Sand impactions represent a subset of large colon impactions, and occur more commonly in regions with sandy soil, or where management practices result in horses having access to sand or gravel (Kilcoyne et al. 2017). Sand impactions can occur with or without concurrent feed impactions.

#### Clinical Signs

***Feed Impaction*** The majority of horses (67–81%) with large colon impactions show mild signs of colic (Plummer 2009). Additional clinical signs in horses with large colon impaction include reduced-to-absent GI sounds and reduced manure production. Vital parameters are often normal, or only mildly abnormal. Many horses with impactions will have a reduced appetite, although those with minimal signs of pain may continue to eat.

***Sand Impaction*** Due to its abrasive nature, sand or gravel within the lumen of the large colon causes irritation and inflammation of the mucosa, which results in colic signs that can range from mild and intermittent, to acute and severe. Additionally, horses with sand enteropathy may have weight loss, or low-volume diarrhea in addition to (or instead of) signs of colic. Generally, clinical signs are similar to those for feed impaction. Horse with severe or longstanding sand impactions may also show signs of endotoxemia due to increased absorption of bacterial toxins across the inflamed colonic mucosa.

#### Diagnostics

***Feed Impaction*** Hematologic analysis in horses with feed impactions are usually unremarkable, although horses that have been impacted for several days can show signs of mild-to-moderate dehydration, and may have mild electrolyte derangements due to decreased feed and water intake. Horses with large colon impactions generally do not have reflux when a nasogastric tube is passed, and abdominal ultrasound is generally unremarkable.

Large colon impactions are best diagnosed on abdominal palpation per rectum. Impactions involving the pelvic flexure can be easily palpated in the left caudal abdomen. Impactions involving the right dorsal and transverse colon are more difficult to palpate, especially in large horses due to their more cranial location. Occasionally, horses with small intestinal strangulation will have a dry, ingesta filled "vacuum packed," large colon on palpation. This should not be confused with a primary large colon impaction, which is characterized by an expanded, ingesta filled large colon, because it can delay treatment. These horses usually have signs of systemic compromise (tachycardia, abnormal mucous membranes, severe pain) absent in horses with primary large colon impactions. Abdominal ultrasound or abdominocentesis are useful in these cases to differentiate strangulating lesions.

***Sand Impaction*** Sand enteropathy occurs without a palpable large colon impaction in about 50% of cases (Kilcoyne et al. 2017). In 21% of horses with intraluminal sand, auscultation of the ventral abdomen caudal to the xyphoid produces a sound like waves on a beach. A sedimentation test for sand can be performed by suspending feces in water within a rectal sleeve and evaluating the fingertips for sand after 20 minutes. Some horses only shed sand intermittently, so a negative sedimentation test does not definitively rule out sand enteropathy (Hanson and Schumacher 2021b).

Abdominal radiographs are the diagnostic of choice for confirming the presence of sand and for monitoring response to therapy (Niinistö et al. 2014, 2018; Kilcoyne et al. 2017). Multiple studies have been conducted to assess whether the amount or location of sand influences outcome, but results have been equivocal.

### Treatment

***Feed Impaction*** Most large colon impactions (84–98%) respond to medical therapy (Plummer 2009; Hanson and Schumacher 2021b). The mainstay of treatment for large colon impactions is administration of enteral fluids with electrolytes via a nasogastric tube. Several studies have shown that the enteral route is superior to the intravenous route for resolution of large colon impactions (Lopes et al. 2002, 2004; Plummer 2009). Administration of fluid into the stomach activates the gastrocolic reflex, increasing colonic motility. With enteral therapy, fluids are administered directly into the intestinal lumen. In contrast, IV fluids must be secreted into the intestinal lumen. One study evaluating three different enteral fluid protocols showed that increased frequency of fluid administration resolved impactions faster than the same volume administered less frequently. In that study, 10–20 mL/kg (5–6 L for a 500 kg horse) of enteral fluids given every 30–60 minutes resolved impactions faster than the same dose given every two hours (Hallowell 2008).

In addition to water and electrolytes, mineral oil, magnesium sulfate ($MgSO_4$), and DSS have all been used for their perceived laxative effects. Mineral oil (5–10 mL/kg) is commonly used in horses with impactions, despite its limited ability to penetrate a mass of firm ingesta. Its limited efficacy and the risk of causing fatal lipoid pneumonia if inadvertently administration into the lungs limit its usefulness in horses with simple feed impactions. $MgSO_4$ is an osmotic cathartic which increases movement of fluid into the intestinal lumen. Published doses and dosing intervals (0.5–1.0 g/kg in 2 L of water, q12–24 hours) should not be exceeded, especially in dehydrated horses due to the risk of magnesium toxicity. DSS, an anionic surfactant, decreases surface tension which increases water absorption into the impaction. DSS has a narrow therapeutic range, and a high risk of toxicity, and should not be used as first-line treatment. For impactions refractory to routine management, DSS can be considered, but should be dosed cautiously. A wide dose range has been published (16–200 mg/kg), and there are reports of toxicity at doses as low as 50 mg/kg (Plummer 2009; Hanson and Schumacher 2021b).

Additional therapies for large colon impaction include anti-inflammatories (flunixin meglumine 1.1 mg/kg, q12 hours), analgesics (alpha-2 agonists, opioids), and spasmolytics (*N*-butylscopolammonium bromide 0.3 mg/kg IV). Horses with significant dehydration may benefit from IV fluids to replace existing losses and to meet maintenance requirements, while enteral fluids therapy is targeted at breaking up the impaction.

Surgical intervention is warranted in horses with progressive signs of pain, or where cardiovascular parameters are deteriorating. The colon is exteriorized in surgery and placed either on the abdomen with the pelvic flexure between the hind limbs, or onto an enterotomy tray placed on the left or right side of the horse. A full-thickness incision is made into the antimesenteric side of the pelvic flexure, and intraluminal lavage combined with external manual agitation is used to evacuate the colon.

***Sand Impaction*** Recent studies have shown that a combination of psyllium (1 g/kg) and $MgSO_4$ (1 g/kg) given once daily, is superior to either medication given alone for resolving sand impactions (Niinistö et al. 2014, 2018). Horses treated with $MgSO_4$ (alone or with psyllium) may experience self-limiting diarrhea. Mineral oil used alone or in combination with psyllium and $MgSO_4$ has been reported for treatment of sand accumulation. Mineral oil alone does not appear to improve sand clearance (Hotwagner and Iben 2008). However, in our hospital mineral oil is used with psyllium to decrease the frequency with which psyllium forms concretions that block the nasogastric tube. If mineral oil is used, it is essential to ensure correct placement of the tube within the stomach. If feed material is not obtained prior to administering treatment, mineral oil should not be used.

The majority of horses with sand impactions will respond favorably to medical therapy. In 1 study, 75% of horses were successfully managed medically while 25% required surgery. Interestingly, there was no relationship between the amount of sand seen radiographically in that study, and the need for surgery (Kilcoyne et al. 2017). Surgical intervention is recommended in cases where pain is moderate to severe, or persists despite medical therapy. Fifty percent of horses undergoing surgery for sand accumulation had additional lesions found at surgery. Of these, 50% had right dorsal displacement (RDD) of the large colon (Kilcoyne et al. 2017).

### Indications for Referral

Most horses with impactions, especially those without sand, usually respond to medical management on the farm. However, horses with persistent pain despite appropriate analgesic administration, those with progressive gas distension, those with systemic compromise (e.g., hypovolemia, fever, leukopenia), or those intolerant of enteral fluid therapy, may benefit from referral (Box 10.7). Although these cases may ultimately respond to medical therapy, they likely will require a level of management that is impractical in a field setting. These horses may resolve faster, with fewer complications if managed in a referral setting.

**Box 10.7 Indications for referral in horses with obstructive lesions of the large colon**

- Pain despite analgesia.
- Progressive gas distention.
- Systemic compromise.
  - Hypovolemia.
  - Fever.
  - Leukopenia.
- Intolerant of enteral fluid therapy.

### Prognosis

***Feed Impaction*** Prognosis for horses with large colon impactions managed medically is excellent, with a >95% rate of survival to discharge. Survival to discharge for horses managed surgically was 58% (Hanson and Schumacher 2021). The lower survival for surgically treated horses was attributed to tearing or rupture of the large colon that occurred during surgical manipulation.

***Sand Impaction*** Prognosis for horses with sand enteropathy is excellent, with one study showing survival to discharge of 94% regardless of whether horses were managed medically or surgically (Kilcoyne et al. 2017).

Several management strategies have been recommended to prevent sand colic. These include raising feed off the ground to prevent accidental ingestion of sand, and feeding a high percentage of the diet as roughage to increase the bulk of ingesta in the colon. Multiple studies have evaluated using psyllium as a dietary supplement to prevent sand accumulation, but none have shown significant benefits over management changes alone.

### Enterolithiasis

Enteroliths, composed of struvite ($Mg^{2+}$, $NH_4$, $PO_4$) are a rare cause of colic in most of the world. However, they are common in California where they account for 21–29% of surgical colics (Pierce et al. 2010; Kelleher et al. 2014). Enteroliths form when minerals dissolved in the colonic fluid precipitate in concentric layers around a central nidus. They can have smooth or rough exteriors (Figure 10.10). Both diets high in alfalfa (>50%) and lack of access to pasture are associated with an increased risk of enterolithiasis (Hassel et al. 2004; Hassel et al. 2008). Some studies have shown increased prevalence in Arabian and Morgan breeds, while others have not found a breed predilection.

Enteroliths form in the right dorsal colon, and peristaltic movement of the colon propels the enteroliths aborally. The most common sites of obstruction are the junction of the right dorsal and transverse colons, and the small colon due to the decreased luminal size in those areas.

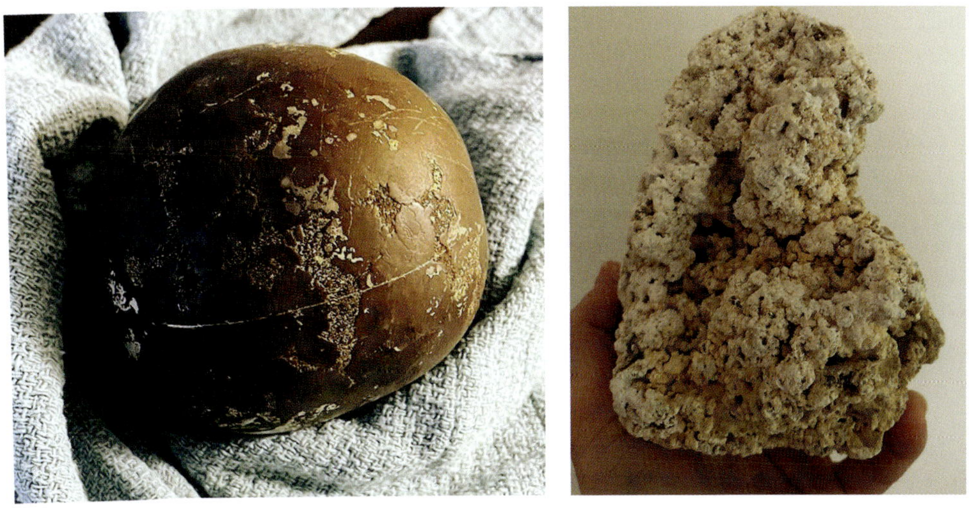

**Figure 10.10** Enteroliths.

***Clinical Signs*** Because enteroliths form over time, most horses with enteroliths are >5 years of age. Colic signs are usually mild to moderate. Horses may have a history of chronic intermittent colic because intermittent obstructions may occur as the enterolith moves with peristalsis. Alternately, movement of the enterolith can cause mucosal irritation which can lead to pain.

Rarely, the pressure of an enterolith against the bowel wall can cause necrosis which can result in signs of endotoxemia. This is more common with small colon enteroliths.

***Diagnostics*** Digital radiography is the diagnostic of choice to detect enteroliths. Sensitivity is 84% with specificity of 96%. Enteroliths in the small colon are less likely to be found radiographically (sensitivity: 61%) compared to those in the large colon (sensitivity: 90%). Increased gas content of the colon decreases the sensitivity of radiographs (Kelleher et al. 2014). Portable x-ray generators are not powerful enough to penetrate the equine abdomen, making diagnosis in the field unrewarding.

***Treatment*** Surgery is the only effective treatment. Euthanasia should be recommended in horses with a radiographically confirmed diagnosis of enterolithiasis without the option for surgery.

Approximately 60% of enteroliths are located in the large colon. For large colon enteroliths, the colon is exteriorized and a pelvic flexure enterotomy is performed. After evacuation of the contents of the colon, a hose is passed through the enterotomy, and advanced to the level of the enterolith. Water is used to float the enterolith, while gentle external manipulation moves it from its original location (usually in the transverse or right dorsal colon) toward the pelvic flexure for removal. The pelvic flexure enterotomy is then closed routinely. If the enterolith is too large to be moved to the pelvic flexure, an enterotomy can be made over the enterolith once it has been moved as far toward the pelvic flexure as possible. In this case, the enterotomy should be made through a tenial band.

Forty percent of enteroliths are located in the small colon. For removal, an enterotomy is made directly over the enterolith through the tenial band. Often the mucosa is adhered to the enterolith and must be carefully detached before the enterolith can be removed. Necrosis of the small colon wall due to the pressure of the enterolith can occur. If the necrotic area is small and does not extend around the circumference of the bowel, it can be inverted and oversewn. However, if the necrotic area encompasses a large part of the circumference of the wall, resection and anastomosis is required. If the enterolith is located in a portion of the small colon that cannot be exteriorized, intraluminal hydration can be used to float the enterolith to a part of the small colon that can be exteriorized. For enteroliths in the aboral small colon, a high enema is used. For enteroliths in the oral small colon, fluid must be introduced through a pelvic flexure enterotomy.

Up to 1/3 of horses will have >1 enterolith (Pierce et al. 2010). Therefore, it is important to palpate the entire gastrointestinal tract to ensure all enteroliths have been found and removed. Enteroliths with flat sides should increase the index of suspicion that there are multiple enteroliths.

***Prognosis*** Complication rates are not different for small colon vs large colon enteroliths. However, one study showed that horses with small colon enteroliths were more likely to have postoperative fever and anorexia compared to those with enteroliths in the large colon. Additionally, more horses with small colon enteroliths had to be euthanized during surgery due to mural necrosis that was inaccessible, or had already led to rupture (Pierce et al. 2010).

Survival to discharge for horses recovered from anesthesia is excellent for horses with both small colon (88%) and large colon (94%) enteroliths. Additionally, 90% of horses that survived long term were able to return to the same or a higher level of activity after surgery (Pierce et al. 2010).

#### Right Dorsal Displacement of the Large Colon

RDD of the large colon is a common cause of colic in the horse. RDDs account for 6–17% of all surgical colics (Smith and Mair 2010; McGovern et al. 2011), and 50% of horses treated surgically for non-strangulating obstructions of the large colon (Whyard and Brounts 2019). The exact cause of RDD is unknown. Theories include abnormal signaling by pacemaker cells located in the pelvic flexure, gas distension and altered motility due to ingestion of soluble carbohydrates, and changes in motility caused by altered fecal microbiota (Whyard and Brounts 2019). Anatomically, as the pelvic flexure and left dorsal and ventral colons move cranially and to the right, the right dorsal and ventral colons are pushed caudally between the cecum and the right body wall.

***Clinical Signs*** Horses with RDD generally have a normal-to-mildly increased heart rate and may have normal to absent gastrointestinal sounds. Because RDD causes simple obstruction, signs of pain are generally mild to moderate. However, colic signs can be more severe in cases where there is substantial gas distension of the displaced colon, or where the colon has been displaced for an extended period of time.

***Diagnostics*** Abdominal palpation per rectum may reveal tight bands coursing horizontally across the caudal abdomen. Inability to palpate the pelvic flexure at its normal location in the mid-ventral abdomen may also be suggestive of RDD. Unfortunately, both of these findings are inconsistent at best. In the author's experience, many horses with palpation findings suggestive of RDD had a different lesion diagnosed at surgery. Conversely, horses where RDD was not expected based on palpation per rectum were found to have RDD at surgery.

Fifty percent of horses with RDD will have an increased GGT, due to compression of the bile duct by the gas distended, displaced colon. A normal GGT does not rule out RDD. However, an elevated GGT in a horse with signs consistent with large colon obstruction should raise the index of suspicion for RDD (Gardner et al. 2005).

***Treatment*** About 60% of horses with a presumptive diagnosis of RDD respond to medical management consisting of withholding feed, enteral fluids, and analgesics (NSAIDs, sedatives). Medical management appears to be more successful in horses without severe gas distention or other signs of systemic compromise. Surgical intervention is recommended in horses that do not respond to medical management. During surgery the large colon is manually repositioned in the correct anatomical location. A pelvic flexure enterotomy may be performed to evacuate the large colon if an impaction is found concurrent with the displacement.

***Prognosis*** Overall survival to discharge for horses with RDD is excellent and is reported between 87 and 100% for both medically and surgically managed horses (Gardner et al. 2005; McGovern et al. 2011; Whyard and Brounts 2019). The majority of horses that recover from surgery (75%) return to their previous level of activity (Whyard and Brounts 2019).

Approximately 40% of horses where RDD was confirmed at laparotomy experienced episodes of colic postoperatively. In one study significantly more horses with surgically corrected RDD that were discharged from hospital underwent a second laparotomy for colic compared to horses with other causes of large colon nonstrangulating obstruction. This supports the theory that abnormal colonic motility plays a role in the pathogenesis of RDD (Smith and Mair 2010; Whyard and Brounds 2019).

#### Left Dorsal Displacement of the Large Colon (Nephrosplenic Entrapment)

The terms "left dorsal displacement (LDD)," and "nephrosplenic entrapment (NSE)," of the large colon are often used interchangeably. An LLD occurs when the colon moves between the left body wall and the spleen, while an NSE occurs when the colon continues to move dorsally and medially until it comes to rest on the nephrosplenic ligament (also called the perirenal fascia), which connects the left kidney to the spleen. Therefore, while all NSEs are LDDs, not all LDDs are NSEs. NSE is diagnosed in 2.7–9% of horses admitted to referral centers for colic (Baker et al. 2011; Lindegaard et al. 2011). Although it has been reported in foals as young as 5 months, NSE occurs most commonly in adult horses, with Warmbloods and geldings overrepresented (Burke and Parente 2016).

***Clinical Signs*** Clinical signs in horses with NSE are similar to those for other obstructive lesions of the large colon. Colic signs are generally mild to moderate, and unless the displacement is of long duration, horses are usually systemically stable with normal vital parameters. Gastrointestinal sounds can range from normal to absent.

***Diagnostics*** Definitive diagnosis of NSE can only be made at laparotomy or necropsy. However, abdominal palpation per rectum and abdominal ultrasound can be useful in horses where NSE is suspected. On palpation per rectum, the colon may be felt within the nephrosplenic space, in the left dorsal abdominal quadrant. This may be difficult or even impossible to appreciate in very large horses where the nephrosplenic space cannot be reached, or in horses where there is significant gas distension of the colon reducing access to the nephrosplenic space. Additionally, in horses with NSE the spleen may be displaced medially or ventrally from its normal position along the left body wall.

Ultrasound of the left paralumbar fossa using a 5–10 mHz, curvilinear probe at a depth of 10–15 cm can also be useful in evaluating horses with suspected NSE. In a normal horse, the left kidney should be visible adjacent to the spleen (Figure 10.11). In horses with NSE, the gas-filled colon will be seen adjacent to the spleen, and the kidney will not be visible.

***Treatment*** Medical management is an appropriate initial option for horses with NSE. In addition to supportive care, several therapies specific to horses with NSE have been reported. Phenylephrine (PE), an alpha 1 receptor agonist, decreases

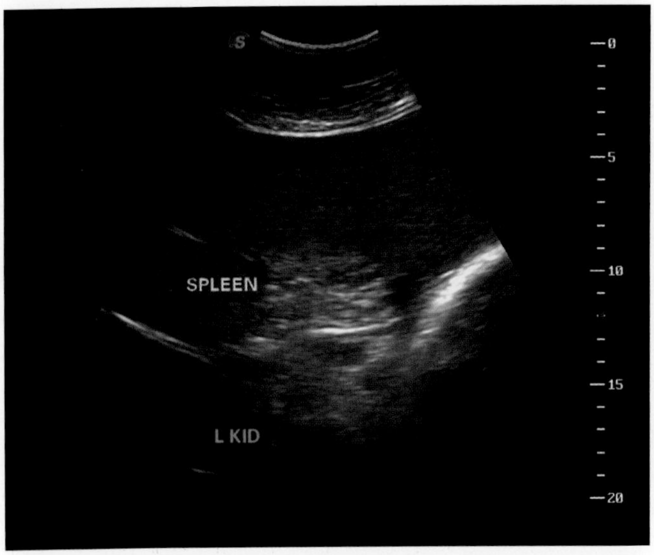


**Figure 10.11** Nephrosplenic window in a normal horse.

splenic area and thickness by 72 and 40%, respectively, for up to 25 minutes (Baker et al. 2011). This may facilitate resolution of NSE by making it easier for the colon to slide off the nephrosplenic ligament. The dose of PE is 3 mcg/kg/min given over 15 minutes, diluted with saline to a total volume of 50–60 mL. This is approximately 20 mg for a 500 kg horse. PE causes systemic vasoconstriction and reflex bradycardia. To avoid syncope, heart rate should be continuously monitored and the rate of administration titrated to maintain a heart rate ≥24 beats/min. PE administration is generally followed by jogging or lunging for 20 minutes to promote movement of the colon off the nephrosplenic ligament. A recent study described fatal hemorrhage in five horses >15 years of age administered PE for treatment of NSE (Fredrick et al. 2010). Owners should be informed of the risks when PE is being used in older horses.

A rolling procedure under general anesthesia has been described which can be done with or without administration of PE (Figure 10.12a–h). Several modifications to the original technique have been described (Boening and vonSaldem 1985; Deen 1990; Baker et al. 2011; Fultz et al. 2013). Briefly, the horse is induced under general anesthesia into right lateral recumbency (Figure 10.12a,b). Hobbles and a hoist are used on either the hind limbs, or all four limbs to rotate the horse into dorsal recumbency, where ballottement of the abdomen is performed for one to two minutes (Figure 10.12c,d). The horse is lowered into left lateral recumbency, rolled into sternal recumbency, and then right lateral recumbency (Figure 10.12e–g). Ultrasound or palpation per rectum is used to assess the success of the procedure (Figure 10.12h). Because all variations of the procedure require a hoist, and multiple people to ballot the abdomen, it is not practical for use in the field.

Overall resolution of NSE using either PE and jogging or rolling is reported to be between 56 and 92% (Fredrick et al. 2010). A study comparing jogging versus rolling for horses with NSE showed significantly better success with rolling (84%) compared to jogging (63%). All horses in that study received PE (Fultz et al. 2013). Another study showed no difference in success for the rolling procedure when PE was added compared to rolling alone (Baker et al. 2011). Therefore, resolution of NSE is more likely with the rolling procedure than jogging, regardless of whether PE is given.

Surgical intervention is recommended for cases of NSE that fail to resolve with medical management, in cases where the horse is becoming systemically unstable, or if a second lesion is suspected in addition to the NSE. The entrapment is corrected by pushing the spleen medially, using the underside of the surgeon's arms. Then the surgeon's hands are used to push the colon laterally, followed by lifting it toward the incision. Once the colon has cleared the ventral margin of the spleen, it is replaced within the abdomen in its correct location, medial to the spleen. Administration of PE intraoperatively may facilitate manual correction by reducing the size and width of the spleen, allowing more room to manipulate the colon into position.

***Closure of the NSS*** The recurrence rate of NSE is reported to be 3.2–21% (Smith and Mair 2010; Baker et al. 2011). For horses who have had ≥2 presumed episodes of NSE, or those where NSE has been confirmed at celiotomy, closure of the nephrosplenic space may be warranted. Standing flank laparoscopy with closure using either suture or a polypropylene mesh has been described. Closure of the NSS prevents recurrence of NSE, but does not prevent any other type of colic, including displacement of the large colon between the spleen and the body wall. Horses with a history of NSE had significantly reduced incidence of colic after closure of the NSS. The reduction in colic episodes after closure was more pronounced in horses where the diagnosis of NSE was confirmed at celiotomy, although this difference did not reach statistical significance (Burke and Parente 2016; Rodriguez et al. 2019).

***Prognosis*** The decision to manage horses with NSE conservatively vs surgically varies by region and clinician preference. Survival to discharge is excellent (84–92%) regardless of whether conservative management or early surgical intervention is chosen (Fredrick et al. 2010; Baker et al. 2011; Lindegaard et al. 2011). A recent meta-analysis (Gillen et al. 2020) comparing medical vs surgical management for NSE showed no significant difference in survival to discharge between groups, with only 11.8% of horses initially managed medically ultimately requiring surgery (Gillen et al. 2020). One study

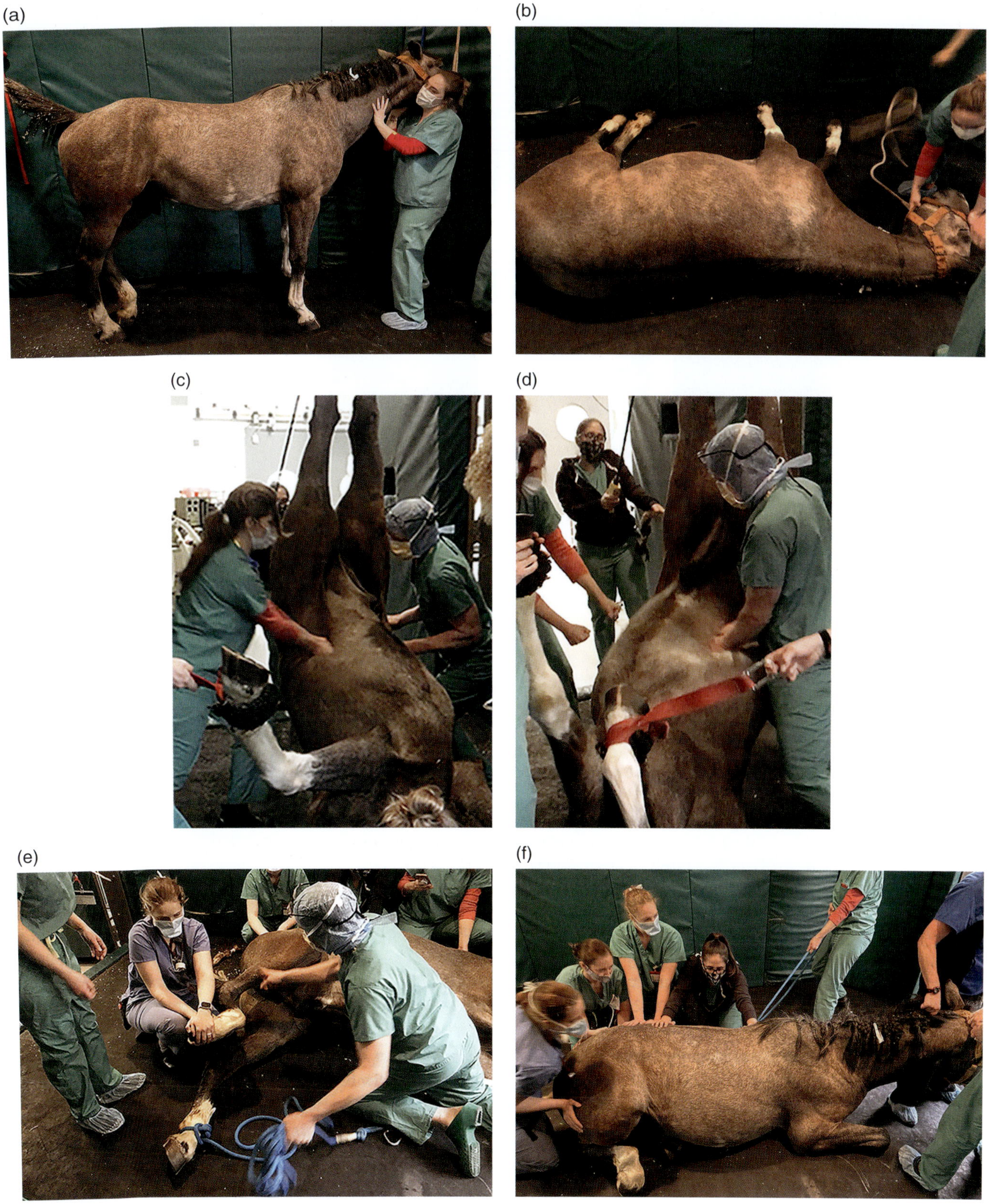


**Figure 10.12** Rolling technique for correction of a nephrosplenic entrapment of the large colon. The horse is induced from the standing position (a) under general anesthesia into right lateral recumbency (b). Note the head elevation and tail tie to facilitate a smooth induction. The horse is then hoisted into dorsal recumbency with the hind-quarters elevated, where ballottement of the abdomen is performed (c,d). Note two people on either side of the horse alternate ballottement of the abdomen to shake the colon free from the nephrosplenic space. Next, the horse is lowered into left lateral recumbency (e) where a rope is attached to the dependent limb to facilitate rolling through sternal recumbency (f) back into right lateral recumbency (g). Rectal palpation (h) or ultrasound may be used to confirm correction of the colonic displacement.

(g)

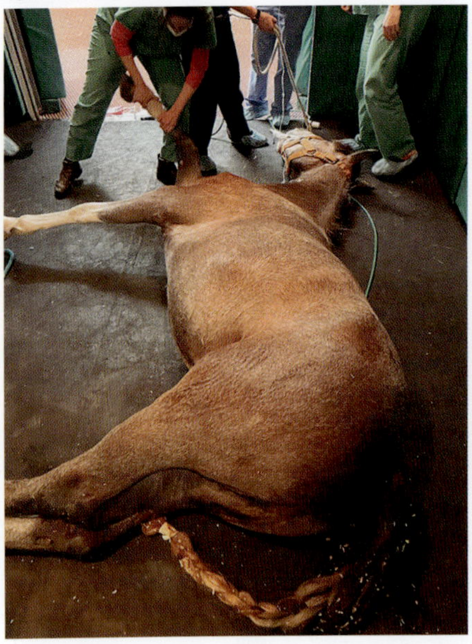

(h)

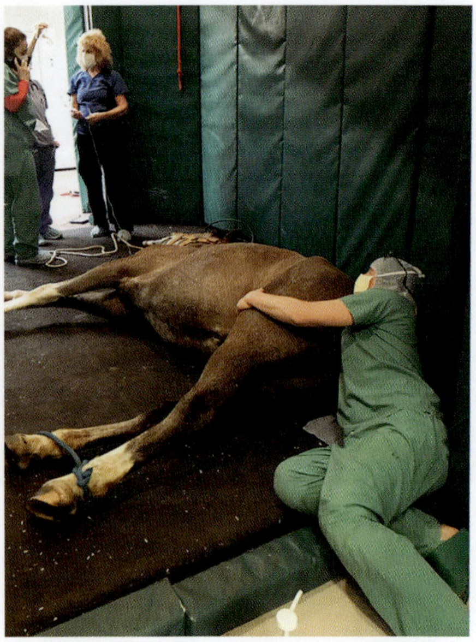

**Figure 10.12** (Continued)

of 142 horses with NSE found that degree of pain, and the presence of gastric reflux and/or gas distension on rectal were significantly associated with the need for surgical intervention (Lindegaard et al. 2011). These studies indicate that the majority of horses with NSE will respond to medical management. However, for horses that will ultimately require surgical correction, prolonged medical management may decrease surgical success. Therefore, frequent reassessment of vital parameters, degree of abdominal distension, and comfort level are essential if medical management is to be pursued.

## Strangulating Lesions

### Large Colon Volvulus

Large colon volvulus (LCV) is one of the most severe and rapidly fatal forms of colic. LCV is diagnosed in 10–20% of surgical colics (Suthers et al. 2013). Although LCV can occur in any horse it is most common in broodmares that have foaled within the last 60 days (Leahy et al. 2018). LCV is rarely diagnosed in ponies. LCV is defined as rotation of the colon around its mesentery, with rotation >360° resulting in a strangulating obstruction and rapid hypoxic damage to tissue.

***Clinical Signs*** Horses with LCV are extremely painful and often appear to be unaware of their surroundings. They can be a danger to themselves, and to anyone trying to work with them. These horses are difficult to keep standing, even with large doses of detomidine and butorphanol, often making a complete colic examination impossible.

***Diagnostics*** A suspected diagnosis of LCV is often made based on clinical signs alone. If the horse can be adequately sedated, abdominal palpation per rectum usually reveals a severely gas distended large colon. If an abdominocentesis can be safely performed, serosanguinous fluid with a high lactate is often obtained, even in horses where the duration of clinical signs is short. This is due to the large volume of tissue affected.

***Treatment*** LCV requires immediate surgery, or euthanasia in cases where surgery is not an option. The volvulus occurs at either the base of the colon, or at the cecocolic ligament. Rotation is usually counterclockwise, with the ventral colon moving medially and dorsally, while the dorsal colon moves laterally and ventrally (Southwood, 2019). To correct the volvulus, the colon must be rotated in the opposite direction of the volvulus. If the volvulus is >360°, the cecum is often displaced and may be difficult to identify, even after correction of the volvulus. Complete resolution of the volvulus is confirmed when the cecum is located lateral to the large colon, and the cecocolic ligament is visible coursing in cranially.

After correction of the volvulus, the surgeon must evaluate the viability of the large colon, and decide if a resection is warranted. Objective means for measuring colon viability intraoperatively is an active area of research. Unfortunately, there is currently no "real-time" test that is both widely available and accurate. Surgeons must rely on subjective measures such as serosal color, bleeding at the pelvic flexure enterotomy site, and pulse quality in the mesenteric vessels. Interestingly, a recent study showed that peripheral venous lactate obtained immediately after manual correction of the LCV was associated with survival. In that study, horses with peripheral lactate >5 mmol/L immediately after correction of the volvulus were 27 times more likely to die than horses with lactate <5 mmol/L (Orr et al. 2020).

***Prognosis*** In one study of a mixed population of horses admitted to a referral hospital in the UK and diagnosed with LCV, 20% of horses did not recover from anesthesia, either due to severity of disease resulting in intraoperative euthanasia, or death under GA. For horses that did recover, abnormal serosal color at surgery, elevated HR 48 hours postoperatively, and colic during the postoperatively period were all associated with decreased survival to hospital discharge (Suthers et al. 2013). In that study, survival to discharge was 71% with long-term survival 48% at one year, and 34% at two years. For horses that survived to discharge but died during the follow-up period, the cause of death was reported as "colic," in 20% of horses (Suthers et al. 2013).

Early recognition and surgical intervention improve survival to discharge. One study of broodmares in Kentucky, where horses lived within one hour of the surgical center, reported a survival to discharge rate of 90%. This is substantially higher than that reported in other studies and indicates that decreased time from onset of colic to surgical correction positively influences outcome (Leahy et al. 2018). In this study, mare fertility after surgery was within ranges previously reported for well-managed Thoroughbred brood mares in Kentucky, indicating that surgery for LCV does not negatively impact future fertility.

## Small Colon and Rectum

There are three main categories of problems associated with the small colon and rectum. The first would be colic-associated problems (most commonly intraluminal obstructions or strangulating obstructions). The second category would be rectal prolapse that may or may not involve the small colon, and the third category would be rectal tears.

### Triage Over the Phone

***Colic Problems*** This will be analogous to any colic problem, with the exception that a description of fever, passage of small volume diarrhea or matted feces, and straining to defecate increases the index of suspicion for small colon (Rhoads et al. 1999; Hanson and Schumacher 2021a). Time elapsed since the horse last passed manure with normal size and might help identify duration of problem.

### Rectal Prolapse

Initial triage should determine duration of prolapse (or when last seen normal), presence of diarrhea or other colic signs, and if horse is actively straining. If safe for owner to do so, could advise owner to apply glycerin to prolapse to reduce any desiccation of tissues while they await veterinarian arrival. Rectal prolapses should be seen as soon as possible or referred for immediate attention if field visit is delayed.

### Rectal Tears

These are typically iatrogenic complications. If there are reports of bleeding or blood at the rectum, it is important to ask if anyone (veterinarian or layperson) has performed rectal procedures on the horse recently, if recent live-cover breeding has occurred or is possible, or if there has been any known trauma to the area. This complaint should be seen as soon as possible or referred for immediate attention if field visit is delayed.

## Triage at the Farm

### History

***Colic Problems*** Important historical details to consider are diet, particularly feeding of alfalfa (in areas prone to enteroliths) or poor-quality feed, known or possible dental problems, history of colitis in this patient or on farm, and recent or prior foaling (if broodmare) (Hanson and Schumacher 2021a). Dietary indiscretion should be considered in foals or young horses.

Duration of colic signs, presence of associated signs (fever, passage of small volume diarrhea or unformed manure, straining), and last witnessed passage of normal manure helps to characterize current colic event.

***Rectal Prolapse*** If not already determined during phone triage, details of duration of prolapse and history of diarrhea or other colic signs should be determined. If horse is a mare of breeding age and there is any possibility of pregnancy, possibility of dystocia or abortion should be determined. Other relevant historical details are deworming history and diet.

***Rectal Tears*** If a pre-existing rectal tear is suspected, then history of recent rectal procedures or evidence of trauma to the perineum should be determined. History of straining might raise index of suspicion for conditions that might cause or predispose to rectal tears.

#### Examination

***Colic Problems*** The examination is similar to any colic workup. It is important to assess for presence of fever and to note presence and degree of abdominal distension, because small colon obstructions are more likely to be complete (Rhoads et al. 1999; Hanson and Schumacher 2021a). Gastric reflux is not unexpected because of the proximity of the small colon to the duodenum via the duodenocolic ligament. Rectal examination has a higher chance of localizing the problem (Rhoads et al. 1999; Hanson and Schumacher 2021a). In general, there will be no or scant manure present, the rectal or small colon lesion will be palpable, or small (+/− large) colon gas distension will be evident; however, rectal impactions are diagnosed by the presence of an expansile, inspissated mass of ingesta within the rectum. With small colon impaction, the rectal mucosa may be edematous and friable. Strangulating lesions may be palpable as a spiral, constriction of the lumen of the small colon. Recognition of a small colon or rectal lesion should prompt referral, because the small diameter of the bowel increases the risk for rupture, horses are often more systemically affected than with comparable lesions in other gastrointestinal locations, and these cases are often refractory to medical therapy due to their aboral location.

***Rectal Prolapse*** The examination should focus on presence of straining and characterizing the type of prolapse and the health of the prolapsed tissue. If the horse is actively straining, caudal epidural anesthesia (Chapter 5, Caudal epidural anesthesia) should be performed to prevent further prolapse of tissues. If the prolapsed tissue is continuous with the anal sphincter, then it is likely a Type I, II, or III (see Table 10.2; Turner and Fessler 1980). If there is a tube of tissue protruding from the anus, it is a Type IV (see Table 10.2; Turner and Fessler 1980). If it is a Type IV, the length of prolapsed intestine should be estimated, because >30 cm prolapse is likely to be associated with avulsion of the mesocolon and subsequent necrosis of the intussuscepted small colon (Ragle et al. 1997). If the prolapsed tissue is viable, then it may be reduced, whereas if it is non-viable, a resection of the exposed tissues will be necessary. Presence of rectal impaction, urinary obstruction, diarrhea, or severe coughing should be noted as conditions predisposing to rectal prolapse. Referral is advised in any case of rectal prolapse, because even if successful reduced, management is complicated by likelihood for recurrence, need for a temporary purse-string suture to maintain reduction, and development of devitalized tissue.

***Rectal Tears*** If a rectal tear (pre-existing or iatrogenic) is suspected during an examination, the owner should be immediately informed of the finding (McMaster et al. 2015). Adequate restraint of the horse should be ensured, which may entail additional sedation or caudal epidural anesthesia. A bare-armed rectal examination should be performed to identify and characterize the tear (see Table 10.2) and remove any manure to length of arm's reach (McMaster et al. 2015). Historical details should be considered with rectal palpation findings to determine if the tear was likely pre-existing or iatrogenic.

### Emergency Triage Steps

#### Patient Stabilization

***Colic Problems*** Small colon colic problems typically do not cause the peracute, severe compromise seen with other colic lesions, even with strangulating lesions (Rhoads et al. 1999; Hanson and Schumacher 2021a). Severe shock in these cases should raise concern for small colon rupture or leakage and septic peritonitis, which can occur relatively quickly in some cases due to the small diameter of the small colon. Respiratory compromise and cardiovascular collapse due to severe gas distension (abdominal compartment syndrome) can be life-threatening in some cases of small colon obstruction when there is complete occlusion of the lumen and gas accumulation in the oral segments of small and large bowel. If the horse

**Table 10.2** Classification of rectal prolapse and rectal tears.

| Classification | Description | Clinical signs |
|---|---|---|
| **Rectal prolapse** | | |
| Type I | Prolapse of rectal mucosa through anus | Circumferential protrusion of mucosa covered mass at anus |
| Type II | Prolapse of all layers of all or part of rectal ampulla | Circumferential protrusion of mucosa covered mass at anus |
| Type III | Type II prolapse with intussusception of small colon into rectum | Circumferential protrusion of mucosa covered mass at anus |
| Type IV | Intussusception of rectum and small colon through anus | Tube of tissue exiting from anus |
| **Rectal tears** | | |
| Grade 1 | Disruption of rectal mucosa and submucosa only | Roughened, superficial defect or flap in rectal mucosa |
| Grade 2 | Defect in rectal muscle layer with intact mucosa | Palpable diverticulum or outpouching covered by smooth, intact mucosa |
| Grade 3A | Disruption of rectal mucosa, submucosa, and muscle at any location except mesorectal attachment with intact serosa | Palpable roughened, deep defect or cavity in the rectum located in the dorsolateral, lateral or ventral circumference |
| Grade 3B | Disruption of rectal mucosa, submucosa, and muscle at the mesorectal attachment | Palpable roughened, deep defect or cavity in the dorsal rectum |
| Grade 4 | Full thickness (all layers) defect in the rectum | Palpable full-thickness defect through the rectal wall with palpation of serosal edge or adjacent serosal surfaces |

has severe abdominal distension compromising breathing, the horse should be trocharized to provide some short-term relief (see Chapter 5, Cecal or Colonic Trocarization).

***Rectal Prolapse*** The biggest urgency for prolapse cases is to prevent further prolapse, especially in Type IV prolapse, and to protect the mucosa from desiccation and injury. If the horse is actively straining, it will be necessary to perform a caudal epidural (see Chapter 5, Caudal epidural anesthesia) and/or resolve the cause of straining (i.e., dystocia). Type IV prolapse may be reducible without caudal epidural anesthesia. If a caudal epidural is used, it is helpful to place a purse-string suture to retain the prolapse prior to referral, which can be done with taking four large circumferential bites around the anus using umbilical tape, leaving two to three fingers width opening, and tying with a bow. If the prolapse is not easily reducible, glycerin, lube with sugar, or hemorrhoid cream should be applied to the exposed mucosa to reduce edema and prevent further desiccation and trauma prior to referral.

***Rectal Tears*** Rectal tears are often iatrogenic complications in otherwise healthy patients (McMaster et al. 2015). The horse often does not require stabilization (further guidelines provided below). Broad-spectrum antimicrobials and non-steroidal anti-inflammatory agents should be administered prior to referral.

### How to Formulate a Diagnostic Plan

***Colic Problems*** The colic workup generally provides much of the diagnostic investigation needed for these cases. A complete blood count can be helpful to assess for systemic inflammation in cases of small colon impaction. Salmonellosis has been associated with small colon impactions, so fecal culture or PCR for this pathogen should be considered as part of biosecurity (Rhoads et al. 1999). Abdominal ultrasound is not generally diagnostic for small colon disease but does help rule out other causes of colic. Abdominocentesis may not be as diagnostic for small colon lesions, even strangulating lesions, but can be helpful for monitoring when debating medical vs surgical treatment. Abdominal radiographs should be considered to characterize gas distension in foals, ponies, or miniature horses, which are too small for rectal examination, and to assess for enteroliths in geographical areas prone to enterolith formation (with the caveat that radiographs are not highly sensitive for small colon enteroliths) (Hanson and Schumacher 2021a). A dental examination should be performed to evaluate for dental problems in cases with small colon impaction.

***Rectal Prolapse*** If the cause of rectal prolapse is not obvious (i.e., dystocia), other causes for straining should be investigated and ruled out (colitis, small colon or rectal impaction, gastrointestinal parasites, urinary tract obstruction or disease). If a Type III or IV rectal prolapse is encountered, it is advisable to evaluate for signs of injury to mesocolonic vasculature (Ragle et al. 1997). Methods of evaluation range from monitoring for signs of sepsis or absence of manure passage, abdominocentesis, or laparoscopic evaluation.

***Rectal Tear*** Once a rectal tear is recognized, emergency treatment (see below) should be considered prior to referral. Complete evaluation of a rectal tear includes direct digital palpation with ungloved hand and endoscopic visualization, and, if more than superficial (Grade 1; see Table 10.2), complete blood count and abdominocentesis and abdominal fluid cytology.

**Emergency Treatment Guidelines Beyond Stabilization**

***Colic Problems*** Referral should be prioritized, because small colon problems tend to be more difficult to treat medically, complicated by other issues (colitis, Salmonella), and are more prone to pressure necrosis and rupture than other locations in the gastrointestinal tract.

***Rectal Prolapse*** Reduction of the prolapse should be prioritized, even if the horse is not actively straining, because this will help protect the mucosa and reduce edema. Referral should be recommended because rectal prolapse is likely to recur and often requires placement of a temporary purse-string suture, which then requires monitoring and management to allow defecation. Surgical resection may be required in selected cases.

***Rectal Tear*** If blood is evident on a rectal sleeve or bleeding is noted after rectal examination, the veterinarian should evaluate for a rectal tear (McMaster et al. 2015). This should be done by ensuring adequate patient restraint (additional sedation, if needed) and performance of a bare-armed rectal examination. If there is any risk of straining, intra-rectal lidocaine or caudal epidural anesthesia should be used to prevent straining. Spasmolytics (e.g., *N*-butylscopolammonium bromide) may make examination more difficult by relaxing and folding the rectal wall. The rectal tear can be identified as a defect in the mucosa, but it can be difficult to determine grade of the tear (McMaster et al. 2015). If a rectal tear occurs as an iatrogenic complication, the owner should be notified immediately, and the horse should be referred to a referral hospital (McMaster et al. 2015). The rectum should be evacuated to the extent of arms reach prior to referral. Packing of the rectum will protect the tear from further fecal contamination during referral (Eastman et al. 2000; McMaster et al. 2015). This can be achieved by placement of caudal epidural anesthesia (see Chapter 5, Caudal Epidural Anesthesia), placement of a lubed stockinette extending from 15 to 20 cm cranial to the tear to the rectum, and lightly filling the stockinette with roll cotton to fill the rectal lumen without packing the tear. The anus should be closed with a purse string or towel clamps to prevent displacement of the rectal packing. Rectal packing may allow up to 8 hours of transport time. Use of spasmolytics may delay further passage of manure if the rectum is not packed, given that immediate transport to a referral hospital is performed and the referral hospital is near (ideally <1–2 hours). If an iatrogenic occurrence, the veterinarian should inform their malpractice insurance provider of the incident as soon as possible after the horse has been referred (McMaster et al. 2015).

## What Can Be Done at the Farm

### Colic Problems

Although enteral fluid and laxative therapy can be performed on the farm, these cases can be difficult to manage medically because of the aboral location of the obstruction and the function of the small colon to absorb water from the ingesta (Hanson and Schumacher 2021a). These cases benefit from concurrent IV fluid therapy, and many cases will require surgical management. Enemas can be useful in management of small colon problems but are associated with a risk of rectal injury or rupture and should be limited to cases without a surgical option or in a referral hospital environment (Hanson and Schumacher 2021a).

### Rectal Prolapse

Although the procedures involved in management of rectal prolapse can be performed in the standing, sedated horse, these problems require close monitoring for recurrence of the prolapse or management of a purse-string suture. For cases with mesocolonic injury secondary to type III or IV rectal prolapse, it is advisable to assess and closely monitor for these injuries, even if surgical management is not feasible or not an option, so that ongoing suffering by the horse is minimized or avoided.

### Rectal Tear

Although small, grade 1 rectal tears can heal with minimal treatment, these iatrogenic complications are often the cause of malpractice claims against the veterinarian (Claes et al. 2008; McMaster et al. 2015). Therefore, it is recommended to refer all rectal tears so that optimal management can be provided and veterinarian liability can be reduced. Even if managed conservatively, rectal tears benefit from close monitoring, re-evaluation, and frequent rectal evacuations (McMaster et al. 2015).

## What Can Be Done at the Referral Hospital

### Colic Problems

Referral hospitals can provide access to full diagnostic capabilities that can aid in accurate diagnosis of a small colon problem and access to surgery if indicated. Even if medical management is feasible, close monitoring and re-evaluation is necessary in these cases. Furthermore, small colon impaction can cause the rectal mucosa to become edematous and friable which increases risk of rectal injury, which is added liability for the treating veterinarian.

### Rectal Prolapse

Facilities to allow a safe environment for caudal epidural anesthesia and rectal procedures may be lacking, and field veterinarians may lack experience in these procedures. Referral hospitals offer the facilities and expertise for these procedures. Close monitoring of the prolapse and capability for surgical resection are available at referral hospitals.

### Rectal Tear

The field veterinarian's liability is reduced by prompt referral to the referral hospital, where thorough evaluation of the tear can be performed. The owner can be provided with best recommendations for management, based on the characteristics of the tear, which may necessitate surgical management and/or frequent manual evacuation of the rectum.

## Advice on How to Decide Between Options When Referral Is Time-Critical

### Colic Problems

If the horse is exhibiting respiratory compromise secondary to abdominal distension, cecal/colonic trocharization should be performed immediately (Chapter 5, Cecal or Colonic Trocharization). Referral should be recommended for management of small colon lesions. If the owner is resistant to referral, medical management can be initiated on the farm, but the owner should be advised of risk of treatment failure and risk of colonic damage or rupture with this option.

### Rectal Prolapse

If the horse is actively straining and a type III or IV prolapse is evident, immediate attempts to prevent straining and reduce the prolapse are necessary to prevent further prolapse. If the prolapse is caused by dystocia, then the dystocia also needs to be addressed as a priority. If actively straining with a type I or II prolapse, referral could be sought without addressing the straining, but there is a risk of progression or development of a type III prolapse. The mucosa should be protected with application of glycerin (even if applied by spray) at a minimum.

### Rectal Tear

If the field veterinarian is unwilling or unable to pack the rectum prior to transport, the next best option would be to evacuate the rectum to arm's length prior to transport to the referral hospital (McMaster et al. 2015). If a rectal tear is suspected and the veterinarian is unwilling to further evaluate, administration of a spasmolytic agent and immediate transport to a referral hospital should be done. In all cases, the owner should be advised of the complication, and the malpractice insurance provider informed (McMaster et al. 2015).

## Important Decisions During Management

### Decision for Hospital Referral vs Farm Management

***Colic Problems*** If a colic presentation is localized to the small colon, referral should be advised. Young horses, including foals, older horses, or horses in areas predisposed to enteroliths would be at highest priority for referral due to a higher prevalence of surgical lesions (Hanson and Schumacher 2021a). Farm management should be attempted if referral is not an option or if the localization is not clear.

***Rectal Prolapse*** Referral should be advised in all cases due to the risk of recurrence and the development of life-threatening complications.

***Rectal Tear*** Referral should be advised in all cases of known or suspected rectal tears, due to the liability incurred by the attending veterinarian (McMaster et al. 2015). If referral is declined, the veterinarian should obtain signed documentation that medical advice has been declined by the owner or agent to reduce their liability.

#### Decision for Medical vs Surgical Treatment

***Colic Problems*** Surgical management is indicated if complete obstruction or strangulation is confirmed or suspected. Medical management can be attempted unless there is progression of clinical signs (pain and gas distension), lack of response to treatment, or deterioration of abdominal fluid cytology suggesting development of intestinal injury (Rhoads et al. 1999; Hanson and Schumacher 2021a).

***Rectal Prolapse*** In general, conservative management is preferred, if feasible. Surgical management is indicated if exposed tissue is necrotic, severely damaged, fibrotic, or irreducible (Turner and Fessler 1980). Laparoscopic assessment and consideration of colostomy are indicated if there is concern for mesocolonic injury.

***Rectal Tear*** Surgical management is required for acute, non-contaminated grade 4 tears, non- to minimally contaminated grade 3 tears, and extensive grade 1 tears (Eastman et al. 2000; Claes et al. 2008; McMaster et al. 2015) (see Table 10.2). Details of surgical management depend on the severity of tear, surgeon's preference, and owner willingness (Eastman et al. 2000; Claes et al. 2008; McMaster et al. 2015). Non-surgical management can be pursued for grade 1 tears, grade 2 tears, and contaminated or extensive grade 3 tears, although this may necessitate intensive management for success (Eastman et al. 2000; Claes et al. 2008; McMaster et al. 2015) (see Table 10.2).

#### How to Manage Important Complications

***Colic Problems*** Manageable complications of small colon lesions include diarrhea, superficial rectal injury, thrombophlebitis, laminitis, recurrent impaction, and peritonitis (Rhoads et al. 1999; Hanson and Schumacher 2021a). Superficial rectal injuries can be minimized by avoidance of or careful rectal examination and fecal softening. Thrombophlebitis and laminitis can be managed by anti-inflammatory therapy, anti-endotoxin therapy, heparin, and local treatments as appropriate (topical anti-inflammatories and hot packing for jugular vein, digital cryotherapy and support for laminitis). Recurrent impaction is managed by small amounts of low bulk feeding and laxative administration. Peritonitis is managed by antibiotic therapy and NSAIDs.

***Rectal Prolapse*** Predominant complications would be recurrence and mucosal injury. Resolution of the underlying cause for the prolapse and prevention of rectal impaction by fecal softening and careful management of indwelling purse-string suture is important to prevent recurrence. Mucosal injury is best prevented by maintaining reduction of the prolapse and prompt treatment if it recurs. Mucosal resection may be necessary if fibrosis causes local stricture. Avascular necrosis secondary to mesocolonic injury is best prevented (rather than managed) by prompt resolution of type III or IV prolapse before long segments are prolapsed.

***Rectal Tear*** Prevention of progression of a tear to grade 4 (full thickness) and prevention of contamination of the tissues with feces are the goals of rectal packing prior to referral or frequent evacuation of tears if medically managed (Eastman et al. 2000; McMaster et al. 2015). Septic peritonitis by translocation, peri-rectal abscessation, or rectal diverticulum formation can be sequelae of contaminated or undermined grade 3 rectal tears (Eastman et al. 2000; Claes et al. 2008; McMaster et al. 2015). Rectal impaction is a sequela of rectal diverticula or large grade 2 tears. Treatment is best managed by prevention of the complications by prompt referral and preventing the tear becoming contaminated and expanded by manure packing. Septic peritonitis requires antimicrobial therapy. Peri-rectal abscesses require drainage and antibiotic therapy. Rectal impactions require fecal softening and/or frequent evacuations.

#### Estimating Prognosis

***Colic Problems*** Small colon lesions have a good prognosis when appropriately managed (Rhoads et al. 1999; Hanson and Schumacher 2021a). This includes prompt surgical treatment when indicated or not responding to medical therapy, because the small diameter makes it more prone to tissue injury. Development of tissue injury or progression to translocation or rupture is associated with a guarded-to-grave prognosis.

***Rectal Prolapse*** Type I or II rectal prolapse have a good prognosis if managed to prevent or resect tissue necrosis (Turner and Fessler 1980). Type IV rectal prolapse have guarded-to-grave prognosis due to the likelihood of mesocolonic injury (Turner and Fessler 1980; Ragle et al. 1997).

***Rectal Tear*** Grade 1 and small grade 2 rectal tears have a good prognosis (Eastman et al. 2000; Claes et al. 2008; McMaster et al. 2015). Large grade 2 and grade 3 tears have a guarded prognosis due to the likelihood of complications and risk of progression (Eastman et al. 2000; Claes et al. 2008; McMaster et al. 2015). Grade 4 tears have a poor prognosis if promptly recognized and treated before abdominal contamination and a grave prognosis if abdominal contamination has occurred (Eastman et al. 2000; Claes et al. 2008; McMaster et al. 2015).

#### Decision for Euthanasia

***Colic Problems*** Septic peritonitis from colonic rupture or leakage and non-response to treatment are indications for euthanasia.

***Rectal Prolapse*** Owner unwillingness to treat a type I or II rectal prolapse, especially if associated with devitalized tissue and recurrent prolapse secondary to unresolved, underlying problems would be indications for euthanasia. Extensive (>30 cm long) or traumatized type IV rectal prolapse should be considered for euthanasia due to likelihood of mesocolonic injury and need for owner commitment to colostomy. Evidence of avascular necrosis secondary to a Type III or IV prolapse is indication for euthanasia.

***Rectal Tear*** Grade 4 rectal tears with abdominal fecal contamination need to be euthanized (Eastman et al. 2000; Claes et al. 2008; McMaster et al. 2015). Euthanasia should be recommended for extensively contaminated or undermined grade 3 rectal tears or if owners decline treatment (Eastman et al. 2000; Claes et al. 2008; McMaster et al. 2015). Euthanasia may be indicated if there is septic peritonitis or abscessation secondary to management of rectal tears or may be elected by owners of horses with recurrent impactions in rectal diverticula (McMaster et al. 2015).

## Colic in the Late-Term Pregnant Mare

### Clinical Signs

Clinical signs are abdominal discomfort. Additional signs to note would be abdominal edema or swelling, presence and character of mammary discharge, and vaginal discharge.

### Triage Over the Phone

In addition to nature and duration of colic signs, the stage of gestation and anticipated or known due date should be determined. These cases should be seen without delay, and if the field veterinarian will be delayed, referral to a hospital should be advised.

### Triage at the Farm

#### History

This is comparable to any colic problem, with added attention to the pregnancy. Stage of gestation and due date should be determined. Parity and past pregnancy or foaling issues should be identified. Prior pregnancy ultrasounds to rule out twinning is helpful information. Observation of recent or rapid changes in the abdominal distension or contour should be asked. The owner's priority for the mare vs the foal should be determined.

### Examination

The colic examination is appropriate for these cases, although parts of this examination are confounded by the presence of a large, gravid uterus. The ventral abdomen should be assessed for edema and swelling. The degree of abdominal distension should be assessed. Mammary development and secretions should be evaluated. Bloody mammary secretions may signify disruption of prepubic tendon (Sprayberry and Lu 2021). Rectal examination should pay attention to the position of the broad ligaments of the uterus. Abdominal ultrasound examination should get a baseline assessment of fetal viability. Late-term pregnant mares may be tachycardic from their pregnancy, but it is difficult to rule out cardiovascular compromise or pain as the cause.

### Emergency Triage Steps

***Patient Stabilization*** Cardiovascular compromise should be addressed with IV fluid therapy. Hyperlactatemia and hemoconcentration are important parameters to correct (Douglas et al. 2021). Hypoxemia is a potential risk for the pregnancy, and intranasal oxygen should be considered if there are any signs of respiratory distress, increased effort, or anemia.

### How to Formulate a Diagnostic Plan

Baseline assessment should include complete bloodwork, including measurement of blood lactate and triglycerides. Abdominocentesis must be ultrasound guided to prevent uterine trauma. Normal ranges for hematologic and peritoneal fluid variables are the same in pregnant and nongravid mares (Van Hoogmoed et al. 1996; Mariella et al. 2014). Abdominal ultrasound should assess abdominal organs, as well as characterize fetal viability and uteroplacental health. Mammary secretions should be collected, and electrolytes measured as a marker of impending parturition (calcium +/− sodium and potassium). Vaginal examination is not routinely performed unless there is vaginal discharge.

### Emergency Treatment Guidelines Beyond Stabilization

Guidelines associated with any colic apply to these cases. If there is any concern for abdominal wall disruption, the mare should be confined, and an abdominal support bandage placed (Ross et al. 2008). Administration of low (0.5 mg/kg) doses of flunixin meglumine should be considered, because endotoxemia is negatively associated with pregnancy maintenance. Altrenogest administration to maintain pregnancy should be considered if the mare is not near term (Douglas et al. 2021). If the mare is intractably painful or in end-stage shock, a terminal caesarian section may be necessary in an attempt to save the foal.

## What Can Be Done at the Farm

Although many of these assessments can be performed in the field, the field veterinarian may not have the same level of confidence in assessing certain parameters (fetal viability) and access to bloodwork results may be delayed. These mares represent high-risk pregnancies and benefit from constant monitoring and ongoing supportive care, which can be more easily provided in a referral hospital.

## What Can be Done at the Referral Hospital

Referral hospitalization allows ready access to all diagnostic modalities and in-hospital analysis of laboratory submissions. Intravenous fluid therapy, parenteral nutrition, intranasal oxygen, and frequent monitoring are readily provided. Ready access to surgical facilities and a team of specialists is helpful when managing uterine torsion, hydrops, and high-risk pregnancies.

## Advice on How to Decide Between Options When Referral Is Time-Critical

Referral should be advised for colicky late-term pregnant mare whenever possible to optimize outcome for the mare and the foal. As with any colic patient, gastric reflux, abdominal discomfort, or cardiovascular compromise are indications for referral. If the mare is intractably painful or in end-stage shock, a terminal caesarian section may be necessary in an attempt to save the foal.

## Important Decisions During Management

### Decision for Hospital Referral vs Farm Management

Referral should be advised whenever possible. If referral is not an option, then field management will have to be attempted (see Chapter 14, Emergency Conditions of the Mare).

### Decision for Medical vs Surgical Treatment

In general, it is preferred to avoid unnecessary surgery in late-term pregnant mares; however, it is also important not to delay surgery, if indicated. General guidelines for management of gastrointestinal lesions are analogous to colic in non-pregnant horses. Decision making for uterine torsion, hydrops, periparturient hemorrhage, and abdominal wall disruption is described in a later chapter (see Chapter 14, Emergency Conditions of the Mare).

### How to Manage Important Complications

The most important complication would be fetal death and abortion. While this is not easily prevented, strategies to prevent endotoxemia, hypoxemia, and hypovolemia should be instituted. Altrenogest administration may be useful in mares that are not near term (Douglas et al. 2021).

### Estimating Prognosis

Prognosis depends on the underlying problem. In general, prognosis for pregnant mares following treatment of gastrointestinal lesions is similar to nonpregnant horses with the exception of mares in late gestation (Douglas et al. 2021). Mares >320 day gestation have a poorer prognosis for survival after uterine torsion, as do mares with tachycardia, and the same may apply broadly to surgical management of gastrointestinal lesions of late-term mares (Chaney et al. 2007). Prognosis for uterine torsion, hydrops, periparturient hemorrhage, and abdominal wall disruption is described in Chapter 14, Emergency Conditions of the Mare. Prognosis for a successful pregnancy is also dependent on the underlying problem but is more guarded in late-term pregnancies than in mid-gestation pregnancy (Douglas et al. 2021).

### Decision for Euthanasia

This is similar to criteria for other colic problems in nonpregnant horses. Abdominal wall disruptions warrant euthanasia if complete or associated with intractable pain or severe shock (Ross et al. 2008; Sprayberry and Lu 2021). Uterine rupture in the late-term pregnant mare, severe hemorrhagic shock from rupture of uterine vessels, or gastrointestinal rupture would also be grounds for euthanasia. Terminal caesarian section may be performed in an attempt to save the foal, although the owner should be advised of cost and prognosis of treating premature neonatal foals.

# Postoperative Colic Problems

## Clinical Signs

Clinical signs are abdominal pain, and special consideration should be given to any changes associated with surgical incisions.

## Triage Over the Phone

Initial phone triage is analogous to any colic problem, with added attention to the type of surgery performed, when it was performed, and any medications the horse is receiving. Postoperative colic is a common complication following colic surgery (French et al. 2002). Any abdominal surgery could be at risk for adhesion formation, and general anesthesia, confinement, and NSAID administration are classically associated with cecal impactions (Aitken et al. 2014). Gastric ulcers or kidney injury can occur following any surgery. Dysbiosis is a consideration with any horse receiving antimicrobial therapy. As with any colic, these cases should be seen without delay, and if the field veterinarian cannot attend to the case quickly, it is prudent to refer for further assessment, ideally to the hospital that performed the surgery.

## Triage at the Farm

### History

If history of surgery not already known or obtained, this information should be determined during history taking. Any medication history and exercise restrictions should be reviewed. Postoperative concerns identified during hospitalization or following discharge should be identified.

### Examination

The colic examination is appropriate for these scenarios. The veterinarian should also pay attention to the patency or any thickening of the jugular veins, evidence of laminitis, and assess surgical incisions for signs of pain, swelling, or dehiscence.

## Emergency Triage Steps

### Patient Stabilization

Patient stabilization is similar to any colic patient. If there is any concern for dehiscence of abdominal incisions, an abdominal bandage should be applied as soon as possible (Hann et al. 2021).

### How to Formulate a Diagnostic Plan

The colic workup will identify specific concerns (fever, gastric reflux, intestinal distension or displacement, laminitis) that will help prioritize subsequent diagnostic tests. Diagnostic workup is similar to any colic problem, with the exception that abdominal ultrasound is especially important to try to characterize the colic problem and assess the integrity of the abdominal incision.

### Emergency Treatment Guidelines Beyond Stabilization

If there is any concern for dehiscence of abdominal incisions, an abdominal bandage should be applied as soon as possible (Hann et al. 2021).

## What Can Be Done at the Farm

This is comparable to any colic problem.

## What Can Be Done at the Referral Hospital

Referral allows for more complete characterization of the colic problem to determine if it is a new problem, recurrence of the previous problem, a complication associated with previous surgery (adhesions, stricture, septic peritonitis) or medications (gastric ulcers, kidney injury). Early referral may allow for successful medical management of certain problems (obstruction caused by stricture or adhesions), which may become refractory to conservative treatment if referral is delayed.

## Advice on How to Decide Between Options When Referral Is Time-Critical

This is similar to any colic problem. Severely compromised or painful horses or horses with dehiscence of abdominal incisions should be referred without delay.

## Important Decisions During Management

### Decision for Hospital Referral vs Farm Management

This decision is similar to any colic problem, with the exception that referral should be pursued, if at all possible, due to the additional possibilities of surgery-related complications. It is preferable to refer to the hospital that performed the surgery for completeness of care.

### Decision for Medical vs Surgical Treatment

In general, this decision process is the same as for any colic. Differences would be that cecal impactions should be prioritized for surgery. Recurrent colics may warrant earlier surgical intervention, and recurrent displacements or volvulus warrant additional surgical procedures (colopexy, resection, or nephrosplenic space ablation [NSEs only]) to prevent additional recurrences. Complete incisional dehiscence requires immediate surgical repair (Hann et al. 2021).

#### How to Manage Important Complications

Certain postoperative colic problems, such as adhesions, intestinal stricture, and recurrent displacements, can be manageable with feeding management (frequent feeding of low bulk feeds).

#### Estimating Prognosis

Prognosis depends on the underlying problem.

#### Decision for Euthanasia

Horses with evisceration through an incisional dehiscence, particularly if the intestine is traumatized or contaminated, are candidates for immediate euthanasia. Other decisions for euthanasia would be similar for other colic problems.

## Peritonitis

### Clinical Signs

Clinical signs for peritonitis will vary on the underlying cause. Peritonitis cases associated with gastrointestinal rupture or leakage are typically associated with severe systemic inflammatory response syndrome (SIRS) and progressing to septic shock (fever or hypothermia, tachycardia, tachypnea, altered mucous membranes, sweating). Peritonitis of other causes is more likely to have obtundation, mild colic signs, and less severe systemic derangements.

### Triage Over the Phone

A history of colic, followed by cessation of pain, and then progression to signs of septic shock (sweating, shaking, obtundation) would be concerning for gastrointestinal rupture. A history of recent abdominal trauma, castration, abdominal surgery, foaling, or breeding, in association with fever, obtundation, inappetence, or mild colic would prompt consideration of peritonitis as a differential diagnosis.

### Triage at the Farm

#### History

If not identified as part of initial phone triage, historical features mentioned above are important to determine. Other considerations would be history of *Corynebacterium pseudotuberculosis* or *Streptococcus equi* subsp. *equi* on the premises (Arndt et al. 2021).

#### Examination

All aspects of the colic examination are relevant for evaluation of peritonitis. Presence of a fever should warrant consideration of peritonitis but does not rule it in or out. Abdominal palpation per rectum may detect a gritty texture to serosal surfaces or collapse of the rectum around the arm and sensation of emptiness in the abdomen in situations of gastrointestinal rupture. Severe clinical derangements consistent with septic shock should warrant concern for gastrointestinal rupture. A vaginal examination should be performed if history of recent breeding or foaling.

### Emergency Triage Steps

#### Patient Stabilization

Patients with a heart rate greater than 80 beats/min or signs of cardiovascular shock will need cardiovascular support (IV fluid therapy). Gastric decompression should be performed in any painful or tachycardic patient but does not rule out presence of gastric rupture.

### How to Formulate a Diagnostic Plan

While there is value to CBC, serum biochemistry analysis, blood L-lactate, and SAA, the essential diagnostic test for peritonitis is abdominocentesis and collection of peritoneal fluid (Henderson et al. 2008; Odelros et al. 2019; Arndt et al. 2021). If peritonitis is diagnosed grossly (altered color, turbid fluid), then a red top tube should be collected for culture and sensitivity, in addition to samples for cytology. Diagnostic imaging (abdominal radiographs and ultrasound) is helpful to identify potential causes.

### Emergency Treatment Guidelines Beyond Stabilization

If peritonitis is diagnosed or suspected, a minimum of systemic antimicrobial therapy should be instituted immediately (typically penicillin and gentamicin until culture results obtained). Supportive intravenous fluid therapy is helpful to improve patient hydration and overall condition. Surgical exploration and management is indicated in cases with abdominal trauma, recent abdominal surgery, uterine tear, and selected other cases (penetrating wire foreign bodies, focal intestinal lesions or neoplasia). Abdominal lavage should be considered in cases of post-surgical peritonitis or notable peritoneal effusion.

## What Can Be Done at the Farm

Emergency support (IV fluid therapy and gastric decompression) can be provided at farm, as well as the initial colic examination. Although abdominocentesis and digital abdominal ultrasonography can be performed on the farm, those diagnostics are usually deferred to the referral hospital. Antimicrobial therapy can be initiated, although it is unlikely that the diagnosis is evident at the farm, and it may affect yield of subsequent peritoneal fluid culture.

## What Can Be Done at the Referral Hospital

If not already performed at the farm, submission of CBC, serum biochemistry, blood L-lactate, +/− SAA, and peritoneal fluid cytology and culture should be performed (Odelros et al. 2019; Arndt et al. 2021). If gastrointestinal rupture is suspected, ultrasound-guided abdominocentesis should be performed to rule out possibility of enterocentesis. Antimicrobial therapy should be initiated, and intravenous fluid therapy considered. If history of recent breeding or foaling, a vaginal examination should be performed. Abdominal ultrasound is warranted in all cases (including transrectal ultrasound assessment of female reproductive tract of recently foaled or bred mares) (Arndt et al. 2021). Abdominal radiographs should be considered, if available (Arndt et al. 2021). Exploratory surgery should be considered in selected cases (post-abdominal surgery peritonitis, penetrating foreign bodies, focal gastrointestinal or abdominal lesions).

## Advice on How to Decide Between Options When Referral Is Time-Critical

Gastric decompression should be performed in all cases. If administration of IV fluids will not delay transport to a referral hospital, then cardiovascular support should be provided in the field. If there is a penetrating abdominal wound, an abdominal bandage should be placed prior to transport to cover the wound to prevent or contain evisceration (see Chapter 7, Penetrating Abdominal Injury).

## Important Decisions During Management

### Decision for Hospital Referral vs Farm Management

If peritonitis is identified or suspected, or if colic or fever is present in any horse following recent castration, abdominal surgery, breeding or foaling, referral should be sought. Any horse with inappetence, fever, or colic that does not resolve with supportive care should be referred for further evaluation, including consideration of peritonitis.

### Decision for Medical vs Surgical Treatment

Medical treatment is the mainstay of most peritonitis cases (Henderson et al. 2008; Odelros et al. 2019; Arndt et al. 2021). Surgical treatment should be considered in any peritonitis case with uterine tear, penetrating full-thickness abdominal trauma, penetrating intestinal foreign bodies, intestinal diverticula, intestinal infarction, or recent abdominal surgery. In general, surgical treatment is more likely in patients with abdominal pain, abnormal or decreasing borborygmi, abnormal or absent feces, presence of gastric reflux, and red peritoneal fluid (Southwood and Russell 2007).

### How to Manage Important Complications

The most important complication associated with peritonitis would be intestinal adhesions, but this appears uncommon in medically managed peritonitis. Adhesions would be best prevented by lavage (via surgery or abdominal drain). Other potential complications include laminitis or antimicrobial associated colitis (consideration of digital cryotherapy and support and enteral administration of pre- or probiotics or DTO-smectite, respectively).

### Estimating Prognosis

Peritonitis associated with gastrointestinal rupture or leakage is grave (Pratt et al. 2003). Prognosis for other cases of peritonitis varies with cases (very good for idiopathic or Actinobacillus peritonitis; fair for Corynebacterium pseudotuberculosis peritonitis or reproductive trauma; guarded for penetrating trauma or intestinal foreign bodies or recent abdominal surgery) (Henderson et al. 2008; Odelros et al. 2019; Arndt et al. 2021).

### Decision for Euthanasia

Euthanasia is indicated for cases of gastrointestinal rupture or leakage, which is typically supported by signs of septic shock and may require surgical exploration to confirm (Pratt et al. 2003). Other potential indications for euthanasia would be non-resolution of signs, development of complications (unmanageable adhesions, severe laminitis or colitis), or unresolvable lesions (neoplasia, inaccessible penetrating foreign bodies).

# Acute Diarrhea

## Introduction

Acute diarrhea can be a life-threatening condition in the horse. Prompt identification of a diagnosis (or suspected diagnosis) of colitis is essential to allow for early intervention, even if a causative agent is not identified at the start of therapy. This section will focus on the general identification, triage, and management of acute diarrhea in adult horses regardless of cause. Information will be presented regarding the most common infectious and non-infectious causes of diarrhea.

## Pathophysiology

Colitis, or primary inflammation of the large intestine, is the most common reason for acute diarrhea in adult horses and will be the focus of this section. Diarrhea (increased fecal water content) secondary to colitis can be due to hypersecretion, increased intestinal permeability, malabsorption, abnormal intestinal motility, or a combination of these. There is a significant difference in the fecal and intestinal microbiome between horses with diarrhea and normal horses, supporting a link between dysbiosis (disturbance of the normal gut flora) and diarrhea (Costa et al. 2012; Rodriguez et al. 2015; Arroyo et al. 2020). Due to the overlap in pathophysiologic mechanisms and clinical signs amongst causes of diarrhea a definitive cause is often not identified, even on post-mortem evaluation (Mendonca et al. 2021). Tables 10.3 and 10.4 summarize the most common causes of acute diarrhea in adult horses. Table 10.5 lists the recommended tests for the diagnosis of infectious causes of acute colitis.

## Evaluation of the Horse with Diarrhea

### Goals

The primary goal of evaluation of acute diarrhea is determining what degree of hydration and circulatory support is needed, which will often dictate whether management in the field or the hospital is recommended. Prevention of complications related to acute colitis is of extreme importance when managing these cases. The diagnosis of a specific etiologic agent often comes secondary to initial stabilization, since treatment of acute diarrhea is relatively consistent regardless of cause.

### History

A thorough history can provide valuable clues to the cause of the diarrhea while waiting for results of diagnostic testing. Collection of historical information should not delay initial stabilization of the patient. Pertinent questions could include:

- Duration of diarrhea, estimate of frequency and volume, description of consistency.
- Any signs of colic or discomfort, and if so severity of signs.
- Any recent fevers.

**Table 10.3** Key features of the main infectious causes of acute colitis in adult horses.

| Cause | Pertinent historical or patient factors | Pathogenesis, transmission | Clinical features | Specific treatment |
|---|---|---|---|---|
| **Infectious** | | | | |
| *Salmonella enterica* ss *enterica* (serovars Typhimurium, Newport, others)<br>Feary and Hassel (2006), Sanchez (2018), and Uzal (2021) | History of stress (colic, hospitalization, surgery) or antibiotic therapy<br>Warmer weather<br>Older horses more susceptible | Fecal–oral route (contaminated feed, water, surfaces, equipment, caretakers)<br>Asymptomatic shedders<br>Shed intermittently in feces | Four syndromes<br>1) Inapparent infection (+/− shedding)<br>2) Depression, fever, anorexia, neutropenia, no diarrhea<br>3) Severe, acute enterocolitis with fever, diarrhea, colic<br>4) Septicemia (foals) | Antibiotics do not improve outcome or decrease shedding<br>If used recommend enrofloxacin or aminoglycosides (less resistance, narrow spectrum) |
| *Clostridium difficile*<br>Baverud et al. (2003), Diab (2013), Feary and Hassel (2006), Jones (2000), Lawler (2008), and Weese et al. (2001) | History of antimicrobial use or stress (surgery, transport, hospitalization) | Spore-forming, endogenous or exogenous sources<br>Healthy foals likely source in environment of breeding farms<br>Pathogenesis due to toxins – toxin A (TcdA) and toxin B (TcdB)<br>Antibiotic-associated and nosocomial diarrhea | Moderate to severe acute fulminant enterocolitis with diarrhea, colic<br>Higher mortality than other causes of acute colitis | Metronidazole if confirmed and until fecal test negative<br>DTO-smectite |
| *Clostridium perfringens*<br>Feary and Hassel (2006), Jones (2000), and Lawler (2008) | More common in foals than adults<br>History of antimicrobial use or stress (surgery, transport, hospitalization) | Spore-forming, endogenous or exogenous sources<br>Type A most common in adults<br>Pathogenesis due to toxins – Type A has alpha toxin and beta2 toxin, enterotoxin unknown significance | Moderate to severe acute enterocolitis with diarrhea, colic<br>Possible cause of anterior enteritis/ duodenitis-proximal jejunitis (DPJ) | Metronidazole if confirmed and until fecal test negative<br>DTO-smectite |
| Potomac Horse Fever (*Neorickettsia* spp.)<br>Bertin (2013), Dutta et al. (1998), Feary and Hassel (2006), Madigan (2000), and Uzal (2021) | Warmer weather (peak incidence July and August)<br>Horses grazing near water or with light source over water bucket | Oral via ingestion of freshwater snails and aquatic insects (intermediate hosts) containing infected trematode<br>Usually sporadic, can be outbreaks | Typhlocolitis with fever (up to 107 °F), mild to severe diarrhea (60% of cases), colic<br>Laminitis (up to 40% of cases, often all 4 ft)<br>Abortion several months after colitis (fetal infection 90–250 day gestation) | Oxytetracycline for 3–5 days<br>Vaccination minimal protection (multiple species/ strains and poor host antibody response) |
| Equine Coronavirus<br>Berryhill (2019), Pusterla et al. (2016), and Uzal (2021) | Colder weather<br>Horses >5 years old<br>Possibly more severe disease in miniature horses | Fecal–oral route<br>Outbreaks common (riding, racing, show horses)<br>Asymptomatic infection and shedding occurs<br>Fecal shedding 3–25 days after disease | Enterocolitis with fever, colic, anorexia (diarrhea uncommon)<br>High mortality, low mortality<br>Increased mortality with intestinal hyperammonemia-associated encephalopathy | Lactulose if encephalopathy |

**Table 10.4** Key features of the main non-infectious causes of acute colitis in adult horses.

| Cause | Pertinent historical or patient factors | Pathogenesis, transmission | Clinical features | Specific treatment |
|---|---|---|---|---|
| Non-infectious | | | | |
| Antimicrobial-associated<br>Arnold (2021), and Khusro (2021) | History of recent antimicrobial administration | Can occur with any antibiotic reported with sulfonamides, ampicillin/amoxicillin, ceftiofur, macrolides, enrofloxacin, tetracyclines, aminoglycosides<br>*C. difficile* often isolated | Enterocolitis with fever and diarrhea<br>Can cause fulminant colitis with sudden death | Stop antibiotic therapy |
| Nonsteroidal anti-inflammatory drug related<br>Cohen (1995) and Davis (2017) | History of recent NSAID administration even at appropriate doses: phenylbutazone, flunixin, meloxicam<br>NSAID administration to anorexic or dehydrated horses increases risk | Prostaglandin inhibition related to drug mechanism of action | Right dorsal colon (RDC) most often affected<br>Necrotizing enterocolitis<br>Severe hypoalbuminemia is common, +/− diarrhea, colic, anorexia<br>Stricture of RDC a possible complication | Remove NSAID therapy<br>Misoprostol<br>Limit roughage intake until protein normal (complete pelleted diet) |
| Cyathostomiasis (small strongyle infestation)<br>Lyons (2000) and Feary and Hassel (2006) | Recent treatment with adulticidal anthelmintics<br>Horses 1–6 years old<br>Late winter/spring<br>Can occur in horses on routine deworming programs | Emergence of encysted larvae from intestine cause of acute diarrhea<br>Fecal egg count often normal (larval stage causes disease) | Chronic diarrhea, weight loss and ill thrift, hypoproteinemia or acute severe typhlocolitis possible<br>High mortality in severe cases | Anthelmintics (moxidectin)<br>Corticosteroids |
| Cantharidin (blister beetle) toxicity<br>Schmitz (1989) and Qualls (2013) | Alfalfa hay feeding | Cantharidin-containing blister beetles in feed<br>Toxic effects include GI, renal, cardiac<br>Demonstration of toxin in urine or stomach contents<br>Severity of signs depends on amount ingested (very low toxic dose) | Colic, anorexia, depression, tachycardia, fever, oral irritation/ulcers, pollakiuria or straining to urinate, synchronous diaphragmatic flutter<br>Sudden death possible<br>Hypocalcemia, hypomagnesemia, azotemia, hematuria, isosthenuria, elevated CK<br>High morbidity and mortality | Gastric lavage<br>Activated charcoal<br>DTO smectite<br>+/− Mineral oil (worse outcome in rat studies)<br>Calcium and electrolyte supplementation |

- Recent medication administration (particularly NSAIDs or antimicrobials).
- Current diet and any changes recently.
- Current turnout and housing scenario (any access to pond or river in the field, any light sources directly over water buckets/troughs, does the horse get turnout on sand or dirt, etc.).
- Recent history of stressful event (transport, hospitalization, etc.).
- Any other horses affected.
- Vaccination and deworming history.
- Reproductive status.
- Concurrent or pre-existing diseases.

#### Triage Over the Phone

The most important aspect of initial contact with the owner regarding acute diarrhea is to determine severity of the horse's overall clinical condition. Horses that are quiet to dull, not eating or drinking, or showing signs of colic, will likely require more stabilization and intervention. Commonly, horses with colitis will not have diarrhea initially in the course of the disease, and therefore the presenting complaint can be lethargy or decreased appetite with or without a fever. In these cases, history, physical examination, and initial bloodwork are critical for developing a working diagnosis of colitis.

#### Triage at the Farm

A thorough physical examination is warranted, with particular attention to vital signs looking for tachycardia (which could indicate pain or hypovolemia) or fever. Gastrointestinal borborygmi may be increased, decreased, or absent; fluidy and hypermotile gut sounds should raise the index of suspicion for colitis. Evidence of hypovolemia or hypovolemic shock can be identified as cool extremities, dark or tacky mucous membranes, prolonged capillary refill time, slow jugular refill, or weak peripheral pulses. Skin tent is unreliable for assessing hydration status in adult horses.

Clinical signs of SIRS, a sequela of endotoxemia secondary to acute colitis, include tachycardia, tachypnea, fever, injected or toxic mucous membranes, and fast capillary refill time. Horses may not pass diarrhea during examination, but fecal staining can be seen on the tail or hind legs. Signs of acute laminitis include elevated digital pulses, heat when touching the hoof wall, or evidence of foot soreness.

In a horse in which no diarrhea is observed, a suspicion for possible colitis can be made with one or more of the following: historical or active fever, lethargy, decreased appetite, hypermotile gastrointestinal sounds, and signs of hypovolemia or systemic inflammation.

## Emergency Triage Steps

### Patient Stabilization

Supportive care in the absence of a definitive diagnosis is essential in cases of acute colitis. Evidence of hypovolemia or hypovolemic shock should be managed with intravenous fluid therapy prior to other interventions. Enteral fluids are appropriate for correcting hypovolemia if the volume of diarrhea is small, or the level of hypovolemia appears mild; intravenous fluids are strongly recommended in more severe cases.

If signs of colic are present or the patient has an elevated heart rate above 60 bpm, nasogastric intubation should be performed to assess for gastric reflux due to ileus or concurrent enteritis. If analgesics are needed, caution should be used with NSAID administration, as the risk of nephrotoxicity from NSAIDs is increased in dehydrated patients. Another option for short-term analgesia in a colicky patient with acute colitis is butorphanol, 0.01–0.06 mg/kg IV or IM (5–30 mg in an average sized horse). Note that the analgesic dose of butorphanol is much higher than that used for sedation alone. Alpha-2 agonists (xylazine 0.2–0.6 mg/kg IV, detomidine 0.004–0.01 mg/kg IV) can be used for sedation and analgesia as needed.

## How to Formulate a Diagnostic Plan

Hematologic and biochemical analysis is used to assess overall systemic status, formulate a treatment plan, and provide prognostic information. Measurement of packed cell volume, total protein, and L-lactate provide information regarding hydration, perfusion, and degree of protein loss via the intestine. A CBC will give evidence of SIRS or endotoxemia, with leukopenia, neutropenia +/− degenerative left shift a common finding in acute colitis. Serum biochemistry can support the diagnosis with hyponatremia, hypochloremia, metabolic acidosis, and hypokalemia or hypocalcemia if inappetence is present. Evaluation of creatinine is key for determining safety of NSAID administration. Acute-phase proteins (fibrinogen, SAA) are unlikely to change the treatment plan but can be used for monitoring over the course of treatment. SAA has been shown to be higher in horses with colitis (Vandenplas et al. 2005; Westerman et al. 2015; Minamijima et al. 2020).

Abdominal palpation per rectum and nasogastric intubation can be useful in cases of diarrhea where colic is also present, to assess for possible primary disease processes causing a secondary diarrhea (such as small colon obstruction/impaction) or complications related to a primary colitis (gastric reflux, colonic distension). Point-of-care abdominal ultrasound can

**Table 10.5** Recommended tests for antemortem diagnosis of infectious causes of acute colitis in adult horses.

| Etiologic agent | Sample type | Diagnostic test | Comments |
|---|---|---|---|
| *Salmonella* spp.<br>Cohen and Woods (1999), Feary and Hassel (2006, Kurkowski (2002), and Pusterla et al. (2010) | Feces, rectal swab, rectal mucosal biopsy<br>Feces, rectal mucosal biopsy | PCR<br>Culture | Highly sensitive and specific; rapid turnaround; serial samples needed (3 samples, 12–24 hours apart)<br>Less sensitive; slower turnaround; provides isolate and susceptibility information; serial samples needed (5 samples, 12–24 hours apart) |
| *Clostridium difficile*<br>Diab (2013), Feary and Hassel (2006, Jones (2000), and Uzal (2021) | Feces<br>Feces | Toxin (TcdA and TcdB) PCR<br>Toxin A/B II ELISA | Highly sensitive; rapid turnaround; possible false positives if asymptomatic carrier<br>Moderate sensitivity; variable performance based on lab |
| *Clostridium perfringens*<br>Feary and Hassel (2006, Jones (2000), and Uzal (2021) | Feces | PCR<br>Toxin ELISA | Highly sensitive; rapid turnaround<br>Only available for enterotoxin which is found in some healthy horses |
| Potomac Horse Fever (*Neorickettsia* spp.)<br>Feary and Hassel (2006) and Shaw and Stampfli (2018) | Feces + EDTA whole blood | PCR | Always submit both samples; blood detection more sensitive early in disease; feces positive later |
| Equine Coronavirus<br>Pusterla et al. (2016) | Feces | PCR | May be negative at first test and positive if retest 24–48 hours later; fecal viral load higher in non-survivors |

identify thickening of colonic or cecal walls or fluid ingesta within the large intestine. Abdominocentesis can be used to diagnose septic peritonitis, which is a less common cause of acute diarrhea.

Definitive diagnosis of infectious causes of acute colitis is dependent on laboratory testing, using feces or whole blood depending on the disease (Table 10.5). Submission of feces and EDTA whole blood for adult diarrhea panels to veterinary diagnostic laboratories is the most comprehensive diagnostic method in cases of acute diarrhea.

## What Can Be Done at the Farm

Cases in which the diarrhea is low volume and the patient has a good appetite and is drinking, can be managed at the farm with enteral fluid support and anti-diarrheal therapies. Administration of continuous IV fluids at the farm is not recommended in colitis cases, both due to the large fluid volumes required as well as the high risk of IV catheter-related complications (thrombophlebitis) in these patients. Acute colitis in horses is a rapidly progressive and potentially fatal condition, so referral to a hospital is indicated in most cases.

## What Can Be Done at the Referral Hospital

Intensive IV fluid therapy, frequent monitoring of hematologic and biochemical parameters, and prevention of complications such as laminitis with continuous distal limb cryotherapy are more easily accomplished in a hospital setting. These cases are extremely dynamic, and frequent monitoring and adjustment of therapies in response to changes in patient status are crucial. Additionally, horses with acute diarrhea should be effectively isolated from other horses for biosecurity purposes, something that may be difficult to achieve on farm.

## Advice on How to Decide Between Options When Referral Is Time Critical

Referral is indicated when patients have signs of hypovolemic shock, SIRS, or endotoxemia. Patients who are anorectic will benefit from hospitalization to allow for either enteral or intravenous caloric supplementation.

## Treatment Recommendations

### Fluid Support

Adult horses with low-volume diarrhea do not necessarily require additional fluid support if hydration parameters are appropriate and they are willing to eat and drink. Enteral fluids via nasogastric intubation are a viable option for fluid support if mild-to-moderate dehydration is present without severe loss of fluids from diarrhea. Maintenance fluid needs (approximately 60 mL/kg/day) can be met via enteral fluids alone, divided into four to five administrations in a 24-hour period. IV crystalloid fluid therapy is indicated for any patient with moderate-to-severe levels of dehydration as indicated on clinical exam or baseline hematology, or for any patient that has profuse diarrhea. Rates of anywhere up to three to four times maintenance may be needed to maintain hydration and perfusion, with bolus administration (20–30 mL/kg) indicated in the acute phase to replace previous fluid losses. Any animal with hyporexia or anorexia should be supplemented with fluids, regardless of clinical status at the time of examination, as these patients are likely to become dehydrated. Rates of fluid administration should be periodically adjusted to maintain hydration without overloading of fluids; this is based on monitoring of PCV, total solids, L-lactate, and heart rate.

Patients with marked hypoproteinemia (total solids less than 4.0 g/dL when rehydrated), or who have a persistently elevated PCV, L-lactate, or heart rate despite fluid therapy, may benefit from colloidal support. The protein-losing enteropathy that occurs with acute diarrhea potentiates loss of intravascular fluid into the extravascular space due to decreased oncotic pressure. Hydroxyethyl starch (HES), a synthetic colloid, has been shown to improve colloid oncotic pressure in hypoproteinemic horses, and is given at a dose of 5–10 mL/kg once in a 24-hour period, at a rate of 0.5–1 L/h (Jones et al. 2001). Side effects of HES in humans and small animal include acute renal injury and coagulopathies, and although these side effects have not been observed in horses, monitoring of creatinine and urine specific gravity is indicated (Schusser et al. 2007). The use of plasma transfusion for colloidal support is often not feasible in adult horses, as the volume of plasma needed to cause a significant improvement in protein levels is financially limiting.

### Adsorbents

Di-tri-octahedral (DTO) smectite (available commercially in powder or paste form for horses) is a natural clay product that decreases fecal water content and has been shown to bind clostridial and other bacterial toxins *in vitro* (Weese et al. 2003, Lawler et al. 2008). Additionally, DTO smectite has been shown to have no effect on the action of metronidazole in horses (Weese et al. 2003). It is best administered to adult acute colitis cases in powder form, at a loading dose of 2–3 pounds in 6 L of water for a 500 kg horse, followed by 1–2 pounds in 3–6 L of water three to four times daily until diarrhea resolves.

### Anti-Endotoxic Therapies

Flunixin meglumine at a low dose (0.25 mg/kg IV q8 hours) is used for anti-endotoxic effects (Werners et al. 2010). Although the overall data for its clinically efficacy is sparse, its use is reasonable in patients with appropriate kidney function. Higher doses of flunixin (0.5–1.1 mg/kg IV q12 hours) also provide anti-endotoxic effects with the addition of anti-inflammatory and analgesic effects. Some evidence suggests that the combination of NSAIDs and the phosphodiesterase inhibitor pentoxifylline (7.5 mg/kg PO q8–12 hours) provides more profound anti-endotoxic effects than flunixin meglumine alone (Werners 2017).

Plasma hyperimmunized against various equine enteric pathogens (*Escherichia coli*, *Salmonella* spp., *Clostridium* spp.) can be administered for anti-endotoxic effects via IgG-mediated complement activation and binding of Gram-negative bacteria, with recommended dosing of approximately 2 L per adult horse (Werners 2017). The data regarding efficacy of plasma administration in equine endotoxemia is conflicting, with *ex vivo* models showing more promising results than *in vivo* in most studies (Wells et al. 1987; Forbes et al. 2012). While some data shows no difference in survival in cases of acute colitis receiving plasma transfusion (Atherton et al. 2011), several retrospective studies have found an association between plasma administration and decreased survival (Arroyo et al. 2019; Sage et al. 2021). The retrospective nature of these studies means that this association with decreased survival is potentially due to case selection, if the sickest patients are more likely to be given additional therapies such as plasma. In summary, enteric hyperimmunized plasma can be utilized in cases of acute colitis, with the understanding that the data regarding its use is relatively weak.

Polymyxin B, a cyclic cationic peptide antimicrobial, binds with the lipid A portion of LPS, rendering it ineffective at triggering an immune response. It has been shown to decrease endotoxin-induced inflammatory activity as well as improve clinical parameters of endotoxemia (Barton et al. 2004; Werners et al. 2010). Although several equine studies have failed to show negative effects at standard dosing (4,000–6,000 IU/kg IV q8–12 hours), nephrotoxicity is a concern, and therefore creatinine and USG should be monitored during administration, and its use should be avoided in horses with an elevated creatinine. Its use could be considered controversial (use of an antibiotic for reasons other than treatment of a bacterial infection), which should be taken into account when deciding whether to use it as a treatment for endotoxemia.

Misoprostol, an E prostanoid receptor agonist (5 mcg/kg PO q12 hour), has been shown *in vitro* to inhibit LPS-induced cytokine production by equine neutrophils and to decrease equine neutrophil adhesion, migration, and respiratory burst (Martin et al. 2017a, b). Clinical efficacy is potentially less promising (Martin et al. 2019). Since misoprostol has useful effects for gastrointestinal mucosal healing, its use in acute colitis could be indicated for gastrointestinal healing, amelioration of protein loss, and anti-endotoxic effects. Clenbuterol hydrochloride, a beta-adrenergic agonist (0.08 mcg/kg PO once), has shown anti-inflammatory effects in horses both *in vivo* and *ex vivo,* including specifically in endotoxin challenges (Cudmore et al. 2013, 2015).

These treatments are summarized in Box 10.8.

## Antimicrobials

The use of antibiotics in cases of acute colitis is only indicated in specific scenarios. Horses in which Potomac Horse Fever (i.e., disease due to *Neorickettsia risticii* or *N. fidlayensis*) is strongly suspected or confirmed should be treated with oxytetracycline (6.6 mg/kg IV q24 hours or 5 mg/kg IV q12 hours). Horses with severe neutropenia (<1,000 neutrophils/μL) could warrant initiation of broad-spectrum antimicrobials to prevent secondary complications from decreased immune function. This decision should be based on the specific case; for instance, a horse with antibiotic-associated diarrhea may be more harmed from antibiotic treatment even when severely neutropenic. In these cases, parenteral antibiotics (potassium penicillin at 22,000 international units/kg IV q6 or procaine penicillin at 22,000 international units/kg IM q12 hours plus EITHER gentamicin at 6.6 mg/kg IV q24 OR enrofloxacin at 5 mg/kg IV q24) are preferred over enteral antibiotics due to a decreased effect on the normal gut microbiota.

Metronidazole (15 mg/kg PO q6–8 hours, or 25 mg/kg PR q6–8 hours) is only indicated in cases of clostridial colitis. The author does not recommend its use in every case of acute colitis in adult horses unless clostridial colitis is confirmed or strongly suspected, and even in these cases it may not be necessary depending on the severity of the clinical disease. Clostridial species are abundant in the gut microbiota of healthy horses (Costa et al. 2012), and giving metronidazole will contribute to dysbiosis. Additionally, there is evidence of increasing resistance of clostridial species to metronidazole (up to 43% of certain isolates in certain geographic locations), so indiscriminate use is discouraged for appropriate antimicrobial stewardship (Feary and Hassel 2006).

## Prebiotics, Probiotics, Fecal Transfaunation

Probiotics refer to live microorganisms that when fed to the host confer a positive health benefit, while prebiotics refer to compounds that induce the growth or activity of beneficial microorganisms. Significant drawbacks of currently available equine probiotics include limited scientific understanding of what organisms are best included and lack of regulatory oversight to ensure the products contain what is advertised on the label (Schoster et al. 2014; Berreta et al. 2021). Several products

**Box 10.8 Anti-endotoxin therapies**

- Flunixin meglumine (0.25 mg/kg IV q8 hours – 1.1 mg/kg q12 hours).
- Pentoxyphylline (7.5 mg/kg PO q8–12 hours).
- Hyperimmunized plasma (2 L per adult horse).
- Polymyxin B (4,000-6,000 IU/kg IVq8–12 hours).
- Misoprostal (5 mcg/kg PO q12 hours).

have been found to contain bacteria with transferrable antimicrobial-resistant genes (Baumgardner et al. 2021). One study found that commercial probiotic administration had no effect on the shedding of Salmonella or incidence of diarrhea in post-operative colic cases (Parraga et al. 1997).

*Saccharomyces boulardii* is a non-pathogenic yeast used in human medicine as an antidiarrheic agent, particularly for *Clostridiodes difficile* diarrhea. A study in horses found that *S. boulardii* decreased the severity and duration of diarrhea in horses with acute enterocolitis, although it only transiently colonized the gastrointestinal tract during the period of administration (Desrochers et al. 2005). A separate study in horses with antimicrobial-associated diarrhea had no improvement in clinical outcome or resolution of signs when given *S. boulardii* (Boyle et al. 2013). Recommended dosage is 50 billion CFU (1,250 mg) per average-sized horse PO q12 hours.

Fecal microbial transplant (FMT) involves the administration of fecal material from a healthy donor to a patient with gastrointestinal upset. A recent study of clinical colitis cases showed a greater reduction in diarrhea score and faster clinical improvement in FMT recipients as compared to cases not treated with FMT (McKinney et al. 2021). A handful of other studies have also shown improvement in clinical disease with FMT administration, although there seems to be wide variation in response between individual horses. Definitive donor criteria are lacking, but current recommendations suggest selecting an adult donor who has no history of gastrointestinal disease or recent medication administration (within the last month, especially antimicrobials or NSAIDs), normal fecal consistency, and is negative for *Salmonella* and *Clostridial* species. A suggested protocol is to collect a fresh pile of feces from the donor (either via abdominal palpation per rectum or passed within the last several hours), mix with several liters of warm water, pass through a strainer, and give via nasogastric intubation. This can be performed once daily for three to seven days. Some resources recommend pre-treating with the proton pump inhibitor omeprazole to avoid acid destruction of the FMT. However, this would take several days of pre-treatment to be effective and has not been demonstrated to be necessary.

## Additional Therapies

Digital cryotherapy (application of ice to the distal limbs) for laminitis prevention is indicated in all cases of acute colitis, particularly those with signs of SIRS/endotoxemia. A study of clinical colitis cases showed that horses treated with prophylactic digital cryotherapy had decreased risk of laminitis (10%) compared to those who were not treated with ice therapy (33%) (Kullmann et al. 2014). Icing needs to be continuous (24/7), initiated before signs of laminitis develop, and continued until the signs of systemic inflammation and endotoxemia resolve. The most effective forms of cryotherapy are those that completely cover the entire foot and distal limb (up to mid metatarsus) in ice.

Lidocaine hydrochloride is used in horses as a continuous intravenous infusion rate for analgesia and gastrointestinal motility (loading dose of 1.3 mg/kg over 15 minutes followed by CRI of 3 mg/kg/h). Additionally, *in vitro* and murine model studies have shown that lidocaine has anti-inflammatory effects. (Cook et al. 2009). For these reasons, lidocaine has potential use in cases of acute colitis in horses, although the evidence confirming its anti-inflammatory properties in vivo in horses is not definitive (Williams et al. 2010). Caution should be used in patients with severe hypoproteinemia; lidocaine is highly protein-bound and therefore these patients are at a higher risk of toxicity.

Horses with acute colitis are at increased risk of coagulopathies, which can lead to complications such as thrombophlebitis and organ dysfunction. In human critical care, administration of anti-coagulants, namely low-molecular-weight heparin, has been associated with decreased time in the intensive care unit and improvement in other outcome variables (Liu et al. 2014). A retrospective study in horses undergoing colic surgery found that horses that received low-molecular-weight heparin had a decreased incidence of laminitis (de La Rebiere de Pouyade et al. 2009). Options for anti-coagulants in horses include low-molecular-weight heparin (enoxaparin 0.35 mg/kg SQ q24 hour or dalteparin 50 units/kg SQ q12 hour for three to five days) or clopidogrel (loading dose 4 mg/kg PO once, then 2 mg/kg PO q24 hours for three to seven days). Low-molecular-weight heparin is preferred over unfractionated heparin due to decreased risk of serious hemorrhage.

## Nutritional Support

Horses with acute colitis and no complicating factors (gastric reflux, abdominal discomfort, etc.) should be allowed and encouraged to eat. It is best to avoid high starch feeds as these ferment in the colon and can potentiate acidosis. The ideal diet for cases of acute colitis is good quality alfalfa or grass hay, or complete pelleted feed (such as a senior feed). If the patient is anorectic or hyporexic, nutritional supplementation is indicated. Horses in good body condition can tolerate three to four days of anorexia, but this does not apply to all patients (such as pregnant or lactating animals, or animals at high risk of hyperlipemia or hypertriglyceridemia). Enteral nutrition is accomplished with nasogastric administration of complete feed as a slurry or Purina Well-Gel®. Horses with acute colitis best tolerate small frequent feedings. If a patient is totally anorectic for 24–48 hours, or will not tolerate enteral feeding, parenteral nutrition is indicated, initially in the form of dextrose supplementation, with transition to partial or total parenteral nutrition if anorexia persists. Addition of psyllium or psyllium-containing products to enteral nutrition protocols should be considered, as this increases short-chain fatty acid production in the equine gut which is helpful for colonic healing and function (Wachtershauser and Stein 2000; Magdesian and Bozorgmanesh 2018).

## Important Decisions During Management

### Decision for Hospital Referral vs Farm Management

Referral of any case of acute colitis for hospitalization is appropriate if the owner is able and willing since these cases are dynamic and can easily become unstable. Patients that are showing signs of SIRS/endotoxemia, dehydration, or hyporexia or anorexia should be referred, if possible, to allow for more intensive supportive care and monitoring.

### Decision for Medical vs Surgical Treatment

Any case of colitis with persistent colic should have a comprehensive workup (nasogastric intubation, abdominal palpation per rectum, abdominal ultrasound, abdominocentesis) to determine the most likely cause. Most causes of abdominal discomfort in acute colitis are not surgical in nature (i.e., ileus, enteritis, gastrointestinal cramping/spasm), and therefore medical management with analgesics is the recommended treatment. However, some cases of colitis can develop more sinister complications that cause abdominal pain, such as colonic infarction. If a patient has intractable abdominal pain and/or an abnormal abdominocentesis (i.e., serosanguinous, elevated L-lactate), infarction of the colon should be suspected, and pursuit of surgical exploration is mainly for diagnostic confirmation, as prognosis for survival is grave in these cases.

### How to Manage Complications

Laminitis has a reported incidence of 11–21% in cases of acute colitis (Staempfli et al. 1991; Cohen and Woods 1999; Kullmann et al. 2014; Luethy et al. 2021). This incidence is even higher, up to 42%, in cases of Potomac Horse Fever (Luethy et al. 2021) and is correlated with decreased survival as compared to horses that do not develop laminitis (Cohen et al 1995; Kullmann et al. 2014). If laminitis develops, methods to decrease loading on the lamellae (impression material, Soft Ride boots, etc.) should be employed. Increased analgesic administration is indicated if signs of laminitis develop, including NSAIDs (flunixin meglumine, phenylbutazone), acetaminophen (20–30 mg/kg PO q12 hour, off set from NSAID administration to increase analgesia), gabapentin (20 mg/kg PO q6–8 hours), or pregabalin (4 mg/kg PO q8 hour), and/or continuous infusions of analgesics (lidocaine, butorphanol, etc.).

Thrombophlebitis is more likely to develop in horses with acute colitis as compared to other hospitalized patients (Dolente et al. 2005). Prevention of thrombophlebitis involves use of long-term catheters made with less thrombogenic material, removal of IV catheters as soon as they are no longer in use for IV fluids or medications, and covering of the catheter insertion site with a neck wrap if needed to prevent fecal contamination. Frequent monitoring of the catheter insertion site and jugular fill is crucial for early identification. Diagnosis is made via clinical examination or ultrasonography, with ultrasound more sensitive for early identification. Treatment with anti-coagulants and/or antibiotics should be considered, with antibiotic therapy used cautiously due to the risk of worsening or return of colitis.

Horses with acute colitis are at risk of organ dysfunction or failure due to hypotension, hypovolemia, SIRS (+/− endotoxemia and sepsis), and disseminated intravascular coagulopathy (DIC). Reports of SIRS in causes of acute colitis estimate prevalence at 57–65% when reported (Johns et al. 2009; Hashimoto-Hill 2011), and one report identified that 32% of colitis cases had subclinical DIC with increased mortality in these patients (Dolente et al. 2002). Monitoring of organ function with serum chemistry, urinalysis, and cardiac troponin I can help identify organ dysfunction, although treatment of these complications when they occur is unrewarding and mainly supportive.

## Estimating Prognosis

Overall survival to discharge for horses hospitalized for acute colitis of any cause ranges from 37 to 75% (Staempfli et al. 1991; Cohen and Woods 1999; Hashimoto-Hill et al. 2011; Petersen et al. 2016; Kovac et al. 2017; Luethy et al. 2021). Data for horses managed in the field is less available, although one report found a survival rate of 66% for horses with acute diarrhea seen in ambulatory practice (Mair et al. 1990). In one study, horses with coronavirus had a higher rate of survival (100%) as compared to Salmonella (70%), Potomac Horse Fever (65.4%), or colitis of unknown cause (69.6%) (Luethy et al. 2021). A history of antibiotic administration has been shown to be associated with a worse prognosis (Cohen and Woods 1999; Kovac et al. 2017). Admission factors associated with decreased survival include tachycardia and increased hematocrit or packed cell volume (Van Duijkeren et al. 1996; Cohen and Woods 1999; Johns et al. 2009; Hashimoto-Hill et al. 2011; Kovac et al. 2017).

A lack of improvement in L-lactate within the first 6–24 hours of treatment is also associated with reduced survival (Hashimoto-Hill et al. 2011; Petersen et al. 2016). Hypoproteinemia is not consistently associated with survival (Cohen and Woods 1999; Kovac et al. 2017; Sage et al. 2021). The first few days of treatment are key in estimating prognosis; in one study 23/41 non-surviving horses died in the first 12 hours of hospitalization (Petersen et al. 2016), and delay of treatment for 24 hours or more after the start of clinical signs was significantly associated with mortality in another (Kovac et al. 2017). Geriatric horses (older than 20 years) were observed to have worse survival compared to young adults (2–12 years of age) in one study (Sage et al. 2021). Data regarding long-term prognosis is sparse, but in a population where follow up was available for 16 of the surviving horses, 14 out of 16 went back to some level of use, and 5 out of 8 racehorses resumed active racing (Staempfli et al. 1991).

## Decision for Euthanasia

Horses that do not respond favorably to treatment within three to five days have a significantly worse prognosis (Van Duijkeren et al. 1996; Kovac et al. 2017). For this reason, a lack of positive response to treatment in this time frame can be an indication for euthanasia, especially if there are financial limitations. In cases of acute colitis where abdominal exploration was elected due to persistent signs of colic, only one out of seven horses survived to discharge (Cohen and Woods 1999). The development of laminitis is associated with a worse prognosis and is a valid reason for euthanasia due to the associated increased mortality (48–57% survival rate) and decreased return to athletic function (Cohen and Woods 1999; Kullmann et al. 2014).

## Carbohydrate (Grain) Overload

### Pathophysiology

Sudden ingestion of large amounts of soluble carbohydrates (corn, barley, etc.) can cause significant disease in the horse for several reasons. Gastric impaction can occur if enough volume is consumed in an extremely short amount of time. The more likely, and more deadly, outcome is excessive fermentation of these carbohydrates within the gastrointestinal tract. The ingestion of large volumes of soluble carbohydrates overwhelms the digestive and absorptive capacity of the small intestine, causing a surge of carbohydrates to be delivered to the large intestine leading to excessive fermentation by Gram-positive lactic-acid-producing bacteria. This in turn causes a lower pH environment within the large intestine, favoring proliferation of Gram-positive bacteria and die-off of Gram-negative organisms and other normal microflora. The end outcome of this process is systemic lactic acidosis, diarrhea, acute colitis, and SIRS/endotoxemia.

### Evaluation of the Horse with Grain Overload

***Goals*** Severity of disease is dependent on volume of grain consumed and the animal's previous diet (if they are somewhat adapted to grain ingestion or not). Gastric lavage, if performed within three hours of ingestion to remove grain from the stomach, can decrease morbidity and improve outcome. This can be followed with administration of adsorbent agents (e.g., activated charcoal). In addition, prevention or management of acute colitis and endotoxemia is necessary in all cases.

***History*** Gathering of historical information is like that for acute colitis, with the addition of specific questions related to the carbohydrate exposure. These include establishing if horses could have accessed high carbohydrate feeds, amount ingested, when it was consumed, the volume consumed, and what exactly was in the product. For example, ingestion of cattle feed by horses could be detrimental from ingestion of soluble carbohydrates and other substances toxic to horses (such as ionophores).

Ingestion of moldy feed stuffs (particularly corn) can also lead to toxicity. Careful questioning of which horses/animals may have been affected is important, since sometimes multiple animals may require medical attention.

***Triage Over the Phone*** Determining the details of consumption prior to arrival is helpful for developing a treatment plan and also ensuring the necessary supplies are available (e.g., activated charcoal). Instruct the client to ensure no further access to grain is available, either for this animal or any others.

***Triage at the Farm*** Assessment of hydration status, and the presence of any clinical signs of systemic inflammation/endotoxemia is vital. Clinical signs of SIRS, a sequela of endotoxemia, include tachycardia, tachypnea, fever, injected or toxic mucus membranes, and fast capillary refill time. Evaluation for signs of acute laminitis is essential, such as elevated digital pulses, heat when touching the hoof wall, or evidence of foot soreness.

Especially if exposure to grain was recent, immediate passage of a nasogastric tube for gastric decompression and lavage is warranted. Administration of IV fluids may be necessary if the patient appears clinically dehydrated, with enteral fluid therapy avoided due to the increased risk of ileus and gastric distension.

## Emergency Triage Steps

### Patient Stabilization

Nasogastric intubation should be performed immediately to allow for gastric decompression if there is a build-up of feed or fluid. Copious gastric lavage should be continued until minimal feed is returned. This can be followed by administration of adsorbent agents such as activated charcoal or DTO-smectite.

Analgesia and control of inflammation in the form of NSAIDs (flunixin meglumine, 1.1 mg/kg IV or PO once) is indicated. Alpha-2 agonists (xylazine 0.2–0.6 mg/kg IV, detomidine 0.004–0.01 mg/kg IV) can be used for sedation and analgesia as needed, particularly if the patient is showing signs of colic.

Signs of dehydration or hypovolemic shock should trigger administration of intravenous fluid boluses to improve perfusion.

### How to Formulate a Diagnostic Plan

Hematologic and biochemical analysis will allow for evaluation of overall systemic status as well as provide information for treatment. Packed cell volume, total solids, and L-lactate can provide information on hydration and perfusion status. Complete blood count will determine if leukopenia +/− neutropenia is present, which would be suggestive of significant acute systemic inflammation. Serum biochemistry may demonstrate a systemic metabolic acidosis as evidence by a decreased pH and bicarbonate or total $CO_2$. Other electrolyte derangements may include hyponatremia and/or hypochloremia if acute colitis is imminent.

Point-of-care abdominal ultrasound can be used to assess stomach size, look for evidence of gastric rupture, and assess for evidence of colitis (thickening of the large intestine or fluidy ingesta). Abdominocentesis is indicated if gastric rupture is suspected.

### What Can Be Done at the Farm

If it can be done safely, nasogastric intubation should always be performed at the farm prior to referral. If the patient is apparently systemically stable, on farm management can be pursued, with administration of adsorbent agents followed by a small period of feed withholding then gradual refeeding. Close monitoring for signs of endotoxemia or laminitis in the days following exposure is necessary.

### What Can Be Done at the Referral Hospital

For patients who are showing signs of SIRS/endotoxemia or significant dehydration, admission to a hospital allows for administration of continuous intravenous fluids and supportive care, in addition to close monitoring. If patients have significant gastric distension, frequent nasogastric intubation for gastric lavage is more easily accomplished at the hospital.

### Advice on How to Decide Between Options When Referral Is Time-Critical

Like other cases of acute colitis, referral is indicated when patients have signs of hypovolemic shock, SIRS, or endotoxemia for intensive supportive care. The presence of gastric reflux, or any suspicion of a gastric impaction, warrants referral due to the need for intravenous fluid and caloric support.

## Treatment Recommendations

Gastric decompression and lavage should be performed using as large bore of a nasogastric tube as is safe for the size of the horse. This lavage should be continued until little to no feed material is returned. If there is concern for a gastric impaction, or suspicion that initial lavage did not return all the feed within the stomach, lavage should be repeated as needed. Depending on the length of time after ingestion of carbohydrates, gastric lavage may be unrewarding, due to the passage of the grain out of the stomach prior to evaluation.

Administration of materials to absorb toxins and metabolites from the intestines should be considered. Activated charcoal can be administered once via nasogastric tube at a dose of 0.5 kg per 500 kg horse. The efficacy of activated charcoal will decrease as the time from carbohydrate ingestion increases. If time since exposure is unknown, use is still recommended. DTO smectite, a natural clay product, binds toxins from multiple different types of enteric bacteria (Hassel et al. 2009), and is therefore useful to mitigate bacterial overgrowth in the large intestine. It is administered at a loading dose of 2–3 pounds in 6 liters of water for a 500 kg horse and should be given separate from (and several hours after) activated charcoal. Doses of 1–2 pounds in 3–6 L of water can be repeated if indicated, particularly if the patient develops diarrhea. DTO smectite is contraindicated in cases of gastric impaction or distension.

The administration of oral sodium bicarbonate (1 g/kg of baking soda via nasogastric tube) to buffer the cecal contents in horses exposed to carbohydrate overload has possible beneficial effects. It has been shown to increase cecal pH and cause a metabolic alkalosis in healthy horses (Taylor et al. 2014). The effects of a single dose lasted for 18 to 24 hours in normal horses; in clinical cases redosing once to twice daily could be considered.

Fluid support, anti-endotoxic therapies, and laminitis prevention are all key cases of carbohydrate overload. The reader is referred to the section on acute diarrhea for specific recommendations regarding these therapies.

## Important Decisions During Management

### Decision for Hospital Referral vs Farm Management

If veterinary attention is solicited shortly after grain ingestion, and the patient is overall systemically stable at the time of examination, management in the field is feasible. Patients who are already showing signs of systemic compromise or complications (dehydration, SIRS/endotoxemia, diarrhea, colic, laminitis, etc.) are best managed in a hospital setting to allow for intensive supportive care and monitoring.

### How to Manage Important Complications

Horses that experience carbohydrate overload are at a high risk of acute laminitis. Management of laminitis is covered in the discussion of acute colitis.

Acute colitis is a likely complication of grain overload, due to the disruption of normal microflora, damage to the intestinal mucosa from acidic pH, and the osmotic effect of the surge of soluble carbohydrates into the large intestine (Sanchez 2018). See the section on management of acute diarrhea for treatment and management recommendations.

Grain overload can cause acute gastric rupture, although this is less common than other causes of primary gastric rupture in horses (Todhunter et al. 1986; Dechant and Winfield 2017). Gastric decompression and lavage is key to preventing this complication, since once it occurs it carries a fatal prognosis.

### Estimating Prognosis

An improved prognosis for survival is expected in horses that ingest smaller amounts of grain, are treated by a veterinarian shortly after ingestion, and that do not develop clinical signs of endotoxemia, laminitis, or severe colitis.

## Decision for Euthanasia

Gastric rupture carries a grave prognosis, so if this condition is confirmed euthanasia is indicated. Horses that develop signs of endotoxemia or acute colitis and fail to show positive response to treatment after the first few days have a worse prognosis for survival. The development of laminitis will potentially lead to long-term unsoundness and has a decreased prognosis for return to athletic function.

### Case Example 10.1 Acute Colic in the Horse

#### Case 1

An 18-year-old Quarter Horse gelding is presented for acute colic (Figure 10.13). He was found down in the stall that morning by the owners when they went to give morning feed. The owners described he had abrasions over his face and was covered in dried sweat when they found him and had knocked his water bucket off the wall. They administered a dose of oral flunixin meglumine while waiting for your arrival and got him up to walk outside. The gelding continued to try to lie down while walking.

On your examination at the farm, you note the gelding is quiet and alert and standing quietly with full-body muscle fasciculations. The gelding has a temperature of 97.7 °F, heart rate of 76 bpm, and respiratory rate of 24 brpm. Mucous membranes are pale pink and tacky with a capillary refill time (CRT) of three to four seconds. Gastrointestinal borborygmi are absent in all quadrants. Juglar refill is prolonged and facial pulses are weak. The gelding's muzzle and distal limbs are cool to the touch.

Nasogastric intubation yields no net reflux, but you obtain a small amount of foul-smelling feed material. Abdominal palpation per rectum demonstrates a few mucus-covered fecal balls within the rectum and dry hard feces palpable in the small colon. The pelvic flexure is palpable on ventral midline with firm dry ingesta.

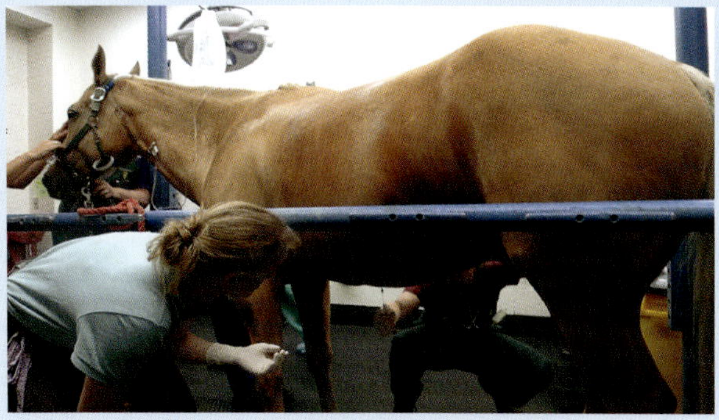

**Figure 10.13** An 18-year-old Quarter Horse gelding presented for acute colic. Immediate referral is recommended when strangulating diseases of the gastrointestinal tract are suspected. Factors to consider for referral include severity of pain, lack of response to sedation or analgesics, abnormal abdominal ultrasound and/or rectal palpation, abnormal abdominal fluid, progressive deterioration despite medical management among other clinical exam findings.

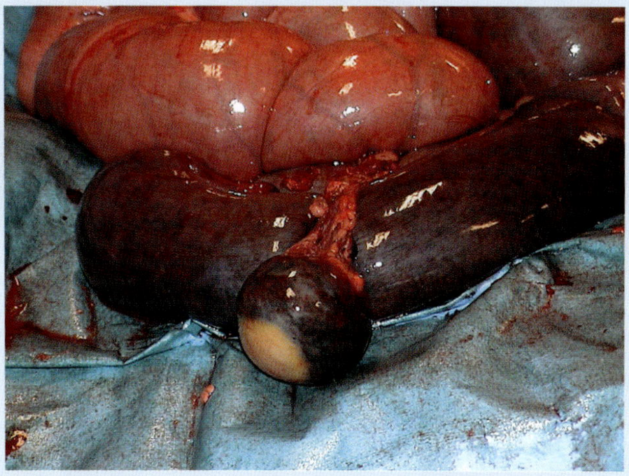

**Figure 10.14** A strangulating lipoma was found in this Quarter Horse. Approximately 10-ft of small intestine (SI) was devitalized requiring resection and anastomosis. Early referral of such problems decreases complications (such as endotoxemia, post-operative ileus, and adhesion formation) and improves outcomes.

What are your differential diagnoses based on initial examination?

The initial evaluation of this patient does not definitively point to a diagnosis. However, the combination of severe pain (history and facial abrasions suggest rolling, tachycardia, muscle fasciculations during examination) and concern for hypovolemic shock (tachycardia, tacky membranes with prolonged CRT, poor jugular refill, weak peripheral pulses and cool extremities) are highly suspicious of a strangulating intestinal lesion. Additionally, when adding in the patient's signalment (middle-age American breed gelding), a SISO (specifically strangulating lipoma) would be a top differential (Figure 10.14). The lack of distended small intestine on abdominal palpation per rectum does not rule out a SISO.

The lack of gastric reflux does not preclude a SISO, and in fact research has shown a positive correlation between lack of gastric reflux at hospital admission and the presence of a SISO. This is due to the delay in back-up of fluid to the stomach from the site of obstruction (the significant length of the horse's small intestine combined with the fact that many strangulating lesions affect the aboral jejunum and ileum).The finding of firm ingesta within the pelvic flexure can be mistaken for a pelvic flexure impaction, which if taken out of context could lead to incorrect treatment with enteral fluids. However, the suggestions of severe pain as well as concern for shock do not fit with a simple large colon impaction. More likely, the dry ingesta within the pelvic flexure is due to lack of normal delivery of intestinal fluids to the colon from the small intestine because of a primary strangulating obstruction.

What is your initial stabilization and triage plan?

Immediate referral is indicated in this case. If there is a delay waiting for transport to the referral facility, an intravenous catheter (14g or larger)) can be placed and an intravenous fluid bolus (10L of crystalloid fluids in a standard-sized adult horse) administered to help address the hypovolemic shock. Enteral fluids are *contraindicated* due to the suspicion of SISO, even though no reflux was obtained. If the patient becomes uncomfortable during examination or while waiting for transport, alpha-2 agonists and/or butorphanol can be administered for sedation and analgesia.

What is Your Plan for Management on the Farm?

This case is one that warrants immediate referral, due to the high suspicion of a strangulating lesion and the need for surgery to correct the lesion. If referral is not an option, additional diagnostics can be performed on the farm to lend support for the diagnosis of SISO. These would include transcutaneous abdominal ultrasound and abdominocentesis. The findings of distended and/or thick-walled small intestine on abdominal ultrasound (Figure 10.15) and serosanguinous abdominal fluid (Figure 10.16a,b) would support a diagnosis of SISO, and again warrant immediate referral.

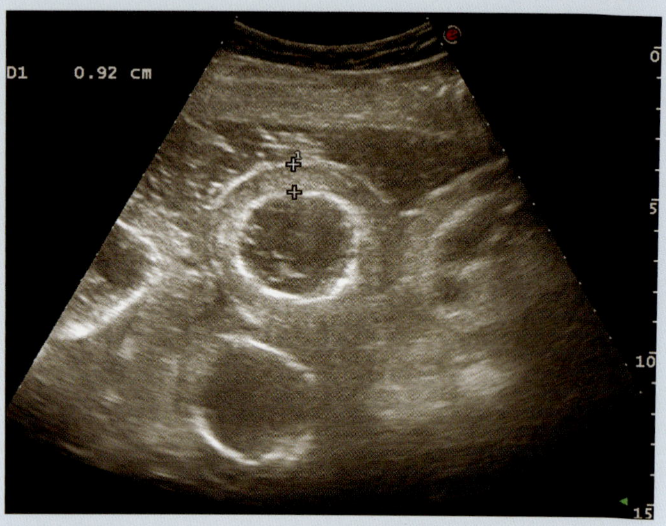


**Figure 10.15** Ultrasound examination of this patient showed multiple loops of distended SI, including the markedly thickened loops shown in this image. Normal wall thickness of the SI is approximately 3mm. Note the abnormal hyperechoic peritoneal fluid (Figure 10.16) in the background consistent with a strangulating lesion.

(a)

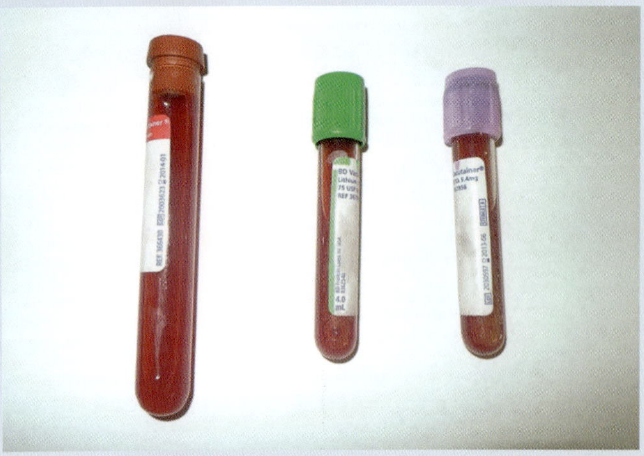

(b)

*Abnormal Abdominocentesis*

*Serosanguinous (ss)*
*– orange, red, dark, opaque, turbid*
*Increased WBC, TPP, RBC*

| | Normal | SISO | Enteritis |
|---|---|---|---|
| Color | clear, yellow | ss | turbid |
| WBC | <5,000 | 15–75,000 | 5–15,000 |
| TPP | <2.5 g/dL | 3–5 g/dL | 3–5 g/dL |
| RBC | None | Increased | None |
| Lactate | 0.7 mmol/L | 2× systemic | PFL = SL |

*PFL – peritoneal fluid lactate SL – systemic lactate*
*SISO – small intestinal strangulating obstruction*

**Figure 10.16** (a) Serosanguinous peritoneal fluid from the horse in this example. The gross changes of red-orange color, increased cloudiness and turbidity reflect the increased red blood cells, nucleated cell count, and total protein of the fluid. (b) Abnormal peritoneal fluid can result from many abdominal problems. Note the comparative peritoneal fluid parameters of SISO and enteritis diseases to normal. In addition to the serosanguinous gross appearance of peritoneal fluid of horses with strangulating lesions, the peritoneal L-lactate is often double compared to systemic values. *These are guidelines only as variability in these parameters occur among horses because of differences in diseases, time of fluid collection, amount and severity of affected intestine among other factors.*

If referral is not an option, and abdominal ultrasound and/or abdominocentesis were not confirmatory of a strangulating lesion, medical management on the farm could be attempted for a brief period (namely intravenous fluid administration, starting with a 10-L crystalloid bolus). If the patient became uncomfortable again when sedation/analgesia wears off, develops gastric reflux, or shows signs of progressive shock despite fluid therapy, then a strangulating lesion is considered to still be the most likely cause of the patient's colic. If referral is not an option, euthanasia is the humane course of action.

What are your triggers for referral?

The initial examination in this patient is suspicious enough for SISO that immediate referral is warranted. Additional findings that would strongly support SISO would include severe pain (rolling, etc.) unresponsive to sedation or analgesia, the presence of gastric reflux, serosanguinous abdominal fluid, or palpable small intestine on abdominal palpation per rectum.

***Source:*** Images courtesy of Rolfe M Radcliffe.

**Case 2**

A 10-year-old Thoroughbred mare is presented for acute colic. The owners noted she was lying down quietly in the stall that morning. When offered grain the mare was eager to eat, but as soon as she finished eating, she would lay back down again. The owners noted there was no manure in her stall from overnight.

On your examination at the farm, the mare is bright and alert and trying to eat grass next to the barn. The mare has a temperature of 99.4 °F, heart rate of 40 bpm, and a respiratory rate of 18 brpm. Mucous membranes are pink and moist with a capillary refill time of approximately two seconds. Gastrointestinal borborygmi are quiet in the dorsal quadrants and normal within the ventral quadrants. Juglar refill and peripheral pulses are normal.

Nasogastric intubation yields no net reflux and retrieves a small amount of fresh grass. Abdominal palpation per rectum yields a small amount of mucous covered feces within the rectum and dry hard feces palpable in the small colon. The pelvic flexure is palpable on ventral midline with hard firm ingesta present, extending cranial within the abdomen past the tips of your fingers. The nephrosplenic space is clear and you can palpate the caudal edge of the spleen against the body wall. The cecal band palpates normally with no cecal distension.

### What Are Your Differential Diagnoses Based on Initial Examination?

The most likely diagnosis based on the abdominal palpation per rectum is a large colon impaction. Although the impaction is present within the pelvic flexure, the fact the impacted ingesta extends further cranially than can be palpated means that more of the colon is likely impacted, and it is possible that the primary site of intraluminal impaction is at the junction of the right dorsal colon and transverse colon (which is too cranial to palpate in most full-sized horses).

A large colon displacement cannot be definitively ruled out, and colonic displacements can often occur concurrently with impactions of the large colon. However, the normal palpation of the spleen and nephrosplenic space and lack of colonic gas distension or tight mesenteric bands makes an LLD of the colon unlikely. Similarly, the lack of colonic distension or tight bands and the ability to palpate the cecal band makes a RDD of the colon unlikely as well.

The patient's relatively mild colic signs and lack of evidence of systemic compromise or shock make a strangulating lesion much less likely in this case.

### What Is Your Initial Stabilization and Triage Plan?

The patient overall appears systemically stable. If the patient becomes uncomfortable during examination, alpha-2 agonists and/or butorphanol can be administered for sedation and analgesia.

### What Is Your Plan for Management on the Farm?

Most large colon impactions can be managed on the farm. The important components of medical management of a large colon impaction such as this one (large based on palpation per rectum) include:

1) Withholding the patient from all hay feeding, and either completely withholding grain or feeding only very small amounts of pelleted feed (max one or two feedings per day of a complete pelleted feed, no more than ½ pound per

feeding, made as a very soupy mash to encourage water consumption). This is appropriate for the current patient as well as most adult horses and should be continued until the impaction is resolved.

   a) There are scenarios where complete withholding of calories is not appropriate (patients at risk for hepatic lipidosis, late gestation pregnant mares, lactating mares); hospitalization may be indicated in these cases.

2) Enteral fluid therapy with water and electrolytes or laxative agents.
   b) Administration of 6–8 L of water with electrolyte powder, ideally repeated two to three times daily (but minimum once daily).
   c) Magnesium sulfate (Epsom salts, 1 pound per day in an average sized horse) is also recommended.
   d) Mineral oil is NOT useful for breaking up a large colon impaction and is therefore not recommended except to be used as a marker of intestinal transit (administered once at the start of therapy).
3) Encourage the patient to drink more water on their own with the use of flavored water (e.g., adding apple juice or a handful of grain to a full bucket of water). Always make sure the patient has a bucket of clean plain water in addition in case they do not want to drink the flavored water.
4) Hand walking of the patient to encourage gastrointestinal motility (a few times a day for 10–15 minutes at a time).

Flunixin meglumine can be administered as needed for pain control, as the resolution of large colon impactions is often uncomfortable due to intestinal cramping.

Repeat abdominal palpation per rectum should be performed daily to assess response to treatment. Owners should be instructed to monitor and track the horse's manure output.

### What Are Your Triggers for Referral?

Some large colon impactions require more aggressive medical management, or even surgical intervention. Indications for referral would include lack of improvement on serial abdominal palpation per rectum, lack of manure production after the first day of treatment, worsening signs of colic, new or increasing gas distension on palpation per rectum, or change in the systemic status of the patient. Additionally, if a patient is one where caloric restriction would potentially be contraindicated (older horse/pony/donkey/etc. at risk for hepatic lipidosis, late gestation pregnant mare, or lactating mare), referral could be indicated for intravenous fluid therapy and dextrose supplementation during treatment of the impaction.

## References


Aitken, M.R., Southwood, L.L., Ross, B.M., and Ross, M.W. (2014). Outcome of surgical and medical management of cecal impaction in 150 horses (1991–2011). *Vet. Surg.* 44: 540–546.

Arndt, S., Kilcoyne, I., Vaughan, B., and Dechant, J.E. (2021). Clinical and diagnostic findings, treatment, and short-term and long-term survival in horses with peritonitis: 72 cases (2007–2017). *Vet. Surg.* 50 (2): 323–335.

Arnold, C., Pilla, R., Chaffin, K. et al. (2021). Alterations in the fecal microbiome and metabolome of horses with antimicrobial-associated diarrhea compared to antibiotic-treated and non-treated healthy case controls. *Animals* 11: 1807. https://doi.org/10.3390/ani11061807.

Arroyo, L.G. et al. (2017). Duodenitis-proximal jejunitis in horses after experimental administration of *Clostridium difficile* toxins. *J. Vet. Intern. Med.* 31: 158–163.

Arroyo, L.G., Gomez, D.E., and Martins, C. (2018). Equine duodenitis-proximal jejunitis: A review. *Can. Vet. J.* 59 (5): 510–517.

Arroyo, L.G., Sears, W., and Gomez, D.E. (2019). Plasma transfusions in horses with typhlocolitis/colitis. *Can. Vet. J.* 60: 193–196.

Arroyo, L.G., Rossi, L., Santos, B.P. et al. (2020). Luminal and mucosal microbiota of the cecum and large colon of healthy and diarrheic horses. *Animals* 10: 1403. https://doi.org/10.3390/ani10081403.

Atherton, R.P., Furr, M.O., McKenzie, H.C., and Desrochers, A.M. (2011). Efficacy of hyperimmunized plasma in the treatment of horses with acute colitis. *J. Equine Vet. Sci.* 31: 19–25. https://doi.org/10.1016/j.jevs.2010.11.013.

Baker, W.T., Frederick, J., Giguere, S. et al. (2011). Reevaluation of the effect of phenylephrine on resolution of nephrosplenic entrapment by the rolling procedure in 87 horses. *Vet. Surg.* 40: 825–829.

Banse, H.E. et al. (2011). Gastric and enteric phytobezoars caused by ingestion of persimmon in equids. *J. Am. Vet. Med. Assoc.* 239 (8): 1110–1116.

Barton, M.H., Parviainen, A., and Norton, N. (2004). Polymyxin B protects horses against induced endotoxaemia in vivo. *Equine Vet. J.* 36: 397–401. https://doi.org/10.2746/0425164044868350.

Baumgardner, R.M., Berreta, A., and Kopper, J.J. (2021). Evaluation of commercial probiotics for antimicrobial resistance genes. *Can. Vet. J.* 62: 379–383.

Båverud, V., Gustafsson, A., Franklin, A. et al. (2003). Clostridium difficile: prevalence in horses and environment, and antimicrobial susceptibility. *Equine Vet. J.* 35: 465–471. https://doi.org/10.2746/042516403775600505.

Bell, R.J.W. and Textor, J.A. (2010). Caecal intussusceptions in horses: a New Zealand perspective. *Aust. Vet. J.* 88 (7): 272–276.

Bergren, A.L., Credille, B.C., Epstein, K.L., and Giguere, S. (2015). Retrospective comparison of gastrosplenic entrapment of the small intestine to other strangulating small intestinal lesions in adult horses. *Vet. Surg.* 44: 535–539.

Berreta, A., Burbick, C.R., Alexander, T. et al. (2021). Microbial variability of commercial equine probiotics. *J. Equine Vet. Sci.* 106: 103728. https://doi.org/10.1016/j.jevs.2021.103728.

Berryhill, E.H., Magdesian, K.G., Aleman, M., and Pusterla, N. (2019). Clinical presentation, diagnostic findings, and outcome of adult horses with equine coronavirus infection at a veterinary teaching hospital: 33 cases (2012–2018). *Vet. J.* 248: 95–100. https://doi.org/10.1016/j.tvjl.2019.05.001.

Bertin, F.R., Reising, A., Slovis, N.M. et al. (2013). Clinical and clinicopathological factors associated with survival in 44 horses with equine neorickettsiosis (potomac horse fever). *J. Vet. Intern. Med.* 27: 1528–1534. https://doi.org/10.1111/jvim.12209.

Bird, A.R., Knowles, E.J., Sherlock, C.E. et al. (2012). The clinical and pathological features of gastric impaction in twelve horses. *Equine Vet. J.* 44 (suppl. 43): 105–110.

Boening, K.J. and vonSaldern, F.C. (1985). Treatment of left dorsal displacement of the large colon in horses by rolling, under general anesthesia. *Tierrartliche-Umschau* 40: 252–254.

Bowlby, C., Mudge, M., Schroeder, E. et al. (2021). Equine inflammatory response to abdominal surgery in the absence of gastrointestinal disease. *J. Vet. Emerg. Crit. Care* 31: 601–607.

Boyle, A.G., Magdesian, K.G., Gallop, R. et al. (2013). Saccharomyces boulardii viability and efficacy in horses with antimicrobial-induced diarrhoea. *Vet. Rec.* 172: 128–128. https://doi.org/10.1136/vr.100833.

Broekman, L.E.M. and Kuiper, D. (2002). Megaesophagus in the horse: a review of the literature and 18 own cases. *Vet. Q.* 24 (4): 199–202.

Burke, M.J. and Parente, E.J. (2016). Prosthetic mesh for obliteration of the nephrosplenic space in horses: 26 clinical cases. *Vet. Surg.* 45: 201–207.

Busoni, V., De Busscher, V., Lopez, D. et al. (2011). Evaluation of a protocol for fast localized abdominal sonography of horses (FLASH) admitted for colic. *Vet. J.* 188 (1): 77–82.

Chaney, K.P., Holcombe, S.J., LeBlanc, M.M. et al. (2007). The effect of uterine torsion on mare and foal survival: a retrospective study, 1985–2005. *Equine Vet. J.* 39 (1): 33–36.

Chiavaccini, L. and Hassel, D.M. (2010). Clinical features and prognostic variables in 109 horses with esophageal obstruction (1992–2009). *J. Vet. Intern. Med.* 24 (5): 1147–1152.

Claes, A., Ball, B.A., Brown, J.A., and Kass, P.H. (2008). Evaluation of risk factors, management, and outcome associated with rectal tears in horses: 99 cases (1985–2006). *J. Am. Vet. Med. Assoc.* 233 (10): 1605–1609.

Cohen, N.D., Carter, G.K., Mealey, R.H., and Taylor, T.S. (1995). Medical management of right dorsal colitis in 5 horses: a retrospective study (1987–1993). *J. Vet. Intern. Med.* 9: 272–276. https://doi.org/10.1111/j.1939-1676.1995.tb01079.x.

Cohen, N.D. and Woods, A.M. (1999). Characteristics and risk factors for failure of horses with acute diarrhea to survive: 122 cases (1990–1996). *J. Am. Vet. Med. Assoc.* 214: 382–390.

Cook, V.L., Jones Shults, J., McDowell, M.R. et al. (2009). Anti-inflammatory effects of intravenously administered lidocaine hydrochloride on ischemia-injured jejunum in horses. *Am. J. Vet. Res.* 70: 1259–1268. https://doi.org/10.2460/ajvr.70.10.1259.

Coronado, F.O. and Beatty, S.S. (2021). Fluid analysis in the equine patient. *Vet. Clin. N. Am. Equine Pract.* 36: e1–e28.

Costa, M.C., Arroyo, L.G., Allen-Vercoe, E. et al. (2012). Comparison of the fecal microbiota of healthy horses and horses with colitis by high throughput sequencing of the V3–V5 region of the 16S rRNA gene. *PLoS One* 7: https://doi.org/10.1371/journal.pone.0041484.

Cudmore, L.A., Muurlink, T., Whittem, T., and Bailey, S.R. (2013). Effects of oral clenbuterol on the clinical and inflammatory response to endotoxaemia in the horse. *Res. Vet. Sci.* 94: 682–686. https://doi.org/10.1016/j.rvsc.2013.01.003.

Cudmore, L., Whittem, T., and Bailey, S. (2015). Anti-inflammatory effects of clenbuterol on equine leukocytes stimulated ex vivo with bacterial toxins. *Res. Vet. Sci.* 34: 5.

Davis, J.L. (2017). Nonsteroidal anti-inflammatory drug associated right dorsal colitis in the horse. *Equine Vet. Educ.* 29: 104–113. https://doi.org/10.1111/eve.12454.

de Bont, M.P. (2018). A novel use for polyamide tie-wraps in the surgical resolution of cecocolic intussusception in a horse. *Equine Vet. Educ.* 30 (5): 255–258.

Dechant, J.E. and Winfield, L.S. (2017). Review of gastric rupture in the horse. *Equine Vet. Educ.* 29: 677–682. https://doi.org/10.1111/eve.12516.

Deen, T. (1990). Correcting left dorsal displacement of the large colon by hoisting and rolling the horse. *Vet. Med.* 85: 284–288.

de La Rebière, D., de Pouyade, G., Grulke, S. et al. (2009). Evaluation of low-molecular-weight heparin for the prevention of equine laminitis after colic surgery. *J. Vet. Emerg. Crit. Care* 19: 113–119. https://doi.org/10.1111/j.1476-4431.2008.00379.x.

Desrochers, A.M., Dolente, B.A., Roy, M.-F. et al. (2005). Efficacy of Saccharomyces boulardii for treatment of horses with acute enterocolitis. *J. Am. Vet. Med. Assoc.* 227: 954–959. https://doi.org/10.2460/javma.2005.227.954.

Diab, S.S., Songer, G., and Uzal, F.A. (2013). Clostridium difficile infection in horses: a review. *Vet. Microbiol.* 167: 42–49. https://doi.org/10.1016/j.vetmic.2013.03.032.

Dolente, B.A., Wilkins, P.A., and Boston, R.C. (2002). Clinicopathologic evidence of disseminated intravascular coagulation in horses with acute colitis. *J. Am. Vet. Med. Assoc.* 220: 1034–1038. https://doi.org/10.2460/javma.2002.220.1034.

Dolente, B.A., Beech, J., Lindborg, S., and Smith, G. (2005). Evaluation of risk factors for development of catheter-associated jugular thrombophlebitis in horses: 50 cases (1993–1998). *J. Am. Vet. Med. Assoc.* 227: 1134–1141. https://doi.org/10.2460/javma.2005.227.1134.

Douglas, H.F., Stefanovski, D., and Southwood, L.L. (2021). Outcomes of pregnant broodmares treated for colic at a tertiary care facility. *Vet. Surg.* 50 (8): 1579–1591.

Dutta, S.K., Vemulapalli, R., and Biswas, B. (1998). Association of deficiency in antibody response to vaccine and heterogeneity of Ehrlichia risticii strains with potomac horse fever vaccine failure in horses. *J. Clin. Microbiol.* 36: 506–512.

Eastman, T.G., Taylor, T.S., Hooper, R.N., and Honnas, C.M. (2000). Treatment of rectal tears in 85 horses presented to the Texas Veterinary Medical Center. *Equine Vet. Educ.* 12 (5): 263–266.

Engelbert, T.A., Tate Jr, L.P., Bowman, K.F., and Bristol, D.G. (1993). Incarceration of the small intestine in the epiploic foramen report of 19 cases (1983–1992). *Vet. Surg.* 22 (1): 57–61.

Espinosa, P., Le Jeune, S.S., Cenani, A. et al. (2017). Investigation of perioperative and anesthetic variables affecting short-term survival of horses with small intestinal strangulating lesions. *Vet. Surg.* 46: 345–353.

Feary, D.J. and Hassel, D.M. (2006). Enteritis and colitis in horses. *Vet. Clin. N. Am. Equine Pract. Adv. Diagn. Manag. Infect.* 22: 437–479. https://doi.org/10.1016/j.cveq.2006.03.008.

Fiege, K., Schwarzwald, C., Furst, A., and Kaser-Hotz, B. (2000). Esophageal obstruction in horses: a retrospective study of 34 cases. *Can. Vet. J.* 41 (3): 207–210.

Fleming, K. and Mueller, P.O.E. (2011). Ileal impactions in 245 horses: 1995–2007. *Can. Vet. J.* 52: 759–763.

Forbes, G., Church, S., Savage, C.J., and Bailey, S.R. (2012). Effects of hyperimmune equine plasma on clinical and cellular responses in a low-dose endotoxaemia model in horses. *Res. Vet. Sci.* 92: 40–44. https://doi.org/10.1016/j.rvsc.2010.10.020.

Fredrick, J., Giguere, S., Butterworth, K. et al. (2010). Severe phenylephrine associated hemorrhage in five aged horses. *J. Am. Vet. Med. Assoc.* 237 (7): 830–834.

French, N.P., Smith, J., Edwards, G.B., and Proudman, C.J. (2002). Equine surgical colic: risk factors for postoperative complications. *Equine Vet. J.* 34 (5): 444–449.

Fultz L.E., Peloso, J.G., Giguere, S., and Adams, A.R. (2013) Comparison of phenylephrine administration and exercise versus phenylephrine administration and rolling procedure for the correction of nephrosplenic entrapment of the large colon in horses: 88 cases (2004–2010). *J. Am. Vet. Med. Assoc.* 242 (8): 1146–1151.

Garcia-Seco, E., Wilson, D.A., Kramer, J. et al. (2005). Prevalence and risk factors associated with outcome of surgical removal of pedunculated lipomas in horses: 102 cases (1987–2002). *J. Am. Vet. Med. Assoc.* 226 (9): 1529–1537.

Gardner, A., Dockery, A., and Quam, V. (2019). Exploratory celiotomy in the horse secondary to acute colic: a review of indications and success rates. *Top. Compan. Anim. Med.* 34: 1–9.

Gardner, R.B., Nydam, D.V., Mohammed, H.O., Ducharme, N.G., and Divers, T.J. (2005). Serum gamma glutamyl transferase activity in horses with right or left dorsal displacement of the large colon. *J. Vet. Intern. Med.* 19: 761–764.

Gayle, J.M., Blikslager, A.T., and Bowman, K.F. (2000). Mesenteric rents as a source of small intestinal strangulation in horses: 15 cases (1990–1997). *J. Am. Vet. Med. Assoc.* 216 (9): 1446–1449.

Gillen, A., Kottwitz, J., and Munsterman, A. (2020). Meta-analysis of the effect of treatment strategies for nephrsplenic entrapment of the large colon. *J. Equine Vet. Sci.* 92: 1–10.

Haddad, R., Corraretti, G., Simon, O., Mair, T., Sutton, A. G., and Kelmer, G. (2022). Small intestinal intussusception in horses: multicentre retrospective report on 26 cases (2009–2020). *Equine Vet. Educ.* 34 (12): e563–e569.

Hallowell, G.D. (2008). Retrospective study assessing efficacy of treatment of large colonic impactions. *Equine Vet. J.* 40 (4): 411–413.

Hann, M.J., Mair, T.S., Gardner, A. et al. (2021). Acute abdominal dehiscence following laparotomy: a multicentre, international retrospective study. *Equine Vet. J.* https://doi.org/10.1111/evj.13498.

Hanson, R.R. and Schumacher, J. (2021a). Diagnosis, management and prognosis of small colon impactions. *Equine Vet. Educ.* 33 (1): 47–56.

Hanson, R.R. (2015). It's not the end: What's new in ileal impactions. *Proceedings: North American Veterinary Conference*, pp. 125–126.

Hanson, R.R. and Schumacher, J. (2021b). Diagnosis, management and prognosis of large colon impactions. *Equine Vet. Educ.* 33 (2): 90–101.

Hashimoto-Hill, S., Magdesian, K.G., and Kass, P.H. (2011). Serial measurement of lactate concentration in horses with acute colitis. *J. Vet. Intern. Med.* 25: 1414–1419. https://doi.org/10.1111/j.1939-1676.2011.00808.x.

Hassel, D.M., Rakestraw, P.C., Gardner, I.A. et al. (2004). Dietary risk factors and colonic pH and mineral concentrations in horses with enterolithiasis. *J. Vet. Intern. Med.* 18: 346–349.

Hassel, D.M., Aldridge, B.M., Drake, C.M., and Snyder, J.R. (2008). Evaluation of dietary and management risk factors for enterolithiasis among horses in California. *Res. Vet. Sci.* 85 (3): 476–480.

Hassel, D.M., Smith, P.A., Nieto, J.E. et al. (2009). Di-tri-octahedral smectite for the prevention of post-operative diarrhea in equids with surgical disease of the large intestine: results of a randomized clinical trial. *Vet. J.* 182: 210–214. https://doi.org/10.1016/j.tvjl.2008.06.016.

Hellstrom, E.A., Ziegler, A.L., and Blikslager, A.T. (2021). Postoperative ileus: comparative pathophysiology and future therapies. *Front. Vet. Sci.* 8: 1–8.

Henderson, I.S.F., Mair, T.S., Keen, J.A. et al. (2008). Study of the short- and long-term outcomes of 65 horses with peritonitis. *Vet. Rec.* 163 (10): 293–297.

Hotwagner, K. and Iben, C. (2008). Evacuation of sand from the equine intestine with mineral oil, with and without psyllium. *J. Anim. Physiol. Anim. Nutr.* 92 (1): 86–91.

Johns, I., Tennent-Brown, B., Schaer, B.D. et al. (2009). Blood culture status in mature horses with diarrhoea: a possible association with survival. *Equine Vet. J.* 41: 160–164. https://doi.org/10.2746/042516409X360208.

Jones, R.L. (2000). Clostridial enterocolitis. *Vet. Clin. N. Am. Equine Pract.* 16: 471–485. https://doi.org/10.1016/S0749-0739(17)30090-1.

Jones, P.A., Bain, F.T., Byars, T.D. et al. (2001). Effect of hydroxyethyl starch infusion on colloid oncotic pressure in hypoproteinemic horses. *J. Am. Vet. Med. Assoc.* 218: 1130–1135. https://doi.org/10.2460/javma.2001.218.1130.

Kelleher, M.E., Puchalski, S.M., Drake, C., and le Jeune, S.S. (2014). Use of digital abdominal radiography for the diagnosis of enterolithiasis in equids: 238 cases (2008–2011). *J. Am. Vet. Med. Assoc.* 245 (1): 126–129.

Khusro, A., Aarti, C., Buendía-Rodriguez, G. et al. (2021). Adverse effect of antibiotics administration on horse health: an overview. *J. Equine Vet. Sci.* 97: 103339. https://doi.org/10.1016/j.jevs.2020.103339.

Kilcoyne, I., Dechant, J.E., and Nieto, J.E. (2016). Comparison of clinical findings and short-term survival between horses with intestinal entrapment in the gastrosplenic ligament and horses with intestinal entrapment in the epiploic foramen. *J. Am. Vet. Med. Assoc.* 29 (6): 660–667.

Kilcoyne, I., Dechant, J.E., Spier, S.J. et al. (2017). Clinical findings and management of 153 horses with large colon sand accumulation. *Vet. Surg.* 48: 860–867.

Kiper, M.L., Traub-Dargatz, J., and Curtis, C.R. (1990). Gastric rupture in horses: 50 cases (1979–1987). *J. Am. Vet. Med. Assoc.* 196 (2): 333–336.

Kovač, M., Huskamp, B., Scheidemann, W. et al. (2017). Survival and evaluation of clinical and laboratory variables as prognostic indicators in horses hospitilized with acute diarrhea: 342 cases (1995–2015). *Acta Veterinaria* 67: 356–365. https://doi.org/10.1515/acve-2017-0029.

Kullmann, A., Holcombe, S.J., Hurcombe, S.D. et al. (2014). Prophylactic digital cryotherapy is associated with decreased incidence of laminitis in horses diagnosed with colitis. *Equine Vet. J.* 46: 554–559. https://doi.org/10.1111/evj.12156.

Kurowski, P.B., Traub-Dargatz, J.L., Morley, P.S., and Gentry-Weeks, C.R. (2002). Detection of Salmonella spp in fecal specimens by use of real-time polymerase chain reaction assay. *Am. J. Vet. Res.* 63 (9): 1265–1268. https://doi.org/10.2460/ajvr.2002.63.1265.

Lawler, J.B., Hassel, D.M., Magnuson, R.J. et al. (2008). Adsorptive effects of di-tri-octahedral smectite on Clostridium perfringens alpha, beta, and beta-2 exotoxins and equine colostral antibodies. *Am. J. Vet. Res.* 69: 233–239. https://doi.org/10.2460/ajvr.69.2.233.

Leahy, E.R., Holcombe, S.J., Hackett, E.S. et al. (2018). Reproductive careers of Thoroughbred broodmares before and after surgical correction of ≥360 degree large colon volvulus. *Equine Vet. J.* 50: 208–212.

LeJeune, S.S. and Whitcomb, M.B. (2014). Ultrasound of the equine acute abdomen. *Vet. Clin. N. Am. Equine Pract.* 30 (2): 353–381.

LeJeune, S.S., Nieto, J.E., Dechant, J.E., and Snyder, J.R. (2009). Prevalence of gastric ulcers in Thoroughbred broodmares in pasture: a preliminary report. *Vet. J.* 181 (3): 251–255.

Lindegaard, C., Ekstrom, C.T., Wulf, S.B., Vendelbo, J.M.B., and Andersen, P.H. (2011). Nephrosplenic entrapment of the large colon in 142 horses (2000–2009): analysis of factors associated with decision of treatment and short-term survival. *Equine Vet. J.* 43 (Suppl. 39): 63–68.

Little, D. and Blikslager, A.T. (2002). Factors associated with development of ileal impaction in horses with surgical colic: 79 cases (1986–2000). *Equine Vet. J.* 34 (5): 464–468.

Liu, X.-L., Wang, X.-Z., Liu, X.-X. et al. (2014). Low-dose heparin as treatment for early disseminated intravascular coagulation during sepsis: a prospective clinical study. *Exp. Therap. Med.* 7: 604–608. https://doi.org/10.3892/etm.2013.1466.

Lores, M. and Ortenburger, A.I. (2008). Use of cecal bypass via side-to-side ileocolic anastomosis without ileal transection for treatment of cecocolic intussusception in three horses. *J. Am. Vet. Med. Assoc.* 232 (4): 574–577.

Lopes, M.A.F., Walker, B.L., White, N.A., and Ward, D.L. (2002). Treatments to promote colonic hydration: enteral fluid therapy versus intravenous fluid therapy and magnesium sulfate. *Equine Vet. J.* 34 (5): 505–509.

Lopes, M.A.F., White, N.A., Donaldson, L. et al. (2004). Effects of enteral and intravenous fluid therapy, magnesium sulfate, and sodium sulfate on colonic contents and feces in horses. *Am. J. Vet. Res.* 65 (5): 695–704.

Luethy, D., Feldman, R., Stefanovski, D., and Aitken, M.R. (2021). Risk factors for laminitis and nonsurvival in acute colitis: retrospective study of 85 hospitalized horses (2011–2019). *J. Vet. Intern. Med.* 35: 2019–2025. https://doi.org/10.1111/jvim.16147.

Lyons, E.T., Drudge, J.H., and Tolliver, S.C. (2000). Larval cyathostomiasis. *Vet. Clin. N. Am. Equine Pract. Emerg. Infect. Dis.* 16: 501–513. https://doi.org/10.1016/S0749-0739(17)30092-5.

Madigan, J.E., Pusterla, N., and Pusterla, N. (2000). Ehrlichial diseases. *Vet. Clin. N. Am. Equine Pract.* 16: 487–499. https://doi.org/10.1016/S0749-0739(17)30091-3.

Magdesian, K.G. and Bozorgmanesh, R. (2018). Nutritional considerations for horses with colitis. Part 2: Parenteral nutrition, new nutritional considerations and specific dietary recommendations. *Equine Vet. Educ.* 30: 608–615. https://doi.org/10.1111/eve.12691.

Mair, T.S. and Smith, L.J. (2005). Survival and complication rates in 300 horses undergoing surgical treatment of colic. Part 1: short term survival following a single laparotomy. *Equine Vet. J.* 37 (4): 296–302.

Mair, T.S., de Westerlaken, L.V., Cripps, P.J., and Love, S. (1990). Diarrhoea in adult horses: a survey of clinical cases and an assessment of some prognostic indices. *Vet. Rec.* 126: 479–481.

Mariella, J., Pirrone, A., Gentilini, F., and Castagnetti, C. (2014). Hematologic and biochemical profiles in Standardbred mares during peripartum. *Theriogenology* 81 (4): 526–534.

Martin, B.B. Jr., Freeman, D.E., Ross, M.W. et al. (1999). Cecocolic and cecocecal intussusception in horses: 30 cases (1976–1996). *J. Am. Vet. Med. Assoc.* 214 (1): 80–84.

Martin, E.M., Till, R.L., Sheats, M.K., and Jones, S.L. (2017a). Misoprostol inhibits equine neutrophil adhesion, migration, and respiratory burst in an in vitro model of inflammation. *Front. Vet. Sci.* 4: 159.

Martin, E.M., Messenger, K.M., Sheats, M.K., and Jones, S.L. (2017b). Misoprostol Inhibits lipopolysaccharide-induced pro-inflammatory cytokine production by equine leukocytes. *Front. Vet. Sci.* 4: 160.

Martin, E.M., Schirmer, J.M., Jones, S.L., and Davis, J.L. (2019). Pharmacokinetics and ex vivo anti-inflammatory effects of oral misoprostol in horses. *Equine Vet. J.* 51: 415–421.

McGovern, K.F., Bladon, B.M., Fraser, B.S.L., and Boston, R.C. (2011). Attempted medical management of suspected ascending colon displacement in horses. *Vet. Surg.* 41: 399–403.

McKinney, C.A., Bedenice, D., Pacheco, A.P. et al. (2021). Assessment of clinical and microbiota responses to fecal microbial transplantation in adult horses with diarrhea. *PLoS One* 16: e0244381. https://doi.org/10.1371/journal.pone.0244381.

McMaster, M., Caldwell, F., Schumacher, J. et al. (2015). A review of equine rectal tears and current methods of treatment. *Equine Vet. Educ.* 27 (4): 200–208.

Mendonça, F.S., Navarro, M.A., and Uzal, F.A. (2021). The comparative pathology of enterocolitis caused by Clostridium perfringens type C, Clostridioides difficile, Paeniclostridium sordellii, Salmonella enterica subspecies enterica serovar Typhimurium, and nonsteroidal anti-inflammatory drugs in horses. *J. Vet. Diagn. Invest.* 10406387211041092: https://doi.org/10.1177/10406387211041091.

Minamijima, Y., Tozaki, T., Kuroda, T. et al. (2020). A comprehensive and comparative proteomic analysis of horse serum proteins in colitis. *Equine Vet. J.* https://doi.org/10.1111/evj.13554.

Niinistö, K., Hewetson, M., Kaikkonen, R. et al. (2014). Comparison of the effects of enteral psyllium, magnesium sulphate and their combination for removal of sand from the large colon of horses. *Vet. J.* 202: 608–611.

Niinistö, K.E., Ruohoniemi, M.O., Freccero, F., and Raekallio, M.R. (2018). Investigation of the treatment of sand accumulations in the equine large colon with psyllium and magnesium sulfate. *Vet. J.* 238: 22–26.

Odelros, E., Kendall, A., Hedberg-Alm, Y., and Pringle, J. (2019). Idiopathic peritonitis in horses: a retrospective study of 130 cases in Sweden (2002–2017). *Acta Vet. Scand.* 61 (18): https://doi.org/10.1186/s13028-019-0456-2.

Orr, K.E., Baker, W.T., Lynch, T.M. et al. (2020). Prognostic value of colonic and peripheral venous lactate measurements in horses with large colon volvulus. *Vet. Surg.* 49: 472–479.

Parraga, M.E., Spier, S.J., Thurmond, M., and Hirsh, D. (1997). A clinical trial of probiotic administration for prevention of salmonella shedding in the postoperative period in horses with colic. *J. Vet. Intern. Med.* 11: 36–41. https://doi.org/10.1111/j.1939-1676.1997.tb00071.x.

Petersen, M.B., Tolver, A., Husted, L. et al. (2016). Repeated measurements of blood lactate concentration as a prognostic marker in horses with acute colitis evaluated with classification and regression trees (CART) and random forest analysis. *Vet. J.* 213: 18–23. https://doi.org/10.1016/j.tvjl.2016.03.012.

Pierce, R.L., Fischer, A.T., Rohrbach, B.W., and Klohnen, A. (2010). Postoperative complications and survival after enterolith removal from the ascending or descending colon in horses. *Vet. Surg.* 39: 609–615.

Pusterla, N., Byrne, B.A., Hodzic, E. et al. (2010). Use of quantitative real-time PCR for the detection of Salmonella spp. in fecal samples from horses at a veterinary teaching hospital. *Vet. J.* 186: 252–255. https://doi.org/10.1016/j.tvjl.2009.08.022.

Pusterla, N., Vin, R., Leutenegger, C. et al. (2016). Equine coronavirus: an emerging enteric virus of adult horses. *Equine Vet. Educ.* 28: 216–223. https://doi.org/10.1111/eve.12453.

Pye, J., Espinosa-Mur, P., Roca, R. et al. (2019). Preoperative factors associated with resection and anastomosis in horses presenting with strangulating lesions of the small intestine. *Vet. Surg.* 48: 786–794.

Plummer, A.E., Rakestraw, P.C., Hardy, J., and Lee, R.M. (2007). Outcome of medical and surgical treatment of cecal impaction in horses: 114 cases (1994–2004). *J. Am. Vet. Med. Assoc.* 231 (9): 1378–1385.

Plummer, A.E. (2009). Impactions of the small and large intestines. *Vet. Clin. N. Am. Equine Pract.* 25: 317–327.

Pratt, S.M., Hassel, D.M., Drake, C., and Snyder, J.R. (2003). Clinical characteristics of horses with gastrointestinal ruptures revealed during initial diagnostic evaluation: 149 cases (1990–2002). *Proc. Am. Assoc. Equine Pract.* 49: 366–370.

Qualls, H.J., Holbrook, T.C., Gilliam, L. et al. (2013). Evaluation of efficacy of mineral oil, charcoal, and smectite in a rat model of equine cantharidin toxicosis. *J. Vet. Intern. Med.* 27: 1179–1184. https://doi.org/10.1111/jvim.12164.

Radcliffe, R.M., Liu, S.Y., Cook, V.L. et al. (2022). Interpreting abdominal fluid in colic horses: understanding and applying peritoneal fluid evidence. *J. Vet. Emerg. Crit. Care* 32 (S1): 81–96.

Ragle, C.A., Southwood, L.L., Galuppo, L.D., and Howlett, M.R. (1997). Laparoscopic diagnosis of ischemic necrosis of the descending colon after rectal prolapse and rupture of the mesocolon in two postpartum mares. *J. Am. Vet. Med. Assoc.* 210 (11): 1646–1648.

Rhoads, W.S., Barton, M.H., and Parks, A.H. (1999). Comparison of medical and surgical treatment for impaction of the small colon in horses: 84 cases (1986–1996). *J. Am. Vet. Med. Assoc.* 214 (7): 1042–1047.

Rodriguez, C., Taminiau, B., Brévers, B. et al. (2015). Faecal microbiota characterisation of horses using 16 rdna barcoded pyrosequencing, and carriage rate of clostridium difficile at hospital admission. *BMC Microbiol.* 15: 181.

Rodríguez, J.M.A., Grulke, S., Salciccia, A., and de la Rebière de Pouyade, G. (2019). Nephrosplenic space closure significantly decreases recurrent colic in horses: a retrospective analysis. *Vet. Rec.* 185 (21): 657–662.

Ross, J., Palmer, J.E., and Wilkins, P.A. (2008). Body wall tears during late pregnancy in mares: 13 cases (1995-2006). *J. Am. Vet. Med. Assoc.* 232 (2): 257–261.

Sage, S.E., Bedenice, D., McKinney, C.A. et al. (2021). Assessment of the impact of age and of blood-derived inflammatory markers in horses with colitis. *J. Vet. Emerg. Crit. Care* 31: 779–787. https://doi.org/10.1111/vec.13099.

Sanchez, L.C. (2018). Disorders of the gastrointestinal system. In: *Equine Internal Medicine*, 4e (ed. S.M. Reed, W.M. Bayly, and D.C. Sellon), 709–842. St. Louis, MO: Elsevier.

Schmitz, D.G. (1989). Cantharidin toxicosis in horses. *J. Vet. Intern. Med.* 3: 208–215. https://doi.org/10.1111/j.1939-1676.1989.tb00859.x.

Schoster, A., Weese, J.S., and Guardabassi, L. (2014). Probiotic use in horses – what is the evidence for their clinical efficacy? *J. Vet. Intern. Med.* 28: 1640–1652. https://doi.org/10.1111/jvim.12451.

Schoster, A., Altermatt, N., Torgerson, P.R., and Bischofberger, A.S. (2019). Outcome and complications following transrectal and transabdominal large intestinal trocarization in equids with colic: 228 cases (2004–2015). *J. Am. Vet. Med. Assoc.* 257 (2): 189–195.

Schusser, G.F., Rieckhoff, K., Ungemach, F.R. et al. (2007). Effect of hydroxyethyl starch solution in normal horses and horses with colic or acute colitis. *J. Veterinary Med. Ser. A* 54: 592–598. https://doi.org/10.1111/j.1439-0442.2007.01007.x.

Scotti, G.B., Lazzaretti, S.S., Zani, D.D., and Magri, M. (2012). Transrectal decompression as a new approach for treatment of large intestinal tympany in horses with colic: preliminary results. *Equine Vet. Educ.* 25: 184–188.

Shaw, S.D. and Stämpfli, H. (2018). Diagnosis and treatment of undifferentiated and infectious acute diarrhea in the adult horse. *Vet. Clin. N. Am. Equine Pract. Recent Adv. Diagn. Manag. Equine Gastrointest. Dis.* 34: 39–53. https://doi.org/10.1016/j.cveq.2017.11.002.

Smith, L.J. and Mair, T.S. (2010). Are horses that undergo an exploratory laparotomy for correction of a right dorsal displacement of the large colon predisposed to post operative colic, compared to other forms of large colon displacement? *Equine Vet. J.* 42 (1): 44–46.

Southwood, L.L. (2019). Chapter 37: Large colon. In: Auer, J.A., Stick, J.A., Kummerle, J.M., and Prange, T. (ed.) *Equine Surgery*, 5e. St. Louis MO: Elsevier. pp. 591–621.

Southwood, L.L. and Wilkins, P.A. (ed.) (2015). *Equine Emergency and Critical Care Medicine*, 1e. Boca Raton, FL: CRC Press.

Southwood, L.L. and Russell, G. (2007). The use of clinical findings in the identification of equine peritonitis cases that respond favorably to medical therapy. *J. Vet. Emerg. Crit. Care* 17 (4): 382–390.

Sprayberry, K.A. and Lu, K.G. (2021). Managing reproduction emergencies in the field, Part 1: injuries in stallions; injury of the external portion of the reproductive tract and gestational condition in the mare. *Vet. Clin. N. Am. Equine Pract.* 37 (2): 339–366.

Staempfli, H.R., Townsend, H.G.G., and Prescott, J.F. (1991). Prognostic features and clinical presentation of acute idiopathic enterocolitis in horses. *Can. Vet. J.* 32: 232–237.

Stephen, J.O., Corley, K.T., Johnston, J.K., and Pfeiffer, D. (2004). Small intestinal volvulus in 115 horses: 1988–2000. *Vet. Surg.* 33(4): 333–339.

Stewart, S.K.T., Hassel, D.M., Martin, H. et al. (2020). Geographic disparities in clinical characteristics of duodenitis-proximal jejunitis in horses in the United States. *J. Equine Vet. Sci.* 93: 1–4.

Stewart, S., Southwood, L.L., and Aceto, H.W. (2014). Comparison of short- and long-term complications and survival following jejunojejunostomy, jejunoileostomy and jejunocecostomy in 112 horses: 2005–2010. *Equine Vet. J.* 46: 333–338.

Suthers, J.M., Pinchbeck, G.L., Proudman, C.J., and Archer, D.C. (2013). Survival of horses following strangulating large colon volvulus. *Equine Vet. J.* 45: 219–223.

Sykes, B.W., Hewetson, M., Hepburn, R.J., Luthersson, N., and Tamzali, Y. (2015). European College of Internal Medicine consensus statement – equine gastric ulcer syndrome in adult horses. *J. Vet. Intern. Med.* 29: 1288–1299.

Taylor, E.A., Beard, W.L., Douthit, T., and Pohlman, L. (2014). Effect of orally administered sodium bicarbonate on caecal pH. *Equine Vet. J.* 46: 223–226. https://doi.org/10.1111/evj.12111.

Todhunter, R.J., Erb, H.N., and Roth, L. (1986). Gastric rupture in horses: a review of 54 cases. *Equine Vet. J.* 18 (4): 288–293.

Turner, T.A. and Fessler, J.F. (1980). Rectal prolapse in the horse. *J. Am. Vet. Med. Assoc.* 177 (10): 1028–1032.

Underwood, C., Southwood, L.L., McKeown, L.P., and Knight, D. (2010). Complications and survival associated with surgical compared with medical management of horses with duodenitis-proximal jejunitis. *Equine Vet. J.* 40 (4): 373–378.

Uzal, F.A., Arroyo, L.G., Navarro, M.A. et al. (2021). Bacterial and viral enterocolitis in horses: a review. *J. Vet. Diagn. Invest.* 10406387211057468: https://doi.org/10.1177/10406387211057469.

van Bergen, T., Wiemer, P., and Martens, A. (2021). Equine colic associated with small intestinal epiploic foramen entrapment. *Vet. J.* 269: 105608.

van Bergen, T., Wiemer, P., Schauvliege, S., Paulussen, E., Ugahary, F., and Martens, A. (2016). Laparoscopic evaluation of the epiploic foramen after celiotomy for epiploic foramen entrapment in the horse. *Vet. Surg.* 45 (5): 596–601.

van Duijkeren, E., Sloet van Oldruitenborgh-Dosterbaan, M.M., Breukink, H.J. et al. (1996). A survey of horses with acute diarrhoea: diagnosis, assessment of the prognosis, and comparison of two antibiotic therapies. *Vet. Q.* 18: 153–156. https://doi.org/10.1080/01652176.1996.9694639.

Vandenplas, M.L., Moore, J.N., Barton, M.H. et al. (2005). Concentrations of serum amyloid A and lipopolysaccharide-binding protein in horses with colic. *Am. J. Vet. Res.* 66: 1509–1516. https://doi.org/10.2460/ajvr.2005.66.1509.

Van Hoogmoed, L., Snyder, J.R., Christopher, M., and Vatistas, N. (1996). Peritoneal fluid analysis in peripartum mares. *J. Am. Vet. Med. Assoc.* 209 (7): 1280–1282.

Varley, G., Bowen, I.M., Habershon-Butcher, J.L., Nicholls, V., and Hallowell, G.D. (2019). Misoprostol is superior to omeprazole-sucralfate for the treatment of equine gastric glandular disease. *Equine Vet. J.* 51: 575–580.

Wächtershäuser, A. and Stein, J. (2000). Rationale for the luminal provision of butyrate in intestinal diseases. *Eur. J. Nutr.* 39: 164–171. https://doi.org/10.1007/s003940070020.

Weese, J.S., Staempfli, H.R., and Prescott, J.F. (2001). A prospective study of the roles of Clostridium difficile and enterotoxigenic Clostridium perfringens in equine diarrhoea. *Equine Vet. J.* 33: 403–409. https://doi.org/10.2746/042516401776249534.

Weese, J.S., Cote, N.M., and Degannes, R.V.G. (2003). Evaluation of in vitro properties of di-tri-octahedral smectite on clostridial toxins and growth. *Equine Vet. J.* 35: 638–641. https://doi.org/10.2746/042516403775696384.

Wells, M.T., Gaffin, S.L., Gregory, M., and Coovadia, Y.Y. (1987). Properties of equine anti-lipopolysaccharide hyperimmune plasma: Binding to lipopolysaccharide and bactericidal activity against gram-negative bacteria. *J. Med. Microbiol.* 24: 187–196. https://doi.org/10.1099/00222615-24-3-187.

Werners, A.H., Bull, S., and Fink-Gremmels, J. (2010). Endotoxaemia: a review with implications for the horse. *Equine Vet. J.* 37: 371–383. https://doi.org/10.2746/0425164054529418.

Werners, A.H. (2017). Treatment of endotoxaemia and septicaemia in the equine patient. *J. Vet. Pharmacol. Ther.* 40: 1–15. https://doi.org/10.1111/jvp.12329.

Westerman, T.L., Tornquist, S.J., Foster, C.M., and Poulsen, K.P. (2015). Evaluation of serum amyloid A and haptoglobin concentrations as prognostic indicators for horses with inflammatory disease examined at a tertiary care hospital. *Am. J. Vet. Res.* 76: 882–888. https://doi.org/10.2460/ajvr.76.10.882.

Whyard, J.M. and Brounts, S.H. (2019). Complications and survival in horses with surgically confirmed right dorsal displacement of the large colon. *Can. Vet. J.* 60: 381–385.

Winfield, L.S. and Dechant, J.E. (2015). Primary gastric rupture in 47 horses (1995-2011). *Can. Vet. J.* 56: 953–958.

Williams, J.M., Lin, Y.J., Loftus, J.P. et al. (2010). Effect of intravenous lidocaine administration on laminar inflammation in the black walnut extract model of laminitis. *Equine Vet. J.* 42: 261–269. https://doi.org/10.2746/042516409X475760.

# 11

# Respiratory Emergencies

*Rebecca C. McOnie, Eileen S. Hackett, and Norm G. Ducharme*

*Department of Clinical Sciences, College of Veterinary Medicine, Cornell University, Ithaca, NY, USA*

## Introduction

Respiratory emergencies are commonly encountered in equine practice. Respiratory distress in the horse is an emergency requiring expedient treatment (Schaer and Orsini 2014). Treatments are often focused on establishing a patent airway and addressing the primary complaint resulting in distress. Knowledge of common etiologies and their specific clinical presentations will assist in triage, treatment, and owner recommendations. Horses in respiratory distress can behave erratically, impacting general occupational safety and complicating treatment. Often, horses present with life-threatening conditions requiring urgent care. Facilitating rapid and appropriate care is the goal of respiratory assessment in the horse. The principles of managing respiratory distress in the horse are presented in Box 11.1 and methods to localize problems in Box 11.2.

## Cornerstones of Emergency Triage

### Establish a Patent Airway

Establishing a patent airway in the case of upper airway obstruction is accomplished by emergency tracheotomy. If the patient is distressed or too anxious to work with safely, a low dose of sedation (e.g., 100–200 mg Xylazine IV) might be required to facilitate efficient tracheotomy. The procedure is described detail in Chapter 5. In the less common instance where upper airway obstruction occurs immediately following extubation (usually resulting from laryngeal paresis or laryngospasm), the patient should be reintubated or tracheotomized to secure the airway. For reintubation, anesthetics are generally required. If re-intubation is not immediately successful and the patient remains distressed, an emergency tracheotomy should be performed without delay. When no sedation or anesthetic agent is readily available, or when it cannot be safely administered to the dysphoric or belligerent patient, it is necessary to wait for the patient to become recumbent prior to performing an emergency tracheotomy. Although the clinician's personal safety is improved by waiting, the likelihood of successful patient outcome is low by this time.

Pulmonary edema and bronchoconstriction play roles in lower airway obstruction. To improve airway patency in these cases, medication administration is recommended. Clenbuterol (0.8 ug/kg PO or IV) can be used to achieve bronchodilation (Constable et al. 2017). Onset of action for the oral formulation is 1–2 h, whereas the IV formulation has a nearly immediate onset of action (Plumb 2015). Furosemide (1 mg/kg IV or IM) is a diuretic that can be used to decrease pulmonary edema and minimize the alveolar diffusion barrier (Constable et al. 2017).

### Oxygen Supplementation

Oxygen supplementation may be beneficial to some horses with respiratory distress and can be administered via nasal cannula (Figure 11.1) or directly into a temporary tracheotomy tube (Sprayberry and Barrett 2015; Wong et al. 2010). The initial rate of supplementation should be 15 L/min in a 500 kg horse, though rates up to 20 L/min are well tolerated (Wilson

*Emergency Triage of the Horse*, First Edition. Edited by Rolfe M. Radcliffe and Jamie J. Kopper.

Companion website: www.wiley.com/go/radcliffe/triage

**Box 11.1 Principles of managing respiratory distress in the horse**

1) Establish a patent airway.
2) Provide oxygen supplementation.
3) Seal and decompress the pleural space.
4) Halt hemorrhage.

**Box 11.2 How to localize respiratory distress in the horse**

1) Recognition of respiratory patterns.
2) Airway endoscopy.
3) Thoracic ultrasonography.
4) Thoracic radiography.

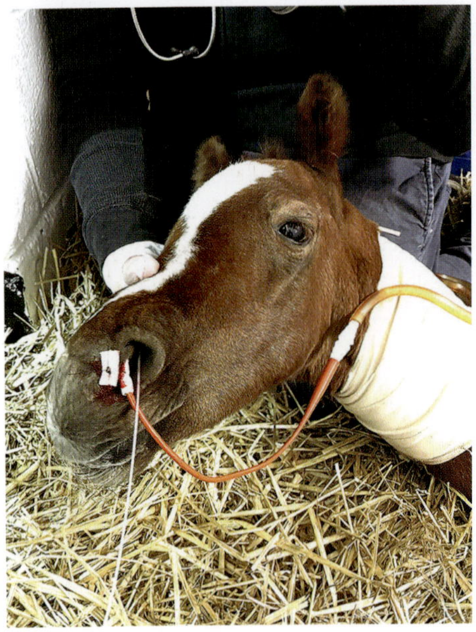

**Figure 11.1** Unilateral nasal cannula placement in a neonatal foal. The red rubber catheter attached to the oxygen source has a small butterfly of medical tape through which suture is securing it to the medial aspect of the nostril. A foal halter or a makeshift brown gauze halter with medical tape can be used to further secure the oxygen tubing to the foal. *Source:* Courtesy of Dr. Amanda Craven.

et al. 2006). Two nasal cannulas can be used to increase inspired oxygen concentration even further. Red rubber catheters (10–20 French) with a tape butterfly should be secured to the nares, so the tip of the catheter is positioned in the rostral nasopharynx. This can be estimated by the distance from the nares to the medial canthus of the eye. A nasopharyngeal oxygen flow rate of 15 L/min via a single cannula in a 500 kg horse would be expected to raise the inspired oxygen and arterial oxygen tension by 2.5 times that of room air. In horses with recurrent airway obstruction, arterial oxygen tension is increased with nasopharyngeal oxygen delivery, though to a lesser degree than in healthy horses (Wilson et al. 2006).

## Seal and Decompress the Pleural Space

To optimize pulmonary function, the pleural space must be sealed and have negative pressure. Pneumothorax or hemothorax impedes lung expansion and ventilation. External thoracic wounds, which can cause both of these abnormalities, should be rapidly evaluated, cleaned and debrided as needed, and sealed to restore the integrity of the thoracic wall (Hassel 2007; Sprayberry and Barrett 2015). Wound care may include partial or complete closure, drain placement, and/or packing; however, it should be completed by placement of an airtight bandage. When a patient presents in severe respiratory distress, wound care should be delayed and an airtight seal should be immediately established, along with placement of a chest tube. A chest tube should be placed to address pneumothorax (caudodorsally) or hemothorax (cranioventrally) for decompression of the chest once sealed.

Pulmonary injury without external thoracic wounds can also result in the development of a hemothorax or tension pneumothorax. Although a chest tube can be readily placed to decompress the thorax, these injuries are not easily treated to seal the pleura. Minor trauma does not require direct care and will likely resolve with maintenance of a chest tube. Severe trauma might require thoracotomy or thoracoscopy to stop hemorrhage or excise leaking bronchial trees (Hassel 2007; Sprayberry and Barrett 2015).

Tracheal lacerations can quickly result in marked subcutaneous emphysema that migrates to cause pneumothorax via pneumomediastinum (Byrne and Barakzai 2020). Many tracheal defects are not readily accessible to seal off on an emergency basis. Therefore, emergency tracheotomy caudal to the site of tracheal injury is recommended.

## Halt Hemorrhage

Hemorrhage can develop from numerous anatomic sites – for example: the nasal mucosa, large vessels of the guttural pouch, and pulmonary parenchyma into the lower airway tree or pleural space. Most sites of airway hemorrhage are not readily accessible for direct hemostasis by digital pressure, clamp, or ligature application.

Consequently, supportive care with permissive hypotension, whole blood transfusion (replace at least 50% blood lost if >30% blood volume; i.e., for a 500 kg horse, 30% blood volume = 12 L), colloid therapy (if pressures are otherwise non-responsive), aminocaproic acid (40 mg/kg IV slowly), and stabilization of tissues (rib, skull fractures) to prevent further injury is first line treatment (Divers et al. 2022). In the upper airway, limited mucosal bleeding can be slowed with topical phenylephrine (15 mg in 10–20 mL 0.9% NaCl). Rostral nasal bleeding, skull defects with sinus injury, or thoracic wall hemorrhage can be diminished by packing with gauze lap sponges or chitosan-impregnated gauze (QuikClot combat gauze[1]).

If intra-thoracic hemorrhage is profuse despite supportive therapies, thoracotomy might be required to directly ligate hemorrhaging vessels or excise macerated tissues.

## Localizing the Cause of Respiratory Distress

### Recognition of Respiratory Patterns

When evaluating horses with respiratory distress, careful attention is required. What is the rate of breathing? Is there an associated noise? Differential diagnoses can be refined, and the problem localized based on observation of the respiratory pattern, auscultation of the entire respiratory tract, and the remainder of the physical examination. Upper airway obstructions can be fixed, where the effort is increased on both inspiration and expiration, or dynamic, with an exaggerated effort only detected on inspiration due to pressure-related tissue collapse. Examples of fixed or continuous upper airway obstruction include retropharyngeal or mandibular lymph node abscessation associated with *Streptococcus equi* infections, and profound swelling following snake envenomation of the muzzle. Upper airway obstruction is often accompanied by profound stertor or stridor, as well as nostril flaring and decreased airflow at the nares. Diseases of the intrathoracic airways manifest as dynamic expiratory dyspnea, when the small airways collapse as the patient exhales. Loud expiratory wheezes and muscular development in the accessory respiratory muscles ("heave line") are indications of small airway collapse (Couetil et al. 2020). A paradoxical breathing pattern, in which the abdomen moves passively outward during expiration and inward during inspiration, can ensue with severe diaphragmatic fatigue, cervical spinal cord injury, or phrenic neuropathy. Disease of the pulmonary parenchyma and pleural space will cause reduced pulmonary compliance and increased effort on inspiration. The patient with reduced compliance will adopt a more rapid, shallow breathing (restrictive breathing) pattern in an effort to maintain minute ventilation in the face of reduced functional residual capacity in the lungs and the increased energy required for normal tidal breathing. Pneumonia and pulmonary edema are examples of parenchymal diseases causing reduced compliance (Constable et al. 2017). Any pleural space problem (pneumothorax, septic pleuritis) will also reduce functional residual capacity by reducing the resting lung volume. Flail chest, resulting from dorsal and ventral (segmental) fractures of adjacent ribs, is characterized by paradoxical motion of the thorax during inhalation and exhalation (Hassel 2007; Sprayberry and Barrett 2015). Restrictive diseases can be differentiated by careful auscultation, ultrasound, and thoracic radiography.

### Airway Endoscopy

Endoscopic examination of the airway can be performed in the patient at rest, with or without sedation. In order to accurately evaluate laryngeal function, sedation must not be administered. The use of a standard 1 m endoscope allows assessment of the nasal passages, pharynx, larynx, guttural pouches, and trachea (Byrne and Barakzai 2020). Limited lower airway evaluation can be performed via bronchoscopy with a 2 m pediatric endoscope. Endoscopic evaluation is useful in localizing and identifying causes of upper airway obstruction. Endoscopy additionally allows minimally invasive sampling of tissues or fluids, administration of topical medications (e.g., antifungal medication into guttural pouch), as well as extraction of masses or foreign bodies using forceps, retrieval baskets, or snares. The usefulness of endoscopy can be limited by severe hemorrhage, when the visual field is entirely obscured. However, endoscopy can often be rewarding in identifying a site of slow hemorrhage (e.g., nasal mucosa, sinus drainage angle). It is recommended to commence the endoscopic examination on the less affected laterality to avoid hemorrhage from abbreviating the exam.

### Thoracic Ultrasonography

Thoracic ultrasonography is a valuable modality for effectively evaluating the pleural space, parenchymal surface, pericardium, and myocardium (Lisciandro 2011). It can be used to guide the ideal location for thoracocentesis or chest tube placement, as well as biopsy or aspirate of a mass. The integrity of the ribs and thoracic wall can also be assessed using

1 Teleflex North America, Morrisville, NC, USA.

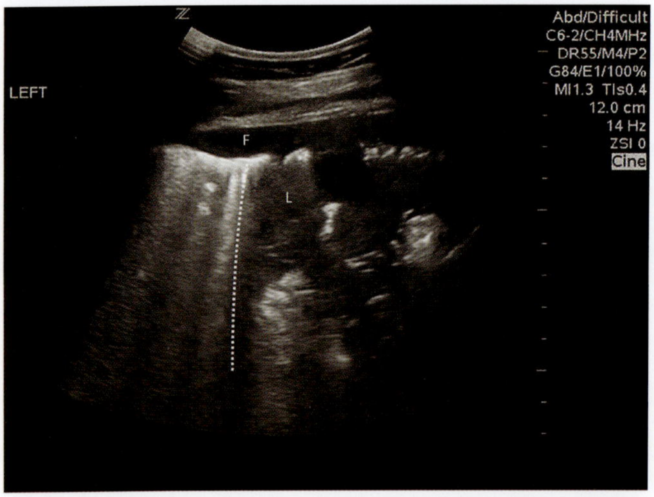


**Figure 11.2** Thoracic ultrasonography revealing a moderate volume of pleural fluid (F) and markedly consolidated, abscessed lung (L, right of the dashed line).

ultrasonography. Normally, a "glide sign" between the pleura and lung should be observed. The glide sign disappears, and static gas shadowing is observed deep to the pleura when gas is present in the thorax. Consolidated or "hepatized" lung and fibrin tags are often observed in conjunction with an accumulation of pleural fluid (Figure 11.2). When the patient is standing, pleural fluid accumulates cranioventrally and is usually easily detected near the $5^{th}$–$8^{th}$ intercostal spaces. Free air in the pleura accumulates caudodorsally. The ribs can be examined transversely and longitudinally to evaluate their structure for fracture margins and displacement. Subcutaneous emphysema will interfere with the ability to examine the thoracic tissues and can result in a reliance on radiographic and clinical findings, or necessitate advanced imaging such as computed tomography (CT). Increasing access and familiarity with ultrasound in general equine practice makes it a valuable diagnostic tool for evaluating and triaging airway disease.

### Thoracic Radiography

Thoracic radiography is useful to evaluate the pulmonary parenchyma, pleural space, mediastinum, thoracic trachea, lymph nodes, and ribs. Radiography is particularly useful in elucidating configuration and displacement in the case of rib fractures, as well as evaluating aeration of the pulmonary parenchyma deep to the pleural surface (Figure 11.3). The feasibility of obtaining diagnostic thoracic radiographs in the field varies with horse size due to the limited power of portable x-ray generators (Constable et al. 2017). A portable x-ray generator and digital radiography system can be useful for thoracic radiography of foals. Lateral and ventrodorsal horizontal beam radiographic views of a recumbent foal can be acquired. Although a full series of diagnostic thoracic radiographs of a mature horse cannot be acquired in the field, a caudodorsal radiograph of the thorax can be beneficial in establishing the diagnosis of pneumothorax when ultrasonography is unavailable. Most referral hospitals have the capability to acquire a complete series of thoracic radiographs, which can aid in making an initial diagnosis and serial monitoring of the patient's condition.

## Emergent Respiratory Problems

### Upper Airway Obstruction and Trauma

*Emergency triage steps:*

**Patient Stabilization**

Multiple equine diseases can manifest as upper respiratory obstruction. However, the cornerstone of treatment for upper respiratory obstruction is immediate tracheotomy followed by therapies targeting the etiology of obstruction. It is prudent to postpone diagnostic testing until after temporary tracheotomy is performed.

Temporary tracheotomy is a procedure that can be performed both in hospital and under field conditions (Box 11.3). The typical site utilized is at the junction of the cranial and middle thirds of the neck, which preserves the cranial third of the neck in case a permanent tracheostomy is subsequently required. There are many types of equine tracheotomy tubes available. "J-shaped" and interlocking tracheotomy tubes are convenient to use, though if significant edema is present ventral to the trachea, an endotracheal tube can be inserted into the tracheotomy site as shorter tubes will easily dislodge with head and neck movement.

(a)

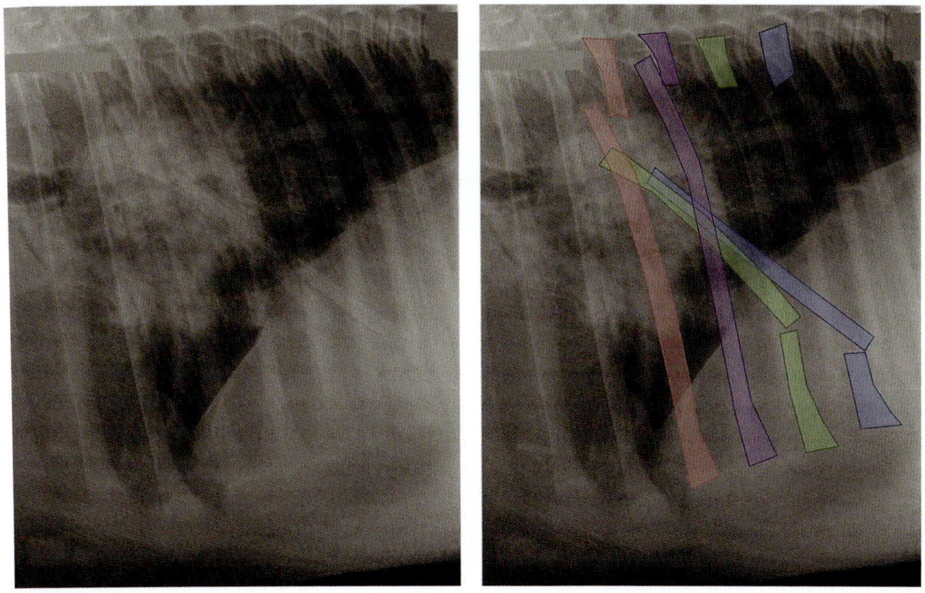

(b)

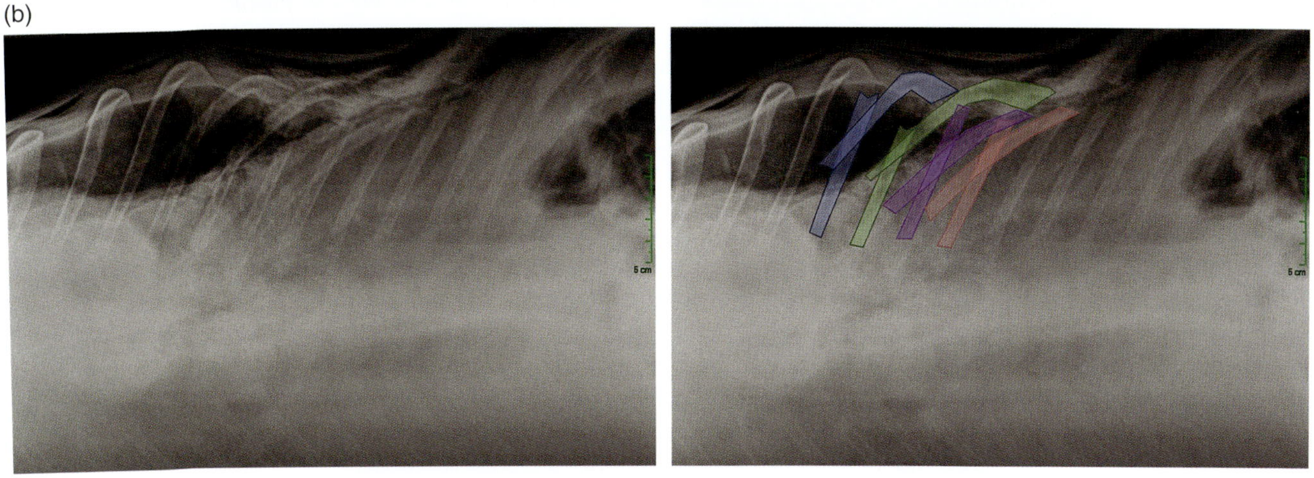


(c)

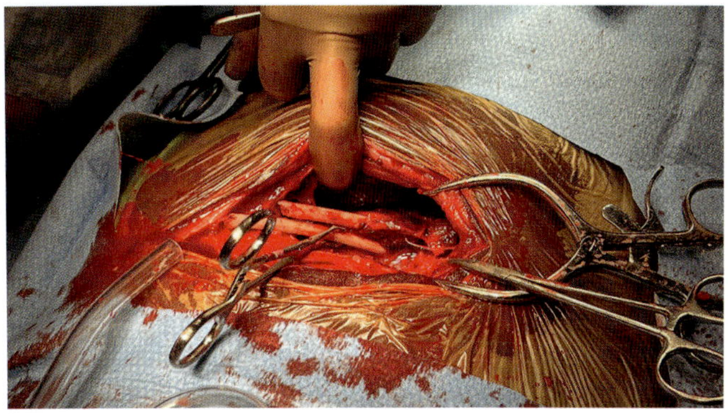

**Figure 11.3** (a) A right lateral, recumbent thoracic radiograph revealing four sequential rib fractures, two of which are segmental and markedly displaced (see blue and green illustrations) and two of which are focal with mild displacement (see purple and pink illustrations). Left-sided pneumothorax and pulmonary opacification (evidence of laceration, contusion) are present. (b) A horizontal beam ventrodorsal thoracic radiograph revealing marked concavity of the thorax at the location of the four adjacent rib fractures. The illustrations are overlaid to highlight the locations of rib fracture and the correlation to the lateral radiographic projection. (c) Intra-operative photograph featuring the displaced ribs penetrating the left lung.

**Box 11.3 Emergency placement of a tracheotomy tube**

1) If circumstances allow, clipping of hair and aseptic preparation should be performed. Lidocaine or another local anesthetic (15–20 mL) can be infiltrated either in a line or an "inverted U" surrounding the proposed surgical site.
2) Following preparation, a 10 cm vertical skin incision is created sharply on ventral midline using a #10 blade and handle.
3) Next, the sternothyrohyoideus muscles are bluntly separated on midline down to the ventral tracheal surface. Palpation of the tracheal surface helps to determine the site for horizontal tracheal incision between two tracheal rings. Incision of tracheal cartilages should be avoided.
4) The tracheal incision, made with a #10 blade, should extend approximately one-third (100°–120°) of the tracheal circumference. Ensure sufficient retraction of the important neurovascular structures abaxial to the site of tracheal incision.
5) Care should be taken to incise the ventral tracheal mucosa to prevent tunneling of the tracheotomy tube in the submucosal region upon insertion, and to avoid laceration of the dorsal tracheal mucosa if a rigid tracheotomy tube is inserted.
6) Airflow will be evident upon penetration of the tracheal mucosa. Lifting the horse's head will widen the distance between tracheal rings and facilitate tracheotomy tube placement.

*Practice tip:* If a tracheotomy tube is not available in an emergency setting, a temporary tube can be made using a 1-gallon hollow plastic jug handle from an empty surgical preparation solution container. Alternatively, a syringe case or barrel of appropriate size with the end transected to form a hollow tube will provide a conduit for air flow until a proper tube can be placed.

Keep a tracheotomy kit assembled and available in an ambulatory vehicle or hospital to allow efficient care of patients in upper airway distress. Scalpel blades loaded on disposable handles are particularly useful in these instances, in addition to a small pack of instruments, including mayo scissors and a Crile forceps. Ideally, several sizes of tracheotomy tubes should be stocked.

### How to Formulate a Diagnostic Plan

A common presentation for respiratory distress in horses is extramural compression of the upper respiratory tract. For example, prominent mandibular and retropharyngeal lymph node enlargement, commonly accompanied by purulent nasal discharge, are hallmarks of *S. equi* infection. In cases of *S. equi* infection, site of lymph node enlargement and abscessation will determine the approach to surgical treatment. Well-demarcated abscesses that are not yet open and draining and compress airway diameter should be drained and sampled for culture and sensitivity. In the submandibular region, ventral surgical drainage is uncomplicated (Boyle et al. 2018). If the retropharyngeal lymph node is the source of abscessation, ultrasound guidance should be used. Short-acting injectable anesthetic can allow rapid and safe surgical drainage in young, poorly compliant horses where careful dissection is required. Upper airway endoscopy and radiography can aid in assessing guttural pouch involvement. Temporary tracheotomy might be necessary in some cases of upper airway obstruction due to *S. equi* abscessation; however, caution should be used. In some cases, the primary site of airway obstruction could be at the location of the tracheo-bronchial lymph nodes and, if this occurs, temporary tracheotomy performed in the cervical region will not improve respiratory function (Boyle et al. 2018). Thoracic radiography can be useful in evaluating this potential cause of obstruction.

Another common problem is arytenoid chondritis which can affect one or both arytenoid cartilages within the larynx (Figure 11.4). Infection of the arytenoid cartilage with and without abscessation results in significant enlargement, decreased motion, and diminished upper airway diameter (Byrne and Barakzai 2020). Uncommonly, chondritis is associated with a foreign body or neoplasia. If respiratory distress results, temporary tracheotomy should be instituted. Laryngeal ultrasound is a useful diagnostic modality for assessing the extent and location of soft tissue and cartilage infection as well as for evaluating for the presence of abscessation that would benefit from surgical drainage. Once the airway is secure, treatments include antibiotics, anti-inflammatories, abscess drainage, and supportive care. Treatment and response to treatment can be guided and evaluated using an endoscope passed transnasally or retrograde through a temporary tracheotomy. Laryngotomy, to establish midline drainage of an arytenoid abscess with transendoscopic guidance, can be performed with the horse standing, under sedation, and with appropriate local anesthesia. Sampling of the abscess with a sheathed swab can allow collection of a useful specimen for culture and sensitivity. Horses can develop persistent deformation of the arytenoid cartilage, or arytenoid chondrosis. In these cases, arytenoidectomy may be necessary to maintain airway function.

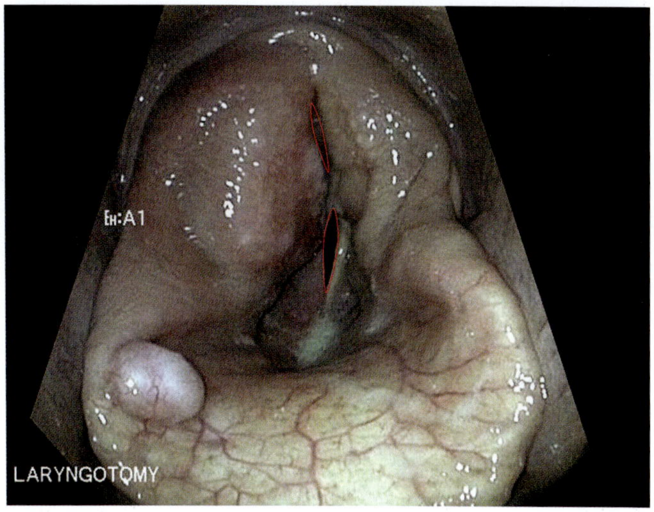


**Figure 11.4** Bilateral arytenoid chondritis causing upper airway obstruction. Airway lumen is outlined in red *Source:* M. Ziad Al-Ani, Robin J.M. Gray.

Upper airway obstruction may also occur acutely during anesthetic recovery. Sources of upper airway obstruction are typically nasal mucosal edema or dynamic laryngeal collapse (Hardcastle et al. 2012; Tute et al. 1996). Nasal edema is more common in horses following surgery in dorsal recumbency, prolonged surgery, or in horses with low colloid osmotic pressure. The placement of nasopharyngeal tubes when the patient is positioned in the operating room can diminish the development of nasal edema. They are recommended for high-risk patients. Horses with significant nasal edema will have increased airway noise both during inspiration and expiration. Treatment of nasal edema is not necessary unless edema is severe and results in significant airway noise or patient distress. If severe, treatments include nasal intubation, nasotracheal intubation, or application of 20–30 mL of topical 1% phenylephrine solution. Phenylephrine solution can be administered by connecting a syringe to a red rubber catheter and inserting this into each nostril. The beneficial effect of topical phenylephrine can be expected within 5–10 minutes of administration.

An intraoperative extended head and neck position as well as peri-neural surgical trauma predisposes horses to laryngeal collapse post-operatively. Horses that develop dynamic laryngeal collapse following anesthetic recovery will have increased airway noise during inspiration. Dynamic laryngeal collapse can be a serious and life-threatening emergency and should be treated with tracheotomy or oro- or nasotracheal intubation upon collapse (Ronaldson et al. 2020). Upper airway endoscopy should be performed to confirm this diagnosis once the patient is stable. Occasionally, horses can have persistent dorsal displacement of the soft palate (DDSP) following standard oro-tracheal intubation. DDSP will likely not result in respiratory distress but can result in a fluttering or gurgling airway noise during expiration. In horses with normal airway function, the soft palate will be replaced easily once swallowing is elicited.

Foals with abnormal guttural pouch ostia are prone to developing guttural pouch tympany. This condition presents uni- or bilaterally in foals with bulbous enlargement noted at Viborg's triangle and stertorous respiration. When bilateral, this condition usually results in respiratory distress necessitating tracheotomy. Upper airway endoscopy of the pharynx and guttural pouches confirms the diagnosis. Definitive treatment can include transnasal placement of an indwelling foley catheter in the guttural pouch, which can also be used rather than tracheotomy if the patient's systemic condition permits. Alternatively, salpingopharyngeal laser fistulation of the guttural pouches can be performed (Bell 2007; Krebs and Schmotzer 2007).

Though relatively uncommon, venomous snakebites to the nose can result in tremendous pain and swelling of the cranial and cervical regions in addition to respiratory distress due to upper airway obstruction (Dickinson et al. 1996). In some cases, nasal cannulas made from syringe cases can be inserted to maintain airway function. In more severe cases, temporary tracheotomy is necessary to secure the airway in the acute phase of disease. Although puncture wounds from snake bites are rarely identified, the development of acute, severe, and painful swelling in a geographical region endemic to venomous snakes should prioritize this diagnosis.

Choanal atresia is a rare congenital condition in which either a membranous, bony, or combination tissue obstructs the flow of air between the nasal passages and the nasopharynx (James et al. 2006; Richardson et al. 1994). The bilateral condition is fatal at birth unless emergency intervention of emergency tracheotomy or orotracheal intubation is performed. Upper airway endoscopy can confirm the diagnosis, as can contrast radiography of the patient's skull. The prognosis is grave for patients affected bilaterally; if the foaling is unattended they are found dead. Establishing an emergency airway

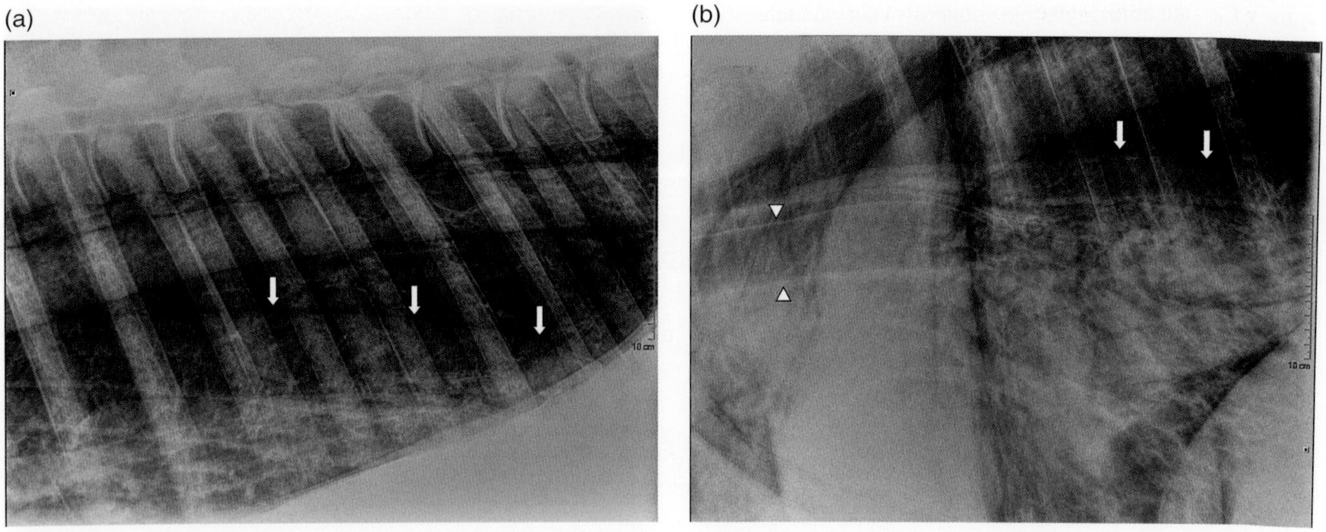


**Figure 11.5** (a) Lateral radiographic view of the caudal thorax demonstrating a pneumothorax. Arrows delineate the margin of collapsed lung. (b) Lateral radiographic projection of the mid-thorax revealing pneumomediastinum in addition to pneumothorax. Arrows delineate the margin of collapsed lung. Arrowheads illustrate the tracheal margin observed as a result of the pneumomediastinum. *Source:* Courtesy of P.N. Goode.

provides the opportunity for surgical treatment. Reports of surgical treatment include transnasal perforation and transendoscopic laser fenestration of obstructing tissue. Complications include stenosis at the surgery site and protracted courses of treatment. Foals with unilateral choanal atresia are not in respiratory distress, and the timing of their surgical treatment is an elective procedure.

Trauma to the cervical region may also be life threatening. Penetrating trauma in the cervical region can result in significant injury to multiple vital structures, including the recurrent laryngeal nerve, vagosympathetic trunk, jugular vein, and carotid artery. Tracheal penetration is often accompanied by emphysema (for additional information on emergency triage of this problem, see Chapter 7). Tracheal rupture or perforation could also lead to pneumomediastinum and pneumothorax, resulting in clinical signs consistent with hypotension and respiratory distress (Byrne and Barakzai 2020). Treatment of respiratory distress secondary to emphysema related to tracheal perforation is often temporary tracheotomy over or caudal to the site of injury. Thoracic ultrasound might not be valuable in the case of extensive emphysema; however, thoracic radiographs can confirm the presence of pneumomediastinum or pneumothorax (Boy and Sweeney 2000) (Figure 11.5). Treatment for tracheal rupture associated with severe clinical signs is surgical repair of the defect. The site of the defect can be confirmed endoscopically. Surgical repair should be performed with the horse in the standing position, unless extensive injury requires resection and anastomosis of the trachea.

### Emergency Treatment Guidelines Beyond Stabilization

***Hospital Referral vs Farm Management*** Often, a horse with moderate airway compression will progress to distress with the stress of trailer transport. In addition to temporary tracheotomy, consider judicious use of anxiolytics such as acepromazine prior to transit and manage the referral to minimize stressors, such as keeping mares and unweaned foals together. Referral centers should be cautioned regarding the case details and recognize that acute decompensation is a risk of transport. Similarly, horses with snake envenomation or traumatic head injuries affecting the airway can have progressive swelling that further compromises airway diameter and are additionally subject to transport risk (Constable et al. 2017).

***Decision for Medical vs Surgical Treatment*** Endoscopy is an important modality for assessment of the upper respiratory tract. A flexible, 1-m scope allows assessment of the nasal passages, ethmoid turbinates, nasal maxillary opening, pharynx, guttural pouches, larynx, and trachea. Most importantly, endoscopy allows for an accurate anatomic and functional evaluation, which is often not possible through other modalities. Endoscopy is essential to the diagnosis of many upper respiratory disorders and is especially helpful in cases of upper respiratory obstruction once temporary tracheotomy has been completed. An accurate understanding of normal anatomy is a skill required for upper airway endoscopy interpretation. Performance of the initial resting examination unsedated is necessary to evaluate laryngeal function. Skull radiographs along with upper airway endoscopy can be evaluated to determine the cause of obstruction or extent of trauma and aid in the decision making for surgical intervention.

***How to Manage Important Complications*** Persistent hemorrhage associated with skull trauma should be managed by packing wounds, supportive care (permissive hypotension, whole blood, colloids), and tying the horse's head at wither height with feed offered in a trough.

Temporary tracheotomy tubes should be monitored closely for obstruction. The silicone tubes should be left without cuff inflation to avoid tracheal mucosal injury and to limit the risk of complete tracheal and tube obstruction by discharge. Therefore, the nickel-plated brass, self-retaining, Pape's model tracheotomy tubes[2] are preferred for safety. Tracheostomy tubes must be checked or changed daily to identify and prevent obstruction from tracheal secretions.

Post-obstruction pulmonary edema, secondary to upper airway obstruction, as well as pneumothorax, which can result from tracheal laceration, are discussed later in this chapter.

***Estimating Prognosis and Decision for Euthanasia*** Prognosis for horses with respiratory distress is highly dependent on the etiology. As with other diseases, limiting the injury-treatment intervals could facilitate the best outcome.

## Lower Airway Obstruction

Lower airway obstruction in the horse is usually associated with chronic inflammation of the airways. Equine asthma describes the three related conditions: inflammatory airway disease (IAD), recurrent airway obstruction (RAO, Heaves), and summer pasture recurrent airway obstruction (SPRAO) (Bond et al. 2018). Patient stabilization is outlined in Box 11.4.

*Emergency triage steps:*

Marked tracheal collapse is another cause of lower airway obstruction in the horse; affected horses often require an emergency tracheotomy (Box 11.3). If feasible, the tracheotomy should be performed caudal to the site of tracheal collapse. In most emergency scenarios, this is unknown, so the tracheotomy should be performed in the mid-to-caudal third of the cervical trachea. Exceptional care should be made to protect vital structures in the vicinity as the tracheotomy is performed; tracheal collapse can increase their mobility and therefore the vulnerability of these structures to injury. Endotracheal tube placement through the tracheotomy will be necessary to increase the diameter of the trachea if the horse's respiratory distress is not alleviated by the tracheotomy alone (Aleman et al. 2008).

### How to Formulate a Diagnostic Plan

Horses with severe asthma can develop an acute respiratory crisis. These horses might have a classic "heave line" or known history of asthma. Wheezes are appreciated on pulmonary auscultation and mucoid nasal discharge is often noted. Thoracic ultrasound, radiographs, bronchoalveolar lavage (BAL), and bloodwork can confirm the diagnosis (Couetil et al. 2020; Marr 2016). An aseptic suppurative BAL and mature, inflammatory leukogram are diagnostic of equine asthma.

**Box 11.4 Patient stabilization for equine asthma**

1) For horses with asthma, treatment includes dexamethasone 0.1 mg/kg intravenously and atropine 0.014–0.02 mg/kg intravenously.
2) Oral albuterol or clenbuterol and inhaled corticosteroid treatment can be helpful once labored breathing is controlled (Cha and Costa 2017). Intranasal oxygen is also helpful.
3) Ensure the horse is housed in a well-ventilated area, offer only soaked or steamed feed, and remove stressors from the environment (Couetil et al. 2020).

2 JorVet, Jorgensen Laboratories, Loveland, CO, USA.

Although tracheal collapse has been reported in a variety of breeds, tracheal collapse in miniature horses and ponies is reported with increased frequency (Aleman et al. 2008). Affected animals commonly make wheezing or honking noises during respiration and often have an elevated expiratory effort. Extra-thoracic tracheal collapse results in inspiratory distress, whereas expiratory respiratory difficulty is associated with intra-thoracic tracheal collapse. A horse can be affected by either or both. Palpation of the cervical trachea might provide an indication of the location and extent of tracheal collapse. Airway endoscopy, ultrasound (to identify tracheal ring fractures), and radiography are beneficial diagnostics for thoroughly evaluating the trachea. Radiograph acquisition should be timed to highlight maximal collapse at end-inspiration (extra-thoracic trachea) and end-expiration (intra-thoracic trachea).

#### Emergency Treatment Guidelines Beyond Stabilization

***Hospital Referral vs Farm Management*** Transport to a referral hospital should be delayed to allow improvement in the patient's condition and eliminate distress by the administration of the above medications. When stable, indications for travel to a hospital include the need for ongoing oxygen supplementation or systemic support, the desire to confirm the diagnosis, or to monitor chronic disease with thoracic radiographs. The desire to further treat or evaluate the patient in the hospital should be weighed against the risk of decompensation during poorly ventilated, stressful transport or hospitalization. Diagnostic evaluation by endoscopy and radiography is indicated in cases of tracheal collapse once the patient's airway has been secured to the greatest possible extent. Intra-thoracic airway collapse cannot be resolved on an emergency basis, so the patient's status should be carefully considered before transport.

***Decision for Medical vs Surgical Treatment*** Lower airway obstruction by bronchoconstriction and poor mucociliary clearance, as observed in equine asthma, is a medically managed disease process. Creating a low-dust environment is imperative to control of equine asthma. Maximal turnout or a well-ventilated stall without shavings or straw (paper pellets or cardboard bedding are appropriate alternatives) should be provided. Inhaled (nebulized) medications can improve airway diameter and clearance; these include albuterol, acetylcysteine, cromolyn sodium, and ciclosenide. Systemically, omega-3 fatty acids and vitamin C can decrease the inflammatory response against environmental allergens.

Medical management of tracheal collapse (avoidance of exercise, stressful conditions, and environmental irritants) might provide relief in the short term for patients early in the course of chondrodysplastic disease (Aleman et al. 2008) or cricoid laryngeal and tracheal cartilage fracture. However, it is unlikely to result in a comfortable outcome for the patient in the long-term. Surgical interventions are possible and can include extra- or intra-luminal stenting. A permanent tracheostomy can be feasible for a patient whose cranial cervical trachea is affected (e.g., due to trauma). The success of surgical intervention likely depends on the location, cause, and extent of tracheal collapse.

***How to Manage Important Complications*** In severe cases of equine asthma, bacterial pneumonia can develop secondary to steroid treatment and poor clearance of the lower airway. Bronchoalveolar lavage can confirm this diagnosis, and culture of the fluid can help to direct treatment. The patient's temperature, CBC, and thoracic imaging should be monitored during treatment with systemic (± nebulized) antibiotics.

***Estimating Prognosis and Decision for Euthanasia*** Control of the clinical signs and progression of equine asthma relies heavily on the appropriate management of the patient on farm. These management practices include offering good quality-soaked or steamed feeds, housing in a well-ventilated area, exercise in an area without excessive dust, and avoidance of dusty bedding to limit the likelihood of acute episodes or respiratory distress (Couetil et al. 2020). Chronically, bloodwork, bronchoalveolar lavage, thoracic radiographs, and ultrasound can be used serially to monitor the patient's progression and more precisely delineate prognosis.

## Pulmonary Parenchyma and Pleural Space Conditions

*Emergency triage steps:*

### Patient stabilization

Intranasal oxygen is recommended during evaluation and initial treatment of patients with presumed pulmonary parenchymal or pleural space conditions. Patient stabilization for pneumothorax is summarized in Box 11.5 (for additional information on emergency triage of thoracic trauma, see Chapter 7).

**Box 11.5 Emergency treatment of pneumothorax has two aims (Hassel 2007; Sprayberry and Barrett 2015)**

1) First, an attempt should be made to surgically repair the chest wound and rib fractures if present, and, if this is not possible or appropriate, to seal the wound with an adherent bandage (Figure 11.6). Clinicians should also attempt to stabilize a flail portion of the chest with a bandage if possible.
2) The second aim of treatment is to evacuate the air from the chest. This can be performed with a sterile teat cannula, needle, or chest tube inserted into the dorsal pleural space following aseptic preparation and local anesthesia. The needle, cannula, or tube is placed in the dorsal $12^{th}$–$15^{th}$ intercostal space, but rib spaces further cranial may also be used.
3) If repeated evacuation of air is needed, a small chest tube can be inserted and sutured in place. A three-way stopcock or Heimlich valve can be fastened to the end of the chest tube for intermittent or continuous removal of air from the chest.

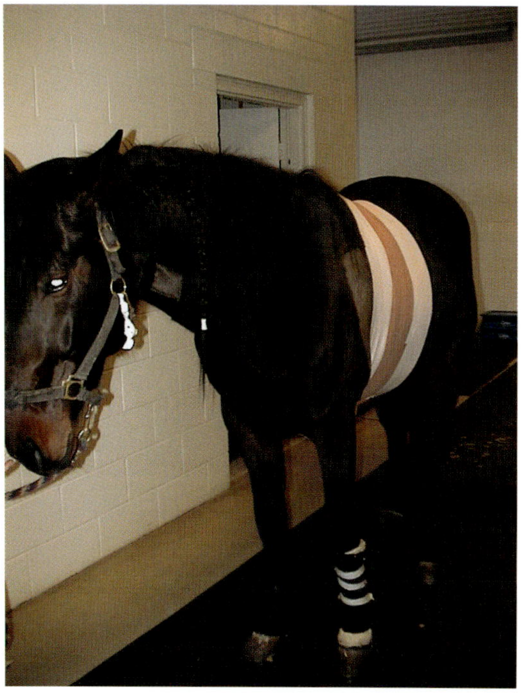

**Figure 11.6** Three year-old Standardbred trotting horse following penetrating thoracic injury. The horse was stabilized via bandaging of the thoracic wound, intranasal oxygen therapy, and removal of pleural air. The horse had internal lung injury associated with displaced rib fractures. Surgical exploration of the thorax was required via thoracotomy under general anesthesia to repair the lung laceration, stabilize the rib fractures, lavage the chest cavity, and close the wound. The horse recovered following surgery and returned to previous performance.

Emergency treatment of pleural fluid accumulation involves the placement of a chest drain on the affected side(s) to allow evacuation of fluid, followed by appropriate further diagnostics, and both targeted and supportive treatments. If placement of the drain is needed near the pericardium, ultrasound guidance is important to prevent inadvertent pericardial and cardiac trauma. Fenestrated chest tubes of various sizes with a blunt trocar (16–32 French Straight Argyle Catheter, Covidien) should be placed in the site of largest fluid accumulation, which is commonly in the $7^{th}$ intercostal space, 2 in. above the point of the elbow. The size of the chest tube may be selected based upon the character of the pleural fluid, with thicker exudate requiring a larger diameter chest tube (Chaffin et al. 2000). Local anesthetic is infiltrated following aseptic preparation. A #10 scalpel is used to create a small skin incision, then a chest tube with a blunt trocar is introduced perpendicular to the chest wall. Firm pressure is needed to insert the chest tube and often, pleural fluid is evident around the sharp trocar prior to removal upon successful placement. Once the majority of the fluid is evacuated, a Heimlich valve can be secured to the chest drain to promote fluid and gas drainage while preventing the ingress of air. The chest tube is secured to the skin using a finger trap suture technique.

Post-obstructive pulmonary edema treatment consists of furosemide diuresis (1 mg/kg IV) and oxygen supplementation. Smoke inhalation, which results from a barn or wildfire, can cause severe pulmonary edema. Oxygen supplementation, diuretic (furosemide) and anti-inflammatory therapy should be initiated (Constable et al. 2017). IV access should be established to manage burn shock if present and provide other directed treatments. Therapy with a nebulized bronchodilator should be considered. Severe heat injury that often accompanies smoke inhalation can cause upper airway obstruction because of direct injury to the upper airway tissues, including secondary edema and mucosal sloughing. See earlier in the chapter for a description of upper airway obstruction stabilization (Marsh 2007).

#### How to Formulate a Diagnostic Plan

Penetrating chest wounds can be life threatening. Clinical manifestation is dependent upon location of the wound and the structures damaged during injury. Pneumothorax should be suspected in wounds through which air movement occurs with each breath. Flail chest is evident by the paradoxical movement of a section of the rib cage during respiration. Pneumothorax can occasionally occur with traumatic cervical trauma, axillary wounds, and other sources of subcutaneous emphysema. Ultrasonographic exam can be used to confirm the presence or absence of pneumothorax (Figure 11.7). Pneumothorax can be ruled out when the caudo-dorsal lung tips or "glide sign" are visible during respiration.

Trauma to the chest and abdomen can result in fluid accumulation and critical emergency. Penetrating trauma and extension of infection into the mediastinal or pleural space regions is rare but can occur. Digital palpation, thoracic radiographs, and ultrasound can assist in discerning the likelihood of mediastinal and pleural involvement (Lisciandro 2011; Sprayberry and Barrett 2015). Thoracocentesis or thoracic drains can be used in conjunction with other therapies to treat these complicated wounds and evaluate the quality of accumulated fluid. Sterile packing of wounds will facilitate contracture and assist in the resolution of other complications such as subcutaneous emphysema (Hassel 2007; Sprayberry and Barrett 2015) and flail chest (Laverty et al. 1996). Respiratory distress can result from significant pleural fluid accumulation. Rapid ultrasound examination of the chest in the 7th and 8th rib spaces at the level of the lower third of the chest wall can confirm the presence of pleural fluid, indicate the amount, and determine bilateral involvement. Conditions resulting in significant pleural fluid accumulation include septic pleuritis, fulminant pleuropneumonia, thoracic esophageal perforation, diaphragmatic hernia, mediastinal neoplasia, and thoracic trauma.

Post-obstruction pulmonary edema is the sudden onset of pulmonary edema following upper airway obstruction and can result in respiratory distress (Constable et al. 2017; Hardcastle et al. 2012; Tute et al. 1996). Forceful inhalation occurring during upper airway obstruction results in increased negative intrathoracic pressure followed by increased venous return, decreased cardiac output, and alveolar fluid transudation. Horses that develop post-obstruction pulmonary edema are distressed, tachypneic, and have auscultable crackles upon examination of the chest bilaterally. Characteristic frothy airway secretions can be evident from the nostrils or tracheostomy site, and decreased oxygen saturation is a common sequela.

#### Emergency Treatment Guidelines Beyond Stabilization

***Hospital Referral vs Farm Management*** The requirement for supportive care including oxygen supplementation, fluid resuscitation, monitoring of thoracic air and fluid accumulation, and caring for indwelling chest tubes will dictate the need for hospitalization. Additionally, surgical intervention for wounds or penetrating foreign bodies may necessitate referral.

***Decision for Medical vs Surgical Treatment*** Thoracic trauma is likely to require surgical intervention when the chest wall is involved. Surgical wounds may be closed if they are acute and clean or sufficiently debrided. Alternatively, they might require drainage, packing, and stent bandaging. Unstable rib fractures might require stabilization to avoid causing

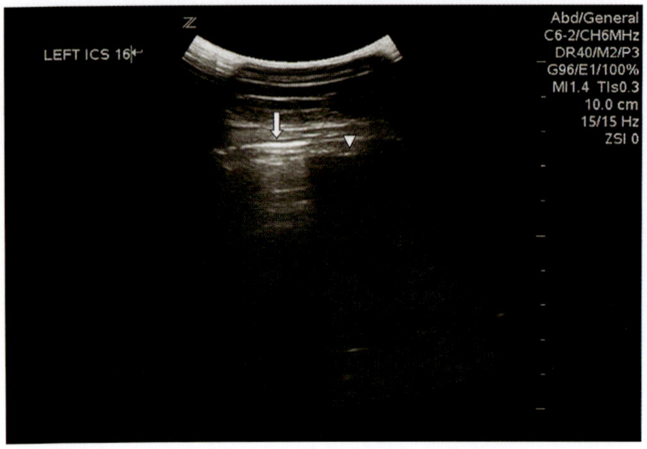


**Figure 11.7** Thoracic ultrasonography revealing a pneumothorax. The arrow demonstrates a hyperechoic line representing the presence of pleural gas. The arrowhead points at the pleural surface, ventral to the dorsal accumulation of gas.

intrathoracic trauma and to permit healing (Hassel 2007; Laverty et al. 1996; Sprayberry and Barrett 2015). Surgery should be performed standing whenever possible to avoid the ventilatory and recovery risks of general anesthesia. However, with severe or deep penetrating injury, general anesthesia is essential, allowing for ventilation control during exploration and repair of thoracic injury. If hemostasis is not feasible by medical means following intra-thoracic trauma, thoracotomy or thoracoscopy might be indicated to evaluate the cause of hemorrhage, apply topical hemostatic agents, or ligate the source of hemorrhage.

***How to Manage Important Complications*** Initial medical treatment of substantial intra-thoracic hemorrhage is recommended. Aminocaproic acid, an antifibrinolytic agent, can be administered at 40 mg/kg IV slowly once, then 20 mg/kg IV slowly every 6 h as needed (Plumb 2015). The medication is administered in 1 L of saline over 20 minutes. Blood transfusion and fluid resuscitation should be aimed at maintaining permissive hypotension (i.e., MAP 60–70 mmHg) (Divers et al. 2022). If the patient's own blood can be aseptically collected from the pleural space, an autotransfusion can be administered.

A persistent pneumothorax can result from substantial pulmonary injury causing leakage of air into the pleural space while the chest cavity is sealed. A large pulmonary laceration might require suture or staple closure via thoracotomy or thoracoscopy to resolve the tension pneumothorax if it cannot be sufficiently managed by supportive thoracic decompression.

Pleuropneumonia with or without a thoracic abscess can develop secondary to thoracic trauma. Sampling of the pleural fluid or abscess for culture and sensitivity testing, establishing drainage via ultrasound guidance, thoracotomy or thoracoscopy with an indwelling drain, and providing lavage in addition to broad spectrum antibiotics may allow resolution of the secondary disease.

***Estimating Prognosis and Decision for Euthanasia*** The patient's prognosis depends on the extent of thoracic wall, mediastinal, and pulmonary injury. Cardiac injury can be acute and rapidly fatal. Extensive hemorrhage can result from severe trauma and require intensive management for survival. Additionally, the ability to control infection, air, and fluid accumulation within the chest influences survival and the rate of complications. Extrathoracic injury may accompany thoracic trauma and significantly decreases the prognosis for survival (Laverty et al. 1996). However, the prognosis for many horses is favorable with appropriate management.

## Synchronous Diaphragmatic Flutter

Synchronous diaphragmatic flutter or "thumps" is associated with the clinical sign of rhythmic movement of the flank resulting from diaphragmatic contraction synchronous with the heartbeat. For this reason, caretakers of horses with this condition often seek care for a primary respiratory disorder as the respiratory pattern is so extraordinary and the horses often exhibit grunting and appear to be in distress. Synchronous diaphragmatic flutter can occur in athletic horses following exertion or in horses with severe systemic disease resulting in marked ionized hypoglycemia, hypomagnesemia, or both (Constable et al. 2017). Patient stabilization of horses with synchronous diaphragmatic flutter is outlined in Box 11.6.

*Emergency triage steps:*

### How to Formulate a Diagnostic Plan

Point-of-care evaluation of peripheral ionized calcium is a key first step to confirm synchronous diaphragmatic flutter in horses that display characteristic signs of this disorder. Timely evaluation is especially indicated in horses considered at higher risk of this disorder such as those participating in endurance riding events, lactating mares, or horses with severe enterocolitis with associated electrolyte disturbances.

**Box 11.6 Patient stabilization for synchronous diaphragmatic flutter**

1) Treatment is immediate administration of 0.5–1 mL/kg (0.58 mEq/kg) of calcium gluconate given intravenously by slow infusion.
2) Higher doses, or repeated dosing, might be required depending on response to therapy. Respiratory function should begin to improve immediately upon intravenous infusion of calcium (Constable et al. 2017).

### Emergency Treatment Guidelines Beyond Stabilization

***Hospital Referral vs Farm Management*** Underlying conditions resulting in hypocalcemia will dictate referral in individual cases. The need for continuous supplementation can necessitate referral.

***Decision for Medical vs Surgical Treatment*** Use care in discriminating this disorder from a primary respiratory disorder or other condition resulting in distress, such as colic or myopathy.

***How to Manage Important Complications*** Following initial triage and acute correction of hypocalcemia, continued assessment and treatment is required to address the underlying condition resulting in the disturbance.

***Estimating Prognosis and Decision for Euthanasia*** The prognosis is dependent on the primary cause of the disorder. Adequate supplementation of calcium should resolve the condition for those patients without a persistent cause of calcium deficiency. Careful management of patients with ongoing calcium losses is required to avoid relapse.

## Hemorrhage from the Nostrils

*Emergency triage steps:*

### Patient stabilization

Blood can appear at the nostrils (epistaxis) for a variety of reasons, including because of nasal injury, foreign bodies or masses, skull and sinus trauma, guttural pouch mycosis, and pulmonary hemorrhage (Archer 2008). The extent of patient stabilization required will depend on the volume of blood loss as well as the type and severity of trauma (Box 11.7).

### How to Formulate a Diagnostic Plan

Airway endoscopy is a useful diagnostic tool for localizing the source of hemorrhage, except when profuse bleeding obliterates any ability to visualize tissues. If this is the case, the hemorrhage is often localized to the guttural pouches or lungs. When blood originates from the nasal mucosa, the nasomaxillary sinus drainage angle, or the ethmoids, skull radiographs can be useful in revealing bone trauma or masses. Fluid accumulation in the guttural pouches can also be noted radiographically. Depending on the stability of the skull, patient's systemic and neurologic status as well as the need for further information, skull CT may be a necessary next step (Tietje et al. 1996). Hemorrhage originating from the trachea or lower airway should be further assessed with thoracic ultrasound and radiographs. Hemorrhage from the guttural

**Box 11.7 Patient stabilization guidelines for horses with epistaxis**

1) In cases of nasal or skull trauma, evaluate airflow through the nares and rule out the need for an emergency tracheotomy. Evaluation of the patient's neurologic status should be made to estimate the potential for cerebral involvement when skull trauma is noted (Feary et al. 2007).
2) Intravenous access should be secured with catheter placement to administer fluid resuscitation. An immediate crystalloid fluid resuscitation bolus of 10–20 mL/kg is generally recommended with marked hemorrhage.
3) Further fluid therapy should be aimed at maintaining permissive hypotension (MAP 60–70 mmHg) if hemorrhage remains uncontrolled (Divers et al. 2022). Otherwise, fluid therapy with crystalloids, whole blood, hypertonic saline and/or colloids should be directed at correcting losses and ensuring adequate perfusion. Aminocaproic acid can be a useful adjunct to decrease hemorrhage.
4) If severe bleeding is perceived to be imminently fatal, as is sometimes the case in guttural pouch mycosis, bilateral temporary ligation of the common carotid arteries can be attempted (Woodie et al. 2002). Anecdotally, in cases of active, severe guttural pouch hemorrhage, ligation of the ipsilateral common carotid artery has also been successful in providing life-saving hemostasis without risking bilateral vagal/recurrent laryngeal nerve damage. Either procedure can occasionally sufficiently slow bleeding to save the patient's life while emergency assessment and further surgical intervention can be initiated.
5) Intranasal oxygen (15 L/min) will be beneficial until lower airway disease is ruled out and adequate perfusion is established.

pouches, pharynx, and trachea generally exits via both nostrils, whereas hemorrhage originating more rostral from the ethmoids, sinus drainage angle, or other structures is most commonly unilateral. When guttural pouch hemorrhage is mild, it can also be unilateral.

## Emergency Treatment Guidelines Beyond Stabilization

***Hospital Referral vs Farm Management*** Acute epistaxis without known trauma is an indication for emergency upper airway endoscopy and evaluation of the guttural pouches. If this cannot be performed on farm, the patient should be stabilized and transported for evaluation. The volume of blood loss should be estimated prior to shipping and the patient should be transported so that their head can be positioned for adequate nasal drainage to avoid aspiration of blood.

***Decision for Medical vs Surgical Treatment*** Guttural pouch mycosis should be treated with surgical intervention (arterial occlusion by balloon catheter, coils, or nitinol plugs) when fungal plaques cover or are in very close proximity to the major vessels of the guttural pouch (Freeman 2015). Whether the procedure is performed standing or under general anesthesia will depend on the patient's systemic condition, the surgeon's comfort, available facilities/equipment, and surgical team familiarity with a specific protocol. Medical treatment, including topical anti-fungal ointment, guttural pouch fenestration, housing and feeding management changes are reasonable alternatives when fungal plaques are present in the guttural pouch but not directly attached to major vessels. Medical management may also be required for treatment of concurrent dysphagia by dietary adjustment, the use of an indwelling feeding tube, or judicious vocal cord injection bulking.

Skull trauma is commonly addressed with surgical excision of small bone fragments or internal fixation of substantial fractures or those close to the orbit. Lavage is often required to remove blood clots from the paranasal sinus and reduce the risk of a secondary sinusitis.

Hemorrhage from the lower airway can be an indication for surgery when abnormal lung (e.g., neoplasia) is identified and can be excised via thoracotomy or thoracoscopy. However, many of these cases deteriorate rapidly, despite medical support, without the opportunity for surgical intervention.

***How to Manage Important Complications*** Uncontrolled hemorrhage can precipitate marked anxiety, striking, and seizures, all of which have the potential to cause injury to the clinician, handler, and other personnel. Manage the patient to keep those working with the horse safe. Use sedation as needed, ensure a patent airway, and provide adequate fluid resuscitation. An IV jugular catheter with an extension set is useful for rapid administration of medication or fluids in these cases.

***Estimating Prognosis and Decision for Euthanasia*** With appropriate surgical intervention, horses affected by guttural pouch mycosis over vital vessels have a fair prognosis for survival when intervention is initiated before severe hemorrhage occurs (Freeman 2015). The prognosis for survival is negatively impacted by dysphagia and the likely sequela of aspiration pneumonia (Lepage 2024).

The prognosis associated with lower airway hemorrhage is tied to its etiology. For example, exercise-induced pulmonary hemorrhage (EIPH) has a good prognosis for resolution by controlling exercise and treating the patient with furosemide. However, acute lower airway bleeding due to neoplasia or thoracic trauma has a poor prognosis for survival (Marr 2016).

### Case Example 11.1 Upper Respiratory Distress

***Respiratory Emergency:***

*Patient: 5-year-old Dutch Warmblood mare*

History: Mid-May of first show season; recently returned from week-long show. Decreased appetite and quiet attitude over the past 48 h. Owner reports fever and swelling around the throatlatch. Increasing respiratory noise over the past 24 h. Outstretched neck and nostril flaring recently noted by farm hand. Emergency evaluation requested for acute worsening of upper respiratory noise and effort.

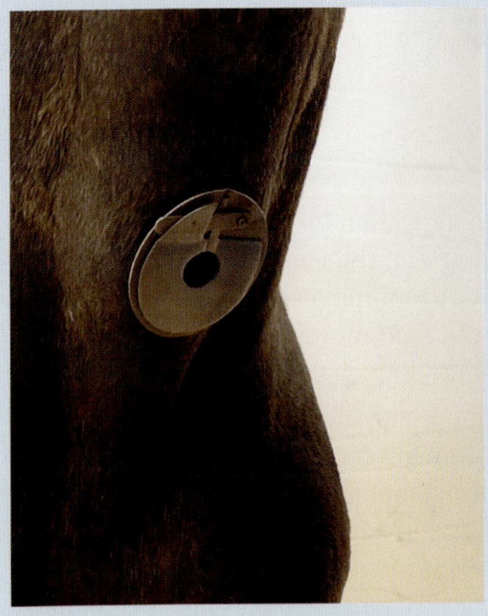

**Figure 11.8** Temporary tracheotomy site with a self-retaining papes (JorVet, Jorgensen Laboratories, Loveland, CO, USA) model tracheotomy tube.

*Step 1: Patient Stabilization:*
Rapidly evaluate and provide immediate stabilization.

1) Have a high index of suspicion for infectious disease based on history. Wear gloves at a minimum for personal protective equipment.
2) Recognize respiratory distress based on outstretched neck, nostril flaring and respiratory noise. Rapid evaluation of mucous membranes and respiratory effort (chest excursion, rate) is performed.
3) Localize respiratory obstruction to the upper airway by listening for upper airway noise (stertor or stridor), evaluating for diminished nasal airflow as well as a palpation of the head and throat.
4) Ensure adequate restraint and perform an emergency tracheotomy to establish a patent airway. Secure a tracheotomy tube (Figure 11.8).
5) If available, provide oxygen through the tracheotomy site.
6) When a patent airway has been established, complete the remainder of the physical examination.

*Step 2: Formulating a diagnostic plan:*
Once the horse is stable, further assess the airway to better localize and elucidate the cause of obstruction.

- Upper airway endoscopy is the priority diagnostic for patient evaluation (Figure 11.9). The guttural pouches should be evaluated particularly when diffuse pharyngeal swelling, lymph node swelling, or dysphagia are identified. Guttural pouch sampling can be performed for *Streptococcus equi equi* PCR and culture. A PCR test usually provides a more rapid positive test result than sample culture for *S. equi*. Retrograde endoscopy via the tracheotomy site can be performed to complement normograde endoscopy.
- Once endoscopy is performed, radiography should be considered to further evaluate a focal site of concern (likely pharynx), or more fully evaluate the upper airway if endoscopy is equivocal (Figure 11.10a,b). Radiography is also useful in identifying metallic foreign bodies that can act as a nidus for abscessation and swelling.
- Laryngeal area and palpable external abnormalities such as wounds or lymph node swelling can be evaluated with ultrasound.
- Following a significant upper airway obstruction, the lower airway should be evaluated by ultrasound for secondary pulmonary edema.

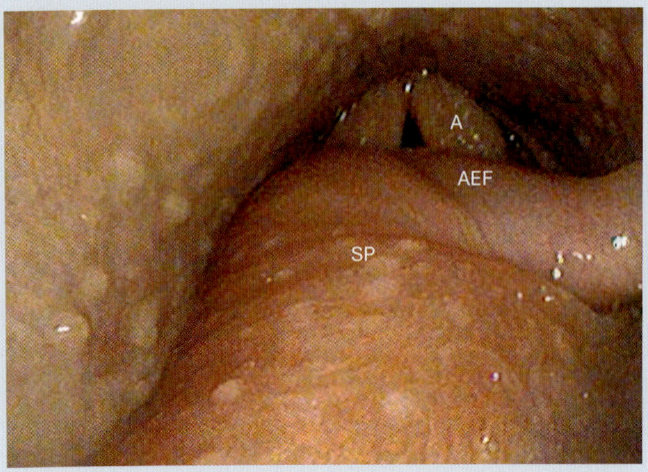


**Figure 11.9** Endoscopy revealing minimal airway due to marked soft-tissue swelling. The soft-tissue enlargement is resulting in distortion of the tissues, including dorsal displacement of the soft palate, partial entrapment of the right aryepiglottic fold, and dorsal pharyngeal collapse. A, left arytenoid; SP, caudal margin of the soft palate, dorsally displaced; AEF, right aryepiglottic fold entrapping the displaced epiglottis.

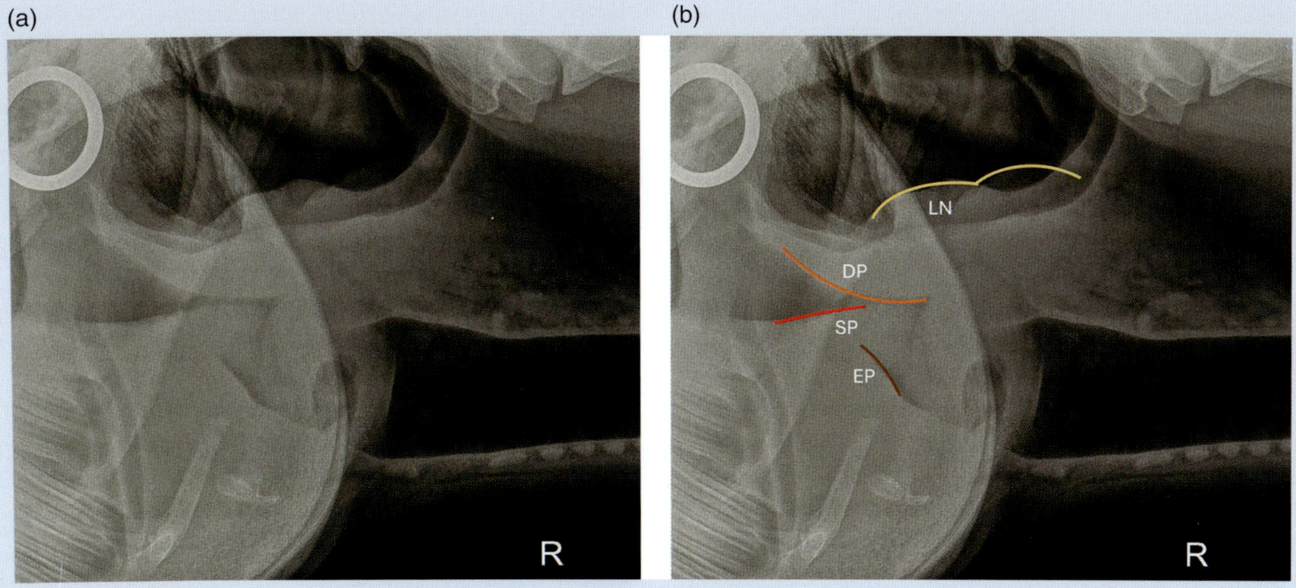


**Figure 11.10** (a) Lateral radiograph of the pharyngeal region of a horse demonstrating marked soft-tissue swelling associated with the soft palate, ventral aspect of the guttural pouch, and laryngeal region as well as presumptive retropharyngeal lymphadenopathy. (b) LN, retropharyngeal lymph node location, enlarged dorsal margin demarcated by yellow line; DP, dorsal pharynx ventrally deviated margin outlined by orange line; SP, dorsally displaced caudal soft palate dorsal margin highlighted in red; EP, epiglottic dorsal margin demarcated by brown line.

- Bloodwork such as a complete blood count and serum biochemistry should be considered to evaluate the patient's systemic health, and inflammatory response to infection. Alternatively, abbreviated bloodwork such as serum amyloid A, a packed cell volume, and total solids, along with a lactate can be performed in the field.
- The patient should be evaluated for dysphagia related to diffuse pharyngeal swelling or direct guttural pouch injury. It is often not possible to immediately evaluate for dysphagia if the horse is inappetent due to stress or pyrexia.

If endoscopy, ultrasound, radiography, or abbreviated bloodwork are not feasible in the field, move to Step 3.

*Step 3: Emergency treatment guidelines:*

Following stabilization with a patent airway and diagnostic evaluation with upper airway endoscopy at a minimum, further specific treatment is indicated. When diffuse pharyngeal swelling and airway collapse is identified with no underlying cause apparent, upper airway infection (± GP infection, lymph node abscessation) with *S. equi* is often later confirmed on PCR. Oral medications should generally be avoided due to the likelihood of dysphagia accompanying pharyngeal swelling.

Due to the necessity for parenteral medications, fluid administration and serial upper airway endoscopy, referral for hospitalization is often necessary.

- Provide anti-inflammatory therapy with a non-steroidal anti-inflammatory drug to diminish the soft-tissue swelling and alleviate pain. Severe swelling can alternatively be treated with dexamethasone. Consider concurrent gastroprotectants when the patient will tolerate oral medications.
- If they are present, lance and drain abscessed mandibular lymph nodes contributing to pain and airway compression. If a mandibular abscess associated with a historical penetrating wound, foreign body or dental disease is present, lance and drain the abscess. Debride the abscess and remove any foreign material. Probe the depths of the abscess to evaluate for tracking near the airway.

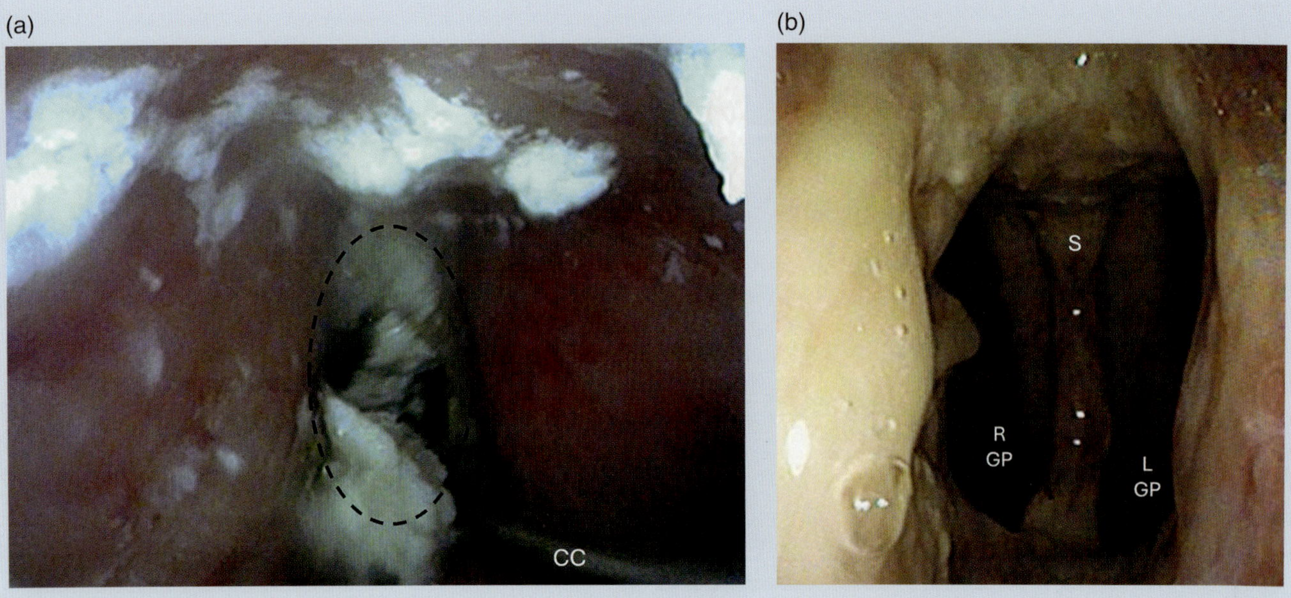


**Figure 11.11** (a) Removal of caseous debris from the guttural pouches assisted by manipulation of a chambers catheter (CC) through a laser-created nasopharyngeal guttural pouch fenestration (margin approximated by dashed black line). (b) Guttural pouch fenestration three weeks post-operatively with healing tissue margins. S, guttural pouch septum; L GP, opening into the left guttural pouch; R GP, opening into the right guttural pouch.

- Manage the tracheotomy site with once or twice daily wound care and cleaning of the tracheotomy tube. Apply a thick ointment, such as petroleum jelly, to the skin around the wound to avoid serum scald and to improve ease of cleaning.
- Lavage guttural pouches as needed if *S. equi* infection is confirmed and discharge is present (Figure 11.11a). Consider nasopharyngeal guttural pouch fenestration if guttural pouch entry or lavage is not feasible due to ostia dysfunction from chronic disease (Figure 11.11b).
- Provide supportive care such as intravenous fluids for resuscitation and maintenance until the patient is able and willing to drink independently. Feed mashes of a complete feed in soup consistency at the level of the ground for ease of intake and to avoid aspiration.
- If pulmonary edema is identified, administer furosemide as needed and avoid fluid overload.
- Antibiotic administration should be considered judiciously. In most cases where a horse has profound airway distress and malaise, as well as an indwelling tracheotomy tube, systemic antibiotic administration is recommended. Penicillin is the medication of choice to treat *S. equi* in this scenario. However, if pharyngeal swelling has resulted from infection and abscessation associated with another etiology, broad-spectrum antibiotic administration, is likely warranted. Culture and susceptibility of a sample from the site of concern is recommended.

*Step 4: Assessment and monitoring:*

If treatment in the field is elected, owners must be able to monitor and care for a tracheotomy site. Additionally, the horse must not be dysphagic and tolerate oral medications. On farm, patient isolation to ensure biosecurity is imperative to avoid disease outbreak.

In a hospital environment, monitoring and care can be readily titrated to the patient's progress.

- Routine assessment to include physical examination and evaluation of respiratory effort, rate, and nasal discharge.
- Monitor appetite and ability to consume feed and water without aspiration.
- Modify wound assessment at the site of temporary tracheotomy, as well as site of abscess drainage if applicable.
- Serial upper airway endoscopy to evaluate extent of swelling and airway lumen diameter. Evaluate patient's response to and tolerance of occlusion of the tracheotomy site when an adequate airway lumen is observed. Remove the tracheotomy tube when sufficient upper airway patency is restored.
- Sample and treat guttural pouch if persistent drainage is noted. Chronic infection can result in chondroid formation.

*Step 5: Decision making during triage:*

Recognition of respiratory distress and localization of the obstruction to the upper airway is imperative for a rapid, life-saving decision to provide an emergency tracheotomy and secure a patent airway. A horse should not be shipped for referral in respiratory distress; an airway should first be established. Recognize presentations of infectious disease and take appropriate biosecurity precautions to prevent dispersion to other animals.

Once an airway is secured and the horses distress is relieved, diagnostics such as upper airway endoscopy, radiography, and ultrasonography can be performed on farm if they are available. Alternatively, immediate referral should be considered to evaluate the cause of airway obstruction. Additional considerations for referral should include the horse's systemic condition, including endotoxemia and hypovolemia. High fever and dysphagia can also be more readily managed in hospital, including the administration of parenteral rather than oral medications. When infectious disease is considered a likely cause of upper airway swelling and occlusion, the ability to isolate the patient on farm and maintain appropriate biosecurity should also be factors when considering referral.

Most horses that have pharyngeal swelling and airway compression associated with *S. equi* have a good prognosis for resolution and return to function. Pharyngeal swelling and airway compression can also result from abscessation related to penetrating wounds, foreign bodies, and dental disease. These differentials can be evaluated with diagnostic imaging.

Complications associated with treatment include local wound infection or emphysema associated with the temporary tracheotomy site. Routine wound care, cleaning of the tracheotomy tube once or twice daily, and systemic antibiotic treatment can help maintain wound health. Spread of *S. equi* infection to nearby, susceptible horses is likely, making biosecurity a concern for on-farm care or return to the farm following hospitalization. *S. equi* can cause chronic guttural pouch infection that produces nasal discharge and chondroid formation. These potential complications can be addressed by ensuring the patient eats at the level of the ground for adequate guttural pouch drainage and providing guttural pouch lavage in the acute stages of disease; nasopharyngeal or cervical guttural pouch fenestration is sometimes needed to establish adequate drainage and remove chondroids in cases of chronic disease.

## References


Aleman, M., Nieto, J.E., Benak, J., and Johnson, L.R. (2008). Tracheal collapse in American miniature horses: 13 cases (1985–2007). *J. Am. Vet. Med. Assoc.* 233 (8): 1302–1306.

Archer, D. (2008). Differential diagnosis of epistaxis in the horse. *In Pract.* 30: 20–29.

Bell, C. (2007). Pharyngeal neuromuscular dysfunction associated with bilateral guttural pouch tympany in a foal. *Can. Vet. J.* 48 (2): 192–194.

Bond, S., Leguillette, R., Richard, E.A. et al. (2018). Equine asthma: integrative biologic relevance of a recently proposed nomenclature. *J. Vet. Intern. Med.* 32 (6): 2088–2098.

Boy, M.G. and Sweeney, C.R. (2000). Pneumothorax in horses: 40 cases (1980–1997). *J. Am. Vet. Med. Assoc.* 216 (12): 1955–1959.

Boyle, A.G., Timoney, J.F., Newton, J.R. et al. (2018). Streptococcus equi infections in horses: guidelines for treatment, control, and prevention of strangles-revised consensus statement. *J. Vet. Intern. Med.* 32 (2): 633–647.

Byrne, C.A. and Barakzai, S.Z. (2020). Equine emergency upper airway management. *Equine Vet. Educ.* 32: 325–334.

Cha, M.L. and Costa, L.R. (2017). Inhalation therapy in horses. *Vet. Clin. Equine* 33: 29–46.

Chaffin, M.K., Carter, G.K., and Dabareiner, R.M. (2000). How to place an indwelling chest tube for drainage and lavage of the pleural cavity in horses affected with pleuropneumonia. *AAEP Proceedings* 46: 145–149.

Constable, P.D., Hinchcliff, K.W., Done, S.H., and Grunberg, W. (ed.) (2017). Diseases of the respiratory system. In: *Veterinary Medicine*, 845–1090. Elsevier.

Couetil, L., Cardwell, J.M., Leguillette, R. et al. (2020). Equine asthma: current understanding and future directions. *Front Vet. Sci.* 7: 450.

Dickinson, C.E., Traub-Dargatz, J.L., Dargatz, D.A. et al. (1996). Rattlesnake venom poisoning in horses: 32 cases (1973–1993). *J. Am. Vet. Med. Assoc.* 208 (11): 1866–1871.

Divers, T.J., Radcliffe, R.M., Cook, V.L. et al. (2022). Calculating and selecting fluid therapy and blood product replacements for horses with acute hemorrhage. *J. Vet. Emerg. Crit. Care* 32: 97–107.

Feary, D.J., Magdesian, K.G., Aleman, M.A., and Rhodes, D.M. (2007). Traumatic brain injury in horses: 34 cases (1994–2004). *J. Am. Vet. Med. Assoc.* 231 (2): 259–266.

Freeman, D.E. (2015). Update on disorders and treatment of the guttural pouch. *Vet. Clin. North Am. Equine Pract.* 31 (1): 63–89.

Hardcastle, M.R., Pauwels, F.E.T., and Collett, M.G. (2012). Clinicopathologic observations on laryngoplasty failure in a horse. *Vet. Surg.* 41: 649–653.

Hassel, D.M. (2007). Thoracic trauma in horses. *Vet. Clin. Equine* 23: 67–80.

James, F.M., Parente, E.J., and Palmer, J.E. (2006). Management of bilateral choanal atresia in a foal. *J. Am. Vet. Med. Assoc.* 229 (11): 1784–1789.

Krebs, W. and Schmotzer, W.B. (2007). Laser fenestrated salpingopharyngeal fistulas for treatment of bilateral guttural pouch tympany in a foal. *Equine Vet. Educ.* 19: 419–423.

Laverty, S., Lavoie, J.P., Pascoe, J.R., and Ducharme, N. (1996). Penetrating wounds of the thorax in 15 horses. *Equine Vet. J.* 28 (3): 220–224.

Lepage, O.M. (2024). Guttural pouch mycosis: a three-step therapeutic approach. *Vet. Sci.* 11 (1): 41.

Lisciandro, G.R. (2011). Abdominal and thoracic focused assessment with sonography for trauma, triage, and monitoring in small animals. *J. Vet. Emerg. Crit. Care* 21 (2): 104–122.

Marr, C.M. (2016). Cardiac and respiratory disease in aged horses. *Vet. Clin. Equine* 32: 283–300.

Marsh, P.S. (2007). Fire and smoke inhalation injury in horses. *Vet. Clin. Equine* 23 (1): 19–30.

Plumb, DC (2025). Plumb's veterinary drugs. Educational Concepts, LLC. dba Brief Media. http://resolver.library.cornell.edu/misc/10758189 (accessed May 2025).

Richardson, J.D., Lane, J.G., and Day, M.J. (1994). Congenital choanal restriction in 3 horses. *Equine Vet. J.* 26 (2): 162–165.

Ronaldson, H.L., Monticelli, P., Smith, R., and Adami, C. (2020). Acute life-threatening laryngeal dysfunction in a draft horse recovering from general anesthesia: a case report. *J. Equine Vet. Sci.* 91: 103–109.

Schaer, D.B. and Orsini, J.A. (2014). Respiratory system. In: *Equine Emergencies Treatments and Procedures*, 4e (ed. J.A. Orsini and T.J. Divers), 450–484. St. Louis: Elsevier.

Sprayberry, K.A. and Barrett, E.J. (2015). Thoracic trauma in horses. *Vet. Clin. Equine* 31: 199–219.

Tietje, S., Becker, M., and Bockenhoff, G. (1996). Computed tomographic evaluation of head diseases in the horse: 15 cases. *Equine Vet. J.* 28: 98–105.

Tute, A.S., Gleed, R.D., Credille, K.M. et al. (1996). Negative pressure pulmonary edema as a post-anesthetic complication associated with upper airway obstruction in a horse. *Vet. Surg.* 25: 519–523.

Wilson, D.V., Schott, H.C. 2nd, Robinson, N.E. et al. (2006). Response to nasopharyngeal oxygen administration in horses with lung disease. *Equine Vet. J.* 38 (3): 2019–2023.

Wong, D.M., Alcott, C.J., Wang, C. et al. (2010). Physiologic effects of nasopharyngeal administration of supplemental oxygen at various flow rates in healthy neonatal foals. *Am. J. Vet. Res.* 71 (9): 1080–1088.

Woodie, J.B., Ducharme, N.G., Gleed, R.D., and Soderholm, L.V. (2002). In horses with guttural pouch mycosis or after stylohyoid bone resection, what arterial ligation(s) could be effective in emergency treatment of a hemorrhagic crisis. *Vet. Surg.* 31 (5): 498.

# 12

# Cardiovascular Emergencies

*Cristobal Navas de Solis*[1] *and Katharyn J. Mitchell*[2]

[1] *Department of Clinical Studies - New Bolton Center, University of Pennsylvania School of Veterinary Medicine, Kennett Square, PA, USA*
[2] *Department of Clinical Sciences, College of Veterinary Medicine, Cornell University, Ithaca, NY, USA*

## Dysrhythmias – Diagnosis and Treatment

### Emergency Triage Steps

#### Recognition of Dysrhythmias – Bradycardias, Tachycardias (How to Read ECGs)

Assessment of the cardiovascular system is an essential part of the physical examination in a critically ill patient. Frequently patients present with tachycardia or tachyarrhythmia while occasionally we see patients with pathological bradycardia. It is important to be able to differentiate a sinus rhythm from an atrial, junctional, or ventricular rhythm (Figures 12.1a–c, 12.2 and 12.3a,b). Recording an electrocardiogram (ECG) is key to determining if the rhythm is normal or abnormal which will then guide treatment. The process of how to record an ECG is covered in Chapter 2. Table 12.1 presents the author's approach to analyzing an ECG (Mitchell 2019, 2020). A case example of a patient presenting with a tachyarrhythmia is found in Appendix 12.3 (online).

Treatment will vary depending on the origin of the rhythm (atrial, junctional, or ventricular) and the heart rate. In the emergency situation, treatment is focused on (1) **improving cardiac output**, (2) **controlling the ventricular rate,** and (3) **converting the rhythm back to a sinus rhythm** (Box 12.1).

It is also important to decide if there is underlying structural cardiac disease leading to the dysrhythmia, if the dysrhythmia is secondary to systemic disease (e.g., systemic inflammatory response syndrome [SIRS], hemorrhage or electrolyte derangements) or if the dysrhythmia is considered a "primary" problem. It will be difficult to control the rhythm if there is severe underlying structural disease while treatment of any systemic problems will play an important role in restoration of a sinus rhythm (van Loon 2019).

***Patient Stabilization*** An intravenous (IV) catheter should be placed and IV fluids considered if there is evidence of poor cardiac output (high heart rate, azotemia, poor peripheral perfusion, abnormal mentation). Large volumes of IV fluids should be avoided until it can be determined if myocardial dysfunction or cardiac failure is present, but a **targeted approach to fluid therapy** with small boluses (e.g., **10 mL/kg**) can be helpful and repeated if necessary.

***Diagnostic Plan*** An ECG is *essential* to accurately diagnose the rhythm present and for monitoring the response to therapy. Point-of-care blood work to assess hydration, perfusion, and monitor for cardiac injury is indicated (PCV/TP, lactate, creatinine, electrolytes, and cardiac troponins). A focused rapid assessment of the cardiovascular structures (EFATE, CRASH, or similar protocol) (Bevevino et al. 2023; Eberhardt and Schwarzwald 2022) to investigate for underlying structural disease and monitor cardiac function should be performed. Non-invasive blood pressure (NIBP) measurements from the tail can be useful to monitor and guide therapy.

***Emergency Treatment Guidelines*** The indications for treatment of dysrhythmias are found in Table 12.2. Rate and rhythm control should be attempted if there is evidence of **hemodynamic instability**, **rapid ventricular rate (>100 bpm)**, **extreme bradycardia (<20 bpm)**, **polymorphic or multiform QRS complexes**, **evidence of R-on-T phenomena,**

*Emergency Triage of the Horse*, First Edition. Edited by Rolfe M. Radcliffe and Jamie J. Kopper.

Companion website: www.wiley.com/go/radcliffe/triage

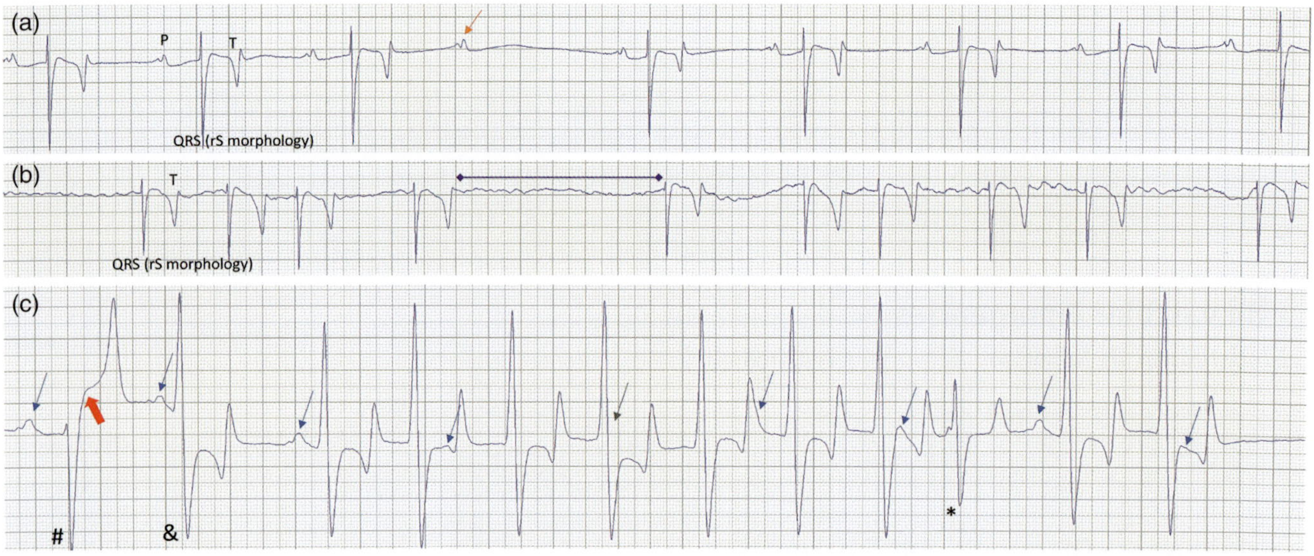


**Figure 12.1** (a) A modified base–apex ECG recording from a horse in normal sinus rhythm (showing the typical equine short R, tall S [rS] QRS morphology). The baseline rhythm is regular until **a second-degree AV block is observed** (orange arrow), where there is a P wave but no subsequent QRS-T. Progressive lengthening of the PQ interval is also observed in the last 5 complexes. The atrial rate is 34/min while the ventricular rate is 30/min. Paper speed 25 mm/s, gain 10 mm/mV. (b) A modified base–apex ECG recording from a horse with an irregularly irregular rhythm. The RR interval is constantly changing, no P waves are observed, but the QRS-T morphology is very appropriate and similar between complexes (showing the typical equine rS morphology). An undulating baseline is present – where fibrillation (f) waves are observed (purple line). **This is atrial fibrillation (AF).** The ventricular response rate is appropriate (approx. 38/min). Paper speed 25 mm/s, gain 10 mm/mV. (c) A modified base–apex ECG recording from a horse with a tachyarrhythmia. The RR interval is variable and the QRS-T morphology differs (three different QRS-T morphologies are present, marked #, &, *). P waves are present but there are variable PQ intervals and P waves are seen wandering in and out of the QRS-T complexes, indicating AV dissociation (observed P waves – blue arrows, presumed hidden in QRS – gray arrow). The ventricular rate is 90/min while the atrial rate is 68/min. **This is a multiform (or polymorphic) accelerated idioventricular rhythm (sometime called slow ventricular tachycardia).** The red arrow indicates ST segment elevation, which can be a marker for myocardial ischemia in other species. Paper speed 50 mm/s, gain 10 mm/mV.

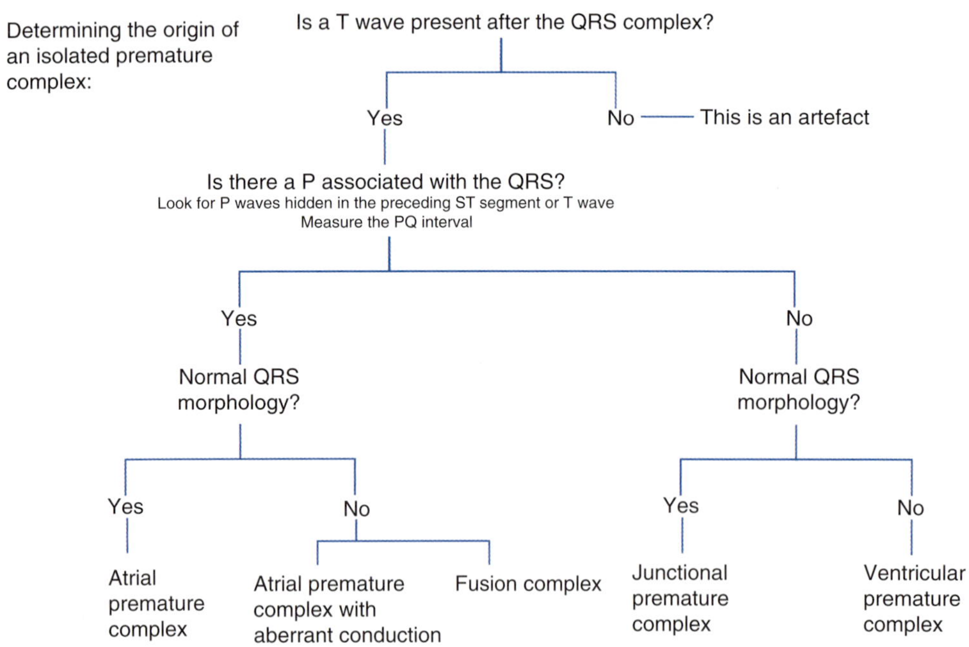


**Figure 12.2** Decision tree algorithm to determine the origin of a premature complex identified on an ECG recording. A fusion complex is a normal complex fused with a complex of ventricular origin. Determining the origin of the rhythm is vital for implementing the most appropriate anti-arrhythmic therapy.

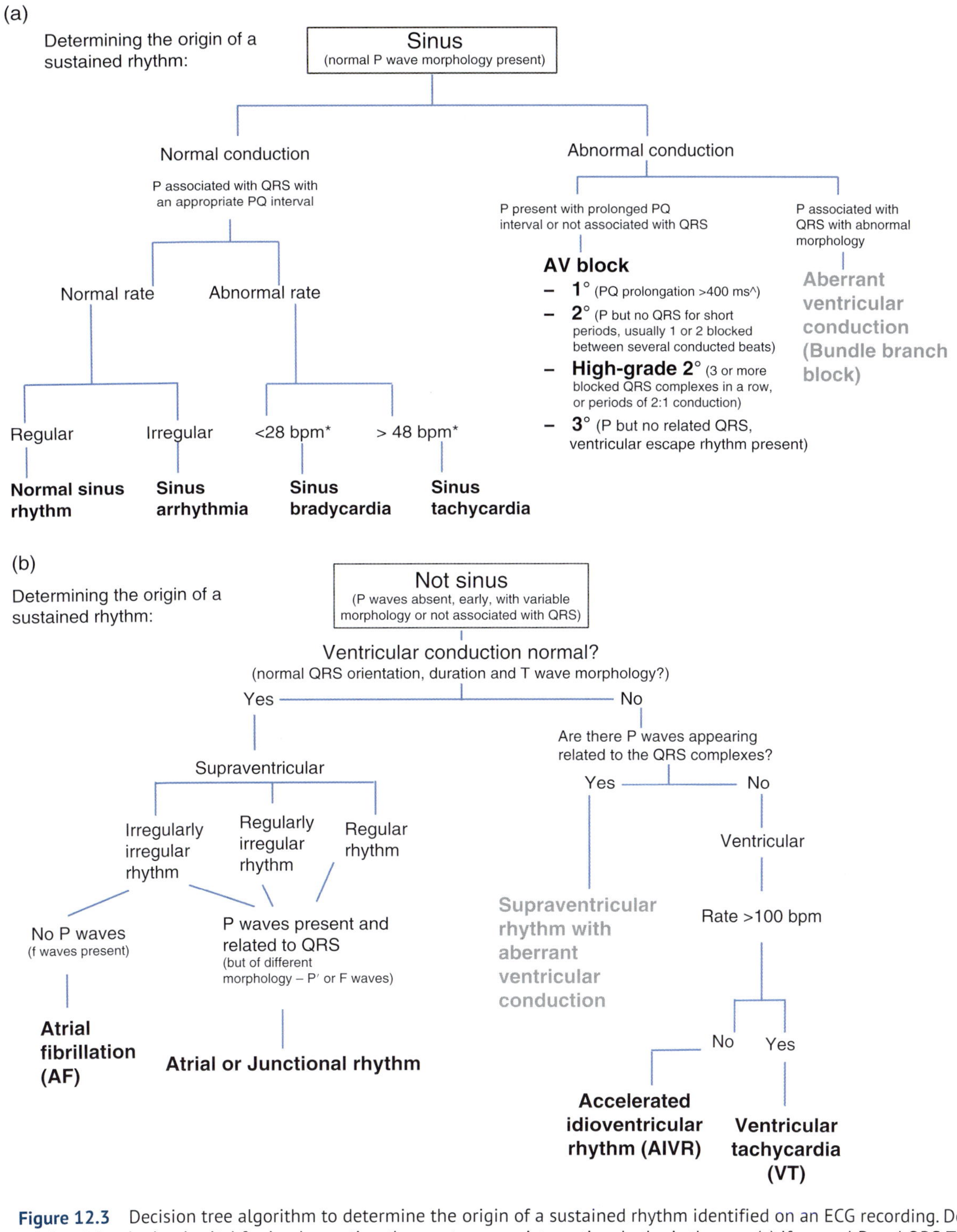


**Figure 12.3** Decision tree algorithm to determine the origin of a sustained rhythm identified on an ECG recording. Determining the origin of the rhythm is vital for implementing the most appropriate anti-arrhythmic therapy. (a) If normal P and QRS-T wave morphology is present, the rhythm is considered likely originating from the sino-atrial node. ^, the PQ interval is dependent on size/body weight, a cut-off of 400 ms is appropriate for a 500 kg horse. *, the HR is dependent on size/bodyweight, these cut-offs apply to the average-sized 500 kg horse. (b) If the rhythm appears to originate from a non-sinoatrial node location, it may be supraventricular (atrial or junctional) or ventricular in origin. AV, atrioventricular; AF, atrial fibrillation; VT, ventricular tachycardia; AIVR, accelerated idioventricular rhythm; F, flutter; 1°, 1st degree; 2°, 2nd degree; 3°, 3rd degree; ms, milliseconds; bpm, beats per min.

**Table 12.1** A step-by-step approach to analyze an ECG and recognize abnormalities.

| | |
|---|---|
| Step 1. | Assess the overall quality of the recording.<br>• The P-QRS-T complexes should be clearly visible and free of obvious artifacts.<br>• Analysis should not be performed if the recording quality is poor, as misdiagnosis of the rhythm is possible. |
| Step 2. | Identify the paper speed (typically 25 or 50 mm/s) and calculate the overall heart rate.<br>The heart rate can be divided into three broad categories, normal (28–48 bpm), bradycardic (<28 bpm), or tachycardic (>48 bpm).<br>Most digital systems will perform an RR interval analysis and calculate the instantaneous heart rate automatically. |
| Step 3. | Assess if the rhythm is regular or irregular.<br>• If the rhythm is irregular, is there any underlying pattern (regularly irregular) or is there no pattern (irregularly irregular)?<br>• Are there pauses, premature complexes, or both? |
| Step 4. | Identify the most normal P-QRS-T complexes (if present) and then compare them to the abnormal complexes.<br>• Is there a P for every QRS?<br>• Is there a QRS for every P?<br>• Do they appear related (similar PR intervals) or dissociated (varying PR intervals)?<br>• Is the morphology of all P-QRS-T complexes similar or different?<br>• Are the QRS complexes of similar polarity and duration (ms). With the modified base–apex lead placement (described in Chapter 4) normal horses should have an rS or S morphology.<br>• Are all T waves the same or is there variation in T wave morphology that could be caused by secondary T wave changes (i.e., if the preceding QRS is abnormal, then likely the following T wave is abnormal as well) or superimposition of other waves (e.g., a P wave within the preceding T wave)?<br>• Identify if any R-on-T phenomena present |
| Step 5. | Measure the PR, QRS, and QT intervals.<br>• Are they similar or varying? |
| Step 6. | Define the rhythm.<br>• Is this a disorder of abnormal impulse formation, abnormal impulse conduction, or both?<br>• Is the rhythm primarily sinus in origin? If no, are the abnormal complexes of **atrial**, **junctional**, or **ventricular** origin? See Figures F1–3.<br>• Is the rhythm sustained, paroxysmal, or intermittent?<br>• What is the timing and frequency of occurrence of abnormal beats? |
| Step 7. | If unsure about the rhythm diagnosis or interpretation of the clinical relevance, seek a second opinion from a person experienced at equine ECG interpretation. |

**Box 12.1 Treatment goals for emergency stabilization**

- Improving cardiac output.
- Controlling the ventricular rate.
- Converting the rhythm back to a sinus rhythm.

or ***torsade de pointes*** as these findings indicate a high risk for the rhythm becoming life-threatening. In most cases, treatment in the field is difficult to achieve due to the lack of availability of appropriate monitoring and medication. Therefore, referral to a hospital facility is frequently indicated in these cases.

***Controlling the Ventricular Rate*** It can be difficult to determine if a rhythm is sinus or non-sinus in origin, particularly at high ventricular rates. In these cases, **attempting to slow the ventricular rate** can be helpful to determine the presence of P waves, associations between P and QRS complexes, and to measure the atrial rate. In the short term (and in the absence of fulminant heart failure), small doses of an **alpha 2 agonist** (e.g., xylazine 0.25 mg/kg IV) can facilitate slowing of the AV conduction for a short period of time, allowing a more accurate ECG diagnosis. Some horses with tachyarrhythmias will be

**Table 12.2** When to treat a dysrhythmia – indications for treatment.

- Is there evidence of hemodynamic instability?
  - Poor peripheral perfusion (cold extremities, weak pulses).
  - Delayed jugular filling, jugular pulsation, jugular distension.
  - Prolonged capillary refill time.
  - Reduced urine output.
  - Dull mentation.
  - Weakness.
  - Collapse/syncope/recumbency.
  - Low systemic blood pressure.
  - Laboratory evidence of reduced perfusion (e.g., hyperlactatemia or azotemia).
- Ventricular rate is consistently high (>100 bpm) or extremely low (<20 bpm).
- Polymorphic or multiform ventricular complexes.
- Evidence of impaired cardiac function on echocardiography.
- *R-on-T phenomena.*
- *Torsade de pointes.*

quite anxious and this can contribute to their rapid ventricular rate, so small doses of **acepromazine** (0.005–0.01 mg/kg IV) can help reduce anxiety and sympathetic stimulation, therefore slowing ventricular conduction (measure NIBP first and don't use if profound hypotension already present). It the rhythm is determined to be supraventricular in origin, attempts can be made to slow AV node conduction for longer periods of time (e.g., **digoxin or sotalol**, see Table 12.3) to improve cardiac output and hemodynamic stability until rhythm control can be attempted.

In cases of bradycardia, attempts should be made to **increase the sinus rate** and **improve AV node conduction**. The use of medication is usually a temporary measure, with the definitive treatment being placement of a pacemaker if no underlying structural reason for the bradycardia is detected and the bradycardia does not resolve. The medications used to treat bradycardia are summarized in Table 12.4. In some cases, a temporary pacemaker lead may need to be placed intravenously, prior to permanent pacemaker implantation (van Loon et al. 2020).

***Controlling the Rhythm*** Once the horse is stabilized and the origin of the rhythm determined, efforts can be made to convert the horse back into a sinus rhythm. While there are many anti-arrhythmic medications available, the practicalities and monetary considerations of treating horses often weighing in excess of 500 kg, make the list considerably shorter. It should be remembered that most anti-arrhythmic medications have the potential to be pro-arrhythmic. Continuous ECG monitoring during therapy is important to recognize adverse events and detect changes in the underlying rhythm.

For confirmed supraventricular dysrhythmias, there is also the possibility of transvenous electrical cardioversion (TVEC) in addition to pharmacological conversion. This can be performed at some referral institutions, and should only be considered once the patient has been stabilized and it has been determined that there are minimal underlying structural changes (Decloedt et al. 2021; Van Steenkiste et al. 2019).

Most ventricular tachyarrhythmias will require treatment, but some of the slower accelerated idioventricular rhythms can be monitored and the abnormal rhythms will resolve once the underlying systemic disease (e.g., hemorrhage, SIRS, endotoxemia, electrolyte derangements) have been treated (Mitchell 2017; Navas de Solis 2020; Williams and Mitchell 2023).

## Important Decisions During Management

### Decision for Hospital Referral

If the patient is hemodynamically unstable, then rapid referral is usually indicated, as these patients require intensive treatment and ongoing monitoring. Most referral facilities have access to a larger range of medication and the ability to provide continuous monitoring.

**Table 12.3** Treatment options for horses with supraventricular or ventricular dysrhythmias.

| Drug | Drug class | Dose recommendations | Dose for 500 kg bwt | Comments |
|---|---|---|---|---|
| **First-line medication for short duration *rate* control if the rhythm is *supraventricular*** | | | | |
| Xylazine | $\alpha_2$ agonist | 0.25 mg/kg bwt slowly IV, repeat once if required | 125 mg IV over 2–3 min | Adverse effects: muscle tremors, bradycardia with AV blocks, reduced respiratory rate, sweating, and ataxia.<br>Contraindications: Preexisting cardiac dysfunction, hypotension or shock, pathological ventricular dysrhythmias, respiratory dysfunction, severe hepatic or renal insufficiency, and seizures. |
| Diltiazem | Class IV $Ca^{2+}$ channel blocker | 0.125 mg/kg over 2 min IV, repeated every 10 min to effect, up to 1.25 mg/kg total dose | 62.5 mg IV over 2 min; total dose 625 mg | Titrate to effect. Use diltiazem doses >0.5–1.0 mg/kg with caution.<br>Adverse effects: Hypotension, tachycardia, sinus arrhythmia, bradycardia, sinus arrest, high-grade AV block, negative inotropism, and exacerbation of heart failure (unless secondary to SVT or AF with rapid ventricular response).<br>Contraindications: Hypotension, bradycardia, SA or AV block, ventricular systolic dysfunction, severe heart failure, cardiogenic shock, and β blocker. |
| Esmolol | Class II $\beta_1$ blocker | 50–100 μg/kg bwt IV slowly over 3–5 min, up to 500 μg/kg total dose | 25–50 mg IV slowly | Ultra-short acting, use incremental doses up to a total dose of 500 μg/kg.<br>Adverse effects: hypotension, bradycardia, and collapse.<br>Contraindications: weakness, bradycardia, AV block, hypotension, negative inotropism, and exacerbation of heart failure. |
| Metoprolol | Class II $\beta_1$ blocker | 0.02–0.06 mg/kg bwt IV q4–6 h | 10–30 mg IV slowly | Short acting (hours).<br>Adverse effects and contraindications: see Esmolol. |
| **First-line medication for longer duration *rate* control if the rhythm is *supraventricular*** | | | | |
| Digoxin | Digitalis glycosides | 0.0022 mg/kg q12 h IV<br>0.011 mg/kg q12 h PO | 1.1 mg IV<br>5.5 mg PO | TDM: peak (1–2 h) and trough (12 h) concentrations at steady state should fall within 0.8–2.0 ng/mL (1–2.6 nmol/L).<br>Adverse effects: Depression, anorexia, colic, diarrhea, sinus bradycardia, AV block, and supraventricular and ventricular dysrhythmias (bigeminy).<br>Contraindications: AV block, diastolic ventricular dysfunction, pre-existing digitalis toxicity, myocarditis, and ventricular dysrhythmias. |
| Sotalol | Class II/III $K^+$ channel and β blocker | 1 mg/kg bwt PO q12 h for 1 d, continue at 2–3 mg/kg bwt PO q12 h | 500 mg initial dose<br>1–1.5 g per maintenance dose | Good oral bioavailability.<br>Generally well tolerated, even with chronic oral administration.<br>Dosage should be gradually reduced before discontinuing medication.<br>Adverse effects: QT prolongation, ventricular dysrhythmias, and sweating.<br>Contraindications: Preexisting QT prolongation. Use with caution in patients with reduced-poor systolic function, uncorrected hypokalemia or hypomagnesemia. |

**Table 12.3** (Continued)

| Drug | Drug class | Dose recommendations | Dose for 500 kg bwt | Comments |
|---|---|---|---|---|
| Atenolol | Class II<br>$\beta_1$ blocker | 0.12 mg/kg bwt PO q12 h initially increasing to 0.25 mg/kg bwt PO q12 h if well tolerated. Can increase up to 1 mg/kg bwt PO q12 h if needed. | 60 mg per dose initially, then 125 mg per dose | Variable bioavailability. Dosage should be adjusted on an individual basis. Dosage should be gradually reduced before discontinuing medication.<br>Adverse effects: Sweating, depression, lethargy, weakness, bradycardia, AV block, hypotension, negative inotropism, and exacerbation of heart failure.<br>Contraindications: Bradycardia, high-degree AV block, and untreated heart failure. |
| Propranolol | Class II<br>$\beta_1/\beta_2$ blocker | 0.38–0.78 mg/kg bwt PO q8 h | 190–390 mg per dose | Variable bioavailability. Dosage should be adjusted on an individual basis. Dosage should be gradually reduced before discontinuing medication.<br>Adverse effects: Depression, lethargy, weakness, bradycardia, AV block, hypotension, negative inotropism, exacerbation of heart failure, and bronchoconstriction (aggravation of recurrent airway obstruction).<br>Contraindications: Bradycardia, high-degree AV block, untreated heart failure, and bronchopulmonary disease. |
| **First-line medication for *rhythm* control – atrial fibrillation – supraventricular tachycardia (confirmed)** | | | | |
| Quinidine sulfate | Class $I_A$<br>$Na^+$ channel blocker | 22 mg/kg bwt PO by NGT q2 h for up to four doses or until converted, adverse or toxic effects, or plasma quinidine concentration >4 µg/mL. Do not exceed six doses PO q2 h.<br>Continue q6–8 h until converted, adverse or toxic effects, or total dose of 180 mg/kg.<br>**Stop therapy if:** QRS duration exceeds more than 25% of its pretreatment value, plasma quinidine exceeds 5 µg/mL, significant adverse reaction or signs of toxicity are observed. | 11 g per dose | *Use with caution*<br>Adverse effects: Commonly, depression, diarrhea, colic, ataxia, and nasal mucosal swelling. Less commonly paraphimosis, urticarial, and laminitis. Accelerated AV conduction, tachycardia, QRS and QT prolongation, VT, *torsade de pointes*, hypotension, negative inotropism, exacerbation of heart failure, cardiovascular collapse, and sudden death.<br>TDM: Therapeutic range 2–5 µg/mL [6.2–15.4 µmol/L] 1–2 h after PO administration.<br>Contraindications: Ventricular tachyarrhythmias, *torsade de pointes*, untreated heart failure, preexisting QRS or QT interval prolongation, complete AV block, and digitalis intoxication. Use with caution in patients with hypokalemia, hypomagnesemia, hypoxia, or acid-base disorders.<br>If therapy with quinidine sulfate is chosen, an IV catheter should be placed and the emergency drugs required to treat any adverse effects should be available immediately adjacent to the stall, with the appropriate drug doses calculated for the patients weight.<br>Transvenous electrical cardioversion (TVEC) could be considered in cases where quinidine sulfate therapy is contraindicated, and there is no underlying relevant structural heart disease or heart failure. |

(*Continued*)

**Table 12.3** (Continued)

| Drug | Drug class | Dose recommendations | Dose for 500 kg bwt | Comments |
|---|---|---|---|---|
| **Second-line medication for *rhythm* control – atrial fibrillation – supraventricular tachycardia (confirmed)** | | | | |
| Quinidine gluconate | Class $I_A$<br>$Na^+$ channel blocker | 1–2.2 mg/kg bwt IV q10 min or 0.1–0.22 mg/kg bwt/min CRI up to 12 mg/kg bwt total dose | 500 mg–1.1 g q10 min or 50–110 mg/min CRI; total dose 6 g | *Use with caution*<br>See above. For use in acute cases only (<7 day duration).<br>#Not available in all regions of the world. |
| Amiodarone | Class III<br>$K^+$ channel blocker | 5 mg/kg bwt/h IV for 1 h, followed by 0.83 mg/kg bwt/h for 23 h, subsequently 1.9 mg/kg bwt/h for 30 h or to effect | 2.5 g for first hour, then 415 mg/h for the next 23 h, then 950 mg/h for additional 30 h | Also class I, II, and IV effects.<br>Adverse reactions: Hind limb weakness, weight shifting, *torsade de pointes*, SA and AV nodal inhibition, bradycardia, and hypotension. Prolonged treatment may affect the lungs, liver, heart, thyroid gland, GI tract, eyes, skin, and nerves.<br>Contraindications: Sino-atrial node dysfunction, bradycardia, AV block, and cardiogenic shock. |
| Procainamide | Class $I_A$<br>$Na^+$ channel blocker | 1 mg/kg bwt/min IV, up to 20 mg/kg bwt total dose | 500 mg/min; total dose 10 g | For use in acute cases only (<7 day duration).<br>Adverse events: Hypotension, QRS and QT prolongation, negative inotropism, dysrhythmia, GI, and neurologic disorders (similar to but generally less severe than quinidine).<br>Contraindications: Untreated heart failure, prolonged QRS or QT interval, complete AV block, and digitalis intoxication.<br>Use with caution in patients with hypokalemia, hypomagnesaemia, or acid-base disorders. |
| Propafenone | Class $I_C$<br>$Na^+$ channel blocker | 0.5–1.0 mg/kg bwt in 5% dextrose slowly IV over 5–10 min<br>2 mg/kg bwt PO q8 h | 250–500 mg IV over 5–10 min<br>1 g PO q8 h | Not commonly available.<br>Adverse effects: GI and neurologic disorders, bronchospasm, neg. inotropism, exacerbation of heart failure, AV block, QRS and QT prolongation, and dysrhythmias.<br>Contraindications: Structural heart disease, heart failure, and SA or AV node dysfunction. |
| **First-line medications (intravenous) for *rhythm* control if the rhythm is *ventricular*** | | | | |
| Lidocaine (lignocaine) | Class $I_B$<br>$Na^+$ channel blocker | 0.25–0.5 mg/kg bwt slow IV, repeat in 5–10 min to effect, up to 1.5 mg/kg bwt total dose; followed by 0.05 mg/kg bwt/min CRI | 125–250 mg per bolus up to total dose of 750 mg; CRI 25 mg/min | Adverse effects: Uncommon at therapeutic doses. Overdose can lead to ataxia, muscle tremors, CNS excitement, dysrhythmias, and collapse.<br>Contraindications: SA, AV or intraventricular block, and bradycardia. Caution with hypovolemia, liver disease, shock, and heart failure. |
| Magnesium sulfate | Physiologic $Ca^{2+}$ and $K^+$ channel blocker. Activator of membrane $Na^+/K^+$ ATPase | 2–6 mg/kg bwt/min IV to effect, up to 55–100 mg/kg bwt total dose | 1–3 g/min; total dose 27–50 g | Adverse effects: Rare, but overdose may lead to CNS depressant effects, weakness, trembling, bradycardia, and hypotension. Very high doses cause neuromuscular blockade with respiratory depression and cardiac arrest.<br>Contraindications: Bradycardia, SA and AV block, and renal failure. |

**Table 12.3** (Continued)

| Drug | Drug class | Dose recommendations | Dose for 500 kg bwt | Comments |
|---|---|---|---|---|
| **Second-line medications (intravenous) for *rhythm* control if the rhythm is *ventricular*** | | | | |
| Procainamide | Class $I_A$ $Na^+$ channel blocker | 1 mg/kg bwt/min IV, up to 20 mg/kg bwt total dose | 500 mg/min; total dose 10 g | As described above. |
| Amiodarone | Class III $K^+$ channel blocker | 5 mg/kg bwt/h IV for 1 h, followed by 0.83 mg/kg bwt/h for 23 h, subsequently 1.9 mg/kg bwt/h for 30 h or to effect | 2.5 g for first hour, then 415 mg/h for the next 23 h, then 950 mg/h for additional 30 h | As described above. |
| Propafenone | Class $I_C$ $Na^+$ channel blocker | 0.5–1.0 mg/kg bwt in 5% dextrose slowly IV over 5–10 min | 250–500 mg IV over 5–10 min | As described above. |
| Metoprolol | Class II $\beta_1$ blocker | 0.02–0.06 mg/kg bwt IV q4–6 h | 10–30 mg per dose | As described above. |
| Quinidine gluconate | Class $I_A$ $Na^+$ channel blocker | 1–2.2 mg/kg bwt IV q10 min or 0.1–0.22 mg/kg bwt/min CRI up to 12 mg/kg bwt total dose | 500 mg–1.1 g q10 min or 50–110 mg/min CRI; total dose 6 g | As described above. |
| Bretylium tosylate | Class III $K^+$ channel blocker | 3–5 mg/kg bwt IV, repeat up to 10 mg/kg bwt total dose | 1.5–2.5 g per dose; total dose 5 g | # Difficult to obtain.<br>Use in cases of refractory life-threatening VT/VF. Also indirect anti-adrenergic effects.<br>Adverse effects: Excitement, GI disorders, hypotension, tachycardia, and dysrhythmias.<br>Contraindications: Preexisting hypotension. |
| **Second-line medications (oral) – *rhythm* control if the rhythm is *ventricular*** | | | | |
| Sotalol | Class II/III $K^+$ channel and $\beta$ blocker | 1 mg/kg bwt PO q12 h for 1 d, continue at 2–3 mg/kg bwt PO q12 h | 500 mg initial dose<br>1–1.5 g per maintenance dose | As described above. |
| Phenytoin | Class $I_B$ $Na^+$ channel blocker | 20 mg/kg bwt PO q12 h for three to four doses or until signs of sedation, followed by 10–15 mg/kg bwt PO q12 h maintenance dose | 10 g loading dose<br>5–7.5 g per maintenance dose | Maintenance dose varies between horses.<br>TDM: 5–10 µg/mL.<br>Adverse effects: Sedation, lip and facial twitching, gait deficits, excitation, seizures, and dysrhythmias. Hepatotoxicity with chronic use.<br>Contraindications: SA or AV block and sinus bradycardia. |
| Propafenone | Class $I_C$ $Na^+$ channel blocker | 2 mg/kg bwt PO q8 h | 1 g per dose | As described above. |
| Propranolol | Class II $\beta_1/\beta_2$ blocker | 0.38–0.78 mg/kg bwt PO q8 h | 190–390 mg per dose | As described above. |
| Metoprolol | Class II $\beta_1$ blocker | 2–4 mg/kg bwt PO q8–12 h | 1–2 g per dose | As described above. |
| Quinidine sulfate | Class $I_A$ $Na^+$ channel blocker | 22 mg/kg bwt PO by NGT q2 h for up to four doses or until converted, adverse or toxic effects, or plasma quinidine concentration >4 µg/mL. Do not exceed six doses PO q2 h. | 11 g per dose | *Use with extreme caution*<br>As described above. |

AF, atrial fibrillation; AV, atrio-ventricular; Bwt, bodyweight; CNS, central nervous system; CRI, continuous rate infusion; GI, gastrointestinal; IV, intravenous; kg, kilogram; NGT, nasogastric tube; PO, per oral; SA, sino-atrial; SVT, supraventricular tachycardia; TDM, therapeutic drug monitoring; VF, ventricular fibrillation; VT, ventricular tachycardia.

**Table 12.4** Therapeutic interventions for bradycardia.

| Drug | Drug class | Dose recommendations | Dose for 500 kg bwt | Comments |
|---|---|---|---|---|
| **Bradyarrhythmias causing hypotension (sinus arrest, sinus bradycardia, high-grade or complete AV block). These medications should be used to provide confirmation of the dysrhythmia (based on a failure to respond appropriately to the medication) and to provide temporary therapy until a longer-term solution can be found (i.e., pacemaker implantation).** | | | | |
| Dobutamine | $\beta_1$-adrenergic, $\beta_2$- and $\alpha_1$-adrenergic<br>Preferred over dopamine | 1–5 μg/kg bwt/min CRI, titrate to effect or adverse reaction | 500–2500 μg/min CRI | Adverse effects: Tachycardia, ventricular dysrhythmias, vasoconstriction, and hypertension (at doses >4 μg/kg bwt/min).<br>Contraindications: Ventricular dysrhythmias, tachycardia, and atrial fibrillation (risk of severe tachycardia due to accelerated atrio-ventricular conduction). |
| Dopamine | $\beta_1$ -adrenergic, dose dependent dopaminergic, and $\alpha$1-adrenergic | 1–5 μg/kg bwt/min CRI, titrate to effect or adverse reaction | 500–2500 μg/min CRI | |
| N-butylscopolammonium bromide (or hyoscine N-butylbromide) | Anticholinergic (vagolytic) | 0.05–0.2 mg/kg bwt IV | 25–100 mg IV | Short duration of action (30 min).<br>Adverse effects: Transient tachycardia, decreased GI motility, and mydriasis.<br>Contraindications: Tachycardia, tachyarrhythmia, heart failure, and GI disease. Do not use in animals with glaucoma. |
| Atropine | Anticholinergic (vagolytic) | 0.01–0.02 mg/kg bwt IV or IM | 5–10 mg IV or IM | Adverse effects: Constipation, ileus, colic, bradycardia (at very low doses), tachycardia, dysrhythmias, and CNS effects (stimulation, drowsiness, ataxia, seizures, respiratory depression). Glycopyrrolate is slightly less arrhythmogenic and rarely results in CNS effects.<br>Contraindications: Tachycardia, tachyarrhythmia, heart failure, GI disease, and colic. |
| Glycopyrrolate | Anticholinergic (vagolytic) | 0.005–0.01 mg/kg bwt IV | 2.5–5 mg IV | |
| Theophylline | Phosphodiesterase and adenosine receptor inhibitor | 12 mg/kg bwt PO loading dose, then 5 mg/kg bwt PO q12 h<br>Sustained release formulation: 20 mg/kg bwt PO loading dose, then 15 mg/kg bwt PO q24 h | 6 g PO loading dose, then 2.5 g PO q12 h<br>10 g PO loading dose, then 7.5 g PO q24 h | Positive chronotropic and inotropic medication.<br>Adverse effects: narrow therapeutic window; tachycardia, tachyarrhythmias, CNS excitation, and seizures.<br>Contraindications: do not use with erythromycin, cimetidine, or fluoroquinolones. |

AV, atrio-ventricular; Bwt, bodyweight; CNS, central nervous system; CRI, continuous rate infusion; GI, gastrointestinal; IV, intravenous; kg, kilogram.

### Decision for Medical vs Surgical Treatment

Cardiac dysrhythmias are treated medically, although they may occur in some surgical patients, particularly while undergoing anesthesia. Recognition and appropriate treatment of cardiac dysrhythmias in these surgical patients is critical to improving their morbidity and mortality while undergoing anesthesia or during recovery.

### How to Manage Important Complications

Complications of dysrhythmias result from decreased cardiac output or deterioration of the rhythm to a life-threatening and untreatable dysrhythmia (e.g., ventricular fibrillation). It is important to **maximize cardiac output** by **optimizing preload**, **normalizing the heart rate,** and **improving systolic function** while monitoring for dangerous rhythms (e.g., short-coupling intervals, R-on-T phenomena, QT prolongation).

#### Estimating Prognosis and Decision for Euthanasia

If the rhythm deteriorates rapidly, sudden death is possible. If there is evidence of severe underlying structural cardiac disease the prognosis for long-term survival is considered guarded and treatment is not recommended in most situations. It is possible that attempted conversion to a sinus rhythm in cases that have substantially impaired cardiac function will precipitate the development of congestive heart failure (CHF). Euthanasia should be considered in patients with signs of congestive heart failure that are refractory to emergency treatment or when the clinical condition of the horse becomes dangerous to itself and those handling it (e.g., frequent episodes of collapse).

#### What Can Be Done on Farm?

Most important is recognition of a cardiovascular abnormality on clinical examination. If there is the possibility to quickly record an ECG of good quality to confirm the diagnosis this is a bonus. In most of these cases, a comprehensive evaluation of the cardiovascular system is necessary to decide about the most appropriate therapy (including echocardiography, telemetric continuous ECG monitoring, measurement of NIBP, blood work including cardiac troponins, etc.); therefore, referral is frequently necessary.

#### What Can Be Done at a Referral Hospital?

A thorough evaluation of the cardiovascular system is necessary to identify any underlying pathology and decide on the most appropriate therapy. This will include echocardiography, telemetric continuous ECG monitoring, measurement of NIBP, blood work including cardiac troponins and electrolytes. In addition, most anti-arrhythmic therapy is also pro-arrhythmic, so close monitoring of the cardiac rhythm is required during therapy, to identify any worsening of the dysrhythmias. There are situations where the cardiac dysrhythmias are secondary to underlying structural heart disease, and this will alter the prognosis and likelihood of response to therapy.

#### How to Decide the Most Appropriate Course of Action?

If the horse has **clinical signs** that the dysrhythmia is **hemodynamically relevant** (see Table 12.2) then **immediate treatment or referral** for appropriate treatment is indicated. If the horse appears hemodynamically stable (e.g., heart rate is fairly appropriate, normal mentation, and good peripheral perfusion) then you can consider referral for evaluation as a less emergent situation.

## Congestive Heart Failure

CHF is the clinical scenario in which the heart is unable to pump enough blood to meet the requirements of tissue perfusion and oxygen delivery or can only do so from an elevated filling (venous) pressure. The problem can arise from abnormal filling or ejection. Left- or right-sided heart failure caused by valvular insufficiency is the most common cause of CHF, and filling problems are rare in the horse.

The most common **signs** (Box 12.2) in horses presenting in CHF are tachycardia, tachypnea, murmurs that are often (but not always) grade $\geq 3/6$, abnormal lung sounds (crackles), jugular distention or pulses, ventral edema, or poor body condition score. Murmurs are more common in the left side of the chest and systolic. A discussion on common murmurs and how to differentiate them is found in Appendix 12.1 (online). Muffled heart sounds; abnormal mucous membranes or fever are less commonly described signs.

**Box 12.2 Clinical signs of congestive heart failure (CHF)**

- Tachycardia.
- Tachypnea.
- Murmurs that are often grade $\geq 3/6$.
- Abnormal lung sounds (crackles).
- Jugular distention or pulses.
- Ventral edema.
- Poor body condition.

## Emergency Triage Steps

### Patient Stabilization

Urgent medical therapy is needed to stabilize horses in CHF. The initial approach to the most common presentations of CHF includes **diuretics** to decrease preload, angiotensin-converting enzyme **(ACE) inhibitors** to reduce preload and afterload and **inotropes** to improve systolic function. It is common that horses in CHF will present with atrial fibrillation (AF) and an increased heart rate. The medications commonly used in treatment of CHF are described in Table 12.5.

**Table 12.5** Therapeutic treatment options for congestive heart failure.

| Drug | Drug class | Dose recommendations | Dose for 500 kg bwt | Comments |
|---|---|---|---|---|
| **Diuretics** | | | | |
| Furosemide | Loop diuretic | 1–2 mg/kg IV initially, repeat as indicated<br>0.12 mg/kg/min CRI if further diuresis is indicated after initial bolus (Johansson et al. 2003)<br>Long term management: 1–2 mg/kg IV or IM q 6–12 h | 500–1,000 mg<br>60 mg/min CRI<br>500–1,000 mg | Induces rapid diuresis (within 15 mins) after administration. Titrate dose based on clinical progression. Oral absorption is poor. If longer-term management is required then intramuscular administration is advised.<br>Adverse effects: hypovolemia, hypokalemia, hyponatremia, hypomagnesemia, metabolic acidosis, azotemia.<br>Contraindications: Pericardial effusion causing cardiac tamponade. Caution in patients with pre-existing renal disease. |
| Torsemide | Loop diuretic | 0.5–1 mg/kg PO q 12 h | 250–500 mg | Advantage of higher oral bioavailability than furosemide, with less hypokalemia and longer half-life.<br>Adverse effects: hypovolemia, hypokalemia, hyponatremia, hypomagnesemia, metabolic acidosis, azotemia. Doses of 4 mg/kg are reported to cause excessive diuresis and dehydration.<br>Contraindications: Pericardial effusion causing cardiac tamponade. Caution in patients with pre-existing renal disease. |
| **ACE inhibitors** | | | | |
| Benazepril | ACE inhibitor | 0.5–1 mg/kg PO q 12 h | 250–500 mg | Preload and afterload reduction through effects on the RAAS.<br>When used in conjunction with diuretics (e.g., furosemide) can reduce clinical signs of heart failure.<br>Enalapril is not absorbed in horses.<br>Adverse effects: azotemia, cough, bronchoconstriction. Monitor for hypotension when used in conjunction with diuretics. NSAIDs may reduce clinical efficacy of ACE inhibitors.<br>Contraindications: Hyponatremia. Do not use in pregnant animals. Caution in patients with pre-existing renal disease. |

**Table 12.5** (Continued)

| Drug | Drug class | Dose recommendations | Dose for 500 kg bwt | Comments |
|---|---|---|---|---|
| Quinapril | ACE inhibitor | 0.25 mg/kg PO q 24 h | 125 mg | Preload and afterload reduction through effects on the RAAS.<br>When used in conjunction with diuretics (e.g., furosemide) can reduce clinical signs of heart failure. Lower ACE inhibition reported compared to benazepril but anecdotally there is still perceived clinical improvement with its use.<br>Adverse effects: azotemia, cough, bronchoconstriction. Monitor for hypotension when used in conjunction with diuretics. NSAIDs may reduce clinical efficacy of ACE inhibitors.<br>Contraindications: Hyponatremia. Do not use in pregnant animals. Caution in patients with pre-existing renal disease. |
| **Inotropes** | | | | |
| Dobutamine | $\beta_1$ – adrenergic, $\beta_2$ – and $\alpha_1$ adrenergic<br>**Preferred over dopamine** | 1–5 μg/kg bwt/min CRI, titrate to effect or adverse reaction | 500–2,500 μg/min CRI | Long-term therapy not effective due to tolerance. Continuous ECG monitoring recommended. Decrease dose if tachycardia or tachyarrhythmias develop.<br>Adverse effects: Tachycardia, ventricular dysrhythmias, vasoconstriction and hypertension (at doses >4 μg/kg bwt/min)<br>Contraindications: Ventricular dysrhythmias, tachycardia, atrial fibrillation (risk of severe tachycardia due to accelerated atrio-ventricular conduction) |
| Digoxin | Digitalis glycosides | 0.0022 mg/kg q 12 h IV (Sweeney et al. 1993)<br>0.011 mg/kg q 12 h PO | 1.1 mg IV<br>5.5 mg PO | TDM: peak (1–2 h) and trough (12 h) concentrations at steady state should fall within 0.8–2.0 ng/mL (1–2.6 nmol/L)<br>Adverse effects: Depression, anorexia, colic, diarrhea, sinus bradycardia, AV block, supraventricular and ventricular dysrhythmias (bigeminy)<br>Contraindications: AV block, diastolic ventricular dysfunction, pre-existing digitalis toxicity, myocarditis, ventricular dysrhythmias. |
| Pimobendan | Phosphodiesterase-3 inhibitor<br>Inodilator | 0.25 mg/kg PO q 12 h | 125 mg | No clinical data on its use in horses with CHF. Concurrent use with calcium channel blockers or beta blockers may attenuate effects of pimobendan.<br>Adverse effects: Dysrhythmias.<br>Contraindications: Hypertrophic cardiomyopathies, valvular stenosis. |

Bwt, bodyweight; Kg, kilogram; CNS, central nervous system; AV, atrio-ventricular; CRI, continuous rate infusion; GI, gastrointestinal; IV, intravenous; ACE, angiotensin converting enzyme; RAAS, renin angiotensin aldosterone system; TDM, therapeutic drug monitoring; CHF, congestive heart failure.

## Emergency Treatment Guidelines

### Diuretics

Decreasing preload is often the most important component of CHF treatment in the horse. Diuretics decrease congestion and slow the progression of the disease by decreasing ventricular filling pressures (Redpath and Bowen 2019).

**Furosemide,** a loop diuretic, given intravenously achieves rapid diuresis (within 15 minutes) and is short acting (approximately two hours) (Hinchcliff and Muir 3rd 1991).

**Torsemide** is another loop diuretic that has the main advantage of a high bioavailability after oral administration (Agne et al. 2018). Other potential advantages are less potassium loss, a half-life that allows dosing every 12 h and less renin–angiotensin–aldosterone system activation than more frequent doses of furosemide.

### ACE Inhibitors

**Benazepril** is given mainly for its preload- and afterload-reducing properties and overall benefits of blunting the renin–angiotensin–aldosterone system. Effects on echocardiographic measurements have been shown in horse (Afonso et al. 2017, 2013). Other ACE inhibitors like quinapril have been used in the horses with perceived clinical benefit despite a lower reported percentage of ACE inhibition in experimental conditions. Enalapril is not absorbed in the horse. For many, benazepril is the ACE inhibitor of choice in most clinical scenarios.

### Inotropes

**Digoxin** is a cardiac glycoside that traditionally has been used for its positive inotropic and rate-controlling effects. One of its main uses is to slow the ventricular response rate in AF, a common scenario in the horse with CHF. Digoxin has arrhythmogenic effects and can cause anorexia and dull mentation.

**Dobutamine** is the most widely used positive inotrope with weak positive chronotropic and vasoconstrictive effects. Due its short half-life a constant rate infusion (CRI) is needed.

**Pimobendan** is an inodilator very frequently used in small animals with valvular disease or CHF. Information about the efficacy in the equine clinical setting is lacking, but pimobendan has been shown to have positive chronotropic and inotropic effects in healthy horses after IV administration (Afonso et al. 2016).

**Other therapies** less commonly used are:

**Sedation** - Sedatives such as acepromazine (0.005–0.01 mg/kg IV or IM) or butorphanol (0.01–0.1 mg/kg IV or IM) can be given to treat anxiety associated with dyspnea. Blood pressure, heart rate, and respiratory rate should be monitored. Acepromazine induces vasodilation and blood pressure should be monitored to prevent severe hypotension and lower doses should be used initially.

**Vasodilators** - Calcium channel blockers such as amlodipine and the indirectly acting vasodilators like prazosin and isoxsuprine have not been evaluated for the management of equine cardiovascular disease and are used anecdotally following doses adapted from small animals (Redpath and Bowen 2019). Hydralazine (0.5–1.5 mg/kg PO q 12 h) and milrinone (0.5 μg/kg bolus then 0.5–5 μg/kg/min CRI) have been rarely reported in the horse.

**Oxygen** supplementation can be administrated via nasal cannulas at 5–10 L/min when tissue oxygenation is assessed as poor. Pleural or peritoneal drainage may be needed if effusions can contribute to respiratory distress or poor ventilation. These scenarios are rare in the horse.

Sildenafil, spironolactone, nitroglycerin (glyceryl trinitrate), bronchodilators, or beta blockers could play a role in some cases of CHF, but their use is **not common** in equine CHF.

### Diagnostic Plan

**History:** Assessing the clinical **history** is a key component. Exercise intolerance, murmurs, increase in respiratory rate or effort, and tachycardia are commonly found in the history of horses with CHF. Occasionally the first sign of heart failure that owners detect is severe pulmonary edema and foamy nasal discharge.

**Clinical Pathology:** Clinicopathological findings are often absent or non-specific. Assessing renal function is recommended due to potential for kidney injury due to poor renal perfusion and the frequent importance of renal function in the pharmacology of drugs used to treat CHF.

**Rhythm Assessment:** Sinus tachycardia is the most common **rhythm**, while AF is also a common finding. Loss of atrial booster pump function at the time of AF development can be a tipping point for horses with long standing moderate-to-severe valvular disease and trigger signs of CHF due to the sudden loss of atrial function. Other bradyarrhythmias and tachyarrhythmias that can cause low output cardiac failure or syncope are described in the dysrhythmia section. Telemetric ECG monitoring is useful in acute CHF to monitor rhythm and rate response to therapy.

**Imaging** is an important piece of the investigation of CHF. Ultrasound is often key and Point of Care Ultrasound **(POCUS)** is more frequently being utilized to quickly evaluate the cardiovascular system (Bevevino et al. 2023; Eberhardt and Schwarzwald 2022). Common echocardiography findings are cardiac chamber enlargement, pulmonary artery larger than the aorta, pericardial effusion, and changes in echogenicity of the valves. The detailed echocardiographic changes associated with different cardiac diseases (Schwarzwald 2019) are beyond the scope of this chapter, but POCUS findings that are high yielding and can aid in triage are relevant to all equine practitioners evaluating emergencies. More details can be found in Appendix 12.2 (online). Radiographs are less commonly performed in horses to evaluate cardiac disease when compared to other species due to the less frequent availability and limited information obtained when compared to echocardiography and ultrasound. A diffuse interstitial to broncho-interstitial pattern, consistent with pulmonary edema and cardiomegaly, are the common findings when radiographs are performed in horses in CHF.

## Important Decisions During Management

### Decision for Hospital Referral

Hospital referral may be indicated for horses requiring intensive treatment or advanced diagnostics (Box 12.3).

### Decision for Medical vs Surgical Treatment

Surgical treatment is not relevant to the management of CHF in the horse. There are exceptional descriptions of pericardiectomy in horses, but this is reserved for rare cases.

## How to Manage Important Complications

If a patient initially stabilizes with appropriate emergency treatment, attention should be placed primarily on maintaining cardiac output while watching for organ dysfunction. Acute kidney injury is a common side effect of both CHF and aggressive treatment with diuretics, ACE inhibitors and inotropes. Laminitis, gastrointestinal injury, or central nervous system dysfunction can also occur secondary to CHF and its treatment.

## Estimating Prognosis and Decision for Euthanasia

The prognosis for horses with CHF is poor. In a case series with 14 horses presented in CHF 7 were euthanized after initial evaluation, 5 died within a year, and 2 were lost to follow up (Davis et al. 2002), and all horses in a case series of severe mitral regurgitation died or were subjected to euthanasia within a year due to the severity of their MR and/or lack of response to therapy (Reef et al. 1998). Pharmacological and monitoring advances in the last 20 years mean that stabilization and short-term therapy are currently a feasible option in many horses. The prognosis for return to athletic function after CHF due to valvular or congenital heart disease is very poor and guarded to fair when acute CHF develops due to pericardial, myocardial disease or dysrhythmias that is amenable to treatment. Euthanasia is a fair option in horses in CHF for which appropriate treatment and monitoring are not option. Natural death in horses with untreated and unmonitored CHF is agonal and should be avoided at all costs.

### What Can Be Done at the Farm

Triage and emergency treatment of horses in CHF can be performed on farm. Therapy and monitoring can be performed on farm in many scenarios when the evaluation and monitoring can be provided by ambulatory veterinarians.

**Box 12.3 A horse may need referral to a hospital if it:**

- Needs intensive therapy that cannot be provided on farm such as CRIs or oxygen.
- Needs intense or frequent monitoring that cannot be provided on farm.
- Needs advanced diagnostics (echocardiography) and this is not available on farm.
- Needs expertise that cannot be provided on farm.

#### What Can Be Done at a Referral Hospital

The possibility of round-the-clock monitoring and delivery of CRI medications are the main advantages of treating CHF in a hospital setting. The frequent presence of cardiologists or large animal internists with cardiac expertise is also an advantage although these experts can be available for ambulatory appointments in some regions.

#### How to Decide the Most Appropriate Course of Action?

Ultimately, the decision for referral or not will involve discussion with the owners about their financial situation, estimated prognosis and likelihood of a successful outcome, coupled with the severity of clinical signs that the patient is exhibiting. For cases of CHF where the underlying disease process can resolve (e.g., CHF secondary to overdose of sedation), advanced diagnostic testing and intensive monitoring and labor-intensive treatments (e.g., CRI's of medication) will be required, which are more easily handled in the referral setting than on farm. If severe underlying disease is suspected or known (e.g., pre-existing progressive mitral valve regurgitation), then the prognosis for horses with CHF is very poor and euthanasia is often indicated. The stress of transport to a referral institution can often worsen the clinical signs and cause the patient unnecessary distress.

## Bacterial Endocarditis

### Emergency Triage Steps

#### Patient Stabilization and Emergency Treatment Guidelines

**Bacterial endocarditis** is a valvular disease that deserves special consideration. The patient stabilization and treatment of the consequences of the valvular insufficiency may be similar than the stated above and the evaluation and treatment of the septic process is described below.

#### Diagnostic Plan

The common clinical and clinicopathological signs of active bacterial endocarditis are fever, shifting lameness, synovial effusion, increase in acute-phase proteins (fibrinogen and SAA), hyperglobulinemia, leukocytosis, neutrophilia, and anemia. The presence of nodular, vegetative valvular lesions or diffusely thickened valves and less commonly with other endocardial areas (e.g., chordae tendinea) supports a diagnosis of bacterial endocarditis, but there is overlap between the appearance of bacterial endocarditis and valvular degeneration.

Blood cultures are important in the workup of horses with suspected endocarditis. Bacteremia can be intermittent, and several blood cultures may be needed. There is not a stablished protocol in the horse and three cultures at least one hour apart have been described. Antimicrobial therapy based on culture and sensitivity and using bactericidal IV antibiotics is the first choice. Broad-spectrum coverage should be initiated promptly, and this often implies an empirical choice before culture and sensitivity results are received or after a negative culture is obtained in horses that the rest of the clinical presentation suggests bacterial endocarditis. Penicillin and gentamicin are common empirical choices when culture and sensitivity are not available or when cultures are negative and infective endocarditis is suspected. *Actinobacillus* spp., *Pasteurella*, and *Streptococcus* spp. are commonly described infectious agents associated with bacterial endocarditis (Henderson et al. 2020; Maxson and Reef 1997; Porter et al. 2008).

#### Other Treatments

The use of platelet aggregation inhibitors (clopidogrel 4 mg/kg, once, then 2 mg/kg, q24h) (Watts et al. 2014) is a reasonable adjunct therapy, but the benefits are unproven or controversial. The main benefit of the use of platelet aggregation inhibitor may be to halt the growth of the endocarditis lesion while the main counterargument is the potential benefit of platelets antibacterial effects.

### Important Decisions During Management

Endocarditis associated with the mitral or aortic valve is more common in the horses and carries is grave prognosis. Endocarditis associated with the tricuspid or pulmonic valve also occurs, has a better prognosis, but this is still guarded.

## Myocardial Injury and Myocarditis

Myocardial disease is relatively uncommonly reported in the horse although perhaps under-recognized.

### Emergency Triage Steps

#### Patient Stabilization

Therapy for myocardial injury is aimed at treating the underlying cause and managing the sequelae and is a combination of the principles described for treating dysrhythmias, CHF, and intoxications. Corticosteroids, Vitamin E, selenium, or antibiotics are used in selected cases in which inflammation, oxidative damage, nutritional deficiency, or infections are associated with the case. Positive inotropic agents could aggravate ventricular dysrhythmias and are contraindicated in horses with an ionophore or cardiac glycoside intoxication and therefore should be used with caution (Decloedt 2019).

***Diagnostic Plan*** Toxic insults and myocarditis may be the most common clinical problems in the emergency setting. Myocardial fibrosis, fatty and fibrofatty infiltrates are also reported and can trigger dysrhythmias or sudden death. The clinical interpretation of myocardial fibrosis is however complicated by the fact that this can be found also in necropsies of horses dead or euthanized due to known non-cardiac causes.

The multiple causes of myocardial disease have been recently reviewed and viral diseases (herpesviruses, influenza or equine viral arteritis) or bacterial diseases (*Streptococcus* spp., *Staphylococcus* spp., *Clostridium chauvoei*, *Borrelia burgdorferi*, Piroplasmosis, Leptospirosis, or *Neorickettsia risticiii*) can be suspected. Fungal disease or parasite migration have been rarely described. Intoxications from Ionophores (monensin, lasalocid, salinomycin) or plants containing cardiac glycosides such as *Digitalis* spp. (foxglove), *Taxus* spp. (yew), *Pimelea* spp., *Nerium oleander*, *Adonis aestivalis* (summer pheasant's eye), *Rhododendron,* etc. have been reported. Other intoxications with cardiac signs are: *Malva parviflora* (marshmallow), atypical myopathy/seasonal pasture myopathy caused by ingestion of hypoglycin-A from seeds of maple trees (*Acer* spp.), White snakeroot (*Ageratina altissima*), cantharidin (blister beetle), sodium fluoroacetate rodenticides, or heavy metals.

Other diseases that can be associated with myocardial insults are nutritional diseases (vitamin E/selenium deficiency), neoplasia (lipoma, pulmonary carcinoma, hemangioma/hemangiosarcoma, lymphoma/lymphosarcoma, melanoma, mesothelioma), systemic disease (systemic hypertension, pheochromocytoma/catecholamines), genetic disease (glycogen branching enzyme deficiency), tachycardia-induced cardiomyopathy, trauma, immune-mediated processes, amyloidosis, hypoxia, or hemorrhage.

Myocardial disease is often subclinical but can present as poor performance, exercise intolerance, sudden death, CHF, weakness, syncope, persistent tachycardia, or cardiac dysrhythmias. Murmurs are uncommonly but could occur due to abnormal filling patterns or to stretching of the atrioventricular valve annulus.

Echocardiography can show abnormal myocardial function, dimensions, or morphology or could be normal. Hyperechoic areas in the myocardium often represent myocardial fibrosis, while dilated cardiomyopathy is rare in the horse and, if recognized, is probably a sequela to a previous episode of myocarditis or myocardial injury/necrosis. Tissue Doppler imaging may be a more sensitive way to detect systolic or diastolic dysfunction than standard 2D echocardiography. Many of the imaging aspects of myocardial disease may be harder to detect with POCUS with the exception of moderate or severe hypertrophy or pseudohypertrophy. A hypertrophic appearance (increased relative wall thickness) can occasionally be seen during myocardial injury (due to edema or cellular infiltration), but a similar appearance can be seen due to dehydration (pseudohypertrophy) (Navas de Solis et al. 2013; Underwood et al. 2011).

#### Cardiac Troponins

Cardiac troponins are part of the cardiac muscle contractile apparatus and are specific markers of damage. Cardiac troponins (cTn) I and T are currently the most used and sensitive markers of myocardial damage. The half-life of cTns after experimental injection of recombinant cTns and after exercise (Kraus et al. 2013; Rossi et al. 2019) was 0.47 and 6.4 h. Peak concentration of cTns has been described at 3–6 h after exercise (return to normal after 24 h) and 24–72 h after monensin administration (Kraus et al. 2010). On many occasions, ongoing damage and elimination are likely to overlap, and the effective half-life may be longer than that described experimentally. It is important to recognize that cTns can increase in systemic diseases such as endotoxemia (Nostell et al. 2012), hemorrhage (Navas de Solis et al. 2015), or colic (Díaz et al. 2014), without the presence of primary myocardial injury.

Cardiac troponin I is most commonly measured in horses in most countries, but recently cardiac troponin T assays have been reported and validated (Ven Der Vekens et al. 2015). The reference range is specific for each cTnI assay and uniform for cTnT. Ultrasensitive cTnT, Roche Diagnostics assays, architect STAT High Sensitivity Troponin I (Abbott), Dimensions Vista Troponin I (Siemens) or Stratus CS Acute Care cTnI Cal Pak, (Siemens), have been reported. A point-of-care analyzer (iStat) has been used in several studies with apparently adequate performance to distinguish horses with and without myocardial insults, but formal validation of this assay is currently not available (Rossi et al. 2018; Shields et al. 2016).

### Important Decisions During Management

Stall rest for at least one month after myocardial injury is recommended and monitoring of the cardiac rhythm at rest and during exercise after the recovery period is often indicated.

The prognosis depends on the severity of the myocardial injury, the degree of myocardial dysfunction, development of any dysrhythmias, and presence and degree of subsequent myocardial fibrosis. Horses with mild myocardial injury can fully recover, but the damage can be life-threatening in some cases.

## Pericardial Disease

Pericardial disease is rarely identified in the horse and can be associated with infectious (bacterial, viral), neoplastic (lymphoma, mesothelioma) or immune-mediated diseases or develop secondary to CHF or pleuropneumonia (Worth and Reef 1998). Bacterial pericarditis can be caused by a variety of etiologic agents, with *Actinobacillus* spp. or opportunistic bacteria associated with exposure to eastern tent caterpillars being most frequently reported. Effusive or fibrino-effusive pericarditis are most common forms, but dry pericarditis can also occur and is more difficult to recognize. Pericarditis can cause cardiac compression (tamponade) due to increased pericardial pressure reducing ventricular filling, or less severe diastolic dysfunction. Because of the lower right-sided pressures, the main consequence is impaired venous return to the right heart, resulting in clinical signs of right-sided CHF including jugular vein distension, pulsation, and formation of peripheral edema.

### Emergency Triage Steps

#### Patient Stabilization

Treatment is dependent on the cause and often includes drainage of pericardial fluid if tamponade is present, anti-inflammatory and antibiotics (broad spectrum, e.g., penicillin/gentamicin), and rest. After drainage, often an indwelling catheter is left to perform pericardial lavage, provide local antibiotic therapy, and avoid adhesions.

It is important to recognize that *diuretics are contraindicated* with pericardial effusion, as a rapid decrease in preload may compound the existing impaired filling and worsen clinical signs.

#### Diagnostic Plan

Clinical signs of pericardial disease are initially non-specific and often depend on the amount and rate of pericardial fluid accumulation and the underlying disease. Common signs include history of respiratory disease, fever, lethargy, exercise intolerance, tachycardia, venous distension jugular pulses, ventral edema, pleural or peritoneal effusions. Classically described cardiac auscultation includes muffled heart sounds or friction rubs.

Echocardiography is the most useful tool for diagnosis and assisting therapy and monitoring. Pericardial fluid analysis, with aerobic and anaerobic culture, can help narrow the list of differential diagnoses.

### Important Decisions During Management

The prognosis is favorable for idiopathic pericarditis but guarded or poor for bacterial pericarditis or neoplasia. Early diagnosis and appropriate, aggressive therapy can allow full recovery and return to athletic function in some cases.

## Cardio-Pulmonary Resuscitation

Cardio-pulmonary resuscitation (CPR) is required when patients suffer from cardio-pulmonary arrest (CPA). In general, CPR in horses should be approached in the same systematic manner as in humans and small animals; however, there are some important considerations (Fletcher et al. 2012). The size of patient will dictate the type of chest compressions and the effectiveness of any attempts at defibrillation. In general, the clinician should remember the CPR basics of ABCD: **A – airway, B – breathing, C – circulation,** and **D – drugs** to be administered. Prompt recognition of the need for CPR, and rapid delivery of basic life support (BLS) and advanced life support (ALS) is critical for CPR to have a successful outcome. The clinical scenario in which the CPA occurred is also important for determining the likelihood of return to spontaneous circulation (ROSC) (e.g., a patient under general anesthesia vs a patient that has collapsed in the field setting or a neonate that has arrested during parturition) (Conde Ruiz and Junot 2018; Duggan et al. 2022; Hopster et al. 2016; Wiechert-Brown et al. 2023).

It is very helpful to have discussed the client's wishes for CPR prior to any emergency or elective procedure that has the potential to result in CPA. Having your team aware of the CPR code status (e.g., green for full CPR including ALS, orange for BLS only and red for do not resuscitate) prior to starting a procedure can allow for timely provision of CPR in an emergent situation, without the need to first contact the owners to get permission. Performing CPR comes with additional costs and risks that the owners should be aware of.

Regular veterinary care team trainings should include running a CPR code so that all members of the care team are familiar with the CPR guidelines and understand their role when an animal suffers from CPA. Preparation and familiarity with the treatment guidelines are critical to performing successful CPR.

### Emergency Treatment Guidelines

Graphical algorithms describing the basic and advanced life support steps for performing CPR in adult horses and foals are found in Figures 12.4 and 12.5, respectively. These can be printed out and placed on a crash cart for quick reference during emergencies. The common emergency medications used during CPR are found in Table 12.6.

If a patient is found unresponsive, the presence of breathing and a heart beat should be evaluated quickly by auscultation of the heart. Palpation of a peripheral pulse can be difficult in the emergency setting and therefore should not be relied upon. If no heart beat is appreciated, external chest compressions should be started immediately. The patient should be in lateral recumbency (preferably right lateral) with the head and neck extended. Forcefully compress the chest just behind the elbow with the resuscitator's knees or hands (if the patient is small). The pulse strength can be monitored to estimate the effectiveness of the compressions, in addition to direct measurements of arterial pressures if available.

If the patient is not breathing, an airway should be obtained either through naso-tracheal or oro-tracheal placement of an endotracheal tube. If this is not possible, an emergency tracheostomy should be performed, and the endotracheal tube placed directly in the trachea. The endotracheal tube's cuff should be inflated, and the tube attached to a demand valve, ambu bag (if the patient is small) or anesthetic machine with rebreathing bag, to provide ventilation. A tidal volume of 10 mL/kg is appropriate (5 L for a 500 kg horse), and the demand valve or rebreathing bag should be compressed to provide between 20 and 40 cm $H_2O$. If no pressure sensor is available, the amount of chest excursion should be visually evaluated. If arterial oxygenation can be monitored, room air is preferred over 100% $O_2$, but in the absence of such monitoring, 100% $O_2$ is appropriate.

One cycle of BLS is two minutes duration. During this time, maintain regular chest compressions (approx. 30–60/min for an adult, 90–120/min for a foal) and provide interposed ventilation (4–6/min for an adult, 10/min for a foal). Every two minutes the compressor should change out, to avoid fatigue and reduced efficacy. Chest compressions in adult horses will not provide sufficient flow to support life but may aid to prolong life in order to facilitate distribution of resuscitative drugs to vital tissues.

If the equipment is available to provide ALS, an ECG should be placed to monitor the cardiac rhythm, end-tidal $CO_2$ measured to assess the effectiveness of compressions, and IV catheter placed, and reversal of any anesthetic, sedative, or analgesic agents should be performed. End-tidal $CO_2$ is used to monitor for ROSC due to increasing pulmonary blood flow associated with effective cardiac output; values above 15 mmHg have been associated with more positive CPR outcomes in small animals.

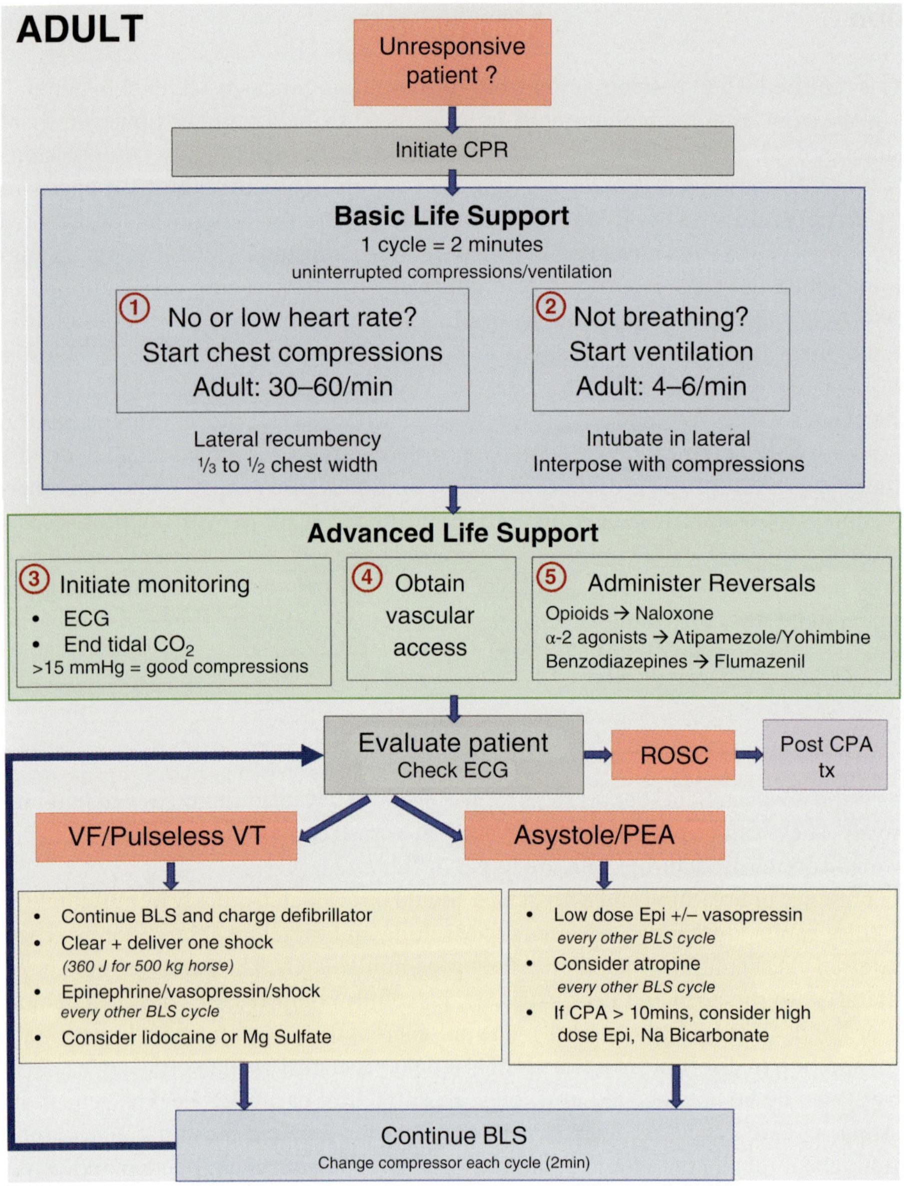


**Figure 12.4** Cardio-pulmonary resuscitation (CPR) algorithm for adult horses. CPR, cardio-pulmonary resuscitation; BLS, basic life support; ALS, advanced life support; ECG, electrocardiogram; α-2, alpha 2; CPA, cardio-pulmonary arrest; ROSC, return of spontaneous circulation; VF, ventricular fibrillation; VT, ventricular tachycardia; PEA, pulseless electrical activity; Epi, epinephrine; Na, sodium; J, joule; Mg, magnesium.

Every two minutes, the patient should be evaluated for ROSC, including a pulse check and ECG rhythm check. Administration of low-dose epinephrine alternating with vasopressin (if available) is recommended every second cycle of BLS if ROSC has not occurred.

If a defibrillator is available and ventricular fibrillation (VF) or pulseless ventricular tachycardia (VT) is present, an attempt at external defibrillation can be made in smaller patients with a size similar to or smaller than an adult human. Successful defibrillation of horses up to 341 kg has been described using custom-made defibrillators, but the default settings and safety mechanisms of commercial defibrillators do not allow to replicate this experience in most settings. It is important to use the electrode gel on the defibrillator paddles and ensure everyone is clear of the horse before defibrillation is attempted. *Do not use* a defibrillator if *alcohol* is present on the skin of the animal, as this poses a fire hazard.

In the case of VT or VF, or after a 6 minute period (3 × BLS cycles) of unsuccessful CPR in the absence of an ECG/hemodynamic monitoring, a dose of lidocaine or magnesium sulfate could be given if several cycles of BLS have not shown any ROSC. If a horse has been in CPA for more than 10 minutes, the chances of successful CPR are very low.

If the patient does show signs of spontaneous circulation, it is important to provide appropriate IV fluid support, monitoring of systemic blood pressure and cardiac output with vasopressor assistance if required. Cerebral edema is a common sequalae of CPA; therefore, close monitoring and treatment (e.g., mannitol) may also be necessary.

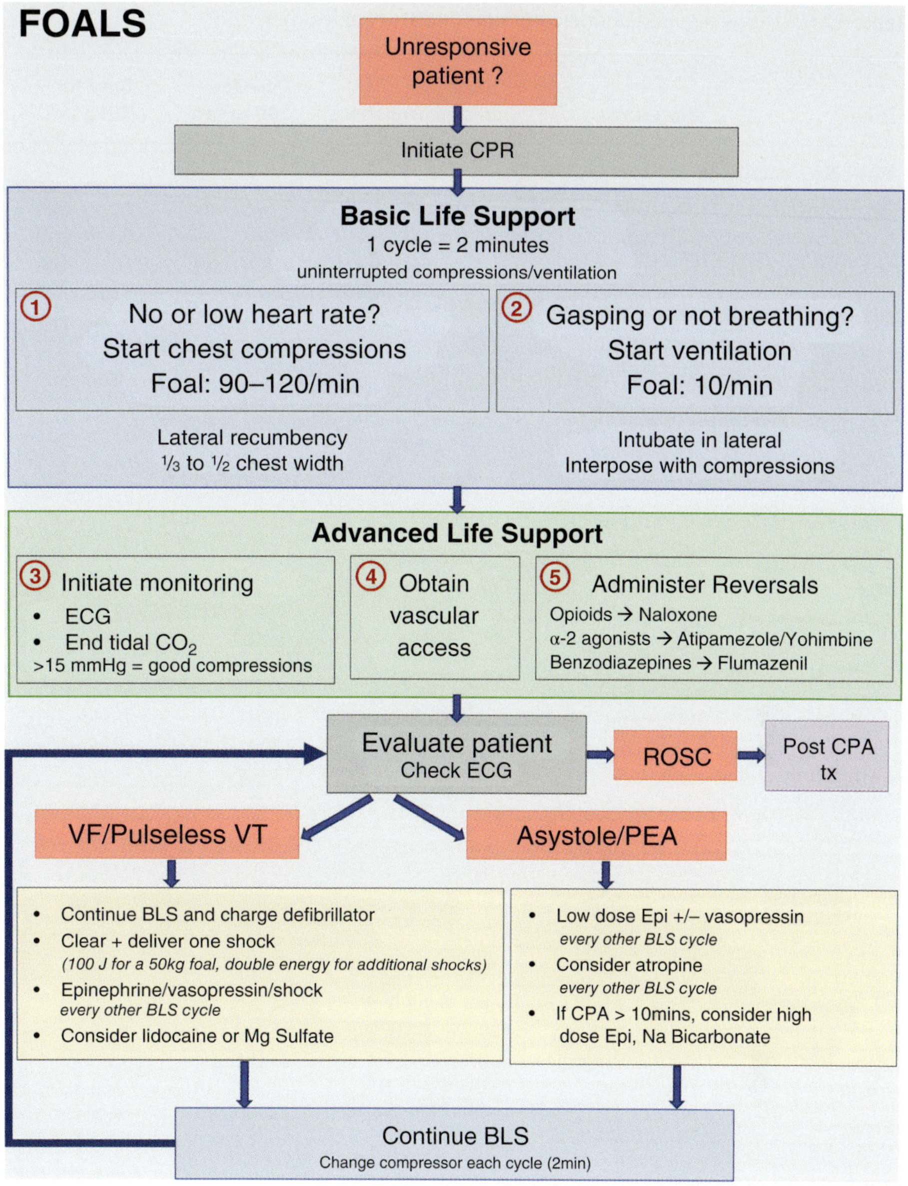


**Figure 12.5** Cardio-pulmonary resuscitation (CPR) algorithm for foals. CPR, cardio-pulmonary resuscitation; BLS, basic life support; ALS, advanced life support; ECG, electrocardiogram; α-2, alpha 2; CPA, cardio-pulmonary arrest; ROSC, return of spontaneous circulation; VF, ventricular fibrillation; VT, ventricular tachycardia; PEA, pulseless electrical activity; Epi, epinephrine; Na, sodium; J, joule; Mg, magnesium.

## Important Decisions During Management

### Decision for Hospital Referral

In the situation of CPR, the decision regarding referral is based upon the availability of appropriate post-resuscitation care and monitoring. If the CPR is successful, the patient is still likely to require intensive care for a period of time and when this cannot be provided locally, then referral to an appropriate hospital facility is indicated.

### How to Manage Important Complications

Depending on the reason for CPA and the speed at which ROSC occurs, there may be important sequalae particularly involving the central nervous, cardiovascular, gastrointestinal, and renal systems. Altered mental state, seizures, renal failure, cardiac injury, decreased cardiac function, dysrhythmias, thoracic trauma (e.g., fractured ribs, lung laceration), and gastrointestinal dysfunction are all possible consequences of CPR, and intensive supportive care is indicated when signs of organ dysfunction are present.

**Table 12.6** Drugs required during cardio-pulmonary resuscitation (CPR).

| Drug | Drug class | Dose recommendations | Dose for 500 kg bwt | Dose for 50 kg bwt | Comments |
|---|---|---|---|---|---|
| **First-line medication during CPR** | | | | | |
| Epinephrine (Adrenaline)<br>1 : 1,000; 1 mg/mL | Non-selective adrenergic agonist | Low dose: 0.01 mg/kg bwt IV<br>High dose: 0.1 mg/kg bwt IV | Low dose: 5 mL<br>High dose: 50 mL | Low dose: 0.5 mL<br>High dose: 5 mL | β-adrenergic at lower doses, $\alpha_1$-adrenergic at higher doses<br>Avoid high doses of epinephrine during CPR where possible<br>Indications: ventricular fibrillation/ pulseless ventricular tachycardia, ventricular asystole, cardiopulmonary resuscitation (use every other cycle, alternate with vasopressin if available)<br>Adverse effects: muscle tremors, excitability, arrhythmias, VF. Overdoses can lead to hypertension, dysrhythmias, renal failure, pulmonary oedema, cerebral hemorrhage<br>Contraindications: non-anaphylactic shock, dysrhythmias, hypertension |
| Arginine Vasopressin (Antidiuretic hormone)<br>20 IU/mL | $V_1$ receptor agonist | 0.8 IU/kg bwt IV bolus | 400 IU (20 mL) IV bolus | 40 IU (2 mL) IV bolus | Indications: ventricular fibrillation/ pulseless ventricular tachycardia, ventricular asystole, cardiopulmonary resuscitation. Alternate with epinephrine during CPR (use every other cycle)<br>Adverse effects: myocardial infarction, sweating, decreased gastrointestinal perfusion, hypertension<br>Contraindications: hypertension, heart failure, renal failure, seizures |
| Atropine<br>15 mg/mL<br>(note concentration) | Anticholinergic (vagolytic) | 0.01–0.02 mg/kg bwt IV or IM | 5–10 mg (0.3–0.7 mL) IV or IM | 0.5–1 mg (0.03–0.07 mL) IV or IM | Indications: bradycardia, high grade 2nd degree AV block, ventricular asystole (use every other cycle)<br>Adverse effects: Constipation, ileus, colic, bradycardia (at very low doses), tachycardia, dysrhythmias, CNS effects (stimulation, drowsiness, ataxia, seizures, respiratory depression) Glycopyrrolate is slightly less arrhythmogenic and rarely results in CNS effects<br>Contraindications: Tachycardia, tachyarrhythmia, heart failure, GI disease, colic |
| Lidocaine (Lignocaine)<br>20 mg/mL | Class $I_B$<br>$Na^+$ channel blocker | 0.25–0.5 mg/kg bwt slow IV, repeat in 5–10 min to effect, up to 1.5 mg/kg bwt total dose; followed by 0.05 mg/kg bwt/ min CRI | 125–250 mg (6.3–12.5 mL) per bolus up to total dose of 750 mg (37.5 mL); CRI 25 mg/ min | 12.5–25 mg (1.3–2.6 mL) per bolus up to a total of 75 mg (3.8 mL); CRI 2.5 mg/min | Indications: VT/VF<br>Adverse effects: Uncommon at therapeutic doses. Overdose can lead to ataxia, muscle tremors, CNS excitement, dysrhythmias, and collapse.<br>Contraindications: SA, AV, or intraventricular block, bradycardia. Caution with hypovolemia, liver disease, shock, and heart failure. |

**Table 12.6** (Continued)

| Drug | Drug class | Dose recommendations | Dose for 500 kg bwt | Dose for 50 kg bwt | Comments |
|---|---|---|---|---|---|
| Magnesium sulfate | Physiologic $Ca^{2+}$ and $K^+$ channel blocker. Activator of membrane $Na^+$/$K^+$ ATPase. | 2–6 mg/kg bwt/min IV to effect, up to 55–100 mg/kg bwt total dose | 1–3 g/min; total dose 27–50 g | 100–300 mg/min; total dose 2.75–5 g | Indications: VT/torsade de pointes<br>Adverse effects: Rare, but overdose may lead to CNS depressant effects, weakness, trembling, bradycardia, hypotension. Very high doses cause neuromuscular blockade with respiratory depression and cardiac arrest.<br>Contraindications: Bradycardia, SA and AV block, renal failure. |
| Amiodarone | Class III $K^+$ channel blocker | 5 mg/kg bwt IV slow bolus | 2.5 g IV slow bolus | 250 mg IV slow bolus | Indications: VT/VF<br>Also class I, II and IV effects.<br>Adverse reactions: Hind limb weakness, weight shifting, *torsade de pointes*, SA and AV nodal inhibition, bradycardia, hypotension. Prolonged treatment may affect lungs, liver, heart, thyroid gland, GI tract, eyes, skin, and nerves.<br>Contraindications: Sino-atrial node dysfunction, bradycardia, AV block, cardiogenic shock. |
| Naloxone | Opioid antagonist | 0.01–0.03 mg/kg bwt IV | 5–15 mg IV | 0.5–1.5 mg IV | Indications: reverse opioids. Monitor for effect as duration of action is shorter than opioids, so redosing may be required<br>Adverse reactions: Rare, wide safety margin, may cause seizures at very high doses<br>Contraindications: Pre-existing cardiac abnormalities, patients with opioid dependency |
| Flumazenil | Benzodiazepine antagonist | 0.01 mg/kg bwt slow IV | 5 mg slow IV | 0.5 mg slow IV | Indications: reverse benzodiazepines<br>Adverse reactions: Seizures.<br>Contraindications: If benzodiazepines were initially given to control seizures, use caution when considering reversal as further seizure activity may occur |
| Atipamezole | $Alpha_2$ receptor antagonist | 0.05 mg/kg bwt slow IV | 25 mg slow IV | 2.5 mg slow IV | Indications: reverse $alpha_2$ receptor agonists<br>Adverse reactions: reversal can occur rapidly, patients may become aggressive or excited<br>Contraindications: Not recommended in pregnant or lactating animals (lack of safety data) |

Bwt, bodyweight; Kg, kilogram; CNS, central nervous system; SA, sino-atrial; AV, atrio-ventricular; CRI, continuous rate infusion; GI, gastrointestinal; VT, ventricular tachycardia; VF, ventricular fibrillation; IV, intravenous; CPR, cardio-pulmonary resuscitation.

#### Estimating Prognosis and Decision for Euthanasia

Unfortunately, very few resuscitation attempts are successful in equine patients with the exception of the immediate post foaling period or in systemically healthy horses under general anesthesia. However, the logistics of performing effective CPR on a 500 kg animal and the size limitations with successful external defibrillation in larger patients during ALS means that many animals will not survive despite our best resuscitation efforts. If an animal does have rapid ROSC, then the prognosis for survival is improved; however, delayed ROSC will be associated with a larger number of complications and likely multiple organ dysfunction. Owners should be warned of this guarded prognosis, particularly when involving critically ill patients.

If you are performing field or hospital-based anesthesia, or in a practice that sees a number of neonates, it is recommended to organize an emergency kit with CPR equipment and coordinate regular training sessions with your staff to practice running a "code." Evidence from human and small animal practice shows that CPR is more effectively performed when the team is well trained and prepared.

#### What Can Be Done on Farm?

Given the urgency of CPA, if it occurs on farm, then CPR will be performed immediately in the field. Often only BLS can be provided in the ambulatory setting. Performing adequate CPR is exhausting, particularly if there is only a small number of people available to help.

#### What Can Be Done at a Referral Hospital?

A referral hospital may have more capacity to provide ALS, with ECG and end-tidal $CO_2$ monitoring, a larger team of people and possibly access to a defibrillator. If ROSC occurs, then the patient will likely still require intensive care with regular monitoring, that is easier to provide in a referral setting.

#### How to Decide the Most Appropriate Course of Action?

In the setting of CPA, the decision to refer will likely be made if ROSC occurs, although this happens very uncommonly after CPR in large animals. If an animal is considered at high risk of having CPA, then referral before this occurs is warranted.

## Blood Coagulation Disorders

Emergencies of coagulation in the horse can be divided into those of hypocoagulation, resulting in the clinical sign of hemorrhage, or hypercoagulation, where excessive clotting or inappropriate thrombosis within the vasculature is evident (Dallap 2004; Epstein 2014; Hurcombe et al. 2022).

The normal process of hemostasis can be divided into three main components – primary hemostasis, with the formation of a platelet plug; secondary hemostasis (formation of a mesh containing cross linked fibrin); and fibrinolysis, which is the process of breaking down the cross-linked fibrin. The formation of blood clots, or thrombi, is common when there is injury or inflammation within the vasculature, primarily aimed at limiting blood loss or the spread of infection in the local tissues. To counterbalance the formation of clots, there are inhibitory and fibrinolytic pathways that aim to limit clot formation to avoid damage to healthy tissue. Balance is required between the pro- and anti-coagulation activity, and dysfunction of either system can promote excessive bleeding or clotting.

### Emergency Triage Steps

Patients can present on emergency with obvious clinical signs of excessive hemorrhage (e.g., a wound that will not stop bleeding, epistaxis, progressively enlarging hematoma) but if the hemorrhage is contained within a body cavity (e.g., abdomen, thorax, pericardium, bladder) then the clinical signs consistent with hypovolemia will be evident, but the source of the hemorrhage may not be obvious without further investigations.

Patients with hypercoagulability may have more subtle or variable clinical signs, depending on the location and size of the thrombi. The signs may be related directly to the clot (e.g., palpable mass in a jugular vein consistent with a thrombus) or a result of obstruction to blood flow (e.g., distension of the venous vasculature and edema of the soft tissues distal to venous thrombus). Arterial thrombi will result in ischemia of the tissue being supplied by that artery (e.g., cranial mesenteric artery thrombosis result in ischemia to the gastro-intestinal tract, resulting in colic signs).

### Patient Stabilization

Rapid recognition and stabilization of patients with excessive bleeding is critical. If the hemorrhage is external, then appropriate bandaging and splinting (where indicated) is the first step to preventing further bleeding. If epistaxis is present, it is essential to keep the patient's head in a neutral-to-slightly elevated position, horses can fatally bleed out quickly from upper respiratory tract origin hemorrhage when the head is held in a low position. Keeping the patient calm (and therefore lowering heart rate and blood pressure) can help minimize ongoing hemorrhage.

Internal hemorrhage is more difficult to stabilize, with the first step keeping the patient calm to prevent further bleeding. Patients experiencing severe blood loss can become quite anxious as hemorrhagic shock develops. Careful sedation may be necessary to keep the patient quiet and prevent worsening injury to themselves or the people working to stabilize them. *Be aware* that boluses of alpha$_2$ agonists can cause *transient increases in systemic blood pressure*, which can worse hemorrhage. Alpha$_2$ agonists should be administered slowly over 2–3 mins, to reduce this effect.

### Diagnostic Plan

If the patient is hemodynamically unstable, then minimal diagnostic evaluation is indicated in the first instance, and you should prioritize lifesaving emergency treatment measures. These unstable patients will have clear evidence of hemorrhagic shock on physical examination, with heart rates >80 bpm, respiratory rates >30 bpm, cold patchy sweating, muscle fasciculations, pale or gray tacky mucus membranes with prolonged capillary refill time, poor jugular filling, and prolonged skin tent. They can have dull mentation with no interest in their environment but could also be anxious and agitated. Gut sounds are typically decreased to absent and extremities cold with weak, thready peripheral pulses. Some patients with hemorrhagic shock appear colicky, pawing, kicking at their abdomen, shifting weight, and trying to lie down. Patients with signs of hemorrhagic shock need urgent but controlled volume expansion to restore cardiac output and maintain critical organ perfusion.

When the patient is fairly stable, then you will have more time to perform a diagnostic evaluation and make decisions regarding the most appropriate treatment. If a clear cause for the hemorrhage is known or can be identified (e.g., trauma) then the diagnostic plan is to stabilize and treat the primary problem and the consequences of the excessive hemorrhage. When the cause of the excessive hemorrhage is not obvious, then further investigations will be necessary, and the decision should be quickly made if this is possible in the field, or if referral is indicated.

Patients with excessive coagulation will likely require more extensive diagnostic evaluation to determine the underlying cause and severity of the disease process.

### Emergency Treatment Guidelines

***Excessive Bleeding*** In the field setting, emergency treatment for excessive hemorrhage is first aimed at restoring the circulating blood volume to maintain cardiac output and critical organ perfusion. Crystalloids are the easiest fluid to start with in the emergency setting, while a quick determination of whether blood products are also indicated should also be made, as these fluids take time to acquire and administer.

The current recommendations for the treatment of hemorrhagic shock are goal directed, with a starting bolus of hypertonic saline at a rate of 4 mL/kg given rapidly IV, followed by a balanced isotonic crystalloid fluid (e.g., Hartmann's solution or Plasmalyte A) at 20 mL/kg given over 30 minutes using a large bore catheter placed in the jugular vein (Crabtree and Epstein 2021; Epstein 2014; Fielding 2014; Fielding and Magdesian 2011; Pantaleon 2010; Pantaleon et al. 2007). Reassessment of heart and respiratory rate, membrane color, and signs of peripheral perfusion should be performed regularly to monitor for any improvement and to guide decisions about the need for further fluid therapy.

When there is evidence of hypocoagulability (e.g., petechia or ecchymoses on mucus membranes, bleeding from catheter or venipuncture sites) then it is highly likely that blood products (fresh frozen plasma or whole blood) will be required to provide support for the coagulation system.

Antifibrinolytics (e.g., aminocaproic acid (20–40 mg/kg diluted in 1 L of 0.9% NaCl IV) or tranexamic acid (5–25 mg/kg diluted in 1 L 0.9% NaCl IV)) is frequently used in the face of excessive hemorrhage, despite a paucity of evidence that horses have increased fibrinolysis and inappropriate break down of clots as a cause for the bleeding.

***Excessive Clotting*** If excessive clotting occurs in the arterial side of the vasculature, then the clinical signs will likely be more severe, but the origin of the thrombosis may not be immediately clear and referral will likely be indicated to perform more advanced diagnostics and provide emergency treatment (e.g., local or systemic anti-coagulant, anti-platelet, and thrombolytic therapy).

Venous thrombosis is typically less immediately life threatening, most commonly involving the jugular vein, where it needs to be determined if there is just thrombosis, or if it is complicated by concurrent infection (thrombophlebitis). Treatment usually involved anti-coagulation and anti-platelet therapies (e.g., aspirin 11 mg/kg PO SID or clopidogrel 4 mg/kg PO loading dose, then 2 mg/kg PO SID, enoxaparin 40–80 IU/kg SC SID), and if infection is present, appropriate anti-microbial therapy will also be indicated (Epstein 2014).

## Important Decisions During Management

### Decision for Hospital Referral

If the patient is hemodynamically unstable, then rapid referral is usually indicated, as these patients require intensive treatment and ongoing monitoring. Most referral facilities have access to a range of blood products (e.g., fresh frozen plasma and universal blood donors) and technical support for thawing, collecting, and administering these products where necessary.

### Decision for Medical vs Surgical Treatment

If the source of hemorrhage is known or located and is not responding to conservative therapy, then surgical intervention may be required to stop further hemorrhage. Examples where surgical intervention can provide rapid resolution for the hemorrhage would include epistaxis from guttural pouch mycosis, where ligation of the common carotid arteries can be lifesaving or in a horse with excessive hemorrhage following castration – standing laparoscopic ligation of the spermatic cord will immediately stop further hemorrhage. Careful consideration of the pros and cons should be given to surgical procedures that require general anesthesia, particularly the risk of prolonged hypotension, and the patients should be appropriately stabilized before general anesthesia is considered.

In cases of excessive thrombosis, surgical intervention is rarely indicated, especially in the emergent situation.

### How to Manage Important Complications

Excessive hemorrhage resulting in hemorrhagic shock is associated with complications associated with critical organ damage (e.g., acute renal failure, laminitis, gastrointestinal, myocardial dysfunction). It is important to recognize the potential for these complications and warn owners, as complications like laminitis can take several days to develop clinical signs. These complications can be mitigated by rapid recognition of excessive hemorrhage and instigation of early and appropriate therapy, including referral.

Thrombosis of large arterial vessels is likely to result in ischemia and subsequent dysfunction of the tissues directly supplied by those arteries which could lead to signs of organ failure. While these types of thromboses are rare, they are highly consequential; therefore, rapid referral is indicated.

### Estimating Prognosis and Decision for Euthanasia

If the patient has severe clinical signs involving hemodynamic instability and the failure of multiple organs then the prognosis will be poor to hopeless and euthanasia is indicated, as these patients can rapidly deteriorate, suffer pain and distress, and die suddenly. If the clinical signs are less severe or respond quickly to appropriate emergency treatment and the patient can be stabilized, then the prognosis can be better, but the possibility of delayed organ failure (e.g., laminitis) should be made clear to the owners. If the excessive hemorrhage is the result of a genetic disorder, then the prognosis is guarded for long-term management, but if an underlying toxicity or systemic disease is identified and can be treated, then the prognosis may be more favorable.

### What Can Be Done on Farm?

Basic life-saving measures can be performed on farm, including bandaging, packing, or splinting of wounds to prevent further hemorrhage. Additionally, the placement of an IV catheter and administration of hypertonic saline or a bolus of crystalloids may provide enough cardiovascular support to allow time for referral. However, the time taken and availability of equipment and appropriate support on farm to perform these treatments should be factored into the decision making. If the distance to the referral hospital is short, then it may make more sense to proceed with referral, while if the journey is likely to be several hours, then stabilization before transport will be a better option if available.

### What Can Be Done at a Referral Hospital?

Most referral hospitals can provide intensive care, continuous monitoring and have access to a wider range of therapeutic interventions and treatments. This could include monitoring of coagulation function testing, access to a variety of blood products, regular assessment of the effect of therapy (e.g., NIBP monitoring), and early identification of any complications (e.g., anuria, laminitis).

### How to Decide the Most Appropriate Course of Action?

Ultimately, the decision for referral or not will involve discussion with the owners about their financial situation, prognosis and likelihood of a successful outcome, coupled with the severity of clinical signs that the patient is exhibiting. For most emergent disorders of the coagulation system, advanced diagnostic testing and intensive monitoring and labor-intensive treatments (e.g., blood transfusions) will be required, which are more easily handled in the referral setting than on farm.

## References


Afonso, T., Giguere, S., Brown, S.A. et al. (2017). Preliminary investigation of orally administered benazepril in horses with left-sided valvular regurgitation. *Equine Vet. J.* 50: 446–451.

Afonso, T., Giguère, S., Rapoport, G. et al. (2016). Cardiovascular effects of pimobendan in healthy mature horses. *Equine Vet. J.* 48: 352–356.

Afonso, T., Giguere, S., Rapoport, G. et al. (2013). Pharmacodynamic evaluation of 4 angiotensin-converting enzyme inhibitors in healthy adult horses. *J. Vet. Intern. Med.* 27: 1185–1192.

Agne, G.F., Jung, S.W., Wooldridge, A.A. et al. (2018). Pharmacokinetic and pharmacodynamic properties of orally administered torsemide in healthy horses. *J. Vet. Intern. Med.* 32: 1428–1435.

Bevevino, K.E., Cohen, N.D., Gordon, S.G., and Navas De Solis, C. (2023). Feasibility of a point-of-care ultrasound protocol for cardiorespiratory evaluation of horses in different clinical settings. *J. Vet. Intern. Med.* 37 (3): 1223–1232.

Conde Ruiz, C. and Junot, S. (2018). Successful cardiopulmonary resuscitation in a sevoflurane anaesthetized horse that suffered cardiac arrest at recovery. *Front Vet. Sci.* 5: 138.

Crabtree, N.E. and Epstein, K.L. (2021). Current concepts in fluid therapy in horses. *Front Vet. Sci.* 8: 648774.

Dallap, B.L. (2004). Coagulopathy in the equine critical care patient. *Vet. Clin. North Am. Equine Pract.* 20: 231–251.

Davis, J.L., Gardner, S.Y., Schwabenton, B., and Breuhaus, B.A. (2002). Congestive heart failure in horses: 14 cases (1984–2001). *J. Am. Vet. Med. Assoc.* 220: 1512–1515.

Decloedt, A. (2019). Pericardial disease, myocardial disease, and great vessel abnormalities in horses. *Vet. Clin.: Equine Pract.* 35: 139–157.

Decloedt, A., Van Steenkiste, G., Vera, L. et al. (2021). Atrial fibrillation in horses part 2: diagnosis, treatment and prognosis. *Vet. J.* 268: 105594.

Díaz, O.M., Durando, M.M., Birks, E.K., and Reef, V.B. (2014). Cardiac troponin I concentrations in horses with colic. *J. Am. Vet. Med. Assoc.* 245: 118–125.

Duggan, M., Schofield, W., and Vermedal, H. (2022). Successful cardiopulmonary resuscitation in an adult horse following cardiovascular collapse on recovery from general anaesthesia in the Trendelenburg position. *Equine Vet. Edu.* 34: e98–e105.

Eberhardt, C. and Schwarzwald, C.C. (2022). Focused cardiac ultrasound examination in the emergency and critical care equine patient: training for non-specialist veterinarians and evaluation of proficiency. *J. Vet. Intern. Med.* 36: 1471–1480.

Epstein, K.L. (2014). Coagulopathies in horses. *Vet. Clin. North Am. Equine Pract.* 30 (437–52): ix.

Fielding, C.L. and Magdesian, K.G. (2011). A comparison of hypertonic (7.2%) and isotonic (0.9%) saline for fluid resuscitation in horses: a randomized, double-blinded, clinical trial. *J. Vet. Intern. Med.* 25: 1138–1143.

Fielding, L. (2014). Crystalloid and colloid therapy. *Vet. Clin. North Am. Equine Pract.* 30: 415–425, viii-ix.

Fletcher, D.J., Boller, M., Brainard, B.M. et al. (2012). RECOVER evidence and knowledge gap analysis on veterinary CPR. Part 7: clinical guidelines. *J. Vet. Emerg. Crit. Care (San Antonio)* 22 (Suppl 1): S102–S131.

Henderson, B., Diaz, M., Martins, C. et al. (2020). Valvular endocarditis in the horse: 20 cases (1993–2020). *Can. Vet. J.* 61: 1290–1294.

Hinchcliff, K.W. and Muir, W.W. 3rd (1991). Pharmacology of furosemide in the horse: a review. *J. Vet. Intern. Med.* 5: 211–218.

Hopster, K., Tüensmeyer, J., and Kästner, S.B.R. (2016). Resuscitation attempts in a foal with sudden cardiac arrest in the early recovery period. *Equine Vet. Edu.* 28: 241–244.

Hurcombe, S.D.A., Radcliffe, R.M., Cook, V.L., and Divers, T.J. (2022). The pathophysiology of uncontrolled hemorrhage in horses. *J. Vet. Emerg. Crit. Care (San Antonio)* 32: 63–71.

Johansson, A.M., Gardner, S.Y., Levine, J.F. et al. (2003). Furosemide continuous rate infusion in the horse: evaluation of enhanced efficacy and reduced side effects. *J. Vet. Intern. Med.* 17: 887–895.

Kraus, M.S., Jesty, S.A., Gelzer, A.R. et al. (2010). Measurement of plasma cardiac troponin I concentration by use of a point-of-care analyzer in clinically normal horses and horses with experimentally induced cardiac disease. *Am. J. Vet. Res.* 71: 55–59.

Kraus, M.S., Kaufer, B.B., Damiani, A. et al. (2013). Elimination half-life of intravenously administered equine cardiac troponin I in healthy ponies. *Equine Vet. J.* 45: 56–59.

Maxson, A.D. and Reef, V.B. (1997). Bacterial endocarditis in horses: ten cases (1984–1995). *Equine Vet. J.* 29: 394–399.

Mitchell, K.J. (2017). Practical considerations for diagnosis and treatment of ventricular tachycardia in horses. *Equine Vet. Edu.* 29: 670–676.

Mitchell, K.J. (2019). Equine electrocardiography. *Vet. Clin.: Equine Pract.* 35: 65–83.

Mitchell, K.J. (2020). *ECG Interpretation in Equine Practice*. CABI.

Navas De Solis, C. (2020). Ventricular arrhythmias in horses: diagnosis, prognosis and treatment. *Vet. J.* 261: 105476.

Navas De Solis, C., Dallap Schaer, B.L., Boston, R., and Slack, J. (2015). Myocardial insult and arrhythmias after acute hemorrhage in horses. *J. Vet. Emerg. Crit. Care (San Antonio)* 25: 248–255.

Navas De Solis, C., Slack, J., Boston, R.C., and Reef, V.B. (2013). Hypertensive cardiomyopathy in horses: 5 cases (1995–2011). *J. Am. Vet. Med. Assoc.* 243: 126–130.

Nostell, K., Brojer, J., Hoglund, K. et al. (2012). Cardiac troponin I and the occurrence of cardiac arrhythmias in horses with experimentally induced endotoxaemia. *Vet. J.* 192: 171–175.

Pantaleon, L.G. (2010). Fluid therapy in equine patients: small-volume fluid resuscitation. *Compend Contin. Educ. Vet.* 32: E1–E6; quiz E7.

Pantaleon, L.G., Furr, M.O., Mckenzie, H.C., and Donaldson, L. (2007). Effects of small- and large-volume resuscitation on coagulation and electrolytes during experimental endotoxemia in anesthetized horses. *J. Vet. Intern. Med.* 21: 1374–1379.

Porter, S.R., Saegerman, C., Van Galen, G. et al. (2008). Vegetative endocarditis in equids (1994–2006). *J. Vet. Intern. Med.* 22: 1411–1416.

Redpath, A. and Bowen, M. (2019). Cardiac therapeutics in horses. *Vet. Clin.: Equine Pract.* 35: 217–241.

Reef, V.B., Bain, F.T., and Spencer, P.A. (1998). Severe mitral regurgitation in horses: clinical, echocardiographic and pathological findings. *Equine Vet. J.* 30: 18–27.

Rossi, T.M., Kavsak, P.A., Maxie, M.G. et al. (2018). Analytical validation of cardiac troponin I assays in horses. *J. Vet. Diagn. Invest.* 30: 226–232.

Rossi, T.M., Kavsak, P.A., Maxie, M.G. et al. (2019). Post-exercise cardiac troponin I release and clearance in normal Standardbred racehorses. *Equine Vet. J.* 51: 97–101.

Schwarzwald, C.C. (2019). Equine echocardiography. *Vet. Clin.: Equine Pract.* 35: 43–64.

Shields, E., Seiden-Long, I., Massie, S. et al. (2016). Analytical validation and establishment of reference intervals for a 'high-sensitivity' cardiac troponin-T assay in horses. *BMC Vet. Res.* 12: 1–11.

Sweeney, R.W., Reef, V.B., and Reimer, J.M. (1993). Pharmacokinetics of digoxin administered to horses with congestive heart failure. *Am. J. Vet. Res.* 54: 1108–1111.

Underwood, C., Norton, J.L., Nolen-Walston, R.D. et al. (2011). Echocardiographic changes in heart size in hypohydrated horses. *J. Vet. Intern. Med.* 25: 563–569.

Van Der Vekens, N., Van Dievoet, M.A., De Puydt, H. et al. (2015). Analytical validation of a high-sensitivity cardiac troponin T assay in horses. *J. Vet. Diagn. Invest.* 27: 504–509.

Van Loon, G. (2019). Cardiac arrhythmias in horses. *Vet. Clin.: Equine Pract.* 35: 85–102.

Van Loon, G., Van Steenkiste, G., Vera, L., and Decloedt, A. (2020). Catheter-based electrical interventions to study, diagnose and treat arrhythmias in horses: from refractory period to electro-anatomical mapping. *Vet. J.* 263: 105519.

Van Steenkiste, G., De Clercq, D., Vera, L. et al. (2019). Sustained atrial tachycardia in horses and treatment by transvenous electrical cardioversion. *Equine Vet. J.* 51: 634–640.

Watts, A.E., Ness, S.L., Divers, T.J. et al. (2014). Effects of clopidogrel on horses with experimentally induced endotoxemia. *Am. J. Vet. Res.* 75: 760–769.

Wiechert-Brown, S.A., Di Concetto, S., Hepworth-Warren, K.L. et al. (2023). Successful cardiopulmonary cerebral resuscitation incorporating defibrillation in a filly with neonatal maladjustment syndrome following a routine anaesthetic procedure. *Equine Vet. Edu.* 35: e77–e85.

Williams, E. and Mitchell, K.J. (2023). Diagnosis and management of accelerated idioventricular rhythms in horses. *Equine Vet. Edu.* 35 (8): 409–412.

Worth, L.T. and Reef, V.B. (1998). Pericarditis in horses: 18 cases (1986–1995). *J. Am. Vet. Med. Assoc.* 212: 248–253.

# 13

# Diseases of the Urinary Tract

*Jamie J. Kopper and Jarrod Troy*

*Department of Veterinary Clinical Sciences, College of Veterinary Medicine, Iowa State University, Ames, IA, USA*

## Urinary Bladder Prolapse

Urinary bladder prolapse is rare in equids and typically follows abdominal contractions or straining (Donaldson 1973; Haynes and McClure 1980; Kumas and Maden 2013; Pascoe and Pascoe 1988; Schott and Woodie 2019a). Although typically diagnosed in mares, scrotal herniation of the bladder is reported (Noone 1966). In mares, two types of bladder prolapse are reported, extrusion or eversion (Donaldson 1973; Haynes and McClure 1980; Kumas and Maden 2013; Pascoe and Pascoe 1988; Schott and Woodie 2019a). **Extrusion** occurs when the bladder passes through a vaginal tear with the serosal surface observed externally and frequently contains urine (Donaldson 1973; Haynes and McClure 1980; Kumas and Maden 2013; Pascoe and Pascoe 1988; Schott and Woodie 2019a). **Eversion** occurs when the urinary bladder everts through the urethral orifice with external observation of luminal mucosa and ureteral orifices (Donaldson 1973; Haynes and McClure 1980; Kumas and Maden 2013; Pascoe and Pascoe 1988; Schott and Woodie 2019a). Everted bladders may contain portions of the gastrointestinal tract as the intestinal viscera follow the everted urinary bladder through the urethral orifice (Haynes and McClure 1980). Prolapsed bladders are frequently edematous and can necrose if left untreated (Donaldson 1973; Haynes and McClure 1980; Kumas and Maden 2013; Noone 1966; Pascoe and Pascoe 1988; Schott and Woodie 2019a).

### Diagnosis

Bladder extrusion: Identify bladder serosal surface exiting a vaginal tear. The bladder commonly contains urine. Detection of vaginal tears may happen only after bladder decompression and reduction.

Bladder eversion: Identify bladder luminal mucosa and the ureteral orifices. Gastrointestinal contents may be contained within the everted bladder.

**Treatment**: Manual reduction *and/or* vaginal repair. Treat underlying cause if necessary.

*In the field*:

*Equipment:*

- Alpha-2 agonists ± butorphanol tartrate.
- Caudal epidural equipment.
- Tail-wrapping material.
- Transrectal palpation materials.
- Aseptic scrub preparation.
- Isotonic fluid (commonly 0.9% NaCl) 2–4 L.
- Sterile gloves.
- 18–20 g 1.5″ (3.81 cm) needle.

*Emergency Triage of the Horse*, First Edition. Edited by Rolfe M. Radcliffe and Jamie J. Kopper.

Companion website: www.wiley.com/go/radcliffe/triage

- 30″ (76 cm) extension set.
- 60 mL syringe.
- Absorbable monofilament suture (0–1 USP; 0.4–0.5 mm).
- Needle drivers, thumb forceps, and Mayo scissors.

*Patient Preparation:*

- Sedate with xylazine hydrochloride or detomidine hydrochloride intravenously for standing procedure. Butorphanol tartrate can be utilized for more profound sedation if needed. (See **Anesthesia in Emergency Medicine.**)
- Perform caudal epidural to reduce straining and facilitate bladder reduction. (See **Advanced Clinical Triage Procedures.**)
- Evacuate manure from rectum.
- Wrap and secure tail so it does not interfere with procedure.
- If possible, aseptically prepare the gluteal region adjacent to vulva. Avoid contact between the bladder and aseptic scrub. Rinse with physiologic saline.
- Lavage bladder with isotonic sterile fluid to remove contaminants.
- Palpate bladder to determine if the bladder is extruded (coming from a vaginal tear) or everted (coming from the urethral orifice).
- Bladder palpation includes identifying if bladder contains urine (extrusion) or potentially gastrointestinal contents (rarely reported in eversion [Haynes and McClure 1980]).

*Bladder extrusion treatment:*

- If present, evacuate urine from the extruded bladder using an 18–20 g 1.5″ (3.81 cm) needle and 60 mL syringe. If large volumes require evacuation a 30″ (76 cm) extension set can be connected to the needle and the syringe used to provide negative pressure creating a siphon.
- Following urine evacuation remove the needle. The puncture site does not typically require suture closure.
- Manually direct the bladder into the vaginal tear and reduce into abdomen.
- Repair the vaginal tear in a continuous horizontal mattress pattern using absorbable monofilament suture (0–1 USP; 0.4–0.5 mm) everting the tissue into the vaginal vault. Avoid inclusion of bladder or any abdominal contents within the closure.
  - A reproductive retractor (e.g., Aanes retractor) may be necessary.

*Bladder eversion treatment:*

- Palpate bladder ensuring no gastrointestinal viscera are contained within the everted bladder.
- Gently invert bladder into urethral orifice by gently lifting and advancing the everted tissue toward the urethral orifice.

*Management post-reduction of urinary bladder:*

- Antibiotic administration depending on contamination level (7–14 days).
- Anti-inflammatory/analgesic.
- Treat underlying cause (e.g., colic; cystitis) or perineal laceration repair when appropriate.

*Referral decision*:

- Urinary bladder prolapse is non-reducible.
- Urinary bladder appears necrotic.
- Everted urinary bladder contains gastrointestinal viscera.
- Vaginal tear repair unfeasible or requires a large animal reproductive retractor for repair.

*Referral hospital*:

- Vaginal tear repair unfeasible in field or reproductive retractor required.
- A combination exploratory celiotomy under general anesthesia and external manual reduction may be necessary for bladder reduction. Manually retract bladder into peritoneal cavity with simultaneous external reduction via an assistant.
  - Gastrointestinal viscera can also be reduced in this manner permitting bladder eversion reduction (Haynes and McClure 1980).

- Urinary bladder necrosis partial cystectomy removing necrotic portion. See Cystorrhaphy in the Ruptured Bladder section of this chapter.
- Post-reduction management similar to in the field or post-operative management for cystorrhaphy in cystectomy cases.

## Obstructive Urolithiasis (Urethrolithiasis)

Obstructive urolithiasis results from uroliths lodging within the urethra causing bladder distension, tenesmus, urine dribbling, posturing to urinate, and/or colic signs (Holt and Pearson 1984; Laverty et al. 1992; Schott and Woodie 2019b; Trotter et al. 1981). Untreated obstructive urethrolithiasis may result in bladder rupture or urethral rupture (Holt and Pearson 1984; Laverty et al. 1992; Schott and Woodie 2019b; Trotter et al. 1981).

**Diagnosis:**

- Observe urethral distension distal to anus combined with perineal urethral pulsation or urolith palpation (commonly at the ischial arch).
  - Transrectal palpation frequently reveals bladder distension and precise palpation of bladder trigone is critical (frequently uroliths obstruct at this location).
- Urinary catheter placement may aid in identification of urethral obstruction.
- Urolith palpation may not be possible when obstruction occurs in the distal urethra.
- Urethral endoscopy or percutaneous ultrasonography is helpful to identify the obstruction and its location.

**Treatment:** Perineal urethrotomy (PU) for urine diversion and/or urolith removal

In the field or in hospital: PU (Schott and Woodie 2019b)

*Equipment:*

- Alpha-2 agonists ± butorphanol tartrate
- Caudal epidural equipment
- Tail-wrapping material
- Transrectal palpation materials
- Male urinary catheter materials
- Aseptic scrub preparation
- Sterile gloves
- #10 or #15 scalpel blade
- Scalpel handle, Allis tissue forceps, and thumb forceps

*Patient Preparation:*

- Sedate with xylazine hydrochloride or detomidine hydrochloride intravenously for standing procedure. Butorphanol tartrate can be utilized for more profound sedation if needed. (See **Anesthesia in Emergency Medicine.**)
- Perform caudal epidural for perineal desensitization. (See **Advanced Clinical Triage Procedures.**)
- Evacuate manure from rectum.
- Wrap and secure tail so it does not interfere with procedure.
- The perineal region should be aseptically prepared to accommodate the PU procedure described below.
- Prepare penile urethra for urinary catheter placement advancing to the level of the ischial arch or more proximal if possible.
  - If not possible in distal urethrolithiasis cases, the distended urethra is palpable at the ischial arch and may be manually stabilized for incision creation.
- Use local anesthetic at PU site if caudal epidural fails or not performed.

*Perineal Urethrotomy (PU):*

- Create a 6–8 cm longitudinal midline skin incision in the perineum starting 4–6 cm ventral to anus ending distal-to-ischial arch.
- Continue the incision dividing through subcutaneous tissues, paired retractor penis muscles, and bulbospongiosus muscle.

- Continue the incision through corpus spongiosum penis exposing urethra. Plentiful hemorrhage frequently occurs but typically resolves spontaneously over 10–30 minutes.
- Continue incision through urethra into urolith or urinary catheter.
  - Urine outflow will be encountered in distal urethrolithiasis cases
- Allis tissue forceps or thumb forceps are helpful for urolith removal if present.
  - Urolith spiculation is common, which causes urethral mucosa adherence requiring careful manipulation during removal.

*Post-PU Management:*

- Evaluate for hydronephrosis via transcutaneous renal ultrasonography.
- Cystoscopy aids in identifying bladder trauma, necrosis, or additional uroliths.
- The PU site commonly heals in 2–3 weeks with wound management. Petroleum jelly applied distal to the PU site and hindlimbs will reduce urine scald.
- Antibiotics 7–14 days or as needed.
- Anti-inflammatory/analgesic 3–5 days or as needed.

*Referral decision*:

- PU for urinary diversion in obstructive urolithiasis is critical and should be performed as soon as possible.
- Distal urethrolithiasis treatment following PU.

## Ruptured Bladder

Uroperitoneum is a medical emergency frequently requiring surgical intervention. Patient stabilization is crucial prior to surgery; electrolyte management must occur to improve the patient's anesthetic status and avoid fatal electrolyte derangements.

### Diagnosis

Uroperitoneum should be suspected in any euvolemic horse (foal or adult) that is not urinating. Diagnosing uroperitoneum in the horse can involve using multiple diagnostics as described below and summarized in Box 13.1 including transrectal palpation of the abdomen, transcutaneous abdominal ultrasound, serum biochemistry analysis (SBA), and peritoneal fluid analysis.

#### Transrectal Palpation of the Abdomen

Although rare, uroperitoneum is reported in adult horses. In adult horses with uroperitoneum due to bladder rupture, the bladder should not be readily palpable. Large volumes of free peritoneal fluid may or may not be appreciable.

#### Transcutaneous Abdominal Ultrasound

The severity of peritoneal effusion depends on the duration of time from bladder rupture to evaluation and the patient's hydration status. Except in very acute assessments, transcutaneous abdominal ultrasound should reveal large volumes of hypoechoic peritoneal effusion.

**Box 13.1 Tools for diagnosis of uroperitoneum**

- Transrectal palpation (adults).
- Transcutaneous abdominal ultrasound.
- Serum biochemical analysis.
  - Hyponatremia, hypochloremia, hyperkalemia, azotemia.
- Peritoneal fluid analysis.
  - Elevations in potassium, creatinine, and UN compared to SBA.
  - Calcium carbonate crystals (adults).

#### Serum Biochemistry Analysis (SBA)

Serum electrolytes will begin mimicking urine electrolyte concentrations including hyponatremia, hypochloremia, hyperkalemia, and azotemia (elevated creatinine and urea nitrogen (UN)).

#### Peritoneal Fluid Analysis

Peritoneal fluid electrolyte analysis collected via abdominocentesis will reveal sodium and chloride concentrations lower than SBA results and higher potassium, creatinine, and UN concentrations. Classically, peritoneal fluid creatinine and UN will be twice the respective SBA concentrations; however smaller discrepancies can occur and should be interpreted considering the entire clinical picture.

## Stabilization

Immediate stabilization goals focus on correcting life-threatening electrolyte derangements and diverting urine to prevent propagation of electrolyte derangements prior to surgical intervention or referral. Hyperkalemia is of the most immediate concern as it can result in cardiac arrest.

#### Hyperkalemia

Serum potassium concentrations >5.5 mEq/L warrant immediate treatment and meticulous monitoring.

An ECG should be performed for cardiac electrical monitoring of changes consistent with hyperkalemia including peaked T waves, shortened QT intervals, lengthened PR interval, loss of p waves, and widened QRS complexes which can progress to asystole.

Treatment of hyperkalemia aims to reduce serum potassium levels and increase cardiac threshold voltage reducing the risk of cardiac arrest. Table 13.1 includes treatment options for hyperkalemia that can be added to 1 L or 5 L bags of 0.9% NaCl or 0.45% NaCl. Ideally, the intravenous fluids (IVF) should not contain supplemental potassium. Additionally, after establishing urine diversion, fluid therapy promoting diuresis should reduce serum potassium levels. Fluid therapy should aim to replace fluid deficits followed by maintenance to twice maintenance rates.

#### Urine Diversion

Urine diversion to prevent the perpetuation of hyperkalemia as the patient is rehydrated should be performed. In patients with a ruptured bladder, this can be accomplished by two means: (1) placement of an indwelling urinary catheter and/or (2) percutaneous abdominal drain placement. Even though the bladder is ruptured, a urinary catheter often diverts significant urine volume as it exits the ureters. Additionally, the urinary catheter may drain urine from the peritoneum, as the urinary catheter is essentially placed intra-peritoneally depending on the size of the defect in the bladder. Temporary abdominal drains can be placed using a teat canula or thoracic trochar catheter as described in Table 13.2 and depicted in Figure 13.1.

Maintenance of indwelling urinary catheter and/or abdominal drain(s) is critical as they can serve as a source of contamination possibly resulting in peritonitis. Additionally, broad-spectrum antimicrobials should be initiated prophylactically.

## When to Refer

- Surgical intervention following patient stabilization.
- Indwelling abdominal drain(s) or urinary catheter maintenance is best accomplished in a hospital setting to decrease the risk of contamination.

**Table 13.1** Medications for treatment of hyperkalemia.

| Drug | Dosage | Mechanism of action | Per 1 L for 50 kg foal | Per 5 L for 500 kg adult |
|---|---|---|---|---|
| 23% Calcium gluconate | 0.25–0.5 mL/kg IV over 5–10 minutes | Does not lower serum potassium<br>Increases cardiac threshold voltage | ~12–25 mL | ~125–250 mL |
| 50% Dextrose | 0.35–0.5 g/kg IV over 3–5 minutes | Promotes translocation of potassium intracellularly | 35–50 mL | 350–500 mL |
| 8.4% Sodium bicarbonate | 1–2 mEq/kg over 15 minutes | Promotes translocation of potassium intracellularly | 50–100 mL | 500–1000 mL |

**Table 13.2** Placement of an abdominal drain in a foal.

Placement of an abdominal drain – foal.

1) Using ultrasound guidance identify a large volume of peritoneal fluid located along the ventral abdomen.
2) Clip and aseptically prepare the chosen location.
3) Using 2% lidocaine locally desensitize the skin and subcutaneous tissue.
4) Using aseptic technique and a #15 blade create a stab incision through the skin, subcutaneous tissue, and into (but not through) the rectus abdominus.
5) Aseptically introduce a 16 french thoracic trochar catheter or teat canula into the stab incision advancing through remaining rectus abdominus into the peritoneum. If using a thoracic trochar catheter, carefully advance the catheter off the trochar (Figure 13.1).
6) If using a thoracic trochar catheter, secure the catheter using a purse string pattern with monofilament suture.
7) Ideally, for drains left in place, attach a closed system collection bag, or a Heimlich valve, onto the catheter preventing peritoneal contamination and pneumoperitoneum.

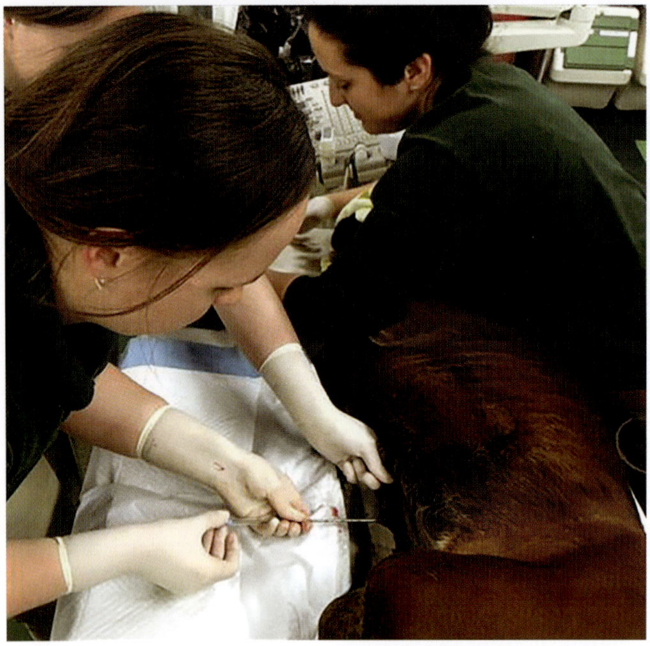

**Figure 13.1** Depiction of chest tube advancement off stylet during abdominal drain placement in a foal with uroperitoneum.

## Urinary Bladder Rupture Surgical Intervention

Ruptured urinary bladder surgical intervention should occur after patient stabilization and aids in uroabdomen resolution (Adams et al. 1988; Richardson 1985; Schott and Woodie 2019a). Cystorrhaphy or cystoplasty is typically performed at a referral hospital in dorsal recumbency under general anesthesia (Adams et al. 1988; Richardson 1985; Schott and Woodie 2019a).

*Patient Preparation:*

- General anesthesia with patient placed in dorsal recumbency.
- A urinary catheter is placed for urine outflow and intraoperative lavage
- Clean and close the male prepuce with sutures or apply caudal retraction with Backhaus towel clamps.
- Aseptically prepare the ventral abdomen for a ventral midline incision extending to the mammary gland (females) or caudal prepuce (males).
- Oversew external umbilicus if present prior to aseptic preparation.

*Equipment:*

- Urinary catheter.
- Aseptic scrub preparation.
- Exploratory celiotomy instrument pack & drapes ± Doyen intestinal forceps.

*Treatment cystorrhaphy:*

- Create a 15–18 cm midline incision 2–5 cm cranial to the umbilicus and extending caudally. Continue incision through skin into the peritoneal cavity.
  - If the external umbilicus is present create a fusiform incision around the umbilicus. Avoid cutting the umbilical vein or arteries during incision creation.
  - In males, direct the caudal extent of the incision 2–4 cm paramedian to the prepuce (Schott and Woodie 2019a). Paramedian diversion may not be necessary if the prepuce is directed caudally via towel clamps (Schott and Woodie 2019a).
- Collect peritoneal fluid for culture and then evacuate fluid via suction.
- Identify the bladder rupture location.
  - Evaluate the urachus, when present for rupture location.
  - Ligate and transect the umbilical vein and umbilical arteries to facilitate bladder evaluation in foals.
- Place stay sutures after locating the rupture to facilitate exposure.
- Excise rupture margins, if feasible, avoiding the stay sutures. (If unfeasible see treatment cystoplasty below.)
  - Excised margin culture and histopathology may be beneficial in septic foals (Adams et al. 1988).
  - In foals, excise urachus as well.
- Close the rupture using a double layer closure avoiding bladder lumen penetration.
  - Use absorbable monofilament or coated multifilament USP 2–0 or 3–0 (0.3 or 0.2 mm) suture on a taper-point needle.
  - The first layer may be an interrupted or continuous pattern.
  - The second layer should be a continuous-inverting pattern.
- Following closure, distend bladder with sterile physiologic saline evaluating for leakage.
- Lavage the peritoneal cavity with warm, sterile physiologic saline following by suction.
  - If not already present, consider place an indwelling abdominal drain.
- Close the ventral midline incision routinely.

*Treatment cystoplasty:*

- Indicated in foals with bladder ruptures where margin viability is unclear allowing for resection of the bladder apex including the rupture site.
- Ventral midline incision similar to cystorrhaphy.
- Ligation of umbilical vein and arteries.
- Stay sutures placed laterally at proposed transection site.
- A Doyen forceps is placed transversely across the bladder and the bladder apex transected proximal to the Doyen forceps (Doyen forceps should leave with the excised portion).
  - Remove any urine from bladder if necessary following transection.
- Remove the excised bladder portion and Doyen forceps.
- Close the bladder as described for cystorrhaphy, assess for leakage, and close ventral midline incision routinely.

*Post-operative cystorrhaphy or cystoplasty management:*

- Continue uroabdomen stabilization as described above.
- Maintain a urinary catheter for bladder decompression for 2–3 days. Remove if straining to urinate.
- Antibiotic administration for 3–5 days to reduce surgical site infection or as guided by patient culture and assessment.
- Anti-inflammatory/analgesic administration for 3–5 days or as needed.

## Acute Kidney Injury (AKI)

Acute kidney injury (AKI) occurs with an abrupt, but potentially reversible, reduction in renal blood flow, glomerular filtration rate (GFR), and/or urine output. AKI can occur for several reasons including iatrogenic toxicities (i.e., aminoglycosides, non-steroidal anti-inflammatory drugs/NSAIDs, oxytetracycline, bisphosphonates), hypoxemia (i.e., hypovolemia, hypotension), other toxicities (i.e., pigmenturia, acorn toxicity, cantharidin toxicity), or any combination of risk factors.

**Box 13.2 Indications of an acute kidney injury**

- Elevations in serum creatinine and urea nitrogen.
- Loss of concentrating ability of urine (i.e., isosthenuria).

## Diagnosis

A diagnosis of AKI can be achieved utilizing SBA, urine tonicity assessment (urine specific gravity [USG]), urine reagent strip analysis, and/or urine sediment examination (SE) (Schott and Esser 2020) also summarized in Box 13.2.

**Serum biochemistry analysis (SBA):** Commonly, AKI is first noted as azotemia on an SBA. It is important to remember that by the time a patient is azotemic they have lost approximately ~60% of functioning nephrons; thus, this is not a sensitive means to diagnose AKI. In horses with AKI, serum creatinine increases more rapidly than urea nitration (UN) resulting in a UN:creatinine ratio < 10:1. Given that single timepoint serum creatinine concentration is an insensitive indicator of renal function utilizing serial blood work and monitoring for increases in creatinine by >0.3 mg/dL while still within the reference interval may be a more sensitive means for monitoring renal function compared to assessing for absolute azotemia.

**Urine tonicity, USG:** With hypovolemia or dehydration, horses with AKI may be azotemic and urine may be concentrated (earlier stage; acute) or progress to isosthenuria (later stage). Isosthenuria may be present despite hypovolemia or dehydration, indicating loss of urine concentrating abilities. USG readings can be divided into three categories: (1) urine that is more dilute than serum/hyposthenuria (USG <1.008), (2) urine that is the same concentration as serum (USG 1.008–1.014), and (3) urine that is more concentrated than serum (USG >1.014). With early AKI the urine may be concentrated but progresses to isosthenuria with increased loss of functioning nephrons.

**Reagent strip analyses** can be helpful, but some reagent strip pads should be interpreted with caution. Normal equine urine is alkaline (Wood et al. 1990), resulting in false trace protein results (Edwards et al. 1989). Protein pad readings of greater than trace should be further investigated with a urine protein-to-creatinine ratio (normal <0.5), as proteinuria may indicate glomerulonephritis. Positive glucose pad results need to be interpreted alongside serum glucose measurements, as hyperglycemia (>160–180 mg/dL) can result in glucosuria (Link 1940). Glucosuria without hyperglycemia is indicative of proximal tubule dysfunction. Positive results for blood on urine reagent strips do not distinguish between the different types of pigmenturia (i.e., myoglobin, red blood cells, hemoglobin). Pigmenturia is specifically discussed later in this text.

**SE** may reveal intact red blood cells indicating renal tubular necrosis or hematuria. Granular casts, indicative of acute tubular injury, may also be observed on SE. A more detailed description of performing an equine urine SE is described elsewhere (Schott and Esser 2020).

## Treatment

Treatment for AKI relies on (1) removing nephrotoxic insult, if possible, (2) correcting dehydration, restoring euvolemia, and/or correcting hypotension, and (3) supporting adequate renal function.

1) When possible, discontinue nephrotoxic medications. If the horse requires medication(s), consider changing it to change to a less nephrotoxic substitute (i.e., changing antimicrobial class). Nephrotoxic plants should be removed and if experiencing pigmenturia the underlying disease process should be treated.
2) Restoring and maintaining adequate kidney perfusion is important for renal function and also mitigates drug (i.e., NSAIDs) nephrotoxic effects if discontinuation is unfeasible. In severely dehydrated or hypovolemic cases, IVF are preferrable because the gastrointestinal tract is also likely hypoperfused and incapable of adequate fluid absorption. If bolusing IVF it is important to monitor urination frequency ensuring the horse is not oliguric or anuric, which is indicative of acute renal failure (ARF) (see below). In a dehydrated horse, a common fluid resuscitation approach involves administering 10–20 mL/kg IVF boluses until urination occurs. If 60 mL/kg of IVF have been administered without urination, the patient should be reassessed for signs of fluid retention (i.e., edema, tachypnea, adventitious pulmonary auscultation) indicating ARF (see below).
3) After resolving the initial fluid deficit, it is important to maintain euhydration to support adequate renal perfusion. This may take the form of intravenous, enteral, or rectal fluid therapy. Given the relatively sodium and chloride rich IVFs available in volumes feasible for equine veterinary practice, utilization of enteral or rectal fluids has advantages. Horses with severe AKI requiring continuous IVFs are best treated in a 24–7 hospital.

**Monitoring** AKI response to therapy includes serial evaluation of azotemia, serum electrolytes, and USGs. If the azotemia is secondary to an acute injury the serum creatinine may decrease by 50% per 24 h after the instigating source is removed and the kidneys are adequately supported with fluid therapy.

**When to refer:** Many AKI cases require continuous rate fluid infusions or frequent fluid administration via nasogastric intubation which is easiest accomplished in a 24–7 hospital.

## Acute Renal Failure (ARF)

ARF occurs during an abrupt severe reduction in GFR which can be due to the same causes as AKI, but now results in oliguria or anuria.

Ideally, patients at risk for developing ARF should be monitored for evidence of AKI with sequential USGs and SEs looking for the presence of urine casts and blood. This allows treatment of AKI before progression into ARF. Continuous IVF therapy and serial monitoring is vital when treating ARF in horses.

### Treatment

Treatment of ARF is aimed at nephrotoxin removal, if present, and restoring patient euvolemia if necessary. Urination frequency should be carefully monitored. If the horse is not urinating several judicious fluid boluses (10–20 mL/kg) can be administered ensuring that the patient has adequate volume and hydration status. During these boluses the patient should be monitored meticulously for pulmonary edema (i.e., increased respiratory rate, bronchovesicular sounds). If the patient appears euvolemic following IVF but still has not urinated diuretic agents can be attempted but are controversial. Commonly used diuretics include furosemide (1 mg/kg bolus or 0.12 mg/kg loading dose followed by a 0.12 mg/kg/h continuous rate infusion [Johansson et al. 2003]) or mannitol (0.25–1 g/kg of 20% mannitol administered over 15–20 minutes). If urinations cannot be established, additional treatment can include dialysis at a referral institution; however, prognosis is generally poor.

After establishing urination, treatment relies upon supporting euvolemia and adequate renal perfusion. Earlier theories of providing excessive IVF volumes to "flush the kidneys" are becoming less prevalent for two reasons. First, excessive IVF volumes increase the kidney workload by processing the excessive fluid administration. Second, if using commercial IVF, electrolytes are provided in far excess requiring excretion by the kidneys.

Serum electrolytes, particularly potassium, should be monitored serially. Ideally, azotemia improves with a 50% reduction in creatinine per 24 h of therapy. Nephrotoxic drug use should be minimized when possible.

**When to refer:** Any horse with suspicion or identification of oliguria or anuria.

## Pigmenturia

Abnormally colored urine or pigmenturia results from one of three conditions: (1) hematuria (bleeding in the upper or lower urinary tract), hemoglobinuria (due to intravascular hemolysis), or myoglobinuria (due to a myopathy and breakdown of muscle tissue). With centrifugation of blood and urine in microhematocrit tubes you can determine the cause of pigmenturia, as shown in Figure 13.2. After centrifugation, patients with **hematuria** will have clear urine supernatant with a pellet of red blood cells and normal appearing serum in hematocrit tubes, patients with **hemoglobinuria** will have hemolyzed serum and the urine will remain pigmented post centrifugation, and patients with **myoglobinuria** will have normal appearing serum and pigmented urine. Depending on the degree of hemolysis, horses with hemoglobinuria may have significant anemia and hyperbilirubinemia, whereas patients with myoglobinuria will have notably elevated CK and AST on SBA.

**Hematuria** (Table 13.3) can be the result of multiple pathologies associated with hemorrhage derived from one or both kidneys (i.e., idiopathic renal hematuria, neoplasia, coagulopathy), the urinary bladder (i.e., ulcerative cystitis, neoplasia, cystolith), the urethra (i.e., geldings, stallions; urethral rent), or vagina (i.e., mares; vaginal varicosities). Infrequently, renal hematuria results in significant blood loss.

**Diagnostic evaluation** for sources of hematuria can begin with careful abdominal palpation per rectum evaluating the bladder for cystolith evidence, bladder wall thickness, and the size and/or texture of the caudal pole of the left kidney. Transcutaneous ultrasonographic evaluation can be performed to assess both kidneys for abnormalities (i.e., nephrolith and neoplasia). Additionally, cystoscopy can be performed. First, aseptically collect a urine sample and empty the bladder

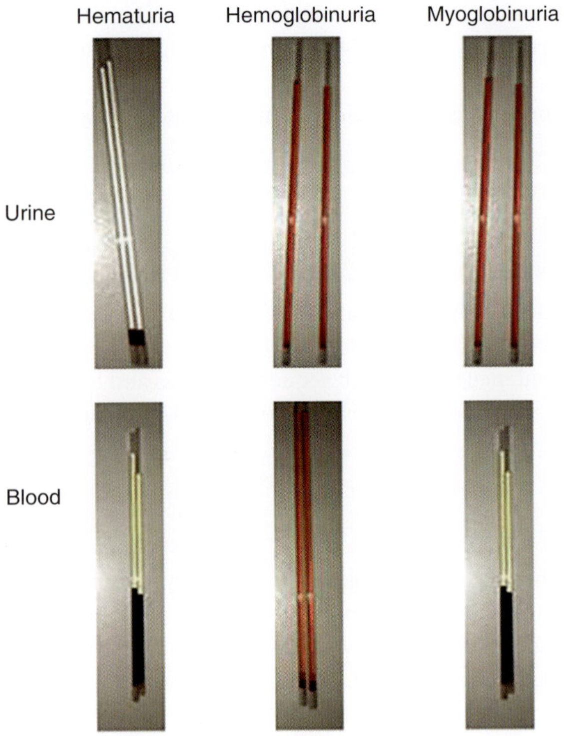


**Figure 13.2** Determining the source of pigmenturia using serum and urine samples in the horse.

using a urinary catheter. Then, while advancing the endoscope the urethra (geldings, stallions) or vagina (mares) can be carefully evaluated followed by the accessory sex glands (geldings, stallions) and bladder. Observation of both ureters allows for the assessment (and even individual collection) of urine coming from each individual ureter.

**Treatment** is dependent on the cause of hematuria. Cystoliths require removal – which can be performed via perineal urethrostomy (gelding, stallion; see obstructive urolithiasis section in this chapter) or by hand (mare). Urethral rents typically resolve with conservative management which can be accomplished by performing a complete or incomplete perineal urethrostomy. Those needing surgical intervention should be referred. Treatment of ulcerative cystitis should be guided by urine culture and sensitivity with re-evaluations prior to discontinuation of antimicrobials.

**Hemoglobinuria** (Table 13.4) results from intravascular hemolysis, frequently from primary immune mediated hemolytic anemia, secondary immune-mediated hemolytic anemia, infectious agents, or toxin ingestion.

**Diagnostic evaluation** for hemoglobinuria includes a careful history (i.e., toxin and infectious disease exposure, concurrent medications) and infectious disease testing (i.e., equine infectious anemia testing, piroplasmosis testing, *Cornybacterium pseudotuberculosis* synergistic hemolysis inhibition test, *Streptococcus equi equi* M protein titer). IgG- and IgM-bound red blood cells can be identified by flow cytometry which supports a diagnosis of primary or secondary immune mediated hemolytic anemia but does not differentiate between the two conditions. Ultimately, primary immune-mediated hemolytic anemia is a diagnosis of exclusion. If secondary immune-mediated hemolytic anemia is suspected concurrently administered medications should be discontinued.

**Treatment** for primary or secondary immune mediated hemolytic anemia relies on immunosuppression and supportive care. Treatment for secondary immune-mediated hemolytic anemia also includes the removal of inciting sources (i.e., concurrently administered medications, treatment of underlying infectious disease).

Immunosuppression is frequently accomplished administering dexamethasone (0.05–0.1 mg/kg IV or IM q24 h, ideally administered in the morning) followed by a gradual tapering with dexamethasone or switching to prednisolone (1–2 mg/kg PO q24 h).

Supportive care includes fluid therapy and possibly a blood transfusion depending on the severity of anemia. Hemoglobin damages renal tubular cells, thus ensuring euvolemia and adequate hydration is critical to renal function. Fluid therapy may be accomplished intravenously, enterally, or rectally as described in **Part 4.B**.

**Table 13.3** Differential diagnoses, diagnostic tools, and treatments for hematuria.

| Diagnosis | Diagnostic tool | Treatment |
|---|---|---|
| Urethral rent | Cystoscopy | Rest, perineal urethrostomy |
| Cystolith | Abdominal palpation per rectum, transrectal ultrasound, cystoscopy | Removal |
| Vaginal varicosities | Exam +/− speculum | Monitoring, ligation |
| Ulcerative cystitis | Cystoscopy, urine culture, biopsy | Antimicrobials based on culture & sensitivity, anti-inflammatory medication |
| Renal neoplasia | Transcutaneous ultrasound, biopsy | Nephrectomy |
| Idiopathic renal hematuria | Cystoscopy, diagnosis of exclusion | Monitoring, nephrectomy |
| Coagulopathy | Coagulation profile, history | Supportive care, vitamin K, history dependent |

**Table 13.4** Differential diagnoses, diagnostic tools, and treatment for hemoglobinuria.

| Hemoglobinuria | Diagnostic tool | Treatment |
|---|---|---|
| Primary immune-mediated intravascular hemolysis | Diagnosis of exclusion, direct coombs test, flow cytometry for IgM and/or IgG antibodies bound to RBCs | *Immunosuppression:*<br>• Example: Dexamethasone: 0.1 mg/kg IV or IM q24, then slowly taper |
| Secondary immune-mediated intravascular hemolysis | Direct coombs test, flow cytometry for IgM and/or IgG antibodies bound to RBCs, history (drug use) and/or positive infectious disease testing (i.e., *Corynebacterium pseudotuberculosis*, *Streptococcus equi equi*) | Stop any concurrently administered medications if possible.<br>*Immunosuppression:*<br>• Example: Dexamethasone: 0.1 mg/kg IV or IM q24, then slowly taper |
| Equine infectious anemia | Coggins test | Contact state veterinarian |
| Piroplasmosis | cELISA and complement fixation test for *Babesia caballi* and *Theileria equi.* | Contact state veterinarian |
| *Pistacia* spp. leaf ingestion | History, pasture evaluation | Supportive care |
| *Acer rubrum* (Red maple) leaf ingestion | History, pasture evaluation | Supportive care |

**Table 13.5** Differential diagnoses, diagnostic tools, and treatment for myoglobinuria.

| Myoglobinuria | Diagnosis | Acute treatment |
|---|---|---|
| Exertional rhabdomyolysis | History, elevation in CK, AST on blood work | Rest<br>Analgesia<br>Fluid therapy |
| Recurrent exertional rhabdomyolysis | History, elevation in CK, AST on bloodwork, exercise challenge test, genetic testing, muscle biopsy | Rest<br>Analgesia<br>Fluid therapy<br>Long-term management depending on diagnostic test results |
| Myosin heavy-chain myopathy, immune-mediated myositis | Elevation in CK, AST on bloodwork, Genetic testing | Rest<br>Analgesia<br>Fluid therapy<br>Immunosuppression: Dexamethasone (0.05 mg/kg) for 3 days, followed by prednisolone (1 mg/kg for 7–10 days) tapered by 100 mg/week over 1 month. |
| Polysaccharide storage myopathy (PSSM) | Elevation in CK, AST on bloodwork, Genetic testing<br>Muscle biopsy | Rest<br>Analgesia<br>Fluid therapy<br>Long-term diet and exercise management |
| Seasonal pasture myopathy | History<br>Serum, plasma, urine for acylcarnitine and uric organic acid concentrations | Anti-inflammatory medication<br>Anti-oxidants (vitamins E, C)<br>Fluid therapy |
| Myofibrillar myopathy | Muscle biopsy | Rest<br>Analgesia<br>Fluid therapy<br>Long-term diet and exercise management |

**Myoglobinuria** (Table 13.5) can occur with several different disease processes. Ultimately, myoglobinuria is the result of rhabdomyolysis or acute muscle injury.

**Diagnostic evaluation and treatment** for causes of rhabdomyolysis are described in detail in **Chapter 8**. As with hemoglobinuria, assuring adequate hydration and euvolemia via fluid therapy (Chapter 28) is imperative to preserve renal function in myoglobinuria cases.

**When to refer:** Horses with significant anemia or pigmenturia resulting in the need for continuous fluid therapy are best treated in a 24–7 care facility.

**Case Example 13.1 Urinary Tract Rupture**

A 3-day-old 50-kg Quarter Horse colt is presented for a 12-h history of lethargy and decreased nursing (Figure 13.3). There was no history of dystocia, and the mare passed her placenta completely within three hours. The foal stood, nursed well post-foaling, had a normal post-foaling examination, and a reported IgG >800 mg/dL. On evaluation you observe that foal appears dull and has no interest in nursing from the mare who is streaming milk from the teats. Your physical examination reveals pink, slightly tacky mucous membranes with a capillary refill time of <2 seconds, normal eye sclera bilaterally, a heart rate of 120 bpm, respiratory rate of 60 brpm with normal bronchovesicular sounds bilaterally, decreased gastrointestinal sounds in all quadrants, and a temperature of 101.2 °F. Facial arterial pulses are strong and synchronous with the heartbeat on palpation. The umbilicus appears and palpated normal with no discharge or drainage observed. Limb palpation of joints and tendon sheathes is normal with no pain response observed. Abdominal palpation reveals no significant abnormalities.

*Stall side bloodwork and serum biochemistry analysis (SBA) reveal the following abnormalities or pertinent values:*

Packed Cell Volume (PCV): 28% (RR: 30–40%).
Total Solids (TS): 5.4 g/dL (RR: 5–6 g/dL).
L-Lactate: 2.0 mmol/L (RR < 2 mmol/L).
Glucose: 150 mg/dL (RR: 70–170 mg/dL).
Potassium: 6 mEq/L (RR: 2.6–4.5 mEq/L).
Sodium: 130 mEq/L (RR: 137–145 mEq/L).
Chloride: 90 mEq/L (RR: 102–114 mEq/L).
Creatinine: 2.2 mg/dL (1.0–1.8 mg/dL).
BUN: 29 mg/dL (14–21 mg/dL).

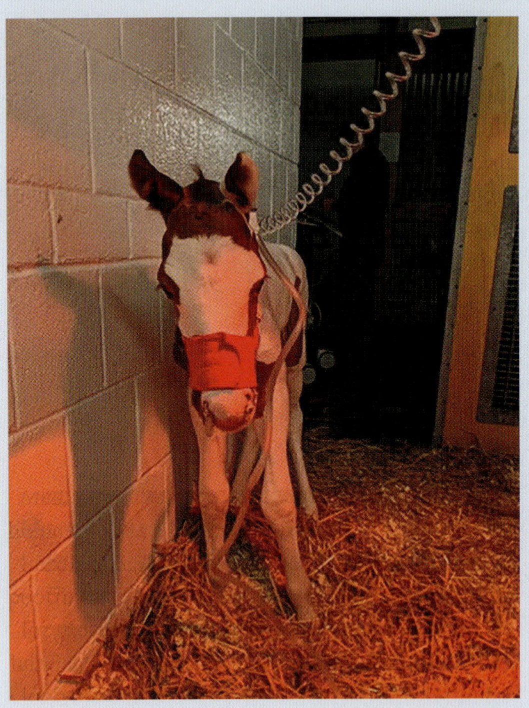

**Figure 13.3** A 3-day-old 50-kg Quarter Horse colt is presented for a 12-h history of lethargy and decreased nursing. Note the foal is being stabilized with appropriate fluid therapy to correct hyperkalemia and urine diversion prior to surgery for a ruptured bladder and secondary uroabdomen.

Transcutaneous abdominal ultrasound reveals a marked amount of hypoechoic fluid within the abdominal cavity with the gastrointestinal tract floating within the fluid and no visualization of the urinary bladder (Figure 13.4). Both kidneys can be observed and appear normal. No other significant findings are observed.

You obtain peritoneal fluid via abdominocentesis using aseptic technique. A copious amount of peritoneal fluid was obtained that was pale yellow with the following pertinent results:

L-lactate: 1.8 mmol/L (<2 mmol/L).
Total protein: <2 g/dL (<2 g/dL).
Potassium: 6.9 mEq/L (2.6–4.5 mEq/L).
Sodium: 122 mEq/L (RR: 137–145 mEq/L).
Chloride: 85 mEq/L (RR: 102–114 mEq/L).
Creatinine: 4.6 mg/dL (1.0–1.8 mg/dL).
BUN: 60 mg/dL (14–21 mg/dL).

*Does this foal have evidence of uroperitoneum likely secondary to a ruptured bladder?*

a) Yes, there is evidence that this foal has a ruptured bladder based on this foal's physical examination, SBA, transcutaneous abdominal ultrasound, and peritoneal fluid analysis. This foal's overall physical examination is unremarkable except for its dull mentation; in these cases, it is important to pursue further hematologic evaluation. In this case the SBA shows hyperkalemia, hyponatremia, hypochloremia, and azotemia. Transcutaneous abdominal ultrasound reveals hypoechoic fluid which when combined with the SBA is consistent with ruptured bladder (Figure 13.4). The SBA and peritoneal fluid analysis results are consistent with ruptured bladder as the peritoneal creatinine/BUN are twice that reported in the SBA. Additionally, peritoneal fluid analysis revealed a higher potassium with a lower sodium/chloride when compared to SBA.

*What are your first stabilization steps and considerations?*

a) Hyperkalemia treatment: This foal will need treatment for its hyperkalemia and reduce the risk of cardiac arrest. This can be accomplished by placement of an IV jugular vein catheter for administration of isotonic fluids that, ideally, do not contain potassium with the addition of 23% calcium gluconate (12–25 mL/1 L bag of fluids for a 50-kg foal), 50% dextrose (30–50 mL/1 L bag), or 8.4% sodium bicarbonate (50–100 mL/1 L bag) (Table 13.1). Once treatment for hyperkalemia has been initiated urine diversion should occur.
   i) An electrocardiogram (ECG) should be placed whenever possible to monitor electrical changes consistent with hyperkalemia.

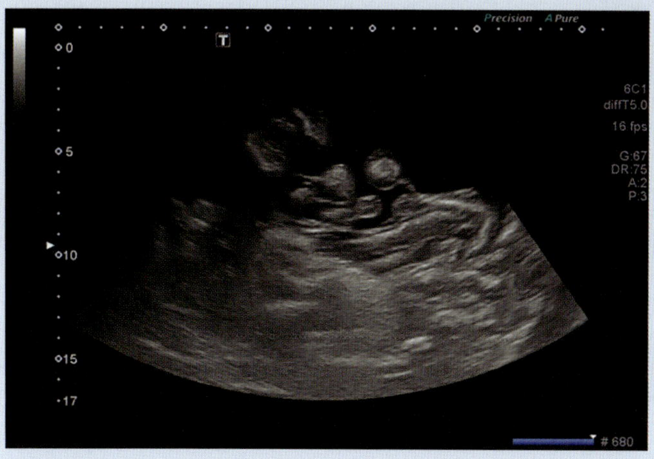


**Figure 13.4** Transcutaneous abdominal ultrasound reveals a marked amount of hypoechoic fluid within the abdominal cavity with the gastrointestinal tract floating within the fluid. Note, the urinary bladder was not visible on ultrasound, consistent with bladder rupture. Emergency triage of such cases to stabilize the patient is the priority prior to surgical repair of the ruptured bladder.

b) Urine diversion: Following initiation of hyperkalemia treatment, the urine should be diverted from the peritoneum to stop the perpetuation of hyperkalemia as the patient is rehydrated. This can be accomplished via:
   ii) Indwelling urinary catheterization.
   iii) Percutaneous abdominal drain placement (Table 13.2).

   Following hyperkalemia stabilization and urine diversion the foal can be treated with surgical intervention for a ruptured bladder. Additionally, indwelling abdominal drain(s) or urinary catheter management is best accomplished in a hospital setting to decrease the risk of contamination and ascending infection.
c) Surgical intervention: Only after patient stabilization occurs should surgical intervention be performed as it aids in uroabdomen resolution. Typically, cystorrhaphy or cystoplasty is performed under general anesthesia at a referral hospital.

## References


Adams, R.A., Koterba, A.M., Cudd, T.C., and Baker, W.A. (1988). Exploratory celiotomy for suspected urinary tract disruption in neonatal foals: a review of 18 cases. *Equine Vet. J.* 20 (1): 13–17.

Donaldson, R.S. (1973). Eversion of the bladder in a mare. *Vet. Rec.* 92 (15): 409–410.

Edwards, D.J., Brownlow, M.A., and Hutchins, D.R. (1989). Indices of renal function: reference values in normal horses. *Aust. Vet. J.* 66 (2): 60–63.

Haynes, P.F. and McClure, J.R. (1980). Eversion of the urinary bladder: a sequel to third-degree perineal laceration in the mare. *Vet. Surg.* 9 (2): 66–71.

Holt, P.E. and Pearson, H. (1984). Urolithiasis in the horse-a review of 13 cases. *Equine Vet. J.* 16 (1): 31–34.

Johansson, A.M., Gardner, S.Y., Levine, J.F. et al. (2003). Furosemide continuous rate infusion in the horse: evaluation of enhanced efficacy and reduced side effects. *J. Vet. Intern. Med.* 17 (6): 887–895.

Kumas, C. and Maden, M. (2013). Bladder eversion caused by chronic cystitis in an Arabian racehorse: a case report. *J. Equine Vet. Sci.* 34: 329–332.

Laverty, S., Pascoe, J.R., Ling, G.V. et al. (1992). Urolithiasis in 68 horses. *Vet. Surg.* 21 (1): 56–62.

Link, R.P. (1940). Glucose tolerance in horses. *J. Am. Vet. Med. Assoc.* 97: 261–263.

Noone, J.P. (1966). Scrotal herniation of the urinary bladder in the horse. *Irish Vet. J.* 20: 11–12.

Pascoe, J.R. and Pascoe, R.R.R. (1988). Displacements, malpositions, and miscellaneous injuries of the mare's urogenital tract. *Vet. Clin. North Am. Equine Pract.* 4 (3): 439–450.

Richardson, D.W. (1985). Urogenital problems in the neonatal foal. *Vet. Clin. North Am. Equine Pract.* 1 (1): 179–188.

Schott, H.C. and Esser, M.M. (2020). The sick adult horse: renal clinical pathologic testing and urinalysis. *Vet. Clin. North Am. Eq. Pract.* 36 (1): 121–134.

Schott, H.C. and Woodie, J.B. (2019a). Bladder. In: *Equine Surgery*, 5e (ed. J.A. Auer, J. Stick, J.M. Kummerle, and T. Prange), 1129–1145. St. Louis, MO: Elsevier.

Schott, H.C. and Woodie, J.B. (2019b). Urethra. In: *Equine Surgery*, 5e (ed. J.A. Auer, J. Stick, J.M. Kummerle, and T. Prange), 1145–1155. St. Louis, MO: Elsevier.

Trotter, G.W., Bennett, D.G., and Behm, R.J. (1981). Urethral calculi in five horses. *Vet. Surg.* 10 (4): 159–162.

Wood, T., Weckman, T.J., Henry, P.A. et al. (1990). Equine urine pH: normal population distributions and methods of acidification. *Equine Vet. J.* 22 (2): 118–121.

# 14

# Reproductive Emergencies

*Soon Hon Cheong[1], Mariana Diel de Amorim[1], and Maia R. Aitken[2]*

[1] *Department of Clinical Sciences, College of Veterinary Medicine, Cornell University, Ithaca, NY, USA*
[2] *Department of Clinical Studies - New Bolton Center, University of Pennsylvania School of Veterinary Medicine, Kennett Square, PA, USA*

## Emergency Conditions of the Mare – Prepartum

### Monitoring the Pregnant Mare

Equine pregnancy length can vary, with gestation in mares ranging from 320 to 360 days. It is common practice to use 340 days as the expected due date. While pregnancy examinations after the initial fetal heartbeat examination (typically at around 25 days of gestation) or following fetal sexing are not routinely performed, serial transrectal and transabdominal ultrasound examinations throughout gestation can significantly increase the chances of early detection and intervention in cases of pregnancy problems such as placentitis (Renaudin et al. 1997; Troedsson 2007).

A commonly performed examination in late pregnant mares is the measurement of the Combined Thickness of the Uterus and Placenta (CTUP). In normal horses, the thickness of the CTUP increases by about 1–2 mm/month as gestational age increases. Further, the thickness of CTUP in normal horses should be less than 8 mm between 271 and 300 days, less than 10 mm between 301 and 330 days, and less than 12 mm from 331 days onward. The CTUP measurement is often increased in mares with ascending placentitis, and mares with a history of previous placentitis or high-risk pregnancies should receive routine prenatal exams as part of their management during pregnancy (Troedsson 2007). CTUP evaluation is not a definitive test as some mares with placentitis may not have increased CTUP and increased CTUP may be caused by edema unrelated to placentitis (Renaudin et al. 1997; Morris et al. 2007; Kimura et al. 2018).

Another crucial assessment for late pregnant mares is the measurement of fetal heart rate. Fetal heart rates tend to decrease as the mares' gestational age increases. During a normal pregnancy, a mare at Month 9 of gestation typically has a fetal heart rate of $92 \pm 9$, while a mare in the last month of gestation has a fetal heart rate of $79 \pm 9$ (Nagel et al. 2010). Fetal heart rate is highly dynamic and can be temporarily accelerated due to fetal activity or depressed during uterine contractions depending on various factors. Monitoring the fetal heart rate should be performed over a period of at least a few minutes to observe if there is significant variability. If a low (<60 bpm) or high (>120 bpm) fetal heart rate is detected, the fetus should be re-assessed after several hours or the next day. Transabdominal ultrasonography can also be used to determine the presentation of the foal (anterior or posterior), particularly in high-risk pregnancies. Preplanning before foaling can greatly increase the likelihood of discovering and managing complications and other problems of parturition in the mare.

To predict when a mare is likely to foal, daily visual inspection of the vulva for any abnormal secretions and monitoring of the mammary glands for premature lactation should be part of routine broodmare farm management. Daily evaluations of mammary secretions are frequently used to monitor mares for foaling readiness. Mammary calcium titration tests, water hardness tests, or pH values are used alone or in combination to assess the mare's readiness for foaling. Calcium levels above 250 ppm indicate that the mare has a 98% chance of foaling within the next 72 h, and a pH below 6.5 typically indicates that foaling may occur within the next 24 h (Canisso et al. 2013; Korosue et al. 2013). Inversion of the sodium and potassium ratios can also be used to predict impending foaling but is generally more expensive to measure.

*Emergency Triage of the Horse*, First Edition. Edited by Rolfe M. Radcliffe and Jamie J. Kopper.

Companion website: www.wiley.com/go/radcliffe/triage

Quiet observation of the foaling process is critical for the early identification of any complications that may require timely intervention. Many foaling facilities have a veterinarian on-site or nearby who can assess and treat foaling problems and determine if referral to a surgical facility is necessary.

## Managing the High-Risk Pregnant Mare

High-risk pregnant mares include those with a history of previous pregnancy complications such as placentitis, hydropsical conditions, abdominal wall disease, previous dystocias, broad ligament hematoma, uterine tears, uterine torsion, or cesarean sections. Additionally, older maiden or multiparous mares and those with poor body score conditions are also at higher risk.

To increase the odds of foal survival, mares with high-risk pregnancies should be foaled out in a facility with a nearby referral hospital setting where the mare and fetus can be monitored frequently and intervention applied in a timely manner.

Regular prenatal examinations are highly recommended for mares with previous pregnancy problems. These include the evaluation of the CTUP, fetal heart rate, and foal presentation in the last trimester of pregnancy as described earlier to determine if there are any signs of impending issues.

Any detectable abnormalities on physical examination or ancillary tests should prompt the clinician to perform further diagnostic tests and institute appropriate treatment. The general goal for managing high-risk pregnancies is to maintain the pregnancy until term or for as long as possible to increase the chance of foal survival – unless pregnancy termination is deemed necessary to save the mare's life, such as in cases of abdominal wall disease or hydropsical conditions, or late twin diagnosis.

## Uterine Torsion

Uterine torsion in mares usually occurs in the third trimester of pregnancy, but not usually at term. If a pregnant mare presents with colic signs, uterine torsion should be considered a possible cause in the third trimester. Diagnosis can be achieved through transrectal palpation of the broad ligament. In normal mares, the broad ligaments do not cross the midline. In mares with uterine torsion, one of the broad ligaments crosses the midline dorsally, while the other broad ligament can be followed going ventral to the uterus.

Uterine torsions often occur before the foal can survive outside the uterus. Thus, the primary goal of initial treatment is to correct the uterine torsion and maintain the pregnancy until the foal is due.

Emergency triage plan: If a mare exhibits signs of systemic compromise, it's important to stabilize the mare and administer pain control. Once stable, the mare can be referred for surgical correction or on-farm correction can be attempted.

Important decisions during management: One of the most important decisions to make during management is to determine the direction of the uterine torsion. The direction of torsion is usually described when viewed from the back of the animal and is either a "clockwise" torsion (when the left broad ligament crosses the midline dorsal to the uterus and goes toward the right) or a "counterclockwise" torsion (when the right broad ligament crosses the midline dorsal to the uterus and goes toward the left side).

The uterine torsion can be resolved by surgical correction (from either a ventral midline incision under anesthesia or a standing flank incision) or by rolling the mare (similar to the Scheffer method for correcting uterine torsion in cattle). We do not generally recommend performing the flank incision surgery at the farm due to concerns about restraint and hygiene. The benefits of rolling the mare are lower cost and lower requirements for standing surgical facilities and instruments. The risk for rolling the mare is the possibility of rupturing the uterus, rupturing vessels, not being able to resolve the torsion, and general anesthetic risk, including myositis and recovery injuries. There is also a need for sufficient personnel to monitor the mare and to roll the mare physically. Therefore, rolling mares is a realistic option for lighter breeds, but draft mares should not be rolled if possible.

If the torsion is severe and chronic, there is a reasonable chance that correcting the uterine torsion will result in reperfusion injury. It may not be possible to save all mares, especially those with a severely compromised uterus. If any systemic compromise is detected, including high lactate, starting treatment to minimize reperfusion injury may be advisable before correcting the torsion.

On-farm management: If a referral is not an option for the mare with uterine torsion, the realistic treatment option will be to roll the mare (Guthrie 1982; Wichtel et al. 1988).

To resolve uterine torsion by rolling the mare, the concept is to have the mare "catch up" with the torsed uterus. The mare should be anesthetized and dropped on her right side if she has a clockwise torsion and dropped on her left side if she has a counterclockwise torsion. The process is to have the mare in lateral recumbency; then, the mare is rolled onto her back and to the other side. Once the mare is rolled, repeat transrectal palpation to determine if the torsion is corrected. If the torsion is corrected, reverse the anesthetic and allow the mare to recover. If the torsion persists, then proceed to roll the mare onto sternal recumbency and repeat the procedure. Some mares will have more than 360° torsion and require more than a single roll to resolve. If there is no progress after several rolls, additional rolls are not likely to be effective and surgical correction is recommended.

If rolling is successful, mares are often treated with a dose or more of an NSAID. Most practitioners will choose to put the mare on altrenogest, but there is no evidence that this is necessary. If the mare is supplemented with altrenogest, this should be tapered and discontinued at around 320 days of gestation.

Referral hospital management: Mares should be stabilized prior to surgery. Surgical correction via standing flank laparotomy on the side toward the rotation is recommended for mares having uncomplicated torsion of the uterus prior to 320 days of gestation (Spoormakers et al. 2015). With longer gestational lengths, other techniques including midline or flank laparotomy under general anesthesia or vaginal correction of uterine torsion yield similar results for mare survival. When a gastrointestinal lesion is also suspected, ventral midline celiotomy allows for excellent visualization and assessment of both the intestinal tract and uterus (Jung et al. 2008). However, regardless of the stage of gestation, when correction of uterine torsion is attempted under general anesthesia, there may be an increased risk of hypoxemia to the fetus associated with positioning and effects of the anesthetic. The flank approach may be performed with the mare standing and sedated (Pascoe et al. 1981). This procedure may be an option if the mare is comfortable enough to remain standing. The flank incision is made on the right side for a clockwise torsion and on the left side for a counterclockwise torsion; however, bilateral flank incisions may be required to resolve the uterine torsion in challenging cases. Additionally, the instillation of sterile isotonic fluids into the abdominal cavity to "float the uterus" can aid in the correction of the torsion. The fluid should be removed by suction from the abdominal cavity after uterine torsion correction.

After uterine torsion correction, the mare should be treated as a high-risk pregnancy as there is a higher likelihood of parturition complications, and the foal is also more likely to require intervention. The mare can be foaled out at the farm if experienced personnel are available to intervene if necessary.

Conclusion/Summary: All mares that present for colic that are in mid-to-late-term gestation should be examined for uterine torsion. Correction of the torsion can be accomplished by rolling or by surgery, either ventral midline or by standing flank surgical approach. The goal is to correct the torsion and support the mare to continue carrying the foal to term. Recurrence of torsion after correction is rare but possible. Foaling should be supervised as the risk of dystocia and neonatal compromise is higher than for a typical mare. The prognosis for the mare is excellent with surgical treatment especially if occurring before 320 days in gestation (Chaney et al. 2007). The prognosis for the foal is guarded as the foal must survive both the initial uterine insult as well as the subsequent risks at parturition.

## Hydrops of the Fetal Membranes

Hydropsical conditions in mares typically occur during the last trimester of pregnancy, with most cases appearing around 250 days of gestation. Although rare, some cases may develop closer to term. Of all the hydropsical conditions, hydrallantois is the most common, accounting for 90% of cases, while hydramnios represents the remaining 10%. For the purpose of this chapter, our focus will be on hydrallantois, as it requires urgent stabilization and treatment due to the rapid accumulation of fluid.

Emergency triage plan: When a mare is suspected to have hydrallantois, a thorough evaluation should be conducted to assess her ability to walk, respiratory rate, heart rate, and pain level. The severity of the condition is typically proportional to the amount of allantoic fluid accumulation, which can cause dyspnea, high heart rates, and difficulty ambulating. Abdominal girth typically increases by more than 4 cm/day, making early diagnosis and intervention crucial to prevent pre-pubic tendon rupture or abdominal wall disease.

Additionally, it is important to evaluate the position of the mammary gland and examine the color of the mammary secretions. Frank blood from both mammary glands is indicative of a complete pre-pubic tendon tear, which may require immediate attention.

Unfortunately, saving the foal in such cases is rare, and pregnancy termination is often the only viable treatment option. However, the prognosis for the mare depends greatly on the quality of care she receives and the timing of referral to a hospital setting. Valuable animals should be referred early due to the rapid and daily increase of allantoic fluid accumulation, and the intensive care required to manage these patients.

Important decisions during management: The prognosis for a foal with hydrops is grave, especially if the condition develops earlier in gestation. Therefore, the priority should be to save the mare and intervene early to prevent potential complications such as pre-pubic tendon rupture or ventral abdominal wall disease. However, there is a chance for foal survival in rare cases of late-term pregnancies with mild-to-moderate hydrops.

If the pre-pubic tendon is still intact, the prognosis for future pregnancies in the mare is good. However, in thoroughbred mares that do not allow for artificial reproductive techniques, consideration should be given to the potential involvement of the pre-pubic tendon.

Approximately 50% of cases diagnosed with hydrops are associated with placentitis, and some mares may retain their placenta following induced parturition or controlled vaginal delivery of the foal. While the recurrence of a hydropsical condition is possible, many mares with previous hydrops have gone on to have subsequent normal pregnancies and foals. Nonetheless, future pregnancies should be considered high-risk, and closer monitoring is recommended.

On-farm management: If referral to a hospital is not possible, management of hydrops can be attempted in the field. The preferred treatment option is the termination of pregnancy through slow transcervical drainage of allantoic fluid and fetal extraction, which has been shown to improve outcomes for mares compared to other methods such as repeated prostaglandin injections, cervical dilation, and fetal removal (Mitchell et al. 2019).

It is important to consider the potential for a severe hypovolemic shock as placental fluids are expelled rapidly during the procedure. Venous access for fluid replacement or hypertonic saline should be readily available in case of an emergency. To avoid hypovolemic shock, clinicians should administer replacement intravenous fluids during drainage of allantoic fluid. Once the majority of the allantoic fluid is drained and the fetus is within reach, vaginal delivery can be performed (Figure 14.1). Euthanasia solution should be available as the foals are typically extracted still alive but have no chance of survival in the vast majority of hydrops cases. Retained fetal membranes is a common complication, which can also be treated and managed in a field setting as described further in this chapter. Mares should be placed on antimicrobials and anti-inflammatory drugs to prevent infection and reduce inflammation.

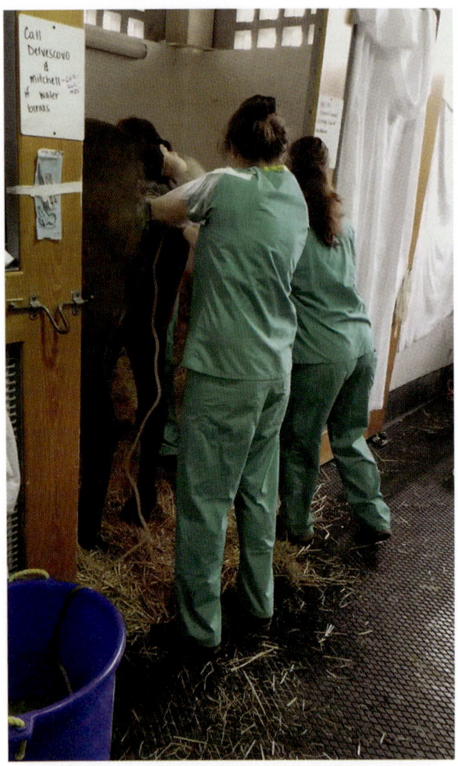

**Figure 14.1** Hydrops treatment by slow transcervical drainage of fetal fluids using a chest cannula attached to tubing. The mare should have aggressive fluid replacement therapy through multiple large catheters, and the fluid drained slowly while dilating the cervix. The foal can then be delivered via assisted vaginal delivery.

Referral hospital management: After a diagnosis of hydroallantois, it is important to formulate a plan for further diagnostic workup and management of the condition. The CTUP should be evaluated, and the severity of fetal fluid accumulation estimated using transrectal and transabdominal ultrasound. Additionally, the integrity of the abdominal wall should be evaluated by assessing mammary secretions and performing a ventral wall transabdominal ultrasound for any muscle wall defects. It is worth noting that the majority of mares with hydroallantois have marked ventral abdominal wall edema.

Since most cases of hydroallantois occur early in gestation and fetal life is incompatible outside of the uterus, it is important to plan for terminating the pregnancy while maintaining body fluid homeostasis during drainage of allantoic fluid. Slow drainage of allantoic fluid while replenishing fluid intravenously is preferred to decrease the risk of hypovolemic shock. It is also recommended to consider bilateral venous access for fluid replacement and access for resuscitation drugs or hypertonic saline, if needed. Slow drainage of placental fluids transcervically can be carried out over a couple of hours. Once the allantoic fluid has decreased significantly and the foal is within reach, a systematic fetal extraction can be safely performed. In cases where the placenta is easily detached, the foal should be humanely euthanized, and the placenta removed. If the mare has retained fetal membranes, appropriate management should be provided, and antimicrobials and nonsteroidal anti-inflammatory drugs (NSAIDs) should be considered for pain management.

Ventral abdominal wall edema in mares with hydrallantois may become more pronounced following treatment, and the mammary gland should be monitored for any displacement or changes in the color of mammary secretions that could indicate the development of pre-pubic tendon rupture.

Conclusion/Summary: Hydrops is a rare condition of pregnancy in the mare. Importantly, if managed appropriately and if the pre-pubic tendon is intact, the prognosis for the mare's survival is good. However, because of the rapid fluid accumulation and interference with normal placental function, the foal has a poor prognosis for survival. To reduce the risk of hypovolemic shock, slow drainage of allantoic fluid transcervically with intravenous fluid replacement is imperative.

It is worth noting that the prognosis for future pregnancies is good if no abdominal wall muscles have been involved. Therefore, careful evaluation of the abdominal wall during diagnosis and management of hydrops is crucial. Early detection and intervention can greatly increase the chances of successful hydrops management and future breeding soundness.

## Body Wall Rupture

Excessive weight gain during the last trimester of pregnancy, such as in twin pregnancy, hydropsical condition, fetal giants, recent trauma, or idiopathic reasons, can lead to body wall disease in mares. Among the various forms of ventral abdominal wall disease, tearing of the pre-pubic tendon is the most severe.

The pre-pubic tendon provides critical support to the abdominal wall. Tearing of this tendon can result in severe complications such as ventral herniation, compromised body wall integrity, and even death. Therefore, it is essential to monitor mares during pregnancy, particularly those at risk of excessive weight gain, to prevent the occurrence of body wall disease and associated complications.

Emergency triage plan: When dealing with potential body wall rupture in mares, it is essential to consider several factors such as pain level, ventral wall edema, ability to walk, breed, and gestational age. Bloody mammary secretions and cranial displacement of the glands may indicate pre-pubic tendon rupture.

Mares with this condition tend to be extremely painful, and foaling assistance is required due to muscle wall disruption. Differential diagnoses of pain and colic signs in a periparturient mare may include intestinal colic, uterine torsion, or hydropsical conditions.

Physical examination, abdominal ultrasound, and colic workup can aid in diagnosis. Additionally, ancillary blood work such as creatine kinase (CK) and aspartate transferase (AST) can help diagnose muscle tearing or damage.

Early detection and management of body wall rupture are critical to prevent complications such as ventral herniation and compromised body wall integrity. Therefore, careful monitoring and prompt intervention are necessary to ensure the health and well-being of the mare and foal.

Important decisions during management: The prognosis for future pregnancies in mares with body wall disease is often poor and contraindicated. However, for horses in which registries allow the use of assisted reproductive technology, they can still be used as embryo transfer donors or for transvaginal oocyte aspiration.

When managing a mare with body wall disease, it is crucial to understand the client's expectations and prioritize the health and safety of both the mare and the foal (Ross et al. 2008). Ideally, the foal should be maintained in utero until the foal is as close to term as possible to maximize the foal's prognosis especially if the foal is not yet at term, while balancing the risk of further disruption of the body wall disease. Fetal maturation and induction of parturition should be considered in mares that exceed 320 days of gestation.

In cases where pre-pubic tendon rupture has not yet occurred, and the mare's life is more valuable, termination of pregnancy and assisted delivery of the foal may be necessary. It is essential to assess the degree of muscle wall tearing and pre-pubic tendon involvement through palpation and transabdominal ultrasound to make informed decisions on the animal's welfare, the continuation of pregnancy, and the risk of evisceration.

Careful management and monitoring of mares with body wall disease are crucial to prevent complications and ensure the best possible outcome for both the mare and the foal. Regular veterinary consultations, diagnostic testing, and prompt intervention can make a significant difference in the prognosis and overall health of the animals involved.

On-farm management: To reduce the risk of evisceration in mares with ventral abdominal wall edema, consider using a belly band or hernia belt for abdominal support. It is best to confine mares to a small stall or paddock to limit physical activity. Pain management should also be a priority, with non-steroidal anti-inflammatory drugs administered to keep animals comfortable. Due to weakened muscle contractions, mares will require foaling assistance, so a foaling plan should be in place to ensure safe delivery.

Referral hospital management: Stall confinement and the use of abdominal bandages or hernia belts can reduce the risk of evisceration. Pain management is crucial, and non-steroidal anti-inflammatories, intravenous lidocaine, and/or morphine may be necessary to keep the mare comfortable. Continuous monitoring of abdominal muscle disruption via transabdominal ultrasound is necessary to understand the progression of the disease and to formulate a plan for the mare and foal. Blood work for CK and AST should be monitored during hospitalization to assess the degree of muscle damage and myonecrosis. Mares in late-term gestation should have their calcium and pH levels in mammary secretions monitored (if not bloody) to determine when they may be ready to foal. Induction of parturition or abortion may be necessary to save the mare depending on the degree of abdominal wall tearing and whether there is the involvement of the pre-pubic tendon. Assistance will be required at foaling due to a lack of abdominal contractions.

Conclusion/Summary: The goal of the treatment of mares with body wall tears is to resolve the cause of the tear which is excess abdominal stretching and weight. It is crucial to localize the muscle wall tearing and determine whether the pre-pubic tendon is involved or not to decide if abortion or continuation of pregnancy is appropriate. Additionally, animal welfare should be considered while managing pain and maintaining the mare's comfort level. The use of assisted reproductive technologies such as embryo transfer or transvaginal aspiration of oocytes should be used in mares where breed registries allow, as future pregnancies in the mare following abdominal wall injury carries significant risk.

## Premature Signs of Impending Parturition (Placentitis or Abortion)

Mares typically display external signs of approaching parturition during the last month of pregnancy, such as the enlargement of mammary glands, relaxation of pelvic ligaments, and vulvar elongation. As the due date approaches, the mare's mammary gland secretion undergoes specific changes, such as an increase in calcium and potassium levels, a decrease in sodium levels, and a decrease in pH. The teat ends may also appear waxed, or milk may leak from the teats. However, if these signs of impending parturition are observed well before the expected due date, it could indicate a pregnancy compromise, and the mare should be evaluated promptly.

Emergency triage plan: The mare should be evaluated to determine if there are any signs of disease, followed by a pregnancy and fetal assessment. Two of the primary concerns are abortion and placentitis. Abortion may be due to an infectious agent, including Equine Herpes Virus-1, which is a contagious disease of concern, or leptospirosis which may be zoonotic, and biosafety precautions are warranted if infection by these agents is suspected. Placentitis is not considered to be a contagious condition, even though it is also caused by infectious agents.

Evaluation of the mare should include a complete history, a thorough physical exam, possible blood collection and submission for laboratory diagnostics, and evaluation of the pregnancy. The goal of the mare exam is to determine if any systemic signs of disease can result in the development of imminent labor signs.

Pregnancy evaluation should consist of a transrectal palpation and ultrasound, transabdominal ultrasound, and possibly a vaginal examination. The transrectal palpation exam can identify fetal viability by fetal movements, identify the location, size, and characteristics of the uterus, and any other abnormalities of the reproductive tract or other viscera. Transrectal ultrasound can be used to evaluate fetal viability and signs of placentitis, including the CTUP, evaluate the characteristics of the fetal fluid, which should be clear for the allantoic fluid and slightly echogenic for amniotic fluid, and any other abnormalities such as placental detachment or abnormal structures. A transabdominal ultrasound examination should be performed if nocardioform placentitis is suspected, as the exudate and placenta separation is localized at the dependent portion of the placenta. Transabdominal ultrasound is also valuable to determine fetal viability by observing fetal heartbeats, fetal orientation, and if there are any other abnormalities.

- Vaginal examination: not always necessary and carries some risk of contamination and initiating labor
- Laboratory diagnosis: Bloodwork such as complete blood count and serum chemistry may not have significant changes. Some markers of inflammation, such as serum amyloid A, may be increased in mares with placentitis. Endocrine changes in mares with placentitis include a decrease in circulating estradiol 17-Beta. Pregnancy in mares is normally maintained by pregnanes such as 5-alpha-dihydro progesterone and in cases of placentitis, total progestogens are still usually adequate for pregnancy maintenance although there may be a shift toward other progestogens. Healthy mares in mid-to-late gestation have very low progesterone concentration. Mares with placentitis have a reduced ability to convert pregnenolone, which is the first product of sex-steroid hormone synthesis from cholesterol to pregnanes that maintain pregnancy in normal mares resulting in higher circulating pregnenolones. Pregnenolone is very similar to progesterone in molecular structure, and most antibodies used to measure progesterone have strong cross-reactivity with pregnenolone resulting in higher apparent progesterone reading in commercial assays. Rising 'progesterone' concentrations using commercial progesterone assays may indicate decreased placental function and the potential risk of abortion or preterm labor. This can be a warning sign that the mare is at risk of losing the pregnancy. We have used the progesterone tests to determine the response

to antibiotic treatments, as successfully treated mares often have a drop in the progesterone concentration, which rises again when the mare is close to foaling.

Important decisions during management: As the foal only becomes viable outside of the uterus around 320 days in gestation, the goal for any management of fetal compromise of a preterm foal is to keep the foal in the uterus as long as possible to allow the foal to reach maturity. It is possible for foals to be viable before 320 days in gestation especially foals from mares with chronic placentitis. This may be due to the chronic stress from placentitis inducing early maturation of the foal. It is important to have a plan on how to manage the foal after it is delivered, as foals from mares with placentitis often require medical interventions.

An important decision is to determine if there is a significant risk of pregnancy loss. For example, with mares having placentitis, serial monitoring of the fetus is recommended, and if the fetus dies *in utero*, the goal switches to remove the fetus in the safest way possible for the mare.

On-farm management: Placentitis: In situations where referral is not an option, placentitis can be managed at the farm. The primary treatment for placentitis is antibiotics.

We recommend starting the mare on broad-spectrum antibiotics such as procaine penicillin G (22,000 IU/kg IM b.i.d.) and gentamicin (6.6 mg/kg IV s.i.d.). If the mare does not respond to this combination of antibiotics, doxycycline (10 mg/kg PO b.i.d) or enrofloxacin (5 mg/kg IV s.i.d) may be attempted. If the mare improves clinically, oral antibiotics, such as trimethoprim sulfadiazine (30 mg/kg PO b.i.d.), may be continued.

Anti-inflammatory drugs, such as flunixin meglumine (1.1 mg/kg IV/PO s.i.d), or firocoxib (0.3 mg/kg PO loading dose, 0.1 mg/kg PO s.i.d) during the acute phase may be beneficial. Pentoxifylline (8.5 mg/kg PO b.i.d) is also often included in the treatment of placentitis.

Hormones: Estradiol cypionate (10 mg IM q3 days for three treatments) has been shown to improve foal outcomes. Altrenogest is widely used at double the typical dose (0.088 mg/kg PO s.i.d) to treat mares with placentitis, but there is limited evidence of its efficacy (Curcio et al. 2017).

Referral hospital management: Close monitoring of the fetus is possible in a referral hospital using frequent transabdominal ultrasound, fetal electrocardiography, and monitoring of hormones. Additionally, referral to a hospital will allow the use of stronger intravenous antibiotics, which is especially beneficial during the early stages of treatment. The ability to provide neonatal intensive care is a critical factor for the decision to refer a mare with placentitis to a hospital.

Antibiotics: Potassium penicillin G (22,000 IU/kg IV q6 h – given slowly) and gentamicin (6.6 mg/kg IV s.i.d.) are good options for the initial treatment. Otherwise, antibiotics, anti-inflammatory drugs, and hormone treatments are similar to those described for on-farm treatment.

Conclusion/Summary: Placentitis is a common problem in foaling mares, typically characterized by early mammary gland development. The goal is to treat the mare with antibiotics and supportive treatment to maintain the pregnancy for as long as possible to allow the foal to develop to a stage where it can be viable. The prognosis for the mare is generally good, but the prognosis for a viable foal is guarded even with an initial positive response to treatments.

## Abortion

Mares may abort at any stage of gestation; the later the gestation stage, the higher the risk of dystocia. Abortion may be due to infectious or non-infectious causes, and it is critical to be aware that some infectious causes of abortion have important consequences. The most important differential for abortion is Equine Herpesvirus-1 (EHV1). This is because the EHV1 virus can spread to other horses, resulting in severe clinical consequences and even death. Another important differential for mid-to-late-term abortion is leptospirosis which can be zoonotic. Thus, it is prudent to approach equine abortion cases with precautions until EVH1 and possibly leptospirosis are ruled out. This may mean having some isolation protocols in the hospital or to perform the procedures and interventions away from other horses if possible. Mares aborting from EHV1 are usually not shedding from the respiratory system by the time the mare aborts. The placenta and vaginal discharge are the main source of the virus and the more appropriate sample to submit for testing.

Emergency triage plan: Assess the situation, determine if the mare has delivered the fetus and fetal membranes, and assess if the location for the examination is appropriate for the examination and biosecurity concerns.

Ensure the mare is systemically stable. If the mare has not yet delivered the fetus, the goal would be to deliver the aborting fetus with as little trauma to the mare as possible. The delivery can be relatively easy or complicated depending on the gestational age and any abnormalities of the foal, such as contracted limbs or a wry neck. The perineum should be cleaned, and a vaginal examination performed to evaluate the caudal reproductive tract of the mare and the fetal disposition. If a fetal malposture cannot be corrected via manipulations, a fetotomy may be required to correct the malposture.

Retained fetal membrane is a relatively common condition after abortion. If the mare has already aborted the fetus and some fetal membranes, it is important to perform a careful placental evaluation to determine if there is a missing piece and if there are obvious abnormalities of the fetal membranes and foal. Treatment for retained fetal membranes will be discussed in more detail later in this chapter. The mare should be monitored closely for signs of metritis and other systemic diseases for a week post-abortion.

If the cause of abortion is due to an infectious agent, the mare may be showing other clinical signs and should be evaluated carefully.

Important decisions during management: If the aborting mare still has the fetus retained and vaginal manipulations on the farm are not progressing, it may be beneficial to refer the mare. If the mare is systemically compromised, it is another reason to refer the mare to a hospital. It is strongly recommended to submit all aborted fetuses and fetal membranes for further diagnostics unless the cause of abortion is obvious. Obvious conditions include twinning and umbilical cord torsions. The cause of abortion is important to know, especially if there are other pregnant mares on the farm. For infectious causes, other mares may also be at high risk for abortion.

Conclusion/Summary: Abortion may be due to infectious diseases such as EHV1 and should be treated as a possible infectious disease until proven otherwise. Management of the mare includes ensuring the aborted fetus is delivered with minimal trauma to the mare, the fetal membranes are completely passed, and the mare should be monitored closely for metritis and other systemic signs of disease.

## Premature Placental Separation

Premature placental separation in mares during parturition is often identifiable by a distinct sign called a "red-bag" delivery. This occurs when the chorioallantois, which is red, remains intact and protrudes from the vulva during birth. Normally, the pressure from uterine contractions will cause the chorioallantois to rupture at the cervical star, releasing allantoic fluid or "water-breaking," and the foal will be covered in the amnion, a white fetal membrane.

However, if the placenta separates prematurely, the chorioallantois will not rupture, but rather protrude from the vulva during parturition. This can cause a serious condition for the foal, as it leads to a lack of oxygen supply or hypoxia and increases the chances of fetal death or neonatal maladjustment syndrome. In cases where a red-bag delivery is not observed, it can still be diagnosed following parturition during placenta evaluation by examining the cervical star. An intact cervical star without other evidence of chorioallantois rupture confirms a red-bag delivery.

Emergency triage plan: If the owner reports a red-bag delivery, the ideal thing to do is to advise the owner to cut the chorioallantois and deliver the foal. This is one instance where speed of delivery is truly critical, and waiting for the veterinarian to arrive would lead to poorer outcomes. The foal should be evaluated and given assistance as needed.

Important decisions during management: There are other differentials for a red structure protruding during parturition and other differentials if a red structure protrudes not during parturition. A prolapsed bladder or bladder eversion may occur. In the case of prolapsed bladder, there is usually a large vaginal tear that results in the bladder protruding from the vulva. The surface of the bladder is smooth, and taking a sample of the fluid content to be analyzed can confirm a prolapsed bladder. Bladder eversion can be observed to arise from the urethral opening. It is difficult to ask the owner to confirm if it is indeed the chorioallantois or a different structure but asking the owner to describe the appearance of the surface of the red structure, and if a cervical star is present can greatly increase the confidence that it is indeed a red-bag delivery.

Conclusion/Summary: Premature placental separation during mare parturition is identifiable by a "red-bag" delivery, which occurs when the chorioallantois remains intact and protrudes from the vulva. This condition can result in hypoxia and other serious complications for the foal, making prompt diagnosis and treatment crucial. Premature separation of the placenta presents with the chorioallantois protruding from the vulva during parturition. The chorioallantois should be ruptured immediately, and the foal delivered and treated as necessary.

## Dystocia

Dystocia is perhaps one of the most stressful emergencies in equine practice because the appropriate intervention and timeliness can significantly influence the outcomes for the mare and the foal (Embertson 1999). Emotions are also usually high as multiple lives are at stake. We will not go through all the permutations of obstetrical manipulations but will highlight key considerations when managing equine dystocia.

The first rule of obstetrics is to be clean and minimize contamination of the uterus. Contamination can lead to infections that are potentially life-threatening and thus, we strongly recommend taking sanitary precautions during obstetrical examinations. It is not absolutely necessary to have everything sterile, but an aseptic technique is preferable. It is acceptable to use clean obstetrical sleeves and either disinfected or clean obstetrical equipment if sterilized equipment is not available. The perineum should be cleaned prior to any vaginal examinations. If possible, the tail should be wrapped and ideally tied to the side to minimize hair being brought into the vagina during manipulations.

The equine reproductive tract is very sensitive to trauma from obstetrical manipulations. Repeated examinations will cause some trauma, but there are some tips to minimize the trauma. First, the amnion is a slippery membrane that protects the vagina from direct contact with the foal. Obstetrical examinations should ideally be performed with the amnion acting as a barrier between your arms and the reproductive tract. The amnion should be used whenever possible to prevent direct contact of the foal with the vagina. The only exception is when examining the reproductive tract for lacerations or tears. It may not be possible to perform all the obstetrical manipulations from within the amnion. Using lubricants and minimizing the number of times and duration of obstetrical manipulations will reduce bruising. Also, minimizing the force used for foal delivery can reduce trauma to the reproductive tract.

Lubricants should be used for any obstetrical examination, but it may be prudent to calibrate the amount of lubricant introduced into the vagina, especially if there are any concerns of a vaginal or uterine laceration or if a cesarean section is a possibility. In these cases, we recommend holding off on infusing large amounts of lube, with only the amount of lubricant required for minimizing reproductive tract trauma used during the initial examination and manipulation stages.

An obstetrical examination should begin with a general assessment of the caudal reproductive tract, especially to determine if the reproductive tract is sufficiently dilated to allow for vaginal delivery of the foal. This is accomplished by applying pressure to determine the "give" of the reproductive tract. The cervix should be assessed to determine if it is fully or partially dilated. A fully dilated cervix will be hardly perceptible and consist of the junction between the vagina and uterus. A partially dilated cervix may feel like a constriction or a flap of tissue between the vagina and uterus. The cervix of a mare can be manually dilated, but this often results in trauma, especially if improperly done, and it is advisable to use drugs whenever possible. Prostaglandin E2 can be used to stimulate cervical dilation. Then the evaluation of the foal should include an assessment of size, presentation, position, posture, and viability.

The nomenclature to describe the fetal state within the uterus in veterinary medicine comprises a description of the *presentation, position, and posture. Presentation* is the orientation of the long axis of the foal relative to the long axis of the mare. If the long axis of the foal is parallel to the long axis of the mare and the foal is facing the vaginal opening, the foal is considered to be in longitudinal, anterior presentation. Similarly, if the long axis of the foal and mare is parallel, but the foal is oriented in the same direction as the mare, the foal will present with the hind end to the vaginal opening and is considered to be in longitudinal, posterior presentation. If the long axis of the foal is perpendicular to the long axis of the mare, the foal is in a transverse presentation, and this will result in a difficult dystocia to correct. The *position* of the foal is the relationship between the foal within its longitudinal axis relative to the mare, and it is described as the relationship between the dorsum of the foal relative to the pelvic bone of the mare closest to the dorsum of the foal. In a normal position, the foal is oriented in its long axis with the dorsum of the foal closest to the sacrum of the mare, resulting in a dorso-sacral position. If the foal is upside-down with the dorsum of the foal closest to the pubis of the mare, the foal would be in a dorso-pubic position. If the foal is oriented on its side, the foal would be in dorso-iliac position. Finally, the *posture* of the foal is the relationship of the foal extremities relative to the normal foaling posture, which in an anterior presentation foaling would involve the head and both front feet extended toward the vaginal opening, or if the foal is in posterior presentation, a normal posture would be for both hind legs to be extended toward the vaginal opening. Abnormalities of the posture are described by the flexion or deviation of a particular joint or point. One of the most common malposture in foals is a lateral deviation of the head and neck. Malpostures of the limbs are named for the most descriptive abnormality. For example, an elbow flexion would also involve the flexion of the shoulders, but just saying elbow flexion is sufficient. This nomenclature is important as it allows an accurate description of the obstetrical findings among veterinarians.

Foals can be delivered in anterior presentation or posterior presentation. It is essential that the foal is in normal posture prior to attempted delivery. If the foal is in transverse presentation, it is recommended to convert the foal to the posterior presentation. This eliminates the need to worry about the head and neck posture and, more importantly, eliminates the risk of the hindlegs being engaged in the reproductive tract in anterior presentation, i.e., the foal being in "dog-sitting" or "hurdling" posture and preventing successful delivery. The recommendation to choose posterior over anterior presentation for the correction of transverse presentation is counterintuitive, yet effective.

Uterine contractions of the mare can be forceful and hamper attempts of repulsion and mutation of the foal. In these situations, an epidural injection can be administered to reduce the straining; however, epidural use may cause undesired recumbency in the mare. This may become problematic if initial manipulations are unsuccessful, and referral is necessary. In some situations, general anesthesia is required to control uterine contractions and allow manipulations to be accomplished safely. Anesthesia is most often performed at a referral hospital; however, controlled vaginal delivery is also possible at the farm if referral is not an option.

Emergency triage plan: The mare should be assessed to determine if there are systemic problems. The mare may require sedation, and an epidural may reduce straining. A thorough obstetrical examination should be performed. Based on the findings of the obstetrical examination, the options for delivery and the initial prognosis for successful delivery should be discussed with the client.

Important decisions during management: Every dystocia is unique, and no single approach works for all cases. To increase the likelihood of a successful outcome, the veterinarian should be aware of the wishes of the client, including the value of the mare and foal, the viability of the foal, and the availability of a referral hospital. Having this information prior to or at the onset of the parturition increases the success for all parties. As the timing of the correction of the dystocia directly affects foal survival, time management becomes essential, both on the farm and at the referral hospital (Byron et al. 2003). It is advisable when managing dystocia to inform an observer of the ideal time frame and have them keep track of time (i.e., 10 minutes for assisted manipulations) as the veterinarian's focus is on the manipulations and correction of the dystocia. The exact timing will depend on the availability and option for referral and the individual case. If significant progress is being made by vaginal manipulations, such as the successful correction of maldisposition within the examination and manipulation time frame, additional time should be allotted to allow for vaginal delivery either by assisted or controlled delivery (Figure 14.2).

On-farm management: The initial examination of equine dystocia is often performed at the farm. In some situations, the owners will opt to transport the mare directly to a referral hospital without a veterinarian assessing the mare at the farm. Some owners are comfortable performing obstetrical examinations and attempting delivery of the foal, and some mares may have

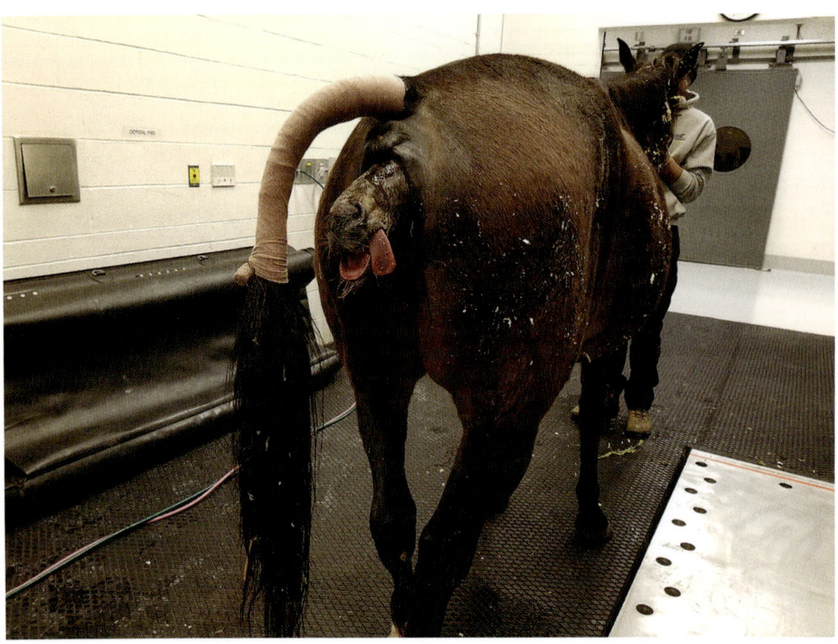

**Figure 14.2** Nose of foal protruding from vulva is very likely to be due to malposture of the foal in anterior presentation, dorsosacral position, and bilateral shoulder flexion posture. Resolution of this condition requires the repulsion of the foal head to make space to reach the forelimbs, then converting bilateral shoulder flexion to bilateral carpal flexion by pulling the carpus across under the sternum then pulling the carpus cranially. Bilateral carpus flexion can then be corrected, and the foal delivered by assisted vaginal delivery which was successful in this case or by controlled vaginal delivery. Alternatively, fetotomy is an option by cutting the limb ideally at the level of the shoulders for non-viable foals, and cesarean section for viable foals.

had extensive manipulations prior to your involvement. In these cases, it is prudent to carefully examine the reproductive tract for any tears, especially if there is more bleeding than anticipated. If the owner is reasonably skilled and is able to correctly identify the foal to be in a dorso-pubic position or any abnormalities in the position or posture of the foal, it is recommended that the mare is walked and not allowed to go down, if possible, until the veterinarian arrives. The reasoning for this recommendation is to reduce the frequency and strength of the mare's uterine contractions resulting in the foal being pushed against the reproductive tract when the disposition is not correct, as this will result in a rapid reduction of foal viability.

There are three main options for delivering the foal at the farm namely (i) assisted vaginal delivery, where the foal is delivered vaginally; (ii) controlled vaginal delivery, where the mare is anesthetized to allow safer vaginal manipulations and delivery; (iii) fetotomy which is only indicated if the foal is dead, where the foal is cut using a fetotomy wire or Gigli wire in the uterus usually to correct malposture; (iv) the final option for delivering a foal at the farm is a terminal Cesarean section where the mare is euthanized and the foal extracted from the uterus. This procedure is indicated when the foal is alive, but the mare has an untreatable condition; this is a salvage procedure to try and save the foal.

Referral hospital management: Time management is essential for successful outcomes of equine dystocia, as prolongations in stage II will negatively affect the survival of the foal (Byron et al. 2003; Norton et al. 2007). A mare that presents to the hospital for management of dystocia should be rapidly assessed to determine the cause of the dystocia and subsequent interventions. Simultaneously, a quick assessment of the mare's systemic stability, including point-of-care blood work (PCV/TS, lactate, stall side chemistry), is recommended. Given the high likelihood that either controlled vaginal delivery or Cesarean section may be performed, an intravenous catheter is placed upon arrival, following initial mare assessment. As these mares have typically undergone assisted vaginal attempts at the farm, the time spent on this approach to delivery in the hospital setting should be minimal. An important consideration during dystocia is foal survival. Ex utero intrapartum treatment (EXIT) is recommended if the foal's muzzle is available, i.e., palpable within the pelvic canal or external, to allow nasotracheal intubation and ventilation. Upon identification of nares, a 7-10 mm internal diameter long endotracheal tube is inserted through the nares with one hand, while the other hand palpates the cranial esophagus to confirm placement within the trachea. The tube is secured by inflating the cuff, capnography is attached, and the foal is then ventilated for the duration of correction of the dystocia. With this EXIT procedure in mind, the following flow chart outlines a suggested timing for interventions.

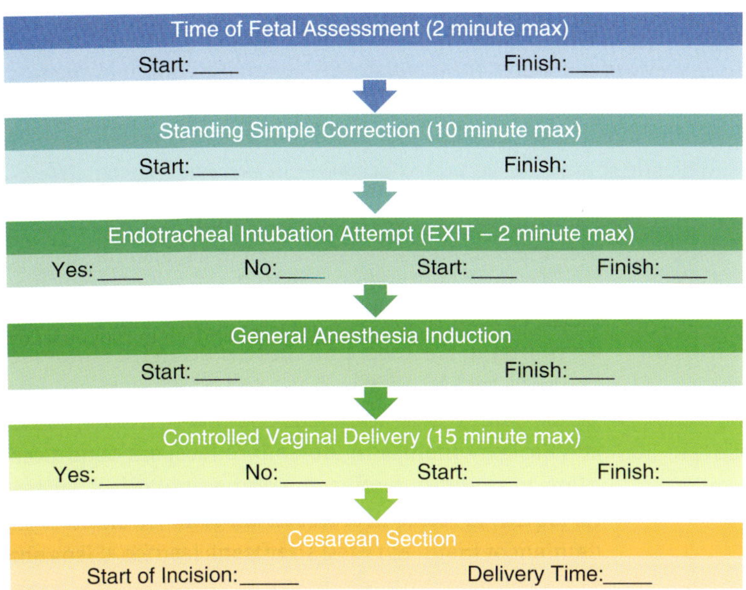


The above flowchart has suggested time frames for each of the procedures; however, the individual case and the clinician representing the interests of the client will dictate the amount of time spent on each. For example, if assisted vaginal delivery attempts were already made at the farm by an experienced veterinarian or owner, the decision might be made to anesthetize the mare immediately following the initial assessment and EXIT procedure. Or if the fetal presentation or posture is such that a muzzle is not available, intubation will not occur. Two additional options that are not listed in the flowchart are fetotomy and terminal cesarean section. As described above, fetotomy would be indicated in dystocia with a non-viable foal, where a cesarean section is not an option for the client, most often due to cost concerns. Terminal cesarean section may be indicated in dystocia, where the mare has an underlying condition, as a salvage procedure for the viable foal. It is important for clients to be aware that mare survival rates are high following controlled vaginal delivery, cesarean section, and fetotomy. Fertility rates following these procedures are also good provided that a skilled specialist is involved (Carluccio et al. 2007; Abernathy-Young et al. 2012). Following correction of the dystocia, it is common for mares to retain their fetal membranes; see the section on Metritis and Retained Fetal Membranes. This should be managed aggressively as this can result in high morbidity and mortality for the mare.

Conclusion/Summary: Successful outcomes following dystocia can be attained, with attention placed on the timing of stage II labor, as this is the single most important determinant of foal survival. As previously mentioned, each dystocia is unique as it pertains to the reason for dystocia, the wishes of the client, the value of the mare and foal, and the viability of the foal. Mare survival and fertility can be attained.

For equine ambulatory practitioners, it is advisable to make arrangements with local bovine practitioners, who are skillful in obstetrics, to have their assistance during equine dystocia cases ahead of time. Often the resolution of difficult dystocia will require significant medical management of the mare and obstetrical expertise; thus, having more skilled personnel increases the likelihood of success. Many equine ambulatory practitioners are not comfortable with performing fetotomies and may not even have the equipment necessary. These multi-veterinarian arrangements for equine dystocia management are especially useful if there are no nearby referral hospitals.

## Emergency Conditions of the Mare – Postpartum

### Periparturient Hemorrhage

Most cases of periparturient hemorrhage occur in the immediate postpartum period. However, it should be noted that mares can have episodes of hemorrhage in the weeks leading up to parturition as well as in the first week postpartum. In the immediate postpartum period, mares may experience various conditions such as vaginal lacerations, uterine tears, and broad ligament hematoma/rupture. Less likely is damage to a gastrointestinal structure during parturition (small colon or small intestine) that results in mesenteric bleeding. The severity of blood loss may vary depending on the extent of the tear. Of these conditions, a ruptured uterine artery can result in the most serious consequences, especially when direct hemorrhage occurs into the peritoneal cavity or into the uterus, which can result in acute and fatal blood loss. While periparturient hemorrhagic conditions tend to affect older mares, typically those over 18 years old, mares of any age may be affected (Dolente et al. 2005; Arnold et al. 2008).

Emergency triage plan: Mares can exhibit a range of symptoms after foaling, including systemic shock, stumbling, and pale mucous membranes. Less commonly, they may present with excessive vaginal bleeding. If a mare shows tachycardia, tachypnea, pale mucous membranes, and increased capillary refill time, there is a strong suspicion of post-foaling blood loss. However, hemorrhage associated with the reproductive tract may not be straightforward to diagnose. Mares may also display colic signs that vary from mild to severe, restlessness, and may not have pale mucous membranes. Therefore, any mare that displays signs of discomfort postpartum should be assessed quickly for signs of hemorrhage. Clinical signs of acute severe hemorrhage may include acute abdominal pain, agitation, restlessness, tachycardia, tachypnea, prolonged capillary refill time, poor pulse quality, muscle fasciculations, sweating, vocalization, weakness, and ataxia.

The priority in such cases is to stabilize the patient to reduce hypovolemic shock and decrease blood loss. This should be done while a diagnosis of the source of bleeding is being made. If the source of bleeding can be identified, the focus should be to facilitate hemostasis. If accessible, lacerations of the reproductive tract may be clamped or ligated. Topical administration of phenylephrine and application of pressure to the site of bleeding may be helpful to control the bleeding. Alternatively, application of hemostatic granules and pressure may also control bleeding. However, for the majority of severe, acute cases of hemorrhage, the source of bleeding is often inaccessible, and treatment is focused on mitigation strategies such as clot stabilization, minimizing clot disruption, and blood transfusion.

Important decisions during management: A quick assessment of the mare's systemic status is essential. If a mare exhibits any of the signs of systemic shock: poor pulse quality, poor capillary refill time, tachycardia, tachypnea, cold extremities, hyperlactatemia, with or without pale mucous membranes, there may be a major ruptured vessel or artery, which could result in fatal hemorrhage. Mares that are bleeding may thrash around from pain or collapse. It is crucial to prioritize the safety of personnel in such situations.

It is recommended to keep the foal in a safe environment where it does not get injured if the mare collapses or tries to go down. Ideally, this is in an area where the mare can still see the foal. It is also crucial to maintain a calm and quiet environment to minimize stress for the mare. If a referral is an option, the first step is to stabilize the animal before transportation. Of note, administration of synthetic colloids should be avoided for the mare that has severe uncontrolled hemorrhage as they may have negative effects on coagulation.

On-farm management: The initial steps in managing a hemorrhagic mare should include a quick assessment of her condition and stabilization of the patient. Pain management and/or sedation may be required for examination, and xylazine and/or butorphanol are recommended for this purpose. Acepromazine should be used with caution or in small amounts to reduce the risk of further hypotension and possible collapse. Aminocaproic acid may be initiated as a bolus treatment (40 mg/kg instilled into 1 L of isotonic crystalloid fluids, intravenously). A constant rate infusion of aminocaproic acid may be used given the medication's short half-life, but this is not advisable in the farm setting. Yunnan Baiyao, a traditional Chinese herbal supplement, (8 mg/kg PO q6 h), can also be used as a hemostatic agent.

In cases where the source of bleeding has been located and the hemorrhage has been controlled, and where intravenous fluid resuscitation is required, hypertonic saline (4 mL/kg) may be administered, followed by isotonic crystalloid fluids. See chapter on IV fluid administration. It should be noted that if hemorrhage is severe and uncontrolled (hemoperitoneum), hypertonic saline and IV fluid boluses should be avoided or used with caution to avoid a rapid rise in blood pressure and clot disruption. In such a situation, permissive hypotension is preferable, by administering isotonic crystalloid fluids at a maintenance rate (1 L/h in a 500 kg horse).

Once patient stabilization is achieved, it is crucial to keep the mare in a quiet environment to decrease the chance of excitement and higher blood pressure that may disrupt the clot. Further diagnostic examinations can then be performed including transabdominal ultrasound to identify swirling echoic fluid (blood) in the peritoneal cavity or intrauterine fluid. A careful manual examination of the vagina, cervix, and uterus should be performed to detect any potential tears. Transrectal palpation should be postponed or performed with caution to avoid clot disruption. Stall confinement for a minimum of two weeks is recommended following stabilization.

Referral hospital management: Upon arrival at a referral hospital, the mare should be examined carefully to determine if severe periparturient hemorrhage has occurred, as other forms of postpartum pain (i.e., colic) can mimic one another. Quick assessment of heart rate, respiratory rate, capillary refill time, mucous membrane color, and attitude can be used in conjunction with packed cell volume (PCV), total solids, and peripheral lactate to assess blood loss. In the initial phases of hemorrhage, tachycardia, tachypnea, and hyperlactatemia occur. As hemorrhage continues, hypoproteinemia (or even relative hypoproteinemia in the face of hemoconcentration) will be present. Changes in PCV and mucous membrane color should not be anticipated in the acute phase of hemorrhage, and these drops in PCV will occur as late as 12–24 h following acute hemorrhage. During this initial assessment, an intravenous catheter should be placed to facilitate administration of medications, fluids, and or blood. Once the diagnosis of hemorrhage is made, careful examination of the reproductive tract, abdominal cavity, and gastrointestinal tract should be performed to determine a source of bleeding and whether further intervention is required. While uterine artery hemorrhage is the most common reason for postpartum hemoperitoneum, bleeding associated with damage to a gastrointestinal structure can also occur during parturition and this usually requires exploratory celiotomy to correct. Careful palpation per rectum by experienced veterinarians is not contraindicated and is often essential in the ultimate diagnosis of postpartum problems.

During this comprehensive assessment, mares should be stabilized. The exact stabilization regarding IV fluid administration or blood transfusion will depend on the severity of hemorrhage. Aminocaproic acid loading dose of (40 mg/kg in 1 L of isotonic crystalloids) and 20 mg/kg q6 h maintenance dose can be used as an anti-fibrinolytic agent to stabilize clots. Tranexamic acid 5–25 mg/kg IV q12 h is an alternative to Aminocaproic acid. Yunnan Baiyao (8 mg/kg PO q.i.d) can also be used as an adjunctive treatment.

Blood transfusion should be considered in the case of severe acute hemorrhage. Transfusion triggers in acute cases include a blood lactate >4 mmol/L, PCV <20%, and oxygen extraction ratio of >40%. In an emergency situation, a cross-match is not necessary and will take valuable time during which blood may be given. Ideal donors are Standardbred geldings who are fully vaccinated and free of disease. The maximum volume that an appropriate donor can give is approximately 20%

of their blood volume (see Chapter 28, Fluid Therapy for Horses). Intravenous crystalloid fluid therapy should be managed carefully depending on the state of hemostasis. In uncontrolled bleeding cases, fluid therapy should be administered carefully with the goal of hypotensive resuscitation (goal of MAP <70 mmHg) so that organ perfusion is achieved without clot disruption. Noninvasive arterial blood pressure can be measured and monitored with a tail cuff. The mare should be handled as little as possible and kept quiet to prevent elevations in blood pressure and dislodging of the clot(s).

Conclusion/Summary: Complete uterine artery rupture in mares can lead to peracute and often fatal hemorrhage. However, other sources of reproductive and gastrointestinal bleeding associated with parturition may occur. The most common of these are uterine or vaginal tears and broad ligament hematoma. All of these may cause significant blood loss and hypovolemic shock but generally present a fair to good prognosis in most cases and future fertility can be reasonable (Arnold et al. 2008). The first goal of management is diagnosis of the problem and severity of the blood loss as this will determine specific management plans for the individual mare.

Importantly, early recognition and prompt management of these conditions are crucial for a successful outcome. Therefore, regular monitoring of postpartum mares and prompt intervention in case of any concerning clinical signs are vital in preventing severe complications.

## Uterine Prolapse

Although uncommon in the mare, uterine prolapse most commonly occurs immediately postpartum and often can be fatal due to uterine artery rupture, septic shock, or septic peritonitis secondary to uterine trauma. Predisposing factors for a uterine prolapse may include dystocia, anesthesia, retained fetal membranes, twin abortions, or rarely, increased abdominal pressure secondary to gastrointestinal disease (colic). Uterine atony and hypocalcemia have been suggested as potential etiology and can be exacerbated by traction or weight of the fetal membranes causing inversion (Figure 14.3).

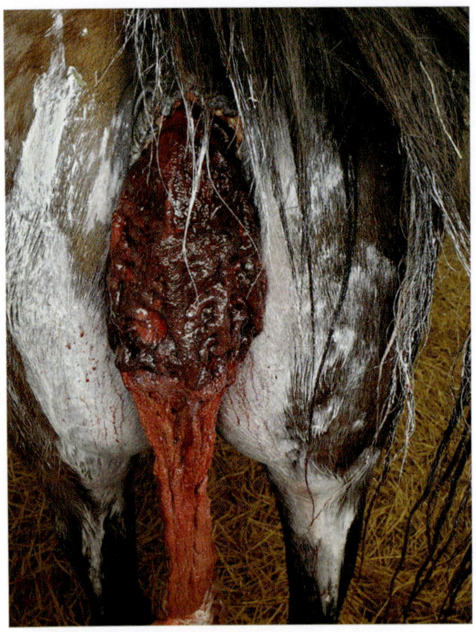

**Figure 14.3** Partial uterine prolapse secondary to retained fetal membranes. A thorough physical examination is important to determine if there is internal hemorrhage that needs to be addressed. If possible, detach the fetal membranes from the uterus, clean the uterus, and examine for any lacerations. An epidural may be helpful to reduce straining during reduction. The uterus must be completely replaced, or the mare will likely have a recurrence of uterine prolapse. Uterine lavage after replacement may be helpful to ensure complete reduction. It is useful to increase uterine muscular tone after replacement to hold the uterus in place as a flaccid uterus is easier to invert and prolapse.

Emergency triage plan: The mare should be assessed for systemic signs of acute blood loss. The uterus should be elevated as quickly as possible to avoid increased tension on the broad ligaments and uterine arteries. This can be accomplished with an assistant holding a sterile garbage bag, clean sheet or towels as a hammock, or a clean tray to support the most ventrally hanging parts of the uterus. It should then be evaluated for any lacerations. Following cleaning using sterile saline and removal of any gross debris, any full-thickness lacerations should be repaired. If the uterus was directly observed to prolapse and is immediately assessed, it may be replaced into the abdomen immediately without additional local anesthesia. However, more often, an epidural is required to provide desensitization and reduce straining during replacement.

If the uterus is edematous, the use of sugar or other hyperosmotic compounds can be used to reduce the size of the uterus prior to attempting reduction. It is also helpful to elevate the uterus to above the level of the vagina to allow gravity to assist in the reduction of the prolapsed uterus. The use of a prolapse tray can be helpful for this purpose.Once the prolapse is replaced it is imperative to ensure that the uterus is completely replaced. If even a small portion of the uterine horn tips is not corrected, straining may occur and the uterus may prolapse again. Lavage of the replaced uterus may help ensure complete reduction of the tips of the uterine horns. Additionally, clean glass bottles or a disposable vaginal speculum may be used to carefully reach and reduce the tips of the horns.

Important decisions during management: Due to the risk of damage to the uterine artery, it is ideal to minimize mare movement until the prolapse has been corrected. If the mare has a foal at her side, keeping the foal in view will minimize her anxiety, decrease vocalization, and may reduce straining. It is important to consider that uterine prolapse itself has an excellent prognosis for survival and future fertility. However, the damage to the uterine artery, or the uterus itself during prolapse, or during correction (i.e., inadvertent tearing), greatly affect the mare's survival. As such, prompt, gentle intervention is critical for successful outcomes.

On-farm management: As mentioned, if possible, the mare should be examined where she was found prolapsed to avoid additional tension on the broad ligaments during walking/transport. The prolapse should be immediately supported by one or more assistants to minimize additional trauma and also reduce edema formation. Quick assessment of her systemic stability should be performed, paying attention to degree of tachycardia and capillary refill time. The mare may require sedation for complete uterine evaluation and reduction. Alpha-2 agonists (xylazine, detomidine) and butorphanol are common medications. An epidural is recommended to facilitate examination and replacement. This is especially useful for repair of any full-thickness lacerations.

Careful but rapid examination of the endometrium should occur to assess for damage, lacerations, gross debris, or fetal membranes. Laceration repair should occur after careful cleaning of the uterus, using absorbable suture such as polyglactin 910 size 1. Any fetal membranes should be carefully removed from the endometrium. If the fetal membranes are firmly attached, they should be trimmed to avoid additional tension on the endometrium following replacement of the uterus. Cleaning of the uterus can be accomplished with sterile saline lavages and digital removal of any gross debris, dilute povidone iodine solution can be used for severely contaminated uterus. Sugar, dextrose solutions, or hypertonic saline solutions may be applied to the endometrial surface to reduce edema if present. Following cleaning and repair, if necessary, the uterus is replaced into the abdominal cavity. Lifting of the uterus by assistants using sheets or towels will facilitate the replacement by the veterinarian. Care should be taken to avoid inadvertent penetration of the uterine wall during replacement. Complete replacement of the uterine horns should be confirmed. Often the use of a disposable vaginal speculum or clean glass bottle can help the veterinarian reach the tips of the uterine horns. Uterine lavage with sterile saline (3–10 L) may aid in removal of any lingering contamination as well as fully expand the uterine horns. Once the uterus is replaced, 10–20 IU of oxytocin should be administered intravenously to aid in uterine contraction.

Depending on the length of time of prolapse, the degree of contamination, and the integrity of the uterus, systemic antimicrobials and anti-inflammatories may be used. Systemic antimicrobials are indicated for uterine prolapses with uterine lacerations or those with retained fetal membranes. Following reduction of the prolapse, daily uterine lavages may be performed as needed for the management of continued retained fetal membranes or removal of debris.

The mare should be monitored closely following reduction of the prolapse for signs of systemic compromise and hemorrhage. Clinical signs may include acute abdominal pain, agitation, restlessness, tachycardia, tachypnea, prolonged capillary refill time, poor pulse quality, muscle fasciculations, sweating, vocalization, weakness, and ataxia. If signs of hemorrhage occur, see section above on Periparturient Hemorrhage.

Referral hospital management: Management of the uterine prolapse in a referral setting is similar to the on-farm management, with the added ease of additional assistants or tools (sterile garbage bags, trays) to aid in the support and replacement of the uterus. The transport of a mare with a uterine prolapse is a decision to be made with caution as the prolapse is ideally treated on site. Should a uterine prolapse occur to a mare that is already hospitalized, the steps described above should be followed.

Conclusion/Summary: Uterine prolapse is an uncommon condition of the postpartum mare that can result in fatal uterine artery rupture. Replacement on site prior to referral is preferred if a veterinarian is readily available to attend to the animal.

## Metritis and Retained Fetal Membranes

Retained fetal membranes in mares is defined as the failure of the placenta to detach within three hours after foaling. Prolonged retention of the fetal membranes beyond this time frame can lead to serious complications such as metritis, systemic compromise, and even the development of laminitis.

Metritis is a common complication associated with retained fetal membranes and can develop due to several factors, including contamination of the uterus with pathogenic bacteria during foaling, obstetrical manipulation, or poor uterine involution. Importantly, metritis can also occur independently of retained fetal membranes and be caused by other factors such as prolonged labor, dystocia, or other forms of trauma to the uterus.

Early recognition and prompt management of retained fetal membranes and associated complications are crucial for a successful outcome. Therefore, routine monitoring of postpartum mares and prompt intervention in case of any concerning clinical signs are essential in preventing severe complications.

Emergency triage plan: When veterinarians are called to examine a foal for a routine post-foaling exam and IgG levels, it is crucial that they also perform a post-foaling examination on the mare. Inquiring about the fetal membranes may provide some insight, but the veterinarian may need to evaluate the placenta to fully assess the mare's condition. Placental tears and discoloration are common when examinations are done many hours after parturition. To properly evaluate the placenta, it should be displayed into an "F" shape, and the tip of each horn should be examined to determine if there are any significant pieces missing. The non-pregnant horn is the most common piece to be retained.

A physical examination of the mare will help assess systemic compromise. Mares that have retained fetal membranes for more than 12 h often have an elevated rectal temperature and a toxic line on their mucus membranes. They may also be anorexic and have elevated heart and respiratory rates. Inspection of the vulva may reveal an obviously attached placenta.

Transrectal palpation and ultrasound can be used to evaluate uterine involution (i.e., rugae) and the amount of intrauterine fluid. A long placenta tag may be visualized through transrectal ultrasound but cannot always be detected. Vaginal palpation should be performed to determine if there are any tears and if any placenta can be felt at that level. The uterus should also be inspected carefully by palpation using the full length of your arm to see if a placenta tag is present in either of the horns. Within the first 24 h post-foaling, the tip of the uterine horn may not be within reach. Filling the uterus with fluids may help dilate the uterine lumen and make any placenta tags easier to identify.

It is important to start treatment for retained fetal membranes as soon as possible. The longer a mare retains the fetal membranes, the sicker she will become and the more support she will need. Differential diagnoses in a mare postpartum with fever should include retained fetal membranes, metritis, and uterine tears causing peritonitis.

Important decisions during management: Retained fetal membranes can occur in any breed but draft horses are predisposed, and management should be identified and treated promptly in all cases.

Additionally, the management of retained fetal membranes should be based on individual cases rather than just the duration of retention. Some mares may show signs of metritis and laminitis earlier than others and may require more intensive management even if the fetal membranes have not been retained for a long period of time.

It is also important to note that while referral to a hospital may be beneficial in some cases, it is not always necessary and may not be feasible for all owners. Management options should be discussed with the owner and based on the individual case.

On-farm management: If the fetal membranes have been retained for only 3–6 h from foaling, oxytocin can be given (2–5 IU, IV or IM).

*Intact fetal membranes can be treated via*:

- The Dutch method, which includes infusing fluid through the umbilical vessel to dilate placenta vessels for easier detachment.
- Burns technique in which a large volume of fluid (tap water or saline with 0.5% iodine solution) is instilled in the allantoic space of the placenta in order to distend the placenta for detachment.
- Uterine lavage with large volumes of fluid can be performed with the goal to dilate the uterus and help the placenta detach.
- Slow peeling of the placenta can sometimes be performed. This technique should be performed by experienced veterinarians as it is critical to detach the fetal membranes gently and slowly. The risks associated with improper physical placental removal include tearing of the placenta, leaving a small tip of the uterine horn, hemorrhage, tip of uterine horn inversion, and uterine prolapse.

*When only a portion of the fetal membranes are retained*:

- Depending on the size of the piece left behind a Burns technique may not be possible, leaving uterine lavage and possibly manual detachment of the retained fetal membranes.

Uterine lavage should be continued for a few more days after the fetal membranes have been removed with the goal to decrease the bacterial load and treat the metritis.

NSAIDs can be administered to help with pain and for antitoxic effects.

Antimicrobial therapy should be initiated, especially if the placenta has been retained for more than six hours. The initial treatment of choice is sulfadiazine/trimethoprim at 30 mg/kg, twice daily, orally.

Frequent oxytocin doses can be administered, starting at 2–5 IU IV or IM.

Some veterinarians may use much larger doses of oxytocin (up to 120 IU) in combination with high dose of xylazine (up to 500 mg), followed by a uterine lavage 30 min after administration in cases where a faster resolution is prioritized over mare discomfort from large dose of oxytocin such as farm that are far away or in cases where resources to manage cases are limited. While this approach is not generally recommended, it may be an option in some situations. Mares with toxic lines in their mucus membranes will benefit from referral for 24-h management and critical care treatment, including IV fluid therapy, broad-spectrum antibiotics, and ice boot therapy.

Referral hospital management: In addition to the above-mentioned treatments, mares with retained fetal membranes may also benefit from supportive care and the treatment of endotoxemia and its sequelae. This can include providing intravenous fluids and electrolytes, to help maintain hydration and electrolyte balance. Anti-inflammatory medications, including NSAIDs or lidocaine CRI, can also be administered to help reduce pain and inflammation. In addition, digital cryotherapy in the form of ice boots is recommended prior to the development of endotoxemia as a preventative measure against laminitis. Additional specific anti-endotoxic therapies may be administered as needed: polymyxin B, misoprostol, ethyl pyruvate, and clenbuterol, among others.

Frequent uterine lavages in any of the techniques mentioned above will be performed two to three times daily until the placenta is retrieved and for a few days after to continue to treat the metritis and decrease the bacterial load.

Intravenous broad-spectrum antimicrobials therapies will be initiated with Penicillin G potassium (22,000 IU/kg, every six hours) and gentamicin (6.6 mg/kg, once daily). Metronidazole can be added if there is suspicion of anaerobic infection.

Bloodwork, especially white blood cell count, can be monitored closely during treatment to assess the severity of metritis and endotoxemia. In some cases, surgical intervention may be necessary if the retained fetal membranes cannot be removed by other means or if there are complications such as uterine tears or hemorrhage.

Overall, the management of retained fetal membranes in mares can be challenging and requires a multi-faceted approach that addresses both the immediate and long-term consequences of the condition. With timely and appropriate treatment, however, many mares will make a full recovery and go on to have successful breeding careers.

Conclusion/Summary: Retained fetal membranes can lead to metritis, which is a bacterial infection of the uterus. The longer the fetal membranes remain in the uterus, the greater the chance of infection, and the more severe the infection may become. Metritis can then lead to endotoxemia, or the presence of segments of Gram-negative bacteria (endotoxin) within the bloodstream. Endotoxemia and the subsequent systemic inflammatory response by the body cause a variety of clinical signs and may lead to the development of laminitis. Mares with retained fetal membranes are especially at risk for the development of laminitis that may be life-threatening. Therefore, prompt diagnosis and aggressive treatment of retained fetal membranes are essential to prevent the development of metritis and endotoxemia, and subsequent laminitis.

## Postpartum Eclampsia

Hypocalcemia is a rare condition in mares post-partum. The condition is caused by a sudden decrease in serum ionized calcium levels, which can lead to muscle tremors, weakness, and even death if left untreated. In mares, it is most commonly seen in draft breeds and may be associated with high milk production. Treatment involves the administration of calcium and supportive care.

Emergency triage plan: Hypocalcemia tetani should be suspected with a mare, with a foal at her side, presents with signs such as wooden horse stance, prolapse of the third eyelid, muscle tremors, salivation, stiffness of the gait, cardiac arrhythmia, and/or recumbency. Differential diagnoses include tetanus, endotoxemia, colic, and laminitis.

Important decisions during management: Timely recognition of the condition and correction of the calcium deficit is imperative for mare survival. Foal nursing should be discontinued until the mare is stabilized and management of properly balanced feeding for the postpartum mare is instituted.

On-farm management: Stabilization of the acute hypocalcemia can be instituted at the farm with slow intravenous fluid administration of 20% calcium borogluconate diluted (1 : 4) in saline to effect. Monitor the cardiac rate and rhythm for the presence of arrhythmias.

Referral hospital management: Serum-ionized calcium should be measured so calcium correction per albumin concentration can be performed, accordingly. Treatment may be repeated if needed. An electrocardiogram should be used to monitor the cardiac rhythm while calcium administration is being performed.

Conclusion/Summary: Hypocalcemia tetani in the postpartum period is exceedingly rare, and early diagnosis will lead to a fast recovery once treatment is initiated.

## Other Reproductive Emergencies

### Mare Reproductive Trauma

Reproductive trauma occurs most commonly during foaling. Trauma to the reproductive tract may be due to insufficient dilation of the reproductive tract during foaling, the foal may cause perineal body lacerations by pushing the foot into the perineal body when in a "foot-nape" posture or completely through the perineal body into the rectum causing a recto-vaginal fistula or third-degree perineal laceration, and iatrogenic trauma from obstetrical manipulation resulting in cervical or uterine tears. Even normal unassisted foaling may result in reproductive tract trauma with bruising or mild lacerations, and the severity and likelihood of trauma increase with prolonged labor or obstetrical manipulations.

Another cause of reproductive trauma is during breeding. Mares may have Caslick's or reconstructive surgery of the perineum that is not sufficiently opened and tears may occur during breeding. Some injuries result from trauma when the stallion's penis lacerates the vagina or uterine wall (Tulleners et al. 1985). The first indication of breeding injury is often the presence of blood on the penis after mating.

Mares can also suffer trauma of the reproductive tract from kicks or bites from other horses, resulting in lacerations of the vulva or vestibule.

Emergency triage plan: The general triage plan for reproductive trauma is to assess the mare's systemic state and then assess the extent of the injury. The mare should be stabilized, especially if there is a major bleed from the injury. As discussed earlier in this chapter, reproductive tract trauma may result in life-threatening blood loss, especially injuries that occur during foaling.

All mares should be carefully examined for reproductive tract trauma especially after significant obstetrical manipulations. Some veterinarians advocate for the assessment for laceration be performed without gloves or sleeves to increase the sensitivity of the examinations to changes in the surface character. Any lacerations detected should be carefully examined to determine the extent of the injury in size and depth, and if the laceration is a full-thickness uterine or vaginal tear as this will significantly affect the prognosis and treatment plan (Javsicas et al. 2010).

Perineal body lacerations, including recto-vaginal fistulas, are not typically repaired at the time of injury. As long as there is no significant amount of bleeding, the injury is usually allowed to initially heal by secondary intention to identify tissues that will slough and the tissues that will be able to hold surgical corrections. A typical timeline for surgical repair of perineal body lacerations is between four and six weeks post foaling. Prior to surgery, it is important to start the mare on a diet to soften the stool, especially if a rectal defect repair is required. Surgical repairs can be performed in one or two stages; however, these may be scheduled and are not emergencies.

Breeding injuries may occur anywhere in the mare reproductive tract including in the dorsolateral portion of the cranial vagina, in the uterine body, or in the caudal vagina. Similar to the examination of the reproductive tract at parturition for lacerations, the extent of the laceration should be determined. Visual examination of the caudal reproductive tract is often performed using a speculum, while the uterus may be inspected via endoscopy.

If there is a large full-thickness tear in the vagina or uterus, other organs may prolapse through the laceration resulting in bladder prolapse, or intestinal evisceration out of the vulva. Clearly, the prognosis is significantly poorer if intestines are prolapsed out of a reproductive tract laceration. Any prolapsed viscera in a mare should be cleaned and replaced if possible, or at least protected from injury and drying out prior to referral. Abdominocentesis is an important diagnostic step to determine the likelihood of a full-thickness tear, and the presence of frank blood in the abdomen suggests a full-thickness tear. It is prudent to perform an abdominocentesis in every mare that had a dystocia and obstetrical manipulations prior to performing uterine lavage. Further, transabdominal ultrasound examinations performed after uterine lavage may help determine if there is an increase or change in the appearance of the abdominal fluid. Peritoneal fluid evaluation is also important to diagnose peritonitis which is a common sequela to reproductive tract trauma. Partial-thickness reproductive tract lacerations may also lead to peritonitis as bacteria may translocate across the damaged vaginal or uterine wall into the peritoneal cavity.

Important decisions during management: Perhaps the most important determination of any reproductive tract trauma is if there is a full-thickness tear that communicates with the peritoneal cavity. If there is a full-thickness tear, the extent and risk of contamination needs to be considered while making a therapeutic plan. The laceration does not need to be full thickness to result in peritonitis from bacterial translocation; however, the degree of peritonitis is often much more severe if uterine content directly enters the peritoneal cavity.

In postpartum mares with full-thickness vaginal or uterine tears, the lochia is an important source of potential abdominal contamination. This is further complicated if there is simultaneous retention of fetal membranes which is not uncommon.

When trauma is associated with significant hemorrhage and retained fetal membranes, one must balance preventing further bleeding with removal of the fetal membranes. Overly aggressive reproductive manipulation may lead to further hemorrhage or contamination of the abdominal cavity, while lack of treatment to metritis systemic illness and other complications. Any uterine lavage should be performed carefully with low volumes to minimize the risk of dislodging the clots and filling the abdomen with uterine fluid. It is imperative to minimize any additives to the uterine flush fluid such as povidone iodine or other disinfectants, and the use of lubricants should be confined to small amounts of sterile lube. Appropriate fluid resuscitation is necessary to maintain organ perfusion, especially if NSAIDs are being used to control pain and inflammation.

A differential for bleeding into the abdominal cavity is bleeding into the uterine lumen. Mares with severe bleeding from a uterine laceration or following cesarean section can result in a large amount of blood pooling within the uterine lumen. The uterine lumen is large during the early postpartum period and large amounts of blood loss into the uterus can result in hemorrhagic shock. These mares may present with copious blood and blood clots discharging from the vulva of the mare. Any uterine evaluation or lavage should be performed with care with low volumes to minimize the risk of dislodging the clot.

An important decision point for reproductive trauma is the determination if the bleeding is stable and contained or poorly controlled. Hemorrhage into the abdominal cavity and uterus is most concerning as these spaces are large and horses often progress to hemorrhagic shock. However, bleeding into the retroperitoneal space is often controlled as the space is smaller and confined. Following acute hemorrhage, most horses have an increase in heart and respiratory rates, a decrease in PCV and total solids (often after 12–24 h), and increasingly dull mentation. These parameters should stabilize if the bleeding in under control. A continuously worsening clinical presentation indicates ongoing blood loss and may require whole blood transfusion or other measures.

Peritonitis may also develop following reproductive tract injury and must be managed. Both conservative medical and surgical options are possible and early interventions will increase the likelihood of a good outcome.

On-farm management: It is possible to attempt to manage reproductive tract trauma at the farm if referral is not an option. The outcome will depend on the severity of trauma and if the treatments successfully prevent side effects of the trauma such as shock, infection, pain, and organ dysfunction. The mainstays of treatment include ensuring clots are stable and no significant continuous bleeding is occurring as discussed earlier. Management of shock and cardiovascular support, broad-spectrum antibiotics and abdominal lavage to manage peritonitis, anti-inflammatory drugs and other pain control, and supporting gastrointestinal function.

Referral hospital management: Uterine and full-thickness vaginal tears can be managed with both medical and surgical management. However, surgical exploration of the abdomen and primary repair of the uterine tear is the gold standard, especially in cases with septic peritonitis. Post-surgical management including abdominal lavage, systemic broad-spectrum antibiotics, anti-inflammatory drugs, pain control, and cardiovascular support are the foundation of treating major reproductive injury of the mare. Conservative management can also be performed at a referral hospital.

Conclusion/Summary: Severe reproductive tract trauma in mares maybe life-threatening, making accurate and timely diagnosis crucial to initiate appropriate treatment and improve outcomes. While good outcomes are possible with surgical and/or conservative medical management even for relatively severe injuries, there are times where the mare's condition deteriorates, and euthanasia becomes necessary.

## Mastitis

Mastitis, a condition characterized by inflammation of the mammary gland, is relatively rare in mares. However, it can occur in certain situations, such as during the weaning process or as a result of iatrogenic factors. Iatrogenic mastitis can be caused by the introduction of pathogenic bacteria while milking mares or by nursing foals, or by trauma to the mammary gland secondary to the use of muzzles on foals. The most common pathogen associated with mastitis in mares is *Streptococcus equi* subspecies *zooepidemicus*.

Emergency triage plan: Assessing a mare's systemic condition is an important step in diagnosing mastitis. Mares with this condition may exhibit signs such as pain during nursing or milking, an enlarged and inflamed mammary gland, fever, and swelling or heat in the affected area.

In more severe cases, mares may develop endotoxemia or exhibit abnormal results on a complete blood count, such as leukocytosis or neutropenia. The milk may also contain clumps of purulent material or appear visually discolored or abnormal.

Cytological evaluation of a smear of the mammary secretions can be helpful in identifying the presence of neutrophils and intracellular bacteria. Additionally, the California Mastitis Test (CMT) may be performed to assess the severity of the inflammation and infection.

Overall, a thorough assessment of the mare's condition, including a physical exam, blood work, and milk analysis, can help diagnose and guide treatment for mastitis.

Important decisions during management: The severity of the mastitis and systemic condition of the animal should dictate if a referral is appropriate.

On-farm management: Prompt treatment of mastitis is crucial to prevent complications and minimize the spread of infection. Anti-inflammatory and broad-spectrum antimicrobial drugs should be initiated as soon as possible, while waiting for culture results from mammary secretions.

Initial treatment may involve the use of sulfadiazine/trimethoprim, but the choice of antimicrobial may need to be adjusted based on the results of culture and sensitivity testing, or if there is a poor response to treatment.

Intramammary antimicrobial infusion can also be used in conjunction with systemic antimicrobial therapy to provide direct treatment to the affected area. It's essential to follow proper administration techniques to ensure the best possible outcomes and minimize the risk of complications.

Overall, timely and appropriate treatment with a combination of anti-inflammatory and antimicrobial therapies is essential for successful management of mastitis in mares.

Referral hospital management: Stabilization of the patient and close monitoring of the serial complete blood cell count are critical in cases of severe mastitis. The intensity of treatment will depend on the systemic compromise of the animal and may require additional measures such as intravenous fluid therapy, ice boots to reduce inflammation, and endotoxic treatment in mares with signs of endotoxemia.

NSAIDs and broad-spectrum antimicrobials such as penicillin G potassium and gentamicin are commonly used to treat mastitis initially. However, it's crucial to adjust the antimicrobial therapy based on the results of culture and sensitivity testing to ensure the most effective treatment.

In addition to these measures, other supportive therapies may be necessary, such as nutritional support and pain management. Close monitoring of the mare's condition is essential to assess the response to treatment and identify any potential complications.

Overall, a comprehensive approach that includes stabilization, intensive treatment, and close monitoring, combined with appropriate antimicrobial therapy based on culture and sensitivity testing, is crucial for successful management of mastitis in mares.

Conclusion/Summary: Although mastitis is relatively uncommon, it can occur at any time, but it's most often encountered during the dry-off period. To ensure effective treatment, antimicrobial therapy should be adjusted based on the results of culture and sensitivity testing.

In some cases, acute mastitis may be iatrogenic and result from dysphagic foals wearing muzzles while housed together with mares. These foals may cause mammary gland trauma and introduce bacteria during nursing, leading to infection in their dams.

It's essential to identify and address any risk factors for mastitis, such as poor hygiene practices or inadequate milking techniques. Early detection and prompt treatment are crucial for successful management of this condition.

Overall, a proactive approach that includes preventative measures, close monitoring, and appropriate treatment based on culture and sensitivity testing is essential for the successful management of mastitis in mares.

## Emergency Conditions of the Stallion

### Scrotal Enlargement

Scrotal enlargement is a clinical sign often associated with scrotal trauma or the presence of additional tissue or fluid within the scrotum. Clinical signs are often variable and are dependent upon the underlying case of the scrotal enlargement. Various causes of scrotal enlargement include inguinal hernias, spermatic cord torsion, testicular/scrotal hematoma, orchitis, epididymitis, testicular/scrotal abscess, hydrocele/hematocele, and testicular neoplasia. Close examination of the area, using ultrasonography, in combination with careful physical examination of the horse will determine subsequent treatment. The two most painful conditions of scrotal enlargement include acquired inguinal/scrotal hernia of intestinal contents and spermatic cord/testicular torsion. These two conditions often result in the horse displaying colic signs and are both emergencies (Figure 14.4).

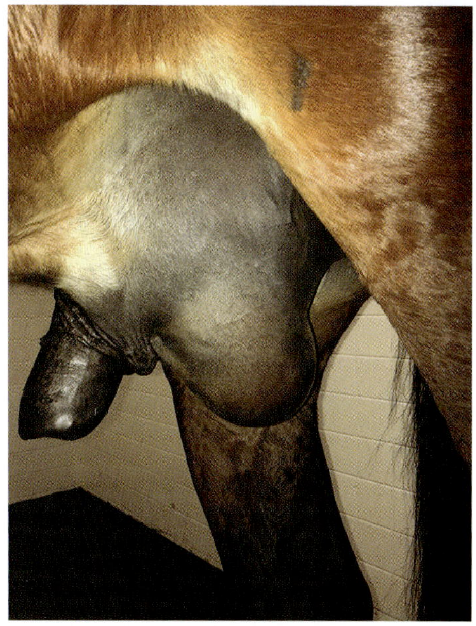

**Figure 14.4** Unilateral scrotal swelling due to an inguinal hernia. Diagnostics by palpation and ultrasonography will aid in differentiating inguinal hernia from spermatic cord torsion and other causes of scrotal enlargement. *Source:* M. Ziad Al-Ani, Robin J.M. Gray.

Emergency triage plan: The colicky horse with scrotal enlargement should have a thorough physical examination in addition to a full colic workup to rule in or out inguinal herniation. This includes careful palpation per rectum to assess the internal inguinal rings. Palpation of the scrotum, testicle, and spermatic cord can aid in the diagnosis of inguinal hernia as well as spermatic cord torsion. Scrotal ultrasonography is indicated for scrotal enlargement to assess for the presence of fluid, echogenicity of the fluids, presence of intestine, or parenchymal enlargement. In general, fine-needle aspirate is not recommended as inadvertent enterocentesis, or introduction of environmental bacteria into a sterile hematoma can occur.

Important decisions during management: Hemicastration may be considered undesirable by the client. However, this procedure should be considered a viable option to preserve fertility of the stallion in cases of a 360° spermatic cord torsion, most cases of acquired inguinal hernia, severe cases of testicular trauma, and refractory cases or orchitis and epididymitis. In these instances, inflammation within the scrotal and testicular tissue alters thermoregulation and may result in permanent damage to both the affected testicle as well as the contralateral unaffected testicle. This may result in reduced fertility or sterility of the stallion. In the case of acquired inguinal hernia, hemicastration and inguinal ring closure prevents recurrence of the hernia. In the months following hemicastration, if the unaffected testicle was normal prior to hemicastration, it will resume normal spermatogenesis following a complete cycle.

On-farm management: On the farm, careful examination to diagnose the cause of scrotal enlargement should occur as the diagnosis of inguinal hernia or testicular torsion should be managed at a referral hospital as soon as possible. Sedation and analgesia are often required to allow full examination of these painful conditions. Alpha-2 agonists and butorphanol are ideal medications for these purposes. Acepromazine should be avoided or used with extreme caution due to the anecdotal association with paraphimosis. Ultrasonographic examination of the testicle in the sedated stallion is often indicated. Orchitis and epididymitis may be managed with broad-spectrum antimicrobials and NSAIDs. Refractory cases should be referred.

Referral hospital management: Acquired inguinal hernia is a surgical emergency that is traditionally managed via a ventral midline celiotomy to relieve the herniation and assess the bowel to determine if resection of the affected bowel is indicated. At the time of surgery, depending on the extent of herniation and the damage to the parietal tunic and inguinal rings, hemicastration and inguinal ring closure is often indicated. In a select few cases, hemicastration may be avoided with subsequent closure of the rings via a follow-up laparoscopic surgery.

Spermatic cord torsion is also a surgical emergency that is corrected via hemicastration of the affected testicle. It is important to note that 180° torsion of the spermatic cord and testicle, with the tail of the epididymis oriented cranially, can be a normal variation of testicular position and does not typically affect perfusion to the testicle, nor cause discomfort to the stallion.

Conclusion/Summary: Acute scrotal enlargement is an emergent condition of the stallion and requires immediate attention to diagnose whether strangulation of the testicle or intestines has occurred. If these conditions have occurred, prompt referral to a hospital setting is indicated to minimize the risk of resection of intestines as well as maximize the stallion's long-term fertility.

## Phimosis and Paraphimosis

*Phimosis* is the inability to protrude the penis from the preputial cavity. It most often occurs secondary to trauma or disease of the tissues surrounding the penis, prepuce, and scrotum. Acute phimosis is often managed with local therapy aimed at reducing inflammation of the penis and sheath with cold hydrotherapy and NSAIDs.

*Paraphimosis* is the inability to retract the penis back into the preputial cavity and is associated with several conditions: trauma, debilitation, administration of sedation or phenothiazine tranquilizers, general anesthesia, or any condition that results in swelling of the preputial or penile tissue.

Emergency triage plan: Following examination of the penis to rule out priapism, the triage of paraphimosis is focused toward resolving edema formation, replacing the penis within the preputial cavity, and retention of the penis within the prepuce. Once replaced, administration of NSAIDs and walking the horse may encourage resolution of swelling. Focal ultrasonographic examination of the penile tissue can diagnose hematomas or fluid pockets that may require drainage prior to replacement of the penis.

Important decisions during management: Aside from trauma-related paraphimosis, the condition is often not painful. Treatment should focus on early replacement of the penis within the preputial cavity as well as treatment of the underlying condition. If the penis remains dependent or incompletely supported, swelling may persist or worsen, and penile paralysis may occur.

On-farm management: If the paraphimosis has occurred as a result of trauma, sedation is indicated for full evaluation of the injured area. An elastic compression bandage can be applied to the penis to reduce edema and facilitate replacement. Start wrapping at the glans and progress proximally up the penis, leaving the wrap in place for 20–30 minutes. Following compression, emollients may be applied to the penis (i.e., silver sulfadiazine cream) and the penis replaced. The penis may be retained within the prepuce via a purse string suture or placement of a probang (Figure 14.5). A purse string suture can be placed within the outer preputial ring using ¼-in. umbilical tape. A probang can be constructed using PVC pipe, a ball of roll cotton, and an exam glove. The penis is replaced and the probang inserted into the preputial cavity and secured against the ventral abdominal wall. The horse will be able to urinate through the purse string suture, or around the probang. Alternatively, if the penis cannot yet be replaced within the preputial cavity, a sling constructed of porous fabric, such as lace, can be fashioned to support the penis against the body wall and minimize edema. Cold water hydrotherapy may also help reduce swelling, especially if the penis cannot be maintained within the prepuce.

The penis should be evaluated every two to three days to assess swelling and function. Through this time, NSAIDs may be administered to manage inflammation, and antimicrobials are indicated if there is cellulitis or if surgical drainage was performed. Full treatment may take one to two weeks.

Referral hospital management: Horses may be managed in the hospital as was described for on the farm treatment. The advantage of hospitalization includes frequent monitoring of the patient and frequent adjusting of the methods of penile retention. This ability cannot be underscored, as appropriate retention within the prepuce is essential for successful management. Cases of refractory paraphimosis, chronic paraphimosis, or those that have resulting penile paralysis may ultimately require a partial or full phallectomy.

Conclusion/Summary: Acute paraphimosis has a good prognosis for full recovery if treated quickly and appropriately. Penile paralysis may result from direct penile trauma or secondary to ineffective support of the penis.

## Trauma of the Penis

Traumatic injuries to the penis of stallions often occur during breeding or semen collection by artificial vagina. One common breeding injury is when mares kick, resulting in acute traumatic injuries to the penis or scrotum. Abrasions from the tail hair that is introduced with the penis into the vagina during breeding or sudden movements by the mare may also cause penile injury. Similarly, improper mounting of the phantom during semen collection using an artificial vagina may cause awkward bending of the penis, leading to trauma. Insertion of the penis into an artificial vagina when the glans penis has begun belling can result in lacerations on the distal third of the penis, with blood often observed dripping from the penis after collection.

Other causes of traumatic injuries to the penis include accidents, such as jumping over fences, resulting in scrapes, abrasions, lacerations, swelling, or other injury. Trauma to the penis may lead to the formation of a hematoma, which can occur anywhere on the penis, yet often on the dorsal aspect.

Emergency triage plan: A comprehensive physical examination is crucial when assessing a horse with penile trauma. Early intervention is vital, as it can minimize the severity of the injury. To prevent excessive swelling, hydrotherapy may be utilized, while anti-inflammatory medication can be administered to manage pain and further reduce swelling.

(a) (b) (c)

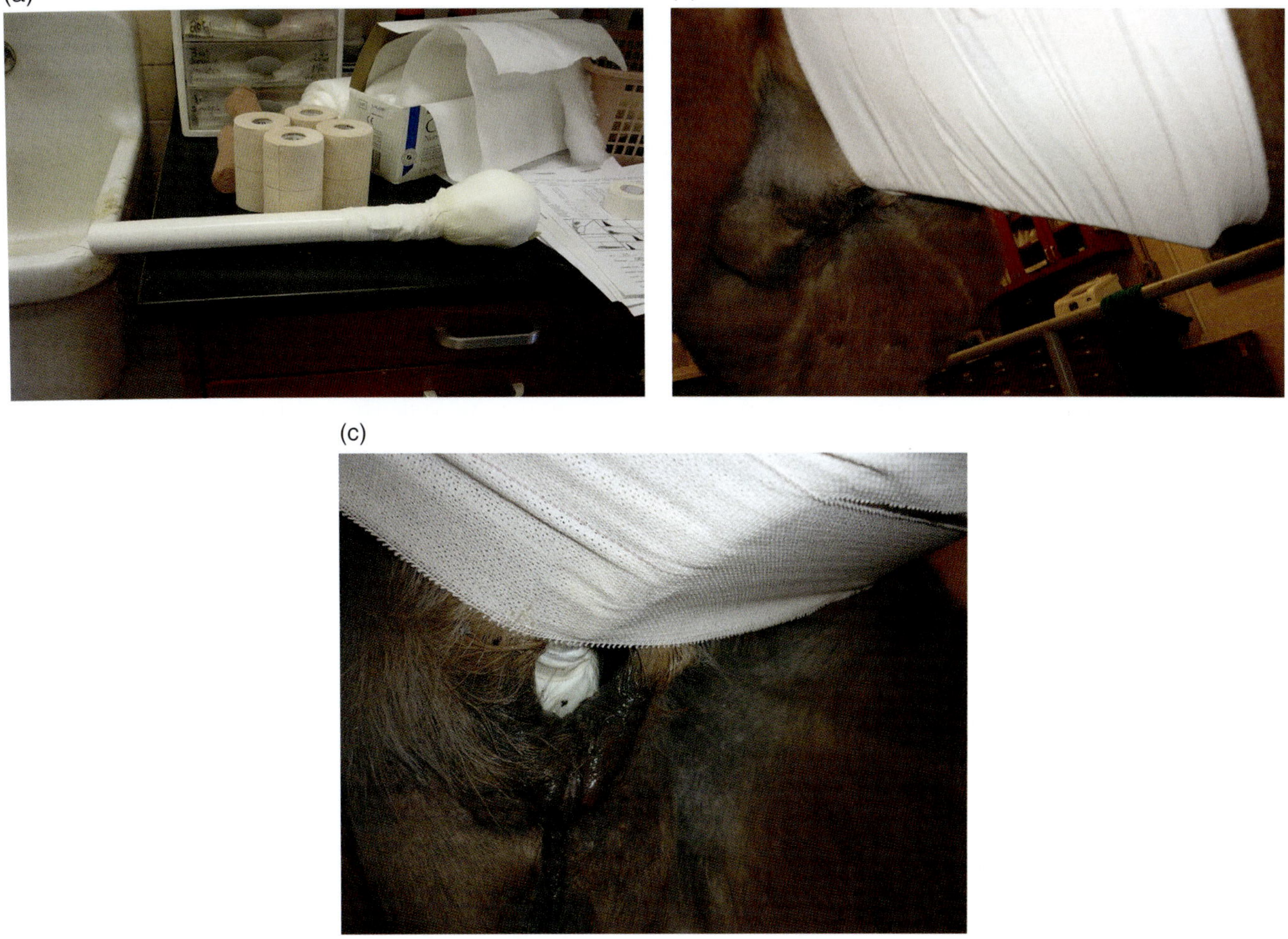

**Figure 14.5** Probang apparatus for retaining the penis in the prepuce. (a) Probang constructed from PCV pipe, roll cotton, latex gloves, secured with elastic tape. The size and construction can vary depending on the patient but commonly a 2–3-in. diameter PVC pipe that is between 35 and 80 cm long enough to be able to secure the probang in place. (b) Probang in place. The penis is cleaned and replaced into the prepuce, then the probang instrument is inserted with the cotton ball side into the prepuce to retain the penis in the prepuce. Elastic tape is used to secure the PVC end of the device in place at the ventral midline. (c) Another view of the probang in place. Note the position of the cotton ball end just within the prepuce and there is enough space between the cotton end and the preputial opening for the horse to urinate.

In cases where the penis cannot be retracted into the prepuce, wrapping it with elastic materials or tight stockinette can provide effective compression to minimize swelling. Massaging the swollen penis and prepuce and applying hyperosmotic treatments, such as sugar or glycerin, topically can also aid in reducing swelling. Other supportive treatments, such as applying petroleum jelly, lanolin, and nitrofurazone, can help prevent desiccation of the penis and minimize cracks (Figure 14.6).

Important decisions during management: Penile trauma can result in the formation of a large hematoma or paraphimosis, leading to secondary damage to the penile tissue due to pressure on the nerves. This can also cause the epithelium of the penis to dry out, resulting in cracks and lacerations that may lead to infections. If the penis cannot be retracted into the scrotum, it may be beneficial to refer the stallion for more intensive management. In cases where conservative management at the farm is unsuccessful, or the chronic injury is worsening, surgical correction may be necessary to address the problem effectively.

On-farm management: Regular cold-water hydrotherapy and NSAID treatments are viable options for managing penile injuries on the farm. However, large hematomas may prevent the penis from retracting into the prepuce, leading to potential epithelial damage and infections. In these cases, antibiotic treatments may also be required. Preventing secondary damage to the penis can be achieved by ensuring it is either retracted into the prepuce or kept in place using a

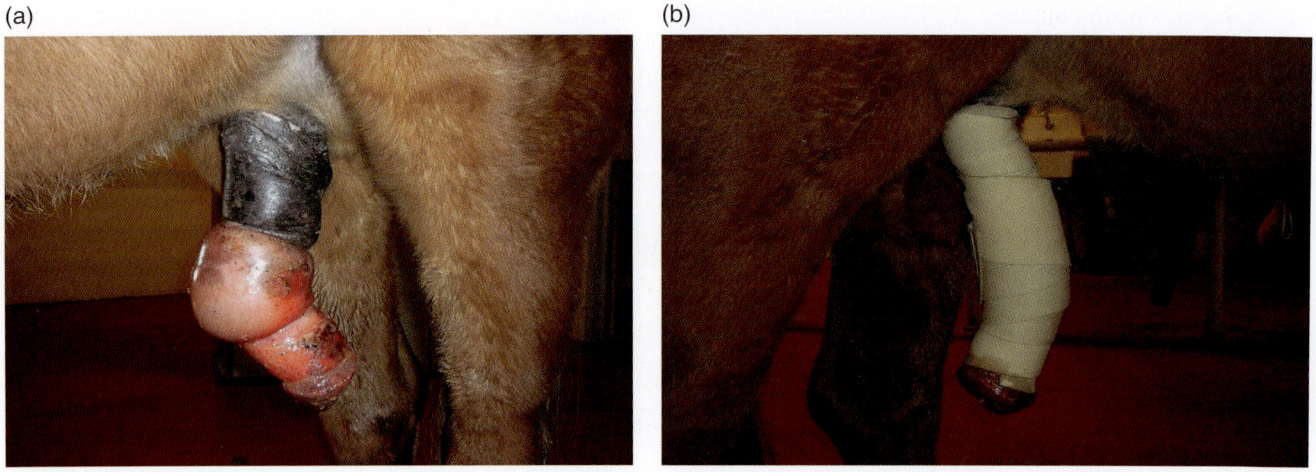

Figure 14.6 Paraphimosis (a) Chronic paraphimosis in a mature Quarter Horse gelding secondary to debilitation. It is important to differentiate paraphimosis from priapism. In the case of paraphimosis, the triage plan will be to reduce edema and replace the penis into the prepuce. (b) Compression bandage applied to a penis with paraphimosis to reduce edema. Hematoma or excessive swelling can occur anywhere; however, it is most common on the dorsal aspect of the penis. Swelling can be reduced with a combination of manual massage, application of hyperosmotic treatments such as sugar or glycerin, and compression by wrapping the penis in elastic material starting from the distal end of the penis.

probang apparatus. If the penis can be retracted, a purse-string suture can be used to prevent it from drying out and accumulating damage. The use of a probang can also facilitate the management of penile trauma.

It is important to keep the stallion away from mares and provide adequate time for recovery. Sexual rest is recommended after the initial injury, which may prove challenging for stallions with a full book of mares to breed.

Referral hospital management: The management of penile injury at a referral hospital is similar to that on the farm. Core treatments include hydrotherapy and NSAIDs, while antibiotics may be necessary if there is evidence of infection. Frequent treatments are possible, and if the condition worsens to a paraphimosis that does not respond to conservative medical treatment, surgical resection of the damaged tissue can be considered as an option.

Conclusion/Summary: Penile injuries should be treated as soon as possible to prevent accumulation of damage to the penile tissue. Hydrotherapy and NSAIDs are the main treatment with supportive care provided as necessary.

## Penile Prolapse and Priapism

Priapism, or persistent erection without sexual stimulation, requires emergency treatment for resolution of the condition without phallectomy. Even with immediate management, surgical intervention may be required. Priapism is most commonly associated with the administration of acepromazine, but it has also been associated with general anesthesia, neuropathy, trauma, debilitation, strangles, exhaustion, spinal injuries, viral infections, and severe colitis (Feary et al. 2010; Driessen et al. 2011). It occurs when arterial inflow or venous outflow are altered, resulting in persistent erection of the corpus cavernosum.

Emergency triage plan: Physical examination of the horse with manual examination of the penis reveals either full or partial erection of the corpus cavernosum. Notably, the corpus spongiosum remains flaccid. The condition can be easily visually misidentified as a dropped penis following sedation, especially in cases of partial erection. However, manual examination of the penis confirms a firm erection of the corpus cavernosum, without erection of the corpus spongiosum penis or corpus spongiosum glandis.

Important decisions during management: Though this is a rare condition, the prognosis for priapism is guarded to poor for return to breeding function, even with prompt treatment.

On-farm management: Following diagnosis, the only documented treatment to be effective in some cases is the administration of benztropine mesylate (16 mcg/kg IV slowly). This anticholinergic medication acts to decrease parasympathetic tone in order to suppress erectile activity. If improvement or resolution does not occur, the horse should be transported to a referral facility for intracorporeal treatment.

Referral hospital management: Intracorporeal treatment is the next step for managing cases of priapism. Alpha adrenergic agonists may be injected directly into the corpus cavernosum penis (CCP) to stimulate smooth muscle contraction. Should erection persist, the most aggressive therapy is to lavage the CCP with sterile heparinized saline to remove the stagnant blood and venous congestion. This procedure should be performed under general anesthesia, though standing lavage may be an option. Large-gauge (14-ga) needles are inserted proximal to the glans penis in the CCP as ingress needles, with egress needles placed in the CCP at the level of the ischium. Lavage should remove blood clots and stagnant blood until fresh arterial blood appears from the egress needles. Instillation of 10mg of 1% phenylephrine into the CCP at the end of the procedure may maintain a flaccid CCP. CCP lavage may be unsuccessful in resolving the priapism. In these refractory cases, partial phallectomy, with or without a Bolz phallopexy, is indicated.

Conclusion/Summary: Priapism is a rare condition caused by altered blood flow to the CCP. Most commonly it is associated with the use of phenothiazine tranquilizers but has been associated with numerous other conditions. It requires immediate attention to decrease the risk of impotence in breeding animals. Despite aggressive medical management, surgical intervention is often necessary.

## Post-Castration Complications

Routine castration has one of the highest complication rates of any surgical procedure, if postoperative swelling is considered. Such complications include swelling, drainage, fever, scirrhous cord, omental herniation, post-castration hemorrhage, and post-castration evisceration (Moll et al. 1995; Shoemaker et al. 2004; Kilcoyne et al. 2013). The two most emergent complications are those of severe bleeding and evisceration immediately following castration. Severe hemorrhage is typically from the testicular artery, though hemorrhage can also occur from the scrotal vessels in older males or the external pudendal artery and vein. Hemorrhage is usually not noted until the horse stands from recovery, when the blood pressure rises and blood drains from the incision. Post-castration hemorrhage should also be considered if the drops of blood from the site are too numerous to count or if there is a constant stream of blood. Alternatively, if the source of bleeding has retracted into the peritoneal cavity, external hemorrhage may not be evident. In these cases, careful examination of the quiet-to-dull gelding post-castration should occur as bleeding into the abdominal cavity may be a rare cause of the clinical signs.

Post-castration evisceration is another potentially fatal complication of castration that requires immediate surgical intervention at a referral hospital (van der Velden and Rutgers 1990; Thomas et al. 1998).

Emergency triage plan: In the event that a newly gelded horse stands up from a castration with either immediate hemorrhage or intestinal contents protruding from the surgical site, immediate referral is indicated. Post-castration hemorrhage may be successfully managed at the farm with exploration of the surgical site and appropriate ligation. However, evisceration necessitates immediate action on the farm to save the animal. Prior to referral, the owner or veterinarian should wrap the animal with a clean bed sheet around the abdomen to keep the intestine compressed against the body (Figure 14.7). Alternatively, with small amounts of herniated omentum or intestine, the tissue may be replaced into the scrotum and the castration site closed prior to referral.

Important decisions during management: Though both of these serious complications are rare, identifying whether a horse has a referral option prior to encountering such a complication will determine the next steps of triage. Two important considerations are: (i) eviscerated tissue needs support to prevent excessive tension on the mesenteric vasculature and to prevent the horse from stepping on his own intestine, and (ii) the absence of external hemorrhage does not indicate that hemorrhage is controlled as bleeding may occur into the abdomen.

On-Farm Management:

Hemorrhage: If hemorrhage is noted immediately following castration, the gelding should be re-anesthetized (or anesthetized if the castration was a standing procedure) to locate the source of hemorrhage. This typically involves examining the subcutaneous tissues and locating the spermatic cord. If the cord is the source of bleeding, placing 1–2 large-gauge transfixation ligatures around the cord (#1–2 USP absorbable suture) with or without repeat application of emasculators. The area is typically packed for the recovery. The gelding should be managed with broad-spectrum antimicrobials and restricted from exercise. If the source is not localized, the site should be packed, and the packing secured in place with large-gauge sutures. Ideally, the gelding would be then transported to a referral hospital for further surgical exploration. It is of critical importance that the source of hemorrhage be located and ligated as the spermatic cord and testicular

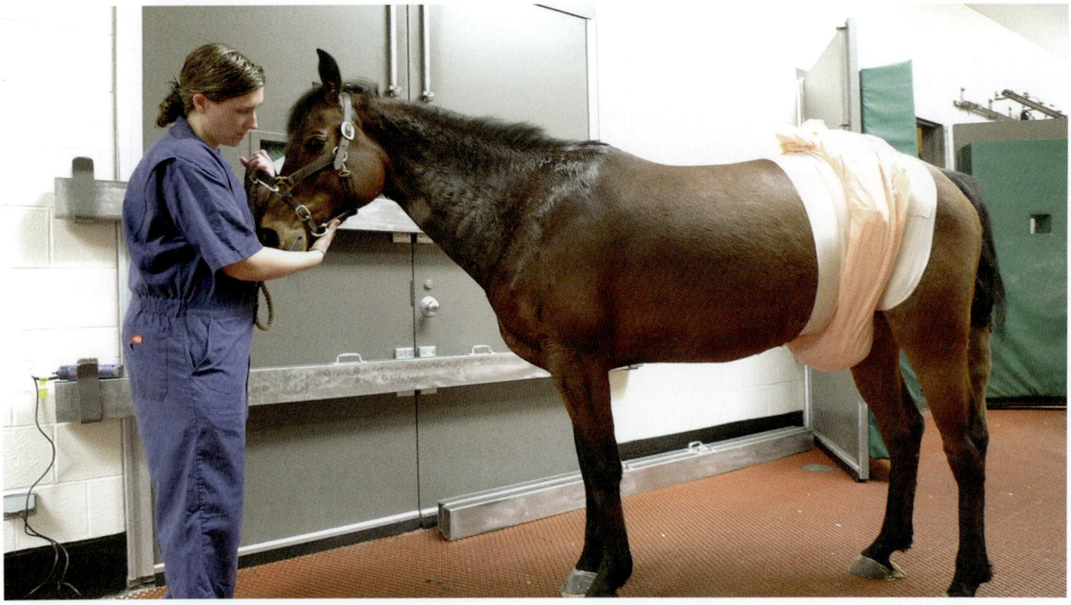

**Figure 14.7** Emergency triage on the farm for post-castration evisceration requires quick action. The veterinarian or owner should support the eviscerated intestine with a sling to prevent further damage. If possible, use a non-adherent layer such as a clean plastic sheet or garbage bag to directly cover the intestine followed by a sheet tied over the back to support the intestine up against the body. Without support, the intestine will often continue to eviscerate and fall to the ground and be stepped on by the horse.

artery can recoil into the abdomen, resulting in possibly fatal hemorrhage without any signs of further external blood loss. In some cases of moderate hemorrhage, the scrotal space may be packed successfully without referral to a hospital setting. However, close monitoring of the patient for clinical signs of continued bleeding–both external and internal–is recommended.

Evisceration: If any portion of intestine is visible at the surgical site following castration, the gelding should be referred to a hospital setting (Figure 14.8a). Though small eviscerations can be managed with intestinal lavage and replacement in a field setting, this procedure and closure of the inguinal ring is ideally performed under strict aseptic conditions. In the event of evisceration, the bowel should be supported with a sling. This would ideally be constructed with a non-adherent material such as a clean garbage bag, which can be supported with a sheet or towel tied up over the back (Figure 14.7). Alternatively, the gelding can be anesthetized for immediate transport to the referral hospital while maintained under general anesthesia. This method avoids further trauma to the eviscerated bowel.

Referral hospital management: Once the gelding arrives at the hospital, quick assessment of the systemic status should occur, paying attention to signs of cardiovascular compromise. If not already in place, an intravenous catheter should be placed, and the horse prepared for general anesthesia. Intravenous fluids may be indicated for cardiovascular support, though caution should be exerted if uncontrolled hemorrhage is present. Following induction of anesthesia, the intestine should be lavaged with sterile crystalloid fluids to remove debris and contamination (Figure 14.8b). If the horse arrives anesthetized on the trailer, he should be transported to the operating room for immediate exploratory celiotomy and inguinal ring closure. While evisceration typically occurs from a single inguinal ring, closure of both rings should be considered in these cases to prevent recurrence during the recovery period. Depending on the extent of injury and the contamination of the affected bowel, resection and anastomosis may be warranted. In the case of severe contamination, resection and anastomosis of the bowel prior to reduction of the evisceration will reduce contamination of the peritoneal cavity and the risk of subsequent septic peritonitis. Intra-abdominal lavage may be indicated following resolution of the evisceration and inguinal ring closure.

Geldings with such severe post-castration complications are at risk of postoperative complications such as surgical site infection or septic peritonitis (evisceration) and should be monitored closely for both.

Conclusion/Summary: While serious complications following castration are rare, they can be immediately life-threatening. Prompt action, including stopping hemorrhage or protecting eviscerated intestine, decreases the morbidity and mortality of these complications.

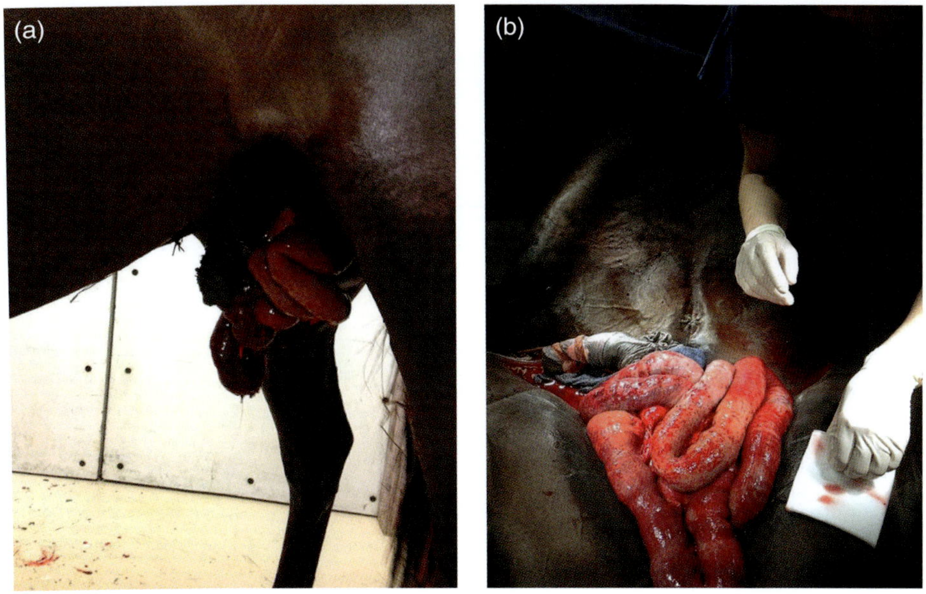


**Figure 14.8** Post-castration evisceration. (a) Evisceration following castration upon arrival to a referral hospital. Emergency triage is to lavage the eviscerated intestines, cover and keep the intestines wrapped against the body using a protective covering such as a clean plastic bag or bed sheets, and refer immediately to a referral center. (b) Evisceration post-castration after induction of anesthesia and lavage of the bowel with sterile saline. If referral is not an option, small eviscerations can be managed in the field. The eviscerated content should be lavaged, examined for damage, replaced through the inguinal canal, and closed under general anesthesia.

### Case Example 14.1 Body Wall Tear

*Patient: 10-year-old pregnant multiparous Standardbred mare at term gestation.*

*History: For the past two days worsening discomfort and inappetence. In the morning, the mare was showing signs of colic which were flank watching and stretching, did not eat which was out of character for this mare, and the mare had sudden increase in ventral edema. The mare was referred for further evaluation.*

*Emergency triage steps:*

#### Step 1 Patient Stabilization

*Provide immediate stabilization steps:*

1) *Pain management.*
2) *Provide abdominal support.*
3) *Administer fluids, other supportive care.*

*Perform a quick, yet focused patient assessment to evaluate the following:*

1) *Heart rate and perfusion status.*
2) *Determine the presence and extent of body wall tear.*
3) *Determine if there is uterine torsion or other cause of late pregnancy colic.*
   - Body wall tears can be painful and progress quickly. Applying abdominal support can delay progression of body wall tears.
   - Other causes of colic in the late pregnant mare may be confused as a body wall tear especially if the mare has ventral edema which can be normal.
   - Excessive weight of a late pregnant uterus especially in cases of twins or hydrops can exacerbate the condition and expedient relief of excessive weight by delivery of the fetus can improve prognosis for mare survival.

### Step 2 Formulating a Diagnostic Plan

Once the horse is stable and other causes of colic are ruled out, evaluate the extent of the body wall tear, and determine the fetal viability and maturity.

1) *Prepubic tendon rupture.*
2) *Herniation/evisceration.*
3) *Muscle enzymes.*
4) *Fetal biometric evaluations.*
5) *Other signs of pregnancy abnormalities.*
   - Prepubic tendon rupture is a severe body wall tear which results in the cranial displacement of the mammary glands (Figure 14.9) and often have bloody mammary secretions. Herniation into body wall tears or evisceration carries grave prognosis.
   - Muscle enzymes can be used to diagnose mild tears and be used to monitor progress but does require submission of blood to laboratories.
   - Resolution of fetal delivery is a key milestone for body wall tear case management, and there are many factors that are important considerations when deciding the best course of action. Ideally, foals should be at least 315 days in gestation before being delivered to maximize the likelihood of a viable foal, but some pregnancies may have to be terminated to save the mare. Therefore, information on fetal biometrics and other signs of abnormalities such as hydrops or placentitis can affect prognosis of a viable foal.

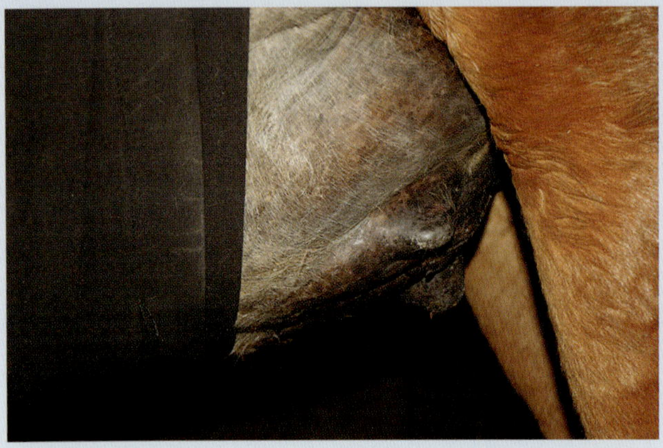

**Figure 14.9** Cranial and lateral displacement of the teats of the mammary glands indicating prepubic tendon rupture.

### Step 3 Emergency Treatment Guidelines

Following initial stabilization and diagnostic evaluation, further specific treatment is indicated.

- Pain management. Keeping the mare as comfortable as possible is key to successful case management. NSAIDs are an important component of pain management, but it is unlikely to be sufficient in more severe cases. Opioids and intravenous lidocaine can improve pain management but may be more difficult to manage in field conditions.
- Abdominal support such as belly bands (Figure 14.10) or hernia belts can delay progression of body wall tears.

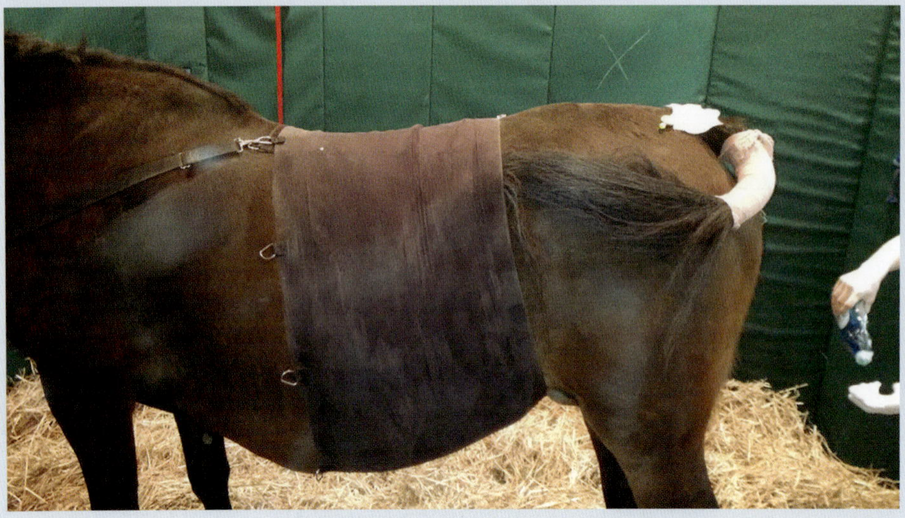

**Figure 14.10** Abdominal support can help delay progression of disease. This mare also has an epidural and is being prepared for parturition induction and assisted delivery.

- Keeping mares quiet and confined to small stalls or paddocks can limit physical activities.
- Ultimately, body wall tear cases must address the increased body weight from pregnancy that is a primary risk factor for body wall tears. Some mares may be stable enough to carry the foal for an extended amount of time to be able to obtain a viable foal, but often delivery of the fetus should be expedited to save the mare.
- Delivery of the fetus. Abdominal contractions should be minimized, and the foaling be assisted to reduce the risk of worsening the body wall tears. A foaling plan is critical to maximize the likelihood of a successful delivery. This may include induction of parturition.

### Step 4 Assessment and Monitoring

Guide clinicians through patient monitoring.

Patients should be monitored for progression of body wall tears, pain management, and fetal viability and maturity.

- Routine assessment of heart rates, respiratory rate, signs of colic, and attitude should be performed to assess pain management.
- The degree of mammary displacement or body wall tear should be monitored.
- Serial foal evaluations of fetal heartrate and maturity.

### Step 5 Decision Making During Triage

There are many factors that influence decision making in cases of body wall tears.

- Following stabilization, referral is recommended for horses that are not imminently due, have poorly controlled pain, premature foal, or other systemic conditions.
- In general, body wall tears are not amenable to surgical corrections and the goal is to salvage the foal and/or mare if possible.
- The mare should not carry future pregnancies but may be an embryo or oocyte donor for breeds that allow assisted reproductive technology
- Worsening body wall tears and uncontrolled pain have poor prognosis and may indicate terminal cesarean section if the foal is at least 315 days in gestation.
- Mares with hydrops, twins, or worsening body wall tears may need to abort the pregnancy to save the mare. Foals may be born alive and have to be euthanized if the foals are premature or have abnormalities. Some cases of severe disease early in gestation may result in loss of both the mare and foal.

## References

Abernathy-Young, K.K., LeBlanc, M.M., Embertson, R.M. et al. (2012). Survival rates of mares and foals and postoperative complications and fertility of mares after cesarean section: 95 cases (1986–2000). *J. Am. Vet. Med. Assoc.* 241 (7): 927–934. https://doi.org/10.2460/javma.241.7.927.

Arnold, C.E., Payne, M., Thompson, J.A. et al. (2008). Periparturient hemorrhage in mares: 73 cases (1998–2005). *J. Am. Vet. Med. Assoc.* 232 (9): 1345–1351. https://doi.org/10.2460/javma.232.9.1345.

Byron, C.R., Embertson, R.M., Bernard, W.V. et al. (2003). Dystocia in a referral hospital setting: approach and results. *Equine Vet. J.* 35 (1): 82–85.

Canisso, I.F., Ball, B.A., Troedsson, M.H. et al. (2013). Decreasing pH of mammary gland secretions is associated with parturition and is correlated with electrolyte concentrations in prefoaling mares. *Vet. Rec.* 173 (9): 218. https://doi.org/10.1136/vr.101658.

Carluccio, A., Contri, A., Tosi, U. et al. (2007). Survival rate and short-term fertility rate associated with the use of fetotomy for resolution of dystocia in mares: 72 cases (1991–2005). *J. Am. Vet. Med. Assoc.* 230 (10): 1502–1505. https://doi.org/10.2460/javma.230.10.1502.

Chaney, K.P., Holcombe, S.J., LeBlanc, M.M. et al. (2007). The effect of uterine torsion on mare and foal survival: a retrospective study, 1985–2005. *Equine Vet. J.* 39 (1): 33–36. https://doi.org/10.2746/042516407x159862.

Curcio, B.R., Canisso, I.F., Pazinato, F.M. et al. (2017). Estradiol cypionate aided treatment for experimentally induced ascending placentitis in mares. *Theriogenology* 102: 98–107. https://doi.org/10.1016/j.theriogenology.2017.03.010.

Dolente, B.A., Sullivan, E.K., Boston, R. et al. (2005). Mares admitted to a referral hospital for postpartum emergencies: 163 cases (1992–2002). *J. Vet. Emerg. Crit. Care* 15 (3): 193–200. https://doi.org/10.1111/j.1476-4431.2005.00136.x.

Driessen, B., Zarucco, L., Kalir, B. et al. (2011). Contemporary use of acepromazine in the anaesthetic management of male horses and ponies: a retrospective study and opinion poll. *Equine Vet. J.* 43 (1): 88–98. https://doi.org/10.1111/j.2042-3306.2010.00107.x.

Embertson, R.M. (1999). Dystocia and caesarean sections: the importance of duration and good judgement. *Equine Vet. J.* 31 (3): 179–180.

Feary, D.J., Moffett, P.D., Bruemmer, J.E. et al. (2010). Chemical ejaculation and cryopreservation of semen from a breeding stallion with paraphimosis secondary to priapism and haemorrhagic colitis. *Equine Vet. Educ.* 17 (6): 299–304. https://doi.org/10.1111/j.2042-3292.2005.tb00396.x.

Guthrie, R.G. (1982). Rolling for correction of uterine torsion in a mare. *J. Am. Vet. Med. Assoc.* 181 (1): 66–67.

Javsicas, L.H., Giguère, S., Freeman, D.E. et al. (2010). Comparison of surgical and medical treatment of 49 postpartum mares with presumptive or confirmed uterine tears. *Vet. Surg. VS* 39 (2): 254–260. https://doi.org/10.1111/j.1532-950X.2010.00645.x.

Jung, C., Hospes, R., Bostedt, H. et al. (2008). Surgical treatment of uterine torsion using a ventral midline laparotomy in 19 mares. *Aust. Vet. J.* 86 (7): 272–276. https://doi.org/10.1111/j.1751-0813.2008.00315.x.

Kilcoyne, I., Watson, J.L., Kass, P.H. et al. (2013). Incidence, management, and outcome of complications of castration in equids: 324 cases (1998–2008). *J. Am. Vet. Med. Assoc.* 242 (6): 820–825. https://doi.org/10.2460/javma.242.6.820.

Kimura, Y., Haneda, S., Aoki, T. et al. (2018). Combined thickness of the uterus and placenta and ultrasonographic examinations of uteroplacental tissues in normal pregnancy, placentitis, and abnormal parturitions in heavy draft horses. *J. Equine Sci.* 29 (1): 1–8. https://doi.org/10.1294/jes.29.1.

Korosue, K., Murase, H., Sato, F. et al. (2013). Comparison of pH and refractometry index with calcium concentrations in preparturient mammary gland secretions of mares. *J. Am. Vet. Med. Assoc.* 242 (2): 242–248. https://doi.org/10.2460/javma.242.2.242.

Mitchell, A.R.M., Delvescovo, B., Tse, M. et al. (2019). Successful management of hydrallantois in a Standardbred mare at term resulting in the birth of a live foal. *Can. Vet. J. = La Revue Veterinaire Canadienne* 60 (5): 495–501.

Moll, H.D., Pelzer, K.D., Pleasant, R.S. et al. (1995). A survey of equine castration complications. *J. Equine Vet. Sci.* 15 (12): 522–526. https://doi.org/10.1016/S0737-0806(07)80421-7.

Morris, S., Kelleman, A.A., Stawicki, R.J. et al. (2007). Transrectal ultrasonography and plasma progestin profiles identifies feto-placental compromise in mares with experimentally induced placentitis. *Theriogenology* 67 (4): 681–691. https://doi.org/10.1016/j.theriogenology.2006.05.021.

Nagel, C., Aurich, J., and Aurich, C. (2010). Determination of heart rate and heart rate variability in the equine fetus by fetomaternal electrocardiography. *Theriogenology* 73 (7): 973–983. https://doi.org/10.1016/j.theriogenology.2009.11.026.

Norton, J.L., Dallap, B.L., Johnston, J.K. et al. (2007). Retrospective study of dystocia in mares at a referral hospital. *Equine Vet. J.* 39 (1): 37–41.

Pascoe, J.R., Meagher, D.M., and Wheat, J.D. (1981). Surgical management of uterine torsion in the mare: a review of 26 cases. *J. Am. Vet. Med. Assoc.* 179 (4): 351–354.

Renaudin, C.D., Troedsson, M.H., Gillis, C.L. et al. (1997). Ultrasonographic evaluation of the equine placenta by transrectal and transabdominal approach in the normal pregnant mare. *Theriogenology* 47 (2): 559–573. https://doi.org/10.1016/s0093-691x(97)00014-9.

Ross, J., Palmer, J.E., and Wilkins, P.A. (2008). Body wall tears during late pregnancy in mares: 13 cases (1995–2006). *J. Am. Vet. Med. Assoc.* 232 (2): 257–261. https://doi.org/10.2460/javma.232.2.257.

Shoemaker, R., Bailey, J., Janzen, E. et al. (2004). Routine castration in 568 draught colts: incidence of evisceration and omental herniation. *Equine Vet. J.* 36 (4): 336–340. https://doi.org/10.2746/0425164044890625.

Spoormaker, T.J.P., Graat, E.A.M., Ter Braake, F. et al. (2016). Mare and foal survival and subsequent fertility of mares treated for uterine torsion. *Equine Vet. J.* 48 (2): 172–175.

Thomas, H.L., Zaruby, J.F., Smith, C.L. et al. (1998). Postcastration eventration in 18 horses: the prognostic indicators for long-term survival (1985–1995). *Can. Vet. J. = La Revue Veterinaire Canadienne* 39 (12): 764–768.

Troedsson, M.H. (2007). High risk pregnant mare. *Acta Vet. Scand.* 49 (S1): S9. https://doi.org/10.1186/1751-0147-49-S1-S9.

Tulleners, E.P., Richardson, D.W., and Reid, B.V. (1985). Vaginal evisceration of the small intestine in three mares. *J. Am. Vet. Med. Assoc.* 186 (4): 385–387.

van der Velden, M.A. and Rutgers, L.J. (1990). Visceral prolapse after castration in the horse: a review of 18 cases. *Equine Vet. J.* 22 (1): 9–12. https://doi.org/10.1111/j.2042-3306.1990.tb04194.x.

Wichtel, J.J., Reinertson, E.L., and Clark, T.L. (1988). Nonsurgical treatment of uterine torsion in seven mares. *J. Am. Vet. Med. Assoc.* 193 (3): 337–338.

# 15

# Neurological Emergencies of the Horse

*Sarah F. Colmer and Amy L. Johnson*

*Department of Clinical Studies - New Bolton Center, University of Pennsylvania School of Veterinary Medicine, Kennett Square, PA, USA*

## Acute Ataxia

Ataxia (incoordination) manifests in abnormal movement of any combination of the affected animal's head, neck, trunk, or limbs. Deficits may arise from pathology in the brain, spinal cord, or both. There are three classifications of ataxia in the horse, including general proprioceptive (GP) or "spinal" ataxia, special proprioceptive or "vestibular" ataxia, and cerebellar ataxia. These clinical signs and categorizations are visible in Table 15.1 for reference.

Identifying neurologic deficits is best done in a methodical fashion so as not to overlook various aspects of the central and peripheral nervous systems. Signs of ataxia are often most noticeable during gait evaluation with changes of speed or direction. **The authors recommend the following order of examination operations when performing a neurologic evaluation** (also summarized in Box 15.1):

- **Step 1: Mentation and behavior assessment**
  - Assess for appropriate mentation (awareness, responsiveness) vs obtundation to stupor.
    - Obtundation and stupor may be attributable to forebrain or brainstem disease.
    - Horses with substantial behavioral abnormalities (head pressing, compulsive walking) likely have forebrain disease.
- **Step 2: Physical examination**
  - May be particularly important in cases of trauma, recumbency, etc.
  - If horse is severely ataxic, take care to clear area of unnecessary persons and pets.
  - Perform examination in safe space (open area, soft footing).
  - Check for fever – increases suspicion for infectious etiology (i.e., viral encephalitis) which may indicate need for personal protective equipment and biosecurity protocols.
- **Step 3: Cranial nerve examination**
  - Descriptions of cranial nerves and associated tests to assess function are listed below in Table 15.2.
  - Deficits most typically indicate abnormalities in the brainstem or peripheral damage to the nerves.
- **Step 4: Gait evaluation**
  - **NOTE:** various aspects of the gait evaluation may need to be modified based on the severity or characteristics of the clinical signs being displayed.
  - Walk in straight line.
  - Trot in straight line – identify obvious lameness that may contribute to gait abnormalities.
  - Walk in serpentines.
  - Walk with head elevated in straight line.
  - Walk while pulling the tail in either direction.
  - Walk in tight circles to the left and right.
  - Walk up and down a hill.
  - Walk up and down a hill with head elevated.
  - Walk backward.

*Emergency Triage of the Horse*, First Edition. Edited by Rolfe M. Radcliffe and Jamie J. Kopper.

Published 2026 by John Wiley & Sons, Inc.
Companion website: www.wiley.com/go/radcliffe/triage

**Table 15.1** Clinical signs associated with the three forms of ataxia in the horse.

| General proprioceptive (spinal) ataxia | Special proprioceptive (vestibular) ataxia | Cerebellar ataxia |
|---|---|---|
| Delayed protraction | Leaning, drifting, falling to one side | Spasticity in movement |
| Excessive limb abduction | Head tilt with asymmetric ataxia | Tremor (may worsen with intention) |
| Excessive limb adduction | Wide-based stance | Loss of balance |
| Hoof wall scuffing | Nystagmus | Loss of coordinated menace response |
| Knuckling onto dorsal aspect of hoof | Circling | Wide head and neck excursion |
| Overreaching/floating aspect to stride | | |

**Box 15.1 Steps to performing a neurological assessment**

- Physical examination.
- Assessment of mentation.
- Cranial nerve examination.
- Gait evaluation.
- Neurolocalize general proprioceptive/spinal ataxia (or other type of ataxia).

**Table 15.2** Cranial nerve examination.

| Nerve | Function | Test | Lesions cause |
|---|---|---|---|
| 1) Olfactory | Smell | Not assessed | N/A |
| 2) Optic | Vision | Pupillary light reflex (PLR), dazzle reflex, menace response | Blindness (lack of menace), lack of PLR and dazzle |
| 3) Oculomotor | Pupillary constriction, extraocular muscles | PLR, eye position, palpebral fissure size | Lack of PLR (and presence of mydriasis), ptosis, lateral and ventral strabismus |
| 4) Trochlear | Extraocular muscle (dorsal oblique) | Eye position | Dorsomedial strabismus |
| 5) Trigeminal | Sensory to head and face, motor to muscles of mastication | Palpebral and more diffuse facial sensation, mandibular excursion | Lack of palpebral reflex and response to facial stimulation, masseter and temporalis atrophy, decreased jaw tone, dropped or deviated jaw |
| 6) Abducent | Extraocular muscles (retractor bulbi and lateral rectus) | Normal globe retraction, lateral globe movement | Medial strabismus, absence of globe retraction during corneal reflex |
| 7) Facial | Facial expression muscles, salivary and lacrimal gland parasympathetic function | Facial symmetry (ears, eyelids, muzzle) | Loss of palpebral reflex and blink, ptosis, ear droop, muzzle deviation (nose pull to normal side), lip droop, dry eye |
| 8) Vestibulocochlear | Hearing, posture, balance | Head and eye position, physiologic nystagmus, response to sound | Abnormal balance/posture/leaning, head tilt, pathologic nystagmus, loss of physiologic nystagmus, deafness |
| 9) Glossopharyngeal | Pharynx | Swallow | Dysphagia, dorsal displacement of the soft palate |
| 10) Vagus | Pharynx and larynx | Swallow, laryngeal movement | Dysphagia, dorsal displacement of the soft palate, laryngeal paralysis |
| 11) Spinal accessory | Cervical muscles, esophagus, larynx | Normal cervical musculature | Cervical muscle atrophy |
| 12) Hypoglossal | Tongue | Tongue tone, strength, symmetry | Tongue muscle atrophy, poor tongue tone, dysphagia |

**Table 15.3** Neurolocalization of spinal ataxia.

| C1-C5 | C6-T2 | T3-L3 | L4-S2 |
|---|---|---|---|
| All four limbs affected | Thoracic limbs often more affected than pelvic limbs | Pelvic limbs affected | Pelvic limbs affected |
| Longer stride length (UMN) in all four limbs | Shorter stride length (LMN) in forelimbs, longer stride (UMN) pelvic limbs | Normal stride length forelimbs, longer stride (UMN) pelvic limbs | Normal stride length forelimbs, shorter stride (LMN) pelvic limbs |
| Inconsistent limb placement all four limbs | Inconsistent limb placement in all four limbs; front limbs might buckle and appear weak | Inconsistent limb placement (UMN) pelvic limbs | Pelvic limbs often placed cranially under body with tendency to buckle or crouch |
| Increased tone and reflexes (UMN) in all four limbs | Thoracic limb tone and reflexes decreased (LMN); pelvic limb tone and reflexes increased (UMN) | Thoracic limbs normal; pelvic limb tone and reflexes increased (UMN) | Pelvic limb tone and reflexes decreased (LMN) |
| Horse might be recumbent with difficulty lifting head and neck | Horse might be recumbent; able to lift head and neck | Horse might "dog sit" | Horse might "dog sit" |

- **Step 5: Neurolocalize general proprioceptive/spinal ataxia:** See Table 15.3
  - **Upper motor neuron signs:** Paresis characterized by a long stride, spasticity, postural deficits, and increased tone
  - **Lower motor neuron signs:** Paresis characterized by a shorter stride, weakness, trembling, muscle atrophy (over time), and decreased tone
- **COMMON CAUSES OF ACUTE ATAXIA**: a non-exhaustive list, summarized in Box 15.2
  - **Equine protozoal myeloencephalitis (EPM)**
    - EPM is caused by coccidia species *Sarcocystis neurona* or *Neospora hughesi*. Horses are the dead-end host for *S. neurona*, infected from consuming contaminated water or feed sources containing opossum feces. **Importantly, most horses exposed to the pathogen do not develop clinical disease.** Clinical signs can be acute or chronic and involve any combination of brain, brainstem or spinal cord-associated deficits, and therefore EPM can mimic most neurologic conditions. Affected animals most commonly exhibit gradual progression of signs but can also experience sudden exacerbations.
    - **History**: EPM can be more common on some farms due to environmental factors; if the farm has a history of high numbers of affected horses over time, this may make EPM more likely. However, outbreaks of EPM typically do not occur, and remember that the horse itself does not spread the disease.
    - **Evaluation**: Mentation can be affected. Ataxia ± cranial nerve signs ± muscle atrophy; can be asymmetric, but does not have to be. Horses with EPM can have a variety of cranial nerve deficits, not limited to dysphagia, facial nerve paralysis, and head tilt. Ataxia can be so severe that horses become recumbent.
    - **Diagnostic techniques**
      1) *Immunodiagnostic testing:* Negative *S. neurona* and *N. hughesi* serology (Either IFAT – UC Davis, or SnSAG 2/4/3 ELISA – Equine Diagnostic Solutions) = high negative predictive value unless signs are very acute and horse has not had time to seroconvert. The positive predictive value of *S. neurona* serology is low, i.e., a "false positive" result is common without testing concurrently alongside cerebrospinal fluid (CSF).

**Box 15.2 Common causes of acute ataxia**

- Equine protozoal myeloencephalitis (EPM).
- Cervical vertebral stenotic myelopathy (CVSM, "Wobblers").
- Sidewinder Syndrome.
- Temporohyoid osteoarthropathy (THO).
- Equine Herpes Myeloencephalopathy (EHM).

NOTE: proof of intrathecal antibody production, established by documenting high levels in the CSF compared with systemic circulation, is best performed with CSF and serum paired titer ratio or specific antibody index (SnSAG 2/4/3 ELISA or IFAT).

- **Treatment options**
  - *Antiprotozoal medications:*
    1) Ponazuril (paste): Dose by weight; loading dose = 3× body weight (BW) day 1, then 1× BW dose daily for at least 28 days.
    2) Sulfadiazine and pyrimethamine (liquid): 20 mg/kg/1 mg/kg PO Q24h for 90 days.
       NOTE: Do NOT administer this medication to pregnant mares: risk of blood dyscrasias and fetal malformation
    3) Diclazuril (pellet): 1 mg/kg PO Q24h for at least 28 days.
  - *Anti-inflammatories:*
    1) Decrease inflammation associated with infection and parasite die-off, first 3–5 days of treatment.
       Flunixin meglumine: 1.1 mg/kg Q12-24 h.
       Dexamethasone: 0.1–0.2 mg/kg Q24h, tapered quickly over 3–5 days (caution if previous history of laminitis or endocrinopathy).
  - *Supportive medications:*
    Vitamin E: antioxidant: 2000–5000 IU/day PO; testing serum vitamin E concentrations is recommended to guide supplementation (normal range = 2–10 ppm).
    Ophthalmic medications: as needed for horses with facial nerve paralysis/recumbent patients.
- **Prognosis**: Fair for horses diagnosed early in disease; worsens with recumbency. Horses that respond in the first few weeks of treatment have more favorable outcomes. Residual deficits are possible if improvement plateaus.
- **What can be done at the farm**
  *Diagnosis*: EPM serology (limited predictive value), CSF and serum paired immunodiagnostics if practitioner comfortable to perform CSF centesis.
  *Treatment*: antiprotozoals, anti-inflammatories, supportive medications.
- **What can be done at the referral hospital**
  ***Diagnosis*: CSF collection and exclusion of other potential differential diagnoses.**
  *Management*: Enteral or parenteral nutrition and intravenous fluid therapy if horse is unable to consume/swallow feedstuffs/water; slinging if needed.
- **When to refer**: If desire for more definitive diagnosis with CSF centesis if practitioner unable to perform on farm; if horse is recumbent, experiencing seizures, or dysphagic to the point of requiring supplemental nutrition and hydration.

– **Cervical vertebral stenotic myelopathy (CVSM or "Wobbler")**
- CVSM results in spinal cord compression associated with narrowing of the vertebral canal, most often due to congenital or developmental bony malformation or osteoarthritis.
- **Signalment and history**: Young male racehorses are overrepresented, as well as older performance horses. History of recent trauma may make acute ataxia attributable to CVSM more likely. Horses may have a history of rapid growth.
- **Evaluation**: Mentation is generally appropriate and no cranial nerve abnormalities are observed. Ataxia is typically symmetric and present in all four limbs. Horses may exhibit limited neck range of motion and may be sensitive to cervical palpation.
- **Diagnostic techniques**
  *Survey radiographs*: Inter- or intra-vertebral minimum sagittal diameter ratios of <50%, malarticulation, and enlargement/irregularity of articular process joints increase suspicion.
  *Myelography*: Performed using iohexol in subarachnoid space administered under general anesthesia; use to demonstrate compression if >50% of dorsal contrast column is attenuated with corresponding reduction in ventral contrast column.
  *Computed tomography*: best performed after myelography to identify dorsolateral/lateral compression.
- **Treatment options**
  1) *Paced diet and exercise restriction*: If diagnosed <1 year of age, may decrease disease progression; repeat radiographs recommended every 6–12 months to assess for improvement in relative size of vertebral canal.
  2) *Anti-inflammatories* may improve signs if acute onset associated with trauma: dexamethasone: 0.1–0.2 mg/kg IV Q24h, phenylbutazone: 2–4 mg/kg Q12h, flunixin meglumine: 1.1 mg/kg Q12h.

3) *Surgery*: Arthrodesis or, in certain cases, foraminotomy; can variably improve clinical signs in appropriate surgical candidates.
   Targeted intraarticular or perineural steroid injections using ultrasound guidance – can improve clinical signs transiently but do not address underlying compression or instability.
- **Prognosis**: Variable depending on degree of ataxia, age, number of affected sites or comorbidities. Does not typically improve without intervention.
- **What can be done at the farm:**
  - *Diagnostics*: survey radiographs to increase suspicion.
  - *Treatment*: systemic anti-inflammatories, paced diet and exercise restriction, targeted injections using ultrasound guidance.
- **What can be done at a referral center**
  - *Diagnostics*: more conclusive survey radiographs (better able to visualize caudal cervical region); myelography ± computed tomography.
  - *Treatment*: surgical arthrodesis or foraminotomy, targeted injections using ultrasound guidance.
- **When to refer**: If horse is recumbent, if cervical radiographs cannot be obtained caudally due to horse size/generator power, if advanced imaging (myelography and/or CT) is desired, if surgical arthrodesis or foraminotomy is being considered.

– **"Sidewinder syndrome"**
- **Signalment and history**: These horses exhibit an acute, abnormal three-track "crab walking" gait and are often older. Association with both neurologic and musculoskeletal conditions such as EPM, coxofemoral osteoarthritis, and thoracolumbar osteoarthritis has been reported.
- **Evaluation**: The gait abnormality is often typified by the pelvic limbs drifting or tracking consistently to one side, with the horse walking on three tracks (e.g., LH, LF/RH, RF). More severely affected horses might circle or spin in place, with the pelvic limbs leading and the thoracic limbs moving in place. Paresis and proprioceptive deficits may be observed with neurologic etiologies.
- **Diagnostic techniques**
  - Can be a diagnostic challenge; an etiology may not be determined.
  - *CSF analysis*: The syndrome has been associated with an EPM diagnosis (see "EPM," pages 329–330).
  - *Imaging*: ultrasound, radiographs, and/or nuclear scintigraphy to look for coxofemoral disease or other thoracolumbar or pelvic pathology.
- **Treatment options**
  - *Anti-inflammatories*: Phenylbutazone (2–4 mg/kg Q12h) or flunixin meglumine (1.1 mg/kg Q12h); ultrasound-guided intraarticular injections of coxofemoral joints if indicated based on imaging.
  - *Anti-protozoal medication*: If EPM positive (see "EPM", pages 329–330).
- **Prognosis**: Largely poor prognosis. Treatment of EPM positive horses may improve signs. Spontaneous resolution or improvement is possible, but signs might recur. Complete, permanent resolution is unlikely.
- **What can be done at the farm**
  - *Diagnostics*: Serology, ultrasound of coxofemoral joints.
  - *Treatment*: Anti-inflammatories, anti-protozoal medications, ultrasound-guided thoracolumbar or coxofemoral injections.
- **What can be done at referral center**
  - **Diagnostics**: Advanced diagnostics including nuclear scintigraphy, CSF centesis, ultrasonography of coxofemoral joints and thoracolumbar region.
  - *Management*: sling assistance.
- **When to refer**: if sling assistance required, horse is a danger to handlers, advanced diagnostic testing desired.

– **Temporohyoid osteoarthropathy ("THO")**
- THO is associated with enlargement/sclerosis/fracture of the stylohyoid bone, tympanic bulla and/or petrous temporal bone. It most frequently causes facial nerve paralysis or vestibular signs/ataxia.
- **Signalment and history**: Horses are often older, though any age can be affected. Signs are typically acute.
- **Evaluation**: Affected horses may exhibit difficult prehension or odynophagia during cranial nerve evaluation. Facial nerve paresis/paralysis (ear/eyelid droop, poor eyelid tone, ptosis, muzzle deviation, lip droop) and vestibulocochlear deficits (head tilt, nystagmus, vestibular ataxia, deafness) may be observed. Corneal ulcers are common.
- **Diagnostic techniques**

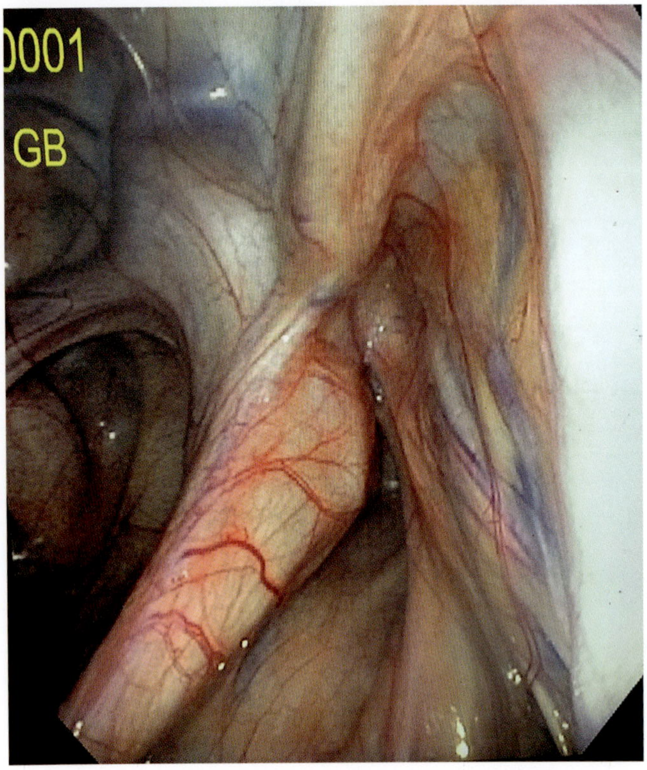


**Figure 15.1** Endoscopy revealing abnormal enlargement of temporohyoid articulation. *Source:* Courtesy of Dr. Kathryn Timko, DVM, DACVIM-LAIM.

  - *Endoscopy*: of guttural pouch to identify asymmetric enlargement of temporohyoid articulation (Figure 15.1).
  - *Computed tomography*: More sensitive; may also reveal ceratohyoid enlargement, petrous temporal bone, and stylohyoid fractures.
- **Treatment options**
  - *Therapeutic*: stall rest, anti-inflammatories (flunixin meglumine: 1.1 mg/kg Q12h), broad-spectrum antimicrobials for possible infectious component (trimethoprim sulfamethoxazole: 30 mg/kg PO Q12h).
  - *Surgical*: Ceratohyoidectomy, basihyoid-ceratohyoid disarticulation.
  - *Management*: temporary or permanent tarsorrhaphy if CN 7 deficits, appropriate ophthalmic treatment (triple antibiotic ointment, lubricant).
- **Prognosis**: Medical and surgical treatment can both result in partial or complete recovery; however, horses are always at risk for acute worsening without surgical intervention. Relapse is more likely with temporal bone fracture. Treatment is recommended for several weeks until signs improve.
- **What can be done at the farm**
  - *Diagnostics*: endoscopy.
  - *Medical treatment*: as described above.
  - *Management*: tarsorrhaphy.
- **What can be done at referral center**
  - *Diagnostics*: computed tomography (CT).
  - *Surgical treatment*: ceratohyoidectomy, basihyoid-ceratohyoid disarticulation.
- **When to refer**: If surgery is desired; if CT is desired; if ataxia is severe enough to require sling support.

– **Equine herpesvirus type 1 myeloencephalopathy (EHM)**
- EHM manifests secondary to vascular endothelial thrombosis of the spinal cord and, less commonly, the brain, and is incredibly infectious and contagious to other equids via spread of respiratory droplets.
- **History and signalment**: many horses have a history of fever, though it can be missed. Other horses on the farm with abortion, respiratory and/or neurologic signs should increase index of suspicion. Some horses become clinical after stress (transport, competition, etc.). The rapid progression of signs increases suspicion of EHM.

- **Examination**: Acute, typically symmetric ataxia that can rapidly progress to full recumbency; pelvic limbs often worse than thoracic limbs. May dog sit ±dribble urine. May exhibit decreased tail and anal tone. Some horses also exhibit cranial nerve signs and obtundation.
- **Diagnostic techniques**
  - *PCR*: nasopharyngeal swabs + whole blood (5× 3 mL EDTA tubes); ideal diagnostic.
  - *CSF analysis*: CSF may appear xanthochromic (yellow) and exhibit high total protein with normal cell count.
  - **NOTE: If EHM is suspected and/or diagnosed, it is a reportable disease in most states. The state veterinarian should be contacted immediately.**
- **Treatment options**
  - *Supportive care*: See *management*.
  - *Anti-inflammatories*: If horse is severely affected/recumbent, consider non-steroidal anti-inflammatories (flunixin meglumine: 1.1 mg/kg Q12h, phenylbutazone: 2–4 mg/kg Q12h) or steroids (dexamethasone: 0.1 – 0.2 mg/kg IV Q24h).
    - **NOTE:** NSAIDs may lower pro-inflammatory state and decrease platelet activation (Pusterla et al. 2022).
  - *Anticoagulant*: low-molecular-weight heparin: 80 U/kg Q24h. May prevent thrombotic sequelae (Stokol et al. 2018).
  - *Antivirals*: Of unknown efficacy, but might be helpful. Valacyclovir: 30 mg/kg PO Q8-12h; can be administered to affected horses or those that came into contact/at risk of exposure in outbreak scenario.
  - *Antimicrobials*: If concern for cystitis in wake of bladder catheterization; broad-spectrum: trimethoprim sulfamethoxazole (30 mg/kg PO Q12h).
- **Management**
  - *Bladder catheterization*: If bladder distension evident ultrasonographically and horse not urinating, may need to perform 3–4X daily.
  - *Nutritional/hydrational support*: May require grain slurry/powdered nutrition slurry (i.e., Purina WellGel, etc.).
    - Nasogastric intubation (can be left indwelling if needed and in appropriate monitoring situation).
    - Low-bulk diets ideal in cases of fecal incontinence.
  - Intravenous fluid therapy with electrolyte/dextrose supplementation.
  - *Recumbency change*
    - Should perform minimum of 2X/day; may require sling support.
  - **NOTE**: If outbreak occurs, quarantine farm for 21–28 days after last case per state veterinarian recommendations, using PPE and isolating infected cases. Monitoring non-affected horses twice daily for fever may enable detection of disease prior to clinical signs. Test all horses in contact with infected horses
- **Prognosis**: variable. Rapid progression and recumbency are associated with poorer outcomes. Full recovery is possible in some cases.
- **What can be done at the farm**
  - *Diagnosis*: nasal swabs and blood PCR.
  - *Treatment*: supportive care, antiviral therapy.
  - *Biosecurity*: Personal protective equipment (PPE) to limit spread both on and off the farm.
- **What can be done at referral center**
  - *Diagnosis*: CSF analysis.
  - *Management*: slinging, intensive nursing care, intravenous nutrition/hydration support.
  - *Biosecurity*: isolation.
- **When to refer**: if clinical signs are rapidly progressive, if EHM is suspected, if biosecurity is not possible on the farm.

**NOTE:** Contact state veterinarian prior to transport, particularly if crossing state lines.

## Encephalitis

- **Viral encephalitides (Rabies, WNV, EEE, WEE).**
  - Acute ataxia accompanied by **fever** ± behavior change increases suspicion for viral encephalitides. **Importantly, fevers can often be missed/not be present with these diseases, and as such, their absence does not rule out viral encephalitis.** See Table 15.4 for signalment and history, evaluation and diagnostics, treatment, and prognosis.

**Table 15.4** Common viral encephalitides.

| Disease | Signalment and history | Evaluation | Diagnostics | Treatment | Prognosis |
|---|---|---|---|---|---|
| Rabies | • Often have history of "colic" signs or lameness<br>• Highly unlikely if vaccinated<br>• Can present with evidence of self-mutilation or with history of pruritis | • Extremely variable signs<br>• **Use PPE if suspected**<br>• **Reportable disease** | • No antemortem confirmatory diagnostics<br>• Submit head (remove with handsaw) to state lab in bag; refrigerate if necessary.<br>• Carefully disinfect equipment used that has come into contact with any fluids | • None | • Uniformly fatal |
| West Nile virus - WNV | • Ask for vaccine history, though duration of protection is unclear. May require multiple annual vaccinations in endemic areas<br>• Seasonal (mosquito vector) | • Acute ataxia, often worse in hind limbs<br>• Fasciculations of muzzle, tongue, head and neck possible<br>• Signs of encephalitis possible (abnormal mentation, cranial nerve signs) | • CSF analysis<br>– ± xanthochromia<br>– ± increased NCC (mononuclear pleocytosis)<br>• Serum or CSF IgM Capture ELISA<br>• PCR / IHC on brain tissue | • Anti-inflammatories<br>– Dexamethasone (0.1–0.2 mg/kg Q24h)<br>– Flunixin meglumine (1.1 mg/kg Q12h)<br>– Phenylbutazone (2–4 mg/kg Q12h)<br>• Hyperimmune plasma – not documented to change outcome or severity of disease<br>• Supportive care | • Variable<br>• Recumbency and rapid progression = poorer prognosis |
| Eastern equine encephalitis - EEE | • Ask for vaccine history.<br>• Cases usually sporadic<br>• Seasonal (mosquito vector) | • Transient fever often missed<br>• obtundation, blindness, head pressing and bruxism | • Serum or CSF IgM ELISA<br>• PCR/IHC on brain tissue | • Anti-inflammatories<br>– Dexamethasone (0.1–0.2 mg/kg Q24h)<br>• Supportive care | • High mortality (up to 100%)<br>• Recumbency = poorer prognosis |
| Western equine encephalitis - WEE | • Ask for vaccine history.<br>• Cases usually sporadic<br>• Seasonal (mosquito vector) | • Transient fever often missed<br>• obtundation, blindness, head pressing and bruxism | • Serum or CSF IgM ELISA<br>• PCR/IHC on brain tissue | • Anti-inflammatories<br>– Dexamethasone (0.1–0.2 mg/kg Q24h)<br>• Supportive care | • Variable; 20–50% mortality |

- **What can be done at the farm**
  - *Therapeutics*: anti-inflammatories.
  - *Biosecurity*: PPE.
  - *Diagnostics*: CSF analysis, serology, nasal swabs.
- **What can be done in a referral hospital**
  - *Management*: sling support, intravenous nutrition/hydration support.
  - *Biosecurity*: isolation.
- **When to refer:** Viral encephalitis should be referred when the horse is recumbent, if sling assistance is needed, if appropriate biosecurity cannot be maintained on the farm, and if neurologic signs are rapidly progressive.

## Bacterial Meningitis

### Introduction

Bacterial meningitis is generally uncommon in horses and is most often reported in septic foals that have a history of failure of the transfer of passive immunity (FTPI) and may also be bacteremic on blood culture. Adult horses exhibit meningitis less frequently, with etiologies suspected most often associated with hematogenous infection, infection secondary to skull fracture, or associated with infection of nearby tissues (sinuses, periorbital tissues, lymph nodes, guttural pouch) (Smith et al. 2004). *Borrelia burgdorferi*, the causative agent of Lyme neuroborreliosis, can also cause bacterial meningitis in adult equids (Divers et al. 2018). If no clear source of meningitis is identified in the adult horse, immunodeficiency syndromes (such as common variable immunodeficiency, or CVID) may be suspected.

- **Signalment and history**
  - Most common in foals; inquire if history of FTPI, blood culture status.
  - Less common in adults; ask if history of infection or fracture of the skull (sinusitis, ocular tissues, lymph nodes, guttural pouch, otitis) or history of chronic, recurrent infections that might suggest CVID.
- **Evaluation**: The most common clinical signs associated with meningitis are fever, neck stiffness/soreness, lethargy, anorexia, and general weakness. Some horses will exhibit preferentially low head carriage. Meningitis can be secondary to brain abscesses/can also spread or be secondary to encephalitis – assess for intracranial signs.
- **Diagnostic techniques**
  - *CSF analysis*: Most commonly exhibit a neutrophilic pleocytosis (>5 cells/μL) ± intracellular bacteria ± elevated total protein (>90 mg/dL). CSF fluid PCR assay for *Streptococcus equi* may be helpful. Paired CSF and serum Lyme multiplex assay for antibody levels against *Borrelia* outer surface proteins (OSP), as well as Borrelia PCR can be used to identify Lyme neuroborreliosis. CSF culture and sensitivity is recommended, though is often negative.
    - **NOTE: Risk of cerebral herniation secondary to high intracranial pressure in the face of CSF centesis has been documented in humans and may occur in some equids with meningitis/encephalitis.**
  - *Clinicopathology*: Blood culture and sensitivity relevant/likely to be positive in foals, and may more likely be positive than CSF culture. CBC most commonly exhibits a mature neutrophilia ± left shift. Biochemical profile may exhibit hyperglobulinemia. Fibrinogen and SAA are often elevated.
    - **NOTE: Hypoglobulinemia and/or lymphopenia in a horse with meningitis increases suspicion for immunodeficiency**
- **Therapeutic options**
  - *Broad-spectrum antimicrobials*: Start empirical antimicrobials immediately. Choose based on CNS penetration: fluoroquinolones, tetracyclines (minocycline > doxycycline), some cephalosporins, potentiated sulfonamides, rifampin, chloramphenicol, among others (Dowling 1999; Sinner and Tunkel 2004)
    - Ceftiofur should be used at high dose (4–6 mg/kg Q12h) in order to achieve CSF penetration, but alternative cephalosporins like ceftriaxone (25–50 mg/kg IV or IM Q12h) or ceftazidime (20–50 mg/kd IV Q6-Q12h) may be better options.
    - Can adjust antimicrobial protocol later based on results of culture and sensitivity.
    - **NOTE: Enrofloxacin should be avoided in foals due to concerns for cartilage damage.**
    - **NOTE: In areas where Borrelia is endemic, suitable antimicrobial coverage should be considered (cephalosporins, penicillin, tetracyclines).**
  - *Anti-inflammatories and analgesia*
    - Flunixin meglumine (1 mg/kg Q12h) OR phenylbutazone (2–4 mg/kg Q12h).
    - Dexamethasone (0.1–0.2 mg/kg IV Q24h).
    - *For additional pain management*: pregabalin (4 mg/kg PO Q8-12h), gapabentin (up to 30 mg/kg PO Q8h) or acetaminophen (20 mg/kg PO Q12h).
  - *Management*
    - Hyperosmolar crystalloids may reduce cerebral edema if concerned that encephalitis is present: Mannitol (0.5–1 g/kg IV as 20% mixture) OR hypertonic saline (2–4 mL/kg IV bolus, then crystalloid).
    - *Supportive supplementation*: Vitamin E (2,000–5,000 IU/day PO), Coenzyme Q10 (1,000 mg/day PO).
- **Prognosis:** Fair-to-poor for bacterial meningitis, with survival rates in adult horses ranging from 0% to 60% (Mitchell et al. 2006; Smith et al. 2004). Survival and full recovery is possible with early initiation of appropriate antimicrobial therapy. The survival rate in foals is low (Sanchez et al. 2008; Viu et al. 2012). The presence of comorbidities and/or nature of inciting infectious event may affect prognosis.

- **What can be done at the farm**
  - *Diagnostics*: clinicopathology.
  - *Treatment*: antimicrobials, anti-inflammatories.
- **What can be done at referral center**
  - *Diagnostics*: CSF analysis.
  - *Treatment*: intravenous antimicrobials.
  - *Management*: continuous intravenous fluids, parenteral nutrition.
- **When to refer**
  - If patient is a foal, if patient is recumbent, if patient requires continuous intravenous nutrition/hydration support.

## Trembling in Horses

Neurologic and neuromuscular causes of trembling in horses are varied, and non-neurologic disease like pain or shock can also be considered depending on history and case details. Below is a non-exhaustive description of common neurologic and neuromuscular causes of equine trembling (summarized in Box 15.3).

- **BOTULISM**
  - *Clostridium botulinum* is a Gram-positive, spore-forming organism that produces toxin leading to flaccid paralysis. It occurs with varying geographic commonality, and in endemic areas, type B toxoid vaccination is recommended and protective against type B (three doses at four week intervals, then annually; pregnant mares should also receive a booster 2–4 weeks prior to foaling). Horses with botulism almost always acquire the disease in one of three ways: ingestion of preformed toxin with feedstuffs ("food-borne" botulism in adults), ingestion of spores that germinate in the gastrointestinal tract and subsequently release toxin ("toxicoinfectious" botulism in foals), or through the contamination of wounds yielding bacterial growth and toxin release ("wound" botulism) (Whitlock and McAdams 2006).
    - **Signalment and history:** identify vaccination status, particularly if in endemic area (Mid-Atlantic United States most common region). Many owners may report "colic"-like signs (i.e., inappetence, lethargy, recumbency, trembling).
      - Foals: toxicoinfectious etiology most common.
      - Adults: ingestion of preformed toxin in feedstuffs most common.
    - **Evaluation:** Many horses exhibit weakness in limbs that may globally progress. Trembling and fasciculations often start in the triceps but can progress. May have decreased tail and anal tone. May begin as increased frequency of recumbency progressing to an inability to rise.
      - *Cranial nerve abnormalities*: dysphagia is most common; may also see decreased eyelid and tongue tone, ptosis, and mydriasis.
      - **HOW TO: "Grain test": Observe ability to consume one cup grain in under two minutes;** many horses with botulism are incapable.
    - **NOTE: Minimize stress and stimulation which can worsen signs**
      - Keep management area dark and quiet.
      - Maintain in stall/confined space.
      - Minimize the horse's activity.
    - **Diagnostic techniques**
      - Typically diagnosed based on clinical signs, vaccination history, and endemic geography.
      - Diagnosis can be achieved in some cases by PCR or culture of feces, feed, gastrointestinal or wound content, or soil under hay feeders. Mouse bioassay (MBA) can confirm presence of toxin but samples often require culture enrichment prior to MBA and access to assay may be limited.

**Box 15.3 Common causes of trembling horses**

- Botulism.
- Tetanus.
- Equine Motor Neuron Disease.

- **Therapeutic options**
  - *Anti-toxin*: Administer intravenous botulism antitoxin as soon as possible (1 unit/500 mL/500 kg horse).
  - **HOW TO**: administer slowly using transfusion filtration set. Start at one drop/second and slowly increase with q5-minute TPR to ensure no transfusion reaction until open flow rate.
  - Sources of botulism antitoxin include local veterinary teaching hospitals or can be obtained from Lake Immunogenics (NY; type A/B/C antitoxin) or Plasvacc (CA; type B antitoxin).
  - **NOTE:** antitoxin only binds circulating toxin, not that which has already bound at motor end plate; signs may progress after antitoxin administration in some horses.
  - **NOTE: antibodies are not cross-protective against types. If type A botulism is suspected, ensure antitoxin contains antibodies against type A.**
- *Antimicrobials*: important if aspiration pneumonia has developed. Consider broad-spectrum options: trimethoprim sulfamethoxazole (30 mg/kg PO Q12h). May need to be administered via nasogastric tube if dysphagic.
  - **NOTE**: Avoid aminoglycosides, procaine penicillin, tetracyclines which can potentiate neuromuscular weakness.
    - **Management**
- *Nutritional/hydrational support*: Usually require grain slurry/alfalfa meal/powdered nutrition slurry (i.e., Purina WellGel, etc.). Parenteral nutrition may be needed if horse does not tolerate enteral feeding (difficult to intubate or develops ileus and reflux).
    - Nasogastric intubation (can be left indwelling if needed and in appropriate monitoring situation).
  - Intravenous fluid therapy with electrolyte/dextrose supplementation
- *Minimize aspiration risk*: If dysphagic, remove feedstuffs and water to prevent aspiration pneumonia. Muzzle if necessary. Hungry horses may even attempt to swallow bedding looking for feedstuffs.
- *Recumbency change:*
  - Should perform minimum of 2×/day; may need sling to accomplish depending on size.
  - **NOTE:** Remember to minimize stress during this process as much as possible. **Slings can be used to assist weak horses to stand but then should be removed so that the horse can choose to lie down when tired. Horses should not be forced to remain standing in slings.**
- *Wound debridement:*
  - As needed if wound botulism suspected.
- *Mechanical ventilation:*
  - Typically only pursued in foals.
    - **Prognosis:** A retrospective study of adult horses treated for botulism at a referral center showed an overall survival rate of 48% (Johnson et al. 2015). Horses that maintained the ability to rise without assistance were substantially more likely to survive. Survival rates in foals are higher than in adult horses. A retrospective study of 30 foals treated for botulism at a referral center had an overall 96% survival rate among treated foals (Wilkins and Palmer 2003).
    - **What can be done on the farm**
- *Treatment*: antitoxin, antimicrobials
- *Management*: nasogastric intubation of nutrition/hydration support, wound debridement
  - **What can be done at referral center**
    - *Management*: Frequent enteral feedings, intravenous partial or total parenteral nutrition, sling support, surgical wound debridement (if wound botulism present), mechanical ventilation, down horse care.
  - **When to refer:** if antitoxin administration not feasible on the farm or if a horse or foal requires repeated or continuous parenteral nutrition, is recumbent, is in respiratory distress and may require mechanical ventilation or requires round-the-clock nursing/supportive care, sling assistance.
- **TETANUS**
  - *Clostridium tetani* is an anerobic bacterium that releases exotoxin resulting in tetany. It is typically associated with a wound, though in many cases the inciting wound may not be identified on physical examination. Vaccination is recommended and protective (2-dose series of toxoid with a 4- to 6-week interval between doses, then annually). Progression of signs to recumbency or dyspnea is associated with a grave prognosis.
    - **Signalment and history:** identify vaccination status and wound history (including recent surgical procedures).
    - **Evaluation: t**rembling/fasciculations, general stiffness, a "sawhorse" stance, third eyelid protrusion, trismus (inability to open the jaw), recumbency and rigidity, difficulty with prehension/swallowing, raised tailhead.
    - **Diagnostic techniques**
      - Typically diagnosed based on clinical signs and vaccination history.
      - Culture of wounds (may be difficult to achieve in most circumstances).

- **Therapeutic options**
  - *Antitoxin*: (100–200 U/kg IV or IM once).
  - *Antimicrobials*: Potassium penicillin – 22,000–44,000 IU/kg IV Qh6 ± metronidazole 15 mg/kg PO Q8h.
  - *Muscle relaxants/sedation:*
    - Acepromazine: 0.02–0.05 mg/kg IM or IV Q6h.
    - Other drugs to consider: trazodone, diazepam, midazolam, phenobarbital, gabapentin, pregabalin.
- **Management**
  - *Nutritional/hydrational support*: May require grain slurry/powdered nutrition slurry (i.e., Purina WellGel, etc.). Parenteral nutrition may be needed if completely dysphagic
    - Nasogastric intubation (can be left indwelling if needed and in appropriate monitoring situation).
    - Intravenous fluid therapy with electrolyte/dextrose supplementation.
  - *Recumbency change*
    - Should perform minimum of 2×/day; may need sling to accomplish depending on size.
    - **NOTE:** Remember to minimize stress during this process as much as possible.
  - *Wound debridement*
    - As needed.
- **Prognosis:** Recumbency and/or dyspnea severely worsen prognosis. Mortality is reported in up to 80% of cases. Horses that maintain the ability to stand have improved prognosis. Improvement may take weeks.

– **What can be done on the farm**
- *Treatment*: antitoxin, antimicrobials.
- *Management*: nasogastric intubation of nutrition/hydration support, wound debridement.

– **What can be done at referral center**
- *Treatment*: intravenous antimicrobials.
- *Management*: frequent enteral feedings, intravenous partial or total parenteral nutrition, sling support, surgical wound debridement (if wound present), mechanical ventilation.

– **When to refer:** if a horse or foal requires continuous parenteral nutrition, is recumbent, is in respiratory distress and may require tracheostomy or mechanical ventilation, or requires round-the-clock nursing/supportive care, sling assistance.

- EQUINE MOTOR NEURON DISEASE

– **Signalment and history:** Often diagnosed in horses with limited or poor-quality pasture and/or with chronically low serum vitamin E concentration (normal range = 2–10 ppm). May have history of profound recent weight loss and/or muscle atrophy.

– **Examination:** Generalized symmetrical weakness, trembling/fasciculations, increased recumbency, symmetric muscle atrophy, poor body condition. May exhibit pigment retinopathy (brown lipofuscin deposits that also can be seen with other vitamin E-associated disorders like eNAD/EDM).

– **Diagnostic techniques**
- ***Serum vitamin E concentration*: collect blood using no-additive (red-top) tube, protect from light.**
- *Muscle biopsy*: sacrocaudalis dorsalis medialis (SCDM) (tailhead).
- **How to**: Sedate with detomidine/butorphanol. Clip and prepare site aseptically. Collect from base of tailhead (careful not to take muscle from too far cranial or abaxial – incision should be 1 cm abaxial to midline). Block subcutaneous tissue with lidocaine. A single small (~4–5 cm) skin/subcutaneous incision should be made, dissecting the fascia to expose the muscle. Two parallel ~2–3 cm vertical incisions in the muscle are then made, connected at the top or bottom, undermined from attachments and then removed with final incision at top or bottom to release muscle. Allow to sit in room air for five minutes then place in formalin and submit for evaluation.

– **Therapeutic options**
- *High-dose vitamin E supplementation*: (5,000–10,000 IU daily); Recheck serum levels in one month; adjust supplementation to maintain >4 ppm.
- *Co-enzyme Q10*: added antioxidant support; 1,000 IU/day.

– **Prognosis:** Unfortunately in many cases by the time of diagnosis, return to function is unlikely, however with vitamin E supplementation, horses can stabilize.

– **What can be done at farm and referral center:** vitamin E, SCDM muscle biopsy.

– **When to refer:** If muscle biopsy is not obtainable on the farm.

# Traumatic Brain Injury

## Introduction

Traumatic brain injury (TBI) can have immediate and delayed-onset consequences as damage to neural tissues is perpetuated by secondary swelling. Mechanisms of damage may include fractures of the calvarium (i.e., frontal/parietal fractures if point of impact (POI) was the dorsal aspect of the skull OR basilar fractures from the poll being the POI (Figure 15.2), intracranial hemorrhage and cerebral edema).

### History

- **Signalment and history**
  - Common histories: kicks from other horses, collisions with objects/buildings/fences, and falls over obstacles or into ditches/flipping over backward.
  - Obtain details about event if witnessed, including time since event.
- **Evaluation**
  - Head trauma: epistaxis, aural bleeding; carefully palpate cranium for any evidence of fracture.
  - Assess respiratory function: laryngeal dysfunction can occur secondary to brain injury. Head swelling/edema can restrict airflow and necessitate tracheostomy. Brainstem damage can also yield abnormal respiratory patterns.
  - Ophthalmologic evaluation: **Fixed, dilated pupil (mydriasis) = poor prognostic indicator** and can be suggestive of midbrain dysfunction or optic nerve damage secondary to basilar skull fractures.
    - Perform fundic exam: retinal detachment possible following head trauma; pallor of optic disc may become apparent after multiple weeks.
  - Perform a neurologic evaluation.
    - General mentation/demeanor.
    - Cranial nerve evaluation.
    - Examine for head tilt.
    - Observe for ataxia.
  - Observe for CSF leakage: Can be associated with fractures to frontal bone, sinuses, ethmoids, cribriform plate (Nout-Lomas 2022).
  - Evaluate for other trauma: lacerations, hematomas, fractures.
  - Recumbency
    - Paresis or paralysis as well as recumbency are poor prognostic indicators.
- **Diagnostic techniques**
  - *Skull radiographs*: look for fracture, fluid lines (blood in sinuses).
  - *CSF centesis*: may be useful to rule out alternative neurologic diagnoses.

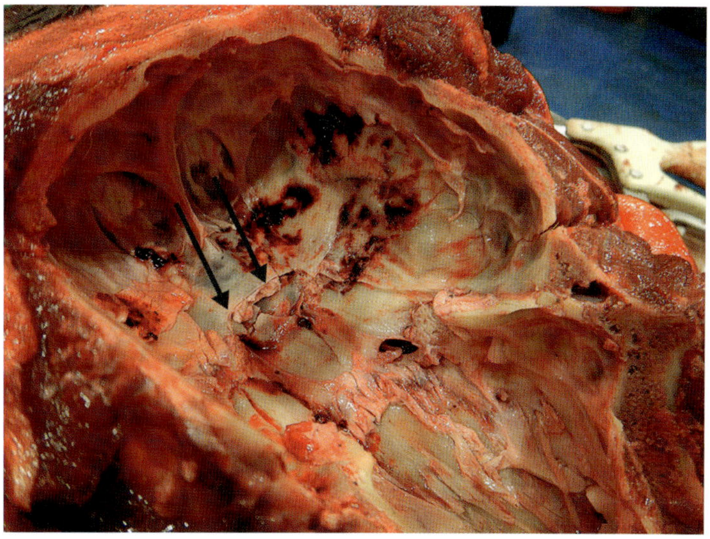

Figure 15.2 Ventral calvarium with brain and pituitary removed from horse with basilar skull fracture. Arrows illustrating severed optic nerve at optic chiasm as consequence of comminuted fractures.

 - *Guttural pouch endoscopy*: may see bleeding associated with rectus capitus rupture and basioccipital bone fracture.
 - *Repeat neurologic evaluation*: *essential* for prognostication, particularly with regard to vision.
- **Therapeutic options**
 - *Establish airway*: intubation, ventilation, supplemental oxygen, tracheostomy if necessary.
 - *Maintain circulating blood volume and red blood cell (RBC) mass if hemorrhage occurred*: intravenous fluids and blood transfusion as necessary.
 - *Seizure control*: diazepam (0.1–0.5 mg/kg IV) for adult, 5–20 mg IV for foal; midazolam (0.04–0.2 mg/kg IV), phenobarbital (5 mg/kg IV bolus, repeated if necessary to control seizures up to 20 mg/kg in first 12–24 h, levetiracetam 32 mg/kg IV or PO q12h).
 - *Address shock*: hypotension is associated with poor outcomes. Goal = maintain mean arterial pressure > 80–90 mmHg with IV fluids and pressors.
 - *Reduce cerebral edema*: with hyperosmolar crystalloids; mannitol (0.5–1 g/kg IV as 20% mixture), hypertonic saline (2–4 mL/kg IV bolus, then crystalloid).
   - **NOTE: Administering cold fluids can be helpful in maintaining hypothermia which is recommended in head trauma cases.**
   - **NOTE: Avoid glucose administration; can increase lactic acid production.**
 - *Sedation*: Avoid xylazine if possible which may increase intracranial pressure (ICP)
 - *Anti-inflammatories*: Flunixin meglumine (1.1 mg/kg Q12h), phenylbutazone (2–4 mg/kg Q12h), Dexamethasone (0.1–0.2 mg/kg IV Q12h first 24h, then Q24h).
 - *Pain management*: Pregabalin (4 mg/kg PO Q8-12h), gapabentin (5–30 mg/kg PO Q8-12h), acetaminophen (20 mg/kg PO Q12h).
 - *Antimicrobials*: broad-spectrum; use if fractures/bleeding/hematoma suspected: trimethoprim sulfamethoxazole (30 mg/kg PO Q12h), minocycline (4 mg/kg PO Q12h).
 - *Fracture repair*.
- **Management**
 - *Supplementation*: vitamin E (5,000 IU/day PO), magnesium sulfate (15–30 mg/kg/h IV).
 - *Head elevation*: cross-tie head, elevate feed buckets/hay racks.
 - *Maintain hypothermia:* may use bags of ice/cold IVF.
 - *Ophthalmic care*: if corneal ulceration from trauma/CN VII deficit, maintain with appropriate medications (triple antibiotic ophthalmic ointment Q6h).
 - *Oxygen therapy*: Flow-by if needed acutely; hyperbaric oxygen therapy for longer-term.
- **Prognosis:** Associated with severity of the initial insult; worsens with progression of signs (i.e., vision loss or recumbency). Maintaining the ability to stand and see and retaining appropriate mentation are positive prognostic indictors. Importantly, blindness due to basilar skull fractures is often immediate and permanent.
- **What can be done at farm –**
 - *Diagnostics*: skull radiographs, guttural pouch endoscopy.
 - *Treatment*: **i**mmediate stabilization, anticonvulsant therapy, fluid resuscitation, anti-inflammatories, antimicrobials.
- **What can be done at referral center –**
 - *Diagnostics*: skull radiographs with high-power generator, skull CT, CSF centesis.
 - *Treatment*: blood transfusion, advanced imaging, surgical fracture repair.
 - *Maintenance*: continuous intravenous fluid therapy/nutrition, oxygenation, parenteral antimicrobial administration, sling support.
- **When to refer:** Horses with traumatic brain injury should be referred immediately if there is an option. Rapid therapeutic intervention has been associated with more favorable outcomes. Referral should also be considered if advanced imaging is desired and if fractures are suspected that may benefit from surgical correction.

## Spinal Cord Injury

Spinal cord injury (SCI) most often occurs with various equestrian sports including racing and jumping, or collision with fixed objects. Cervical spinal injuries are considered the most common SCI in horses (Feige et al. 2000; Tyler et al. 1993), though lumbar fractures are most common in racehorses. Foals can exhibit vertebral pathologic fractures associated with osteomyelitis (Stewart et al. 2007). SCI can occur in the absence of fracture with subluxation or contusion. Recovery of the spinal cord and amelioration of clinical signs can be rapid when a fracture is not present.

- **Signalment and history:** Obtain details about event if witnessed, including time since event and duration, character, and progression of ataxia.
- **Evaluation**
  - Carefully palpate neck/back for pain, heat, swelling, crepitus.
  - Assess respiratory function- phrenic nerve damage C4-C7: may affect respiration.
  - Perform a neurologic evaluation.
    - Assess mentation.
    - Ability to stand/recumbency.
      - If standing, evaluate posture and gait; if ataxic, neurolocalize.
      - If recumbent, evaluate ability to maintain sternal position; if not, increases concern for upper cervical pathology.
      - Assess cutaneous trunci reflex with hemostat, pen, etc.; identify if region where reflex not present; may aid in specifically localizing site of pathology.
      - Assess for sensation of pain with hemostat (i.e., in distal limbs). **NOTE: absence of nociception is associated with poor prognosis.**
      - Observe for Horner syndrome: Trauma or pathology in T1-T3 region; characterized by sweating of face/neck/trunk, miosis, ptosis, and third eyelid protrusion ipsilateral to lesion.
  - Evaluate for additional potential trauma: lacerations, hematomas, fractures, head trauma.
- **Diagnostic techniques**
  - *Survey vertebral radiographs*: Often limited in field, particularly caudal cervical region. Investigate for evidence of fracture, subluxation.
  - *Myelography*: Often limited to cervical region unless equid is small.
  - *CT/MRI*: Size of gantry may limit anatomic region imageable.
  - *CSF centesis*: If intrathecal hemorrhage and not iatrogenic, may be associated with vertebral fracture and poor prognosis; neutrophilia may be present if osteomyelitis (i.e., foals with *Rhodococcus equi*).
- **Therapeutic options**
  - *Maintain circulating blood volume and red blood cell mass*: control hemorrhage, intravenous fluids, blood transfusion as necessary.
  - *Establish airway*: intubation, ventilation, supplemental oxygen, tracheostomy, if necessary.
  - *Address shock*: Hypotension is associated with poor outcomes. Goal = maintain mean arterial pressure > 80–90 mmHg with IV fluids and pressors.
  - *Anti-inflammatories*: Flunixin meglumine (1.1 mg/kg Q12h), phenylbutazone (2–4 mg/kg Q12h), dexamethasone (0.1–0.2 mg/kg IV Q24h)
  - *Pain management*: pregabalin (4 mg/kg PO Q8-12h), gabapentin (5–30 mg/kg PO Q8-12h), acetaminophen (20 mg/kg PO Q12h).
  - *Antimicrobials*: broad-spectrum; use if open fractures/wounds: trimethoprim sulfamethoxazole (30 mg/kg PO Q12h), minocycline (4 mg/kg PO q12h).
  - *Fracture repair.*
- **Management**
  - *Manually evacuate bladder/rectum if needed*: Bladder catheterization (serial or indwelling).
  - *Nutritional and hydrational support as needed.*
  - *Slinging/changing of recumbency*: If not in face of displaced vertebral fractures/subluxations.
  - *Surgical decompression*: **NOTE: Undergoing general anesthesia is a risk for horses with respiratory compromise or displaced fractures which can worsen in induction or recovery.**
  - *Ophthalmic care*: if corneal ulceration from trauma/CN VII deficit, maintain with appropriate medications (triple antibiotic ointment Q6h).
  - *Supplementation*: Vitamin E (5,000 IU/day PO), magnesium sulfate (15–30 mg/kg/h IV).
- **Prognosis: NOTE: Horses that improve rapidly following onset of acute SCI have fair-to-good prognosis. Partial or full improvement can take weeks to months depending on the severity and nature of the lesion. Paralysis and/or recumbency significantly negatively impact prognosis. Absence of pain response is a poor prognostic indicator.**
- **What can be done at the farm**

  - *Diagnostics*: cervical vertebral column radiographs, CSF centesis.
  - *Treatment*: immediate stabilization, fluid resuscitation, anti-inflammatories, antimicrobials
- **What can be done at referral center**
  - *Diagnostics*: advanced imaging (spinal radiographs with in-hospital high-power generator, myelography, CT).
  - *Treatment*: blood transfusion, pain management, surgical fracture repair.
  - *Maintenance*: continuous intravenous fluid therapy/nutrition, oxygenation, parenteral antimicrobial administration, sling support.
- **When to refer:** Horses should be referred if recumbent. Referral should also be considered if advanced imaging is desired and if fractures are suspected that may benefit from surgical correction.

## Seizures

- Seizures always originate in the forebrain of the affected horse and can occur secondary to trauma, metabolic derangement, infectious, iatrogenic, neoplastic or toxic causes, and in some cases can be idiopathic in origin (Table 15.5). Seizures are often characterized by sudden tonic–clonic activity of muscle.
  - **Signalment and history**
    - Identify chronicity, severity, and any comorbidities which may aid in identifying seizure etiology. Ask if medication administration precipitated seizure.
    - In some cases, the horse may have exhibited abnormal mentation (restlessness, distraction, dullness) prior to the seizure (known as the prodromal phase or "pre-ictal") as well as similar abnormality after the seizure (postictal phase). Loss of menace response and ataxia are common post-ictal findings.
  - **Examination**
    - Categorize seizure episode if possible.
      - Focal vs generalized
      - Focal: localized signs such as isolated facial or limb twitching.
      - Generalized: diffuse signs over the whole body.
      - Status epilepticus: sustained seizure activity lasting longer than five minutes.
    - IF horse is safe to handle, a comprehensive physical examination should be performed; potential for self-induced trauma, particularly if generalized seizures.
- **Diagnostic techniques**
  - *CSF analysis*: cytological evaluation, paired CSF and serum titers for EPM and Lyme.
  - *Clinicopathology*: Hematology, biochemical profile (including electrolytes, liver values), ammonia (if available), serology (EPM, Lyme, viral encephalitides): paired with CSF if applicable; samples for toxicology evaluation (i.e., heavy metal testing, etc., if available).
  - *Imaging*: Skull radiographs and/or CT, MRI.
- **Therapeutic options**
  - *Anti-convulsant therapy*: Table 15.6 repeat dosing may be necessary.
  - *Sedation:* if needed; xylazine and detomidine may increase intracranial pressure, while acepromazine may decrease seizure threshold in the horse.
- **Management**
  - *Establish intravenous access*: particularly important if repeat seizure episodes.
  - *Create safe environment*: place head bumper if horse having repeated episodes with recumbency/thrashing/head pressing; maintain in padded stall if needed. Remove water buckets, feed tubs. Minimize number of people in stall/space with horse during and immediately after seizure.
  - *Anti-convulsant therapy* if multiple seizure episodes are identified; Table 15.6.
  - *Anti-inflammatories:*
    - Flunixin meglumine: 1.1 mg/kg Q12h.
    - Dexamethasone: 0.1–0.2 mg/kg Q24h.
    - *Antiprotozoal medications* (if EPM suspected) – see "*EPM*" section, pages 329–330 for details.
- **Prognosis:** Variable based on etiology. If etiology is extracranial and treatable, prognosis is more favorable. In many cases, a definitive source of seizures is not reached. As seizure activity increases in severity, duration, or number of episodes, prognosis likely worsens.

**Table 15.5** A non-exhaustive list of differential causes for seizures in horses.

| Category of disease | Causes |
|---|---|
| Developmental | • Dandy-walker-like syndrome<br>• Hydrocephalus |
| Iatrogenic | • Adverse drug reaction<br>– Enrofloxacin<br>– Intravenous doxycycline<br>– Dewormers<br>– Associated with iohexol administration (myelogram)<br>• Air embolus<br>– Catheter-associated<br>– Injection<br>• Intracarotid injection |
| Idiopathic | • Open |
| Infectious | • Abscess<br>• Encephalitis<br>• Meningitis<br>• Parasitic |
| Metabolic | • Hepatoencephalopathy<br>• Hyperammonemia<br>• Various electrolyte derangements<br>– Hypocalcemia<br>– Hypoglycemia<br>– Hypomagnesemia<br>– Hyponatremia<br>– Hypernatremia |
| Neoplastic | • Primary intracranial neoplasm<br>• Secondary intracranial neoplasm |
| Traumatic | • Bleeding<br>• Edema<br>• Fracture<br>• Ischemia/hypoxia |
| Toxic | • Arsenic<br>• Lead<br>• Organophosphate<br>• Strychnine<br>• Various molds |

- **What can be done at the farm**
  - *Diagnostics*: clinicopathologic investigation, skull radiographs, ± CSF centesis, video monitoring.
  - *Treatment*: anticonvulsants, anti-inflammatories.
  - *Management*: head bumper, padded area, heavily bedded stall.
- **What can be done at referral center**
  - *Diagnostics*: CSF centesis, video monitoring, CT, MRI, electroencephalography (EEG).
  - *Management*: Intravenous CRI, sling support.
- **When to refer – Refer ONLY after the horse is not actively seizing, given the propensity for the horse to harm itself on a trailer *en route* to a referral center and the potential risk to people accompanying the horse.** Refer if repeated seizure episodes that necessitate multiple administrations of anti-convulsant, if horse is dangerous to itself and handlers, if episodes become longer in duration/increased in frequency/severity, if horse is recumbent and therefore requires changes of recumbency/hoisting, evidence of obvious head trauma detected or owner interested in pursuing advanced imaging/diagnostics.

**Table 15.6** Anti-convulsant therapy in the horse.

| **Emergency anti-convulsant therapy** | | | |
|---|---|---|---|
| **Medication** | **Dose** | **Notes** | |
| Diazepam | • 0.1–0.5 mg/kg IV (adult)<br>• 5–20 mg IV (foal) | • Initial dose can be repeated as needed | |
| Midazolam | • 0.04–0.2 mg/kg bolus<br>• 0.01–0.04 mg/kg/h CRI | • Initial dose can be repeated as needed<br>• If CRI desired it should be started after bolus dose | |
| Guaifenesin | • 90–130 mg/kg | | |
| Pentobarbital | • 3–10 mg/kg IV | • Administer slowly to effect | |
| Phenobarbital | • 5–15 mg/kg IV | • Administer slowly to effect<br>• Risk of respiratory depression | |
| Propofol | • 4 mg/kg IV (foal) | | |
| **Maintenance anti-convulsant therapy** | | | |
| **Therapy** | **Dose** | **Route of administration** | **Frequency** |
| Phenobarbital | 5–11 mg/kg | PO | Q12-24h |
| Potassium bromide | up to 60–90 mg/kg | PO | Q24h |
| Levetiracetam | 32 mg/kg | PO | Q12h |

## Dysphagia

Inability of a horse to effectively obtain and subsequently swallow feed material or water; can result from abnormalities in prehension, mastication or swallowing. Pathology may involve central or peripheral (cranial nerve) neurologic disease, or problems with teeth, lips, mouth, tongue, pharynx, mandible, or esophagus.

- **History**: Three categories for the causes of dysphagia have been historically established as painful, neurogenic, and obstructive (Baum et al. 1988a, b; Cohen 1993), and differentials for each can be viewed in Table 15.7. The most common causes of dysphagia are not neurogenic but rather pain-associated or obstructive.
  - Inquire if horse experienced episodes of dysphagia in the past, has access to certain plants, etc., during turnout, or if the horse has had endoscopic evaluations in the past.
  - Vaccination history can be useful when prioritizing differentials, i.e., the likelihood of viral encephalitis or botulism as sources for dysphagia in the affected animal.
  - Diet: if forage is in the form of round bales or silage, increases suspicion for botulism.
- **Examination**
  - **NOTE:** if the history includes a short duration of clinical signs (less than one week) and a clear cause for the dysphagia is not identified, gloves should be worn when performing an oral examination due to a possibility of rabies.
  - *Neurologic evaluation*: Dysphagia associated with lesions of the brainstem is often accompanied by ataxia. Observe for any muscle fasciculations that may be associated with neuromuscular conditions (i.e., botulism).
    - Observe the horse's ability to grab, prehend and swallow feedstuffs.
      - Observe for quidding (dropping feed) or balling up feedstuffs (without actually swallowing).
    - Pay particular attention to cranial nerve involvement.
      - Trigeminal nerve: CN 5 – (facial sensation and muscles of mastication).
      - Facial nerve: CN 7 – (facial muscles outside of mastication, i.e., lips, etc.).
      - Glossopharyngeal nerve: CN 9 – (pharyngeal and cranial esophageal function).
      - Vagus nerve: CN 10 – (pharyngeal, laryngeal, and esophageal function).
      - Hypoglossal nerve: CN 12 – (motor to tongue).
  - *Physical examination*: Investigate the skull/maxilla/mandible for any palpable fractures or visible hematomas associated with trauma.
  - *Dental evaluation*: Place a speculum for safe, comprehensive evaluation of dentition. Observe for fractures, abscessation, sharp points, or waves in dentition. Observe for glossitis/lingual foreign bodies.

**Table 15.7** Non-exhaustive list of sources of dysphagia in the horse.

| Pain-associated | Neurogenic | Obstructive |
|---|---|---|
| Dental disease (tooth root abscess, periodontal disease, worn, missing or broken teeth) | Guttural pouch mycosis | Pharyngeal disease (abscess, neoplasia, foreign body) |
| Foreign body/glossitis/tongue trauma | Toxicity: metals (lead, etc.), plants (yellow star thistle, Russian knapweed, moldy corn, etc.) | Esophageal obstruction (choke, stricture, diverticulum, megaesophagus) |
| Strangles/lymphadenopathy | Viral encephalitides (EEE, WEE, VEE, rabies) | Dorsal displacement of the soft palate |
| Snake bite | Other encephalitides (verminous, bacterial, fungal) | Rostral displacement of the palatopharyngeal arch |
| Fracture of skull/mandible | Meningitis | Guttural pouch tympany |
| Neoplasia/mass | Hepatoencephalopathy | Epiglottic cyst |
| | Otitis (secondary damage to CN VII) | Follicular hyperplasia/pharyngitis |
| | Brainstem disease (trauma, neoplasia, abscess) including equine protozoal myeloencephalitis and Lyme neuroborreliosis | Fourth branchial arch defect (foals) |
| | Neonatal maladjustment syndrome | Guttural pouch empyema |
| | White muscle disease | |
| | Botulism | |
| | Temporohyoid osteoarthropathy | |

- **Diagnostic plan**
  - *Blood collection*: hematology, biochemical profile, ammonia (if available).
    - Optional: serology (EPM, Lyme) – ideally paired with CSF.
  - *Imaging*: Skull and esophageal radiographs, CT, ultrasound of the tongue (when foreign body suspected), swallow study with contrast radiography or fluoroscopy.
  - *Endoscopy* of airway, guttural pouches, and esophagus.
  - *CSF centesis*: cytology, total protein; EPM, Lyme immunologic testing – ideally paired with serum.
- **Therapeutic plan:** largely dictated by the cause of the dysphagia.
  - *Broad-spectrum antimicrobials*: to treat aspiration pneumonia: trimethoprim sulfamethoxazole (30 mg/kg, Q12h) + metronidazole (15 mg/kg PO Q8h to Q6h); can be given via NGT. If intravenous route is elected due to dysphagia, a common intravenous combination is potassium penicillin G (22,000 IU/kg, Q6h) and gentamicin (6.6 mg/kg, Q24h).
  - *Treat inciting cause*: Botulism antitoxin (see *botulism* section), EPM treatment (see *EPM* section), address dental concerns if present, etc.
- **Management**
  - *Nutritional/hydrational support*: May require grain or alfalfa meal slurry/powdered nutrition slurry (i.e., Purina WellGel etc). Parenteral nutrition may be needed if completely dysphagic.
    - When calculating caloric needs for the horse, digestible energy is calculated as $DE = 155\,(BW)^{0.75}$ where BW = body weight in kg; a 500 kg horse requires approximately 16,400 kcal/day. Horses with dysphagia may be in catabolic states and require more than maintenance digestible energy.
    - Nasogastric intubation (can be left indwelling if needed and in appropriate monitoring situation; Repeat nasogastric intubation may be irritating to the pharynx, larynx, and esophagus, and an indwelling tube may both decrease irritation and be more practical if the patient is less tolerant of intubation).
    - Intravenous fluid therapy with electrolyte/dextrose supplementation.
    - Esophagostomy tube may be placed.

- *Minimize aspiration risk*: If dysphagic, remove feedstuffs and water, as risk of aspiration pneumonia very high. Muzzle if necessary. Hungry horses may even attempt to swallow bedding looking for feedstuffs.
- **Prognosis:** Variable depending on etiology; if neurogenic dysphagia is suspected, management is often unfulfilling given the general poor prognosis affiliated with most associated conditions. Owners should be informed of these expectations early in the case management process.
- **What can be done at the farm**
  - *Diagnostics*: blood collection, imaging (radiographs), endoscopy, CSF centesis.
  - *Treatment*: antimicrobials, antiprotozoals, antitoxin, address dental concerns.
  - *Management*: serial or continuous nasogastric intubation, Intravenous fluid therapy.
- **What can be done at a referral center**
  - *Diagnostics*: computed tomography, barium swallow study.
  - *Management*: esophagostomy, continuous IVF, parenteral nutrition, parenteral antimicrobials.
- **When to refer:** In general, neurogenic causes of dysphagia should always be referred to a tertiary care facility when possible due to intensive management needs. Referral is strongly indicated if the horse in question is recumbent (i.e., as a sequela to botulism).

## Urinary Incontinence

The involuntary passage of urine (incontinence) has been reported in a variety of circumstances, both neurogenic and non-neurogenic (Table 15.8). This section will focus mainly on neurogenic causes of urinary incontinence. Disorders of the bladder and urethra can result in urinary incontinence, as can abnormalities anywhere along the nerve supply to these organs. Urinary incontinence can be the result of either upper motor neuron (UMN) or lower motor neuron (LMN) disturbances. UMN derangements can result in disinhibition of the urethral sphincters leading to an increase in their tone and difficulty voiding urine, while lower motor neuron pathology can cause paralysis of the detrusor muscle and minimize tone of the bladder and urethral sphincters, both scenarios resulting in lack of urine voiding control (Furr and Sampieri 2007).

- **History**
  - Owners or managers will typically observe urine dribbling from either the vulva or penis. Dribbling may be continuous or may be sporadic or periodic (Mair 2022).
  - Acute-onset urinary incontinence may present more commonly as a consequence to trauma of the sacral or coccygeal region or equine herpesvirus-1 myeloencephalopathy (EHM). As such, obtaining a thorough history and investigating for accompanying neurologic signs (or lack thereof) will enable a practitioner to determine a need for appropriate biosecurity implementation (as should be the case for EHM-associated urinary incontinence, for example).

**Table 15.8** Neurogenic and non-neurogenic causes of urinary incontinence.

| Neurogenic | Non-neurogenic |
|---|---|
| Sabulous cystitis (secondary to neurogenic bladder dysfunction) | Trauma to urethral sphincter (such as that in postpartum mares) |
| Trauma (sacral or coccygeal region) | Congenital abnormalities (patent urachus, ectopic ureter) |
| Equine herpesvirus-1 myeloencephalopathy (EHM) and other viral encephalitides | Cystitis and/or urethritis |
| Equine protozoal myeloencephalitis (EPM) | Neoplasia |
| | Polyuria |
| Spinal neoplasia (particularly melanoma in gray horses) | |
| Polyneuritis equi | |
| Toxicities (Sudan grass toxicity, sorghum toxicity) | |
| Idiopathic bladder paralysis | |

- Medical history
  - Previous neurologic disease?
  - Reproductive history if relevant (i.e., postpartum mare, history of dystocia during lifetime can predispose years later).
- **Examination**
  - If horse has accompanying neurologic signs that render it severely ataxic or recumbent or has fever, respiratory infection or limb edema, referral to a tertiary care facility is recommended in light of both supportive care needs and (if EHM is a concern) appropriate biosecurity protocols. However, always contact state vet prior to shipping horse that is an EHM suspect.
  - UMN sources of bladder pathology often present with other severe clinical signs such as recumbency. LMN urinary incontinence may be accompanied by altered anal sphincter tone, reduced perineal sensation, reduced tail tone, atrophy of hind limb musculature (Figure 15.3) and pelvic limb paresis. UMN and LMN causes of urinary incontinence are typically managed in the same manner.
  - Observe for urine scald in region of vulva and perineum (mares) (Figure 15.4) or the ventral abdomen (geldings and stallions) and limbs.
  - Observe for urine dribbling that occurs during exercise or coughing (if present) as a consequence of increasing abdominal pressure.
  - Observe for obvious evidence of trauma along dorsal midline, particularly in sacral/coccygeal regions.
  - Observe the horse for evidence of ataxia or paresis (sudden onset increases suspicion of EHM).
  - Observe the horse for accompanying cranial nerve abnormalities (can be seen with polyneuritis equi or EPM), particularly facial nerve or vestibulocochlear nerve abnormalities.
  - *Palpation per rectum*: note bladder size, tone and if horse is reactive to palpation.
  - *Reproductive examination*: if relevant (i.e., postpartum mare).
- **Diagnostics**
  - *Blood collection*: hematology, biochemical profile (including electrolytes, liver values, creatinine), ammonia (if available), vitamin E, serology (EPM, Lyme) – ideally paired with CSF.
  - *Nasal swab + blood submission for EHV PCR testing*

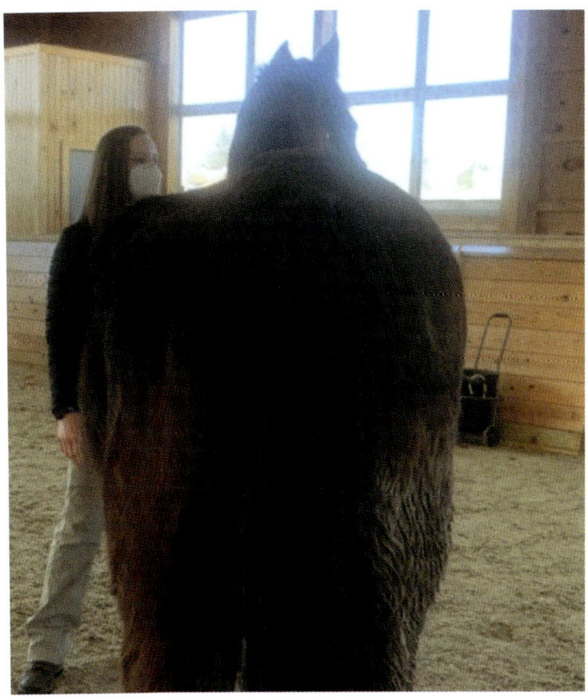

**Figure 15.3** Horse with urinary incontinence accompanied by profound left-sided gluteal muscle atrophy.

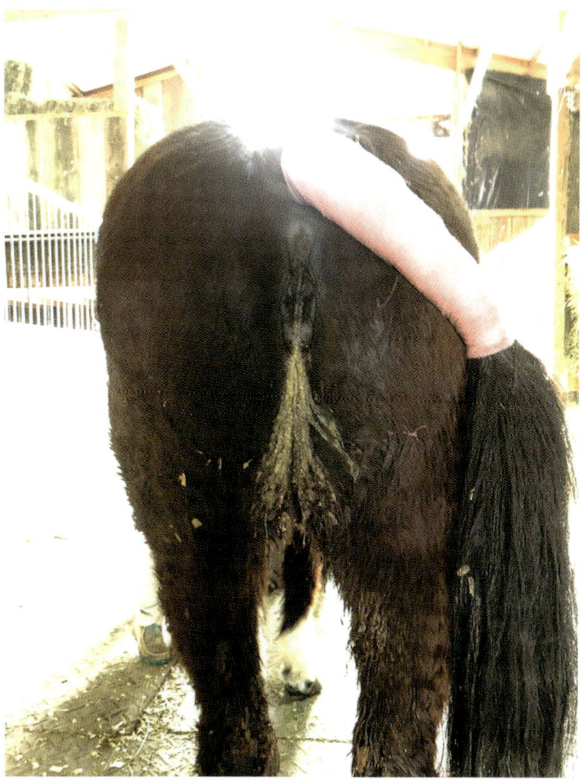

**Figure 15.4** Mare with urinary incontinence and severe urine scald. *Source:* Courtesy of Dr. Kathryn Timko DVM DACVIM-LAIM.

    - If concurrent fever/other signs of EHM.
    - 5× 3 mL EDTA tubes + nasal swabs.
  - *Imaging*
    - Sacral/coccygeal radiographs.
    - Ultrasonography of the urinary tract.
      - Transabdominal & transrectal.
  - *Urinalysis & urine culture* (if sterile sample can be obtained)
    - May reveal evidence of cystitis (>$10^4$ colony-forming units/mL).
  - *Endoscopy (of lower urinary tract)*
    - Evaluate anatomy.
    - Assess urethral sphincter tone.
    - Observe for material in the bladder.
    - Assess for irritation of bladder mucosa (cystitis) which can cause and be caused by bladder atony.
  - CSF centesis: cytology, total protein, EPM, and Lyme testing.
- **Therapeutic options**
  - *Bladder catheterization*
    - If palpation per rectum reveals a taut, full bladder and the clinician has concerns for potential bladder rupture (± ultrasonography increases this suspicion), catheterization and removal of bladder contents in an effort to ameliorate or avoid overdistension should be attempted. Indwelling catheterization is not recommended in light of possible infection.
    - **HOW TO:**
      - *Step 1*: Sedate the horse as needed. Particularly for stallions and geldings, use of acepromazine to encourage "dropping" of the penis can aid in facilitating the passage of a urinary catheter.
      - *Step 2*: Clean the perineum or sheath/exterior of the penis using dilute betadine solution or water to minimize introduction of bacteria/ascending infection.
      - *Step 3*: Using sterile gloves and technique and applying sterile lubricant, gently pass a stallion catheter into the urethra until urine is obtained.
      - *Step 4*: Acquisition of a sterile urine sample can be obtained at this time.
      - *Step 5*: Allow urine to flow until it discontinues. If endoscopy is being utilized, a suction system can be applied to facilitate urine removal, as can a dosing syringe.
      - *Step 6 (optional)*: Depending on the contents of the bladder, lavage may be necessary to evacuate concretions and thick contents that may be present from chronic bladder dysfunction.
  - *Therapeutic support:*
    - Treatment and management of urinary incontinence can be limited regardless of the cause of the clinical signs. This is possibly due in part to the likelihood that by the time horses with urinary incontinence are seen by clinicians, permanent detrusor dysfunction may have already occurred (Mair 2022). See Table 15.9 for pharmacologic options and dosing information.
- **Management**
  - *Quarantine*: If EHM is suspected. See *Equine herpes myeloencephalopathy* section.
  - *Husbandry*: Maintaining a clean and dry perineal region as well as limbs is one of the most difficult aspects of managing cases of urinary incontinence, particularly in regard to mares. This can require attention to these regions multiple times a day, and involve frequent bathing and drying to prevent or at least minimize urine scald.
  - *Periodic bladder lavage*: as needed.

**Table 15.9** Pharmacologic options for managing urinary incontinence in horses.

| Therapy | Dose | Route of administration | Frequency | Note |
|---|---|---|---|---|
| Bethanechol | 0.2–0.4 mg/kg | PO | Q6-12h | Efficacy not reported |
| Phenoxybenzamine | 0.2–0.7 mg/kg | PO | Q6-8h | Decreases urethral resistance |
| Prazosin | 5 mg | PO | Q8h | Decreases urethral resistance |

- **Prognosis:** Prognosis for resolution of urinary incontinence is generally poor, but can vary with the inciting etiology. Some horses with EPM or acute trauma may improve with treatment and time.
- **What can be done at the farm**
  - *Diagnostics*: radiographs, ultrasonography, urine culture and sensitivity, CSF analysis, blood collection, nasal swab.
  - *Treatment*: bladder lavage/catheterization, therapeutics, treatment for inciting cause, antimicrobial administration if infection suspected.
- **What can be done at referral center**
  - *Diagnostics*: cystoscopy, nuclear scintigraphy.
  - *Management*: quarantine (if EHV suspected), supportive care (as needed, i.e., if horse becomes recumbent, etc.)
- **When to refer:** suspicion of EHM, recumbency/need for sling support, need for nutritional/hydrational support

**Case Example 15.1 Neurologic Disease**

A 500 kg, 6-year-old Quarter Horse mare is presented for evaluation. The owner heard crashing sounds coming from the horse's stall and came over to find the horse down and thrashing. The mare eventually staggered to a standing position and was noticed to have developed a right-sided head-tilt, prompting the owner to seek veterinary evaluation.

*During your physical examination and initial neurological evaluation, you identify the following:*

- Bilateral spontaneous nystagmus with fast phase to the left.
- Right-sided ptosis.
- Right-sided ear droop.
- Left-sided muzzle deviation.

*A gait evaluation is performed, during which you identify the following:*

- Wide-based stance.
- Circling to the right.
- Difficulty turning to the left.
- Leaning to the right.
- No evidence of deficits in proprioception.
  - *What type of ataxia is being described above? What is your top differential diagnosis?*
    - ***Vestibular ataxia****; the forementioned description of posture and gait as well as abnormal nystagmus are typical for peripheral vestibular disease. There is no mention of gait abnormalities consistent with general proprioceptive (spinal) ataxia such as delayed protraction, excessive limb adduction, scuffing of the toes, overreaching or "floating" aspect to stride,* etc. *There is also no mention of intention or head tremors or marked spasticity, such as what might be expected in cases of cerebellar ataxia. In this case, this horse can be neurolocalized to the right peripheral vestibular system. Facial paralysis (cranial nerve VII) often accompanies peripheral vestibular disease (cranial nerve VIII) due to the proximity of these two nerves within the petrous temporal bone. The cranial nerve deficits are primarily right-sided, and peripheral vestibular disease tends to produce nystagmus with a fast phase away from the side of the lesion (in this case, fast phase to the left, lesion on the right). Without other cranial nerve deficits in additional to CN VII and CN VIII, nor other signs of intra-cranial disease (abnormal mentation, other cranial nerve abnormalities, proprioceptive ataxia), a working diagnosis of peripheral vestibular disease is supported. Of note, horses with THO are typically deaf on the affected side, with minimal likelihood of return of hearing.*
    - ***Temporohyoid osteoarthropathy (THO)*** *is the top differential diagnosis in this case. This is a progressive condition classified by bony thickening with fusing of the stylohyoid bone to the petrous temporal bone. The etiology of this condition may lie in infectious sources (otitis, for example) and/or degenerative joint disease (osteoarthritis). An act as simple as swallowing or chewing or as severe as head trauma from falling/a kick by another horse can lead to onset of signs associated with THO. Another important differential diagnosis for THO is equine protozoal myeloencephalitis.*
  - *What is your on-farm diagnostic plan for the horse above?*
    - ***Guttural pouch endoscopy****: generally, affected horses will require sedation in order to safely pursue endoscopy. It is important to remember that these horses may be very painful and thus fractious, particularly if the onset of their disease is the result of a fracture. Fighting the operator of the endoscope may result in further discomfort, which sedation may minimize. Visualizing the ipsilateral guttural pouch (in this case, the right guttural pouch) may enable the diagnosis to*

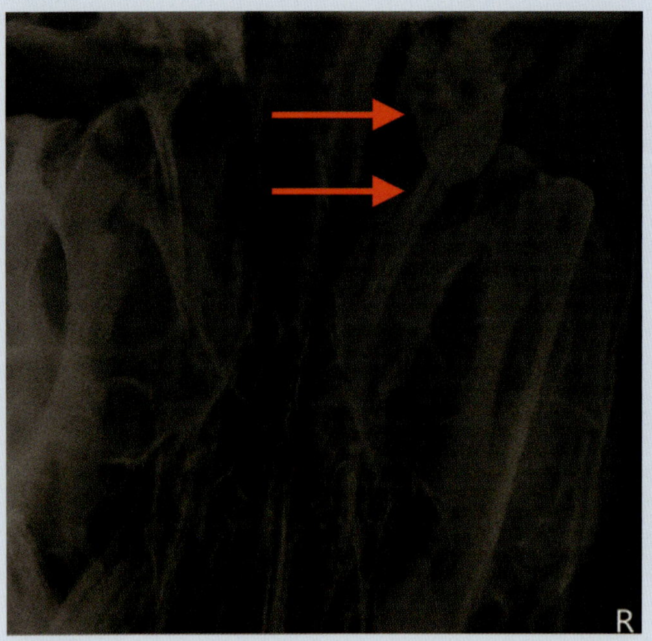


**Figure 15.5** Severe right temporohyoid osteoarthropathy (THO) as evidenced by marked, smooth osseous proliferation surrounding the right temporohyoid articulation (top arrow) and moderate, diffuse thickening of the right stylohyoid bone (bottom arrow).

*be made on the basis of identifying enlargement of the proximal stylohyoid bone. Having someone manually place pressure in the region of the intermandibular space while scoping the pouch may enable the viewer to appreciate stiffness and lack of mobility of the affected joint and/or may cause the horse to become more painful. Importantly, not all horses with THO will present with obvious abnormalities visible on endoscopy. Also important, some horses with abnormalities on guttural pouch endoscopy (or other skull imaging) might not be clinically affected.*

- ***Radiographs**: on the farm, DV radiographs that are well-centered may enable identification of enlargement/asymmetry/abnormality in the silhouette of the proximal stylohyoid bone (Figure 15.5).*
- *Ultimately, computed tomography (CT) may be the most informative diagnostic test available for THO (but is of course not available in farm scenarios and requires referral/transport).*

- *What will be your stabilization/management/therapeutic plan for this case?*

*Horses diagnosed with THO often can improve, though improvement may take weeks of management, and horses may plateau in their signs (ataxia, cranial nerve deficits) without full recoveries.*

- ***Stall rest**: stall rest is the safest approach for horses afflicted with vestibular ataxia given their tendency to fall and lean as a consequence of poor balance. Those handling these horses should be informed of risks of handling. Stall rest may also be best for horses with THO in general, as keeping these horses quiet is ideal while potential fractures heal.*
- ***Keep environment well-lit**: keeping the lights on will help horses with vestibular ataxia visually compensate for their deficits. Darkness may exacerbate the severity of the vestibular ataxia. With this in mind, some horses being referred to tertiary-care facilities may benefit from waiting until daylight before shipping.*
- ***Ensure ability to chew and swallow** and address as needed; some horses with THO may be limited in their ability to chew and swallow, often due to pain. While some horses may be able to prehend normally, others may require mash or gruel options, while still others may require parenteral nutrition (necessitating referral). Keep in mind that nasogastric intubation can engender pain and worsen fractures in horses with THO.*
- ***Ophthalmic care**: Horses with cranial nerve VII deficits may have inappropriate eyelid tone/lack of palpebral reflex and thus be subjected to chronic and severe corneal ulceration. Treatment of corneal ulcers should be considered in these cases, and for those without improvement in their palpebral reflex and continued ulceration, temporary, or permanent tarsorrhaphies should be discussed. Corneal ulceration due to facial nerve paralysis is an ophthalmic emergency and failure to immediately address the invariably infected ulcer and protect the cornea through constant lubrication or tarsorrhaphy increases risk of development of a melting ulcer and subsequent loss of the globe.*

- ***Antimicrobials**: Because it is thought that THO can have infectious origins in some cases (otitis, for example), broad-spectrum antimicrobial treatment is usually initiated. Antibiotic treatment can also protect against ascending bacterial meningoencephalitis should a full-thickness skull fracture be present. Trimethoprim sulfamethoxazole is a commonly used choice.*
- ***Pain management**: Anti-inflammatories (flunixin meglumine, phenylbutazone) can be useful as analgesics.*
- ***Consider referral**: If surgery is an option, it is generally recommended sooner than later. Referral may also be necessary to reach a diagnosis (if CT is needed or the practitioner is not comfortable performing endoscopy or radiographs on the ataxic horse), or if the management of the horse cannot be feasibly continued on the farm (parenteral nutrition, hydration, sling support, ophthalmic care).*

## References


Baum, K., Halpern, N., Banish, L. & Modransky, P. (1988a). Dysphagia in horses: the differential diagnosis. II. *The Compendium on Continuing Education for the Practicing Veterinarian*, USA.

Baum, K., Modransky, P., Halpern, N. & Banish, L. (1988b). Dysphagia in horses: the differential diagnosis. I. *Compendium on Continuing Education for the Practicing Veterinarian*, 10, 1301–1304.

Cohen, N.D. (1993). Neurologic evaluation of the equine head and neurogenic dysphagia. *Vet. Clin. North Am. Equine Pract.* 9: 199–212.

Divers, T.J., Gardner, R.B., Madigan, J.E. et al. (2018). Borrelia burgdorferi infection and Lyme disease in North American horses: a consensus statement. *J. Vet. Intern. Med.* 32: 617–632.

Dowling, P.M. (1999). Clinical pharmacology of nervous system diseases. *Vet. Clin. North Am. Equine Pract.* 15: 575–588.

Feige, K., Fürst, A., Kaser-Hotz, B., and Ossent, P. (2000). Traumatic injury to the central nervous system in horses: occurrence, diagnosis and outcome. *Equine Vet. Edu.* 12: 220–224.

Furr, M. and Sampieri, F. (2007). Differential diagnosis of urinary incontinence and cauda equina syndrome. *Equine Neurol.* 119–125.

Johnson, A.L., Mcadams-Gallagher, S.C., and Aceto, H. (2015). Outcome of adult horses with botulism treated at a veterinary hospital: 92 cases (1989–2013). *J. Vet. Intern. Med.* 29: 311–319.

Mair, T. (2022). Urinary incontinence and urinary tract infections. *Vet. Clin. North Am. Equine Pract.* 38: 73–94.

Mitchell, E., Furr, M.O., and Mckenzie, H.C. (2006). Bacterial meningitis in five mature horses. *Equine Vet. Edu.* 18: 249–255.

Nout-Lomas, Y.S. (2022). Traumatic nervous system injury. *Vet. Clin. North Am. Equine Pract.* 38: 363–377.

Pusterla, N., Hussey, G.S., and Goehring, L.S. (2022). Equine herpesvirus-1 myeloencephalopathy. *Vet. Clin. North Am. Equine Pract.* 38: 339–362.

Sanchez, L.C., Giguère, S., and Lester, G.D. (2008). Factors associated with survival of neonatal foals with bacteremia and racing performance of surviving thoroughbreds: 423 cases (1982–2007). *J. Am. Vet. Med. Assoc.* 233: 1446–1452.

Sinner, S.W. and Tunkel, A.R. (2004). Antimicrobial agents in the treatment of bacterial meningitis. *Infect. Dis. Clin. N. Am.* 18 (581–602): ix.

Smith, J.J., Provost, P.J., and Paradis, M.R. (2004). Bacterial meningitis and brain abscesses secondary to infectious disease processes involving the head in horses: seven cases (1980–2001). *J. Am. Vet. Med. Assoc.* 224: 739–742.

Stewart, A., Salazar, P., Waldridge, B. et al. (2007). Computed tomographic diagnosis of a pathological fracture due to rhodococcal osteomyelitis and spinal abscess in a foal. *Equine Vet. Edu.* 19: 231–236.

Stokol, T., Serpa, P.B.S., Brooks, M.B. et al. (2018). Subcutaneous Administration of low-Molecular-Weight Heparin to horses inhibits ex vivo equine herpesvirus type 1-induced platelet activation. *Front Vet. Sci.* 5: 106.

Tyler, C.M., Davis, R.E., Begg, A.P. et al. (1993). A survey of neurological diseases in horses. *Aust. Vet. J.* 70: 445–449.

Viu, J., Monreal, L., Jose-Cunilleras, E. et al. (2012). Clinical findings in 10 foals with bacterial meningoencephalitis. *Equine Vet. J. Suppl.* 100–104.

Whitlock, R.H. and Mcadams, S. (2006). Equine botulism. *Clin. Tech. Equine Pract.* 5: 37–42.

Wilkins, P.A. and Palmer, J.E. (2003). Botulism in foals less than 6 months of age: 30 cases (1989–2002). *J. Vet. Intern. Med.* 17: 702–707.

# 16

# Emergency Problems of the Eye

*Kelly Knickelbein*[1] *and Nicole Scherrer*[2]

[1] *Department of Clinical Sciences, College of Veterinary Medicine, Cornell University, Ithaca, NY, USA*
[2] *Department of Clinical Studies - New Bolton Center, University of Pennsylvania School of Veterinary Medicine, Kennett Square, PA, USA*

## Ophthalmic Basics

### Ophthalmic Examination

A proper ophthalmic examination starts with observation. Horses that have been previously examined or medicated can be sensitive to people near their head. For this reason, a more accurate interpretation of blepharospasm will be possible from a distance, preferably from outside of the stall. Observation from a closer distance will allow evaluation of facial and globe symmetry. Palpation can be used to investigate any asymmetry noted and to characterize the texture and sensitivity of the globe. Retropulsion is performed by pushing the globe back into the orbit through closed lids. It is important to note that this should not be performed if there is any threat of globe rupture. Resistance to retropulsion suggests the presence of a retrobulbar mass. Retropulsion of the contralateral eye at the same time (using an index finger on each eye to palpate through a closed upper eyelid) can provide a baseline for the individual patient. This technique can be used to help distinguish between changes in globe size and globe position (e.g., exophthalmos which would be associated with abnormal retropulsion and buphthalmos which would be associated with normal retropulsion). Lastly, when retropulsion of the globe is performed, the third eyelid is displaced within the orbit and therefore passively elevates to cover the globe.

Reflexes and responses should be evaluated after the initial observation. The menace response is commonly used in vision evaluation, though at times may be difficult to interpret. If there is a question regarding an animal's vision a maze test can be performed. This involves obstacles that the horse is encouraged to walk through or guide around. Completion of the menace response requires an intact visual and motor cortex, including cranial nerves II (optic nerve) and VII (facial nerve). Keep in mind that this is a protective response that is learned and may not be present in animals less than two weeks of age. To perform this test the veterinarian should touch the periocular area once or twice to first stimulate the palpebral reflex. This should be followed by movements that create visible motion without creating stimulation of aural or tactile senses. The menace response should be evaluated throughout the horse's monocular visual field. For the horse this extends approximately 150° (starting directly behind the horse) leaving a small section perpendicular to the forehead that requires binocular vision. The dazzle reflex is a very simple test that, similar to the menace response, evaluates the function of the retina, CN II, and CN VII. When a focal light source is directed toward the eye the horse should respond by blinking. After vision is fully assessed the focal light source is used to evaluate pupil size and pupillary light reflexes (PLR). Pupil symmetry can be evaluated by standing approximately six feet in front of the horse with a focal light directed at the center of the horse's head to visualize both tapetal reflexes simultaneously. The normal horse pupil is round when dilated and oval shaped when constricted with the horizontal axis being longer than the vertical axis. After pupil symmetry is evaluated PLR should be evaluated individually. This is done by directing the focal light into each eye from approximately 2–3 cm. When the light is directed into one eye both pupils should constrict (direct/indirect reflex). It is normal for the equine pupil to respond slowly with vertical movement being more noticeable than horizontal movement. The palpebral reflex is stimulated when the medial or lateral canthus is touched. A normal response is complete closure of the eyelids. Failure of this reflex occurs if there is damage to either the trigeminal (CN V) or facial nerve (CN VII) or if the eyelids are unable to close properly (e.g., trauma). Incomplete lid closure for any reason can predispose the horse to exposure keratopathy and other related consequences.

*Emergency Triage of the Horse*, First Edition. Edited by Rolfe M. Radcliffe and Jamie J. Kopper.

Companion website: www.wiley.com/go/radcliffe/triage

Following evaluation of the ocular reflexes and responses, examination of the globe is performed. A dark area of the barn is ideal for this stage of the examination; towels can be used to cover windows. If a barn is unavailable, the examination can be performed in the evening to provide a better examination environment.

Generally, examination is easiest if started on the less painful eye. There is no strict order of examination; however, the order should be consistent for each individual examiner to not miss important abnormalities. Most frequently the examination begins with the adnexa. This is best done with a direct focal light. Common abnormalities are tumors (sarcoids, squamous cell carcinoma) and tarsal margin irregularities.

Purkinje–Sanson reflections can be used to examine the cornea, anterior chamber, iris, and lens. Reflections can be used to examine the clarity and location of any abnormalities. Opacities can be further investigated with the use of slit lamp biomicroscopy. Transillumination can be used to evaluate the anterior chamber by directing a focal beam at a 45° angle to the corneal surface. This method of observation will allow for evaluation of aqueous flare and cells within the anterior chamber. To evaluate the entire lens pharmacological dilation is necessary. 1% tropicamide is most commonly used because it is effective in 20–30 minutes and has a shorter duration (~4–8 h) than atropine (Gelatt et al. 1995).

The horse's fundus can be seen using either direct or indirect ophthalmoscopy and ideally should be examined with both techniques. Indirect ophthalmoscopy requires a focal light source and handheld lens. This technique provides a wide field of view; however, the image visualized is upside down and backwards. Conversely, direct ophthalmoscopy (diopter wheel set at 0 to −3) provides an upright image with a very magnified view (approximately 15 times that of indirect ophthalmoscopy). Either technique can recognize important abnormalities such as retinal detachment, optic nerve atrophy, or chorioretinitis. The nontapetal fundus is often overlooked but is more often affected than the tapetal fundus with lesions such as chorioretinitis and chorioretinal scarring (Cutler et al. 2000). Two common patterns of chorioretinal scarring are peripapillary (butterfly lesions) and multifocal (bullet hole lesions).

The components of an ophthalmic exam are summarized in Box 16.1.

## Sedation

A brief ophthalmic examination on a non-painful and willing patient may be possible without sedation (Box 16.2). If sedation is needed for a brief examination, xylazine (0.3–0.5 mg/kg IV) is typically adequate. If the eye is fragile, extremely painful, or a standing procedure is necessary, detomidine (0.01–0.02 mg/kg IV) is recommended. Acepromazine (0.03–0.05 mg/kg IV) or butorphanol (0.01–0.02 mg/kg IV) can be used to complement either alpha-2 agonist. Due to the potential for unpredictable head movements with butorphanol, it should be avoided in patients undergoing standing procedures during which trauma to the globe is possible. In a fractious patient, morphine can be given as an adjunct to sedation (0.1–0.2 mg/kg IV slowly). The horse must be sedated prior to giving morphine to avoid the excitement phase. An important side effect of

**Box 16.1 Components of an ophthalmic examination**

- Observation.
- ± Retropulsion of the globe.
- Menace response.
- Dazzle reflex.
- Pupillary light reflex.
- Palpebral reflex.
- Examination of the anterior segment.
- Fundic examination.

**Box 16.2 Ideal medications to facilitate ophthalmic examinations**

- Xylazine.
- Detomidine.
- Acepromazine.
- Morphine.

alpha-2 agonist and opioid administration is gastrointestinal stasis, and manure production should be monitored closely (Merritt et al. 1998; Thibault et al. 2019).

## Preparation

Preparation of the periorbital and periocular tissues should be performed prior to any procedure, including administration of local anesthesia. Dilute betadine solution is created by adding 10% betadine solution to sterile saline at a 1:50 dilution. The periorbital tissue is cleaned by soaking gauze with the dilute betadine solution and wiping the skin. Dilute betadine is also safe for the ocular surface and can be irrigated onto an anesthetized cornea via a syringe attached to a needle that has been broken off at the hub.

## Local Anesthesia

The auriculopalpebral nerve block is the most common periocular block performed. It reduces motor input to the orbicularis oculi muscle resulting in temporary paralysis of the upper eyelid. The block can be applied to facilitate examination and procedures. In a painful eye, an auriculopalpebral block is recommended to avoid pressure on the eye from the horse blinking and resisting examination. If corneal damage is present, contraction of the orbicularis oculi muscle can cause further damage to the globe. This block is unnecessary in cases of facial nerve paralysis because the horse's ability to close the eyelids is diminished or absent. The auriculopalpebral nerve block can be performed by injecting 2–4 mL of local anesthetic perineurally. There are three locations at which this block can be performed: the depression at the base of the ear, at the highest point of the caudal zygomatic arch, or at the lowest point of the zygomatic arch temporal to the orbital rim (Figure 16.1).

To desensitize the medial two-thirds of the superior eyelid, the supraorbital foramen, where the supraorbital (frontal) nerve exits, can be palpated by placing your index finger at one canthus and your ring finger at the other canthus. The middle finger will then naturally lie at the supraorbital foramen. Local anesthetic can be instilled in this area at a volume of 2 mL.

The most common topical ophthalmic anesthetics are tetracaine and proparacaine. The benefits of tetracaine are that it does not require refrigeration and is more effective at anesthetizing the equine cornea (Sharrow-Reabe and Townsend 2012). In the absence of these ophthalmic anesthetics, the injectable anesthetics lidocaine and bupivacaine can be used. Mepivicaine is reported to be a poor corneal anesthetic (Pucket et al. 2013). If topical anesthetics are ineffective, subconjunctival mepivacaine, lidocaine, or bupivacaine can be used. Subconjunctival anesthetics can be administered using a 25–27 gauge needle and a 1 mL syringe. Approximately 0.5 mL of an anesthetic is injected into the subconjunctival space adjacent to the lesion.

Retrobulbar anesthesia is commonly used in equine ophthalmology. The most common reason for performing a retrobulbar block is enucleation, for which a 4-point retrobulbar block provides excellent desensitization. A 20-gauge 3.5″ spinal needle with the stylet removed is bent to mimic the curvature of the bony orbit. This needle is passed transcutaneously around the globe at 4 points (the medial and lateral canthi, dorsally, and ventrally) and then guided within the orbit up to the level of the hub. Anesthetic (typically mepivacaine for its quick onset and long duration of action) is injected slowly once the needle is in place (10 mL per site). If the goal is corneal anesthesia with the intent to maintain the globe, a retrobulbar block via the supraorbital fossa is appropriate (McKinney 2021). This is performed using a straight 20–22 gauge 2.5–3.5″ spinal needle. It is directed behind the globe through the supraorbital fossa. The needle will initially cause dorsal deflection of the globe followed by a pop through the fascia and return to normal globe position.

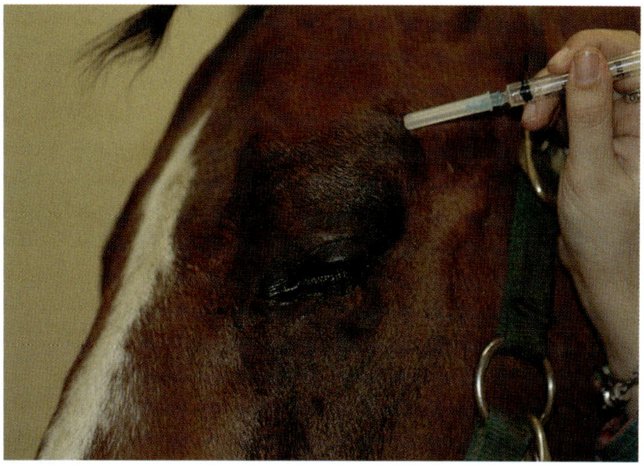

**Figure 16.1** The tip of the needle points to where the auriculopalpebral nerve can be palpated as it crosses over the zygomatic arch temporal to the orbit.

## Orbital Abscess/Cellulitis

Cases of orbital abscess or cellulitis are often accompanied by severe discomfort, blepharoedema, and chemosis. Depending on the severity of the disease, exophthalmos and strabismus may be seen as well (Hubert 1996).

### Emergency Stabilization

Often a complete ophthalmic examination is not possible due to pain and swelling of the eyelids and conjunctiva. If there is an external wound, a swab for aerobic and anaerobic bacterial cultures should be collected. The wound should be explored, lavaged with dilute betadine solution, and if possible, drainage should be established.

### Diagnostic Plan

After a complete ophthalmic examination, the eyelids and orbital tissue can be further assessed with ultrasound. This can help to detect a foreign body and help determine if a mass is present (Hubert 1996). Ultrasound-guided sample acquisition is ideal and is especially important if initial empiric treatment has failed to result in improvement. If possible, drainage should be established with ultrasound guidance under deep sedation or anesthesia.

It is important to remember that with any retrobulbar abnormality, exophthalmos can present as an acute problem. Subtle changes associated with retrobulbar neoplasia and arteriovenous malformations can often seem acute. Advanced imaging such as computed tomography (CT) is necessary to help determine the most likely differentials, extent of disease, and prognosis.

### Treatment

Initial treatment with systemic anti-inflammatories (flunixin meglumine, 1.1 mg/kg IV or PO q12h) and broad-spectrum antibiotics (trimethoprim sulfamethoxazole, 30 mg/kg PO q12h) generally results in significant improvement within 24 h. Depending on the severity of the swelling a systemic steroid may be indicated in place of or in addition to a systemic non-steroidal to avoid blindness from irreversible damage to the optic nerve. If initial treatment fails, diagnostics including imaging (orbital ultrasound, head CT), culture/sensitivity, and biopsy collection should be considered.

The need for referral is dependent on the veterinarian's comfort with periorbital ultrasound and response to initial treatment.

## Orbital Fractures

A horse with head trauma can have a wide variety of clinical signs that include a completely normal appearance to severe ataxia or even obtundation. Horses have a complete bony orbit which helps to protect the eye in the case of a traumatic event. The rim of the equine orbit comprises the frontal bone dorsally, lacrimal bone medially, zygomatic bone ventrally, and temporal bone laterally. The components of the dorsal orbital rim, especially the zygomatic process of the frontal bone and the zygomatic arch, are at highest risk for traumatic fracture due to their prominence (Gilger 2010). Depending on the location and severity, fracture of the orbital bones can cause extensive damage to the globe. Clinical signs that can be seen with orbital fractures include blepharospasm, blepharoedema, chemosis, bony asymmetry, crepitus, emphysema, enophthalmos, exophthalmos, strabismus, and epiphora.

The most common causes of orbital fractures include rearing in a confined space (41.7%), kick to the head (33.3%), and collision with an object (25%) (Gerding et al. 2014). According to Gerding et al., injuries sustained from a kick to the head are more likely to result in a major complication (enucleation or euthanasia). Interestingly, a fracture is more likely to occur when kicked by a shod hoof (70.6%) in comparison to an unshod hoof (23.5%) (Joss 2019).

### Emergency Stabilization

Following any trauma to the head the horse should undergo a thorough physical examination prior to an ophthalmic examination. If neurologic status is in question, a neurologic examination should be performed prior to the ophthalmic examination. Sedation should be given cautiously and only after a complete physical examination to ensure the patient is stable following the head trauma. Recall that the onset of neurologic signs can be delayed hours in some cases of head trauma (Dallap Schaer 2007; Ragle 1993). The author prefers a short-acting sedative like xylazine. Access to reversal is ideal. An exaggerated response to sedation can be a sign of a traumatic brain injury.

Following an acute injury, full assessment of the globe may be difficult due to the degree of periorbital swelling or entrapment of the globe in a recessed position. Affected horses are generally extremely painful, and early administration of analgesics will help facilitate an easier examination. The goal of the initial examination is to determine the extent of the orbital fractures and if there are accompanying ocular problems. Possible ocular issues include nasolacrimal duct obstruction or transection, facial nerve paralysis, entrapment of extraocular muscles in fractures, corneal ulceration, uveitis, hyphema, and corneal perforation. Gerding et al. reported that corneal ulceration was the most common ocular complication secondary to orbital fracture (7/18). A thorough examination of both eyes is extremely important as vision loss in the contralateral eye will significantly impact the horse's overall prognosis. A thorough neuro-ophthalmic examination including assessment of the menace response, palpebral, dazzle, and direct/indirect PLR should be performed.

### Diagnostic Plan

A complete ophthalmic examination can help determine what abnormalities need to be addressed. In a painful eye, an auriculopalpebral nerve block is recommended to avoid pressure on the eye from the horse blinking. If corneal damage is present, contraction of the orbicularis oculi muscle can cause further damage to the globe. The auriculopalpebral block can be performed by instilling 2–4 mL of 1% lidocaine or 2% mepivacaine over the zygomatic arch. The palpebral branch of the nerve can be palpated in this area. It is important to remember that this block is motor only and no desensitization will occur.

In some cases, digital palpation of the orbit can allow for diagnosis of an orbital fracture (Gerding et al. 2014). This can be done with a combination of external palpation and palpation through the conjunctiva after application of a topical anesthetic. Palpation should be performed very cautiously until a complete assessment of the globe can be performed as to prevent worsening of a deep corneal ulceration or perforation. Palpation in combination with diagnostic imaging is the gold standard. Skull radiographs can be difficult to interpret due to superimposition of tissue and bone. CT or magnetic resonance imaging (MRI) can provide an accurate three-dimensional image of the skull and is considered the gold standard to determine if surgical intervention is necessary. CT is preferable for bony changes and therefore is the better modality for surgical planning.

### Treatment

Non-displaced fractures can be managed medically with systemic anti-inflammatories. Associated skin lacerations or sinus involvement are situations in which broad-spectrum systemic antimicrobials are warranted, as fractures into the sinus are considered open fractures due to the presence of normal bacteria and fungal flora.

Displaced fractures that impinge on the globe, extraocular muscles, or nasolacrimal duct should be surgically stabilized. Fractures can be repaired via closed or open reduction and in some cases use of internal fixation is necessary (Caron et al. 1986). Internal fixation can be achieved with stainless steel wire sutures or an implant. It is important that if surgical repair is elected that it be performed prior to callus formation which usually occurs in 7–10 days. It has been shown that early repair of orbital fractures will result in a more cosmetic outcome (Caron et al. 1986). If corneal ulceration, severe uveitis, or hyphema is present, placement of a subpalpebral lavage (SPL) is ideal as patient discomfort can make manual application of medications directly to the eye difficult. Specific topical treatment for these conditions is discussed in the sections below.

Following head trauma, a primary reason for referral is the hospital's ability to continuously monitor if any neurologic concerns are present or develop. If referral is not an option video monitoring at the farm may be possible to set up. In a case of trauma without neurologic abnormalities, referral should be considered if the bony fragments are displaced and/or interfering with the globe. If surgery is not an option and the globe is intact, the prognosis for long-term comfort is good; however, vision is likely to be reduced.

## Eyelid Emergencies

The most common eyelid emergency is an eyelid laceration. While generally an obvious diagnosis, some small lacerations may be missed by the owners and the accompanying signs are blepharoedema, chemosis, and ocular discharge. Entropion is an eyelid emergency that is almost exclusively seen to affect the inferior eyelid of foals.

### Emergency Stabilization

The most important and the first step is to carefully assess the globe. If the globe is not ruptured, the cornea should be generously lubricated to prevent development of or worsening of a corneal ulcer. Without an appropriate upper and lower eyelid, tear film distribution will be abnormal and corneal ulceration can develop as a secondary problem even if it is not initially present. Lubrication should be continued frequently (every 2–4 h) until the eyelid laceration can be repaired.

### Diagnostic Plan

Once the globe is confirmed to be stable, it is important to anesthetize the ocular surface and palpate the conjunctival fornices to rule out any foreign bodies. A complete ophthalmic examination with fluorescein stain should always be performed.

### Treatment

Treatment for an eyelid laceration is a two-layered primary closure. Most lacerations can be repaired standing with proper sedation and local blocks. Sedation with an alpha-2 agonists (xylazine or detomidine) ± acepromazine is sufficient in most patients. An auriculopalpebral nerve block can be performed to immobilize the upper eyelid. Steps for performing an eyelid laceration repair are demonstrated in Figure 16.2. For a fresh laceration, the cut edges should be debrided with a scalpel. If the laceration is chronic, aggressive debridement of any granulation tissue is required. It is important to preserve any eyelid skin and conjunctiva. There are 3 steps to eyelid closure: deep sutures placed in the subcutaneous/orbicularis oculi muscle and not penetrating the conjunctival surface (5–0 polyglactin 910), figure-8 suture (5–0 nylon) at the eyelid margin, and skin sutures (5–0 nylon). The deep sutures should be placed in a horizontal simple interrupted pattern instead of the standard vertical (superficial to deep) pattern. This keeps the suture at one level of depth making it less likely to penetrate the conjunctiva and rub on the corneal surface. The figure-8 suture is used to achieve ideal eyelid margin apposition and should appose only the 5–10 mm closest to the eyelid margin. The remainder of the wound should be closed with simple interrupted or cruciate skin sutures. Adjunctive medical therapy should include the administration of a tetanus toxoid booster, a systemic broad-spectrum antibiotic, and a systemic non-steroidal anti-inflammatory.

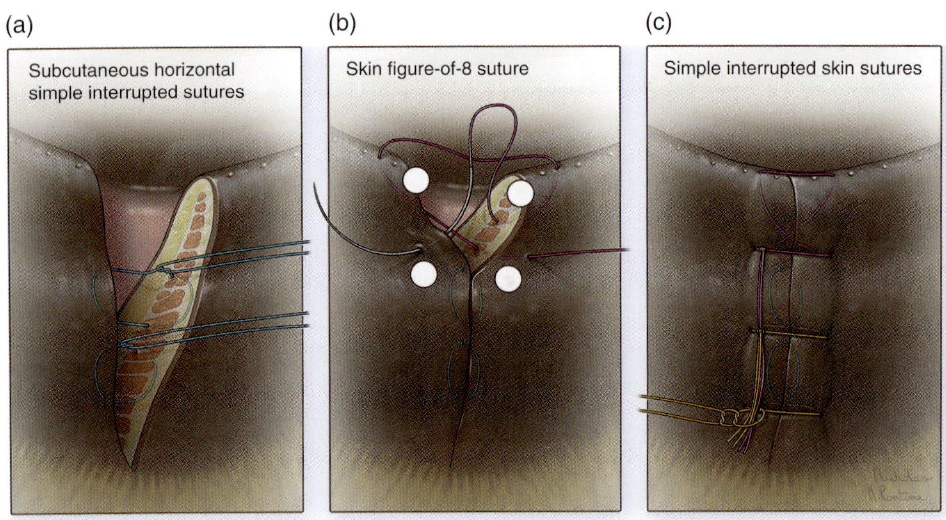


**Figure 16.2** Steps to an eyelid repair. (a) The first step of eyelid laceration repair is placing horizontal simple interrupted sutures within the subcutaneous tissue to appose the two sides of the laceration. It is important that these sutures do not involve the conjunctiva. (b) The second step of eyelid laceration repair is the figure-of-8 suture. This suture is a skin suture and apposes the eyelid margin while keeping the knot and free suture ends away from the corneal surface. (1) The first suture bite is placed through the haired skin ~2 mm away from the cut surface and ~5 mm from the eyelid margin and exits through the cut surface. (2) The second bite enters the cut surface on the opposite side of the laceration and exits near the meibomian gland openings ~2 mm from the cut surface. (3) The third bite enters near the meibomian gland openings on the opposite side and exits through the cut surface. It is very important that the suture involving the meibomian gland openings not be on the conjunctival surface at any point or corneal rubbing will occur. (4) The fourth bite enters the cut surface on the opposite side and exits the skin ~2 mm from the cut surface. Bites 1 and 2 and bites 3 and 4 should be mirror images of each other. It is important when tying to not overtighten. Suture tags are left long to incorporate into the other skin sutures to direct them away from the cornea. (c) Simple interrupted skin sutures are placed to finish the skin closure of the laceration. The prior suture tags are tied into the second knot of each suture to direct the tags away from the eye.

Entropion can be corrected by placing temporary tacking vertical mattress sutures in the affected portion of the eyelid to evert the eyelid margin. If the entire inferior eyelid is affected, 4 sutures are usually needed. If only the temporal margin is affected, fewer sutures can be placed. The first bite of the vertical mattress suture should be taken within 5 mm of the eyelid margin in order to achieve appropriate eversion. Depending on the foal's systemic status, a light sedative may be given, and local subcutaneous line block should be performed. A small, non-absorbable suture material (5–0 nylon) should be used. This will cause minimal tissue reaction and irritation. Permanent correction of eyelid entropion is very rarely indicated in the horse. With either condition, if a corneal ulcer is present, it should be managed, as discussed below in the "Injury to the cornea and sclera" section. To avoid stress on a newly repaired eyelid laceration, placement of an SPL may be warranted. Ideally this would be placed in the unaffected eyelid.

Referral is recommended in cases of eyelid laceration repair dehiscence. It is critical that granulation tissue be adequately debrided prior to re-repair of the laceration to allow for appropriate healing.

## Injury to the Cornea and Sclera

Most injuries to the cornea or sclera present with nonspecific signs of ocular disease: blepharospasm, epiphora, and redness. Dependent on duration and severity, a corneal opacity may be present.

In some cases, an ulcer will be present initially but may heal quickly and trap infection within the cornea resulting in a stromal abscess. This condition is characterized by ocular pain, corneal opacity (white, yellow, pink, or red), and often a secondary uveitis.

### Emergency Stabilization

In the case of a painful and possibly fragile eye, it is ideal to place a protective mask to prevent further injury until diagnostics can be performed. The authors prefer the Equine-Medi Lens® (Intrepid International) which is a firm but flexible half cup or the Recovery Visor (Protective Pet Solutions). These masks do not cause moisture build-up and allow for assessment of ocular comfort without the need to remove the mask. A systemic anti-inflammatory should be (flunixin meglumine 1.1 mg/kg) administered.

### Diagnostic Plan

With a possibly fragile globe, it is important that the horse be sedated and an auriculopalpebral nerve block be performed prior to examination. This reduces pressure on the globe and lessens the chance of further injury. The biggest concern following a globe trauma is iris prolapse. If pressure is applied to a fragile globe this can easily lead to permanent vision loss. A fluorescein stain should always be performed. If a corneal ulcer is present, please refer to the section on "Corneal abrasion and ulceration" below. If there is no stain uptake in a painful eye with a corneal opacity, a stromal abscess should be suspected. Unfortunately, there is no widely available diagnostic to confirm suspicion of a stromal abscess. If there is any concern for a stromal abscess, treatment with topical anti-inflammatories should be avoided.

### Treatment

A full-thickness laceration to the cornea or sclera is a surgical emergency. The sooner the laceration is closed, the better the prognosis for vision. Lacerations through the limbus carry a poor prognosis for vision. Referral should always be recommended in the case of a deep or full-thickness corneal laceration.

Treatment of a stromal abscess should include frequent topical antimicrobials that penetrate intact corneal epithelium. Fungi have an affinity for collagen within the deep stroma and Descemet's membrane, so a fungal etiology is often suspected. From cultured surgical samples of stromal abscesses, fungi have been shown to be the most common organisms (de Linde Henriksen et al. 2014). However, bacteria can also cause a stromal abscesses, so coverage with both a broad-spectrum antibiotic and antifungal is indicated. Medications that penetrate an intact corneal epithelium include chloramphenicol and fluoroquinolones (antibiotics) and voriconazole and DMSO/Itraconazole (antifungals). If the abscess is vascularized, administration of systemic itraconazole (3 mg/kg PO BID, Korenek et al. 1994; Foley and Legendre 1992) or voriconazole (4 mg/kg

PO SID) may be worthwhile. Systemic fluconazole is of little benefit as the drug has limited efficacy against the commonly cultured genera, *Aspergillus* and *Fusarium*. (Brooks et al. 1998; Pearce et al. 2009) Topical atropine should be applied to effect to reduce the chance of posterior synechiae, help stabilize the blood ocular barrier, and improve ocular comfort. Administration of atropine as frequently as every six hours has not been correlated with signs of colic or significant reduction in gastrointestinal motility in normal horses (Ekstrand et al. 2022; Ström et al. 2021; Wehrman et al. 2017).

Stromal abscesses should be referred if they are unresponsive to medical management, refractory to appropriate pain medication, or if miosis persists despite atropine administration. Surgical treatment is often successful, with penetrating lamellar keratoplasty reported to be successful in 98.1% cases and deep lamellar endothelial keratoplasty successful in 89.4% (Brooks et al. 2008). Intrastromal injection with voriconazole may lead to resolution without surgery in refractory cases (Smith et al. 2014; Tsujita and Plummer 2013).

## Corneal Abrasion and Ulceration

Corneal abrasions and ulcers are the most common ophthalmic emergency seen in horses (Brooks 2002). Typical clinical signs associated with corneal ulceration or abrasions are epiphora, blepharospasm, or redness.

### Emergency Stabilization

A corneal ulcer is an emergency in any situation. When an ulcer is suspected, the horse should be examined by a veterinarian as soon as possible to determine appropriate treatment.

### Diagnostic Plan

A corneal ulcer is diagnosed with fluorescein stain. Fluorescein stain is water soluble so is absorbed by the hydrophilic corneal stroma. A corneal abrasion will take up only faint fluorescein stain because some epithelial cell layers remain. A true corneal ulcer will take up fluorescein unless all the stroma is gone and only Descemet's membrane remains. Anytime there is a loss of stroma and no stain uptake, there should be concern for a descemetocele, which is a very deep and fragile corneal ulcer. An underlying cause for the ulcer should always be investigated.

A simple corneal ulcer is one that has no signs of infection (no stromal loss or cellular infiltrate) and has been present for less than seven days. A complicated ulcer has stromal loss, cellular infiltrate, or has been present for longer than seven days. Reflex uveitis (miosis, aqueous flare) is often more severe with infected corneal ulcers.

A complicated corneal ulcer can be present for several reasons: infection, persistent mechanical trauma or exposure, or a nonhealing ulcer. Referral should be offered for the majority of complicated ulcers. A complete ophthalmic examination can help to rule out persistent trauma such as a foreign body or distichiae and ectopic cilia (inappropriate position of hairs). The palpebral conjunctiva and eyelid margin near the ulcer should be examined closely with magnification, as should the bulbar surface of the third eyelid.

The next step should be corneal cytology. This can be performed after applying a topical anesthetic. The blunt edge of a scalpel blade should be held at a 45° angle to the corneal surface and cells can be gathered from the ulcer surface by gently scraping, then spreading the cells on a clean slide. Diff-Quik stain can be used to examine the cells present. The number of neutrophils generally correlates with severity of infection. Type of infection can be determined based on the presence of fungal hyphae or intracellular bacteria (Figure 16.3). Culture and susceptibility should be performed; however, results are often delayed and therefore not helpful in making initial treatment decisions.

If cytology shows no signs of infection and there is no stromal loss nor infiltrate, then a nonhealing ulcer is the most likely diagnosis. A nonhealing ulcer is a diagnosis of exclusion. Mechanical trauma from a foreign body or misplaced hair, or exposure from facial nerve paresis/paralysis must be ruled out to reach this diagnosis. In a nonhealing ulcer, the epithelium does not adhere normally to the underlying stroma. These ulcers are always superficial, generally have mild corneal edema without cellular infiltrate and poor vascular invasion.

### Treatment

Simple corneal ulcers should be treated with a prophylactic broad-spectrum topical antibiotic (neomycin-polymyxin B-bacitracin or Terramycin®). A systemic nonsteroidal anti-inflammatory drug (flunixin meglumine 1.1. mg/kg IV or PO q12-24 h) can be given, and comfort should improve quickly as the ulcer resolves.

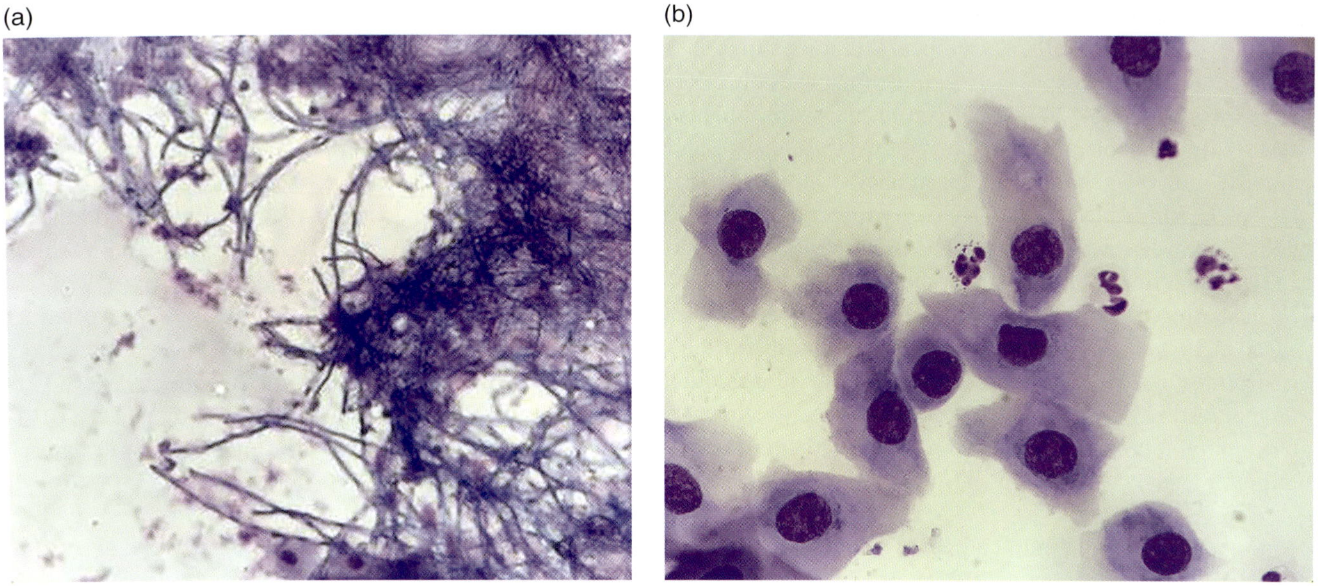


**Figure 16.3** Images of cytology slides collected from corneal ulcers. (a) Large mat of fungal hyphae. (b) Few neutrophils with intracellular cocci surrounded by normal epithelial cells.

Distichiae and ectopic cilia should be treated with cryoepilation, electrocautery, or surgical removal. Treatment can be difficult as it is necessary to destroy or remove the entire hair follicle to prevent regrowth. A foreign body within the conjunctiva can be removed with scissors. Aggressive lavage with sterile saline should be performed after to make sure that all pieces are gone. Facial nerve paralysis should be managed with a partial temporary, split-lid (Divers et al. 2006), or permanent tarsorrhaphy dictated by the underlying cause.

An infected corneal ulcer should be treated with the 5 As (Box 16.3): antibiotic, antifungal, anticollagenase, atropine, and systemic anti-inflammatory (Table 16.1). It is important that a topical anti-inflammatory not be used as they can be delay healing and promote keratomalacia (Flach 2001; Guidera et al. 2001; Hersh et al. 1990; Lin et al. 2000). Due to globe fragility from stromal loss or malacia, placement of an SPL is generally indicated for infected corneal ulcers. SPLs facilitate application of frequent topical medications without manipulation of the eye. Refer to the section on "Subpalpebral Lavage Systems" in the "Advanced Clinical Triage Techniques" chapter (Chapter 5). A guide for medication choices is listed below.

- Topical antibiotics are ideally chosen based on cytology ± culture. For antibiotic choice, if Gram-positive cocci are seen a fluoroquinolone combined with cefazolin is an excellent antimicrobial choice. If Gram-negative rods are seen a fluoroquinolone alone or combined with tobramycin is appropriate (Table 16.1).

**Box 16.3 The 5As for treatment of infected corneal ulcers**

- Antibiotic.
- Antifungal.
- Anticollagenase.
- Atropine.
- (Systemic) Anti-inflammatory.

**Table 16.1** Commonly used antibiotics and their spectrum.

| | |
|---|---|
| Broad spectrum | First line: Triple antibiotic, terramycin<br>Second line: Fluoroquinolones |
| Gram-positive cocci | First line: Triple antibiotic<br>Second line: cefazolin |
| Gram-negative rods | Tobramycin, gentamicin |

- Topical antifungal choice depends on the suspicion for fungal involvement based on clinical appearance, geography, and cytology ± culture results. The clinical literature supports the use of voriconazole as the most effective antifungal for the most commonly seen species in equine fungal keratitis. Recent literature has shown significantly reduced MIC values in vitro for luliconazole in comparison to many antifungals including voriconazole (Roberts et al. 2020). In some areas, DMSO/itraconazole, miconazole, natamycin, and silver sulfadiazine are also good antifungal choices.
- Topical anticollagenases can be applied every 1–4 h based on the severity of keratomalacia. Serum, EDTA, and N-acetylcysteine have anticollagenase properties. Serum has growth factors that may hasten ulcer healing. While EDTA does not have growth factors, it has the benefit of being able to be prepared quickly in the field. Half the volume of an EDTA blood tube is filled with sterile water to create 0.17% EDTA solution that is easy to use in the field.
- Topical atropine frequency should be adjusted based on pupil size. In the author's opinion it can be applied as often as every eight hours. It has been shown that administration of atropine up to every six hours does not have an effect on gastrointestinal motility as assessed by borborygmi frequency and that treatment every six hours followed by every 12 h did not result in evidence of ileus or colic in healthy horses. (Ekstrand et al. 2022; Ström et al. 2021; Wehrman et al. 2017). Once pupil dilation has been achieved, the frequency should be decreased to q12-24 h. Monitoring of the contralateral pupil for evidence of systemic atropinization is indicated.

A nonhealing ulcer should be treated with topical antimicrobials to prevent infection. This includes a broad-spectrum antibiotic (neomycin-polymyxin B-bacitracin or Terramycin) and antifungal (DMSO/itraconazole). Atropine should be applied every 24–72 h as needed to dilate the pupil and improve comfort. A systemic nonsteroidal can be given based on level of discomfort. Unfortunately, appropriate topical treatment alone will not result in proper healing of a nonhealing ulcer. Treatment with a cotton swab debridement can be performed in the field. A recheck should be performed within 5–7 days and if healing remains abnormal, referral for a more aggressive debridement should be offered. Diamond burr debridement has a healing rate of 92% in approximately two weeks (Lassaline-Utter et al. 2014). In cases refractory to diamond burr debridement, a superficial keratectomy is indicated and generally results in healing of the ulcer.

In any case of a corneal ulceration where application of medications is not possible, an SPL should be placed. This can be performed in the field and is described in Chapter 5.

Referral should be strongly advised for any horse that has stromal loss >50%, fibrin or hypopyon within the anterior chamber, or severe miosis (Figure 16.4). Even without these signs, if an ulcer has been present for more than three weeks referral should be strongly considered.

(a) (b)

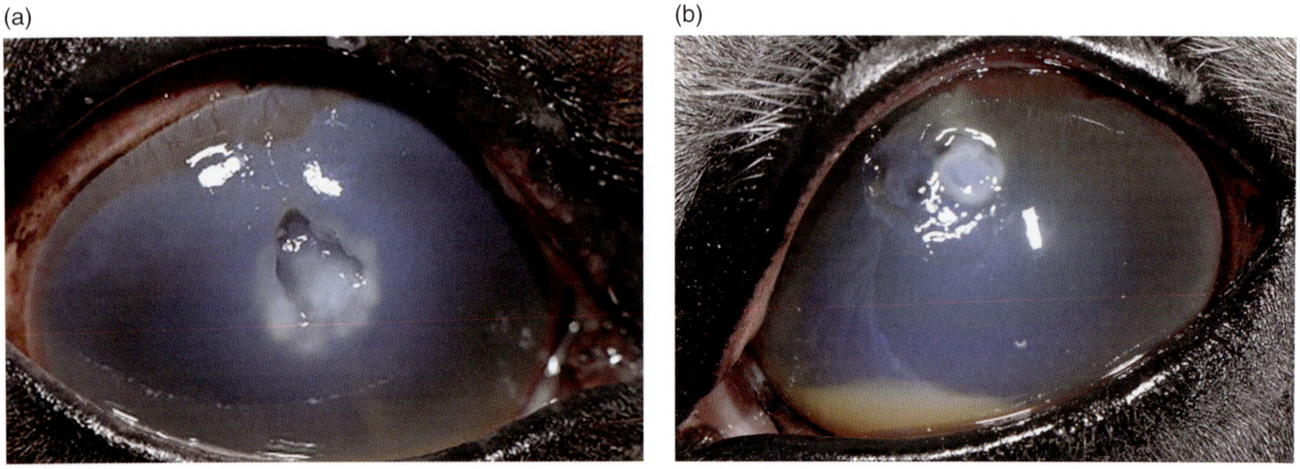

**Figure 16.4** Infected corneal ulcers. (a) Short limbal vessels extending toward an ulcer with >50% stromal loss and cellular infiltrate. (b) A corneal ulcer in the dorsal cornea with stromal loss and cellular infiltrate. Hypopyon can be seen in the anterior chamber.

## Corneal Foreign Bodies

Corneal foreign bodies are usually organic material. Clinical signs seen include blepharospasm, ocular discharge, conjunctival hyperemia, and corneal vascularization. In some cases, corneal foreign bodies are an incidental finding.

### Emergency Stabilization

Pain medication should be given and, if necessary, a protective mask placed to prevent rubbing which may worsen the condition.

### Diagnostic Plan

A sedated ophthalmic examination should be performed to help determine the depth of the corneal foreign body. An auriculopalpebral block should be performed to avoid any pressure applied to the eye until a full-thickness foreign body has been ruled out.

### Treatment

In most cases, superficial foreign bodies can be safely removed with hydropulsion. This is performed with sterile saline or eyewash in a 6-mL syringe attached to a 25-gauge needle with the needle tip removed (Labelle et al. 2014). The syringe is held at a 45° angle and sprayed at the foreign body to dislodge it.

If there is concern that the foreign body penetrates the full thickness of the cornea, referral should recommended. The foreign body may be acting like a seal and manual removal will result in leakage of aqueous humor. In a referral situation, the foreign body can be removed under general anesthesia and the defect can be repaired immediately to reduce complications associated with globe perforation.

## Chemical Injuries

Ocular chemical burns are seemingly uncommon in horses. Associated clinical signs are severe ocular pain, corneal ulceration, corneal edema, and corneal vascularization. Chlorhexidine and other antiseptic scrubs are likely the most common cause of chemical injury to the eyes of horses. Under general anesthesia, scrub from preparation for placement of an arterial catheter or periocular surgical site may get into the eyes. To prevent this severe ocular injury, only dilute betadine solution should be used as an antiseptic around the eye. Fly sprays and other chemical sprays may also lead to ocular surface disease.

### Emergency Stabilization

The first step following chemical exposure to the cornea is copious irrigation with sterile saline. It is important that the fornices are lavaged well to remove all the offending chemical.

### Diagnostic Plan

When a chemical burn is suspected, the owners or veterinary care team should be questioned to try to determine the origin of the exposure. Fluorescein staining should always be performed.

### Treatment

Appropriate corneal ulceration treatment should be started as previously described including topical antimicrobials and atropine. A contact lens can be applied to improve comfort and prevent symblepharon (Christmas 1991). Chemical burns can be incredibly painful. In addition to systemic NSAIDs (flunixin 1.1 mg/kg IV or PO q12h), additional pain management may be needed and may include acetaminophen (20 mg/kg PO q12h) and gabapentin (20 mg/kg PO q8-12h).

Referral should be discussed if pain is not well controlled despite appropriate treatment. Use of a protective mask to prevent rubbing is recommended.

## Anterior Uveitis

Equine Recurrent Uveitis (ERU) is a chronic inflammatory disease that is reported in up to 10% of the equine population. Clinical signs of ERU include blepharoedema, blepharospasm, chemosis, corneal edema, miosis, corneal vascularization, aqueous flare, and anterior chamber fibrin. While ERU is a common cause of anterior uveitis, other etiologies include reflex uveitis, blunt trauma, and underlying systemic infectious disease. Uveitis in foals should always prompt a thorough systemic evaluation, with sepsis and *Rhodococcus equi* infection being the most likely causes in neonates and weanlings, respectively.

### Emergency Stabilization

Systemic and topical anti-inflammatories should be given to reduce intraocular inflammation.

### Diagnostic Plan

A complete ophthalmic examination will help to determine the severity of uveitis and the best treatment plan. Fluorescein stain should always be performed to rule out a corneal ulcer as a cause for the ocular discomfort and inflammation. Ideally, intraocular pressures (IOPs) are measured. Low IOP (<15 mmHg) is typical in horses with uveitis.

All horses with uveitis should undergo a thorough general physical examination and those with evidence of concurrent systemic abnormalities, especially evidence of neurologic disease, should undergo a thorough diagnostic workup.

### Treatment

Treatment of uveitis involves administration of topical and systemic anti-inflammatories. Topical atropine should be given to reduce ciliary spasm and avoid posterior synechiae. Atropine also stabilizes the blood aqueous barrier.

In a severe case of uveitis, systemic flunixin meglumine (1.1 mg/kg IV or PO q12h) and dexamethasone (0.1 mg/kg IV, IM or PO q24h) may be recommended in addition to a topical steroid (neomycin-polymixin B-dexamethasone q12h-q8h) and nonsteroidal medication (0.1% diclofenac q12h-q8h). Atropine should be given as needed for pupil dilation, generally q8-24h. In a mild case of uveitis, the patient may respond to topical medications alone.

Referral should always be offered when uveitis is chronic or recurrent. Options for management of chronic or recurrent uveitis include long-term topical medications, low-dose intravitreal gentamicin, or a suprachoroidal cyclosporine implantation.

## Glaucoma

Glaucoma is a disease that results in vision loss due to loss of retinal ganglion cells. This occurs due to elevated IOP, which is associated with pain. The most common clinical sign of glaucoma in horses is corneal edema. The incidence of glaucoma is reported to be <1%; however, this is likely an underestimation. The majority (~90%) of horses with glaucoma, have glaucoma secondary to ERU (Michau 2017). Risk factors for glaucoma include uveitis, age (>15 years), and breed (Appaloosa) (Curto et al. 2014). Another common cause of glaucoma in horses is secondary to hyphema.

### Emergency Stabilization

For any horse in which glaucoma is suspected, a systemic anti-inflammatory should be administered. Ideally, IOP is evaluated prior to administering pressure reducing medications, though if tonometry is not available then treatment should not be delayed.

### Diagnostic Plan

It is important to determine if the affected eye remains visual, which can be established by assessing the menace response, dazzle reflex, direct/indirect PLR, and ability to navigate obstacles. In any eye with corneal edema, tonometry should be performed. Results are generally similar between the two types of tonometers currently in use (applanation and rebound); however, there is less inter- and intra-user variation with the rebound tonometer (Lewin et al. 2020). Normal IOP in a horse is reported to be 15–30 mmHg (Dwyer 2021). It is important to remember that in an eye with active uveitis the pressure should be low. An eye with aqueous flare and an IOP of 25 mmHg is abnormal and should be treated for both uveitis and secondary glaucoma. Fluorescein staining should always be performed as a cornea with edema is more prone to corneal ulcers.

### Treatment

In an eye with glaucoma, treatment for both uveitis and glaucoma should be initiated. For uveitis treatment, please refer to the section “Anterior uveitis” above. Of note, atropine is generally contraindicated in glaucoma due to the potential for mydriasis and cycloplegia to result in an acute rise in IOP. Initial management of IOP should be with the ophthalmic anti-glaucoma medication combination dorzolamide/timolol ophthalmic solution (or compounded ointment) q12h. Dorzolamide and timolol work synergistically to reduce the production of aqueous humor, and this is currently the most effective anti-glaucoma medication for horses (Michau 2017). Ideally, IOP is monitored during treatment to ensure the desired response. The choice of topical anti-inflammatory depends on the severity of corneal edema present. While appropriate to use a topical steroid (neomycin-polymixin B-dexamethasone) on a mildly edematous cornea, a cornea with more significant edema is likely to develop corneal bullae and subsequent corneal ulceration. In these cases, a topical NSAID (0.1% diclofenac) is a safer choice.

If the horse does not respond to medical management, trans-scleral cyclophotocoagulation (TSCP) can be considered. In this procedure, laser energy is used to damage the ciliary body and reduce aqueous production. At four years after TSCP, 59% of horses for which there was follow-up remained visual (Annear et al. 2010). Anecdotally, a better response is noted when TCSP is performed early in the disease process.

Glaucoma is diagnosed and monitored with tonometry. For that reason, if tonometry is unavailable in the field, referral is indicated. Medical treatment is generally life-long, and enucleation should be recommended for non-sighted eyes.

## Acute Blindness

Blindness is often first noted when a horse begins to bump into things. It is important to remember that this does not mean that vision was normal prior to this moment. Horses do an excellent job at compensating for poor vision until all vision is lost.

### Emergency Stabilization

The most important first step is to ensure that the blind horse and all handlers are safe. A padded stall free of anything loose on the ground is ideal. If the horse remains anxious, trazodone (2.5–10 μg/kg PO q12h) is an excellent anxiolytic. Infectious and potentially transmissible causes of chorioretinitis and encephalitis resulting in blindness (including equine herpesvirus type 1) should be considered, and appropriate precautions taken until ruled out. Most reversible causes of blindness will be improved with systemic anti-inflammatories. Systemic dexamethasone (0.1 mg/kg IV q24h) is a good choice so long as the horse is not predisposed to laminitis.

### Diagnostic Plan

To try to determine the cause of blindness, thorough neuro-ophthalmic and ophthalmic examinations should be performed. Reasons for visual impairment or blindness can include opacity of the cornea, aqueous humor, or lens, retinal detachment or degeneration, optic nerve damage, and cortical disease. It is rare that the cornea or anterior chamber become opaque

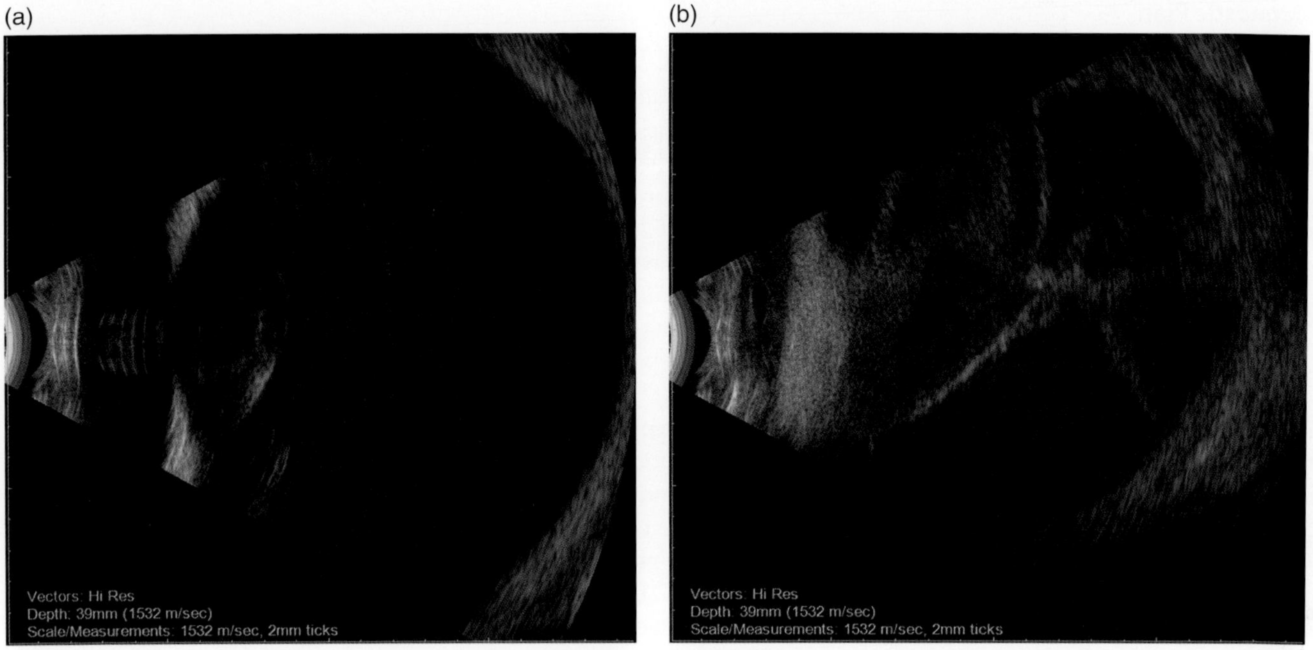


**Figure 16.5** Ultrasound images obtained with a 20 MHz probe of an equine eye with a normal posterior segment (a) and an eye with a retinal detachment (arrowheads) as well as vitreous and subretinal opacities (b).

enough to cause complete blindness. Even an advanced cataract will allow for some degree of light transmission and therefore maintenance of the dazzle reflex and PLRs. Blindness resulting in an absent menace response, dazzle reflex and PLR, is most often caused by abnormalities of the retina, optic nerve, optic chiasm, or brain. An absent dazzle and dilated pupil are very poor prognostic indicators for vision (Dwyer 2021; Millichamp 1992).

Ultrasound can be used to evaluate the position of the retina if it cannot be seen with ophthalmoscopy. Transpalpebral or transcorneal ultrasound can be performed with a linear or microconvex probe at a depth of 4–5 cm (Hallowell and Bowen 2007). Retinal detachment may be difficult to confirm in some cases as the detached retina may be obscured by vitreal opacities. The ultrasonographic appearance of retinal detachment is most often characterized by the classic "seagull sign" (Figure 16.5), in which the retina only remains attached at the optic nerve and ora ciliaris retinae. If the retina is torn and detached, it may not have this classic appearance and may appear more disorganized.

The optic nerve head can be seen with ophthalmoscopy unless the more anterior structures are too opaque. With acute injury, the optic nerve head can look hyperemic and swollen. With more chronic damage, the optic nerve is pale and atrophied. To investigate the entirety of the optic nerve, chiasm, tracts, and brain, advanced imaging is needed (CT or more ideally, MRI). A differential for acute blindness with fixed bilateral mydriasis in older horses is a pituitary tumor compressing the optic chiasm. (Wallace et al. 1996).

## Treatment

Treatment for acute blindness depends on the underlying cause. Acute retinal detachment may respond to aggressive systemic anti-inflammatory treatment. One of the authors has seen vision return as long as two weeks after sudden onset of blindness due to retinal detachment. In the case of optic nerve injury resulting in blindness and mydriasis, the prognosis for return of vision is grave.

Acute blindness is a time-sensitive condition, and referral is recommended in the early stages to attempt to obtain a diagnosis and initiate appropriate treatment.

**Case Example 16.1 Corneal Injury**

**Ocular Emergency**

Presenting complaint: The horse was noted to have squinting and tearing of the left eye the evening prior. No treatments were administered prior to calling the veterinarian.

*Ophthalmic Examination*

When observed from a distance, the left eye was held ~50% open, moderate epiphora was present, and moderate blepharedema of the upper and lower eyelids (Figure 16.6). There were no signs of globe rupture and palpation around the globe was within normal limits. Due to the presence of moderate ocular pain sedation was given (xylazine 0.3 mg/kg IV).

Once the horse was sedated, the complete ophthalmic examination was performed. Moderate hyperemia and chemosis were present. A superficial corneal opacity was seen in the axial cornea that was horizontally elongated (~15 × 5mm) and surrounded by loose epithelial edges. Moderate corneal edema was associated with the opacity. No corneal vessels were seen. The pupil was mildly miotic. Fluorescein stain was applied and confirmed a corneal ulceration.

Problem: Complicated corneal ulcer
Differentials: Infected ulcer, nonhealing ulcer, persistent trauma to cornea

*Diagnostics*

An auriculopalpebral block was performed and topical proparacaine was applied to the cornea. The blunt edge of a blade was used to collect corneal cytology. This revealed few neutrophils but no infectious agents. A dry cotton swab was used to remove the loose epithelial edges. Since no treatment has been administered culture was not performed at this time.

Problem: Infected corneal ulcer

*Treatment*

The horse was difficult to administer medications to, so a subpalpebral lavage was placed in the inferior eyelid after anesthetizing the lower eyelid. Medications (0.1 mL) were given via SPL waiting five minutes between.

- Topical antibiotic: Ofloxacin q4h.
- Topical antifungal: Voriconazole q4h.
- Topical anticollagenase: Serum q4h.
- Topical atropine: q12h.
- Oral anti-inflammatory: Flunixin meglumine 1.1 mg/kg q12h, tapering dose.

Reevaluate in 3–5 days as long as comfort continues to improve.

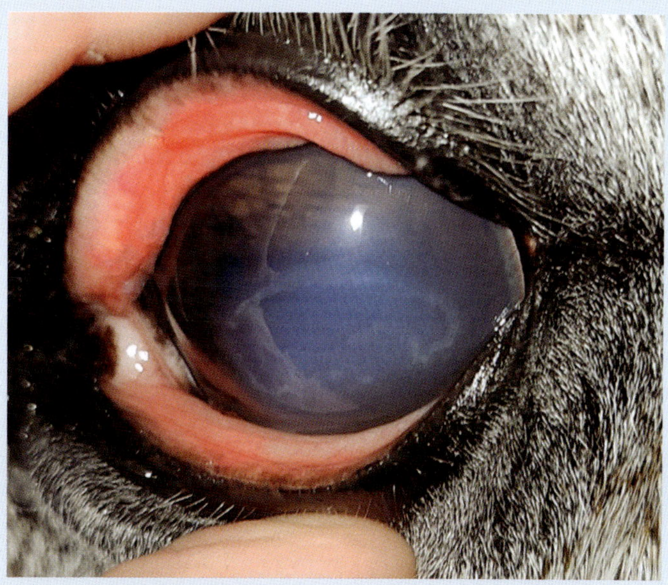

**Figure 16.6** Horse presenting with a history of squinting and tearing of the left eye. Examination revealed moderate ocular pain, epiphora and blepharedema as well as superficial corneal opacity. A corneal ulcer was diagnosed and treated.

## References

Annear, M.J., Wilkie, D.A., and Gemensky-Metzler, A.J. (2010). Semiconductor diode laser transscleral cyclophotocoagulation for the treatment of glaucoma in horses: a retrospective study of 42 eyes. *Vet. Ophthalmol.* 13 (3): 204–209. https://doi.org/10.1111/j.1463-5224.2010.00779.x. PMID: 20500721.

Brooks, D.E. (2002). Equine ophthalmology. *AAEP Proceedings*, 48, p 300–313.

Brooks, D.E., Andrew, S.E., Dillavou, C.L. et al. (1998). Antimicrobial susceptibility patterns of fungi isolated from horses with ulcerative keratomycosis. *Am. J. Vet. Res.* 59: 138–142.

Brooks, D.E., Plummer, C.E., Kallberg, M.E. et al. (2008). Corneal transplantation for inflammatory keratopathies in the horse: visual outcome in 206 cases (1993–2007). *Vet. Ophthalmol.* 11: 123–133.

Caron, J.P., Barber, S.M., Bailey, J.V. et al. (1986). Periorbital skull fractures in five horses. *J. Am. Vet. Med. Assoc.* 188: 280–284.

Christmas, R. (1991). Management of chemical burns of the canine cornea. *Can. Vet. J.* 32: 608–612.

Curto, E.M., Gemensky-Metzler, A.J., Chandler, H.L., and Wilkie, D.A. (2014). Equine glaucoma: a histopathologic retrospective study (1999–2012). *Vet. Ophthalmol.* 17: 334–342.

Cutler, T.J., Brooks, D.E., Andrew, S.E. et al. (2000). Disease of the equine posterior segment. *Vet. Ophthalmol.* 3: 73–82.

Dallap Schaer, B. (2007). Ophthalmic emergencies in horses. *Vet. Clin. N. Am. Equine Pract.* 23: 49–65.

Divers, T.J., Ducharme, N.G., De Lahunta, A. et al. (2006). Temporohyoid osteoarthropathy. *Clin. Tech. Equine Pract.* 5: 17–23.

Dwyer, A. (2021). Ophthalmic emergencies in the field. *Vet. Clin. N. Am. Equine Pract.* 37: 441–460.

Ekstrand, C. et al. (2022). Plasma atropine concentrations associated with decreased intestinal motility in horses. *Front Vet. Sci.* 9: 1–11.

Flach, A.J. (2001). Corneal melts associated with topically applied nonsteroidal anti-inflammatory drugs. *Trans. Am. Ophthalmol. Soc.* 99: 205.

Foley, J.P. and Legendre, A.M. (1992). Treatment of coccidioidomycosis osteomyelitis with ltraconazole in a horse: a brief report. *J. Vet. Intern. Med.* 6: 333–334.

Gelatt, K.N., Gum, G.G., and Mackay, E. (1995). Evaluation of mydriatics in horses. *Vet. Comp. Ophthalmol.* 5: 104–107.

Gerding, J.C., Clode, A., Gilger, B.C., and Montgomery, K.W. (2014). Equine orbital fractures: a review of 18 cases (2006–2013). *Vet. Ophthalmol.* 1–10.

Gilger, B.C. (2010). Diseases and surgery of the globe and orbit. In: *Equine Ophthalmology*, 2e (ed. B.C. Gilger), 93–132. St. Louis: Elsevier Science.

Guidera, A.C., Luchs, J.I., and Udell, I.J. (2001). Keratitis, ulceration, and perforation associated with topical nonsteroidal anti-inflammatory drugs. *Ophthalmology* 108: 936–944.

Hallowell, G.D. and Bowen, I.M. (2007). Practical ultrasonography of the equine eye. *Equine Vet. Edu.* 19: 600–605.

Hersh, P.S., Rice, B.A., Baer, J.C. et al. (1990). Topical nonsteroidal agents and corneal wound healing. *Arch. Ophthalmol.* 108: 577–583.

Hubert, J. (1996). What is your diagnosis? Chronic retrobulbar abscess in a horse. *J. Am. Vet. Med. Assoc.* 209: 1703–1704.

Joss, R. (2019). The risk of a shod and unshod horse kick to create orbital fractures in equine cadaveric skulls. *ZORA* 1–25.

Korenek, N.L., Legendre, A.M., Andrews, F.M. et al. (1994). Treatment of mycotic rhinitis with itraconazole in three horses. *J. Vet. Intern. Med.* 8: 224–227.

Labelle, A.L., Psutka, K., Collins, S.P., and Hamor, R.E. (2014). Use of hydropulsion for the treatment of superficial corneal foreign bodies: 15 cases (1999–2013). *J. Am. Vet. Med. Assoc.* 244: 476–479.

Lassaline-Utter, M., Cutler, T.J., Michau, T.M., and Nunnery, C.M. (2014). Treatment of nonhealing corneal ulcers in 60 horses with diamond burr debridement (2010–2013). *Vet. Ophthalmol.* 1: 76–81.

Lewin, A.C., Liu, C.C., Camacho-Luna, P. et al. (2020). Inter-user and intra-user variation of two tonometers in horses. *Equine Vet. J.* 55: 572–576.

Lin, J.C., Rapuano, C.J., Laibson, P.R. et al. (2000). Corneal melting associated with use of topical nonsteroidal anti-inflammatory drugs after ocular surgery. *Arch. Ophthalmol.* 118: 1129–1132.

de Linde Henriksen, M., Andersen, P.H., Mietelka, K. et al. (2014). Equine deep stromal abscesses (51 cases – 2004–2009)–Part 2: the histopathology and immunohistochemical aspect with attention to the histopathologic diagnosis, vascular response, and infectious agents. *Vet. Ophthalmol.* 17: 1–22.

McKinney, R.A. (2021). The retrobulbar block: a review of techniques used and reported complications. *Equine Vet. Educ.* 33: 332–336.

Merritt, A.M., Burrow, J.A., and Hartless, C.S. (1998). Effect of xylazine, detomidine, and a combination of xylazine and butorphanol on equine duodenal motility. *Am. J. Vet. Res.* 59: 619–623.

Michau, T.M. (2017). Equine glaucoma. *Vet. Clin. North Am. Equine Pract.* 33: 519–540.

Millichamp, N.J. (1992). Ocular trauma. *Vet. Clin. N. Am. Equine Pract.* 8 (3): 521–536.

Pearce, J.W., Giuliano, E.A., and Moore, C.P. (2009). In vitro susceptibility patterns of aspergillus and fusarium species isolated from equine ulcerative keratomycosis cases in the midwestern and southern United States with inclusion of the new antifungal agent voriconazole. *Vet. Ophthalmol.* 12: 318–324.

Pucket, J.D., Allbaugh, R.A., Rankin, A.J. et al. (2013). Comparison of efficacy and duration of effect on corneal sensitivity among anesthetic agents following ocular administration in clinically normal horses. *Am. J. Vet. Res.* 74: 459–464.

Ragle, C.A. (1993). Head trauma. *Vet. Clin. N. Am. Equine Pract.* 9: 171–183.

Roberts, D., Cotter, H.V.T., Cubeta, M., and Gilger, B.C. (2020). In vitro susceptibility of Aspergillus and Fusarium associated with equine keratitis to new antifungal drugs. *Vet. Ophthalmol.* 23 (5): 918–922.

Sharrow-Reabe, K.L. and Townsend, W.M. (2012). Effects of action of proparacaine and tetracaine topical ophthalmic formulations on corneal sensitivity in horses. *J. Am Vet. Med.* 241: 1645–1649.

Smith, K.M., Pucket, J.D., and Gilmour, M.A. (2014). Treatment of six cases of equine corneal stromal abscessation with intracorneal injection of 5% voriconazole solution. *Vet. Ophthalmol.* 17: 79–85.

Ström, L., Dalin, F., Domberg, M. et al. (2021). Topical ophthalmic atropine in horses, pharmacokinetics and effect on intestinal motility. *BMC Vet. Res.* 17: 1–13.

Thibault, C.J., Wilson, D.V., Robertson, S.A. et al. (2019). A retrospective study of fecal output and postprocedure colic in 246 horses undergoing standing sedation with detomidine, or general anesthesia with or without detomidine. *Vet. Anaesth. Analg.* 46: 458–465.

Tsujita, H. and Plummer, C.E. (2013). Corneal stromal abscessation in two horses treated with intracorneal and subconjunctival injection of 1% voriconazole solution. *Vet. Ophthalmol.* 16: 451–458.

Wallace, M.A., Crisman, M.V., Pickett, J.P. et al. (1996). Central blindness associated with a pituitary adenoma in a horse. *Equine Pract.*

Wehrman, R.F., Gemensky-Metzler, A.J., Zibura, A.E. et al. (2017). Objective evaluation of the systemic effects of topical application of 1% atropine sulfate ophthalmic solution in healthy horses. *J. Am. Vet. Med. Assoc.* 251: 1324–1330.

# Part 3

## Specific Problems in Horses and Donkeys

# 17

# Infectious Disease and Biosecurity

*Brandy A. Burgess*

*Department of Population Health, College of Veterinary Medicine, University of Georgia, Athens, GA, USA*

## Zoonotic and Contagious Diseases of the Horse

Exposure to zoonotic and contagious diseases is an eventuality for all equine practitioners. Not only are almost two-thirds of the 1,400 plus infectious human pathogens zoonotic, but so too are nearly three-quarters of newly emerging or re-emerging infectious agents (Taylor et al. 2001). If we want to stop the cycle of transmission, then we need to disrupt the chain of infection (Figure 17.1). While this chain can be broken at any of the six links (pathogen, reservoir, portal of exit, mode of transmission, portal of entry, susceptible host), during emergent situations, we tend to implement strategies targeting the likely mode of transmission (Table 17.1). Fortunately, these prevention efforts can effectively mitigate transmission risks for multiple potential pathogens, even without a microbiological diagnosis.

### Common Modes of Transmission

In general, modes of transmission can be categorized as (i) contact transmission (direct or indirect), (ii) airborne transmission (aerosol or droplet), or (iii) vector-borne transmission.

1) *Contact transmission* can occur by *direct* physical contact or *indirectly* by a *vehicle* or *fomite*. Common vehicles may include blood products, feed/water, urine/feces, or even people with contaminated clothing or hands; and common fomites may include common use equipment such as stethoscopes, keyboards, and cleaning equipment. Prevention efforts to decrease direct contact transmission may include separating individuals and/or using barrier nursing precautions; the addition of hand hygiene and the use of dedicated equipment can further decrease the likelihood for indirect transmission. Salmonellosis is a common infectious disease in horses that is considered contact transmitted (via the fecal–oral route) and may be effectively managed using contact (barrier nursing) precautions.
2) *Airborne transmission* can occur via *aerosols* (particles less than 100 μm in diameter that may remain airborne for a period of time) or *droplets* (larger particles that may travel up to 2 m) generated during coughing, sneezing, and vocalizing, or while performing some diagnostic procedures (e.g., bandage changes, wound irrigation, endoscopy). Prevention efforts to decrease aerosol transmission may include patient isolation (i.e., housing a patient in its own air space) or at least housing at a significant distance from others; while prevention of droplet transmission may include the use of barrier nursing precautions and segregation relative to patient housing and while performing diagnostic or treatment procedures. Equine influenza is a common equine pathogen that is considered airborne transmitted, spreading rapidly through a barn as coughing horses generate both aerosols and droplets.
3) *Vector-borne transmission* can occur when *invertebrates* (e.g., flies, ticks, mosquitos) transmit a potential pathogen. Prevention efforts to decrease this transmission route may include an insect/tick control program and ensuring facilities have no standing water. Vesicular stomatitis, considered to be transmitted by arthropod vectors (e.g., sand flies and black flies), causes disease seasonally among horses in some regions and may be controlled through effective vector management programs.

*Emergency Triage of the Horse*, First Edition. Edited by Rolfe M. Radcliffe and Jamie J. Kopper.

Companion website: www.wiley.com/go/radcliffe/triage

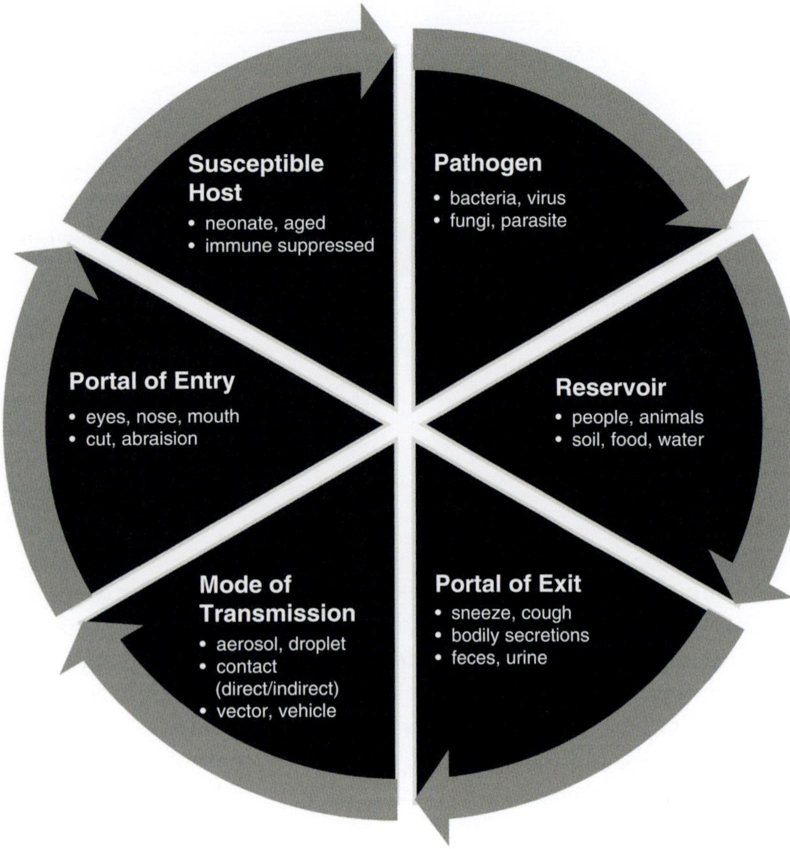


**Figure 17.1** Chain of infection.

**Table 17.1** Standard and transmission-based precautions.

| Standard precautions | Airborne transmission precautions (in addition to standard precautions) |
|---|---|
| • Hand washing (or use of alcohol-based hand rub) after touching potentially contaminated materials<br>• Wearing gloves (as appropriate)<br>• Protect mucous membranes from splashes/sprays<br>• Mask and eye protection<br>• Face shield<br>• Wear protective outerwear (e.g., coveralls, barrier gown)<br>• Care when handling potentially contaminated equipment and linens/towels/halters/lead ropes<br>• Routinely C&D surfaces | **Aerosol transmission precautions**<br>• Airway protection (N95 [requires fit-testing] or PAPR)<br>• Head covering (e.g., bouffant cap)<br>• Isolate patient in negative pressure stall<br>**Droplet transmission precautions**<br>• Wear mask and eye protection or face shield within 3 feet<br>• Impervious barrier gown<br>• Head covering (e.g., bouffant cap)<br>• Segregate patient from healthy/susceptible animals<br>**Contact transmission precautions *(barrier nursing precautions)***<br>• Hand hygiene and gloves<br>• Barrier gown<br>• Footwear covering and/or footwear hygiene<br>• Segregate patient from healthy/susceptible animals<br>• Dedicated equipment (if possible) |

*Source:* Keim and Kaufmann (1999) and Williams et al. (2015).

### Risk Assessment

It is generally recommended to employ standard precautions at all times. However, additional precautions should be utilized based on the likely mode of transmission (as indicated above; see Table 17.1) and while taking stock of the risk for transmission. In other words, perform a risk assessment by considering the agent's prevalence in your practice region (how likely is it to be encountered), the agent's infectiousness (how likely is it to be transmitted), and the consequences of infection (what is the outcome of infection).

Simply put, when you encounter a patient with a potentially infectious and/or zoonotic disease, consider the following:

$$\text{Risk} = \text{Prevalence} \times \text{Infectiousness} \times \text{Consequences}$$

While we can come to a common understanding of an agent's infectiousness and consequences of infection in people and animals, the prevalence will vary by region, season, and over time. See Table 17.2 for a place to start with a risk assessment. Note that agent prevalence is not included in the table as this will vary and is incumbent on the practitioner to be aware of trends in their practice region in a given season or time period.

## Managing Infectious Diseases

The management of infectious diseases in populations is operationalized through the development and implementation of an infection control program (ICP). An ICP comprises all strategies employed to reduce the likelihood of the introduction and transmission of a potential pathogen into and within a premises, facility, or population. It is important to note that each premises or facility is unique in its design, animal population, and level of risk aversion, and that this may change over time. As such, it is important to focus prevention efforts on defined programmatic activities with the goal of reducing rates of adverse outcomes (e.g., healthcare-associated infections) within a facility rather than stipulating practices that must be implemented (e.g., use of footbaths/mats) (Morley et al. 2013). So, while there is a recognized standard of practice relative to infection prevention efforts, specific programmatic activities will necessarily vary by premises/facility. With this in mind, experts have identified key areas for the development and implementation of programmatic activities including (i) managing patient contact, (ii) personal and environmental hygiene, (iii) surveillance, and (iv) education and awareness of personnel (Morley et al. 2013).

### Managing Patient Contact

There are many strategies that can be used to decrease patient contact (both direct and indirect) including (but not limited to) the use of barrier nursing precautions, movement restrictions, and separation or isolation.

1) *Barrier nursing precautions* refers to the use of personal protective equipment/PPE (i.e., disposable gowns, gloves, facial protection), and implementation of footwear hygiene (i.e., footwear covers or use of footbaths or footmats) to create a "barrier" between "clean" and "dirty" (see Table 17.3). Unfortunately, regardless of the PPE used, barrier nursing is difficult to do well with an estimated PPE contamination rate ranging from 25 to 100% (Verbeek et al. 2016). Therefore, there needs to be an investment in time to properly don and doff and to educate personnel on "how" to properly don and doff and "why" it's important, as well as ready access to appropriate PPE. Done well, barrier nursing can decrease the likelihood for transmission of an infectious agent from patient to patient as well as between patients and personnel (or vice versa).
2) *Movement restrictions* are intended to manage the traffic flow of patients and personnel to minimize the potential for contact between infectious disease suspects and the generally healthy patient population. Largely, traffic flow should run from clean to dirty areas and from low to high pathogen risk areas. In addition, time spent in common use areas, such as treatment and diagnostic spaces, should be minimized.
3) *Separation* refers to hospital or facility areas with infection control practices that create separation between high-risk patients or patient groups. Consideration should be given to a patient's immune status and its severity of disease when establishing these. For example, protocols may differ in housing units for adults versus neonates, critical care versus elective surgery patients, infectious versus non-infectious patients, or for hospitalized (inpatients) versus non-hospitalized (outpatients). Note that the ability of a facility to achieve separation is contingent on the physical and operational limitations of the facility and its available resources. Some facilities may have equipment and/or personnel dedicated to these areas to decrease the likelihood for cross-contamination.

**Table 17.2** Contagious and zoonotic disease matrix of equine pathogens.

| **Contagious and zoonotic disease matrix of equine pathogens** | | **Risk assessment** | | | | | | |
|---|---|---|---|---|---|---|---|---|
| **Syndrome** | **Agent/disease** | **Mode of infection** | **Zoonotic disease potential** | **Infection risk to people** | **Consequences in people** | **Infection risk to horses** | **Consequences in horses** | **Environmental persistence** |
| Gastrointe stinal | Anthrax (*Bacillus anthracis*) | A, C | X | H | H | L | H | H |
| | Campylobacteriosis (*C. coli, C jejun*) | C | X | M | M | L | M | L |
| | *Clostridium difficile* | O | X | H | M | L | M | H |
| | *Clostridium perfringens* | O | X | L | M | L | M | H |
| | Coronavirus (not infectious between most host spp) | R, O | | | | H | L | L |
| | *Cryptosporidium* (not all biotypes are zoonotic) | O | X | H | M | H | M | H |
| | Equine coronavirus | R, O | | | | H | M | L |
| | *Giardia* spp. (not all biotypes are zoonotic) | O | X | L | M | L | M | L |
| | Rotavirus (not infectious between most host spp.) | O | | | | M | M | H |
| | Salmonellosis (*Salmonella enterica*) | O | X | M | M | H | M | M |
| Respiratory | Anthrax (Bacillus anthracis) | R, C | X | H | H | L | H | H |
| | *Bordetella bronchiseptica* | R | X | L | L | | | L |
| | *Chlamydophilla psittici* | R | X | M | H | L | H | L |
| | Equine Viral Arteritis | R, C | | | | | | L |
| | Equine Herpesvirus (Type 1 or 4) | R | | | | | | L |
| | Equine Influenza Virus | R | X | L | L | | | L |
| | Hendra virus (Equine morbillivirus) | C, R | X | H | H | H | H | M |
| | *Rhodococcus equi* | R. O | X | L | L | | | L |
| | Strangles (*Streptococcus equi equi*) | R | | | | | | M |
| | Tuberculosis (*Mycobacterium tuberculosis, M. Bovis*) | R, O, C | X | L | H | | | H |

| Recommended precautions[a] | | | | | | | | Nationally notifiable | |
|---|---|---|---|---|---|---|---|---|---|
| Bite/ scratch concern | Human pregnancy concern | Isolation recommended | Face shield recommended | Respiratory protection | Barrier nursing and special | Attention to environmental | Hygiene recommended | Human cases | Animal cases |
| | | X | | X | X | | | X | X |
| | X | X | X | | X | | | | |
| | | X[a] | X[a] | | X[a] | | | | |
| | | | | | X[a] | | | | |
| | | | | | X[a] | | | | |
| | | X[a] | X[a] | | X[a] | | | X | |
| | | | X | | X | | | X | |
| | | | | | X[a] | | | | |
| | | X | X | | X | | | X | X[c] |
| | | X | | X | X | | | X | X |
| | | X | | | X | | | | |
| | X | X | X | | X | | | | X |
| | | X | | | X | | | | X |
| | | X | | | X | | | | X[d] |
| | | X | | | X | | | | |
| | | X | X | | X | | | X | X |
| | | | | | gloves | | | | |
| | | X | | | X | | | | |
| | | X | | X | X | | | X | X |

*(Continued)*

**Table 17.2** (Continued)

| **Contagious and zoonotic disease matrix of equine pathogens** | | **Risk assessment** | | | | | | |
|---|---|---|---|---|---|---|---|---|
| **Syndrome** | **Agent/disease** | **Mode of infection** | **Zoonotic disease potential** | **Infection risk to people** | **Consequences in people** | **Infection risk to horses** | **Consequences in horses** | **Environmental persistence** |
| Skin and soft tissue infections (including surgical site infections) | *Corynebacterium pseudotuberculosis* | C, V | X | L | L | | | H |
| | *Dermatophilus congolensis* | C | X | L | L | | | L |
| | Dermatophytosis (ringworm; Trichophyton spp, Microsporum spp.) (ringworm; *Trichophyton* spp, *Microsporum* spp.) | C | X | H | L | | | M |
| | Multi-drug resistant bacteria | R, O, C | X | M | | | | var |
| | Methicilin-resistant *Staphylococcus aureus* | C | X | M | M | | | L |
| | Methicilin-resistant *Staphylococcus pseudintermedius* | C | | | | | | L |
| | Sporotrichosis (*Sporathrix schenckii*) | C | X | L | M | | | M |
| | Lice and mites | C | X | M | L | | | L |
| Lymph node and other abscesses | *Corynebacterium pseudotuberculosis* | C, V | X | L | L | | | H |
| | Strangles (*Streptococcus equi equi*) | R | | | | | | M |
| | Sporotrichosis (*Sporothrix schenckii*) | C | X | L | M | | | M |
| Fever of unknown origin | Equine Herpesvirus (Type 1 or 4) | R | | | | | | L |
| | Equine Infectious Anemia | V | | | | | | L |
| | Equine Influenza Virus | R | | L | L | | | L |
| | Strangles (*Streptococcus equi equi*) | R | | | | | | M |
| Neurologic | Equine Herpesvirus (Type 1) | R | | | | | | L |
| | Listeriosis (*Listeria monocytogenes*) | R, O, C | X | M | H | | | L |
| | Rabies (rabies virus, Iyssavirus) | R, C | X | M | H | | | L |
| Urinary | Leptosprosis (*Leptospira* spp.) | O | X | M | M | | | L |
| | Multi-drug resistant bacteria | R, O, C | | | | | | var |

| Recommended precautions[a] | | | | | | | | Nationally notifiable | |
|---|---|---|---|---|---|---|---|---|---|
| Bite/ scratch concern | Human pregnancy concern | Isolation recommended | Face shield recommended | Respiratory protection | Barrier nursing and special | Attention to environmental | Hygiene recommended | Human cases | Animal cases |
| | | | | | X | | | | |
| | | | | | gloves | | | | |
| | | | | | gloves | | | | |
| | | | | | | | | | |
| | | | | | | | | | |
| | | var | | | X | | | | |
| | | X | | | X | | | | |
| | | | | | X | | | | |
| X | | | | | gloves | | | | |
| | | | | | X | | | | |
| | | X | | | X | | | | |
| X | | | | | X | | | | |
| | | X | | | X | | | | X[d] |
| | | X | | | | | | | X |
| | | X | | | X | | | | |
| | | X | | | X | | | | |
| | | X | | | X | | | | X[d] |
| | X | X | X | | X | | | | |
| X[b] | | X | | | X | | | | X |
| | X | X | X | | X | | | | |
| | | var | | | X | | | | |

(*Continued*)

**Table 17.2** (Continued)

| Contagious and zoonotic disease matrix of equine pathogens | | Risk assessment | | | | | | |
|---|---|---|---|---|---|---|---|---|
| **Syndrome** | **Agent/disease** | **Mode of infection** | **Zoonotic disease potential** | **Infection risk to people** | **Consequences in people** | **Infection risk to horses** | **Consequences in horses** | **Environmental persistence** |
| Abortion | Brucellosis (*Brucella abortus, B. suis*) | R, O, C | $X_g$ | M | H | | | L |
| | Psittacosis (*Chlamydophila psittaci*) | R | X | M | H | | | L |
| | Equine Herpesvirus (Type 1) | R | | | | | | L |
| | Equine Viral Arteritis | R, C | | | | | | L |
| | Leptospirosis (*Leptospira* spp.) | O | X | M | M | | | L |
| | Listeriosis (*Listeria monocytogenes*) | R, O, C | X | M | H | | | L |
| Oral ulcer/erosion | Vesicular Stomatitis | V | X | L | L | M | L | L |
| Other | Anthrax (*Bacillus anthracis*) | R, C | X | H | H | | | H |
| | Equine infectious anemia | V | | | | | | L |
| | Listeriosis (*Listeria monocytogenes*) | R, O, C | X | M | H | | | L |
| | Multi-drug resistant bacteria | R, O, C | | | | | | var |

[a] Immune compromised people should always take greater precautions, as they are susceptible to infections that the general population is not.

**Subscripts**

$X_a$ = Primary concern is for patients with clinical disease though others shed agent

$X_b$ = Bite hazard

$X_c$ = Only serotypes Gallinarum-Pullorum and Enteritidis

$X_d$ = Only EHV-1 cases with neurological disease are reportable

**Infection risk to people**

L = Low likelihood

M = Moderate

H = Highly infectious

**Infection consequences in people**

L = Low

M = Moderate

H = High consequences

var = variable

**Route of infection**

A = Aerosol

D = Droplet

C = Contact

V = Vector

**Environmental persistence**

L = Low persistence, easily deactivated

M = Moderate

H = Highly persistent/stable

var = variable

**Created by**: Brandy A. Burgess, DVM, MSC, PhD, DACVIM, DACVPM
Paul S. Morley, DVM, PhD, DACVIM

| Recommended precautions[a] | | | | | | | | Nationally notifiable | |
|---|---|---|---|---|---|---|---|---|---|
| Bite/ scratch concern | Human pregnancy concern | Isolation recommended | Face shield recommended | Respiratory protection | Barrier nursing and special | Attention to environmental | Hygiene recommended | Human cases | Animal cases |
| | X | X | X | | X | | | | X |
| | X | X | X | | X | | | X | X |
| | | X | | | X | | | | X[d] |
| | | X | | | X | | | | X |
| | X | X | X | | X | | | | |
| | X | X | X | | X | | | | |
| | | X | | | X | | | X | X |
| | | X | | X | X | | | | X |
| | | X | | | | | | | X |
| | X | X | X | | X | | | | |
| | | var | | | X | | | | |

**Table 17.3** Barrier nursing precautions.

| Personal protective equipment | | Recommendations | Caveats |
|---|---|---|---|
| Barrier Gowns (to protect skin and underlying clothing) | Disposable | • Intended for single use<br>• Wear impermeable gowns with splash/spray hazard | • Generates waste |
| | Re-usable/ washable | • Launder between use<br>• Wear impermeable gowns with splash/spray hazard | • Difficult to doff without cross-contamination |
| Gloves | Exam gloves | • Should not be "cleaned" and reused<br>• Double glove if contamination is expected | • Generates waste<br>• Use does not replace hand hygiene<br>• Glove failures are common and often unrecognized by the wearer |
| Facial protection (to protect mucous membranes of the eyes, nose, and mouth) | Goggles/glasses | • Wear with mask<br>• Use with splash/spray hazard | • Can be cleaned and re-used |
| | Surgical mask | • Use with splash/spray hazard | |
| | Face shield | • Wear with mask<br>• Use with splash/spray hazard | • Can be cleaned and re-used |
| Footwear Hygiene | Disposable shoe covers | • Intended for single use<br>• Covers existing footwear | • Footwear should be easily cleaned<br>• Generates waste |
| | Footmat or footbath | • Should be regularly cleaned and refilled | • Disinfectants can be rapidly inactivated by organic debris<br>• Disinfectants can be damaging to footwear |

4) *Isolation* can be considered a very high level of separation that incorporates separate air space thereby reducing airborne transmission risk. It can also serve to prevent widespread environmental contamination as it effectively minimizes personnel and patient traffic.

Potentially infectious patients should be separated or isolated as soon as is reasonably possible to protect patients and personnel. See Table 17.2 for agent-specific recommendations.

## Personal and Environmental Hygiene

Broadly, hygiene practices are intended to reduce the burden of potential pathogens to a level that is of minimal consequence to personnel, patients, and the hospital. There are multiple practices that can be used in this effort including (but not limited to) hand hygiene, dedicated hospital attire, use of footbaths or footmats for footwear hygiene, and cleaning and disinfection (C&D) protocols.

1) *Hand hygiene*, one of the most important measures to prevent the transmission of zoonotic and contagious disease agents, includes hand washing with soap and water or hand rubbing with an alcohol-based hand sanitizer (Larson 1988; Burke 2003; Anonymous 2004, 2011; Williams et al. 2015). Properly performed, the mechanical action of hand washing or rubbing reduces organic debris and microorganisms on the skin. Frequent *hand washing* may impact skin integrity, predisposing the hands to colonization with potentially pathogenic agents, and reducing compliance with hand hygiene protocols (Larson 1999, 2001). With this in mind, it is prudent to also supply hand moisturizers to promote healthy skin and improve compliance. *Alcohol-based hand sanitizers* (60–95% ethyl or isopropyl alcohol) are a nice alternative that can be as effective as handwashing with the benefit of being available at the point of care, fast acting, have a broad spectrum of activity with a minimal risk for emerging resistance, and tend to not be as compromising to skin integrity (Traub-Dargatz et al. 2006).

*A few important notes regarding hand hygiene:*

- While performing patient management, hand contamination tends to increase over time (Pittet et al. 1999; Traub-Dargatz et al. 2006).
- Alcohol-based hand sanitizers should not be used for alcohol-resistant agents (e.g., parvovirus, spore-forming agents such as Clostridium) (Boyce and Pittet 2002).
- Gloves are an adjunct to hand hygiene, not a replacement for hand hygiene, as glove failure is a relatively common, although often unrecognized, event (Korniewicz et al. 2004; Burrow and Pinchbeck 2006).
- Gloves should not be washed and re-used, even on the same patient, as this compromises glove integrity (Boyce and Pittet 2002).
- Lack of compliance with hand hygiene protocols has been attributed to being too busy or forgetting, compromised skin integrity, and the lack of available supplies (Nakamura et al. 2012; Anderson and Weese 2016).

See Table 17.4 for indications and techniques for performing hand hygiene.

2) *Dedicated attire* refers to clothing and footwear that are not worn outside of the practice environment. This may include the use of a white coat or coveralls over street clothes or the use of scrubs. While there is limited data supporting this practice in veterinary medicine, it makes practical sense to not wear potentially contaminated clothing outside of the clinic or field practice setting. In human healthcare, up to 63% of staff uniforms may be colonized with potentially pathogenic bacteria (Wiener-Well et al. 2011). In the surgical setting, this can be important as both dedicated surgical

**Table 17.4** The practice of hand hygiene.

| Indications for hand washing/sanitizing | Antiseptic hand washing (recommend using products combining soap and a biocide[b]) |
|---|---|
| • At times of arrival or leaving hospital<br>• Before and after every patient contact<br>• After touching surfaces or objects likely to be contaminated<br>• After handling patients likely to be colonized with resistant organisms<br>• Before preparing food or medications for patients<br>• After removing gloves or PPE<br>• After contact with body fluids (e.g., urine, blood, saliva)<br>• After smoking, sneezing, coughing, nose blowing, or use of the restroom<br>**Note:** Gloves should be used as an adjunct to hand washing, not in lieu of hand washing; and are indicated for contact with body fluids, mucous membranes, or non-intact skin[a] | **Technique:**<br>1) Completely wet hands and wrists in running stream of warm water; keep hands lower than elbows to avoid recontamination<br>2) Apply soap–antiseptic combination over front and back of hands<br>3) Rub all surfaces of hands and wrists, interlace fingers, and lather for manufacturers recommended time (15–30 seconds)<br>4) Thoroughly rinse hands in clear running water<br>5) Dry hands thoroughly with disposable towel<br>6) Turn off faucets with towel<br>Alcohol-based hand rubbing (Recommend using products containing 60–95% ethyl or isopropyl alcohol[a])<br>**Technique:**<br>• Place hand disinfectant in readily available locations (e.g., stall side)<br>• Dispense 2–3 mL onto hands (achieves 90% coverage[c])<br>• Rub all hand surfaces for 15 seconds<br>• Let disinfectant dry thoroughly before handling objects<br>**Note:** Not effective in the presence of organic debris or for alcohol-resistant pathogens (e.g., *Clostridium* spp. spores, parvovirus) |
| Hand hygiene in healthcare settings – Hand hygiene basics (Anonymous 2011) | www.cdc.gov/handhygiene/Basics.html |
| Hand hygiene in healthcare settings – Guidelines (Anonymous 2011) | www.cdc.gov/handhygiene/Guidelines.html |

[a] Boyce and Pittet (2002).
[b] Larson (2001) and Williams et al. (2015).
[c] Zingg et al. (2016).

footwear and use of a cover gown over scrubs when not in the surgical suite have been shown to lower contamination in the surgical suite and on surgical scrubs, respectively (Copp et al. 1986; Amirfeyz et al. 2007).

3) *Footmats and footbaths* can be used to improve footwear hygiene and subsequently environmental hygiene. While their use has been shown to reduce contamination, their efficacy is highly dependent on the disinfectant type and frequency of cleaning and refilling, amount of organic debris on footwear and in the footbath/mat, and compliance of personnel (Morley et al. 2005; Dunowska et al. 2006; Hornig et al. 2016). They can, however, be a good way to indicate that personnel are entering a hospital area with a different risk level, and therefore different infection control protocols, and may serve to manage traffic flow.
4) C&D is a multi-step process that can be critical for the disruption of the chain of infection. This process includes the following:
   - Removal of visible organic debris: This is important as the presence of organic debris (e.g., blood, urine, feces) can reduce the efficacy of disinfectants.
   - Scrubbing with a detergent to disrupt biofilms: On a cleanable surface (e.g., sealed concrete), this can result in a significant decrease in bacterial load on a surface (Walters 1967).
   - Rinse and allow to dry: Rinsing is important as some detergents inactive disinfectants; and applying a disinfectant to a dry surface ensures that it will not be diluted by any standing water.
   - Apply disinfectant at an appropriate concentration and contact time: Chemical disinfection is a chemical reaction that can be adversely impacted by the presence of organic debris as well as environmental conditions such as temperature and UV light. On a cleanable surface, a chemical disinfectant can further reduce viable organisms when applied at label indications (Walters 1967).

Commercially available chemical disinfectants are registered with the U.S. Environmental Protection Agency (EPA) and, as such, must be applied as indicated on the label (concentration and contact time), while taking all necessary safety precautions. See Table 17.5 for a summary of efficacy and limitations for the major chemical disinfectant classes.

*A few important notes regarding Cleaning and Disinfection:*

- Routine C&D should be performed throughout a facility, including personnel areas as well as animal housing and treatment areas. Pay attention to corners, under cabinets, cabinet and drawer pulls, keyboards, and faucets.
- Facilities should be well maintained to facilitate C&D – cracks/crevices repaired, wood and concrete should be sealed or replaced with a non-porous option.
- In general, multi-use diagnostic and treatment areas should be cleaned between patients. This includes all equipment such as stocks, buckets, and twitches.
- Enhanced cleaning may be warranted in areas where a suspected or confirmed infectious disease case was housed or managed. This may include use of a higher-order disinfectant, additional cleaning steps, and increased attention to ensure cleaning of high-contact areas such as cabinet/drawer pulls, keyboards, and light switches.

## Surveillance

On the whole, surveillance is the systematic collection, analysis, and interpretation of data. It incorporates monitoring for a pre-specified event that will prompt a predetermined corrective action or mitigation plan. Implementing a long-term surveillance program allows for managers to establish the expected baseline level of a particular event in their facility and/or population, and allows for mitigation efforts to be tailored to a facilities goal and unique risks. There are many types of surveillance including (but not limited to) syndromic, active, and passive.

1) *Syndromic surveillance* is monitoring for non-specific indicators of disease, such as diarrhea without a definitive diagnosis or fever of unknown origin. This type of surveillance requires defining syndromes of interest, but once definitions are developed, it is comparatively easy to perform. This type of surveillance can be useful in emergent situations to ensure patients with potentially contagious disease are appropriately managed (e.g., use of barrier nursing precautions or mandatory testing to rule-out agents of concern). An example of syndromic surveillance is having clients complete an infectious disease questionnaire prior to an appointment or monitoring for fevers in a high-risk animal housing area.

**Table 17.5** Characteristics of chemical disinfectants.

| Disinfectant[a] | Activity in organic debris | Spectrum of activity | Limited activity | No activity | Comments |
|---|---|---|---|---|---|
| Peroxygen | Very good | Gram-positive bacteria<br>Gram-negative bacteria<br>Fungal organisms<br>Enveloped viruses<br>Non-enveloped viruses<br>Protozoa | Cryptosporidium<br>Bacterial spores<br>Mycobacterium | n/a | Considered environmentally friendly<br>Minimally toxic<br>Rapid action<br>Corrosive |
| Phenolic | Very good | Gram-positive bacteria<br>Gram-negative bacteria<br>Enveloped viruses | Fungal organisms<br>Non-enveloped viruses<br>Mycobacterium | Bacterial spores (static)<br>Cryptosporidium | Environmentally unfriendly<br>Irritating to skin/mucous membranes<br>Toxic to cats and pigs<br>Minimal residual activity<br>Non-corrosive |
| Quaternary ammonium | Moderate | Gram-positive bacteria<br>Gram-negative bacteria<br>Fungal organisms<br>Enveloped viruses | Non-enveloped viruses | Cryptosporidium<br>Bacterial spores (static)<br>Mycobacterium | Minimally toxic<br>Minimal residual activity<br>Inactivated by anionic detergents<br>Less effective at low temperatures/pH<br>Non-corrosive |
| Sodium hypochlorite | Poor (rapidly inactivated) | Gram-positive bacteria<br>Gram-negative bacteria<br>Enveloped viruses<br>Non-enveloped viruses<br>Mycobacterium<br>Bacterial spores | n/a | Cryptosporidium | Minimal residual activity<br>Inactivated by cationic detergents/sunlight<br>Less effective at low temp/high pH<br>Chlorine gas if mixed with other chemicals<br>Corrosive to metals |

[a] Follow label directions for appropriate dilutions and safety precautions.
*Source:* Block (2001), Linton et al. (1987), Morley (2002), Morley and Weiss (2009), and Burgess and Traub-Dargatz (2014).

2) *Active surveillance* is purposefully performed to collect primary data on an event of interest. This type of surveillance can result in high-quality data, but can be resource intensive (financially and with respect to personnel time). An example of active surveillance is to purposefully collect fecal samples from all horses with colic for the detection of *Salmonella* or the purposeful collection of environmental samples to look for an agent of concern (e.g., *Salmonella*, carbapenem-resistant *E. coli*).
3) *Passive surveillance* is leveraging existing data that was collected for another purpose. This is considered a secondary data source, and as such, may not be as accurate as data generated from active surveillance, but will be less resource intensive. An example of passive surveillance is to monitor for multi-drug resistant organisms detected in diagnostic samples from your patient population.

Often, surveillance efforts will include a combination of active, passive, and syndromic surveillance, may incorporate monitoring of patients and/or the environment, and may be continuous and/or targeted at high-risk groups, high-risk housing areas, or high-risk time periods. The key here it to establish a surveillance program so that you will be able to perceive an abnormal occurrence of events (e.g., an increase in healthcare-associated infections) and take a rapid, appropriate response to mitigate risks.

### Education and Awareness of Personnel

Managing infectious disease risk in a facility or population is contingent on effective implementation of appropriate policies and practices. Integral to this is providing appropriate training and education, so personnel understand why policies and practices are needed and how to implement them effectively.

1) *Create a safety culture* that stems from developing a shared collection of values and norms within the workplace. A safety culture prioritizes safety, should empower personnel to contribute to this effort, and should be reflected in workplace policies and practices (Clarke 2000).
2) *Communication of risk* to key personnel to ensure that appropriate precautions are taken when managing suspected or known infectious disease cases (or their samples). This may take the form of stall signage, a group text, and/or a listserv posting.
3) *Education and re-education* are integral to effective implementation. The program is only as strong as its weakest link. To gain compliance, personnel should understand the "why" of programmatic activities and demonstrate competence relative to operationalizing policies and practices.
4) *Reporting on programmatic activities* should occur regularly to create awareness around a program's successes and failures. Regular reporting can remind personnel of the importance of infection prevention activities, empower them to make good decisions, and keep them engaged in program refinement and/or development.

Some facilities may create infection control committees to develop policies and practices to manage infectious disease risk in a facility. These committees can encourage participation in program development and/or improvement, and keep personnel engaged. That being said, there should be one person who is regularly evaluating protocols, any data generated by programmatic activities, and who will make tough decisions about patient, population, and facility management relative to infectious disease risk and risk mitigation. The latter is particularly important during times of emergent issues (e.g., an outbreak).

## References

Amirfeyz, R., Tasker, A., Ali, S. et al. (2007). Theatre shoes – a link in the common pathway of postoperative wound infection? *Ann. R. Coll. Surg. Engl.* 89 (6): 605–608.

Anderson, M.E. and Weese, J.S. (2016). Self-reported hand hygiene perceptions and barriers among companion animal veterinary clinic personnel in Ontario, Canada. *Can. Vet. J.* 57 (3): 282–288.

Anonymous (2004). Guideline for hand hygiene in healthcare settings. *J. Am. Coll. Surg.* 198 (1): 121–127.

Anonymous (2011). Hand hygiene in healthcare settings: guidelines. http://www.cdc.gov/handhygiene/Guidelines.html (accessed 1 March 2012).

Block, S.S. (ed.) (2001). *Disinfection, Sterilization, and Preservation*, 5e. Philadelphia, Lippincott: Williams & Wilkins.

Boyce, J.M. and Pittet, D. (2002). Guideline for hand hygiene in health-care settings. Recommendations of the Healthcare Infection Control Practices Advisory Committee and the HICPAC/SHEA/APIC/IDSA Hand Hygiene Task Force. Society for Healthcare Epidemiology of America/Association for Professionals in Infection Control/Infectious Diseases Society of America. *MMWR Recomm. Rep.* 51 (RR-16): 1–45. quiz CE41-44.

Burgess, B.A. and Traub-Dargatz, J.L. (2014). Biosecurity and control of infectious disease outbreaks. In: *Equine Infectious Diseases*, 2e (ed. D.C. Sellon and M.T. Long). St. Louis: Saunders Elsevier.

Burke, J.P. (2003). Infection control – a problem for patient safety. *N. Engl. J. Med.* 348 (7): 651–656.

Burrow, R. and Pinchbeck, G. (2006). Study of how frequently surgeons' gloves are perforated during operations. *Vet. Rec.* 158 (16): 558–561.

Clarke, S. (2000). Safety culture: under-specified and overrated? *Int. J. Manag. Rev.* 2 (1): 65–90.

Copp, G., Mailhot, C.B., Zalar, M. et al. (1986). Covergowns and the control of operating room contamination. *Nurs. Res.* 35 (5): 263–268.

Dunowska, M., Morley, P.S., Patterson, G. et al. (2006). Evaluation of the efficacy of a peroxygen disinfectant-filled footmat for reduction of bacterial load on footwear in a large animal hospital setting. *J. Am. Vet. Med. Assoc.* 228 (12): 1935–1939.

Hornig, K.J., Burgess, B.A., Saklou, N.T. et al. (2016). Evaluation of the efficacy of disinfectant footmats for the reduction of bacterial contamination on footwear in a large animal veterinary hospital. *J. Vet. Intern. Med.* 30 (6): 1882–1886.

Keim, M. and Kaufmann, A.F. (1999). Principles for emergency response to bioterrorism. *Ann. Emerg. Med.* 34 (2): 177–182.

Korniewicz, D.M., Garzon, L., Seltzer, J., and Feinleib, M. (2004). Failure rates in nonlatex surgical gloves. *Am. J. Infect. Control* 32 (5): 268–273.

Larson, E. (1988). A causal link between handwashing and risk of infection? Examination of the evidence. *Infect. Control Hosp. Epidemiol.* 9 (1): 28–36.

Larson, E. (1999). Skin hygiene and infection prevention: more of the same or different approaches? *Clin. Infect. Dis.* 29 (5): 1287–1294.

Larson, E. (2001). Hygiene of the skin: when is clean too clean? *Emerg. Infect. Dis.* 7 (2): 225–230.

Linton, A.H., Hugo, W.B., and Russell, A.D. (ed.) (1987). *Disinfection in Veterinary and Farm Animal Practice*. Oxford: Blackwell Scientific Publications.

Morley, P.S. (2002). Biosecurity of veterinary practices. *Vet. Clin. North Am. Food Anim. Pract.* 18 (1): 133–155, vii. https://doi.org/10.1016/s0749-0720(02)00009-9. PMID: 12064165.

Morley, P.S. and Weese, J.S. (2009). *Biosecurity and Infection Control in Large Animal Practice from Large Animal Internal Medicine*, 4e. St. Louis: Mosby Elsevier.

Morley, P.S., Morris, S.N., Hyatt, D.R., and Van Metre, D.C. (2005). Evaluation of the efficacy of disinfectant footbaths as used in veterinary hospitals. *J. Am. Vet. Med. Assoc.* 226 (12): 2053–2058.

Morley, P., Anderson, M., and Burgess, B. (2013). Report of the third Havemeyer workshop on infection control in equine populations. *Equine Vet. J.* 45 (2): 131–136.

Nakamura, R.K., Tompkins, E., Braasch, E.L. et al. (2012). Hand hygiene practices of veterinary support staff in small animal private practice. *J. Small Anim. Pract.* 53 (3): 155–160.

Pittet, D., Dharan, S., Touveneau, S. et al. (1999). Bacterial contamination of the hands of hospital staff during routine patient care. *Arch. Intern. Med.* 159 (8): 821–826.

Taylor, L.H., Latham, S.M., and Woolhouse, M.E. (2001). Risk factors for human disease emergence. *Philos. Trans. R. Soc. Lond. Ser. B Biol. Sci.* 356 (1411): 983–989.

Traub-Dargatz, J.L., Weese, J.S., Rousseau, J.D. et al. (2006). Pilot study to evaluate 3 hygiene protocols on the reduction of bacterial load on the hands of veterinary staff performing routine equine physical examinations. *Can. Vet. J.* 47 (7): 671–676.

Verbeek, J.H., Ijaz, S., Mischke, C. et al. (2016). Personal protective equipment for preventing highly infectious diseases due to exposure to contaminated body fluids in healthcare staff. *Cochrane Database Syst. Rev.* 4: CD011621.

Walters, A. (1967). Hard surface disinfection and its evaluation. *J. Appl. Bacteriol.* 30 (1): 56–65.

Wiener-Well, Y., Galuty, M., Rudensky, B. et al. (2011). Nursing and physician attire as possible source of nosocomial infections. *Am. J. Infect. Control* 39 (7): 555–559.

Williams, C.J., Scheftel, J.M., Elchos, B.L. et al. (2015). Compendium of veterinary standard precautions for zoonotic disease prevention in veterinary personnel: National Association of State Public Health Veterinarians: Veterinary Infection Control Committee 2015. *J. Am. Vet. Med. Assoc.* 247 (11): 1252–1277.

Zingg, W., Haidegger, T., and Pittet, D. (2016). Hand coverage by alcohol-based handrub varies: Volume and hand size matter. *Am. J. Infect. Control* 44 (12): 1689–1691.

# 18

# Systemic Inflammatory Response Syndrome, Shock, and Sepsis

*Samuel D. Hurcombe*[1] *and Jamie J. Kopper*[2]

[1] *Department of Clinical Studies - New Bolton Center, University of Pennsylvania School of Veterinary Medicine, Kennett Square, PA, USA*
[2] *Department of Veterinary Clinical Sciences, College of Veterinary Medicine, Iowa State University, Ames, IA, USA*

## Definitions, Criteria, Clinical Signs and Patient Stabilization

### Systemic Inflammatory Response Syndrome

*Systemic inflammatory response syndrome (SIRS)* is an exaggerated defense response of the body to noxious stressors such as infection, trauma, surgery, inflammation, ischemia and reperfusion injury, and malignancy. The consequence is an overwhelming inflammatory response leading to non-specific derangements of the cardiorespiratory, thermoregulatory systems, and leucon responses of the patient. Of note, SIRS is a criterion that patients meet, rather than a specific diagnosis. The SIRS criterion was originally designed to serve as an early warning signal with low specificity to identify patients at risk for sepsis or other critical illness that may need more intensive care in an emergency setting. Upon recognizing a patient meets SIRS criteria (Table 18.1), the clinician should next ask themselves what the inciting source is for that patient and what next steps need to be taken.

### Shock

*Shock* can be defined as a potentially life-threatening critical condition characterized by decreased blood flow or perfusion which no longer adequately supplies oxygen and nutrients to the cells leading to metabolic dysfunction of the cells, tissues, and organs. Clinical signs of shock are outlined in Box 18.1. Shock can resolve with treatment or progress to organ failure and death. Several forms of shock can coexist in the same patients, all contributing to cardiovascular collapse and death if overwhelming or left untreated. Shock categories and common clinical examples are described in Box 18.1.

### Sepsis

*Sepsis* refers to a patient with a bacterial infection in their bloodstream and meeting SIRS criteria (i.e., showing clinical signs of illness associated with the infection). It is important to note that a number of apparently healthy patients are bacteremic (i.e., have bacteria in their blood stream) at any given time but are clinically healthy. Sepsis can be divided into several categories including sepsis, severe sepsis, and septic shock depending on the degree of associated clinical signs. Box 18.2 helps delineate the difference between sepsis (sometimes referred to as “early sepsis), severe sepsis, and septic shock.

*Emergency Triage of the Horse*, First Edition. Edited by Rolfe M. Radcliffe and Jamie J. Kopper.

Companion website: www.wiley.com/go/radcliffe/triage

**Table 18.1** SIRS criteria for adults and foals.

| | Adult horse | Newborn foal (birth to 3 days) (Roy et al. 2017) | Neonatal foal (4–14 days) (Wong and Wilkins 2015) | Juvenile foal (15 days–6 months) (Wong and Wilkins 2015) | Weanling foal (7 months to 1 year) (Wong and Wilkins 2015) |
|---|---|---|---|---|---|
| Fever or hypothermia | >101.3 °F (38.5 °C) or <98.6 °F (37 °C) | >102.6 °F (39.2 °C) or <99 °F (37.2 °C) | >102.6 °F (39.2 °C) or <99 °F (37.2 °C) | >102.6 °F (39.2 °C) or <99 °F (37.2 °C) | >102.6 °F (39.2 °C) or <99 °F (37.2 °C) |
| Tachycardia (beats/min) | >52 | > 115 | > 120 | > 96 | > 96 |
| Tachypnea (breaths/min) | >20 | > 56 | > 56 | > 44 | > 20 |
| Leukocytosis, leukopenia, or >5% band neutrophils | >12.5 or <5.0 × $10^3$ | >14.4 or <6.9 × $10^3$ | >12.5 or <4 × $10^3$ | >12.5 or <4 × $10^3$ | >12.5 or <4 × $10^3$ |
| Venous blood lactate level (mmol/L) | >2.06 | >5 | >2.5 | >2.5 | >2.5 |
| Venous blood glucose level (mg/dL) | NA | <50 | <50 | <50 | <50 |
| Mucous membrane color | Normal/ abnormal | NA | NA | NA | NA |

- Foals must meet 3 of the provided criteria, of which one must be an abnormal temperature or leukocyte count (Wong and Wilkins 2015).
- Adults should meet 5–6 of the criteria including an abnormal blood lactate and abnormal mucous membrane color (Roy et al. 2017).

**Box 18.1 Clinical signs of shock, in addition to SIRS criteria**

**Clinical signs of shock**

Altered mental status (dull, agitated, uncharacteristic)

Cool distal extremities (ears, distal limbs, muzzle)

Abnormal mucous membrane color (injected, purple, blue)

Abnormal capillary refill time (prolonged or rapid)

Weakly, absent, or hyperkinetic palpable peripheral pulses (e.g., transverse facial artery)

**Box 18.2 Stages of Sepsis**

**Sepsis**

Patient meets SIRS criteria (see Table 18.1)

Patient has evidence of or is suspected to have a bacterial infection

**Severe sepsis = sepsis criteria *and***

Evidence of organ dysfunction (e.g., elevation in creatinine, elevation in liver enzymes)

Hypotension (i.e., systolic blood pressure <90 mmHg, mean arterial pressure <65 mmHg)

Evidence of hypoperfusion (e.g., elevated blood lactate, poor capillary refill time, cool distal extremities)

**Septic shock = severe sepsis criteria *and***

Hypotension and hypoperfusion despite fluid resuscitation

Of note, the descriptor "endotoxemia" is frequently used in equine practice to describe horses that are suspected to have clinical signs due to systemic side effects of exposure to lipopolysaccharide (LPS), a key component of Gram-negative bacteria. Horses are one of the most exquisitely sensitive species to LPS, containing enough LPS in their gastrointestinal tracts to kill them at any given time. Given that, clinically, horses rarely encounter LPS without the associated bacteria; a more accurate description would likely be Gram-negative sepsis and the horses should be treated as such.

*Patient stabilization for patients with clinical signs of shock*

1) Apply first-aid principles as indicated by overt clinical signs.
   a) Bleeding wound: Apply a hemostat or ligate bleeding vessels, apply a tourniquet or pressure bandage.
   b) Fracture/luxation: Apply a well-padded bandage +/− splint as described elsewhere.
   c) Colic: Pass a nasogastric tube and provide gastric decompression.
   d) ECG assessment: portable ECG devices are becoming accessible to veterinarians. [1]Many of these devices link to an application on your phone and save ECG traces that can be immediately viewed and electronically sent for interpretation.
2) Obtain venous access – jugular venous access is preferred. Large-gauge (10 > 12 > 14 gauge), shorter catheters will optimize the ability to administer large volumes of fluids.
   a) In animals with shock, adequate blood flow is being shunted away from "less critical organs" such as the gastrointestinal tract. Thus, other means of fluid administration (enteral, rectal) are less likely to be effective.
3) Obtain blood for diagnostic tests if indicated.
   a) Diagnostic tests to determine the severity of shock and help guide fluid therapy should include a complete blood count (CBC), serum biochemistry including indicators of liver and kidney function and electrolytes and blood L-lactate. Additional diagnostic tests are aimed at determining the primary cause of shock (i.e., distributive vs. obstructive vs. cardiogenic, etc.).
   b) Additional diagnostic tests to consider include invasive or non-invasive blood pressure measurements.
4) Begin resuscitative fluid therapy: rates/volumes will depend on your physical examination findings.
   Example shock fluid rates
   a) Isotonic replacement crystalloid (Plasmalyte®, Lactated Ringers' Solution, Hartmanns' Solution, Normasol®) up to 80 mL/kg IV in the first hour.
      i) Start with 20 mL/kg IV bolus. Reassess physical examination with special attention paid to heart rate. Re-assess L-lactate if available. For a 500 kg horse, this would be equivalent to a 10 L bolus.
      ii) If the horse remains tachycardic with exam findings of poor perfusion continue with a second 20 mL/kg IV bolus of isotonic replacement crystalloid fluids. Then, reassess exam findings.
      iii) Continue for total of 4 × 20 mL/kg IV boluses (80 mL/kg total) if indicated by physical examination findings.
      iv) Continue with 1–2 times maintenance (2–4 mL/kg/h) until referral or further diagnostics.
   b) Hypertonic saline (7.2% NaCl) may be used once at a dose of up to 4 mL/kg.
      i) The goal with using hypertonic saline is to cause a rapid increase in plasma osmolality leading to fluid recruitment from the intracellular to extracellular spaces (Schnuelle et al. 2022). In the short term (~30 minutes) this provides about a 4× increase in volume versus volume given (i.e., 2 L of hypertonic saline results in an 8 L increase intravascular volume). However, it is important to know that this effect is short lived and if administration of hypertonic saline is not followed by the administration of an appropriate volume of crystalloids after approximately 30–45 minutes the opposite effects will be observed as fluids once again re-distribute.
5) Additional therapeutics may be indicated depending on the patients' underlying condition or presenting complaint and physical examination findings as outlined in Table 18.2.
6) When should I refer?
   a) Many patients showing evidence of shock should be referred to a hospital setting for further evaluation and treatment as many will require intensive 24/7 care. If referral is an option, efforts should be aimed at providing both rapid stabilization as described above and equally rapid transportation using safe transportation practices (i.e., break-away halters, not tying unstable patients, removing dividers, and other obstacles where possible).

1 Eko DUO digital stethoscope, Eko Devices, Inc. Oakland, CA, 94612. AliveCor KardiaMobile, AliveCor, Inc. Mountain View, CA, 94041.

**Table 18.2** Different types of shock and common causes in horses.

| Shock category | Clinical scenario | Additional treatments and diagnostics |
|---|---|---|
| Hypovolemic shock – hemorrhage<br>Hypovolemic shock – dehydration | • External trauma/wound with major vessel breach<br>• Internal trauma (blunt or penetrating trauma)<br>• Guttural pouch mycosis<br>• Middle uterine artery bleed (mares only)<br>• Free water deprivation<br>• Excessive sweating<br>• Enterogastric reflux<br>• Diarrhea<br>• Polyuria | See coagulopathies and hemorrhage in horses and foals |
| Cardiogenic shock | • Sustained ventricular dysrhythmias<br>• Myocardial disease (ionophore, oleander/rhododendron [cardiac glycoside])<br>• Pericardial disease<br>• Cardiac tamponade (pericardial, mediastinal, pleural effusions)<br>• Congenital anomalies<br>• Congestive heart failure (valvular disease) | See cardiovascular diseases |
| Maldistributive/septic shock | • Endotoxemia – various (enteritis, enterocolitis, colitis, typhlocolitis, pneumonia, pleuropneumonia, (endo)metritis, GI ischemia/reperfusion injury, any disease leading to a sustained SIRS state.)<br>• Enterotoxemia – various (toxic shock syndrome, Clostridiosis)<br>• Toxigenic causes | See pressure support in horses and foals |
| Obstructive shock | • Abdominal compartment syndrome (massive intestinal distension, and/or peritoneal effusion) | See diseases of the abdomen |

*Below are steps for triaging and treating adult horses with sepsis*

1) Complete a patient assessment to better understand the degree of systemic compromise:
   a) Complete physical examination
      i) Part of the physical examination should be assessment of blood pressure. If you cannot obtain indirect measurements, a crude assessment can be made by palpating for peripheral pulse pressures (i.e., transverse facial artery in adults, coccygeal or metatarsal artery in foals) and assessing temperature of distal extremities.
   b) Acquisition of basic laboratory work –CBC and serum chemistry.
2) Considering this information, develop a problem list and differential list to determine the likely primary source(s) – unlike foals, adult horses rarely develop sepsis without an underlying disease process.
   a) Examples: Colitis resulting in translocation of enteric bacteria, severe pleural pneumonia resulting in translocation of bacteria.
3) Develop a further diagnostic and treatment plan:
   a) Examples of additional diagnostics:
      i) Thoracic and abdominal ultrasound to better assess possible sources.
      ii) Enteric disease panel if suspect colitis.
      iii) Transtracheal wash if suspect pneumonia.
      iv) Blood cultures – recognize that many blood cultures are negative despite active infection, so a negative culture does not rule out disease.
   b) Additional treatment plan:
      i) Broad-spectrum antimicrobials – if the patient is suspected to be septic, particularly with moderate-to-severe leukopenia, broad-spectrum antimicrobials are usually warranted.
      ii) Anti-inflammatory medications – in many instances, renal function pending, the horse may be undergoing an exaggerated inflammatory response which can be detrimental. Additionally, medications such as flunixin meglumine have been reported to have "anti-LPS" effects and help ameliorate the clinical signs associated with LPS in the horse.

iii) Crystalloid fluid therapy – if the patient is azotemic, dehydrated, or hypotensive use of crystalloid fluids is indicated. In many patients these are given intravenously, but enteral fluid therapy can be considered in some patients. An example fluid plan would be to start with a 20 mL/kg bolus (i.e., 10 L for a 500 kg horse) followed by reassessment of physical examination and perfusion parameters (i.e., has the horse urinated, has the heart rate improved, have peripheral pulse pressures improved). This can be repeated up to 3 times.

iv) Colloid fluid therapy – if the patient has concurrent hypoproteinemia, it may also benefit from colloids (natural or synthetic) to improve the colloid oncotic pressure and help retain crystalloid fluids within the vascular space. Natural colloids (i.e., plasma) may have additional benefits such as administration of immunoglobulins and clotting factors however comes with the risk of transfusion reactions and disease transmission. Synthetic colloids should be used in caution with patients that are azotemic due to a potential risk of acute kidney injury. A starting place for administration of colloids is a 10 mL/kg bolus followed by reassessment of a physical examination and perfusion parameters.

v) Laminitis prophylaxis – many septic horses are at risk for developing laminitis. Depending on your assessment of their risk the use of distal limb cryotherapy (i.e., ice boots) can be considered as prophylaxis.

4) When should I refer?
   a) Management of these horses can be very challenging, time and labor intensive. Thus, horses that require frequent treatment (i.e., continuous fluids, ice boots), do not respond to initial therapy (i.e., remain hypotensive despite initial efforts), or who are at risk for clinical decompensation are all good candidates for referral.

*Below are steps for triaging and treating foals with sepsis*
Additionally, please see the neonatal emergency chapter (Chapter 20) for more detailed information.

5) Complete a patient assessment to better understand the degree of systemic compromise:
   a) Complete physical examination
      i) Part of your physical examination should be assessment of blood pressure. If you cannot obtain indirect measurements, a crude assessment can be made by palpating for peripheral pulse pressures (i.e., transverse facial artery in adults, metatarsal artery in foals) and assessing the temperature of distal extremities.
   b) Acquisition of basic laboratory work –CBC, serum chemistry, and IgG.
   c) Any foal that is failing to nurse, hypoglycemic and lethargic should be presumed to have a component of sepsis unless proven otherwise.
6) Considering this information, develop a problem list and differential list to determine the likely primary source(s) – neonatal foals, unlike adults, commonly develop sepsis due to environmental exposure combined with an incompetent immune system so they may not have an underlying cause.
   a) Examples: failure of passive transfer, umbilical infection
7) Develop a further diagnostic and treatment plan:
   a) Examples of additional diagnostics:
      i) Blood cultures – recognize that many blood cultures are negative despite active infection, so a negative culture does not rule out disease Additionally, the clinician should not wait for the results of the cultures before instituting antimicrobial therapy if sepsis is suspected.
      ii) If joint effusion is present, assessment of the synovial structure for evidence of localized infection (i.e., arthrocentesis, ultrasound)
      iii) Abdominal and thoracic ultrasound to look for complicating factors (i.e., pneumonia, ileus, omphalitis, etc.)
   b) Additional treatment plan:
      i) Broad-spectrum antimicrobials – if the foal is suspected to be septic, broad-spectrum antimicrobials are warranted.
      ii) Dextrose supplementation – foals that are hypoglycemic need dextrose support. In a hypoglycemic crisis (i.e., a foal with severe hypoglycemia and associated clinical signs) a bolus can be administered. However, long-term management is best done as a continuous rate infusion.
      iii) Crystalloid fluid therapy – if the patient is azotemic, dehydrated, hypotensive, or unable to take nutrition by mouth, use of crystalloid fluids is indicated. An example fluid plan would be to start with a 20 mL/kg bolus (i.e., 1 L for a 50 kg foal) followed by reassessment of physical examination and perfusion parameters (i.e., has the foal urinated, has the heart rate improved, have peripheral pulse pressures improved). This can be repeated up to 3 times in a 24 h period, but due to risk of volume overload the patient's need for colloids (i.e., plasma) must be carefully considered as well.

iv) Colloid fluid therapy – if the patient has partial (400–800 mg/dL) or complete (<400 mg/dL) failure of transfer of passive immunity a plasma transfusion is warranted, particularly in a patient with concern for sepsis where immunoglobulins are being actively consumed. A place to start is a 20 mL/kg bolus (i.e., 1 L per 50 kg foal) which can be repeated up to 3 times in a 24-h period with careful attention to signs of volume overload. This volume must be considered with the foal's overall fluid plan and in many instances depending on the number of liters needed, they may be split over 2 days.

v) Nutritional plan – foals that are hypoglycemic need nutritional support in the form of parenteral nutrition (even partial with just dextrose) and may need a feeding tube for enteral nutrition.

vi) Nursing care – recumbent foals and those spending more time down than usual need intensive nursing care including frequent (q2 h) recumbency care and cleanliness care to prevent the development of serious and sometimes life-threatening decubital ulcers. Decubital ulcers can develop rapidly and once they develop easily progress, are challenging to treat and can quickly involve synovial structures.

8) When should I refer?
   a) Management of these foals can be very challenging, labor intensive, and foals can rapidly decompensate. Early referral often results in decreased total cost to the client and improved outcome. Any foal that requires continual therapy, multiple farm visits, or is at risk for decompensation is a candidate for referral.

## Case Example 18.1 SIRS, Shock, Sepsis

### Case 1

A 500 kg mare is presented for further evaluation due to epistaxis secondary to a gunshot wound to the sinuses. On evaluation you note that there is a large (estimated 5 L) pool of blood at her feet with more spread through the pasture with ongoing bilateral epistaxis. On physical examination you note that the mare is dull, has a heart rate of 100 bpm, respiratory rate of 40 breaths/min, and cool distal extremities. The transverse facial arterial pulse is not palpable, jugular refill is prolonged at four to five seconds and distal extremities (ears, distal limbs) are cool to the touch. Borborygmi are decreased throughout, and rectal temperature is 98 °F. Stall-side evaluation reveals the following abnormalities or pertinent values:

Packed Cell Volume (PCV): 25% (RR: 30–40%).
Total Solids (TS): 3.5 g/dL (RR: 5–6 g/dL).
L-Lactate: 7.0 mmol/L (RR <2 mmol/L).
Creatinine: 2.5 mg/dL (1.0–1.8 mg/dL).

1) **Does this horse have evidence of shock?**
   Yes. This horse has evidence of hypovolemic shock due to blood loss secondary to epistaxis. Physical exam findings consistent with this include an altered mentation, tachycardia, tachypnea, poor peripheral pulses, poor jugular refill (indicative of hypotension) cool distal extremities, and hypothermia. Hematologically, this is supported by a hyperlactatemia and azotemia. Although the PCV by itself is not alarming, when considered in combination with the TS this is supportive of severe blood loss as a decrease in PCV often follows a decrease in TS with acute hemorrhage.
2) **What are your first stabilization steps and considerations?**
   a) This horse will need a blood transfusion. Transportation to the nearest hospital capable of a blood transfusion should be arranged. If this is not possible see "coagulopathies and hemorrhage of the foal and horse" for performing a blood transfusion in the field.
   b) While transportation and referral for transfusion is being arranged, rapidly begin the following:
   c) Place a large bore IV catheter in a jugular vein. Begin administering either a 10 L bolus of isotonic replacement crystalloids or 2 mL/kg bolus of hypertonic saline followed by 10 L of crystalloids.
   d) Attempt to stop hemorrhage from the nares. Remember that horses are obligate nasal breathers, thus, if you are going to pack both nostrils first, a tracheostomy must be performed to secure an airway. After securing an airway, using stockinette soaked in 1% phenylephrine HCl (i.e., phenylephrine nose spray) pack the nostril(s). If available, phenylephrine may help provide local vasoconstriction.

**Case 2**

A 50 kg 24-h old foal is presented for further evaluation due to decreased nursing and failure to stand. The owners report that the foal initially met its milestones (standing, nursing), but they have not observed it nurse for the past 12 h.

On evaluation you note that the foal is dull and laterally recumbent. Eyes are sunken with entropion OU. Mucous membranes are purple and tacky with a prolonged capillary refill time of three to four seconds. Jugular refill is poor bilaterally. Heart rate is 140 bpm with a respiratory rate of 20 brpm and a rectal temperature of 98 °F. Distal extremities (ears, hooves) are cool. Coccygeal and metatarsal arterial pulses are not palpable. Stall-side hematological evaluation reveals the following:

PCV: 50%.
Total solids: 4.0 g/dL.
L-Lactate: 9.6 mmol/L.
Blood glucose: <25 mg/dL.
IgG: <400 mg/dL.

1) **Does this foal meet SIRS criteria?**
Yes – this foal is tachycardic, hypothermic, hyperlactatemic, and hypoglycemic.
2) **Does this foal have exam findings consistent with shock?**
Yes, the foal is tachycardic and has a prolonged capillary refill time. Additionally, the foal has cool distal extremities indicating peripheral vasoconstriction and tachycardia with poor peripheral pulse pressures on palpation indicating hypotension. Furthermore, the foal is hyperlactatemic indicating poor tissue perfusion.
3) **Does this foal have evidence of sepsis?**
Yes, the foal is hypoglycemic, hyperlactatemic, and laterally recumbent. At a minimum, based on perfusion parameters (prolonged capillary refill time, poor peripheral pulse pressures, hyperlactatemia) the foal likely has severe sepsis. Depending on its response to fluid resuscitation, it may have septic shock.
4) **What are possible categories for this foal's shock?**
Hypovolemic – dehydration.
Maldistributive – sepsis.
5) **What are your initial stabilization steps for this foal?**
If possible, referral should be recommended due to the intensive care (i.e., 24/7) that critically ill foals often need. While this is being arranged, start the following:
   1) Place an IV catheter in a jugular vein.
   2) Administer a 20 mL/kg bolus of isotonic replacement crystalloid IV fluids (i.e., 1 L for a 50 kg foal) with 5% dextrose.
      a) Half-way through the bolus reassess the blood glucose reading. If >200 mg/dL slow the rate of infusion and switch to isotonic crystalloid fluids without dextrose for subsequent boluses.
      b) Concurrently, administer broad-spectrum antimicrobials*. Some examples include:
         i) Potassium penicillin (22,000 IU/kg IV) and amikacin (25 mg/kg IV).
         ii) Ceftiofur sodium (5 mg/kg IV) +/– amikacin (25 mg/kg IV).
         iii) *If referring, please check with your referral hospital regarding their desire for and type of antimicrobials as resistance patterns vary depending on geographic location.
   3) If referral is not an option, continued fluid therapy should include plasma (no more than 40–60 mL/kg in a day) for immunoglobulin and colloid support and a continuous rate infusion of crystalloid fluids with dextrose to maintain a blood glucose between 80 and 200 mg/dL until the foal is able to nurse adequately.

**Case 3**

A 500-kg 12-year-old Grade gelding is presented for further evaluation in the summertime due to diarrhea and hyporexia. You are practicing in the Midwest. On physical examination you note that the gelding is febrile (103.5 °F), tachycardic (80 bpm), and has a mildly increased respiratory rate (36 brpm). Mucous membranes are injected with a toxic line and a prolonged capillary refill time of four seconds. Peripheral pulse pressures are poor. Jugular refill is poor. The ears and distal limbs are cool to the touch. Watery diarrhea is present in the gelding's tail. Stall-side bloodwork reveals the following abnormalities:

PCV: 60%.
Total solids: 5.0 g/dL.
Blood L-lactate: 5.4 g/dL.

*Additional abnormalities identified on a serum chemistry and a CBC include*

Creatinine: 2.9 mg/dL (reference range: 0.9–1.9).
Blood urea nitrogen (BUN): 50 mg/dL (15–25).
White blood cell count: 2,000/μL (5,000–12,000).
Neutrophil count: 1,000/μL (2,000–6,000) with suspect bands.

1) **Does this horse meet SIRS criteria?**
Yes, the horse is febrile, tachycardic, tachypneic, and leukopenic.
2) **Does this horse have evidence of sepsis?**
Yes, the horse meets SIRS criteria, has abnormally colored mucous membranes, and leukopenia. This horse also meets criteria for severe sepsis based on the presence of organ dysfunction (azotemia) and clinical evidence of hypotension and hypoperfusion based on the tachycardia, poor palpable peripheral pulses, poor jugular refill, cool distal extremities, and hyperlactatemia. Whether or not it is septic shock will depend on if the horse responds to your initial fluid resuscitation.
3) **Does this horse have evidence of shock?**
Yes, Hypovolemic – severe dehydration and potentially maldistributive – sepsis.
4) **What is an initial treatment plan for this patient?**
Fluid therapy – crystalloids: Given that this horse is tachycardic, hemoconcentrated, has physical exam evidence of poor perfusion, and ongoing fluid losses (diarrhea) fluid therapy is warranted. Ideally, this would be given intravenously due to both decreased intestinal function (colitis) and poor perfusion parameters (the intestinal tract is also likely poorly perfused with decreased absorptive capacity). A reasonable starting place would be a 20 mL/kg bolus (10 L) followed by reassessment of perfusion parameters and repeating if necessary.

Fluid therapy – colloids: With hypoproteinemia in the face of hemoconcentration, colloids may be considered as the protein will get lower as the horse is rehydrated.

Antimicrobials: Use of antimicrobials in horses with colitis is controversial due to the risk of further exacerbating dysbiosis. However, in this case, with the geographic location and season making *Neorickettsia risticii* a differential, starting empirical treatment with oxytetracycline (6.6 mg/kg IV q12–24 h) is easily justifiable which is both the treatment of choice for *N. risticii* and a broad-spectrum antimicrobial. In other circumstances, arguments for antimicrobials include fever and leukopenia with neutropenia and arguments against antimicrobials include the aforementioned concerns for exacerbating dysbiosis. Given the nephrotoxicity of oxytetracycline, its use should be combined with fluid therapy as described and monitoring of renal function.

Anti-inflammatory medications: Given evidence of a systemic response to LPS use of flunixin meglumine can be considered and balanced with the risk of nephrotoxicity and decreased intestinal epithelial healing.

Laminitis prophylaxis: Horses that are febrile, tachycardic, and leukopenic are at risk for laminitis. Thus, use of ice boots should be considered.
5) **Is this horse a candidate for referral?**
Yes. Ultimately this is a decision made by you and the owner. However, the labor intensiveness of fluid therapy (and likely on-going needs), risk for laminitis and time involved with ice boots, evidence of shock without knowing if the horse will respond to initial treatments, and biosecurity risks to the farm with watery diarrhea are all good indicators to consider referral.

## References

Roy, M.F., Kwong, G.P., Lambert, J. et al. (2017). Prognostic value and development of a scoring system in horses with systemic inflammatory response syndrome. *J. Vet. Intern. Med.* 31 (2): 582–592.

Schnuelle, M.L., Hopster, K., Toribio, R.E., and Hurcombe, S.D. (2022). Effects of 7.2% hypertonic saline solution on cardiovascular parameters and endogenous arginine vasopressin secretion in euvolemic isoflurane-anesthetized horses. *Am. J. Vet. Res.* 83 (9): ajvr.21.08.0133.

Wong, D.M. and Wilkins, P.A. (2015). Defining the systemic inflammatory response syndrome in equine neonates. *Vet. Clin. N. Am. Equine Pract.* 31 (3): 463–481.

# 19

# Coagulation and Hemorrhage in Horses and Foals

*Rebecca Bishop*[1] *and Pamela Wilkins*[1,2]

[1] *Department of Veterinary Clinical Medicine, College of Veterinary Medicine, University of Illinois Urbana-Champaign, Urbana, IL, USA*
[2] *Department of Comparative Biosciences, College of Veterinary Medicine, University of Illinois Urbana-Champaign, Urbana, IL, USA*

## Overview of Coagulation and Coagulopathy

### Introduction

Normal function and balance of coagulation processes is essential for organ and tissue function. Coagulation disorders can manifest from problems of either inadequate or excessive coagulation, and both are encountered in equine patients. Emergent conditions associated with the coagulation system are listed in Table 19.1. While the mainstay of treatment is identifying and addressing the underlying cause of coagulopathy, the practitioner should be vigilant for and attend to hyper- or hypo-coagulable states present in these, often critically ill, patients.

### Review of Coagulation and Fibrinolysis

Understanding development and diagnosis of coagulopathy requires a fundamental understanding of the physiologic mechanisms of blood clotting and dissolution. **Primary hemostasis** is the initiation of clot formation when platelets in the blood stream interact with subendothelial tissues within vessels. Platelets attach to the endothelium and change shape to form a monolayer along the vessel wall. If there is turbulent blood flow (as in large vessel disruption) or hyperactive endothelium (as in systemic inflammatory conditions, for example, systemic inflammatory response syndrome or SIRS), platelets will continue aggregating and release granules containing clot activating factors (including thrombin, collagen, and thromboxane A2) which promote further platelet activation. Under normal conditions, healthy endothelial cells will produce prostacyclin, which decreases platelet ADP release, preventing unnecessary or excessive platelet aggregation.

**Secondary hemostasis** continues with the activation of soluble coagulation factors, and results in formation of a stable fibrin clot. Secondary hemostasis has been traditionally modeled by the coagulation cascade, consisting of the intrinsic, extrinsic, and common pathways. While the coagulation cascade best reflects in vitro coagulation, the cell-based model of coagulation is a better representation of in vivo coagulation. The cell-based model consists of three overlapping phases: initiation, amplification, and propagation, and includes platelet-associated factors and receptors that are not represented in the coagulation cascade. Ultimately, both models involve the same essential coagulation factors, and result in the conversion of fibrinogen to fibrin, yielding a stable clot.

The **fibrinolysis system** is activated concurrently with the initiation of coagulation. Fibrinolysis is critical for dissolution of blood clots, prevention of excessive fibrin distribution, restoration of nutrient blood flow, and inhibition of excessive clot expansion. The primary actor in fibrinolysis is plasminogen, which is produced in the kidneys and liver. Plasminogen is converted to the active form plasmin by various plasminogen activators and kallikrein. Once activated, plasmin degrades fibrinogen and fibrin to their soluble degradation products (FDPs) and downgrades coagulation by inactivation or degradation of coagulation factors.

*Emergency Triage of the Horse*, First Edition. Edited by Rolfe M. Radcliffe and Jamie J. Kopper.

Published 2026 by John Wiley & Sons, Inc.
Companion website: www.wiley.com/go/radcliffe/triage

**Table 19.1** Common conditions associated with coagulation disorders in horses.

| |
|---|
| **Acute blood loss** |
| Aortic root rupture |
| Uterine artery rupture |
| Guttural pouch mycosis |
| External trauma |
| **Chronic blood loss** |
| Intestinal bleeding (right dorsal colitis) |
| Leptospira pneumonia – foals |
| Renal/urethral hemorrhage (pyelonephritis, idiopathic hematuria renal pseudoaneurysm) |
| Secondary immune mediated hemolytic anemia/IMHA (neoplasia, abscesses including *Rhodococcus equi*, clostridial myositis, drug reaction – penicillin, TMS) |
| Primary IMHA (neonatal isoerythrolysis, autoimmune disease) |
| Equine infectious anemia |
| Piroplasmosis |
| Red maple leaf toxicity |
| **Hypocoagulation** |
| Thrombocytopenia (immune mediated, acquired) |
| Thrombasthenia (abnormal platelet function) |
| Toxicosis (rodenticide, drug reaction) |
| Advanced disseminated intravascular coagulation (DIC) |
| Iatrogenic – dilution of coagulation factors by large volume fluid administration |
| Severe burns |
| Snake envenomation |
| **Hypercoagulation** |
| Thrombocytosis (uncommon) |
| Arteritis/vasculitis |
| Systemic inflammation/SIRS/sepsis |
| Consumptive coagulopathy – DIC |
| Snake envenomation |
| Locally – administration of irritating/hypertonic solutions (phenylbutazone, enrofloxacin) |

## Identification of Coagulation Disorders

Homeostasis between platelet activators and inhibitors, and between clot formation and breakdown, is required for normal function. Abnormalities of coagulation may present as thrombosis (hypercoagulation) or hemorrhage, including bleeding diathesis (hypocoagulation) or hemorrhagic crisis despite normal coagulation functions. In some cases, such as disseminated intravascular coagulation (DIC) associated with severe systemic inflammation, both hypo- and hyper-coagulant states may occur in the patient concurrently. Clinical identification of blood loss or possible coagulopathy is critical to inform the practitioner's diagnosis and treatment plan. General principles of the clinical examination and available diagnostic tests will be reviewed first, followed by more specific discussion of diseases commonly associated with coagulopathy in horses.

## Clinical Examination

Physical examination findings suggestive of acute bleeding or blood loss include tachycardia, tachypnea, pale mucous membranes, cool extremities. Petechiae, ecchymoses, and epistaxis or other indicators of mucosal bleeding suggest disorders of primary hemostasis (Figure 19.1). Horses with disorders of secondary hemostasis may have intracavitary hemorrhage, hematomas, or hemarthrosis.

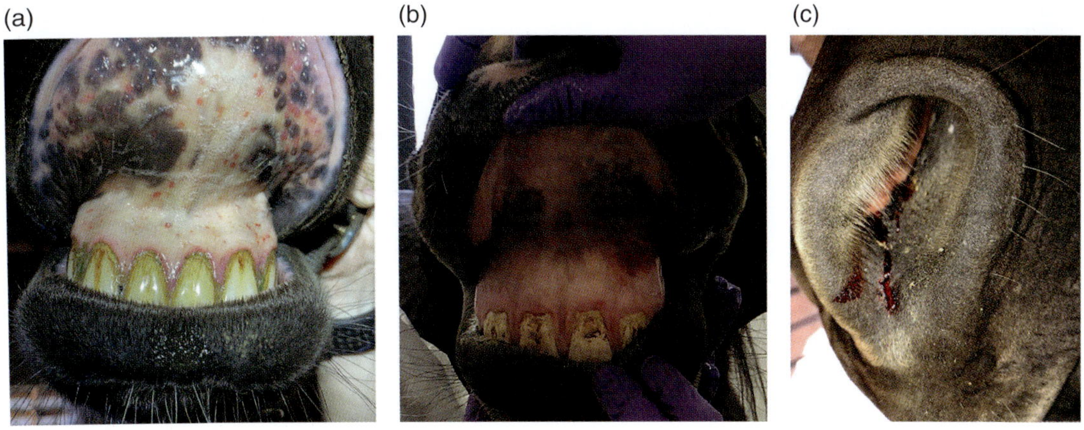

**Figure 19.1** Clinical examination findings suggestive of primary hemostatic disorder include (a) Petechiae on the oral mucous membranes of a Thoroughbred gelding with colitis. *Source:* Courtesy of Dr. Danielle Guilfoyle. (b) Large ecchymoses on gingiva of a 5-year-old Standardbred gelding with purpura hemorrhagica. *Source:* Courtesy of Dr. Kathryn Timko. (c) Spontaneous epistaxis in a 25-year-old grade gelding. *Source:* Courtesy of Ellie Masters.

Clinical signs of hypercoagulability depend on the location (jugular, appendicular, disseminated) and nature (complete, partial, microvascular) of thrombus formation. These may include a palpably thickened or rope-like vein, venous distension proximal to the affected vessel, partial or complete ischemia of tissues distal to the affected vessel, asymmetric cold limbs, hypothermic lameness, worsening colic secondary to mesenteric microvascular thrombosis, or regional edema with petechial or ecchymotic hemorrhage.

## Diagnostic Tests

There is a wide array of diagnostic tests available to assist the practitioner in identifying a cause of, or confirming suspicion of, coagulopathy. While many tests are only available in a clinic or specialized laboratory setting, others are available for use patient- or stall-side (Table 19.2). For all tests, atraumatic venipuncture during blood collection is important to limit contact and/or vessel trauma as activators of coagulation.

### Tests of Primary Hemostasis (Box 19.1)

**Platelet count** is the most basic assessment of primary hemostasis. Horses normally have a lower platelet count than other species (150,000–250,000 platelets/μL), and equine platelets are susceptible to clumping with prolonged storage. As a rule of thumb, if petechiae are present, the expected platelet count is 40,000–60,000 platelets/μL. Clinical bleeding may not be seen until the count is <30,000 platelets/μL and life-threatening hemorrhage may occur at <10,000 platelets/μL. Platelet count is generally measured from whole blood in EDTA (purple top tube) using one of several methods. Platelet counts can be estimated by microscopic examination of a blood smear: with a 100× objective, each platelet seen is equal to approximately 15,000 platelets/μL. If there are more than 10–15 platelets per high-powered field, the platelet count is within normal limits. More quantitative methods include manual count using a hemocytometer or use of an automated hematology analyzer. Regardless of method, a blood smear should be checked for platelet clumps. Warming the blood before analysis may minimize pseudothrombocytopenia due to platelet clumping (Williams and Archer 2016). An advantage of platelet count is that it can be performed with basic laboratory equipment. However, platelet count can be of limited utility due to the artifactual decrease with prolonged storage.

Abnormal platelet function can result in bleeding despite a normal or increased platelet count. The **platelet function analyzer (PFA-100)** tests platelet function in vitro by simulating the platelet adhesion and aggregation that occurs after vascular injury. The PFA-100 has been validated for use in horses (Segura et al. 2005) but must be run within one hours of sample collection. Causes of abnormal platelet function include Glanzmann thrombasthenia, von Willebrand's disease, and drug reactions.

**Template bleeding time (TBT)**, also commonly referred to as buccal mucosal bleeding time (BMBT), is a global assessment of platelet number and function. TBT is performed patient-side and should be considered if there are signs of primary hemostatic dysfunction with a normal or increased platelet count. To perform, a template device is used to create a small,

**Table 19.2** Common tests of coagulation homeostasis. For stall-side tests, manufacturer information included in table footnote.

| Test | Sample type | Stall-side | In house lab | Reference lab | Normal | Considerations |
|---|---|---|---|---|---|---|
| Platelet count | Whole blood in EDTA | | X | X | 150k–250k plt/μL | Platelet clumping may falsely decrease count |
| Template bleeding time (TBT) | In vivo | X[a] | | | 2–6 minutes | Invasive, poor reproducibility |
| PFA-100 | Whole blood | | X | | 60–116 minutes | Must perform w/in 1 h of collection |
| Prothrombin time (PT) | Citrated plasma | X[b] | | X | 16–20 seconds | Artifactually decreased by low fibrinogen |
| Partial thromboplastin time (PTT) | Citrated plasma | | | X | 45–66 seconds | |
| Activated clotting time (ACT) | Whole blood | X[c] | | | | Less sensitive than aPTT; available test not validated |
| Antithrombin | Citrated plasma | | | X | 85–130% | |
| Protein C | Citrated plasma | | | X | Not established | |
| Thrombin-antithrombin complexes (TAT) | | | | | | Typically research settings only |
| Fibrin(ogen) degradation products (FDP) | Citrated plasma | | | X | ≤10 μg/mL | Low sensitivity |
| Fibrinogen | Whole blood in EDTA or citrated plasma | | X | X | 200–400 mg/dL | Confounded by inflammation |
| D-dimers | Citrated plasma | | | X | <500 ng/mL | May be up to 1,000 ng/mL in some healthy horses |
| Sonoclot, TEG, ROTEM | Citrated plasma or fresh whole blood | | X | | Device-specific | High interoperator variability; Must perform in 30–60 minutes of collection |
| VCM-Vet | Fresh whole blood | X[d] | | | See Figure 19.2 | Duration of test limits assessment of clot lysis |

[a] Surgicutt, International Technidyne Corp.
[b] CoaguCheck-XS, Roche Diagnostics.
[c] SCAT-ACT, Haematologic Technologies.
[d] VCM-Vet, Entegrion Inc.

**Box 19.1 Summary of tests assessing primary hemostasis**

- Platelet count
- Platelet function analyzer (PFA-100)
- Template bleeding time
- Clot retraction time

standardized incision on the buccal mucosa, or caudolateral forelimb (Kopp et al. 1985). For the forelimb, hair is clipped at the incision site distolateral to the accessory carpal bone. Blood is absorbed with filter paper held 1–2 mm below the incision, and the time from incision to cessation of bleeding is recorded (normally two to six minutes). Prolonged TBT suggests thrombocytopenia, thrombocytopathia, lack of von Willebrand's factor, or vasculitis. The TBT can be easily performed in the field with minimal equipment. However, the diagnostic utility is limited by poor reproducibility and wide reference range in horses (Segura and Monreal 2008).

**Clot retraction time** is a crude measure of platelet number and function. To perform, whole blood is allowed to clot in a vacutainer tube, and the time to clot formation and subsequent clot retraction is measured. Both times will be prolonged in thrombocytopenia. While quite easy to perform, results are highly variable and this test is not recommended if alternatives are available.

**Box 19.2 Summary of tests of secondary hemostasis**

- Prothrombin time (extrinsic and common pathway)
- Activated partial thromboplastin time (intrinsic and common pathway)
- Activated clotting time (intrinsic and common pathway)

### Tests of Secondary Hemostasis (Box 19.2)

**Prothrombin time (PT)** assesses function of the extrinsic and common coagulation pathways, by measuring the time to clot formation when calcium is added to platelet-poor plasma or anticoagulated whole blood. An increase in time by 20% is considered abnormal. While PT is often performed in a reference laboratory, a stall-side PT assay is available that is comparable to lab-based methods (Berlin et al. 2019). **Activated partial thromboplastin time (aPTT)** measures function of the intrinsic and common coagulation pathways. As for PT, platelet-poor plasma or anticoagulated whole blood is stimulated to clot by addition of activating agent, calcium, and phospholipid. PT and aPTT should be interpreted together, and with consideration of other laboratory findings (Table 19.3). Fibrinogen should be measured concurrently, as low fibrinogen can prolong both PT and aPTT independent of other coagulopathy.

**Activated clotting time (ACT)** is a rapid, stall-side test that uses diatomaceous earth to stimulate the intrinsic and common coagulation pathways. While it has been described as reproducible when used in horses, ACT is susceptible to variations in platelet count, hematocrit, and plasma protease activity (Rawlings et al. 1975), and is less sensitive than aPTT for monitoring heparin anticoagulation (Murray et al. 1997).

### Anticoagulant Testing (Box 19.3)

**Antithrombin** and **Protein C** are critical components of the anticoagulant system that can be measured by chromogenic assays (Topper and Prasse 1996, 1998). Decreased antithrombin and protein C have been associated with hypercoagulability in horses. While one cause of decreased antithrombin is consumption in thrombin formation (as in DIC), it can also be decreased due to failure of production or protein loss (enteropathy, nephropathy, whole blood loss). Interpretation is further complicated as antithrombin is a positive acute-phase protein – that is, it increases in some inflammatory conditions.

**Table 19.3** Guidelines for interpretation of prothrombin time (PT) and activated partial thromboplastin time (aPTT).

| Activated partial thromboplastin time (aPTT) | Prothrombin time (PT): Normal | Prothrombin time (PT): Prolonged |
|---|---|---|
| Normal | | Factor VII deficiency<br>• Over dilution of plasma with citrate<br>• Early vitamin K deficiency/antagonism<br>• Inherited FVII deficiency (dogs)<br>• DIC (cats) |
| Prolonged | Intrinsic pathway deficiency<br>• Difficult venipuncture (artifact)<br>• DIC (early)<br>• Synthetic liver failure<br>• Heparin therapy<br>• Inherited deficiency of intrinsic or contact coagulation factors (rare in horses) | Multiple factor or common factor deficiencies<br>• Vitamin K deficiency/antagonism (anticoagulant rodenticides)<br>• DIC<br>• Liver failure |

**Box 19.3 Summary of tests assessing anticoagulation system**

- Antithrombin
- Protein C
- Thrombin–antithrombin complexes (TAT)

**Box 19.4 Summary of tests assessing clot breakdown**

- Fibrinogen
- Fibrin(ogen) degradation products
- D-dimers

**Thrombin–antithrombin complexes (TAT)** can be measured by sandwich ELISA. TAT are increased with activation of coagulation and establishment of a pro-coagulable state and are associated with DIC and sepsis in humans. Increased TAT has been documented in horses with severe colic, reflective of a hypercoagulable state (Topper and Prasse 1996, 1998). However, measurement of TAT is often impractical in a clinical setting and is potentially overly sensitive, increasing with simple catheter placement (McGovern et al. 2013).

#### Clot Breakdown (Box 19.4)

**Fibrinogen** is produced by the liver and consumed in clot formation. Fibrinogen can be decreased by DIC, liver disease, whole blood loss, or dilutional coagulopathy. Fibrinogen can be measured by a simple heat precipitation method, the von Clauss method, or automated photometric analyzer, and should be included in a standard coagulation profile. Low levels of fibrinogen (<100 mg/dL) have been associated with DIC in humans. However, fibrinogen is also a positive acute-phase protein, and dramatic increases are seen with inflammatory conditions in horses. As DIC in equine patients is often concurrent or secondary to inflammatory conditions, the association between hypofibrinogenemia and DIC is less consistent in horses (Welch et al. 1992; Kw et al. 1993). Fibrinogen should be considered in light of any suspected level of inflammation, and DIC should be considered if the fibrinogen concentration is lower than expected. Increases in fibrinogen are non-specific and not associated with thrombosis or clot lysis.

**Fibrin(ogen) degradation products (FDPs)** are produced when fibrin and fibrinogen are broken down by plasmin. Increased FDPs suggests a hyperfibrinolytic state or dramatic increase in clot formation. FDPs are typically measured by a semi-quantitative test in a laboratory setting. While normal ranges of FDPs have been reported in horses, measurement of FDPs in horses with colic had low sensitivity for diagnosis of DIC (Stokol et al. 2005).

**D-dimer** is a crosslinked dimer of the smallest FDPs that result from degradation of fibrin and are specific for plasmin degradation of fibrin (rather than fibrinogen). D-dimer levels can be measured by semi-quantitative latex agglutination or latex-enhanced turbidometric assays. Increased D-dimer levels are associated with increased fibrinolysis or decreased clearance of products due to liver disease, and may reflect a physiologic response to primary disease or pathologic coagulopathy. Increased D-dimers have been reported in horses with severe colic, in association with DIC (Stokol et al. 2005), and negative prognosis (Monreal et al. 2000; Cesarini et al. 2010; Nikvand et al. 2019).

#### Viscoelastic Monitoring

Viscoelastic tests evaluate clot formation in vitro by assessing changes in viscosity and/or elasticity. Using fresh or citrated whole blood, viscoelastic tests allow evaluation of all phases of clot formation and retraction. These tests are more comprehensive than the previously discussed in vitro tests, and include contributions of both platelets and coagulation factors to clot formation, tracing the entire clot retraction process rather than the endpoint as measured by FDPs or D-dimer. An additional benefit of viscoelastic tests is the ability to detect both hypercoagulable and hypercoagulable states (McMichael and Smith 2011).

Viscoelastic testing requires specialized equipment and either fresh whole blood, called "native" blood, or citrate anticoagulated blood depending on the test. Available viscoelastic testing devices vary in the instrument design and terminology used. **Thromboelastography (TEG)** detects changes in impedance as blood clots within an oscillating cup with a fixed probe, while **rotational thromboelastometry (ROTEM)** and **Sonoclot** detect changes in impedance through a vibrating probe immersed in a stationary blood sample. A variety of protocols for use of TEG, ROTEM, and Sonoclot have been reported, with most utilizing one or more activators to stimulate in vitro coagulation. The **VCM Vet** is designed for field use and requires only fresh whole blood loaded into a specialized warmed test cartridge. Within the test cartridge, two parallel glass discs oscillate to initiate coagulation by contact activation and detect changes in viscosity.

Regardless of the specific test mechanisms, viscoelastic tests generate output as a tracing of clot formation and retraction, with multiple metrics to numerically describe the shape of the trace. Each device uses proprietary terminology (Table 19.4), but the underlying principles of test interpretation are the same. For simplicity, the shared terminology of ROTEM and

**Table 19.4** Terminology for viscoelastic test parameters. While the principles of viscoelastic testing are the same, each device uses proprietary variable output.

| Clot development | ROTEM | TEG | Sonoclot | VCM Vet |
|---|---|---|---|---|
| Time to fibrin formation | Clot time (CT) | Reaction time (R) | SonACT | Clot time (CT) |
| Rate of fibrin formation | Clot formation time (CFT)<br>α angle (α) | Kinetics (K)<br>α angle (α) | Clot rate (CR) | Clot formation time (CFT)<br>α angle (Alpha) |
| Strength of fibrin clot | Maximum clot formation (MCF) | Maximum amplitude (MA) | Peak amplitude | Maximum clot formation (MCF) |
| Fibrinolysis | Lysis at 30 and 60 minutes (LY30, LY60) | Clot lysis at 30 and 60 minutes (CL30, CL60) | $R_3$ | Lysis at 30 and 45 minutes (LI30, LI45) |

VCM Vet will be used in this text. The lag time between the start of the test and fibrin formation [clot time (CT)] is dependent on coagulation factors and hematocrit. The fibrin formation curve is described by the rate of fibrin formation [clot formation time (CFT), alpha angle (α)] and the strength of fibrin clot [maximum clot firmness (MCF)]. The rate and strength of fibrin clot formation is affected by hematocrit, coagulation factors, platelet number, and function. Fibrinolysis is measured as a percent or factor of clot remaining (lysis at 30 and 45 minutes [LI30, LI45]) after CT, and is dependent on the qualities of the fibrin clot as well as the activity of plasmin and its activators in the blood.

Visual assessment of the trace is a quick and easy way to grossly assess if coagulation is normal or abnormal. In a normal horse, the trace has the shape of a white wine glass, while a hypocoagulable sample resembles a champagne flute, and hypercoagulable sample resembles a red wine or coupe glass (Figure 19.2). A hypercoagulable state can also be identified by decreased time to fibrin and clot formation (short CT and CFT), rapid rate of fibrin formation (high alpha), and increased strength of the fibrin clot (high MCF). Low hematocrit or high fibrinogen concentrations can result in a trace that appears to be hypercoagulable. A hypocoagulable state is identified by increased time to fibrin and clot formation (prolonged CT and CFT), slow rate of fibrin formation (low alpha), and decreased strength of the fibrin clot (low MCF). High hematocrit or low fibrinogen concentrations can result in apparently hypocoagulablility.

Fibrinolysis is assessed by the slope in the later part of the tracing (after MCF), reflecting the speed and degree of clot lysis. A hypofibrinolytic state is reflected in increased LI30/LI45, meaning that less clot is remaining, and a hypofibrinolytic state is reflected by decreased LI30/LI45, meaning that a greater percentage of clot is remaining. Clot lysis should be interpreted with consideration for the strength and amount of fibrin clot that formed initially, as a weaker clot will be lysed more rapidly (and a stronger clot lysed more slowly) with normal activity of the fibrinolytic system.

Viscoelastic test results are susceptible to variation in sample type and handling. For traditional viscoelastic tests (TEG, ROTEM, Sonoclot), use of fresh whole blood is associated with greater variability compared to anticoagulated blood. The choice of activator (if used) affects test interpretation, as some stimulate the extrinsic pathway (e.g., tissue factor) while others stimulate the intrinsic pathway of coagulation (e.g., kaolin, ellagic acid). Even with anticoagulated samples, TEG, ROTEM, or Sonoclot should be run at standardized times (30 or 60 minutes), as blood becomes more hypocoagulable with increased storage. For the VCM Vet, fresh unadulterated whole blood must be loaded into the test cartridge within four minutes of collection. Needle gauge and syringe size can also affect the degree of contact activation during sample collection. It is important that standardized protocols for blood collection, test timing, and use of activating agents are standardized within the clinic. The primary patient-specific variable that affects viscoelastic tests results is hematocrit, with high hematocrit resulting in hypocoagulable tracings and low hematocrit resulting in hypercoagulable tracings (McMichael et al. 2011).

Diagnostic utility of viscoelastic testing has been documented in septic foals and adult horses with gastrointestinal disease (Dallap Schaer et al. 2009; Mendez-Angulo et al. 2010; Epstein et al. 2011, 2013). However, despite potential to improve case management and outcome by earlier identification of coagulopathy, the expense and technical expertise required may be a barrier to clinical application in equine practice (Junge et al. 2016; Thane et al. 2017). Cost, ease of use, and repeatability are important considerations for the practitioner selecting a viscoelastic testing device.

The **Sonoclot** has been shown to have better interoperator reliability than TEG (Hett et al. 1995). However, the Sonoclot results are influenced by age, sex, and platelet count (Horlocker and Schroeder 1997), and have variable reproducibility (McMichael and Smith 2011). Additional limitations of Sonoclot are the lack of a standardized protocol and the inability to run more than one sample simultaneously.

(a)

| | | |
|---|---|---|
| CT | 531s | [536–1270] |
| CFT | 1281s | [123–574] |
| Alpha | 17° | [12–51] |
| A10 | 7 | [9–27] |
| A20 | 10 | [18–36] |
| MCF | 13 | [17–39] |
| LI30 | 100% | [97–100] |
| LI45 | 99% | [82–100] |

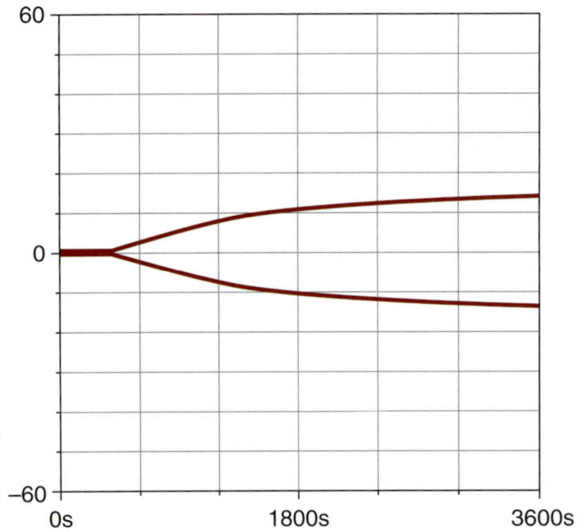


(b)

| | | |
|---|---|---|
| CT | 828s | [536–1270] |
| CFT | 270 | [123–574] |
| Alpha | 38° | [12–51] |
| A10 | 22 | [9–27] |
| A20 | 28 | [18–36] |
| MCF | 29 | [17–39] |
| LI30 | 100% | [97–100] |
| LI45 | 96% | [82–100] |

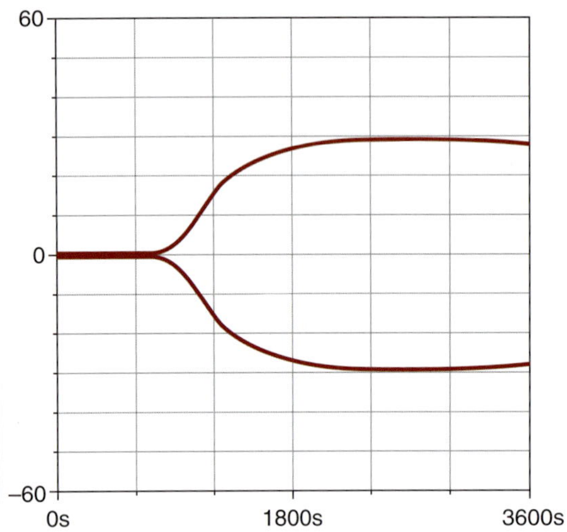


(c)

| | | |
|---|---|---|
| CT | 677s | [536–1270] |
| CFT | 143s | [123–574] |
| Alpha | 51° | [12–51] |
| A10 | 96 | [9–27] |
| A20 | 96 | [18–36] |
| MCF | 96 | [17–39] |
| LI30 | 100% | [97–100] |
| LI45 | 99% | [82–100] |

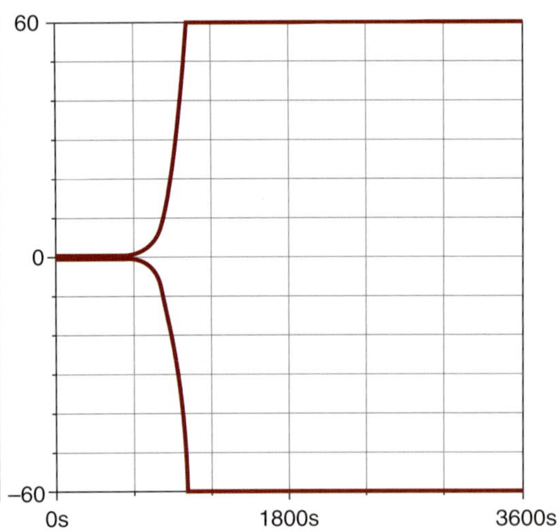


**Figure 19.2** Viscoelastic test outputs from VCM-Vet. Overall impression of coagulation status can be garnered from quick visual assessment of the trace shape, test values, and reference ranges are shown in the adjacent table. (a) Hypocoagulable samples resemble a champagne flute, such as this sample from a post-operative large colon volvulus with clinical signs of DIC. (b) A normal horse's trace resembles a white wine glass. (c) Hypercoagulable samples resemble a red wine or coupe glass, as in this extreme example from a horse with severe fibrinous peritonitis. *Source:* Courtesy of Dr. Rebecca Bishop.

The **TEG** is less costly than ROTEM and has capacity to run two samples concurrently. However, variable protocols limits comparison between studies, or between values obtained at one lab compared to another. Significant individual variation in TEG values may limit diagnostic utility (Mendez-Angulo et al. 2010), and there are no validated definitions of hypercoagulable states for various animal species.

The **ROTEM** is less susceptible to movement or vibration artifacts than TEG or Sonoclot. Additional features include an electronic pipette to decrease interoperator variability, and capacity to run up to four concurrent samples.

Unlike other viscoelastic testing devices, the **VCM Vet** is small, sturdy, and easily transportable to be used stall-side or in the field. Samples are processed in self-contained cartridges, limiting sources of interoperator variability. The VCM Vet has been validated for use in adult horses (Bishop et al. 2023) and foals (Migliorisi et al. 2020), and is readily used for patient-side assessment of coagulation homeostasis. Use of consistent needle and syringe size (18-gauge needle, 3 mL) syringe is recommended as the VCM Vet device is susceptible to variation due to contact activation during venipuncture. Current test software limits the total test duration to one hour, which is insufficient to capture clot lysis in most horses (Bishop et al. 2023).

## Emergency Conditions Associated with Blood Loss

### Acute Blood Loss

While acute large-volume blood loss may be easily apparent to the owner and clinician in the case of external bleeding (Case Example 19.1), as from trauma or guttural pouch mycosis, internal hemorrhage must not be forgotten as a cause of peracute or acute signs of shock. Possible causes of internal bleeding include uterine artery rupture, aortic root rupture, trauma or bleeding from a neoplastic mass. Hemothorax secondary to rib fracture should be considered in neonatal foals with signs of acute internal hemorrhage.

### Recognition of Hemorrhage

- Horses with clinically significant acute hemorrhage will demonstrate signs of shock, including tachycardia, tachypnea, pale mucous membranes, delayed capillary refill time, agitation or depression, sweating, and cold extremities. Blood should be obtained to measure the packed cell volume (PCV) and total protein at a minimum. However, remember that PCV may remain within normal for up to 12 h after onset of acute hemorrhage if intravenous fluids are not administered. Measurement of L-lactate can also be easily performed patient-side to assess the degree of tissue hypoxia. Ultrasonographic examination of the chest and abdomen is useful to identify internal hemorrhage, which appears as mixed echogenicity effusion, often with a swirling or "snow globe" appearance (Figure 19.3). Abdominocentesis can confirm intraperitoneal hemorrhage, although the specific source is often difficult to identify.

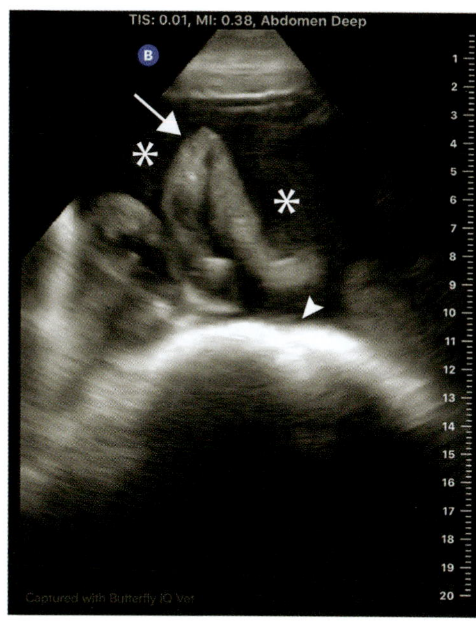


**Figure 19.3** Transabdominal ultrasonographic image from a mare with spontaneous hemoabdomen secondary to splenic neoplasia. Internal hemorrhage appears as a mixed echogenicity effusion (*) with a swirling or "snow globe" appearance when viewed live. Small intestine (arrow) can be seen within the effusion, ventral to the visceral surface of adjacent large intestine (arrowhead). *Source:* Courtesy of Dr. Rebecca Bishop.

### Treatment

The goals of treatment are to control hemorrhage and to restore both blood volume and oxygen-carrying capacity. If bleeding is external, a tourniquet or pressure bandage should be applied until definitive surgical hemostasis can be achieved. Stabilization of a hemorrhagic crisis due to guttural pouch mycosis is challenging; both internal carotid arteries should be temporarily ligated if possible, as ligation of the affected side only results in increased blood flow through the Circle of Willis. The horse should be kept quiet if possible to decrease blood pressure and slow ongoing blood loss. Sedatives, such as alpha-agonists or acepromazine, should be used judiciously with careful consideration for their hemodynamic effects.

### Fluid Resuscitation

Crystalloid fluids are used to restore circulating blood volume, especially in cases of hemorrhagic shock. However, administration of large volumes of crystalloid fluids can dilute platelets and coagulation factors, resulting in impaired clot formation. Synthetic colloids, such as hetastarch, have a similar negative effect on hemostasis through hemodilution (Jones et al. 1997). "Hypotensive resuscitation" or initial conservative administration of crystalloid fluids should be the goal until definitive hemostasis can be established and maintained. Once bleeding is controlled a 20 mL/kg "shock dose" of intravenous crystalloid fluid can be administered. Hypertonic saline (2–4 mL/kg IV bolus) can also be considered if immediate volume resuscitation is needed.

### Blood/Blood Products

An important consideration when attending to a horse with acute hemorrhage is whether – or when – to initiate a blood transfusion. Clinical indications to consider transfusion include: suspected or known large-volume blood loss with signs of shock and decreasing total solids, acute blood loss, and PCV <20%, increased L-lactate (>4 mmol/L) despite volume replacement (indicates tissue hypoxia), or chronic anemia with PCV 10–12% and evidence of tissue hypoxia.

**Fresh whole blood** is the ideal choice to replace acute volume loss (hypovolemic anemia). The volume to be administered should be determined based on the known or estimated volume lost. If the patient presents with acute blood loss with signs of shock, blood volume loss can be estimated at 30%, or 12 L for a 500 kg horse (Table 19.5). Blood transfusion volume is then calculated to replace 25–50% of the known or estimated volume lost; 3–6 L for the 500 kg horse. Remaining blood volume will be compensated by fluid shifts after transfusion. In the case of blood loss into a body cavity, up to 75% of red blood cells (RBCs) will be autotransfused within one to three days. Alternatively, the volume to administer can be calculated from the donor and patient PCV. The maximum volume that can be collected from most blood donor horses is 8 L, and the volume donated should be replaced with crystalloid fluids, especially if more than 3–5 L are collected. Refer to **Chapter 5** for recommendations for blood collection and administration.

A first blood transfusion can be performed without cross-matching. Only two of the 26 equine blood types are strongly antigenic (Qa and Aa), and horses do not develop antibodies to other blood types until after exposure to an antigenic blood type. However, broodmares may be sensitized to other blood types during pregnancy to parturition and are therefore predisposed to adverse reactions. Blood should initially be administered at a slow drip (0.3 mL/kg over the first 10–20 minutes) and the patient monitored for any adverse reaction, including but not limited to increase in temperature, pulse, and respiratory rate (TPR). Measurement and recording of the TPR every 5 minutes for the first 20 minutes of transfusion, and every 15 minutes thereafter is recommended. If there are no signs of an adverse reaction, the rate can be increased for the remainder of the transfusion. If hypovolemic, increase the rate of 20–40 mL/kg/h (10–20 L/h for a 500 kg horse); practically, this equates to an open bolus on most blood administration sets. Blood transfusion sets (Figure 19.4) may develop clogged filters after a few liters and may need to be changed several times during a transfusion, depending on the volume being administered.

**Table 19.5** Calculations to determine volume of blood loss or blood transfusion needed.

| Transfusion volume | |
|---|---|
| **Adult** | **Foal** |
| **Based on estimated 30% blood volume loss:**<br>Body weight (kg) $\times 0.08 \times 0.3$<br>Example: 500 kg $\times 0.08 \times 0.3 = 12$ L<br>Administer 25–50% of calculated volume: $3-6$ L | **Based on estimated 30% Blood Volume Loss:**<br>Body weight (kg) $\times 0.16 \times 0.3$<br>Example: 50 kg $\times 0.16 \times 0.3 = 2.4$ L<br>Administer 25–50% of calculated volume: $0.6-1.2$ L |
| **Based on PCV:**<br>$\text{Body weight (kg)} \times 0.08 \times \frac{PCV_{desired} - PCV_{actual}}{PCV_{donor}}$ | **Based on PCV:**<br>$\text{Body weight (kg)} \times 0.16 \times \frac{PCV_{desired} - PCV_{actual}}{PCV_{donor}}$ |

Adverse reactions occur in 16% of blood transfusions (Hurcombe et al. 2007). Mild adverse reactions, including urticaria/hives, fever, and tachypnea, are most common. In cases of mild adverse reaction, flunixin meglumine (1.1 mg/kg IV) with or without an anti-histamine (diphenhydramine 0.5–1 mg/kg IM, tripelennamine, 1.1 mg/kg IM or hydroxazine 0.5–1 mg/kg PO) can be administered. Acute anaphylaxis is reported in 2% of transfusions and should be treated with epinephrine (0.01–0.02 mL of 0.1 mg/mL solution IV).

**Platelet transfusion** can be indicated for treatment of severe thrombocytopenia (<15,000–30,000 platelets/μL), or known functional platelet abnormalities, especially during prolonged bleeding or if surgical bleeding is expected. Although platelet transfusion would ideally be prepared by plasma apheresis or centrifugation, gravity sedimentation of whole blood will result in a platelet-rich plasma supernatant. Citrate anticoagulant is recommended but can impair platelet function if the appropriate ratio is not used (take care not to underfill the collection bag). Blood should be collected in plastic, as glass containers cause platelet activation.

**Plasma transfusion** should be considered to address clotting factor deficiency or hypoalbuminemia in a patient with apparently adequate oxygen-carrying capacity. Fresh frozen plasma contains immunoglobulins, coagulation factors, and anticoagulant proteins such as antithrombin, protein C, and protein S. For severe hypoproteinemia, the volume of plasma can be calculated from the desired total protein concentration and the protein concentration in the plasma product. Alternatively, the recommended dose of plasma to support coagulation homeostasis is 4 mL/kg body weight, or 2 L for a 500 kg horse (Mudge 2019). Initial administration of plasma should be slow with careful monitoring for signs of reaction, as described for whole blood.

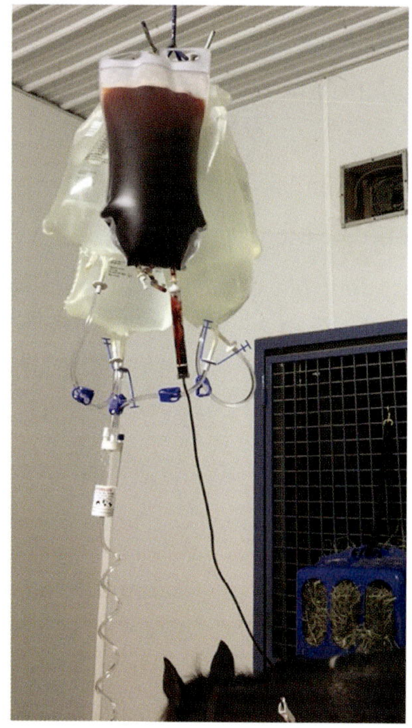

**Figure 19.4** Blood transfusion in progress; clots in the filter of the blood transfusion set may develop and slow transfusion rate. Note that crystalloid fluids are being administered through a separate intravenous catheter. *Source:* Courtesy of Dr. Rebecca Bishop.

#### Adjunctive Coagulation Treatments

A variety of adjunctive treatments are available to support the coagulation and fibrinolytic system in horses in coagulopathic crisis. These treatments are commercially available and reasonably shelf-stable; if kept on hand, emergency treatment can be started while blood donor or referral arrangements are made.

**Aminocaproic acid** and **tranexamic acid** inhibit fibrinolysis by binding plasminogen activators and increasing antiplasmin activity to prevent clot breakdown. Aminocaproic acid is administered in 1L saline over 30–60 minutes, first at a loading dose of 40 mg/kg, followed by 20 mg/kg every 6 h. Tranexamic acid is administered in 1 L saline as a bolus, 20 mg/kg IV every 12 h.

**Yunnan Baiyo** is a traditional Chinese herbal medication that is theorized to cause platelet activation and increase expression of glycoproteins on the platelet surface (Tang et al. 2009). Hemostatic efficacy had been demonstrated in human surgical patients, and anecdotal reports in horses support its use. The reported dose is 8 g (typically one box or bottle) PO every 12 h.

**Formalin** has also been suggested for emergency treatment of acute bleeding, to increase endothelial/platelet adhesion, although no effect on hemostatic variables has been demonstrated in healthy horses (Taylor et al. 2000). The reported clinical dose is 10–100 mL of 10% formalin in 1 L saline administered IV.

**Conjugated estrogens** (Premarin) is used to control bleeding by enhancing platelet activity and decreasing antithrombin activity (Hedges et al. 2007). Its use has been described for humans with uremia and horses with uterine bleeding. The reported clinical dose for horses is 25–50 mg per 500 kg body weight administered IV.

#### Topical Hemostatic Agents

A variety of products are available that exert hemostatic effects by applying pressure or providing scaffold for platelets and coagulation factors. Use of such products has been reported for stabilization of coagulation in traumatic wounds, foot abscesses, castration sites, as well as other surgical applications (Ramey et al. 2021). Gelatin, cellulose-based (Surgicel), collagen-based (Instat, Avitene), and polysaccharide-based (TraumaDex, Arista, Chitosan) products are available in a variety of formulations including impregnated sponges, gauze, or free granules. Some products are absorbed rapidly within hours (Ahuja et al. 2006) or weeks (Schonauer et al. 2004), while others may persist for months to years (Sileshi et al. 2008).

Considerations for use of hemostatic agents include delayed wound healing and potentiation of infection. All products may delay wound healing, aside from the polysaccharide hemispheres (Ahuja et al. 2006). Cellulose-based products have a low pH which may be antibacterial and are preferred for use in contaminated areas (Spangler et al. 2003). Collagen products function as a scaffold for primary hemostasis and are therefore less effective in patients with thrombocytopenia (Boucher and Traub 2009).

## Chronic Blood Loss

Chronic blood loss and anemia may cause presentation with overt signs of tissue hypoxia or may be uncovered in the course of evaluation for non-specific signs such as lethargy, fever, or weight loss. Regardless of the cause, emergency stabilization with blood transfusion should be considered for chronic anemia with a PCV <10–12% and evidence of tissue hypoxia. Specific treatment will be discussed for each major cause of chronic anemia individually.

## Blood Transfusion for Normovolemic (Chronic) Anemia

For normovolemic or chronic anemia, whole blood transfusion should be performed judiciously with consideration for possible volume overload. A safer alternative is **packed Red Blood Cells (RBCs)** to convey oxygen-carrying capacity while minimizing additional volume administration. While packed RBCs are ideally prepared by centrifugation or plasmapheresis, gravity sedimentation is a practical option that capitalizes on the propensity of equine RBCs to rouleaux in solution to generate more concentrated RBCs. Gravity sedimentation is performed by simply allowing RBCs to settle in the collection bag before and during administration. In the case of chronic anemia, the volume to be administered should be calculated from the target and donor PCV (Table 19.5). Assuming a 500 kg patient and donor PCV of 35%, this calculation equates to approximately 6 L to raise the patient's PCV by 5%.

As for acute blood loss, blood should initially be administered slowly while monitoring for signs of adverse reaction. After 20–30 minutes, the remainder of the calculated volume is administered at a rate of 5 mL/kg/h (2.5 L/h). Refer to **Chapter 5** for specific recommendations for blood collection and administration

## Chronic Blood Loss

**Intestinal bleeding** is less common in horses than other species, but right dorsal colitis is occasionally associated with mild anemia (25–30%) (Cohen et al. 1995). Fecal occult blood tests are commercially available, but are of limited to no diagnostic utility in horses (Pellegrini 2005, Rebalka and Lindinger 2021). **Pulmonary hemorrhage** can occur intermittently due to an inhaled foreign body. Mild-to-moderate anemia has also been reported secondary to pulmonary hemorrhage in foals with Leptospira pneumonia (Broux et al. 2012). **Renal/urethral hemorrhage** has been reported due to pyelonephritis (Kisthardt et al. 1999), urethral rents, and isolated cases of renal pseudoaneurysm (Larsdotter et al. 2009) and idiopathic hematuria.

## Immune-Mediated Hemolytic Anemia (IMHA)

IMHA results in anemia due to destruction of red blood cells by the immune system. Causes of primary IMHA in horses include neonatal isoerythrolysis (NI) and auto-immune disease. Secondary IMHA can occur due to neoplasia, abscesses (including *Rhodococcus equi*), clostridial myositis, or drug reaction (most commonly penicillin or Trimethoprim sulfamethoxazole/TMS).

### Treatment of IMHA

Immunosuppression is the mainstay of treatment for secondary or auto-immune IMHA (for neonates, see NI below). Dexamethasone (0.1–0.2 mg/kg IV q24 h) or prednisolone (1–2 mg/kg IV, IM or PO q24 h) is administered and response to treatment monitored. Azathioprine (3 mg/kg PO q24 h) may be added if anemia is refractory to corticosteroid treatment.

### Treatment of Neonatal Isoerythrolysis (NI)

The best treatment for NI is prevention: foals should be withheld from nursing from the mare in the first 24 h of life if the mare has a history of previous NI-affected foals, or if clinical signs are identified early. To ensure passive transfer of immunity, immunoglobulins should be provided by an alternate route (enteral administration of donor colostrum from an unaffected mare within 12 h of birth, or plasma transfusion). Moderately affected foals can be treated with supportive care, exercise restriction, and monitoring. Administration of corticosteroids can be justified in severe cases of NI to decrease removal of the antibody-labeled red blood cells from circulation by the reticuloendothelial system. See **Chapter 20** for emergency stabilization of the neonate.

Signs of hypoxic shock occur around a PCV of 10–12%, and include progressive tachycardia and tachypnea, and decreased venous oxygen tension. Fever may be present. The goal of treatment is to improve tissue oxygenation. Intranasal oxygen insufflation is of limited utility in these cases, as the hemoglobin present in the blood is likely already at maximal oxygen-carrying capacity.

**Blood transfusion** is the mainstay of treatment for hypoxic shock in foals with NI. Ideally blood from a universal donor (Aa and Qa negative) or cross-matched unrelated donor is used for transfusion. Washed RBCs from the mare can be prepared to remove the offending antibody in the plasma by centrifugation, or serial gravity sedimentation with isotonic saline. Blood volume required is calculated as shown in Table 19.5, with a factor of 0.16 reflecting the higher relative circulating volume in neonatal foals. However, large volume infusion should be avoided when possible as >4 L blood transfusion has been associated with liver failure (Polkes et al. 2008). Typical starting volume for an average size foal is 1.8–2.0 L.

## Equine Infectious Anemia (EIA)

EIA is caused by an RNA virus that replicates in monocytes, macrophages, and endothelial cells. The virus is transmitted by biting insects, primarily Tabanid flies (horse and deer flies), as well as contaminated instruments, needles or blood products. Acute EIA infection is associated with anemia, thrombocytopenia, and fever (More et al. 2008). Additional clinical signs include depression, weakness, hemorrhage, peripheral edema, and weight loss in both acute and chronic forms. An inapparent carrier state is also possible. EIA is diagnosed by antibody tests – AGID or ELISA. EIA is reportable, and affected horses must be either placed in life-long quarantine or euthanized.

## Piroplasmosis

Piroplasmosis is caused by the intra-erythrocyte hematoprotozoa *Babesia caballi* and *Theileria equi*. Piroplasmosis is transmitted primarily by ticks, but in utero transmission to the fetus and iatrogenic transmission on contaminated instruments can also occur. The United States and Canada are considered disease-free, although outbreaks have been reported (Short et al. 2012; Ueti et al. 2012). Piroplasmosis is endemic in parts of Mexico, Central and South America, Southern Europe, Asia, and Africa.

### Clinical Signs

Signs of acute piroplasmosis infection include lethargy, fever, petechiae, edema, and hemoglobinuria. Colic, neurologic, and respiratory signs may also occur. Clinical signs typically appear 10–30 days after natural transmission, but as early as 5 days after iatrogenic intravenous transmission.

### Treatment

Treatment of horses with piroplasmosis consists primarily of supportive/symptomatic care. If untreated, horses with *T. equi* will become lifelong carriers, while natural clearance of *B. caballi* can occur. The carrier state is protective against reinfection, and, therefore, elimination is not desired in endemic areas.

In non-endemic areas, Piroplasmosis is reportable and affected horses must be enrolled in an approved treatment program, life-long quarantine, or be euthanized. Definitive treatment consists of imidocarb dipropionate (2.2–4.4 mg/kg IM once or q72 h for four doses), and clearance is confirmed by PCR or serology.

## Red Maple Leaf Toxicity

Ingestion of wilted leaves of the red maple tree (*Acer rubrum*), silver maple (*Acer saccharinum*), and sugar maple (*Acer saccharum*) causes severe acute methemoglobinemia and hemolysis in horses. Leaves of the Pistacia species (not native to North America but found in the southern United States) causes a similar clinical presentation (Bozorgmanesh et al. 2015).

#### Clinical Signs

Consumption of ≥1.5 g leaves/kg body weight will likely cause clinical signs of hypoxia secondary to oxidative damage, hemolysis, and methemoglobinemia. Muddy brown to cyanotic mucous membranes are highly suggestive of methemoglobinemia. Hypoxia results in lethargy, fever, tachycardia, tachypnea, and hemoglobinuria. Other signs include colic, renal insufficiency/acute kidney injury, and laminitis.

#### Treatment

Treatment is primarily supportive, including IV fluids, pain medication, and blood transfusion as indicated by clinical signs. **Mineral oil** or Biosponge may be administered enterally to prevent further toxin absorption if ingestion is acute or has been ongoing. **Antioxidant support** is also recommended, specifically Vitamin C (ascorbic acid; 30–50 mg/kg IV q12 h in saline is preferred, or 9,000 mg/kg PO for 12 weeks), as Vitamin E (α-tocopherol; 800 IU/kg PO q24 h) only reduces hemolysis (O'Callaghan et al. 2015). Anti-inflammatory doses of corticosteroids may also be considered to decrease inflammation and reduce RBC destruction (dexamethasone, 10–20 mg/500 kg horse).

#### Prognosis

Prognosis is guarded (~41% survival) and complications are frequent, including colic, laminitis, acute kidney injury, and DIC (Alward et al. 2006). Corticosteroid administration and lack of fever on admission were negatively associated with survival in this large retrospective study.

## Emergency Conditions Associated with Coagulopathy

### Disseminated Intravascular Coagulation (DIC)

DIC describes disruption of coagulation and fibrinolysis homeostasis secondary to severe systemic inflammation (systemic inflammatory response syndrome or SIRS). In adult horses, DIC is most commonly associated with ischemic or inflammatory conditions of the large colon (large colon volvulus, colitis) resulting in massive systemic release of endotoxin and other pathogen-associated molecular patterns (PAMPs) (Morris and Beech 1983; Welch et al. 1992; Dolente et al. 2002, 2005; Dallap et al. 2003). In foals, DIC primarily occurs in association with SIRS and sepsis. Other causes of SIRS/sepsis include pleuropneumonia, enterocolitis, strangulating intestinal disease, other infectious diseases (EIA, anaplasmosis, and Equine Viral Arteritis), trauma (especially severe burns), Clostridial myositis, and neoplasia.

### Clinical Signs

The early stage of DIC typically manifests as a hypercoagulable state. Multisystemic thrombosis is the most common clinical sign, including jugular thrombophlebitis as well as laminitis and other organ dysfunction. Massive deposition of fibrin throughout microvasculature in the hypercoagulable phase can result in multiorgan failure. As DIC progresses, clotting factors and platelets are consumed, eventually resulting in a hypocoagulable state, which is associated with a poor prognosis. In actuality, the process is not linear, and all systems – activation, coagulation, fibrinolysis, and anticoagulation – can be explosively activated at once in the same patient.

### Diagnosis

Diagnosis of DIC is based on presence of a primary systemic disease that is a risk factor and clinical evidence of hyper- and/or hypocoagulability, supported by one or more clinicopathologic abnormality. Clinical pathology findings consistent with DIC include thrombocytopenia, prolonged PTT and/or aPTT, decreased fibrinogen (or lower than expected for inflammatory state), decreased antithrombin, increased D-dimers or FDPs (Stokol et al. 2005), or abnormal viscoelastic trace. The practitioner should keep in mind that coagulopathy may be subclinical in critically ill horses; screening with coagulation assays or viscoelastic tests, with repeat testing and monitoring, is warranted for patients with critical illness (Figure 19.2). In one study, in 70% of horses with large colon volvulus, at least 3/6 coagulation tests were abnormal without clinical evidence of coagulopathy (Dallap et al. 2003). A similar study in horses with colitis determined that horses with subclinical coagulopathy, recognized with testing, were 8 times more likely to not survive (Dolente et al. 2002).

## Treatment

The mainstay of treatment for DIC is aggressive treatment of the primary underlying disease, along with general supportive care and monitoring (see Chapter 27). Therapy specific to coagulation homeostasis will be addressed here.

### Fluid Therapy

**Crystalloid fluids** should be administered as needed to maintain blood volume and pressure, although aggressive fluid administration can cause dilution of platelets and blood proteins (including clotting factors), resulting in dilutional coagulopathy as well as hypoproteinemia.

**Colloids** are indicated to support circulating blood volume and oncotic pressure in the face of hypoproteinemia and edema. The use of plasma or platelet transfusion in treatment of DIC is controversial, as addition of clotting factors may be "fuel to the fire" in a hypercoagulable state. On the other hand, **fresh frozen plasma** provides antithrombin, commonly decreased in critically ill horses, and is beneficial to coagulation homeostasis. Transfusion is recommended in any horse with active or high risk of bleeding. **Synthetic colloids**, such as hetastarch, should be avoided if there is evidence of existing coagulopathy, as they can cause or worsen coagulopathy in a dose-dependent fashion (Jones et al. 1997; Blong et al. 2013).

### Endotoxemia

Endotoxin-related SIRS is a driving force behind DIC in many critically ill horses. **Polymyxin B** (6,000 IU/kg IV in saline q8–12 h) can be used to prevent or treat endotoxemia by binding to and neutralizing circulating endotoxin. **Flunixin meglumine** is also indicated to decrease the deleterious effects of the inflammatory response to endotoxin. A lower dose of flunixin (0.25–0.5 mg/kg IV) can be used to inhibit production of prostaglandins responsible for hemodynamic effects of endotoxin.

### Anticoagulation

Anticoagulation approaches can be used to limit activation of the coagulation cascade and consumption of coagulation factors in early DIC.

**Heparin** inhibits clot formation by activation of antithrombin. Experimental studies in healthy horses show decreased inflammation following small colon enterotomy (Alonso et al. 2020). However, there are no controlled studies to support the use of heparin in DIC, and use may negate the anti-inflammatory effects of antithrombin (Hoffmann et al. 2006). **Low-molecular-weight heparins** (dalteparin, enoxaparin) are less likely to cause adverse reactions, with a longer half-life, greater inhibition of factor X, and more predictable pharmacokinetics with dose-dependent clearance (Feige et al. 2010). Both are administered subcutaneously every 24 h, dalteparin at 50–100 IU/kg, and enoxaparin at 40–80 IU/kg. **Unfractionated heparins** (calcium heparin, sodium heparin) are more cost-effective and readily available, but injection site swelling with subcutaneous administration is common, and there is an increased risk of iatrogenic hypocoagulation as evidenced by prolonged aPTT and decreased PCV (Feige et al. 2010). Calcium heparin should be administered subcutaneously as a tapering course, beginning with 150 IU/kg once, then 125 IU/kg q12 h for three doses, then 100 IU/kg q12 h. Sodium heparin is administered subcutaneously at 40–80 IU/kg q12 h.

**Aspirin** inhibits platelet activation through inhibition of arachidonic acid and thromboxane. While aspirin does inhibit thromboxane (TXA2) in healthy horses, its effect on platelet aggregation in healthy horses is inconsistent (Brainard et al. 2011). This may be because the role of TXA2 in platelet function is less consistent in horses than in humans (Poole 1993).

**Clopidogrel (Plavix)** mediates anticoagulant effects by decreasing ADP-induced platelet aggregation. The effect on platelets is irreversible resulting in effects that persist until inhibited platelets are replaced, 6 days after treatment is discontinued (Brainard et al. 2011). The recommended dose is a loading dose of 4 mg/kg, followed by 2 mg/kg PO q24 h.

#### Prognosis

Prognosis of DIC is largely dictated by the nature of the primary condition and response to treatment. An increased number of abnormal coagulation tests is associated with worse outcomes (Dallap et al. 2003). In horses with colic, prolonged PT, aPTT, increased TAT or FDPs, decreased antithrombin and protein C, and thrombocytopenia are associated with nonsurvival (Pablo et al. 1983; Johnstone and Crane 1986; Kw et al. 1993; Collatos et al. 1995a, b; Topper and Prasse 1996, 1998; Monreal et al. 2000).

## Immune-Mediated Thrombocytopenia (ITP)

ITP occurs in horses in association with viral infections (EIA), abscessation, neoplasia (especially hemangiosarcoma), drug reactions (trimethoprim-sulfa), or can be idiopathic. Foals may develop ITP due to ingestion of colostral antibodies. ITP in combination with IMHA is called Evan's Syndrome, and occurs most commonly due to abscesses or neoplasia.

### Clinical Signs

Clinical signs of ITP reflect deficiency of primary hemostasis: petechiae, ecchymoses, and epistaxis or other mucosal bleeding. In foals, thrombocytopenia has been documented in conjunction with vesicles and other skin lesions (Perkins et al. 2005).

### Diagnosis

ITP is diagnosed by low platelet count, either by estimation from a blood smear or an absolute count. Mean platelet volume suggests a regenerative response to thrombocytopenia. If ITP is suspected, blood can be tested for antibody-coated platelets or a regenerative platelet response at some reference laboratories (platelet surface associated antibody, Kansas State Veterinary Diagnostic Laboratory). Viscoelastic testing can also be useful for functional assessment of coagulation status and to help direct therapy, as even with low platelet counts some patients will maintain normal coagulation function.

### Treatment

Horses, and especially foals, with severe thrombocytopenia should be stall rested until platelet count is >40,000 platelets/μL to decrease the risk of severe bleeding. The overall goal of treatment is to decrease ongoing platelet destruction and restore platelet function.

#### Immunosuppression

Immunosuppression with dexamethasone (10–80 mg IV or PO q12–24 h) or azathioprine (3 mg/kg PO q24 h) is recommended in adult horses to halt ongoing immune-mediated platelet destruction. In severe thrombocytopenia (<10,000 platelets/μL), dexamethasone and azathioprine can be administered concurrently. Platelet counts should be monitored every three to six days during treatment, and steroids tapered only after the platelet count returns to normal. Corticosteroid administration may not be necessary in foals, as most foals recover with or without steroid treatment (Perkins et al. 2005).

#### Vincristine

Vincristine is a chemotherapeutic drug that also increases platelet release from the bone marrow (Allen et al. 2021). Addition of vincristine is indicated if splenomegaly is identified concurrently with thrombocytopenia, suggesting immune-mediated platelet destruction. The suggested dose regimen is 0.004 mg/kg IV q24 h for three to five days, twice weekly for one to two weeks, and then once weekly until platelet count is stable (Fey and Sasse 1998).

#### Transfusion

Plasma or whole blood transfusion can provide platelets to decrease the immediate risk of bleeding, but may be of little benefit if thrombocytopenia is due to consumption. Whole blood should be collected in a plastic bag to preserve platelet function (recall that glass causes platelet activation). Platelet-rich plasma may also be of benefit if available. Fresh frozen plasma may also help by providing hemostatically functional platelet microparticles if platelets are unavailable.

## Clotting Factor Deficiencies

### Vitamin-K-Dependent Coagulopathy

Warfarin (Coumadin) overdose or anticoagulant rodenticide toxicity causes coagulopathy due to antagonism of vitamin-K-dependent coagulation factors (II, VII, IX, X). Ingestion of moldy sweet clover, and administration of some lactam or beta-lactam antibiotics can also cause vitamin K responsive coagulopathy. Clinical signs reflect derangement of secondary hemostasis, including intracavitary hemorrhage, hematomas, or hemarthrosis.

### Diagnosis

Presumptive diagnosis of warfarin toxicity is based on clinical signs and history of known or suspected ingestion. Prolonged PT and aPTT is supportive, although aPTT may remain normal in early stages of toxicity.

### Treatment

Treatment consists of vitamin K administration, 1 mg/kg or 300–500 mg for an adult horse, subcutaneously q24 h for one week. Second-generation or long-acting rodenticides may require prolonged therapy.

## Heritable Clotting Factor Deficiencies

Heritable clotting factor deficiencies are overall uncommon in horses (Dahlgren et al. 2021) but should be considered as differential diagnoses for horses presenting with signs of coagulopathy, especially when patient signalment matches reports in the literature or no apparent cause coagulopathy is present.

### Hemophilia A

Hemophilia A is an X-linked recessive mutation that results in Factor VIII deficiency. Clinical signs include recurrent bleeding and hematoma formation. Hemophilia A has been reported in male Thoroughbreds, Standardbreds, Quarter Horses, Arabian horses, and Tennessee Walking Horses. Suspicion of Hemophilia A is supported by prolonged aPTT with normal PT and decreased fibrinogen concentration. Definitive diagnosis is by measurement of FVIII:C. FVIII:C levels may also be low or low–normal in carriers.

### Von Willebrand Disease

Von Willebrand Disease, factor VIII-associated deficiency, has been reported in a few Thoroughbreds (Rathgeber et al. 2001) and a single Quarter Horse (Winfield and Brooks 2014). Clinical signs include episodic hemorrhage (epistaxis) and prolonged bleeding from venipuncture or procedure sites. Qualitative deficiencies in platelet function and increased in vivo bleeding time with normal platelet count, PT, and aPTT are supportive. Diagnosis is confirmed by von Willebrand factor assays. Acute or anticipated bleeding can be treated with plasma or cryoprecipitate transfusion to deliver factor VIII, von Willebrand factor, and fibrinogen. Larger volumes are needed for surgical hemostasis than to control mucosal bleeding. Desmospressin (DDAVP) is used in humans and dogs to increase von Willebrand factor release from endothelial cells, but is cost prohibitive in horses.

### Glanzmann's Thrombasthenia

Glanzmann's Thrombasthenia is an autosomal recessive inherited platelet defect such that platelets fail to bind fibrinogen, aggregate, or cause clot retraction. It has been reported in Quarter Horses, Thoroughbreds, Oldenburg warmbloods, and Peruvian Pasos (Fry et al. 2005; Livesey et al. 2005; Macieira et al. 2007; Sanz et al. 2011). Clinical signs include epistaxis, purpura, and gingival bleeding. Failure of the blood clot to retract from the walls of a plain vacutainer tube is a crude test to support suspected diagnosis of Glanzmann's Thrombasthenia. In vitro coagulation tests (PT, aPTT, FDPs) are normal, as secondary hemostasis is unaffected. Viscoelastic testing reveals increased CFT and decreased clot strength. There are two known genetic mutations associated with Glanzmann's Thrombasthenia in horses (Christopherson et al. 2007; Norris et al. 2015). There is no specific treatment; platelet transfusion is required for severe traumatic bleeding or prophylactically for surgical hemostasis.

#### Prekallikrein Deficiency

Kallikrein, the active form of prekallikrein, is involved in feedback amplification for FXIIa activation. Familial prekallikrein deficiency has been identified in Belgian drafts (Geor et al. 1990) and miniature horses (Turrentine et al. 1986). Other factors are involved in FXIIa activation, so clinical signs are often subtle, ranging from clinically normal to abnormal bleeding. Diagnosis is supported by prolonged aPTT with normal PT and fibrinogen, and confirmed by direct measurement of prekallikrein.

### Liver Failure

Liver failure secondary to hepatic necrosis, cirrhosis, and acute hepatitis has been associated with coagulopathy in horses (Lisman and Leebeek 2007). Coagulopathy may occur due to synthetic liver failure (insufficient production of fibrinogen and coagulation factors), vitamin K deficiency (impaired intrahepatic recycling or inadequate absorption), dysfibrinogenemia, platelet dysfunction, or abnormal clearance (increased fibrinolytic activators, FDPs, and D-dimers). Evaluation of coagulation homeostasis by traditional clotting profiles and/or viscoelastic testing is indicated in horses with signs of liver failure, especially before any invasive procedure. However, polycythemia is common in horses with liver failure, which may cause artifactual hypocoagulopathy on viscoelastic testing (McMichael et al. 2011), when in vivo coagulation function is normal.

### Snake Bite

Snake venom includes hemorrhagic toxins that affect coagulation. Depending on the toxin type, coagulopathy may manifest as hypercoagulation, hypocoagulation, or hyperfibrinogenolysis (clots dissolve as they form). In addition to direct coagulopathic affect, other toxins in venom can initiate a systemic inflammatory response resulting in DIC.

#### Diagnosis

Classic clinical signs of snake envenomation include bleeding snake bites, severe swelling, and pain at the location of the bite (Dickinson et al. 1996; Fielding et al. 2011). Coagulopathy typically affects both primary and secondary hemostases, resulting in petechiae, ecchymoses, hemorrhage, and hemolysis. Laboratory abnormalities include pancytopenia, hemolytic anemia, prolonged PT and PTT, hypoproteinemia, and hyperlactatemia.

#### Treatment

Treatment includes antivenin if available and primarily supportive care. Plasma is indicated for treatment of coagulopathy and colloid support. Other supportive care includes non-steroidal anti-inflammatory drugs, crystalloids, and maintenance of airway patency. Corticosteroids are contraindicated as they increase mortality in humans. For additional information on treatment of snake envenomation, see **Chapter 26**.

### Hypercoagulation

Virchow's triad describes the three pillars or requirements for blood clotting: intravascular vessel wall damage, stasis of blood flow, and presence of a hypercoagulable state. Manifestations of hypercoagulation or thrombosis in horses include arteritis/vasculitis, laminitis, pulmonary infarction, iliac thrombosis, and spontaneous or sepsis-associated limb thrombosis in foals. However, by far the most common manifestation in horses is thrombophlebitis, either as a sequela of disease-causing systemic inflammation (e.g., endotoxemia, large colon ischemia, pleuropneumonia, toxic metritis) (Dolente et al. 2005), or perivascular administration of hypertonic or irritating medications (e.g., phenylbutazone, enrofloxacin).

### Clinical Signs

Clinical signs of thrombosis include localized firmness and a cord-like vein, with vascular engorgement proximal to the thrombus if vascular occlusion is complete. Bilateral jugular vein thrombosis is rare, but when present can result in severe swelling of the head and may present in respiratory distress requiring emergency tracheotomy. With iliac or other limb thrombosis, the limb may be cool to the touch distal to the level of thrombus. Septic thrombophlebitis, commonly catheter-associated, presents with heat and pain associated with the swelling, purulent discharge from the catheter site. Systemic signs include intermittent fever, depression, and neck stiffness.

## Diagnosis

### Ultrasound

Ultrasonographic examination of the affected area is useful to confirm the presence and extent of intravascular clot formation, describe the character of the clot, and monitor the progression or response to treatment (Gardner et al. 1991). Ultrasonographic examination of the jugular vein is reasonably easy to learn for the practitioner with some soft-tissue ultrasound experience. A high-frequency linear probe is recommended; however, a transrectal or low-frequency curvilinear probe may be used if a linear probe is not available. Clipping the area, application of coupling gel, and distension of the vein by an assistant facilitate examination. Comparison to the contralateral vein is useful for the inexperienced practitioner. Inflamed vessel walls will be thickened, and perivascular edema may be present, especially with a septic phlebitis. The thrombus appears as a partially or completely occlusive hyperechoic structure, and septic thrombi often are heterogenous with cavitated hypoechoic regions (Gardner et al. 1991). Doppler can be used to determine the extent of blood flow (or lack thereof). Ultrasonographic examination can also be useful to guide sample collection for bacteriologic culture.

### Laboratory Abnormalities

Clinicopathologic abnormalities associated with septic thrombophlebitis include leukocytosis, neutrophilia, and hyperfibrinogenemia. Presence of a hypercoagulable state is supported by changes in clot strength and CFT on viscoelastic testing (Epstein et al. 2011, 2013).

## Treatment

The intravenous catheter, if present, should be removed as soon as phlebitis or thrombosis is suspected. Ideally the catheter is removed aseptically and the tip submitted for bacteriologic culture (Dolente et al. 2005). If any suspicion of phlebitis, alternative veins should be used for venipuncture and medication administration.

### Local Treatment

Heat (to encourage blood flow and fibrinolysis) and icing or hydrotherapy (to reduce inflammation) are recommended 3–4 times daily for the first week. Dimethyl Sulfoxide (DMSO), with or without added antimicrobials such as gentamicin, applied topically is readily absorbed through the skin and may have anti-inflammatory and antithrombogenic effects. Topical diclofenac (Surpass) is a locally effective NSAID and can be combined with other local and systemic treatment.

### Systemic Treatment

Systemic NSAIDs (phenylbutazone or flunixin meglumine) are indicated to reduce pain and inflammation. Antibiotics, either broad spectrum or as directed by susceptibility, are indicated if infection is present or suspected.

### Anticoagulation

If generalized coagulopathy is present or suspected, treatment with heparin, clopidogrel, and/or aspirin is recommended as for DIC (above). Warfarin anticoagulation has also been reported for treatment of jugular thrombophlebitis in horses, but risk of bleeding is high and daily monitoring of PT is required (Scott et al. 1980).

### Thrombolytics

Thrombolytic therapies may be considered to facilitate resolution or recanalization of large thrombi (Dias and de Lacerda Neto 2013). Streptokinase is a nonenzymatic protein that complexes with plasminogen to stimulate clot lysis. It can be administered locally or systemically to promote thrombolysis, although horses should be monitored for anaphylactic reactions (Banerjee et al. 2004). Recombinant tissue plasminogen activator is commonly used for thrombolysis in human patients and may also be useful in horses (Bäumer et al. 2013).

### Surgery

Large occlusive thrombi refractive to medical treatment may necessitate referral for surgical intervention to restore blood flow. Surgical treatments described include phlebotomy (Russell et al. 2010), thrombectomy with Fogarty or other angiographic catheters (Hilton et al. 2008), and venous grafting (Rijkenhuizen and Swieten 1998).

### Prognosis

Prognosis for resolution and long-term function following thrombosis is variable and depends largely on the vessel(s) involved and extent of vascular occlusion. With time, vascular flow is restored by recanalization of the vein and/or development of collateral circulation. In cases of bilateral jugular obstruction, impaired venous return may result in dysphagia and dyspnea. While these sequelae have no apparent effect on performance for pleasure or non-racing athletic performance, they are associated with decreased return to racing for Standardbreds (Moreau and Lavoie 2009). While uncommon, severe complications may occur in horses with septic jugular thrombophlebitis related to migration of septic thrombi, including pleuropneumonia, pulmonary thromboembolism, bacterial endocarditis, and bacteremia.

## Management Decisions in Blood Loss and Coagulopathy

### When to Refer

For the majority of diseases described here, the severity of illness and treatment required is dictated by the underlying cause of blood loss or coagulopathy. For example, horses with severe blood loss, or DIC secondary to systemic illness will need additional treatment for their primary disease, beyond the treatments described here. In other cases – thrombocytopenia, immune-mediated anemia, traumatic hemorrhage – the well-prepared practitioner is likely equipped to handle the case on-farm. Whether a case can be adequately treated on the farm in large part is dependent on what resources are available to the practitioner – including medications/materials, assistance, and time. Providing on-farm intensive care is time-consuming, and the practitioners should ensure compensation is commensurate with their time and effort. Often referral for such cases is in the best interest for all involved and should be recommended.

### Prognosis

Prognosis for disorders of blood loss and coagulopathy is largely determined by the underlying cause. Acute large volume intracavitary hemorrhage and severe systemic illness with DIC are associated with a poor-to-guarded prognosis. Other diseases, such as infections and immune-mediate hemolytic anemia or thrombocytopenia, clotting factor deficiencies, and thrombosis can have a fair-to-good prognosis with appropriate therapy and, in some cases, ongoing management.

### Euthanasia

With the exception of Equine Infectious Anemia, treatment can be offered with variable prognoses as discussed above. For horses with severe hypovolemic or septic crises, if initial stabilization efforts to not improve signs of shock, euthanasia may be the more humane alternative to referral or prolonged attempts at on-farm stabilization. In such cases, practitioners should keep in mind, and counsel owners, that the physiological effects of shock also result in psychological distress and suffering. Additionally, in cases with a poor-guarded prognosis, euthanasia is a reasonable alternative to referral if clients are financially restricted.

**Case Example 19.1 Acute Epistaxis in the Horse**

#### History

A 5-year-old, 450 kg Standardbred gelding is presented for evaluation due to epistaxis following a cart accident during a race. The horse landed on its face and was down for five minutes before being able to stand. Upon standing, epistaxis was noted from the right nostril. The horse was assessed by a veterinarian at the track, administered a dose of flunixin meglumine, and monitored. Due to persistent epistaxis a few hours later and concerns about the volume of blood lost, the horse was referred for further evaluation.

### Triage Exam

On presentation, the horse is quiet but alert and responsive with active but low-volume right-sided epistaxis. The heart rate is 40 beats/min, respiratory rate 16 breaths/min, rectal temperature 100.6 °F. Mucous membranes are pink and most, CRT is <two seconds. The transverse facial arterial pulse is normal and jugular refill is 3 seconds. Extremities are normothermic and digital pulses are within normal limits.

Packed Cell Volume (PCV): 39% (RR: 30–40%).
Total Solids (TS): 6.0 g/dL (RR: 5-6 g/dL).
L-Lactate: 0.4 mmol/L (RR <2 mmol/L).

Question 1: Does this patient have evidence of hypovolemic shock?
No, despite the owner's concern about large volume blood loss, the horse appears to be hemodynamically stable based on the normal TPR, normothermic extremities, and normal arterial pulses/jugular refill. This is further supported by the normal L-lactate and TS. PCV is also within normal limits, although this alone cannot be used to assess acute blood loss, as PCV may remain within normal limits for many hours following hemorrhage.

Question 2: What are your next steps for stabilization and evaluation?

- Place a large bore intravenous (IV) catheter in a jugular vein to secure venous access. Crystalloid fluids and blood transfusion are not indicated at this time, but may be necessary if bleeding continues, horse does not drink, or hypovolemic shock develops.
- Monitor epistaxis, TPR, PCV/TS, and L-lactate for changes suggestive of continued blood loss and hypovolemic shock.
- Evaluate for source of epistaxis – airway and guttural pouch endoscopy, head radiographs

### Additional Diagnostics

Airway endoscopy finds blood in the proximal trachea, but no blood near the carina, suggesting an upper respiratory source of hemorrhage. There is no blood, bruising, or stylohyoid bone fracture identified in either guttural pouch. The ethmoid turbinates appear intact. Bruising is noted in the right dorsal aspect of the pharynx, and active hemorrhage is identified from the right frontomaxillary aperture. There is also a large hematoma, with active bleeding, dorsolaterally within the right nasal passage mucosa at approximately 10–14 cm from the nares.

On palpation of the head, you note crepitus over the right maxilla, caudal and dorsal to the commissure of the lips. You obtain skull radiographs, which identify a minimally displaced fracture of the incisive bone/maxilla rostral to the maxillary cheek teeth.

Question 3: What additional treatment should be considered at this point?

- Continued epistaxis – support coagulation:
  - Aminocaproic acid: 15 g in 1 L saline over 15–20 minutes.
  - Yunnan Baiyo: One box (32 tablets) by mouth every 8 h.
- Serial monitoring of TPR, PCV, TS, and L-lactate to assess need for blood transfusion.
- Maxillary fracture:
  - The fracture is in a location not readily accessible for internal fixation.
  - The fracture has minimal instability and likely will heal with conservative treatment.
  - Offer a soft diet to prevent further disruption of the fracture during prehension and mastication.
- Perform a complete physical examination for other sequelae of the traumatic accident.
  - The patient has a deep carpal wound and multiple superficial abrasions which will need evaluation and treatment.
  - Abdominal and thoracic ultrasound were within normal limits.

### Case Progression

The epistaxis resolves during the first night of hospitalization, but starts again after morning hay meal is offered in a hay net. The volume of hemorrhage is mild–moderate. PCV/TS have decreased to 30% and 5.0 g/dL, respectively, but TPR and L-lactate remain stable. Aminocaproic acid (5 g in 1 L saline every 6 h) and Yunnan Baiyo are continued for a total of 24 and 48 h, respectively. The horse's diet is changed to senior mash and soft chopped hay; epistaxis resolves by evening and does not recur (Figures 19.5–19.7).

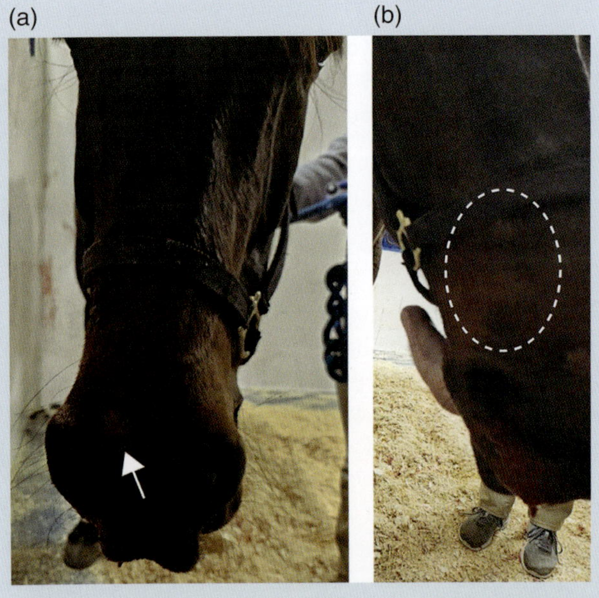


**Figure 19.5** Images of the patient's head at presentation. (a) mild epistaxis and abrasion of the nose (arrow). (b) swelling over the right maxilla (dashed circle).

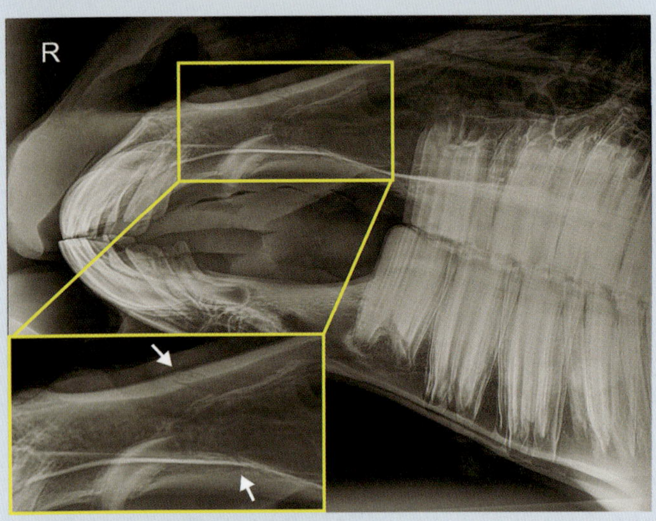


**Figure 19.6** Right lateral to left lateral projection of the rostral skull showing multiple serpiginous lucencies in the maxilla, rostral to the cheek teeth (inset, arrows).

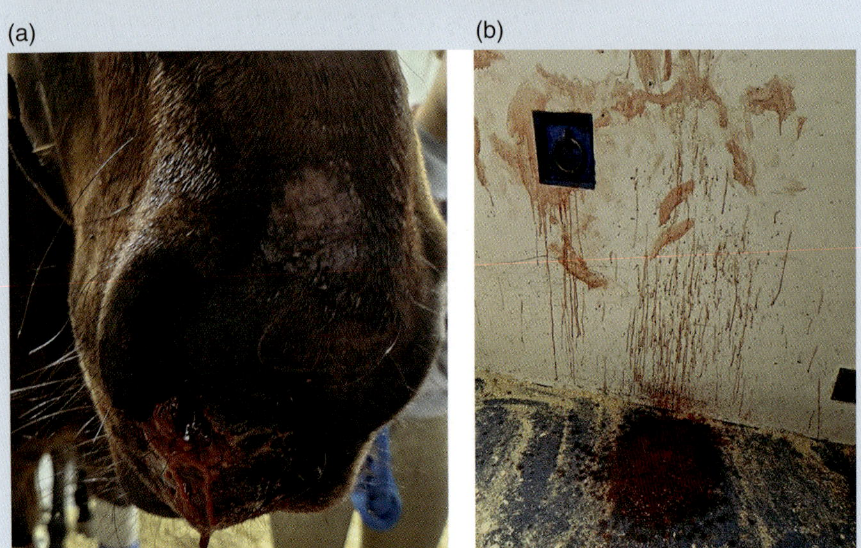


**Figure 19.7** Recurrent right unilateral epistaxis (a) and hemorrhage in stall (b) present on the second morning of hospitalization.

## References

Ahuja, N., Ostomel, T.A., Rhee, P. et al. (2006). Testing of modified zeolite hemostatic dressings in a large animal model of lethal groin injury. *J. Trauma* 61: 1312–1320.

Allen, E.C., Tarigo, J.L., Levine, D.N. et al. (2021). Platelet number and function in response to a single intravenous dose of vincristine. *J. Vet. Intern. Med.* 35: 1754–1762.

Alonso, J.D.M., Schmidt, E.M.S., Eckersall, P.D. et al. (2020). Inflammatory response of healthy horses subjected to small colon enterotomy and treated or not with heparin. *J. Equine Vet. Sci.* 90: 102989.

Alward, A., Corriher, C.A., Barton, M.H. et al. (2006). Red maple (Acer rubrum) leaf toxicosis in horses: a retrospective study of 32 cases. *J. Vet. Intern. Med.* 20: 1197–1201.

Banerjee, A., Chisti, Y., and Banerjee, U.C. (2004). Streptokinase – a clinically useful thrombolytic agent. *Biotechnol. Adv.* 22: 287–307.

Bäumer, W., Herrling, G.M., and Feige, K. (2013). Pharmacokinetics and thrombolytic effects of the recombinant tissue-type plasminogen activator in horses. *BMC Vet. Res.* 9: 158.

Berlin, N., Kelmer, E., Segev, G. et al. (2019). Assessment of the CoaguChek-XS portable prothrombin time point-of-care analyzer for horses. *J. Vet. Diagn. Invest.* 31: 448–452.

Bishop, R.C., Kemper, A.M., Burges, J.W. et al. (2023). Preliminary evaluation of reference intervals for a point-of-care viscoelastic coagulation monitor (VCM Vet) in healthy adult horses. *J. Vet. Emerg. Crit. Care (San Antonio).* 33 (5): 540–548. https://doi.org/10.1111/vec.13317. Epub 2023 Aug 10. PMID: 37561043.

Blong, A.E., Epstein, K.L., and Brainard, B.M. (2013). In vitro effects of three formulations of hydroxyethyl starch solutions on coagulation and platelet function in horses. *Am. J. Vet. Res.* 74: 712–720.

Boucher, B.A. and Traub, O. (2009). Achieving hemostasis in the surgical field. *Pharmacotherapy* 29: 2S–7S.

Bozorgmanesh, R., Magdesian, K.G., Rhodes, D.M. et al. (2015). Hemolytic anemia in horses associated with ingestion of pistacia leaves. *J. Vet. Intern. Med.* 29: 410–413.

Brainard, B.M., Epstein, K.L., Lobato, D. et al. (2011). Effects of clopidogrel and aspirin on platelet aggregation, thromboxane production, and serotonin secretion in horses. *J. Vet. Intern. Med.* 25: 116–122.

Broux, B., Torfs, S., Wegge, B. et al. (2012). Acute respiratory failure caused by Leptospira spp. in 5 foals. *J. Vet. Intern. Med.* 26: 684–687.

Cesarini, C., Monreal, L., Armengou, L. et al. (2010). Association of admission plasma D-dimer concentration with diagnosis and outcome in horses with colic. *J. Vet. Intern. Med.* 24: 1490–1497.

Christopherson, P.W., Santen, V.L., Livesey, L., and Boudreaux, M.K. (2007). A 10-base-pair deletion in the gene encoding platelet glycoprotein iib associated with glanzmann thrombasthenia in a horse. *J. Vet. Intern. Med.* 21: 196–198.

Cohen, N.D., Carter, G.K., Mealey, R.H., and Taylor, T.S. (1995). Medical management of right dorsal colitis in 5 horses: a retrospective study (1987–1993). *J. Vet. Intern. Med.* 9: 272–276.

Collatos, C., Barton, M.H., and Moore, J.N. (1995a). Fibrinolytic activity in plasma from horses with gastrointestinal diseases: changes associated with diagnosis, surgery, and outcome. *J. Vet. Intern. Med.* 9: 18–23.

Collatos, C., Barton, M.H., Prasse, K.W., and Moore, J.N. (1995b). Intravascular and peritoneal coagulation and fibrinolysis in horses with acute gastrointestinal tract diseases. *J. Am. Vet. Med. Assoc.* 207: 465–470.

Dahlgren, A.R., Tablin, F., and Finno, C.J. (2021). Genetics of equine bleeding disorders. *Equine Vet. J.* 53: 30–37.

Dallap Schaer, B.L., Bentz, A.I., Boston, R.C. et al. (2009). Comparison of viscoelastic coagulation analysis and standard coagulation profiles in critically ill neonatal foals to outcome. *J. Vet. Emerg. Crit. Care* 19: 88–95.

Dallap, B.L., Dolente, B., and Boston, R. (2003). Coagulation profiles in 27 horses with large colon volvulus. *J. Vet. Emerg. Crit. Care* 13: 215–225.

Dias, D.P. and De Lacerda Neto, J.C. (2013). Jugular thrombophlebitis in horses: a review of fibrinolysis, thrombus formation, and clinical management. *Can. Vet. J.* 54: 65–71.

Dickinson, C.E., Traub-Dargatz, J.L., Dargatz, D.A. et al. (1996). Rattlesnake venom poisoning in horses: 32 cases (1973–1993). *J. Am. Vet. Med. Assoc.* 208: 1866–1871.

Dolente, B.A., Wilkins, P.A., and Boston, R.C. (2002). Clinicopathologic evidence of disseminated intravascular coagulation in horses with acute colitis. *J. Am. Vet. Med. Assoc.* 220: 1034–1038.

Dolente, B.A., Beech, J., Lindborg, S., and Smith, G. (2005). Evaluation of risk factors for development of catheter-associated jugular thrombophlebitis in horses: 50 cases (1993–1998). *J. Am. Vet. Med. Assoc.* 227: 1134–1141.

Epstein, K.L., Brainard, B.M., Gomez-Ibanez, S.E. et al. (2011). Thrombelastography in horses with acute gastrointestinal disease. *J. Vet. Intern. Med.* 25: 307–314.

Epstein, K.L., Brainard, B.M., Giguere, S. et al. (2013). Serial viscoelastic and traditional coagulation testing in horses with gastrointestinal disease. *J. Vet. Emerg. Crit. Care (San Antonio)* 23: 504–516.

Feige, K., Schwarzwald, C.C., and Bombeli, T. (2010). Comparison of unfractioned and low molecular weight heparin for prophylaxis of coagulopathies in 52 horses with colic: a randomised double-blind clinical trial. *Equine Vet. J.* 35: 506–513.

Fey, K. and Sasse, H.H.L. (1998). Relapsing immune-mediated thrombocytopenia of unknown origin in a stallion. *Equine Vet Educ* 10: 127–132.

Fielding, C.L., Pusterla, N., Magdesian, K.G. et al. (2011). Rattlesnake envenomation in horses: 58 cases (1992–2009). *J. Am. Vet. Med. Assoc.* 238: 631–635.

Fry, M.M., Walker, N.J., Blevins, G.M. et al. (2005). Platelet function defect in a thoroughbred filly. *J. Vet. Intern. Med.* 19: 359–362.

Gardner, S.Y., Reef, V.B., and Spencer, P.A. (1991). Ultrasonographic evaluation of horses with thrombophlebitis of the jugular vein: 46 cases (1985–1988). *J. Am. Vet. Med. Assoc.* 199: 370–373.

Geor, R.J., Jackson, M.L., Lewis, K.D., and Fretz, P.B. (1990). Prekallikrein deficiency in a family of Belgian horses. *J. Am. Vet. Med. Assoc.* 197: 741–745.

Hedges, S.J., Dehoney, S.B., Hooper, J.S. et al. (2007). Evidence-based treatment recommendations for uremic bleeding. *Nat. Clin. Pract. Nephrol.* 3: 138–153.

Hett, D.A., Walker, D., Pilkington, S.N., and Smith, D.C. (1995). Sonoclot analysis. *Br. J. Anaesth.* 75: 771–776.

Hilton, H., Aleman, M., Textor, J. et al. (2008). Ultrasound-guided balloon thrombectomy for treatment of aorto-iliac-femoral thrombosis in a horse. *J. Vet. Intern. Med.* 22: 679–683.

Hoffmann, J.N., Wiedermann, C.J., Juers, M. et al. (2006). Benefit/risk profile of high-dose antithrombin in patients with severe sepsis treated with and without concomitant heparin. *Thromb. Haemost.* 95: 850–856.

Horlocker, T.T. and Schroeder, D.R. (1997). Effect of age, gender, and platelet count on Sonoclot coagulation analysis in patients undergoing orthopedic operations. *Mayo Clin. Proc.* 72: 214–219.

Hurcombe, S.D., Mudge, M.C., and Hinchcliff, K.W. (2007). Clinical and clinicopathologic variables in adult horses receiving blood transfusions: 31 cases (1999–2005). *J. Am. Vet. Med. Assoc.* 231: 267–274.

Johnstone, I.B. and Crane, S. (1986). Haemostatic abnormalities in horses with colic — their prognostic value. *Equine Vet. J.* 18: 271–274.

Jones, P.A., Tomasic, M., and Gentry, P.A. (1997). Oncotic, hemodilutional, and hemostatic effects of isotonic saline and hydroxyethyl starch solutions in clinically normal ponies. *Am. J. Vet. Res.* 58: 541–548.

Junge, H.K., Ringer, S.K., Mayer, N., and Schwarzwald, C.C. (2016). Assessment of method reliability and determination of reference intervals for rotational thromboelastometry in horses. *J. Vet. Emerg. Crit. Care (San Antonio)* 26: 691–703.

Kisthardt, K.K., Schumacher, J., Finn-Bodner, S.T. et al. (1999). Severe renal hemorrhage caused by pyelonephritis in 7 horses: clinical and ultrasonographic evaluation. *Can. Vet. J.* 40: 571–576.

Kopp, K.J., Moore, J.N., Byars, T.D., and Brooks, P. (1985). Template bleeding time and thromboxane generation in the horse: Effects of three non-steroidal anti-inflammatory drugs. *Equine Vet. J.* 17: 322–324.

Kw, P., Mj, T., Jn, M., and Eg, W. (1993). Analysis of hemostasis in horses with colic. *J. Am. Vet. Med. Assoc.* .

Larsdotter, S., Ley, C., and Pringle, J. (2009). Renal pseudoaneurysm as a cause of hematuria in a colt. *Can. Vet. J.* 50: 759–762.

Lisman, T. and Leebeek, F.W.G. (2007). Hemostatic alterations in liver disease: a review on pathophysiology, clinical consequences, and treatment. *Dig. Surg.* 24: 250–258.

Livesey, L., Christopherson, P., Hammond, A. et al. (2005). Platelet dysfunction (Glanzmann's thrombasthenia). *Horses.* 19: 917.

Macieira, S., Rivard, G.-É., Champagne, J. et al. (2007). Glanzmann thrombasthenia in an Oldenbourg filly. *Vet. Clin. Pathol.* 36: 204–208.

Mcgovern, K.F., Lascola, K.M., Smith, S.A. et al. (2013). The effects of hyperglycemia and endotoxemia on coagulation parameters in healthy adult horses. *J. Vet. Intern. Med.* 27: 347–353.

Mcmichael, M.A. and Smith, S.A. (2011). Viscoelastic coagulation testing: technology, applications, and limitations. *Vet. Clin. Pathol.* 40: 140–153.

Mcmichael, M., Smith, S.A., Mcconachie, E.L. et al. (2011). In-vitro hypocoagulability on whole blood thromboelastometry associated with in-vivo expansion of red cell mass in an equine model. *Blood Coagul. Fibrinolysis* 22: 424–430.

Mendez-Angulo, J.L., Mudge, M.C., Vilar-Saavedra, P. et al. (2010). Thromboelastography in healthy horses and horses with inflammatory gastrointestinal disorders and suspected coagulopathies. *J. Vet. Emerg. Crit. Care (San Antonio)* 20: 488–493.

Migliorisi, A., Kemper, A.M., and A., P., Austin, S. M., Bishop, R. C., Mccoy, A. & Wilkins, P. (2020). In-vitro coagulation parameters in healthy and sick foals using the point-of-care (POC) viscoelastic coagulation monitor Vet-VCM. In: Abstracts from the International Veterinary Emergency and Critical Care Symposium, and the European Veterinary Emergency and Critical Care Annual Congress 2020. *J. Vet. Emerg. Crit. Care* 30: S17–S22.

Monreal, L., Anglés, A., Espada, Y. et al. (2000). Hypercoagulation and hypofibrinolysis in horses with colic and DIC. *Equine Vet. J.* 32: 19–25.

More, S.J., Aznar, I., Bailey, D.C. et al. (2008). An outbreak of equine infectious anaemia in Ireland during 2006: Investigation methodology, initial source of infection, diagnosis and clinical presentation, modes of transmission and spread in the Meath cluster. *Equine Vet. J.* 40: 706–708.

Moreau, P. and Lavoie, J.-P. (2009). Evaluation of athletic performance in horses with jugular vein thrombophlebitis: 91 cases (1988–2005). *J. Am. Vet. Med. Assoc.* 235: 1073–1078.

Morris, D.D. and Beech, J. (1983). Disseminated intravascular coagulation in six horses. *J. Am. Vet. Med. Assoc.* 183: 1067–1072.

Mudge, M.C. (2019). Chapter 4 – Hemostasis, surgical bleeding, and transfusion. In: *Equine Surgery*, 5e (ed. J.A. Auer, J.A. Stick, J.M. Kümmerle, and T. Prange). W.B. Saunders.

Murray, D.J., Brosnahan, W.J., Pennell, B. et al. (1997). Heparin detection by the activated coagulation time: a comparison of the sensitivity of coagulation tests and heparin assays. *J. Cardiothorac. Vasc. Anesth.* 11: 24–28.

Nikvand, A.A., Jalali, S.M., Ghadrdan Mashhadi, A. et al. (2019). Clinical, hematologic, hemostatic, and serum biochemical findings related to survival in Arabian horses with colic. *Vet. Clin. Pathol.* 48: 441–448.

Norris, J.W., Pombo, M., Shirley, E. et al. (2015). Association of factor V secretion with protein kinase B signaling in platelets from horses with atypical equine thrombasthenia. *J. Vet. Intern. Med.* 29: 1387–1394.

O'Callaghan, D.K., Schall, S.A., Birmingham, S.S.W., and Lehman, J.S. (2015). Protective effects of ascorbic acid and α-tocopherol on the in vitro oxidation of equine erythrocytes caused by extracts of wilted red maple leaves. *J. Equine Vet. Sci.* 35: 940–946.

Pablo, L.S., Purohit, R.C., Teer, P.A. et al. (1983). Disseminated intravascular coagulation in experimental intestinal strangulation obstruction in ponies. *Am. J. Vet. Res.* 44: 2115–2122.

Pellegrini, F.L. (2005). Results of a large-scale necroscopic study of equine colonic ulcers. *J. Equine Vet. Sci.* 25: 113–117.

Perkins, G.A., Miller, W.H., Divers, T.J. et al. (2005). Ulcerative dermatitis, thrombocytopenia, and neutropenia in neonatal foals. *Animals (Basel)* 19: 211.

Polkes, A.C., Giguère, S., Lester, G.D., and Bain, F.T. (2008). Factors associated with outcome in foals with neonatal isoerythrolysis (72 cases, 1988–2003). *J. Vet. Intern. Med.* 22: 1216–1222.

Poole, A.W. (1993). Thrombosis in the horse: the role of platelets in its pathogenesis and therapy. *Equine Vet Educ* 5: 99–102.

Ramey, D., Mudge, M., Rudolphi, O., and Waxman, S. (2021). Use of an absorbable haemostatic gauze product to control bleeding in 20 horses. *Equine Vet Educ* 33.

Rathgeber, R.A., Brooks, M.B., Bain, F.T., and Byars, T.D. (2001). Clinical vignette. Von Willebrand disease in a Thoroughbred mare and foal. *J. Vet. Intern. Med.* 15 (1): 63–66. https://doi.org/10.1111/j.1939-1676.2001.tb02302.x. PMID: 11215915.

Rawlings, C.A., Byars, T.D., Van Noy, M.K., and Bisgard, G.E. (1975). Activated coagulation test in normal and heparinized ponies and horses. *Am. J. Vet. Res.* 36: 711–713.

Rebalka, I.A. and Lindinger, M.I. (2021). In vitro validation assessment of a fecal occult blood protein test for horses. *J. Equine Vet. Sci.* 104: 103695.

Rijkenhuizen, A.B.M. and Swieten, H.A. (1998). Reconstruction of the jugular vein in horses with post thrombophlebitis stenosis using saphenous vein graft. *Equine Vet. J.* 30: 236–239.

Russell, T.M., Kearney, C., and Pollock, P.J. (2010). Surgical treatment of septic jugular thrombophlebitis in nine horses. *Vet. Surg.* 39: 627–630.

Sanz, M.G., Wills, T.B., Christopherson, P., and Hines, M.T. (2011). Glanzmann thrombasthenia in a 17-year-old Peruvian Paso mare. *Vet. Clin. Pathol.* 40: 48–51.

Schonauer, C., Tessitore, E., Barbagallo, G. et al. (2004). The use of local agents: bone wax, gelatin, collagen, oxidized cellulose. *Eur. Spine J.* 13: S89–S96.

Scott, E.A., Byars, T.D., and Lamar, A.M. (1980). Warfarin anticoagulation in the horse. *J. Am. Vet. Med. Assoc.* 177: 1146–1151.

Segura, D. and Monreal, L. (2008). Poor reproducibility of template bleeding time in horses. *J. Vet. Intern. Med.* 22: 238–241.

Segura, D., Monreal, L., Espada, Y. et al. (2005). Assessment of a platelet function analyser in horses: reference range and influence of a platelet aggregation inhibitor. *Vet. J.* 170: 108–112.

Short, M.A., Clark, C.K., Harvey, J.W. et al. (2012). Outbreak of equine piroplasmosis in Florida. *J. Am. Vet. Med. Assoc.* 240: 588–595.

Sileshi, B., Achneck, H.E., and Lawson, J.H. (2008). Management of surgical hemostasis: topical agents. *Vascular* 16 (Suppl 1): S22–S28.

Spangler, D., Rothenburger, S., Nguyen, K. et al. (2003). In vitro antimicrobial activity of oxidized regenerated cellulose against antibiotic-resistant microorganisms. *Surg. Infect.* 4: 255–262.

Stokol, T., Erb, H.N., De Wilde, L. et al. (2005). Evaluation of latex agglutination kits for detection of fibrin(ogen) degradation products and D-dimer in healthy horses and horses with severe colic. *Vet. Clin. Pathol.* 34: 375–382.

Tang, Z.L., Wang, X., Yi, B. et al. (2009). Effects of the preoperative administration of Yunnan Baiyao capsules on intraoperative blood loss in bimaxillary orthognathic surgery: a prospective, randomized, double-blind, placebo-controlled study. *Int. J. Oral Maxillofac. Surg.* 38: 261–266.

Taylor, E.L., Sellon, D.C., Wardrop, K.J. et al. (2000). Effects of intravenous administration of formaldehyde on platelet and coagulation variables in healthy horses. *Am. J. Vet. Res.* 61: 1191–1196.

Thane, K., Bedenice, D., and Pacheco, A. (2017). Operator-based variability of equine thromboelastography. *J. Vet. Emerg. Crit. Care (San Antonio)* 27: 419–424.

Topper, M.J. and Prasse, K.W. (1996). Use of enzyme-linked immunosorbent assay to measure thrombin-antithrombin III complexes in horses with colic. *Am. J. Vet. Res.* 57: 456–462.

Topper, M.J. and Prasse, K.W. (1998). Analysis of coagulation proteins as acute-phase reactants in horses with colic. *Am. J. Vet. Res.* 59: 542–545.

Turrentine, M.A., Sculley, P.W., Green, E.M., and Johnson, G.S. (1986). Prekallikrein deficiency in a family of miniature horses. *Am. J. Vet. Res.* 47: 2464–2467.

Ueti, M.W., Mealey, R.H., Kappmeyer, L.S. et al. (2012). Re-emergence of the apicomplexan theileria equi in the united states: elimination of persistent infection and transmission risk. *PLoS One* 7: e44713.

Welch, R.D., Watkins, J.P., Taylor, T.S. et al. (1992). Disseminated intravascular coagulation associated with colic in 23 horses (1984–1989). *J. Vet. Intern. Med.* 6: 29–35.

Williams, T.L. and Archer, J. (2016). Effect of prewarming EDTA blood samples to 37°C on platelet count measured by Sysmex XT-2000iV in dogs, cats, and horses. *Vet. Clin. Pathol.* 45: 444–449.

Winfield, L.S. and Brooks, M.B. (2014). Hemorrhage and blood loss-induced anemia associated with an acquired coagulation factor VIII inhibitor in a Thoroughbred mare. *J. Am. Vet. Med. Assoc.* 244 (6): 719–723. https://doi.org/10.2460/javma.244.6.719. PMID: 24568115.

# 20

# Foal Emergencies

*Jenifer R. Gold*

*Gold Equine Medicine Consulting, Florence, MT, USA*

## Introduction

Neonatal foals are extremely vulnerable to systemic disease. *In utero* situations such as placentitis usually lead to a foal born that is systemically ill, making transition from fetus to neonate challenging. Rapid decline and death can occur if early recognition of problems are missed and emergency treatment delayed (Palmer 2005a, Axon et al. 2015; Magdesian 2014).

Neonatal foals need a physical examination to help guide diagnostics, stabilization, and treatment. It is imperative to understand what normal healthy foal behavior and physical examination findings are in order to diagnose clinical abnormalities. The 1, 2, 3 rule is a great way to guide what's normal in the first few hours of life for the foal and mare (Box 20.1).

## Normal Physical Examination

Examination of the newborn foal should start with looking at the mucous membranes; note color of gums, nostrils, ears, and if a filly look at the vulva (Figure 20.1). The gums should be pink and moist. Septic foals can have petechia/ecchymosis, and this doesn't always present just in the gums. The eyes should be examined for congenital issues, signs of difficult parturition (scleral hemorrhage), uveitis, hypopyon, ulceration, entropion presence, sunken eyes, or other issues. Foals don't have corneal sensation for the first several weeks of life, so they can have ulcers without any clinical signs. Evaluate the heart rate, respiratory rate, and gastrointestinal borborygmi. Palpate of ribs for factures particularly along the costochondral junction. Palpate joints and the umbilicus for signs of abnormalities, possible infection (thickened, edematous, swollen, lameness). If the foal is a colt, check for testicles and if any signs of inguinal hernia. Colts can have a persistent frenulum of the penis, so it may take several days for them to drop. A colt typically urinates in the first 8–10 h of life. If the foal is a filly the vulva should be checked for any congenital abnormalities. A filly will typically urinate in the first 12–14 h of life. Check the rectum for any congenital abnormalities. The newborn foal should be stimulated to pass meconium after nursing for the first time.

## Mare History – Pregnancy, Parturition, Passage of Placenta

It is extremely important to try to get a good history on the mare. Did she have any problems peripartum including premature lactation, vaginal discharge, placentitis, placental separation partial or complete, systemic illness, surgery, chronic lameness, laminitis, or metabolic disease? These peripartum issues will increase the risk of the foal being born unhealthy (Axon et al. 2015).

Is the mare primiparous or multiparous? What was the mare's gestational length?

*Emergency Triage of the Horse*, First Edition. Edited by Rolfe M. Radcliffe and Jamie J. Kopper.

Companion website: www.wiley.com/go/radcliffe/triage

**Box 20.1 The 1, 2, 3 rule of normal behavior for the mare and foal**

- A neonatal foal should stand in one hour, nurse in two hours, and the mare should pass the placenta in three hours.
- Between one to five minutes after birth a foal's heart rate should be >60 bpm and respiratory rate should be >20 breaths/min. By one to two hours the heart rate should be 80–120 beats/min and respiratory rate should be 30–40 breaths/min.
- Between 5 and 10 minutes after birth a foal should have a suckle reflex, sit in sternal without support, and start to try to stand in 20 minutes. The foal should shake their head if a finger is stuck in their nostril or ear. Stimulation of the thoracolumbar region (running fingers down the thoracolumbar spine) should cause the foal to throw its front legs forward and attempt to rise off the hind limbs.
- Temperature initially will be 99–100 °F (37.2–37.8 °C) and should rise to 100–102 °F (37.8–38.8 °C) within the first several hours of life. Newborn foals should be able to thermoregulate.

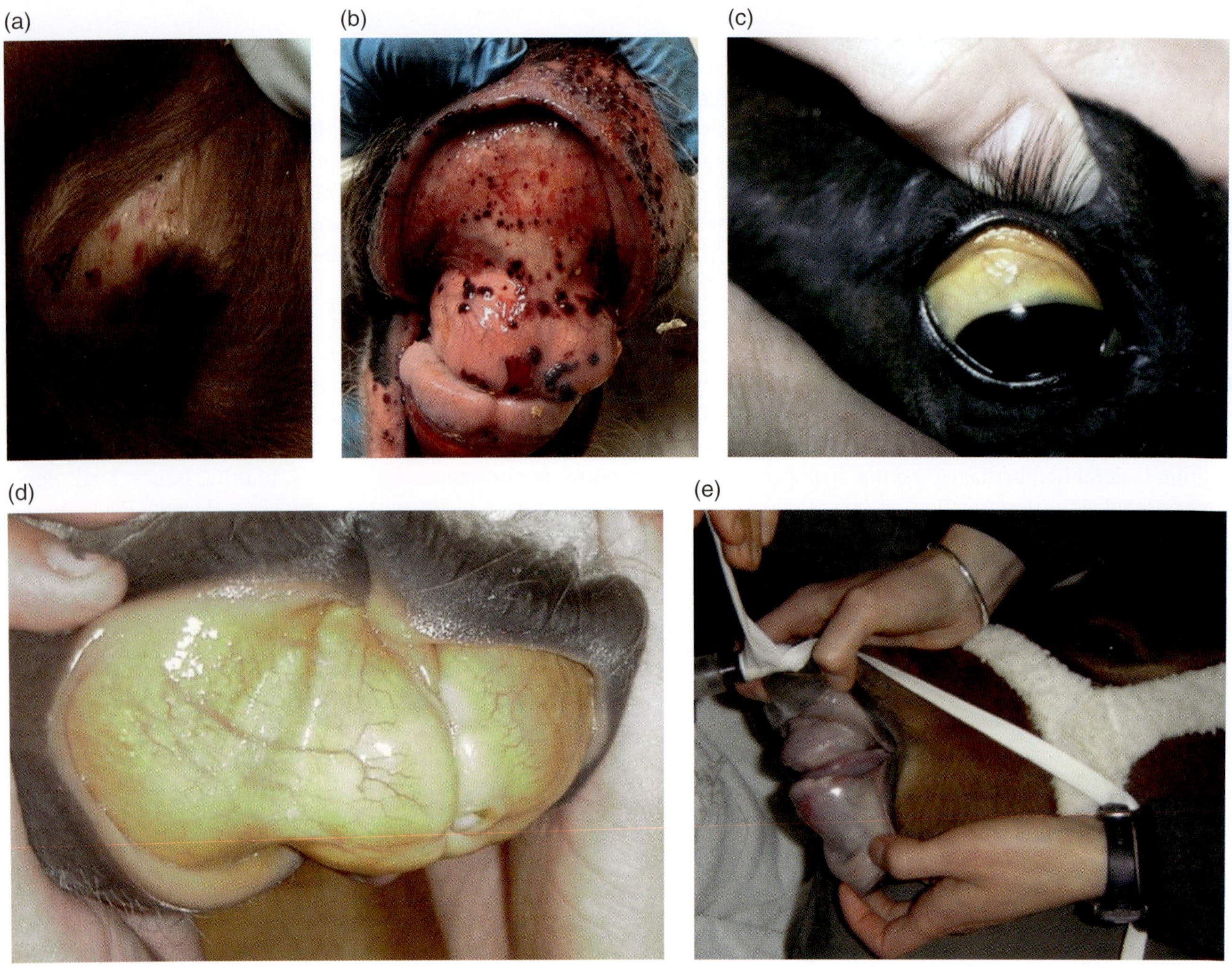


**Figure 20.1** Mucous membranes in diseased foals. (a,b) Petechia in mucous membranes of the mouth and ears – Sepsis alert!!! (c,d) Icteric mucous membranes – possible neonatal isoerythrolysis, EHV-1, sepsis. (e) Cyanotic mucous membranes – respiratory distress, prematurity, sepsis.

Normal gestation duration

- Pony breeds 320–345 days.
- Thoroughbreds 320–360 days.
- Donkeys 360–380 days.

Was the parturition observed?

- Normal Stage 2 parturition lasts 20 minutes.

Did the mare pass her placenta?

- The mare should pass her placenta within three hours following parturition.
- The placenta should weigh 10–12% of the foal's body weight.
- Is the placenta complete-body and both uterine horns present?

All the above are important considerations that along with physical examination findings determine if the foal may have serious problems including sepsis, dysmaturity, immaturity, neonatal encephalopathy (NE), or other diseases. A foal having a high creatinine and blood urea nitrogen concentrations suggests the placenta was abnormal (Bain 2004; Palmer 2005b; Chaney et al. 2010). Such foals should be monitored closely for the first 72 h for signs of NE and/or sepsis.

## The Critically Ill Neonate

It is very important to understand that management of the critically ill neonatal foal takes a lot of time and can be expensive. Many treatments can be done on the farm with experienced caretakers; these treatments include plasma transfusion, initial fluid therapy for stabilization, feeding via nasogastric tube, warming the foal if needed. These types of treatments can be done to stabilize the foal and utilized if only minor issues are noted. If the foal cannot maintain body temperature, cannot rise on its own, cannot nurse or other major problems, the foal should be referred. It should be recognized that equipment, personnel, and specialists in the field of neonatology may often only be obtained at equine critical care units and are frequently needed for the best chance of survival (McDonald et al. 1990; Spurlock and Furr 1990; Magdesian 2004; Palmer 2005b; Sanchez 2005a; Axon 2006; Russell et al. 2008; McKenzie 2018).

## Stabilization of the Critically Ill Neonate

Support of cardiovascular and respiratory systems helps with tissue perfusion and oxygenation.

Some of the critically ill foals need to be stabilized before a complete physical examination. If a foal is obtunded and unable to rise nasal oxygenation and venous access are essential, along with heart rate, respiratory rate, temperature, distal limb temperature and pulse quality, arterial blood gas, glucose, lactate concentrations, and blood pressure if possible (Wotman et al. 2005; Henderson et al. 2007; Russell et al. 2007, 2008; Hackett and McCue 2010; Borchers et al. 2012).

### Cardiovascular Support

Catheters should be placed aseptically in the jugular vein with the foal in lateral recumbency (Figure 20.2). Over-the-wire polyurethane catheters are less thrombogenic, flexible, and easier to place in hypovolemic foals (Figure 20.2). Blood for blood cultures is obtained through the catheter aseptically (Russell et al. 2008). Fluid therapy is the first line of treatment. Positive inotropes and vasopressors may also be utilized in the hospital setting.

### Fluid Therapy: Hypovolemia

Warmed balanced isotonic fluids are administered at 20 mL/kg over 20–30 minutes with clinical re-evaluation of parameters after every bolus. Parameters to evaluate are warming of distal limbs, urination, increase GI borborygmi, improvement of blood gas, and L-lactate concentrations (Magdesian and Madigan 2003; Magdesian 2010).

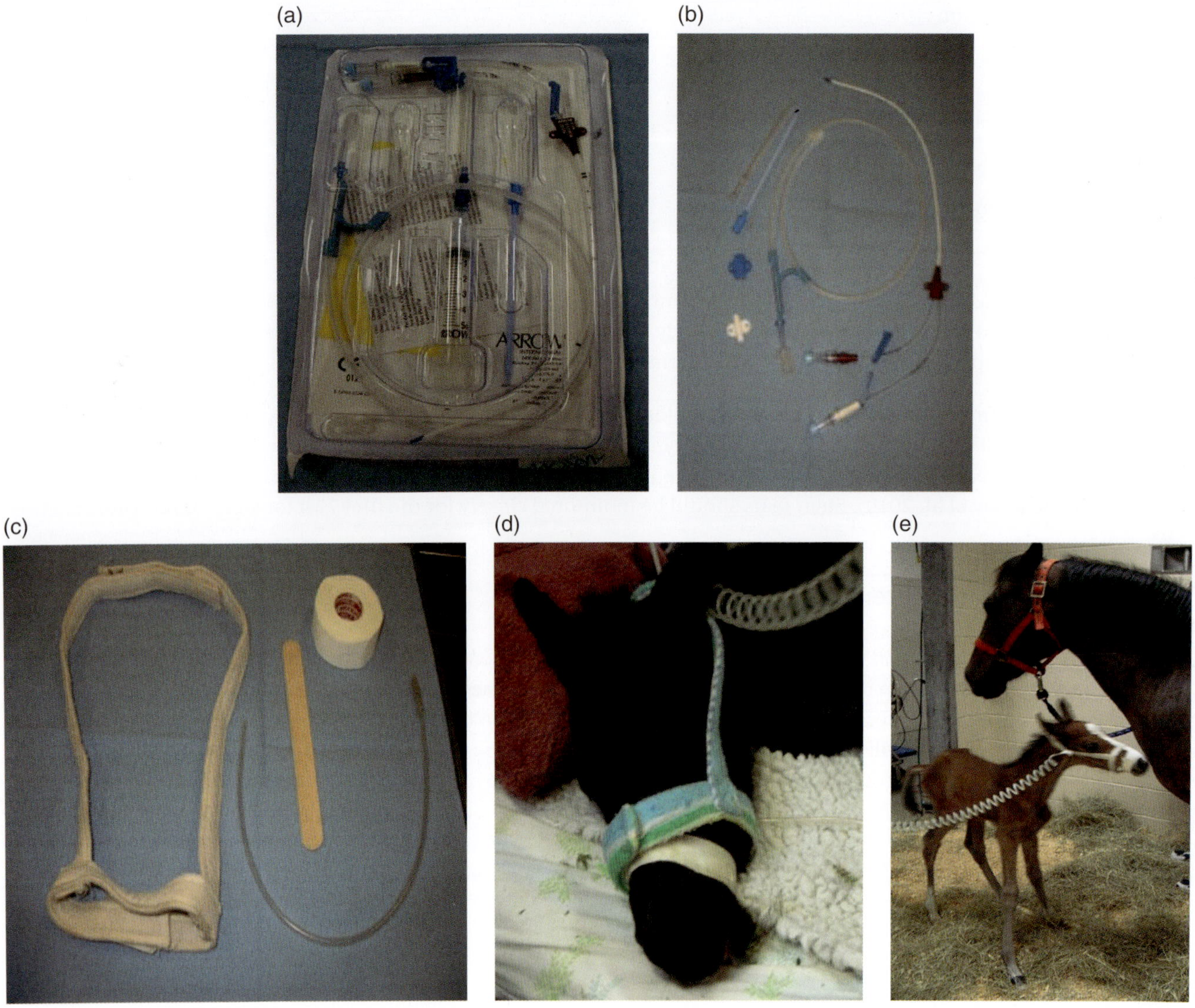


**Figure 20.2** Foal catheter and oxygen insufflation. (a,b) Over the wire catheter. (c–e) Nasal oxygen insufflation.

Monitoring of these parameters will help prevent fluid overload in hypoproteinemia and septic shock situations. Plasma can be utilized as well for its immunoglobulins, coagulation factors, and other protein products. Understanding that plasma may not increase albumin greatly but may help with vascular pressure.

## Fluid Therapy: Dehydration

Once hypovolemia is resolved, the level of dehydration should be ascertained and estimation of fluid replacement therapy. It is critical to remember neonatal foals have a larger interstitial volume (Palmer 2002; Hollis et al. 2010).

Mild (5%) dehydration or 50 mL/kg body weight is difficult to recognize. Clinical signs of moderate (7%) to severe (10%) dehydration or 70–100 mL/kg body weight, respectively, are tacky mucous membranes, slow capillary refill, sunken eyes, decreased urine production. Clinical signs of life-threatening (15%) dehydration or 150 mL/kg body weight are tacky mucous membranes, slow capillary refill, no urine production, tachycardia, tachypnea, sunken eyes, muddy mucous membranes, poor pulse quality, obtundation to unresponsive.

Treatment should include fluid deficit, ongoing losses, and maintenance requirements (Box 20.2). Clinical parameters should be checked frequently to ensure appropriate care.

**Box 20.2 Example fluid therapy calculation for correction of severe dehydration in a foal**

Example: 10% dehydrated 70 kg foal. Fluid deficit is 7 L to be administered over 12 h (583 mL/h). Maintenance would be 2–4 mL/kg/h choosing 3 mL/kg/h would be 210 mL/h + 583 mL/h = 793 mL/h including resuscitation and no ongoing losses. If on the farm, the foal could receive 1,500 mL q2-h boluses.

**Box 20.3 Example fluid therapy calculation for intravenous glucose support in a foal**

Example: 50 kg foal at 4 mg/kg/min = 50 kg × 4 mg/kg/min × 60 minutes = 12,000 mg/h or 12 g/h × 1,000 mL/50 g = 240 mL/h of 5% dextrose in water solution.

Remember glucose solutions should not be given as a bolus. Administration of a bolus may result in electrolyte derangements and further dehydration due to osmotic diuresis. Hyperglycemia is also detrimental to the neurologic status of critically ill neonates. If the foal is hypoglycemic at presentation, begin with a 1% glucose solution (20 mL of 50% dextrose into 1-L balanced polyionic fluids) added to the resuscitation boluses at 4–8 mg/kg/min in two boluses and reassess in one hour. Following resuscitation, a CRI of 5% dextrose at a rate of 4 mg/kg/min should be initiated.

## Glucose Therapy

Critically ill foals need intravenous glucose support (Box 20.3). Checking glucose concentrations should be done stall side and the AlphaTRAK[1] has been validated in foals (Hackett and McCue 2010). A 5% dextrose solution should be used as a constant rate infusion typically beginning at 4 mg/kg/min. This rate can be increased up to 8 mg/kg/min. A solution up to 10% dextrose can be utilized. Aim for glucose concentrations between 60 and 180 mg/dL. Also see Chapter 32 for nutritional information for foals.

## Electrolyte Therapy

Critically ill neonatal foals can have electrolyte derangements with a variety of issues.

Fluid therapy alone many times corrects the abnormalities present. Please see Appendix 4, Emergency treatment protocols.

***Potassium*** Hyperkalemia: Typically, hyperkalemia occurs with a ruptured bladder in equine neonates. It can also be seen with milk replacer mixing error, nutritional myodegeneration, catastrophic muscle injury, or rarely cellular leakage of potassium.

Uroperitoneum typically requires placement of a urinary catheter, drainage of the peritoneal urine, and fluid therapy with 5% dextrose solution. To assist with cardiac stabilization calcium gluconate can be added at a 1 mL/kg IV slowly with 10% calcium gluconate, 1–2 mEq/kg IV or sodium bicarbonate and/or 1 g/kg IV of glucose.

Hypokalemia: Much more common than hyperkalemia. Supplementation should be initiated if the potassium is less than 2.5 mEq/L. Care is needed to not administer potassium too quickly. The rate of administration should <0.5 mEq/kg/h.

*Calculation of approximate K+ supplementation need can be done using the formula*

$$\text{Potassium replacement}\left(\text{mEq}\right) = 0.4 \times \text{body weight}\left(\text{kg}\right) \times \text{potassium deficit in mEq.}$$

***Sodium*** It is not uncommon to see neonatal foals with either hypo or hypernatremia. Both electrolyte abnormalities can cause neurologic dysfunction if too low or too high or not corrected appropriately.

Moderate-to-severe hyponatremia can be corrected up to 115–120 mEq/L quickly and then slowed down to 0.5 mEq/h for the remainder of time until normal range.

Hypernatremia should be handled with care and should not be correctly more quickly than the 0.5 mEq/h.

## Positive Inotropes and Vasopressors

The goal of inotropes/vasopressors is to achieve tissue perfusion, not to achieve a specified blood pressure point. The mean arterial blood pressure should be >60 mmHg but can be achieved at lower values; thus, multiple factors such as L-Lactate concentration should be considered. Dobutamine (3–10 μg/kg/min) and norepinephrine (0.3–1.0 μg/kg/min)

1 AlphaTrak Zoetis Company, Parsippany-Troy Hills, NJ.

are used most frequently, but dopamine (2–15 µg/kg/min) or vasopressin (2–10 µg/kg/min) is also utilized. The goal for the use of these agents is to improve perfusion, pulse pressure, urine production, and arterial blood gas parameters of the foal (Axon et al. 2015).

## Neonatal Clinical Abnormalities

### Prematurity/Dysmaturity

Gestational length can vary greatly in mares. Multiparous mares typically have consistent gestational length from year to year. Thus, a mare that has had a normal foal at 320 days may be premature for another mare/foal. Typically, it is thought however a foal is premature if it is born <320 days gestation. Clinical signs of prematurity or dysmaturity are presented in Box 20.4 (Jeffcott et al. 1982; Ousey et al. 2011; Clothier et al. 2020).

### Diagnostics

*It is important once a physical examination has been performed to*

- Perform Hematology, Biochemistry, Lactate and Glucose concentrations.
- If 12 h + perform IgG concentration value.
- Radiograph carpus/tarsus - Four grades of cuboidal bone ossification include: grade 1: Cuboidal bones visible, but lack ossification, grade 2: All cuboidal bones have some radiographic evidence of ossification, grade 3: The cuboidal bones are small and round, but not fully ossified, grade 4: The cuboidal bones are fully ossified and shaped like an adult (Figure 20.3).

### Clinical Pathology Finding

- Leukopenia: White cell count <6,000 cell/µL, neutropenia with a neutrophil:lymphocyte ratio <1.0.
- Hypoglycemia: Lack of nursing, insulin response contributes to abnormal glucose hemostasis.

**Box 20.4 Clinical Signs foal prematurity and dysmaturity**

- Small body size.
- Silky, fine hair coat.
- Generalized weakness, hypotonia.
- Increased passive range of motion of limbs.
- Flexor tendon and periarticular ligament laxity.
- Incomplete cuboidal bone ossification - typically presents in premature foals.
- Domed forehead.
- Floppy ears.
- Inability to thermoregulate.
- Abnormal neutrophil/lymphocyte counts/ratio.
- Diminished or absent suckle reflex.
- Ineffective suckle reflex.
- Time to stand and nurse abnormal.
- Enteral feed intolerance; colic, diarrhea, reflux.

***Dysmaturity*** is considered in foals that have a prolonged gestation typically >340 days. These foals have similar characteristics of the premature foal except they may also be:

- Larger in size.
- Lack of muscle development.
- Extensor tendon contracture or laxity.
- Longer hair coat.

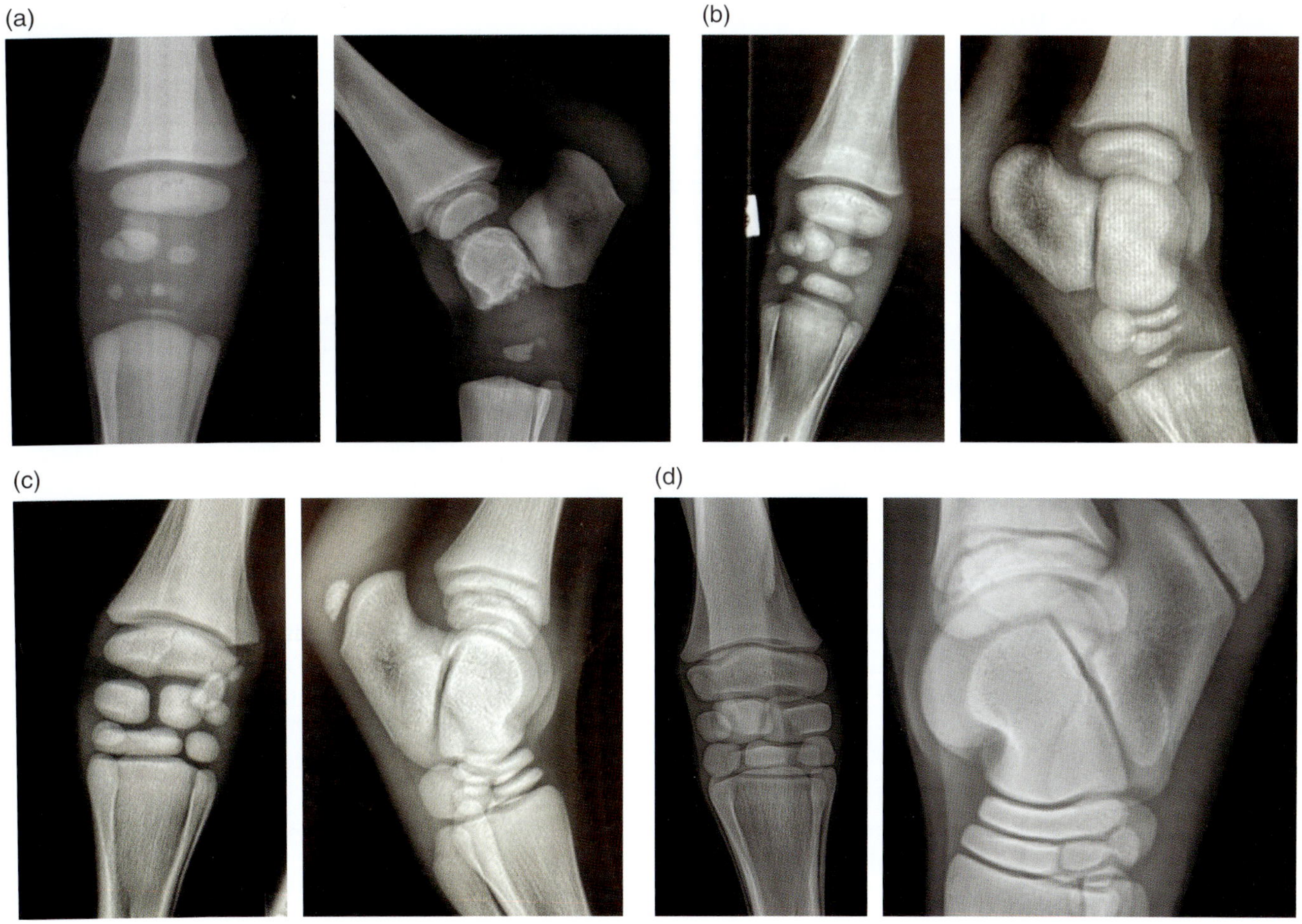


**Figure 20.3** Foal Cuboidal Bone Ossification Grading (DP and Lateral views). (a) Grade 1: Some cuboidal bones visible, lack of ossification. (b) Grade 2: All cuboidal bones have some radiographic evidence of ossification. (c) Grade 3: The cuboidal bones are small and round, but not completely ossified. (d) Grade 4: The cuboidal bones are fully ossified and shaped like an adult.

- Critical-illness-related cortisol insufficiency in some cases.
- Hypoxemia, hypocapnia, respiratory acidosis if immature lung development.
- Hyponatremia, hypochloremia with GI loss or renal immaturity/dysfunction.

## Emergency Triage Steps

- Supportive care: fluid therapy 90–120 mg/kg/day; be careful to not overhydrate!
  - Glucose support 4 mg/kg/min (can go up to 8 mg/kg/minute) using 5% dextrose solution.
- Enteral feeding (normal amount for foal to nurse = 25% of body weight daily) if not sure of GI function, start at 10% of body weight/day divided into smaller feedings
  - For example: Feed every two hours during the day and every three hours overnight for the first two weeks of life.
  - Foals should gain approximately 2 lbs (1 kg) daily.
- Respiratory support: intranasal oxygen therapy 5–10 L/min. $PaO_2$ should be maintained between 80 and 110 mmHg and $SaO_2$ >92%.
- Thermoregulatory support-Bair Hugger[2] or heat lamp.
- Musculoskeletal support depending upon finding of examination.

2 3M Bair Hugger, St. Paul MN.

## Failure of Passive Transfer

This is a common disorder in premature/dysmature foals and sick/critically ill foals. Adequate passive transfer of immunity is >800 mg/dL of serum IgG concentrations, partial failure of passive transfer is 400–800 mg/dL, and complete failure of passive transfer is <400 mg/dL (Chavatte et al. 1998; Sievert et al. 2022).

Best to treat quickly as foals are prone to local and systemic infections.

### Etiology

- Poor quality colostrum: (age of mare >14 years, breed and individual variation, seasonal weather, and climate change).
- Failure of the mare to lactate: systemic illness, fescue toxicosis.
- Premature lactation: placentitis, twins, premature placental separation.
- Failure to nurse: NE, weakness, musculoskeletal abnormalities, gastrointestinal abnormalities/colic, dam rejection.
- Failure to absorb collostral antibodies: enteritis, hypoxic damage of specialized enterocytes.
- Consumption: SIRS/Sepsis.

### Clinical Signs

- Failure of passive transfer does not have specific clinical signs of disease. Rather, foals having failure of collostral antibody protection are more susceptible to local and systemic infections including sepsis.

### Clinical Pathology

- Radioimmunoassay (RIA) – most accurate but is not available for 24 h.
- Glutaraldehyde coagulation or zinc turbidity is quick/easy low specificity.
- Idexx SNAP test higher specificity, similar sensitivity.

### Emergency Triage Steps

- Treatment depends upon environmental conditions and the systemic status of the foal.
- Foals that are healthy with an IgG between 400–800 mg/dL on clean, well-managed farms with little disease may not need treatment.
- Foals with IgG <800 mg/dL that are systemically compromised or unclean environment should be supplemented with immunoglobulins.
- Foals with an IgG <400 mg/dL need immunoglobulin supplementation regardless of environmental conditions or management practices.
- Supplementation of immunoglobulins can be done either orally or intravenously.
- Foals 12–24 h of age can be administered immunoglobulins orally if they have a functional gastrointestinal tract. NOTE: efficacy of oral supplementation decreases after 12 h of age.
- Foals >18 h of age or with gastrointestinal dysfunction require IV administration.
- Immunoglobulin levels should be re-evaluated after supplementation to assure adequate concentrations have been reached.

### Oral Supplementation

- Equine colostrum is the ideal supplement.
  - Administer orally or via nasogastric tube.
  - 1–2 L of good quality colostrum divided into 200–400 mL feedings.

### Intravenous Immunoglobulin Supplementation

- Multiple commercially available products are available that have a guaranteed IgG concentration and are free of anti-equine antibodies (Hollis et al. 2010; Palmisano et al. 2023).

- Typically, 1 L of normal equine plasma containing 1,200 mg/dL will increase a 45 kg foal's IgG concentration approximately 200 mg/dL.
  - 2–4 L of plasma may be required to increase serum IgG concentrations. >800 mg/dL in foals with complete failure of passive transfer.
- Some products are hyperimmune with 2,500 mg/dL.
- Septic foals will typically need more due to IgG consumption and catabolism.
- Fresh frozen plasma should be thawed slowly in warm water.
- Plasma should be administered with a blood administration set with online filter.
- Transfusions should be monitored for any reactions; fever, piloerection, muscle fasciculations, tachycardia/tachypnea, respiratory distress, abdominal pain, collapse.
- Start plasma administration slowly for the first 10–15 minutes and monitor vitals, and if no reaction can be administered at full flow with continued monitoring.
- If any reaction noted stop administration of plasma immediately.
- If respiratory dyspnea/distress administer IV epinephrine (0.01–0.02 mg/kg or 0.3–0.7 mL, 1 : 1,000 concentration for a 50 kg foal-dilute with sterile saline to 3–7 mL at 1 : 10,000).

### Prevention

- Measure IgG at 12–14 h of age post foaling.
- Measure quality of colostrum with a Brix refractometer.
- Good quality colostrum should be >1.060.
- Oral supplementation can be performed at birth if needed.

## Sepsis

Sepsis remains the leading cause of death in sick neonatal foals (Figure 20.4). Sepsis can be asymptomatic and present as acute collapse. Foals with sepsis that progress to septic shock have an increased risk of mortality. Sepsis is the systemic inflammatory response to infection (Taylor 2015; Wong et al. 2018; Eaton 2023; Scalco et al. 2023).

### Etiology

- Foals can become septic *in utero,* during or after parturition.
- *Predisposing factors include*
  - Maternal illness.
  - Placentitis.
  - Premature placental separation.
  - Abnormal gestational length.
  - Failure of passive transfer of immunity.
  - Dirty environmental conditions.
- *In utero* infection is typically caused by placentitis.
- Post parturition infection typically occurs via the GI tract, respiratory, or umbilicus. Translocation of bacteria in the gastrointestinal tract is the most important factor.
- Bacteria involved.
  - Gram-negative bacterial infections predominate.
  - Gram-positive bacterial infections are rising.
  - EHV-1 and equine arteritis virus can also cause sepsis.
  - Bacteria can disseminate throughout the body and localize in different body systems which result in enteritis, meningitis, pneumonia, or septic joints/osteomyelitis.
- If sepsis goes uncontrolled it can lead to septic shock, multiple organ dysfunction, and death.

### Clinical Signs

- Much depends upon severity of illness and the duration, along with the foal's immune system competency.

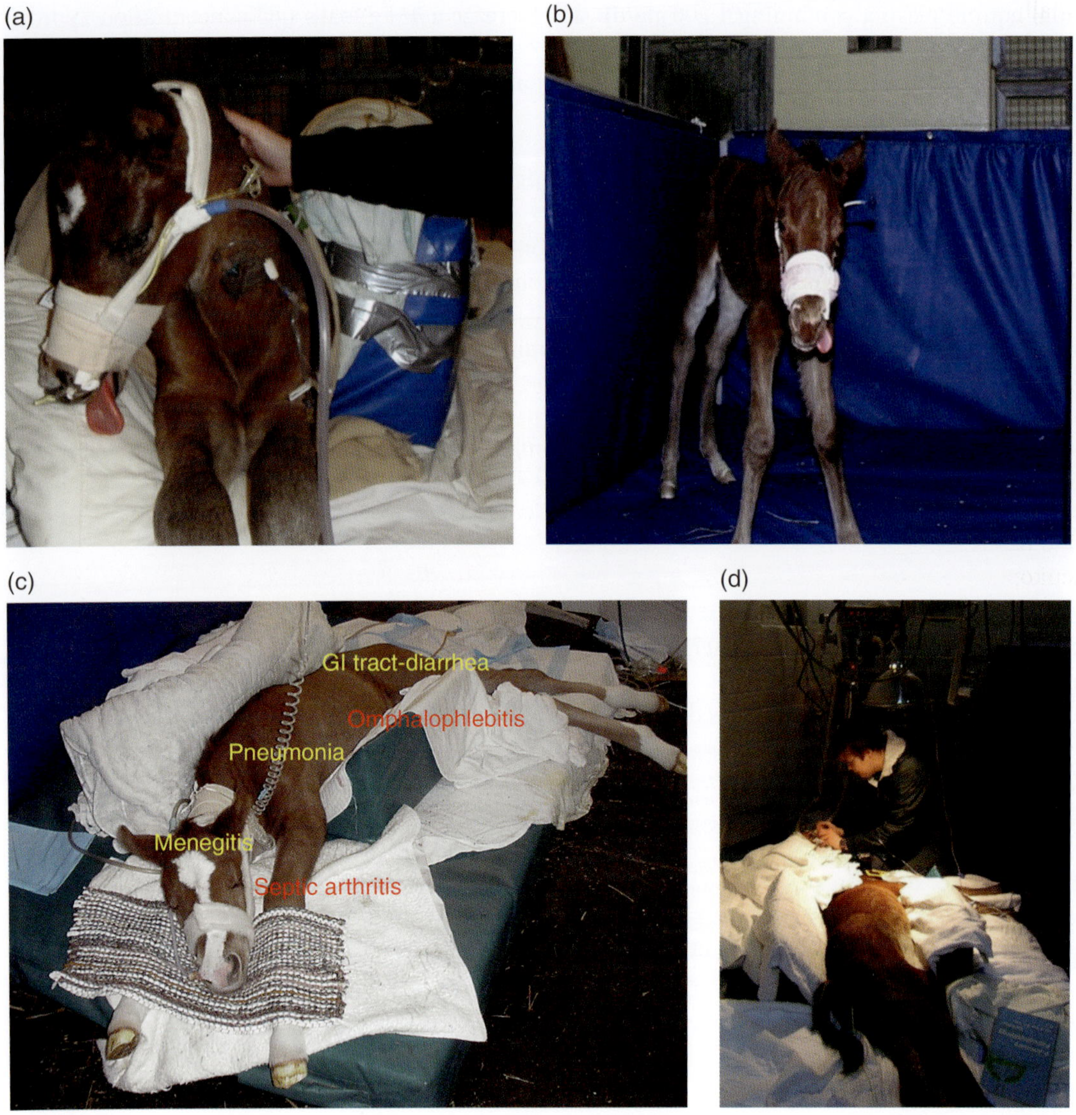


**Figure 20.4** Neonatal sepsis and encephalopathy. (a) Sepsis and (b) encephalopathy. (c) Neontal Sepsis: Possible infection sites. (d) Septic foal on ventilator.

- Clinical signs can be subtle and difficult to determine, however if not treated may lead to septic shock, multiple-organ dysfunction syndrome (MODS), and death.
- Not nursing, obtundation, increased recumbency are all early indicators of sepsis.
- Rectal temperature is variable.
- Hyperemic mucous membranes (Figure 20.1) and coronary band, and scleral injection are all early indicators of sepsis. Cyanotic mucous membranes occur with advanced stages of sepsis and shock.
- Uveitis may be present if *in utero* sepsis.
- Enteritis: clinical signs include diarrhea, reflux, ileus, abdominal distention.
- Pneumonia: signs referred to respiratory system such as tachypnea, dyspnea +/− cough.

## Clinical Pathology Findings

- Azotemia: Increased blood urea nitrogen (BUN) or creatinine can occur due to hypovolemia/dehydration, hypotension, decreased glomerular filtration rate from any cause and or direct renal damage from coagulopathy, ischemia, or cytokine release.

- Fibrinogen: May initially be normal and then increase over time. If >400 mg/dL at birth most likely the foal was septic *in utero*. If a foal is septic and the fibrinogen does not increase it may be indicative of disseminated intravascular hemolysis (DIC).
- Hyperbilirubinemia: Can be seen due to increased red cell turnover, anorexia, hepatic dysfunction, or sepsis associated hemolysis.
- Hypoglycemia: Common finding in septic foals. They typically do not have the reserves to maintain glucose homeostasis.
- Hypovolemia/hemoconcentration: Common finding due to lack of nursing/obtundation.
- Hypoglobulinemia: Can be seen due to failure of passive transfer or consumption of globulins.
- Hypoxemia: A $PaO_2$ <60 mmHg is associated with pulmonary dysfunction, ventilation–perfusion mismatch, pulmonary hypertension, or hypoventilation.
- Metabolic acidosis: Is typically seen due to poor perfusion/hypovolemia, anerobic metabolism. Metabolic acidosis is an arterial pH less than 7.35 or $HCO_3$ <24 mEq/L. Hyperlactatemia contributes to the acidosis.
- L-Lactate: Typically lactate concentrations are higher in neonates than in adult horses for the first 24 h after birth. L-Lactate concentrations are highest just after parturition ($2.3 \pm 0.9$; $4.9 \pm 1.0$; $3 \pm 0.4$ mmol/L in multiple studies). Concentrations then decline to $1.2 \pm 0.3$ mmol/L by 24 h of age. Critically ill neonates with high lactate concentrations that do not respond to resuscitation efforts may have a poor prognosis.
- White cell count: Leukopenia and neutropenia (white cell count <5,000 cells/μL, neutrophils <3,400 cells/μL. Increased band neutrophils (>50 cells/μL). Toxic changes may be present in the neutrophils. Leukocytosis can also occur (>12,000 cells/μL), typically with a neutrophilia.

### Diagnosis

- History of mare and foal, clinical examination findings, clinical pathology results and culture.

### Emergency Triage Steps

- Antimicrobial therapy – broad-spectrum IV bactericidal activity should be started immediately if sepsis is suspected. Minimum of 10–14 days treatment plan.
  - Because of unique physiology, antimicrobial choice and dosing is different for foals compared to adult horses (Magdesian 2017).
  - Potassium penicillin/ampicillin for Gram-positive/some Gram-negative and anaerobes.
  - Aminoglycoside for Gram-negative infections, as long as renal function is good.
  - Ceftiofur Gram-negative/Gram-positive and some anaerobes if questionable renal function.
  - Please do not use Excede in neonatal foals; dosing is different than adults and it's better to use Naxcel than Excede.
  - Many antimicrobial choices may be considered depending upon the clinical problem (Corley and Hollis 2009).
- Immune support - administration of fresh frozen plasma.
- Supportive care - thermoregulation, fluid therapy plus glucose support, enteral support, monitor ins (fluid/enteral going in) and outs (fecal and urine production).
- Blood pressure support using inotropes or vasopressors may be valuable in the hospital setting if foals fail to respond to fluid resuscitation.
- Other treatments depend upon systemic manifestations.

## Neonatal Encephalopathy (NE)

NE results from decreased oxygen and tissue perfusion during the prenatal and perinatal period (Figure 20.4). Multisystemic disease, characterized by dysfunction of the central nervous system (CNS), along with abnormalities of the gastrointestinal tract and or renal system is often associated with NE. If the foal does not have seizures and has mild disease the prognosis tends to be excellent. However, if seizures are present, prognosis tends to be guarded (Vaala 1994, Rossdale 2004, Toribio 2019; Wong 2020; Gold and Wong 2024).

## Etiology

Results from any adverse periparturient occurrence that results in decreased oxygen supply to tissues or other compromise of the fetus. Inflammatory mediators likely also play a role.

- Maternal causes
  - Anemia.
  - Cardiovascular disease.
  - GI compromise – abdominal surgery/colitis.
  - Hypertension due to painful conditions such as laminitis.
  - Hypotension – endotoxemia.
  - Respiratory disease.
- Placental causes
  - Placentitis.
  - Placental insufficiency.
  - Premature placental separation.
  - Reduced umbilical blood flow.
- Parturition causes
  - Cesarean section.
  - Dystocia.
  - Induction of labor.
  - Premature placental separation.
  - Uterine inertia.
- Neonatal causes
  - Anemia.
  - Congenital cardiovascular disease.
  - Dysmaturity.
  - Prematurity.
  - Respiratory disease.
  - Septic shock.

## Clinical Signs

Depends upon the affected organ systems and the length and severity of the insult. Also depends upon when the insult occurred with relation to fetal or neonatal life. Clinical signs of NE are typically seen at birth up to 72 h post-partum.

- Central nervous signs
  - Loss of affinity for mare.
  - Inability to find udder.
  - Loss of suckle reflex.
  - Hyperresponsiveness.
    - Extensor rigidity.
    - Intermittent opisthotonos.
    - Petit mal to grand mal seizures.
    - Hyporesponsive.
- Renal signs
  - Decreased urine production.
  - Isosthenuric urine.
  - Decreased creatinine clearance.
  - Edema development.
  - Anuric renal failure.
- Gastrointestinal tract signs
  - Gas distension and colic.
  - Necrotizing enterocolitis.

  - Hemorrhagic diarrhea.
  - Sepsis.
  - GI rupture.
- Other organ system signs
  - Cardiovascular system.
    - Decreased myocardial function.
    - Arrhythmias.
    - Decreased response of vasculature to endogenous and exogenous adrenergic mediators.
  - Respiratory system
    - Hypoxia, acidemia lead to increased pulmonary resistance.
    - Potential to revert to fetal circulation.
  - Hepatic system
    - Elevated liver enzymes.
    - Elevated bilirubin.
  - Endocrine system
    - Hypocortisolemia.
    - Inappropriate ADH secretion.
    - Abnormal parathyroid hormone secretion.

## Diagnosis

- Clinical signs, as described above, and lack of other disease processes.

## Note of Importance

- NE often occurs with sepsis and prematurity.

## Emergency Triage Steps

Supportive care, nutritional support, fluid therapy, antimicrobials (compromised foals) (Papazian et al. 1993; Wilkins 2005; Giguiere et al. 2007, 2008).

- *Central nervous system*
  - Maintenance of cerebral perfusion/blood pressure with IV fluid therapy.
  - Allopurinol 40 mg/kg PO with two to three of birth, free radical scavenger.
  - Vitamin C 100 mg/kg/day IV, helps with NMDA blockade, free radical scavenger.
  - Magnesium Sulfate 25 mg/kg/h, NMDA blockade.
  - Thiamine 10–20 mg/kg IV q12–24 h cerebral support.
  - Vitamin E 500 IU q24 h PO, antioxidant.
- Seizures
  - Diazepam 0.1–0.44 mg/kg 5–10 mg for a 50 kg foal.
  - Midazolam 0.1 mg/kg IV 3–5 mg for a 50 kg foal, CRI, –0.02–0.1 mg/kg/h.
  - Phenobarbital 2–10 mg/kg IV q12–24 h given slowly to effect, ½ life is about 100 h.
  - Phenytoin 5–10 mg/kg loading dose, 1–5 mg/kg q4 h for first 24 h.
- Nursing care
  - Restrain foal on mattress with foal wall supports, leg wraps, ocular lubricants.
- Feeding
  - If coordinated suckle and swallow, feed via nasogastric tube, go slowly versus the 25% of body weight to make sure GI tract is functioning (provide 10% increasing to 25% body weight daily divided into small feedings (typically q2 h).
- *Gastrointestinal tract*
  - Be cautious when feeding via nasogastric tube.
  - Parenteral nutrition is also an option if GI tract is not functioning appropriately.

- *Renal*
  - Urine specific gravity and volume should be monitored to assess renal function.
  - Catheterization of bladder to allow to monitor ins/outs.
  - Dopamine 2–5 μg/kg/min to enhance urine production.
  - Furosemide 0.25–1.0 mg/kg IV or CRI 0.25–2 mg/kg/h.
  - Monitor electrolytes.

## Neonatal Isoerythrolysis (NI)

Alloimmune hemolytic anemia of newborn foals caused by antibodies against the foal's erythrocytes in the mare's colostrum (Bailey et al. 1987; Vaala 1990; McClure 1997; Divers 2003; Polkes et al. 2008; Sellon and Wilkins 2010). NI is typically seen in foals from multiparous mares and involving factors Aa and Qa. Theses foals will typically not have failure of passive transfer. Owner should be warned that the mare is at risk for having NI foals in the future. Large volume and repeat transfusions can result in liver injury or kernicterus in severe cases. These foals should be monitored closely.

### Etiology

Surface antigens Aa and Qa factors are the most immunogenic factors and cause approximately 90% of NI cases. Donkey factor has been shown in mule foals and can cause problems. The prevalence of NI is low in Thoroughbred and Standardbred horses is low. All mares bred to donkeys are at risk of producing foals that develop NI; however, only 10% of mule foals develop NI. To develop NI the mare must be negative for the type of RBC antigen factor. The mare is exposed to and produces antibodies against RBC antigens. This typically occurs when multiparous mares are exposed to fetal RBCs during previous pregnancies or primiparous mares that have had a blood transfusion or developed placental abnormalities which cause exposure to fetal RBCs. The foal inherits specific RBC antigen from the stallion and the foal ingests and absorbs alloantibodies from the colostrum.

### Clinical Signs

- Normal at birth, develop signs post colostrum ingestion.
- Clinical signs vary depending upon rate and severity of hemolysis and resulting anemia.
- Possible icteric mucous membranes (Figure 20.1).
- Can occur five hours to seven days post-partum.
- Peracute cases occur less than five hours.
- Mild cases
  - Lethargy.
  - Tachypnea.
  - Tachycardia.
  - Pale icteric mucous membranes.
- Severe, acute onset
  - Febrile.
  - Stop nursing.
  - Pigmenturia.
- Peracute
  - Found dead.
  - Multiple organ failure.
  - Seizures.
  - May or may not be icteric.

### Diagnosis

Clinical signs, maternal alloantibodies on foal's RBCs. Foals will be anemic and hyperbilirubinemic. Severely affected foals have increased L-Lactate concentrations, metabolic acidosis, pigmenturia, and elevated liver enzymes, thrombocytopenia, and neutropenia. Hemolytic cross match is the most reliable test. Mix the mares serum with foal's RBCs (minor cross match) strong hemolytic reaction is positive. Alloantibodies responsible for NI are stronger hemolysins than agglutinins; therefore, do not test for agglutination. Jaundiced foal agglutination test (JFA) can be performed in the field and with experienced handlers, as it correlates well with the hemolytic test. JFA – mix the mare's colostrum with foal's blood and look for agglutination. Hemolytic test – Foal RBCs are mixed with mares blood and evidence of clumping/agglutination confirms anti-RBC antibodies are present.

### Emergency Triage Steps

If clinical signs develop before 24 h, colostrum should be withheld from foal and milked out.

If mild hemolysis, no treatment may be needed. In more severe cases a blood transfusion may be necessary along with supportive care.

- If foal is not nursing and hypovolemic
  - Fluid therapy.
  - Oxygen insufflation.
- Decision for blood transfusion
  - Depends upon clinical signs – weakness, tachypnea, tachycardia, and laboratory findings.
  - PCV is unreliable indicator of tissue perfusion.
  - Combination of PCV <12% and hemoglobin <5 g/dL are often used along with clinical signs.
  - Washing mare's RBCs are ideal choice for transfusion.
  - Aa/Qa negative blood donor or Standardbred, Morgan or Quarter Horse gelding with no prior blood transfusions are suitable donors.
- Optimal blood volume

$$\text{PCV}\left(\text{desired}\right) - \text{PCV observed} \times \text{Body weight}\left(\text{kg}\right) \times \text{Blood volume}\left(\text{L/kg}\right)$$

PCV of donor

- 150 mL/kg is blood volume of a 2-day-old foal.
- Can also administer 2–3 L empirically and monitor foal response to treatment.
- Prognosis
  - Favorable prognosis for uncomplicated cases.
  - Foals that continue hemolysis post transfusion are at risk for development of kernicterus and severe degenerative liver disease, which bare a grave prognosis.

### Prevention

NI is preventable. At-risk mares, Aa and Qa-negative mares, and mares that have already had NI foals can be identified. At-risk mares should be screened for anti-RBC antibodies, which are produced during the last month of pregnancy. If anti-RBC antibodies are present a hemolytic or JFA test should be done prior to the foal nursing. If the JFA or hemolytic test is positive, foals should be supplemented with colostrum from another source (tested) and should not nurse from mare for 48 h or as determined by the JFA. The mare should be milked out and the milk/colostrum discarded.

## Pneumonia

Pneumonia is common in sick neonatal foals and a complication of other neonatal disease. Recumbent, weak, obtunded foals may also acquire aspiration pneumonia. Pneumonia is the leading cause of mortality and morbidity in foals and is common in neonates and 1–6-month-old foals. Bacterial pneumonia is the most common; however, viral and fungal infections may contribute (Kosch et al. 1984; Wilkins 2003; Wilkins et al. 2007, 2010a, b; Palmer 2005b; Wong et al. 2010).

### Etiology

Most of the same bacteria/viruses that cause sepsis also cause pneumonia. Older foals often get *Rhodococcus equi or Streptococcus zooepidemicus*. It is common to have anaerobic bacteria involved along with viruses such as Influenza,

EHV-1, EHV-2, EHV-4, adenovirus, and rhinovirus; however, these are usually not primary causes of pneumonia. Environmental and management, parasitic and viral infection are all predisposing factors. Neonates typically get pneumonia due to sepsis, prolonged recumbency, or aspiration during nursing. Foals 1–6 months of age are typically affected via inhalation of organisms in dust or aerosolization. Older foals get acute respiratory dysfunction as well as neonates. The exact cause in older foals in unknown but may be due to dysfunction of the immune system.

### Clinical Signs

- Depends upon the severity, chronicity, and etiology.
- Range of clinical signs
  - Tachypnea.
  - Nostril flare.
  - Increased abdominal push.
  - Febrile.
  - +/− cough.
  - +/− nasal discharge.
- Auscultation
  - Increased inspiratory and expiratory sounds.
  - Increased tracheal rattle.
  - Crackles, wheezes.

### Diagnosis

Physical examination, clinical pathology including serum amyloid A and fibrinogen, ultrasound, radiographs, transtracheal wash, culture and sensitivity, and arterial blood gas analysis.

### Emergency Triage Steps

The aim is to eliminate infection, provide systemic and respiratory support, prevent spread if infectious.

- Antimicrobials broad spectrum.
- Intranasal oxygen insufflation.
- Nebulization.
- Steroidal anti-inflammatory therapy (dexamethasone, 0.2 mg/kg IV q12 h for three days).

## Respiratory Distress

Respiratory distress may be associated with congenital upper airway abnormalities such as choanal atresia and subepiglottic cysts (needs upper airway endoscopy). Rule out fractured ribs by palpation and ultrasound (perform during initial examination to rule out rib fractures).

### Etiology

Overwhelming inflammatory response of the respiratory system elicited by a primary disease process such a sepsis, SIRS, pneumonia, trauma, or other factors.

### Clinical Signs

- Nostril flare.
- Expiratory grunt.

- Rib retraction.
- Increased abdominal effort.

### Diagnosis

Physical examination, history, concurrent disease, arterial blood gas.

### Emergency Triage Steps

- Intranasal oxygen insufflation.
- Steroidal anti-inflammatory therapy (dexamethasone, 0.2 mg/kg IV q12 h for three days).
- If upper airway obstruction – tracheostomy.

## Apnea

Slow respiratory rates or irregular respiratory patterns such as apnea, then tachypnea are all abnormal.

### Etiology

Associated with NE/maladjustment syndrome. Hypoglycemia, hypothermia, and prematurity.

### Clinical Signs

- Irregular breathing pattern.

### Diagnosis

History, clinical findings, ultrasound, and radiographs to rule out other causes, arterial blood gas.

### Emergency Triage Steps

- Caffeine 10 mg/kg loading dose, then 2.5 mg/kg PO or per rectum as needed.
- Doxapram 0.5 mg/kg loading dose than 0.3-0.08 mg/kg/min CRI use for neonatal foals that have hypercapnia without hypoxemia.

## Congenital Heart Disease

When foals are born, 90% have audible murmurs and 96% have a variety of arrhythmias including atrial tachycardia, A–V block, and ventricular premature contractures which typically disappear within 15–20 minutes. Foals with grade III/V or greater murmurs, jugular pulses, cyanosis, peripheral edema, pleural edema, ascites, syncope, weakness, lack of normal growth, and or lethargy are all suggestive of cardiac insufficiency.

### Etiology

Depends upon the type of cardiac problem.

Patent ductus arteriosus (can be seen in normal foals); should not be heard three to four days post-partum.

1) Persistent pulmonary hypertension/ reversion to fetal circulation: This foal needs to be hospitalized.
   a) The transition from fetal to neonatal circulation requires resolution of pulmonary hypertension present in the fetus. Its cause is in its failure of the fetus to make the respiratory and cardiac transition to extrauterine life or reversion of

the foal to fetal circulation in response to hypoxemia and or acidosis. Differentiation of this problem is accomplished through serial arterial blood gas analysis. Differentials are sepsis, bacterial/viral pneumonia, or congenital cardiac malformations. Reversion to fetal circulation should be suspected in a neonatal foal with hypercapnic hypoxemia that continues or worsens. Treatment is correction of acidosis and alleviation of hypoxemia. Initial therapy is intranasal oxygen therapy at 8–10 L/min. Many foals will respond to this right away. Failure to improve or worsening of hypoxemia would require mechanical ventilation.

2) Holosystolic murmur heard left side ICS 3–4: Ventricular septal defect – most frequent congenital cardiac abnormality in large animals. Murmur is noted bilaterally but usually more pronounced on the right-side ICS 3–4.
3) Atrial septal defect – uncommon in foals, typically seen with complex congenital anomalies.
4) Pronounced heart-based murmur: Tetralogy of Fallot – pulmonary valve stenosis, ventricular septal defect, overriding aorta, and right ventricular hypertrophy. Loud murmur grade IV/VI to VI/VI pansystolic murmur with palpable thrill on left heart base.

### Clinical Signs

- Murmur.
- Exercise intolerance.
- Cyanosis.
- Failure to thrive.
- Difficulty nursing.
- Dyspnea.

### Diagnosis

Echocardiography, Ultrasound, Radiographs (ECG detect arrythmias not murmurs).

### Emergency Triage Steps

- Physical examination.
- Echocardiography.

## Dysphagia

Dysphagia is common in foals and can be from multiple issues. Foals may present with milk coming from the foal's nostrils, inability to suckle, or aspiration pneumonia (Holcoombe et al. 2012; Delvoscovo et al. 2021).

### Etiology

Inability to suckle can be caused by NE, severe hyponatremia, botulism, white muscle disease/selenium deficiency, craniofacial malformation, and cranial nerve deficits.

Milk coming from the nostrils can be caused by pharyngeal paralysis due to NE (typically transient), selenium deficiency/white muscle disease, cleft palate, epiglottic cyst, botulism, choke, megaesophagus, branchial arch defect, HYPP, and idiopathic (these foals can drink from a bucket or pan on the ground, may be a breed predisposition).

### Clinical Signs

- Milk coming from nostrils.
- Difficulty nursing.
- Cough.
- Weakness.

### Diagnosis

Physical examination, clinical pathology, endoscopy-before and after nursing, ultrasound, thoracic radiographs, selenium concentrations/glutathione peroxidase, if a Quarter Horse and suspicious of HYPP, genetic testing

### Emergency Triage Steps

If underlying cause is known, treat the underlying cause.

Foals with dysphagia need to be fed via nasogastric tube if too weak to drink voluntarily. If they can drink from a bucket, muzzle foal until offered milk and then place bucket in a dependent position to help minimize aspiration. Most of the foals have a good prognosis unless a fatal congenital issue.

Treat aspiration pneumonia with broad-spectrum antimicrobials.

If HYPP diagnosis, typically foals, will improve with time. Severe cases may be managed with acetazolamide 2 mg/kg PO q12 h.

## Colic

Multiple factors can lead to colic in the neonatal and older foal. Foals may present with or without abdominal distension and display mild-to-moderate or severe pain. Common causes of colic in neonatal foals include meconium impaction, infectious causes/sepsis, NE or congenital issues such as atresia coli or ileocecocolic agangliosis seen in lethal white foals (Sanchez 2005a, MacKinnon et al. 2013).

### Etiology

Meconium impaction – foals should pass meconium (dark brown, hard fecal balls) within the first 24 h of life, followed by more yellow, soft mares milk feces. Meconium impactions are more common in colts as they have a smaller pelvic canal compared to fillies. Atresia coli – suggestive if lack of fecal staining in enema fluid and absence of fecal colored material in rectum. Mucous may be present.

Ileus can happen with NE or sepsis, hypovolemia, prematurity, or shock.

Intussusception may be caused by congenital abnormalities or hypermotile intestine.

Enteritis/colitis can cause ileus in foals with sepsis, bacteremia.

Gastroduodenal ulcers may not be seen in neonates but commonly in older foals.

Peritonitis may occur secondary to ruptured duodenal or gastric ulcer, enteritis, urachal abscess, or other internal umbilical infection.

Chyloperitonitis or peritonitis secondary to presence of chylous effusion.

Intestinal volvulus is also a cause for colic in foals.

### Clinical Signs

- Obtundation.
- Lack of nursing.
- Abdominal distension.
- Rolling.
- Lying on back.
- Tail swishing.
- Posturing to defecate.
- Lack of fecal production.
- Diarrhea.

### Diagnosis

Clinical signs, clinical pathology (depending upon etiology), abdominal ultrasound, abdominal radiographs, abdominocentesis (sterile technique and 20-gauge inch needle or teat cannula), gastroscopy, digital rectal examination.

## Emergency Triage Steps

- Physical examination.
- Digital rectal examination.
- Nasogastric intubation.
- Ultrasound.
- Radiographs.
- Abdominocentesis.
- Clinical pathology, L-lactate, glucose, PCV/TP.
- Gastroscope if indicated.
- Make decision if colic may be managed on the farm or requires referral.

### Meconium Impaction

- Digital rectal exam to suspect or confirm meconium blockage (Fischer and Yarbrough 1995; Pusterla et al. 2004; Sanchez 2005b).
- *Ultrasound findings*
  - Obstruction.
  - Thickening.
  - Excess abdominal fluid.
  - Umbilical structures.
  - Bladder.
- Radiographs can help visualize extent of meconium in rectum/small colon.
- Contrast radiographs 5 mL/kg barium via nasogastric tube serial radiographs 10, 20, 40, 60 minutes, 2 and 4 h post administration.
- Purpose – Finds obstruction, delayed gastric emptying and transit time
- Barium should be gone from stomach in 1.5–2 h. Cecum fills by 2 h, transverse colon by 3 h.
- Initial treatment with enema – ivory soap and a small amount of mineral oil, gravity flow 300–500 mL/50 kg foal. Do not give too many enemas as it can cause horrible rectal irritation, edema, and straining.
- Acetylcysteine retention enema
  - 30 French Foley catheter inserted into rectum and balloon inflated slowly.
  - Administer acetylcysteine slowly and leave in 30–45 minutes with hind limbs and abdomen elevated if possible.
  - Enema can be repeated q12–24 h if needed.
  - Acetylcysteine enema solutions-2 choices
  - 1) 8 g *N*-acetyl-L-cysteine powder, 200 mL water.
  - 2) 40 mL 20% solution of acetylcysteine (mucomyst®), 160 mL water.
  - Foal should start passing feces 5–10 minutes later. If no feces passed further diagnostics are needed and possible referral.
- Surgery is not commonly required for meconium impactions in foals; however, surgery may be indicated when medical management fails, with radiographic evidence of obstruction, and with increasing pain and progressive abdominal distention.

### Enteritis

- Typically seen before development of diarrhea.
- Pyrexia.
- Clinical pathology – leukopenia.
- Ultrasound – thickened small intestine, fluid filled small intestine with minimal motility commonly seen with enteritis.
- Fluid therapy with dextrose.
- Supportive care.
- Broad-spectrum antimicrobials.

### Ileus

- Clinical signs/clinical pathology findings.
- Fluid therapy with dextrose.

- Withhold nursing.
- Lidocaine CRI typically use 0.025 mg/kg/min in foals.

## Foal Diarrhea/Enterocolitis

Diarrhea is one of the most common clinical problems seen in foals. The causes can be infectious or non-infectious and identifying the exact cause can be complicated as many gastrointestinal pathogens can be identified in healthy foals (Hollis et al. 2008). Diarrhea can be mild and self-limiting to life-threatening with severe hypovolemia/dehydration and electrolyte abnormalities (Magdesian 2005; Wong et al. 2010).

### Etiology

Diarrhea in foals results typically from increased secretion and malabsorption. Infectious agents enter different parts of the intestinal tract, and the effects depend on where the organism invades such as the crypts or villous cells, depth of invasion (mucosa/submucosa), and the inflammatory reaction created by the invasion. Exotoxins and endotoxins can be produced by the infectious agents which in turn can alter electrolyte and fluid movement across the mucosa (Table 20.1).

**Table 20.1** Causes of diarrhea in neonatal foals.

| Inciting cause | Age | Comment |
|---|---|---|
| Sepsis | <4 days | Common site for localized infection |
| Neonatal encephalopathy | <4 days | Asphyxia can lead to ileus or necrotizing enterocolitis |
| Foal heat | 6–12 days | Developmental changes in GI tract/microbiome |
| **Nutritional causes** | | |
| Foreign material | Older foals | Sand/dirt |
| Orphan foal | Any age | Milk formulas, inaccurate mixing, overfeeding |
| Lactulose intolerance | Any age | |
| Primary | | Rare |
| Secondary | | Common with small intestinal infections |
| **Bacteria** | | |
| *Clostridium perfringens C* | <4 days | Hemorrhagic diarrhea, ileus, shock, death |
| *Clostridium perfringens A* | <4 days | Transient hemorrhagic diarrhea |
| *Clostridium difficile* | <4 days | Severe watery to hemorrhage diarrhea |
| *Escherichia coli* | <1 month | Frequent cause of sepsis<br>RARELY if ever cause of primary diarrhea |
| *Rhodococcus equi* | 3 weeks and older | Intestinal form, diarrhea, colic |
| *Salmonella* spp. | <4 days<br>All ages | Sepsis<br>Enterocolitis |
| **Viruses** | | |
| Rotavirus Group A | 1–6 months | Common cause of infectious diarrhea |
| Group B | <7 days | Recently identified severe diarrhea |
| Corona Virus | All ages | Typically co-infection with rotavirus or *Clostridium* spp. |
| **Parasites** | | |
| *Cryptosporidium* | <4 days<br>2–3 weeks<br>Older foals | Life threatening in immune compromised foals<br>Prolonged diarrhea<br>Chronic intermittent diarrhea |
| Helminths | 7 days–6 months | Uncommon, *Strongyloides westerii*, cyathostomiasis |

## Clinical Signs

The clinical signs vary widely from mild, self-limiting diarrhea to hemorrhagic enterocolitis seen with clostridial infections or sepsis.

- Pyrexia.
- Obtundation.
- Lack of nursing.
- Hypovolemia/dehydration.
- Signs of colic.

## Diagnosis

Clinical signs, organisms identified, farm history (e.g., previous *Clostridial* spp. infections), Ultrasound findings; thickened loops of small intestine, increased peritoneal fluid, fluid-filled colon, cecum, and/or small intestine. Radiographs especially if worried about sand. Diagnostic evaluation may include Culture/PCR and other testing (Table 20.2).

Clinical pathology changes: Typically seen with sepsis or bacterial infections.

- Leukopenia.
- Left shift.
- Toxic neutrophils.
- Hyperfibrinogenemia.
- Elevated serum amyloid A.
- Hypoproteinemia.
- Hyponatremia/hypochloridemia.
- Metabolic acidosis.

**Table 20.2** Tests for diagnosis of enteric pathogens.

| Pathogen | Procedure | Comments |
|---|---|---|
| *Clostridium difficile* | Culture<br>ELISA for toxins A and B<br>Gram stain of fecal smear<br>PCR for toxigenic genes | Toxin should be identified |
| *Clostridium perfringens* | Culture<br>ELISA for enterotoxin<br>Multiplex PCR | Toxin should be identified |
| *Cryptosporidium* | Acid fast staining<br>Flow cytometry<br>Immunofluorescent antibody assay | Beneficial to have experience identifying stained oocytes |
| Cyathostomiasis | Fecal and larval egg count | |
| *Lawsonia intracellularis* | PCR and immunoperoxidase stain on feces<br>Intestinal biopsy | |
| Rotavirus | Fecal ELISA<br>Fecal latex agglutination<br>Electron microscopy | |
| *Salmonella* spp. | Fecal culture and PCR | Repeat 3–5 cultures necessary |

### Emergency Triage Steps

Stabilization is the first priority.
Strict isolation and hygiene protocols should be in place.
IV Fluid therapy, essential for stabilization.
Correct hypovolemia/dehydration and calculate for ongoing losses.
Plasma transfusion if hypoproteinemia is present.
Antimicrobial therapy:
Broad spectrum for foals <7 days of age.
Older foals, determine inciting cause and select appropriate drug.
Example: If clostridial diarrhea, metronidazole and penicillin are warranted.
Nutrition and gastrointestinal rest are important considerations.
Some foals need to be withheld from milk for several days due to ileus and colic and should receive partial parenteral nutrition (PPN) or total parenteral nutrition (TPN).
Other foals do well with limited nursing, allowing nourishment of the GI tract but in small volumes (allow to nurse for one to two minutes every two hours versus free choice). If limited nursing, foals need to be on IV fluid therapy.

*Other treatments*

Di-tri-octahedral smectite (be aware can cause constipation).
Bismuth subsalicylate and sucralfate.
Cleaning of peri-rectal area and the application of protective cream such as zinc.

## Uroperitoneum

Uroabdomen is not a surgical emergency, but the hyperkalemia caused by a ruptured bladder is life-threatening. Surgical correction of the ruptured bladder should be delayed until the potassium concentration is below 5 mEq/L or less. Please see Chapter 13, *Diseases of the Urinary Tract* and Appendix 4, *Emergency Treatment Protocols.*

The most common places for rupture of the urinary tract occur at the bladder or the urachus. Less frequent places for rupture are extra-abdominal urachus, retroperitoneal ureter, and urethra. Foal with a rupture in the urinary tract are usually less than 7 days of age, although older foals can be affected. No sex predilection is known (Kablack et al. 2000; Wilkins 2004; Dunkel et al. 2005; Vander Werf et al. 2010).

### Etiology

Localized ischemia, sepsis, and necrosis are significant factors leading to rupture of the bladder or other parts of the urinary tract. Other causes may be increased pressure during parturition, congenital defects, urachal infection, or external trauma. The exact pathophysiology is unclear. Although sepsis, or malperfusion are probably the most accurate. Uroperitoneum develops as urine accumulates in the abdominal following rupture of the bladder or urachus.

Disruption of the urinary tract retroperitoneally may end up with urine in the abdomen or it may be retained in the space such as perineal edema, periabdominal or perivaginal edema may occur.

When urine accumulates in the abdominal cavity, equilibrium of urine electrolytes and water across the peritoneal membrane with systemic circulation, leading to hyponatremia, hypochloridemia, and hyperkalemia. Systemic absorption of creatinine results in azotemia. Foals can have such abdominal distension that it leads to respiratory distress and accumulation of pleural fluid, lung atelectasis, or ARDS.

### Clinical Signs

Signs are varied depending upon duration and location of urinary rupture. They may present for suspected meconium impaction due to signs of straining.

- Straining to urinate.

- Dribbling urine.
- Frequent stretching out.
- Abdominal distension.
- Decreased urination.
- Lethargy.
- Obtundation.
- Decreased nursing
- Systemic clinical signs may be seen.
- Subcutaneous edema.

### Diagnosis

Physical examination, abdominal ultrasound (anechoic peritoneal fluid +/− bladder wall or urachal defect). Clinical pathology findings depend upon the duration of the uroperitoneum and potential other clinical issues. Hyperkalemia, hyponatremia, hypochloridemia, azotemia are classic but, if not seen, uroperitoneum should not be discounted. Peritoneal fluid analysis: Peritoneal creatinine-to-serum creatinine ratio greater than 2 : 1 is diagnostic for uroperitoneum. Can also use subcutaneous urine creatinine-to-serum creatinine ratio.

### Emergency Triage Steps

Stabilization of the patient is the key to dealing with ruptured urinary tract/bladder.

- Intravenous fluid therapy using 0.45% NaCl or Lactated Ringers solution with 5% dextrose.
- Urinary catheter placement.
- If potassium is greater than 5.5 mEq/L, then this should be corrected prior to anesthesia/surgery.
- Drain urine from abdomen with teat cannula, or foley catheter, or human peritoneal dialysis catheter.
- Broad-spectrum antimicrobials.
- Nasal oxygen insufflation if respiratory distress.
- Once stabilized, surgical repair may be offered.
- Prognosis depends upon whether foal is septic or otherwise healthy.

## Limb Deformities

A wide variety of flexural limb deformities and angular limb deformities (ALD) occur in foals (Figure 20.5). Some are congenital, while others develop after birth. Most cases of flexural and ALD in the neonatal foal will resolve with time, physical therapy, or medical management. As stated earlier all premature or dysmature foals should have radiographs of the carpus and tarsus to check for the ossification of cuboidal bones (Figure 20.3). For foals with severe deformities, nursing care is extremely important and intensive. Foals with severe flexural limb deformities often have a history of dystocia; therefore, such foals often have NE as well (Adams 1990; Hunt 1997; Auer 2006; Auer and von Rechenberg 2006, Bramlage and Auer 2006).

### Etiology

Flexural limb deformities can be other laxity (hyperextension) or contractural deformities. Laxity tends be seen in premature/dysmature foals that have overall poor muscle tone and increased tendon and periarticular laxity. Full-term foals can be born with tendon laxity, but the exact etiology is unknown.

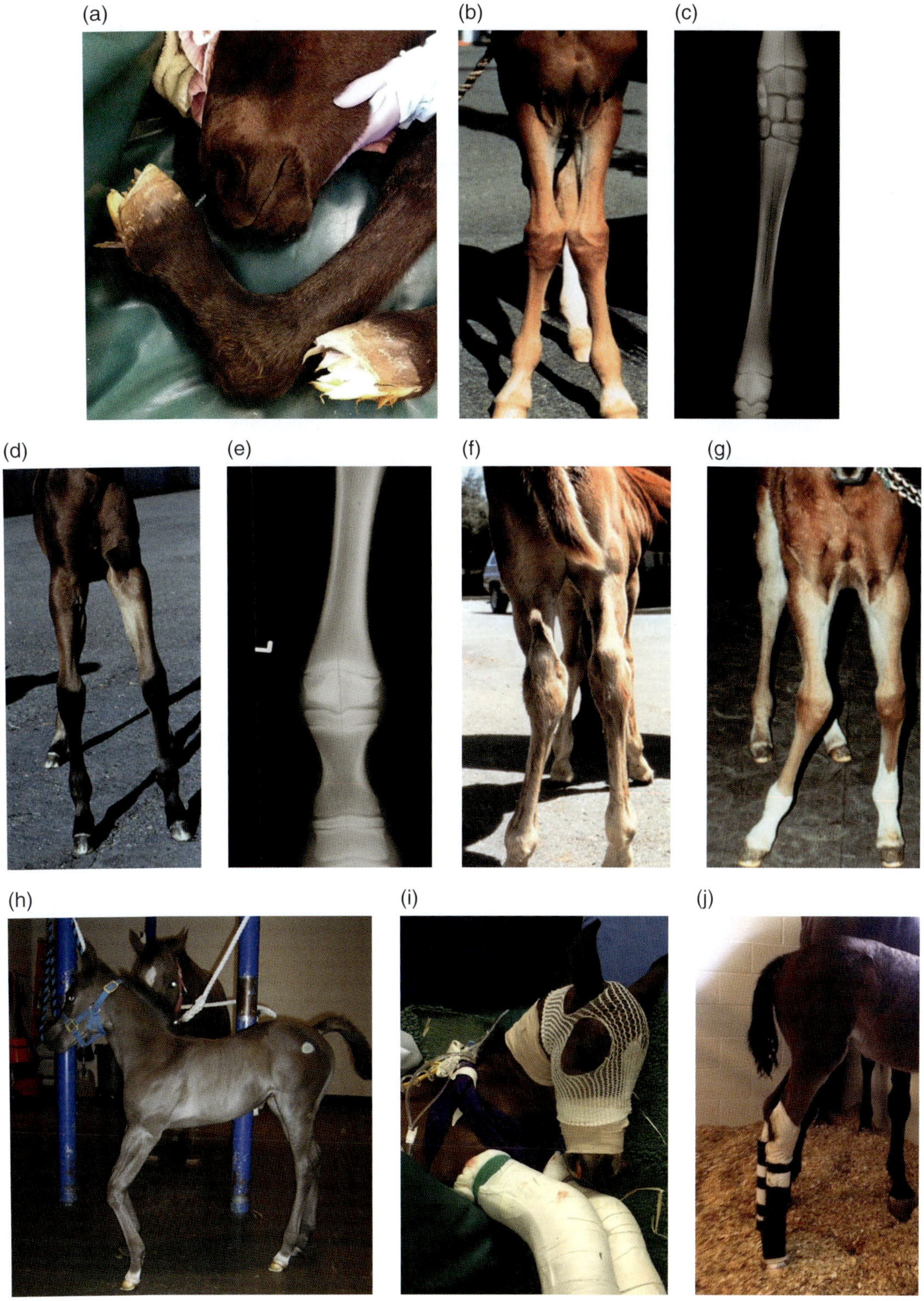


**Figure 20.5** Angular, flexural, and hyperextension limb deformities. (a) Severe hyperextension deformity of the fetlock joint in a neonate. (b,c) Valgus angular limb deformity (ALD) of the carpal joints of young foals. (d,e) Varus angular limb deformity of the fetlock joints of young foals. Windswept angular limb deformity of the tarsal (f) and carpal (g) joints in foals. (h) Moderate flexural (contractural) deformity of the carpal joints in a 1-week-old foal. (i,j) Splints for management of flexural deformities in neonatal foals. *Source:* (h) Courtesy of Dr. Ashlee Watts.

## Clinical Signs

Premature foals with tendon laxity can involve multiple joints. Sometimes the laxity is so severe the foal cannot stand. In normal gestation foals, laxity tends to involve the fetlock joints, which can be in the front or hind limbs or both.

Tendon contracture can be bilateral or unilateral and tends to involve the carpus and fetlock in the front limbs and fetlock in the hind limbs. The presentation of tendon contracture can be mild and able to stand to inability to stand.

Some foals with carpal contracture rupture their common digital extensor tendon which creates swelling on the dorsolateral carpus. Unilateral contracture foals should have a lameness examination as well.

ALD are identified by physical examination and watching the foal move. Hoof wear should be equal and can help identify ALD if the hoof is worn unevenly. Premature foals with ALD typically have periarticular laxity which is confirmed by joint manipulation.

## Diagnosis

Physical examination and manipulation of limbs can help identify laxity, contracture, or ALD.

Lameness evaluation is also important. Radiographs help confirm the diagnosis and provide evidence for the degree of angulation as well as for the identification of incomplete ossification or sepsis (Figure 20.5).

## Emergency Triage Steps

- Laxity
  - Do not splint or bandage as usually it will worsen laxity.
  - Stall confinement and time tend to improve laxity.
  - Small protective wrap over heel bulbs may be needed if laxity is severe.
  - Foals with distal limb laxity may need hoof trimming and heel extensions.
- Contracture
  - Foals with mild-to-moderate contracture may require bandaging, possible splinting, and physiotherapy.
  - Fiberglass cast material or PVC pipe may be used for a splint.
  - Oxytetracycline (44–70 mg/kg IV) diluted in 1 liter of fluids given slowly helps relax tendons.
  - Prior to oxytetracycline administration, check creatinine as oxytetracycline is nephrotoxic.
  - Do not exceed three doses of oxytetracycline administer IV once a day.
  - If no response to oxytetracycline and splinting, consider a cast which should be removed after three to five days.
  - Pain medication is also important; consider acetaminophen at 40 mg/kg orally BID or meloxicam 0.6 mg/kg PO q12–24 h. Butorphanol or buprenorphine can also be used for analgesia. Butorphanol (0.01–0.04 mg/kg IV) Buprenorphine (0.0004–0.01 mg/kg IV or IM).
  - If everything above fails, consider surgery, but the chances of an athletic animal are reduced greatly.
  - Contracture in foals that are rapidly growing may be managed via diet restriction or early weaning.
- Angular Limb Deformity
  - Time.
  - Stall confinement.
  - Proper foot care.
  - Shoes with extension or acrylic hoof extensions can be utilized.
  - Periosteal stripping.
  - Pin or transphyseal bridging for severe deformities.
  - Don't forget fetlock ALD should treated within the first month of life.
- Recumbent foal
  - Development of decubital ulcers.
  - Pressure sores with improper bandaging and splinting.
  - Ensure all underlying tissues are well padded.
  - Splints and bandages should be replaced daily, and limb examined closely for development of sores.

## Septic Arthritis

The typical statement by an owner is "I am sure the foal was stepped on by the mare." Any neonatal foal that becomes acutely lame should have septic arthritis as the top differential unless another cause is identified.

### Etiology

The most common route of septic arthritis in the neonatal foal is via hematogenous spread. Foals that have failure of passive transfer, bacteremia or septicemic have an increased risk of septic arthritis. The common organisms isolated are Gram positive: *Staphylococcus* spp., *Streptococcus* spp., and *Rhodococcus equi*. Gram negative: *Escherichia coli, Actinobacillus equuli, Salmonella* spp., and *Klebsiella* spp. Mixed infections also occur. Anaerobic infection rare but could be caused by Clostridium spp. Blood culture isolates may not be the same as synovial fluid isolates.

### Clinical Signs

- Variable pyrexia.
- Lameness.
- Painful, warm joint effusion.
- Leukocytosis.
- Hyperfibrinogenemia.
- Osteomyelitis seen with fibrinogen >800 mg/dL.

### Diagnosis

Physical examination, lameness evaluation, radiographs, ultrasonography, Arthrocentesis (typically a neutrophilic pleocytosis with increased protein). Typically, synovial fluid leukocyte count >20,000 cells/μL indicates hematogenous acquired septic arthritis, leukocyte count >10,000 cells/μL indicative of infection when combined with clinical signs. Synovial fluid lactate, glucose, and pH are also helpful in evaluating for sepsis. Lactate will increase while glucose and pH will decrease compared to serum/plasma concentrations.

### Emergency Triage Steps

- Systemic broad-spectrum antimicrobials.
- Joint lavage.
- Intraarticular antimicrobials.
- +/− regional limb perfusion.
- +/− arthroscopic surgery.
- If using amikacin for both systemic and intraarticular routes the total dose of amikacin should total and not to exceed 25 mg/kg. Typically, 1/3 dose is delivered via intraarticular or regional limb perfusion routes and 2/3 dose is provided systemically.
- Monitor BUN and Creatinine concentrations with the use of aminoglycosides.
- If more than one joint is affected, prognosis is guarded.

## Maternal Rejection and the Orphan Foal

Rejection of a foal or other circumstances that leave a foal without a dam can be challenging.

Initially orphans are high maintenance due to needing to be fed q2h or more, but this lengthens out as the foal grows (Box 20.5). The most important aspect of an orphan foal is to get colostrum into the foal. Time is of the essence and the colostrum should be administered prior to 12h of age.

## Colostrum

It's good to be prepared for situations when either the mare has poor colostrum, or the foal is orphaned. If possible, it's good to collect good-quality colostrum from a mare that has a foal or one that had a still born foal. Colostrum can be collected and filtered with gauze in a freezer bag or container and frozen for up to two years. Do not microwave colostrum to thaw it as this will damage the antibodies and other proteins!

Colostrum may also be milked from a mare every 2h until 6–12h post parturition. A mare that is nursing a foal can donate 250mL of colostrum after her foal nurses. A single feeding of colostrum is about 450–500mL for a 50kg foal. The foal should have three to four feedings of 500mL of colostrum within the first 8h of life.

## Administration of Colostrum

The colostrum should be warmed in a hot bath of water unless it is obtained right from the mare. The colostrum can be administered via bottle. However, be aware that foals may aspirate, so placement of a nasogastric tube for administration of colostrum may be necessary.

The foal should have the IgG concentrations measured by 12–14h of age. Thus, if inadequate passive transfer of colostral antibodies, the foal can have plasma administered to boost the IgG concentrations.

Substitutes for colostrum are available; however, realistically mare colostrum or plasma are what the foal needs.

## Switching to Solid Feed

Milk-replacer pellets can be offered from the time the foal is one week of age. Slowly work the amount of milk replacer pellets to 2–3lbs a day. Foal creep feed can slowly be introduced at this time, along with hay or pasture when the foal is around a month of age.

Once the foal is eating 4–6lbs of milk replacer or foal creep feed a day, the foal can be weaned off milk. This can happen anywhere from 2 to 4 months of age.

Foals should be turned out with other foals or an older gelding, so they can learn to play and interact with other horses.

### Box 20.5 Feeding the orphan foal

1) Foals drink up to 25% of their body weight. Initially start with 10% of body weight and increase it slowly over the first 10 days of life. A normal foal will drink 15–17 times an hour, then the frequency decreases to 3–4 times an hour. As a guideline, a foal should be fed every 1–2h for the first week of life and then every 4–6h the 2nd week of life. From there, the feeding frequency can decrease, and introduction of milk pellets can be made.
2) Feeding by bucket is easier and faster than bottle feeding. Start by letting foal suckle on a milk – wet finger, then draw him toward the milk bucket. They usually catch on within an hour or two.
3) Once the foal is old enough, milk can be replaced twice a day with the bucket cleaned in between. Foals do well on commercial mare's milk replacers and have growth rates similar to nursing foals.
4) Cow's milk or goat's milk can be used, but neither is ideal. Both goat's and cow's milk are more concentrated than mare's milk, with twice the fat and half the lactose. The protein and mineral content are similar. Cow's milk tends to cause diarrhea, and therefore needs to be diluted, while foals will get impacted with goat's milk. In addition, it's best not to offer calf or lamb milk replacers. The foal should always have freshwater access in the stall along with feed.

## Case Example 20.1 Neonatal Sepsis and Encephalopathy

### Patient: 14-Hour Old Warmblood Colt

History: Born 5 days early, stood within 30 minutes, nursed within 1.5 h, passed meconium. Mare had been dripping milk for 7 days prior to foaling. No colostrum when foal was born. Foal was administered 3 L of plasma prior to presentation. Foal appeared to be nursing well.

By afternoon, mare's udder was full, and the colt wasn't interested in nursing.

At presentation the foal weighed 41 kg. Mucous membranes were pink and tacky, CRT 3 seconds, and sclera were injected. Heart rate was 80 beats/min with no arrhythmias or murmurs noted. Respiratory rate was 24 breaths/min with no abnormal lung sounds or tracheal noise.

Differential Diagnosis: Sepsis and/or neonatal encephalopathy.

Step 1: Patient Stabilization

*Provide immediate stabilization steps (see Chapter 20: Foal Emergencies)*

1) Place over the wire catheter (Figure 20.6a).
2) Supportive care: fluid therapy 90–120 mg/kg/day be careful to not overhydrate!
   a) Glucose support 4 mg/kg/min (can go up to 8 mg/kg/min) using 5% dextrose solution.
3) Obtain blood for PCV/TP, L-Lactate, glucose, blood culture, CBC and biochemistry panel, IgG concentration.
4) Start broad-spectrum antimicrobials.

Perform a focused patient assessment to evaluate

1) Mucous membrane color, petechia or ecchymosis, icterus?
2) Heart rate/respiratory rate/GI borborygmi.
3) Palpation of ribs for fracture.

(a) (b)

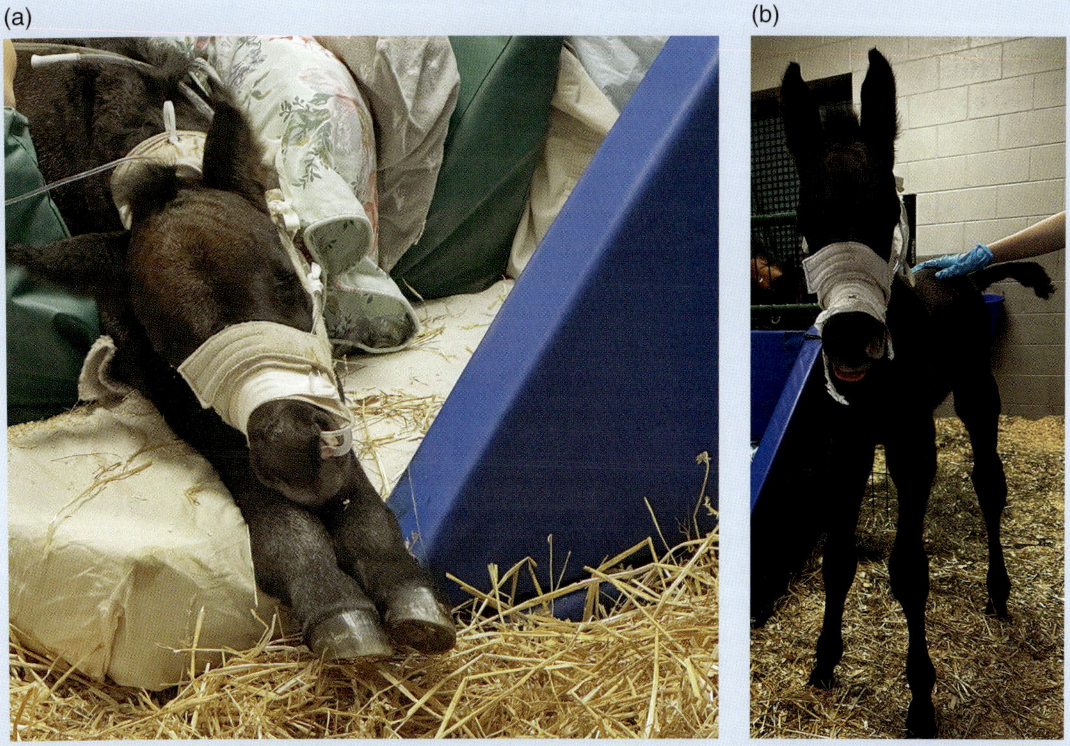

**Figure 20.6** (a) 14-h premature warmblood colt with sepsis and neonatal encephalopathy. An over-the-wire catheter was placed to provide supportive care including IV fluids with dextrose, broad-spectrum antibiotics, and plasma. Enteral feeding with the mare's milk was performed initially via nasogastric tube. (b) The foal responded well to treatment and within 48 h was strong and nursing well.

4) Palpation of joints.
5) Umbilical palpation.
6) Testicles descended.
   - A foal should be considered septic until proven otherwise.
   - Does foal need oxygen support?
   - Can foal be managed on the farm?

The foal was found to still have a low IgG, hyperlactatemia, hypoglycemia, and a leukopenia with a neutropenia and band neutrophils.

Step 2: Formulating a Diagnostic Plan

*Once the foal is stabilized, further evaluation can be performed on the foal utilizing radiographic equipment and ultrasound, and further diagnostic testing*

1) Ultrasound umbilicus.
2) Ultrasound abdomen and thorax.
3) Radiograph carpus and tarsus.
4) Fecal sample for foal diarrhea panel – suspect clostridial infection of bloody diarrhea.
5) IgG immunoglobulin testing for complete passive transfer of colostral antibodies.
6) Blood culture submitted.
7) Treat the foal as if septic.
   a) Broad-spectrum antimicrobials.
   b) Plasma transfusion.
   c) Retest IgG.
   d) Intravenous fluid therapy with dextrose.
   e) Blood pressure monitoring.
   f) Nasogastric tube for small amount of enteral feeding – 10% of body weight.
8) Assessment of glucose, L-Lactate, PCV, and total protein should be performed q4 h.
9) Physical examination assessment – watch for any changes in physical examination parameters.
10) Strongly consider referral as this case is going to be very labor intensive.

The foal had a blood culture obtained and was started on broad-spectrum antimicrobials (ampicillin and amikacin). This foal had a normal umbilicus and normal palpation of joints. He was treated with antimicrobials, plasma, IV fluid therapy, dextrose at 4 mg/kg/min and fed 10% of his body weight of mare's milk via nasogastric tube for the first 24 h. After which the foal started to improve and was nursing well after 48 h of care (Figure 20.6b).

His blood culture came back positive for *E. coli and Klebsiella* sp. The foal was sent home after seven days of hospitalization. The owner was told to make sure to watch for lameness or swelling of joints, umbilical swelling/drainage, and or fever.

## References

Adams, R. (1990). Noninfectious orthopedic problems. In: *Equine Clinical Neonatology* (ed. A.M. Koterba, W.H. Drummond, and P.C. Kosch), 333–366. Philadelphia: Lea and Febiger.

Auer, J.A. (2006). Diagnosis and treatment of flexural deformities in foals. *Clin. Tech. Equine Pract.* 5: 282–295.

Auer, J.A. and von Rechenberg, B. (2006). Treatment of angular limb deformities in foals. *Clin. Tech. Equine Pract.* 5: 270–281.

Axon, J.E. (2006). Assessment of the critically ill neonate. *Proc. 28th Bain Fallon Memorial Lect.* Coffs Harbor 28: 97–110.

Axon, J.E., Russel, C.M., and Wilkins, P.A. (2015). Neonatology. In: *Equine Emergency and Critical Care* (ed. L.L. Southwood and P.A. Wilkins), 551–554. Boca Raton, FL: CR Press, Taylor and Francis Group.

Bailey, E., Conboy, H.S., and McCarthy, P.F. (1987). Neonatal isoerythrolysis of foals: an update on testing. *Proc. 3rd Ann. Conven. Am. Assoc. Equine Pract.* 33: 341–355.

Bain, F.T. (2004). Management of the foal from the mare with placentitis: a clinician's approach. *Proc. 50th Ann. Convene Am. Assoc. Equine Pract.* 50: 162–164.

Borchers, A., Wilkins, P.A., Marsh, P.M. et al. (2012). Admission L-lactate concentration in hospitalized equine neonates: a prospective multicenter study. *Equine Vet. J.* 41: 57–63.

Bramlage, L.R. and Auer, J.A. (2006). Diagnosis, assessment and treatment strategies for angular limb deformities in the foal. *Clin. Tech. Equine Pract.* 5: 259–269.

Chaney, K.P., Holcombe, S.J., Schott, H.C. 2nd et al. (2010). Spurious hypercreatininemia: 28 neonatal foals (2000–2008). *J. Vet. Emerg. Crit. Care* 20: 244–249.

Chavatte, P., Clement, F., Cash, R. et al. (1998). Field determination of colostrum quality by using a novel, practical method. *Proc. 44th Am. Assoc. Equine Pract.* 44: 206–209.

Clothier, J., Small, A., Hinch, G., and Brown, W.Y. (2020). Prematurity and dysmaturity are associated with reduced height and shorter distal limb length in horses. *J. Equine Vet. Sci.* 91: 103129. https://doi.org/10.1016/j.jevs.202J0.103129. Epub 2020 May 22. PMID: 32684267.

Corley, K.T.T. and Hollis, A.R. (2009). Antimicrobial therapy in neonatal foals. *Equine Vet. Educ.* 21: 436–448. https://doi.org/10.2746/095777309X445352.

Delvescovo, B., Mullen, K.R., Eicker, S.W. et al. (2021). The effect of neonatal dysphagia on subsequent racing performance in Standardbred horses. *Equine Vet. J.* 53 (3): 481–487. https://doi.org/10.1111/evj.13326. Epub 2020 Sep 6. PMID: 32725699; PMCID: PMC9511700.

Divers, T.J. (2003). Liver failure and hemolytic anemia. In: *Manual of Equine Emergencies*, 2e (ed. J.A. Orsini and T.J. Divers), 315–338. Philadelphia: Saunders.

Dunkel, B., Palmer, J.E., Olson, K.N. et al. (2005). Uroperitoneum in 32 foals: influence of intravenous fluid therapy, infection, and sepsis. *J. Vet. Intern. Med.* 19: 889–893.

Eaton, S. (2023). Neonatal sepsis – pathology and clinical signs. *Equine Vet. Educ.* 35: 498–503. https://doi.org/10.1111/eve.13796.

Fischer, A.T. and Yarbrough, T.Y. (1995). Retrograde contrast radiography of the distal portions of the intestinal tract in foals. *J. Am. Vet. Med. Assoc.* 207: 734–737.

Giguère, S., Sanchez, L.C., Shih, A. et al. (2007). Comparison of the effects of caffeine and doxapram on respiratory and cardiovascular function in foals with induced respiratory acidosis. *Am. J. Vet. Res.* 12: 1407–1416.

Giguère, S., Slade, J.K., and Sanchez, L.C. (2008). Retrospective comparison of caffeine and doxapram for the treatment of hypercapnia in foals with hypoxic-ischemic encephalopathy. *J. Vet. Intern. Med.* 22 (2): 401–405. https://doi.org/10.1111/j.1939-1676.2008.0064.x. PMID: 18371030.

Gold, J.R. and Wong, D.M. (2024). Neonatal Encephalopathy. In: *Equine Neonatal Medicine* (ed. D.M. Wong and P.A. Wilkins), 895–914. Florida: Wiley Blackwell.

Hackett, E.S. and McCue, P.M. (2010). Evaluation of a veterinary glucometer for use in horses. *J. Vet. Intern. Med.* 24: 617–621.

Henderson, I.S.F., Franklin, R.P., Boston, R.C. et al. (2007). Association of hyperlactatemia with age, diagnosis and survival in equine neonates. *Proc. Am. Assoc. Equine Pract.* 53: 354–355.

Holcoombe, S.J., Hurcombe, S.D., Barr, B.S., and Schott, H.C. II (2012). Dysphagia associated with presumed pharyngeal dysfunction in 16 neonatal foals. *Equine Vet. J.* 44: 105–108. https://doi.org/10.1111/j.2042-3306.2011.00451.x.

Hollis, A.R., Wilkins, P.A., Palmer, J.E. et al. (2008). Bacteremia in equine neonatal diarrhea: a retrospective study (1990–2007). *J. Vet. Intern. Med.* 22: 1203–1209.

Hollis, A., Wilkins, P.A., Tennent Brown, B. et al. (2010). The effect of intravenous plasma administration on fibrinogen concentration in sick neonatal foals. *J. Vet. Intern. Med.* 24: 786. (abstract).

Hunt, R.J. (1997). Noninfectious musculoskeletal disorders of foals. In: *Current Therapy in Equine Medicine*, 5e (ed. N.E. Robinson), 623–627. St Louis: Saunders.

Jeffcott, L.B., Rossdale, P.D., and Leadon, D.P. (1982). Haematological changes in the neonatal period of normal and induced premature foals. *J. Reprod. Fertil. Suppl.* 32: 537–544.

Kablack, K.A., Embertson, R.M., Bernard, W.V. et al. (2000). Uroperitoneum in the hospitalized equine neonate: retrospective study of 31 cases, 1988–1997. *Equine Vet. J.* 32: 505–508.

Kosch, P.C., Koterba, A.M., Coons, T.J. et al. (1984). Developments in management of the newborn foal in respiratory distress. 1: evaluation. *Equine Vet. J.* 16: 312–318.

MacKinnon, M.C., Southwood, L.L., Burke, M.J., and Palmer, J.E. (2013). Colic in equine neonates: 137 case (2000–2010). *J. Am. Vet. Med. Assoc.* 243 (11): 1586–1595.

Magdesian, K.G. (2004). Monitoring the critically ill equine neonate. *Vet. Clin. N. Am. Equine Pract.* 20: 11–39.

Magdesian, K.G. (2005). Neonatal foal diarrhea. *Vet. Clin. N. Am. Equine Pract.* 21: 295–312.

Magdesian, K.G. (2010). Update on fluid therapy in horses. *Proc Central Veterinary Conference*, 28–31 August, Kansas.

Magdesian, K.G. (2014). Neonatology. In: *Equine Emergencies* (ed. J.A. Orsini and T.J. Divers), 527–564. St. Louis, MI: Elsevier.

Magdesian, K.G. (2017). Antimicrobial pharmacology for the neonatal foal. *Vet. Clin. North Am. Equine Pract.* 33 (1): 47–65. https://doi.org/10.1016/j.cveq.2016.12.004. PMID: 28325182.

Magdesian, K.G. and Madigan, J.E. (2003). Volume replacement in the neonatal ICU: crystalloids and colloids. *Clin. Tech. Equine Pract.* 2: 20–30.

McClure, J. (1997). Strategies for prevention of neonatal isoerythrolysis in horses and mules. *Equine Vet. Educ.* 9: 118–122.

McDonald, P.G., Green, M.A., Vaala, W.E. et al. (1990). Nursing care of the neonatal foal. In: *Equine Clinical Neonatalogy* (ed. A.M. Koterba, W.H. Drummond, and P.C. Kosch), 625–652. Philadelphia: Lea and Febiger.

McKenzie, H.C. (2018). Disorders of foals. In: *Equine Internal Medicine*, 2e (ed. S.M. Reed, W.M. Bayly, and D.C. Sellon), 1365–1438. St Louis, MI: Elsevier.

Ousey, J.C., Kölling, M., Kindahl, H. et al. (2011). Maternal dexamethasone treatment in late gestation induces precocious fetal maturation and delivery in healthy Thoroughbred mares. *Equine Vet. J.* 43: 424–429.

Palmer, J.E. (2002). When fluids are not enough – ionopressor therapy. *8th International Emergency and Critical Care Symposium*, 4–8 September, San Antonio, pp 669–673.

Palmer, J.E. (2005a). Neonatal diseases in foals. In: *In: Proc of a workshop on: Uterine Infection in Mares and Women: a Comparative Study II*, Havemeyer Foundation Monograph Series, No. 19, 9–13 November (ed. M.M. LeBlanc, J.F. Wade, and L. Foster). South Carolina. https://www.cabidigitallibrary.org/doi/pdf/10.5555/20083120993.

Palmer, J.E. (2005b). Ventilatory support of the critically ill foal. *Vet. Clin. N. Am. Equine Pract.* 21: 457–486.

Palmisano, M., Javsicas, L., McNaughten, J. et al. (2023). Effect of plasma transfusion on serum amyloid A concentration in healthy neonatal foals and foals with failure of transfer of passive immunity. *J. Vet. Intern. Med.* 37 (2): 697–702. https://doi.org/10.1111/jvim.16647. Epub Feb 24. PMID: 36825688; PMCID: PMC10061169.

Papazian, L., Albanese, J., Thirion, X. et al. (1993). Effect of bolus doses of midazolam on intracranial pressure and cerebral perfusion pressure in patients with severe head injury. *Br. J. Anaesth.* 71: 267–271.

Polkes, A.C., Giguère, S., Lester, G.D. et al. (2008). Factors associated with outcome in foals with neonatal isoerythrolysis (72 cases, 1988–2003). *J. Vet. Intern. Med.* 5: 1216–1222.

Pusterla, N., Magdesian, K.G., Maleski, K. et al. (2004). Retrospective evaluation of the use of acetylcysteine enemas in the treatment of meconium retention in foals: 44 cases (1987–2002). *Equine Vet. Educ.* 16: 133–136.

Rossdale, P.D. (2004). The maladjusted foal. *Proc. 50th Ann. Conven. Am. Assoc. Equine Pract.* 50: 75–126.

Russell, C., Palmer, J.E., Boston, R.C. et al. (2007). Agreement between point-of care glucometry, blood gas and laboratory-based measurement of glucose in an equine neonatal intensive care unit. *J. Vet. Emerg. Crit. Care* 17: 236–242.

Russell, C.M., Axon, J.E., Blishen, A. et al. (2008). Blood culture isolates and antimicrobial sensitivities from 427 critically ill neonatal foals. *Aust. Vet. J.* 86: 266–271.

Sanchez, L.C. (2005a). Equine neonatal sepsis. *Vet. Clin. N. Am. Equine Pract.* 21: 273–293.

Sanchez, C. (2005b). Non-diarrheal disorders of the gastrointestinal tract in neonatal foals. *Vet. Clin. N. Am. Equine Pract.* 21: 313–332.

Scalco, R., de Oliveira, G.N., da Rosa, C.B. et al. (2023). Red blood cell distribution width to platelet ratio in neonatal foals with sepsis. *J. Vet. Intern. Med.* 37 (4): 1552–1560. https://doi.org/10.1111/jvim.16793. Epub 2023 Jun 12. PMID: 37306395; PMCID: PMC10365058.

Sellon, D.C. and Wilkins, P.A. (2010). Neonatal isoerythrolysis. In: *Equine Internal Medicine*, 3rde (ed. S.M. Reed, W.M. Bayly, and D.C. Sellon), 1336–1337. St. Louis: Saunders.

Sievert, S., Schuler, G., Büttner, K., and Wehrend, A. (2022). Comparison of different methods to determine the absorption of colostral IgG in newborn foals. *J. Equine Vet. Sci.* 114: 104008.

Spurlock, S.L. and Furr, M. (1990). Nursing care of the neonatal foal. In: *Equine Clinical Neonatology* (ed. A.M. Koterba, W.H. Drummond, and P.C. Kosch), 671–685. Philadelphia: Lea and Febiger.

Taylor, S. (2015). A review of equine sepsis. *Equine Vet. Educ.* 27 (2): 99–109. https://doi.org/10.1111/eve.12290. Epub 2015 Jan 14. PMID: 32313390; PMCID: PMC7163761.

Toribio, R.E. (2019 Aug). Equine neonatal encephalopathy: facts, evidence, and opinions. *Vet. Clin. North Am. Equine Pract.* 35 (2): 363–378. https://doi.org/10.1016/j.cveq.2019.03.004. Epub 2019 May 11. PMID: 31088699.

Vaala, W.E. (1990). Neonatal anemia. In: *Equine Clinical Neonatology* (ed. A.M. Koterba, W.H. Drummond, and P.C. Kosch), 571–588. Philadelphia: Lea and Febiger.

Vaala, W.E. (1994). Peripartum asphyxia. *Vet. Clin. N. Am. Equine Pract.* 10: 187–218.

Vander Werf, K.A., Beard, L.A., and McMurphy, R.M. (2010). Urinothorax in a quarter horse filly. *Equine Vet. Educ.* 22: 239–243.

Wilkins, P.A. (2003). Lower respiratory problems of the neonate. *Vet. Clin. N. Am. Equine Pract.* 19: 19–33.

Wilkins, P.A. (2004). Respiratory distress in foals with uroperitoneum: possible mechanisms. *Equine Vet. Educ.* 16: 377–380.

Wilkins PA (2005) How to use midazolam to control equine neonatal seizures. *Proceedings of the 51st Annual Convention of the American Association of Equine Practitioners, Seattle, Washington, USA*, pp.279–280.

Wilkins, P.A. (2010a). Perinatal asphyxia syndrome. In: *Equine Internal Medicine*, 3e (ed. S.M. Reed, W.M. Bayly, and D.C. Sellon), 1324–1328. St. Louis: Saunders.

Wilkins, P.A. (2010b). Persistent pulmonary hypertension. In: *Equine Internal Medicine*, 3e (ed. S.M. Reed, W.M. Bayly, and D.C. Sellon), 1319–1320. St. Louis: Saunders.

Wilkins, P.A., Otto, C.M., Dunkel, B. et al. (2007). Acute lung injury (ALI) and acute respiratory distress syndromes (ARDS) in veterinary medicine: consensus definitions. Special commentary. *J. Vet. Emerg. Crit. Care* 17: 333–339.

Wong, D. (2020). Neonatal encephalopathy. In: *Large Animal Internal Medicine* (ed. B.P. Smith, D.C. Van Metre, and N. Pusterla), 281–288. St Louis, MI: Elsevier.

Wong, D.M., Alcott, C.H., Wang, C. et al. (2010). Physiologic effects of nasopharyngeal administration of supplemental oxygen at various flow rates in healthy neonatal foals. *Am. J. Vet. Res.* 9: 1081–1088.

Wong, D.M., Ruby, R.E., Dembek, K.A. et al. (2018). Evaluation of updated sepsis scoring systems and systemic inflammatory response syndrome criteria and their association with sepsis in equine neonates. *J. Vet. Intern. Med.* 32 (3): 1185–1193. https://doi.org/10.1111/jvim.15087. Epub 2018 Mar 26. PMID: 29582480; PMCID: PMC5980351.

Wotman, K., Palmer, J.E., Boston, R.C. et al. (2005). Lactate concentration in foals presenting to a neonatal intensive care unit: association with outcome. American College Veterinary Internal Medicine Scientific Forum. *J. Vet. Intern. Med.* 19: 409.

# 21

# Hepatic and Metabolic Emergencies

*Joy E. Tomlinson*[1] *and Thomas J. Divers*[2]

[1] *Department of Clinical Studies - New Bolton Center, University of Pennsylvania School of Veterinary Medicine, Kennett Square, PA, USA*
[2] *Department of Clinical Sciences, College of Veterinary Medicine, Cornell University, Ithaca, NY, USA*

## Clinical Signs of Liver Disease

Liver disease is common in both adult horses and foals, and clinical signs vary and may affect several body systems. The clinical signs of liver disease in the horse are summarized in Box 21.1.

**Box 21.1 Clinical signs of liver disease in the horse**

- Dullness and inappetence.
- Icterus (Figure 21.1a).
- Photosensitization (Figure 21.1b). Sunburned appearance to white markings.
- Neurologic signs: These are mostly cortical signs of hepatic encephalopathy.
  - Early subtle behavior changes are often missed or can be episodic
  - Playing in the water bucket
  - Yawning
  - Ptyalism
  - Pacing or circling
  - Head pressing (Figure 21.1c)
  - Episodic aggression or violent behavior
  - Responses to stimuli can be exaggerated or reduced
  - Cortical blindness (negative menace, positive pupillary light response)
  - Somnolence, stupor, seizures
  - Ataxia can occur with or without obvious cortical signs
  - Recumbency and coma in the terminal stage
- Discolored urine (Figure 21.1d). Urine can be a dark orange color due to bilirubinuria, which indicates increased conjugated (direct) bilirubin.
- Weight loss. Can indicate chronic disease.
- Respiratory distress due to bilateral laryngeal paralysis - a rare neurologic manifestation.
- Ventral edema – subjectively more common in hyperlipemia.
- Colic. Can be due to gastric impaction, obstructive cholelithiasis, or swelling of the liver and tension on the liver capsule, e.g., with severe hepatic lipidosis.

*Emergency Triage of the Horse*, First Edition. Edited by Rolfe M. Radcliffe and Jamie J. Kopper.

Companion website: www.wiley.com/go/radcliffe/triage

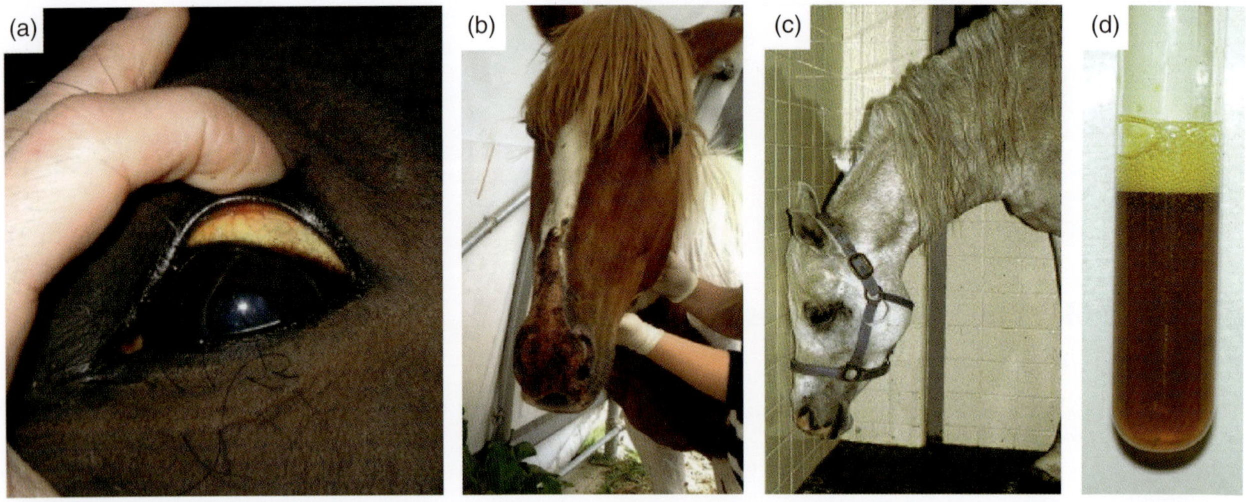


**Figure 21.1** Clinical signs of hepatitis. (a) Icterus of the sclera. (b) Photosensitization of the white markings on the face. (c) Horse with hepatic encephalopathy showing head-pressing behavior. (d) Bilirubinuria with characteristic green-orange foam that builds when the urine is shaken.

## Triage of Neurologic Emergency

Differential diagnoses and triage approach for neurologic emergencies are covered in Chapter 15. If signs are neurolocalized to the forebrain and other signs attributable to hepatic disease are present, hepatic encephalopathy should be considered as a differential diagnosis. Some affected horses may also have ataxia. However, some cases of liver failure are peracute, and there might not be other evidence of hepatitis on clinical examination. Serum biochemistry with liver panel and ammonia is best to confirm the diagnosis, but results are often not immediately available, unless the horse is referred to a hospital with in-house laboratory equipment. Hepatic encephalopathy can occur without blood ammonia being above the normal reference range. Encephalopathy with icterus or bilirubinuria should be presumptively treated for hepatic encephalopathy (see section below) until diagnostics are completed.

Referral should be offered for horses with suspected hepatic encephalopathy or primary hyperammonemia. Horses with hepatic encephalopathy are often difficult to control and can worsen rapidly, endangering the patient and the attending people. Many treatments require intravenous infusions and/or are not stocked by most ambulatory practitioners.

## Triage of Colic Emergency

Differential diagnoses and approach for colic are covered in Chapter 10. If colic is accompanied by fever and icterus, cholangiohepatitis with obstructive cholelithiasis should be considered. Sonography of the liver may be diagnostic. Complete blood count and serum biochemistry can aid in the diagnosis. Emergency referral decision is the same as for most causes of colic. If acute, intractable pain is present, referral is indicated for possible surgical treatment. If colic is less severe, but cholelithiasis is diagnosed, optimal treatment may be achieved with hospitalization and intravenous fluids and medications; however, there is more opportunity to attempt treatment in the field, and this will be a case-by-case discussion depending on severity of disease, owner finances and capabilities, and the veterinarian's availability for daily visits.

## Diagnostic Tests for Liver Disease

Liver disease is diagnosed by serum biochemistry. Standard chemistry panels typically include AST and GGT, which can indicate hepatitis but do not give information regarding liver function. Therefore, specific liver panels are recommended if liver failure is suspected. Urine dipstick can be used in the field to check for bilirubinuria, which may confirm liver failure. However, lack of bilirubinuria does not rule out liver failure, and a small number of horses may have a positive bilirubin test on urine without having liver failure. Recommended tests to determine the cause of hepatitis and the prognosis can include review of patient history and diet, complete blood count with fibrinogen and/or SAA, hepatitis virus PCR, liver ultrasonography, liver biopsy, and gastroduodenoscopy. Liver biopsy is rarely needed on an emergency basis.

## Patient History

- Treatment with equine origin biologic products within the previous 4–12 weeks – increases risk of Theiler's disease.
- Other horses on the farm with hepatitis – suggests exposure to toxin or Equine parvovirus-hepatitis.
- The diet and pasture should be examined for potentially toxic chemicals, pyrrolizidine alkaloid containing plants, alsike clover, fall panicum or Klein grass, moldy feeds, or high water iron content. Ingredients in supplements should be carefully reviewed. Local agricultural extension agents can assist in identifying other less common hepatotoxic plants.
- Recent illness, stressor (e.g., severe weather, herd changes), reduced feed intake, or poor-quality feed, especially in ponies, miniature horses, donkeys, or adult horses with pars pituitary intermediate dysfunction (PPID). These could be triggers for hyperlipemia.
- History of colic, gastrointestinal disease, or fevers. Recurrent low-grade colic and/or inappetence could fit with intermittent biliary obstruction and cholangiohepatitis/cholelithiasis.
- Weight loss, or recently becoming difficult to maintain weight, indicates possible chronic underlying disease, even if clinical presentation otherwise appears acute onset.
- Skin conditions that look like sunburn on white areas, or scratches on the white legs could indicate photosensitization.

## Serum Biochemistry

It is important to choose a panel that includes liver-specific markers including serum bile acids (SBA), direct bilirubin, and triglycerides (TG) (Box 21.2). Many of the standard serum biochemical panels at major commercial laboratories include markers which are not liver-specific in horses and should not be over-interpreted.

### Box 21.2 Serum biochemistry testing in horses with suspect liver disease

#### Hepatocellular enzymes

- AST: liver, muscle, red blood cells. Evaluate in relation to CK (muscle) and other liver enzymes.
- SDH, GLDH: labile, liver specific.
- ALT, LDH: not liver specific in horses.
- Hepatocellular enzymes fall during chronic disease and might not reflect severity of underlying pathology.

#### Cholestatic or induction enzymes

- GGT: liver specific. Biliary remodeling is a consistent response to liver injury. GGT will rise with hepatocellular diseases too. Remains elevated in chronic disease.
- ALP: not liver specific in horses.

#### Functional markers

- Bilirubin
  - Indirect (unconjugated) bilirubin: can be elevated with anorexia, hemolysis, hepatitis, or rarely due to congenital defects in conjugation.
  - Direct (conjugated) bilirubin: elevated due to cholestasis.
  - In primary cholestatic disease, direct bilirubin typically > 25% of total bilirubin.
- Serum bile acids
  - Best test of liver function.
  - Increased due to portosystemic shunt (rare), liver failure, or cholestasis.
  - Elevated bile acids >20 μmol/L indicates poor prognosis with ~50% survival in horses with chronic liver disease. However, some etiologies that cause acute or subacute liver disease are reversible and carry a better prognosis.
  - The degree of elevation of bile acids above 20 μmol/L does not reflect worse prognosis. Degree of elevation of direct bilirubin in horses with high bile acids reflects worse prognosis.
- Triglycerides
  - Hyperlipidemia: increase <500 mg/dL.
  - Hyperlipemia: >500 mg/dL. Serum and plasma are also grossly lipemic.
- Ammonia
  - Marker of hepatic encephalopathy. Degree of elevation does not correlate with severity of signs. Hyperammonemia without liver disease can occur in some horses with intestinal disease.

– *Requires special handling.* Blood should be collected into EDTA or heparin tubes, separated immediately, and the plasma should be frozen. See lab instructions for shipping and labeling. It is often recommended to send a control sample from a normal horse collected and processed the same way to ensure there is not false increase in ammonia from handling.
- Globulins: often increased
- Blood urea nitrogen (BUN): reduced in liver failure
- Albumin: reduced in end-stage liver failure
- Lactate: increased in failure. Lactate is normally metabolized and cleared by the liver.

### Urine Dipstick

- Bilirubinuria: indicates increased direct bilirubin and hepatitis.
- Occult blood: suggests icterus likely caused by hemolysis instead of hepatitis.

### Complete Blood Count and Fibrinogen or Serum Amyloid A (SAA)

Complete blood count and fibrinogen or SAA are indicated to look for evidence of bacterial infection or concurrent disease.

- Hct or PCV: Can remain increased (polycythemia) even after fluid resuscitation. In terminal liver failure, RBC membrane fragility increases and hemolysis can sometimes be observed.
- Hgb, Serum iron, and % saturation: can also be elevated due to polycythemia.
- Leukogram: can be inflammatory if bacterial cholangiohepatitis or concurrent disease. Can show evidence of endotoxemia associated with gut translocation and reduced filtering function of the liver.
- Fibrinogen: can be increased if underlying inflammatory disease, or reduced in liver failure due to lack of production.

### Coagulation Panel

Coagulation panel is not often required during emergency triage.

- PT, PTT: can be increased due to lack of production of clotting factors.

### Viral PCR and In Situ Hybridization (ISH)

- Serum, EDTA plasma, or liver samples are acceptable.
- Equine parvovirus-hepatitis (EqPV-H) PCR: for cases of acute hepatitis/suspect Theiler's disease.
  - Many clinically normal horses are infected; therefore, test results must be interpreted cautiously.
  - Low Ct value indicates high viral load, consistent with parvoviral hepatitis.
  - High Ct value could be an incidental finding.
  - Serial testing showing a rise in Ct as hepatitis improves is a strong indication that EqPV-H caused the hepatitis.
- Equine parvovirus-hepatitis ISH: ISH labels viral nucleic acids in tissue samples and can be useful to distinguish incidental EqPV-H infection versus EqPV-H hepatitis.
- Equine hepacivirus PCR: for cases of chronic hepatitis, which could have acute onset of clinical signs.
  - Many clinically normal horses are infected; therefore, test results must be interpreted cautiously.
  - Serial testing showing chronic infection (>six months) in combination with consistent histopathologic findings and ruling out other causes is required to make a presumptive diagnosis of hepaciviral hepatitis.

### Ultrasonography

- Liver should be visualized on the right side, approximately from the 7th to 16th intercostal spaces, and on the left side in the 6th–9th intercostal spaces. It should be hypoechoic to the spleen and have sharp margins.
- Even in severe disease, the liver can appear normal.
- Hyperechogenicity can be consistent with fibrosis or lipidosis.
- Hypoechogenicity can indicate hepatic necrosis.
- Heteroechogenicity or nodular appearance can indicate infection, fibrosis, or neoplasia.
- Cholangiohepatitis and cholelithiasis can be indicated by distended bile ducts, echoic bile "sludge," and acoustic shadows in bile ducts indicate cholelithiasis (Figure 21.2).

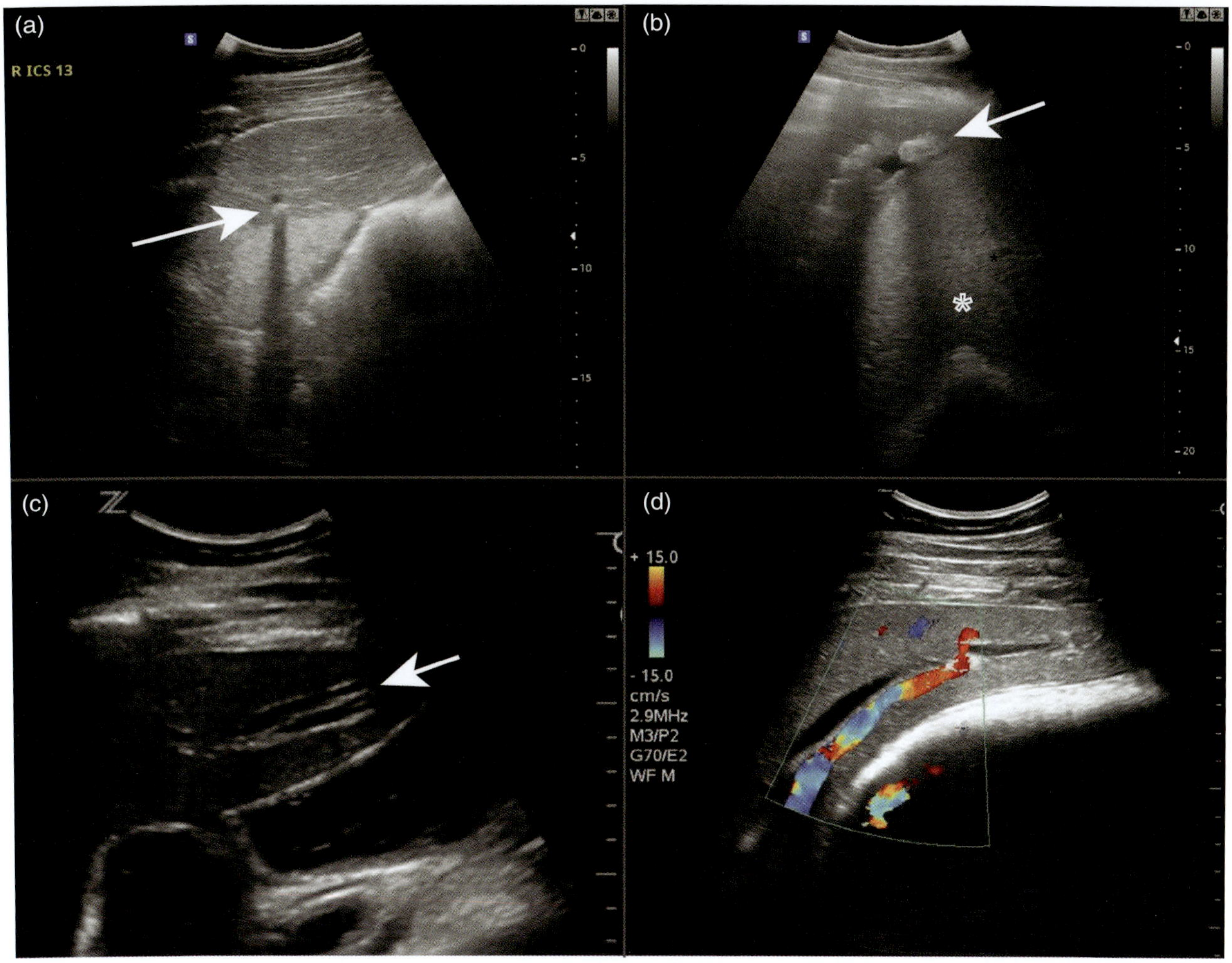


**Figure 21.2** Example images of horses with cholelithiasis. Characteristic findings include observation of choleliths and bile duct distention. (a) Small echoic shadowing cholelith in the right 13th intercostal space (ICS; arrow). (b) Hyperechoic cholelith with minimal shadowing (arrow) in the left cranial abdomen. Note the liver remains hypoechoic to the spleen (*). (c) Parallel ducts indicate a dilated bile duct adjacent to a blood vessel (arrow). (d) Color doppler imaging can be used to confirm flow in vessels and lack of flow in bile ducts.

### Biopsy

- Biopsy is rarely indicated for emergency triage, but it can aid in diagnosis and prognosis.
- In chronic disease, the liver remodels in similar ways in response to multiple underlying causes, and the inciting cause might not be identifiable.
- Samples should be submitted for aerobic and anaerobic culture.
- Liver fibrosis can be indicative of prognosis if graded; however, most histopathology reports include a subjective description without a formalized score or grade. Practitioners are cautioned not to over-interpret any degree of fibrosis to indicate a poor prognosis, and to speak with the pathologist if there is need for clarification on severity and prognosis.

### Gastroduodenoscopy

- If cholelithiasis is suspected or diagnosed sonographically, and the horse presents with colic, duodenoscopy can be performed to examine the duodenal papilla for the presence of an obstructive cholelith, which would require surgical removal.

## Causes of Liver Failure in Horses

Table 21.1 summarizes classic findings with different causes of equine hepatitis. More detailed descriptions of the most common etiologies are below, with treatment and diagnostic plans. Emergency triage steps and patient stabilization guidelines for liver failure are listed in Box 21.3. Recommendations for what can be done on the farm versus in the hospital are presented in Box 21.4.

**Table 21.1** Differential diagnoses for liver failure and characteristic findings. Biochemical values indicated are typical findings for each disease but can vary.

| Disorder | Etiology | Signalment, history | Clinical signs | Biochemical findings |
|---|---|---|---|---|
| Parvoviral hepatitis, aka Theiler's disease | Equine parvovirus-hepatitis | Adult horses<br>Summer to fall, or 4–10 weeks after equine biologic product administration | Encephalopathy common<br>+/− icterus<br>+/− colic<br>Can be found dead | ↑↑↑ hepatocellular (AST >1,000 IU/L)<br>↑ GGT (~100–300 IU/L)<br>Dbili <20% Tbili<br>↑ PT, PTT, SBA<br>+/− ↑ $NH_3$, ↓ blood glucose |
| Hepaciviral hepatitis | Equine hepacivirus | Adult horses | Weight loss, dull, inappetant<br>+/− encephalopathy, icterus | ↑ hepatocellular<br>↑↑↑ GGT (>300 U/L), SBA |
| Chronic active hepatitis | Unknown, suspect immune disorder | Adult horses | Icterus, weight loss, +/− colic, encephalopathy | Variable |
| Cholangiohepatitis/ cholelithiasis | Ascending bacterial infection | Choleliths are more common in middle-aged-to-older horses with cholangiohepatitis<br>+/− history of recent GI disease | Icterus, fever<br>+/− colic, anorexia<br>+/− weight loss | ↑ hepatocellular (AST <1,000 IU/L)<br>↑↑↑ GGT (>300 IU/L), SBA<br>Dbili >20% Tbili<br>Normal PT, PTT, $NH_3$<br>Inflammatory leukogram |
| Hyperlipemia/hepatic lipidosis | Negative energy balance. Conditions that increase energy demand such as concurrent illness, pregnancy, lactation, severe diet | Adult ponies, miniature horses, donkeys, and occasionally horses with PPID.<br>Less commonly late-term pregnant and azotemic mares.<br>Miniature horse foals. | Anorexia<br>Depression<br>Diarrhea<br>Ventral edema | ↑↑ TG +/− lipemic serum<br>Variable ↑ AST > ↑ GGT<br>Often azotemia |
| Pyrrolizidine alkaloid (PA) toxicosis | PA toxins containing plants in the western US. *Crotalaria* (rattlebox) grows in southeastern US but is rarely consumed by horses. | Adult horses in western United States | Hepatic encephalopathy<br>Icterus mild-moderate<br>+/− photosensitization | ↑-↑↑ AST<br>↑↑ GGT<br>↑ SBA, poor prognosis if SBA > 50 μmol/L |
| Tyzzer's disease | *Clostridium piliforme* | 8–42 day old foals<br>Usually single foal affected | Depression, anorexia<br>Hyper- or hypo-thermia<br>Icterus<br>Seizures<br>Diarrhea<br>Death | ↑↑ AST, SDH, bilirubin<br>↓ blood glucose<br>Severe metabolic acidosis |
| Aflatoxicosis | Rare | | | |
| Leukoencephalomalacia | Frequently causes hepatitis but rarely causes failure | | | |

| | | | | |
|---|---|---|---|---|
| External bile duct obstruction | Right dorsal colon displacement or volvulus | | Colic<br>No fever | ↑↑ GGT (>100 IU/L)<br>↑↑ bilirubin (>12 mg/dL)<br>Normal globulin, fibrinogen |
| Portocaval shunt | Congenital defect | >6 week old foal, once eating solid feed | Relapsing episodes of seizure, blindness, coma, other signs of encephalopathy | Normal liver enzymes<br>↑ AST/CK, ↓ blood glucose after seizure<br>↑ $NH_3$, SBA |
| Primary hyperammonemia of Morgan horses | Congenital defect in urea synthesis | Weanling Morgan foals | Poor growth, depression | ↑ liver enzymes<br>Normal/↑ bilirubin<br>↑↑↑ $NH_3$ (>200 µmol/L) |
| Primary hyperammonemia of adult horses | Presumed gastrointestinal dysbiosis and/or increased intestinal permeability | Adult horses, often with colic or diarrhea | Encephalopathy – cortical blindness, circling, head pressing, etc.<br>+/− Colic, diarrhea | ↑↑↑ $NH_3$ (>200 µmol/L)<br>Severe metabolic acidosis<br>↑ blood glucose |
| Alsike clover toxicity | Environmental conditions increases growth of mycotoxin (e.g., *Cymadothea trifolii*) or accumulation of another toxin (e.g., saponin). | Horses grazing in northern US, Canada | Icterus<br>Photosensitization | ↑↑ GGT<br>+/− ↑ AST |
| Panicum spp. toxicity | Unknown toxin | Sporadic cases in horses eating Fall panicum hay (mid-Atlantic states) or Klein Grass (Texas) hay in early fall or winter. | | ↑-↑↑ AST<br>↑↑ GGT |
| Iron toxicity | Primary hemochromatosis, disorder of iron uptake and storage<br>Iatrogenic treatment with iron sulfate | | | |

Dbili, direct bilirubin; GI, gastrointestinal; PPID, pars pituitary intermedia dysfunction; SBA, serum bile acids; Tbili, total bilirubin; TG, triglycerides.

**Box 21.3 Emergency triage and patient stabilization of horses exhibiting fulminant liver failure and hepatic encephalopathy**

- There is no specific antiviral treatment or prevention for parvoviral or hepaciviral infection available currently.
- There is no specific treatment for PA toxicity. Ensure access to toxins is removed for the patient and all other horses on the property.
- The following recommendations are appropriate for any underlying cause of hepatic encephalopathy, including primary gastrointestinal hyperammonemia.
- ***DO NOT USE DIAZEPAM.***
- Tranquilize if needed to control maniacal behavior. Low-dose alpha-2 agonists or barbiturates are indicated (Table 21.2).
- Control cerebral edema if neurologic signs are severe. Mannitol or hypertonic saline, with or without DMSO can be given.
  - **Mannitol** 0.5–1.0 g/kg IV q12–24 h (250–500 g/500 kg horse) give as a 20% solution IV over 20–30 minutes.
  - **Hypertonic saline** 2–4 mL/kg IV (1–2 L/500 kg horse).
  - **DMSO** 0.1–1.0 g/kg IV (50–500 g/500 kg horse) dilute DMSO in 5 L crystalloid and give slowly to prevent hemolysis. RBC of horses in liver failure are more fragile than normal.
- **Begin IV fluid therapy,** especially if the horse is acidotic.
  - **Plasma-Lyte**
    - 1–2.5% **dextrose** to target blood glucose 90–120 mg/dL. Reduces hepatic energy requirements for gluconeogenesis and protein catabolism, thus reducing ammonia production.
    - 40 mEq/L **KCl** to reduce hyperammonemia.
    - Acetate-buffered crystalloid is best. Otherwise, use what crystalloid is available.
    - Replace deficit, then maintain on 80 mL/kg/day (~1.5× maintenance rate).
    - Polycythemia, protein, and lactate may be relatively unresponsive to fluid therapy in some cases of hepatic failure and should not be used to guide resuscitation.
  - **AVOID bicarbonate** unless plasma bicarbonate is <12 mEq/L. Rapid correction of acidosis promotes ionized ammonia, which worsens encephalopathy.
  - **AVOID hetastarch** due to potential effect on coagulation.
- **Reduce blood ammonia**
  - **Neomycin sulfate** 4–8 mg/kg PO q8h (2–4 g/500 kg horse) mixed in molasses. Can be used for 3 days. Can cause diarrhea or nephrotoxicity if used excessively.
  - **Lactulose** 0.1–0.5 mL/kg PO q6–12 h (50–250 mL/500 kg horse).
  - **Lactic-acid-producing probiotics.**
  - **Metronidazole** 10–15 mg/kg PO q12 h (5–7.5 g/500 kg horse) this drug is metabolized by the liver; therefore, this lower-end dose is preferred to avoid toxicity.
  - **Mineral oil** is a less effective alternative, but should be used if the above medications are not available.
  - A combination of neomycin, lactulose, and probiotics is preferred for severe cases. Lactulose alone can be effective in milder cases and can be used for longer treatment. Metronidazole should be used if primary gastrointestinal hyperammonemia is suspected, or can be used as an alternative to neomycin.
- **Treat endotoxemia** if present.
  - **Flunixin meglumine** 0.25 mg/kg PO q8 h (125 mg/500 kg horse). Can use full 1.1 mg/kg dose for the first day, or for longer in cases of cholangiohepatitis.
- **Antioxidants**
  - **Vitamin E** 5,000–7,000 IU/500 kg horse PO q24 h.
  - **Pentoxifylline** 7.5–8.4 mg/kg PO/IV q12–24 h (3.75–4.2 g/500 kg horse).
  - **S-adenosylmethionine** 10–20 mg/kg PO q24 h (5–10 g/500 kg horse).
  - **Acetylcysteine (sterile)** 100 mg/kg in 5–10% dextrose, IV over four hours for acute fulminant or progressive liver disease.
- **Corticosteroids** for relapsing chronic active hepatitis, drug-induced hepatopathy, or acute progressive hepatic failure if other treatments are not effective.
  - **Prednisolone** 1 mg/kg PO q24h (500 mg/500 kg horse) for several weeks, or
  - **Dexamethasone** 0.05–0.1 mg/kg PO/IM/IV q24 (25–50 mg/500 kg horse) decreasing over two to three weeks.

- **Antimicrobials** to treat bacterial cholangiohepatitis and/or to prevent bacteremia. Non-toxic, bactericidal antibiotics such as ceftiofur are preferred.
  - **Ceftiofur** 2.2–5 mg/kg IV/IM q12 h (1.1–2.5 g/500 kg horse)
- **Clotting factors** if coagulopathy and/or hypoalbuminemia are present. 4 liters plasma can be administered for its colloid effect and to replace clotting factors.
- **Minimize stress**
- **Nutrition**
  - Feed small amounts of grain and grass hay frequently. Feeds with high branched chain amino acids, such as beet pulp, milo, sorghum, barley, oats, and corn, are preferred. Avoid alfalfa hay, which has high protein content. Grazing non-legume pasture is acceptable.
- **AVOID nasogastric intubation.** Horses in hepatic failure often have clotting defects. Additionally, swallowing and digesting blood can worsen hepatic encephalopathy. If intubation is required for nutrition or medications, or due to colic, use a small tube and caution.
- **Keep horse out of the sun** to avoid photosensitization.

**Table 21.2** Appropriate sedatives for horses with hepatic encephalopathy. Avoid heavy sedation that would lower the head below the withers, as this could promote cerebral edema.

| Drug | Dose | Dose for 500 kg horse |
|---|---|---|
| Xylazine | 0.2 mg/kg IV | 100 mg |
| Detomidine | 0.005–0.01 mg/kg IV | 2.5–5 mg |
| Detomidine CRI | 0.6 μg/kg/min, decrease by 50% q10 minutes | 0.3 mg/min |
| Pentobarbital | 5.0–11.0 mg/kg IV to effect, q4h or PRN<br>*euthanasia solutions should not be used because they are not sterile and contain other active ingredients | 2,500–5,500 mg |
| Phenobarbital | 12 mg/kg IV loading dose, then 6.6 mk/kg IV q12 h | 6,000 mg loading<br>3,300 mg maintenance |
| Flumazenil | 5–10 mg per horse slow IV | 5–10 mg, efficacy is low |
| Sarmazenil | 0.04 mg/kg IV | 20 mg, efficacy might be low |

**Box 21.4 Recommendations for what can be done on the farm versus in the hospital**

**What can be done at the farm for hepatic and metabolic emergencies**

- Most diagnostic tests, including liver biopsy, and many treatments can be performed on the farm, although hospitalization is often required for optimal treatment. Hepatic encephalopathy, hyperlipemia, and horses with concurrent colic and hepatitis are best referred.

**What can be done at a referral hospital**

- Expertise in treating complex medical cases.
- Medications on hand for stabilization of hepatic encephalopathy.
- Safe facilities for encephalopathic horses.
- Continuous infusion of intravenous fluids, nutrition, and medications.
- Continuous monitoring.
- Liver biopsy.
- Surgical treatment of obstructive cholelithiasis.

**Advice on how to decide between options when referral is time-critical**

- Early referral likely improves prognosis for many causes of hepatic failure in horses.
- If a horse exhibits mild signs of hepatic encephalopathy, early referral should still be offered, as transportation might become difficult to impossible if disease progresses.

**There are two major causes of hepatic failure commonly resulting in hepatic encephalopathy: Theiler's disease and pyrrolizidine alkaloid toxicity.** A newly discovered condition of chronic hepaciviral hepatitis should be added as a differential diagnosis for chronic fibrosing hepatitis which can present with hepatic encephalopathy. Treatment, referral decisions, and prognosis and euthanasia decisions will be described for these conditions together.

## Parvoviral Hepatitis (Theiler's Disease or Serum Hepatitis)

### Summary

**Equine parvovirus-hepatitis is a common equine viral infection, infecting ~15% of horses.** It typically causes subclinical hepatitis, but can occasionally cause severe hepatic necrosis, resulting in acute failure and often death. This severe clinical presentation is known as Theiler's disease and is discussed here.

Horses might have a history of being treated with an equine biologic product in the prior 4–10 weeks. USDA licensed products are now required to test negative for EqPV-H. Therefore, unlicensed equine origin biologic products, such as blood transfusions or allogenic stem cells, are more of a concern. The virus is transmissible between horses nasally and has been identified in nasal, oral, and fecal excretions. A non-biologic form of the disease is seasonal occurring spontaneously in the summer and fall, and there can also be clusters of cases on a single farm.

### Clinical Signs

- Acute onset hepatic encephalopathy.
- Encephalopathy can precede icterus.
- Sometimes, horses are simply found dead. Necropsy might show a small, flaccid, "dish rag" liver.
- Fever is uncommon.

### Biochemical Findings and Diagnostic Criteria

- Primarily hepatocellular. Severe increases in AST, SDH, GLDH. AST often >1,000 IU/L.
- Moderate increases in GGT, ~100–300 IU/L.
- Direct bilirubin usually <20% of total bilirubin.
- Liver ultrasonogram might reveal a small, hypoechoic liver.
- Serum or liver PCR for EqPV-H should show a low Ct value that increases over time after recovery.
- Liver biopsy shows centrilobular to massive hepatocellular necrosis with variable mononuclear inflammation and ductular reaction.

## Pyrrolizidine Alkaloid (PA) Toxicosis

### Summary

**This condition is observed primarily in the western United States, where multiple plants containing PA toxins can be found.** These include *Senecio jacobea* (tansy ragwort), *Senecio vulgaris* (common groundsel), *Cynoglossum officinale* (hound's tongue), and *Amsinckia intermedia* (fiddleneck). *Crotalaria* (rattlebox) also contains PA toxins and grows in the southeastern US, but it is rarely consumed by horses. Typically, chronic low-level ingestion of these toxins in hay results in progressive liver damage; acute disease has been reported but is very rare. Clinical signs begin 1–12 months after ingestion. If disease is caught early and the source of PA toxins is removed, horses can improve. Severe fibrosis on biopsy and serum bile acids >20 μmol/L indicate poor prognosis.

### Clinical Signs

- Although disease is chronic, acute decompensation and hepatic encephalopathy is common.
- Weight loss might be present, suggesting the more chronic course of disease.

- Icterus – mild to moderate.
- Photosensitization can also be present.
- Gastric impaction and laryngeal paralysis are rarely observed.

### Biochemical Findings and Diagnostic Criteria

- Hepatocellular enzyme elevations are variable and can be mild in chronic disease.
- Moderate-to-severe increases in GGT and bile acids.
- Liver ultrasonogram might reveal a hyperechoic liver.
- Liver biopsy shows fibrosis, megalocytosis, and biliary hyperplasia.
- Presumptive diagnosis is based on history of exposure, clinical signs, laboratory evidence of hepatitis, and biopsy findings.

## Hepaciviral Hepatitis

### Summary

**Equine hepacivirus (EqHV), aka Non-primate hepacivirus (NPHV),** is a close relative of Hepatitis C virus (HCV), which causes chronic infection, chronic hepatitis, cirrhosis, and liver cancer in people. There is recent recognition that **EqHV causes a similar condition of chronic infection and chronic hepatitis in horses.** This viral infection might be a cause of what is currently known as "chronic active hepatitis." Because this condition is newly recognized, clear diagnostic criteria and case descriptions are currently lacking. Additionally, infection prevalence is high, and horses can be viremic for many months or years without disease, complicating diagnosis.

### Clinical Signs

- Weight loss and inappetence are common.
- Can develop acute onset hepatic encephalopathy.
- Icterus may not be present.
- Fever is uncommon.

### Biochemical Findings and Diagnostic Criteria

- There is currently no definitive diagnosis. It is essential to rule out other causes of hepatitis, especially treatable causes such as bacterial cholangiohepatitis, before proceeding with a presumptive diagnosis of hepaciviral hepatitis.
- Disease is primarily hepatocellular, but chronic remodeling results in severe increases in cholestatic enzymes.
- Sonographic findings are variable and can be normal. Nodular appearance can indicate cirrhosis.
- Biopsy shows fibrosis, mononuclear portal inflammation, hepatocyte necrosis, and ductular reaction.
- Serum or liver EqHV PCR is sustained positive for months. A single positive result is insufficient to confirm the diagnosis.

## Primary Hyperammonemia of Adult Horses

### Summary

**This is a condition of excessive ammonia production in the gastrointestinal tract and is often associated with concurrent colic or colitis.** It is presumed due to bacterial dysbiosis. Horses exhibit similar clinical signs as hepatic encephalopathy, including ataxia, circling, head pressing, and cortical blindness. Biochemistry reveals hyperglycemia, metabolic acidosis, and hyperammonemia with normal hepatic enzymes. Treatment approach is similar as for hepatic encephalopathy. Supportive treatment with fluids and neomycin or lactulose is often effective. Sodium benzoate (250 mg/kg in 10% dextrose in water IV over one hour) can be beneficial when blood ammonia is >300 µmol/L and magnesium sulfate 1 g/kg PO/NGT can be added to the treatment regime. **Sodium benzoate should not be used in liver disease! Prognosis is fair with supportive therapy.

### Referral Decision

- Refer if hepatic encephalopathy (or primary hyperammonemia) is suspected.
  - Horses with hepatic encephalopathy are often difficult to control and can worsen rapidly, endangering the patient and the attending people.
  - Many treatments require intravenous infusions and/or are not stocked by most ambulatory practitioners.
- Triage before transport can include sedation and treatments for cerebral edema, to reduce blood ammonia, and some IV dextrose or oral corn syrup if blood glucose is low.
- If referral is not an option, the practitioner should institute as many of the above therapies as are feasible and take efforts to counsel owners and handlers on safety measures.

### Prognosis and Euthanasia Decision

- Prognosis is poor to grave for horses with:
  - Theiler's disease. However, horses that survive the first few days typically make a full recovery.
  - PA toxicity and hepatic encephalopathy. Death usually occurs within 10 days of onset of signs.
  - Hemolysis.
  - Severe, bridging fibrosis. However, short-term survival for many months might be possible if encephalopathy is absent or can be controlled with oral medications.
- Euthanasia is indicated when the horse's behavior cannot be safely controlled, body weight cannot be maintained, or the horse progresses into seizures, recumbency, and/or coma.

## Cholangiohepatitis/Cholelithiasis

### Summary

**Ascending bacterial infection of the liver is a common cause of equine hepatitis.** Over time, this can lead to the formation of choleliths and to the development of fibrosis, progressing to liver failure. Choleliths are more common in middle-to-older-age horses. If treated early, cholangiohepatitis has a good prognosis, with resolution in ~80% of cases. Severe fibrosis on biopsy or large choleliths that cannot be accessed surgically indicate poor prognosis.

### Clinical Signs

- Horses most often present with icterus, fever, and anorexia.
- Recurrent colic is more typically associated with cholelithiasis and intermittent bile duct obstruction.
- Obstruction of the common bile duct and/or proximal duodenum can result in acute severe colic.
- Weight loss and photosensitization can be evident.
- Encephalopathy is rare, unless disease is end-stage.

### Biochemical Findings and Diagnostic Criteria

- Primarily cholestatic, with severe increases in GGT, often 300–2,500 U/L, and bile acids.
- Direct bilirubin usually comprises >25% of total bilirubin.
- Mild-to-moderate increases in hepatocellular enzymes AST, SDH, GLDH.
- Inflammatory leukogram with neutrophilic leukocytosis.
- Increased plasma fibrinogen, serum amyloid A, and globulins.
- Sonographic examination might show dilated bile ducts, sludge in the bile ducts, and/or acoustic shadows indicative of stones.
- Increased echogenicity could indicate fibrosis.
- Gastroscopy to evaluate the duodenal papilla might reveal a dilated bile duct opening or a stone obstructing the opening.

- Liver biopsy shows periportal fibrosis, dilation of bile ducts, and inflammation, typically neutrophilic.
- Liver culture is only positive in ~50% of cases. Common flora include Gram-negative enteric aerobes and anaerobes.

### Patient Stabilization of Horses with Suspected Cholangiohepatitis/Cholelithiasis

- Antibiotics: Broad-spectrum coverage is needed. Initial therapy with intravenous penicillin and gentamicin can be followed by long-term oral antibiotics. Ceftiofur or Trimethoprim-sulfamethoxazole are reasonable first-line treatments. Enrofloxacin would be indicated for Gram-negative enterics. Metronidazole should be added for anaerobic coverage, and the lower dosage should be used if hepatic function is compromised. Chloramphenicol is a good broad-spectrum alternative; however, it is also liver metabolized and should be avoided if hepatic function is severely compromised. Treatment should continue until the GGT is normal or for up to six weeks after normalization of GGT.
  - Ceftiofur 3.0 mg/kg IV/IM q12 h.
  - Trimethoprim-sulfamethoxazole 20–30 mg/kg PO q12 h.
  - Enrofloxacin 5–7.5 mg/kg PO/IV q24 h.
  - Metronidazole 15–25 mg/kg PO q8–12 h.
- *Anti-inflammatory, antioxidant*
  - Flunixin meglumine 0.25–1.1 mg/kg PO q8–12 h.
  - Pentoxifylline 7.5–8.4 mg/kg PO/IV q8–12 h.
  - *S*-adenosylmethionine (SAMe) 10 mg/kg PO q24 h *efficacy questioned.
- *Dissolve and pass stones*
  - Dimethyl sulfoxide (DMSO) 1 g/kg as 10% solution IV q24 h for 5–7 days might help dissolve calcium bilirubinate stones.
  - Ursodeoxycholic acid (Ursodiol) 15 mg/kg PO q24 h (or divided q12) increases bile flow.
  - IV crystalloid fluids 90–120 mL/kg/day to increase bile flow.
  - Grazing can be encourage to promote bile flow. Ensure minimal sunlight exposure to prevent photosensitization.
- Treat colic: If the horse is actively showing colic signs, treat with flunixin and sedation as needed.
- **Treat hepatic encephalopathy** as indicated above if present. This is not usually necessary.

### Referral Decision

- Immediate referral is required in cases of intractable colic, as this might require surgical intervention to remove obstructive choleliths.
- If choleliths are suspected or observed sonographically, referral should be offered for optimal medical treatment, including intravenous medications and fluids. Typically, short-term hospitalization will be followed by weeks to months of oral antibiotic therapy.

### Prognosis and Euthanasia Decision

- Prognosis is generally good, with ~80% survival even with elevated bile acids. Most horses either decompensate within the first few days of treatment or recover.
- Severe colic with obstructive cholelithiasis in a location not accessible surgically is a reason for euthanasia.
- Severe fibrosis on liver biopsy indicates poor prognosis for long-term survival. Biopsy results should not be overinterpreted, however, and the decision for euthanasia should be made based on the horse's clinical picture and response to treatment.
- Encephalopathy and increased blood ammonia typically indicate end-stage disease and poor prognosis.

## Hyperlipemia

### Summary

**Hyperlipemia is caused by negative energy balance resulting in excessive mobilization of fat.** Ponies, miniature horses, and donkeys are predisposed to hyperlipemia. Horses with pars pituitary intermedia dysfunction are also at risk. There is typically some inciting cause, such as pregnancy, lactation, or concurrent disease. Severe dietary restriction to promote weight loss in ponies and miniature horses with equine metabolic syndrome has occasionally induced hyperlipemia. Donkeys that are "pining," when removed from herd-mates, may become anorexic and develop hyperlipemia.

## Clinical Signs

- Horses typically present with anorexia and depression.
- This may be accompanied by diarrhea and/or ventral edema.
- Encephalopathy and icterus are uncommon.
- Horses can also show evidence of an underlying disease condition which precipitated the negative energy balance and may have a history of recent rapid weight loss.

## Biochemical Findings and Diagnostic Criteria

- Whitish discoloration of the plasma or serum (hyperlipemia) can confirm the diagnosis stall-side but may not be present.
- Increased serum TG.
- Variable increases in hepatocellular enzymes and GGT are observed.

## Patient Stabilization of Horses with Hyperlipemia

- **Nutrition is the single most important aspect of treating hyperlipemia.** Enteral nutrition can be initiated on the farm, but *referral is typically required* for a combined treatment with IV and oral nutrition. Early treatment improves prognosis.
  - *Immediate triage*
    - 60 mL corn syrup PO q2 h, or
    - Nasogastric intubation with 0.5 g/kg glucose as a 15% solution, 10–20 g KCl, and 1–2 pounds complete feed slurry.
  - *Continued enteral feeding*
    - An indwelling nasogastric tube can be used for frequent feedings q2–4 h until TG begin to drop and appetite returns.
      - Day 1: 50% of daily energy (DE) requirement, ~15 kcal/kg.
      - Day 2: 75% of DE requirement, ~22 kcal/kg.
      - Day 3+: 100% of DE requirement, ~30 kcal/kg if feeding is tolerated without reflux or diarrhea.
      - Even 14–24 kcal/kg/day is likely to be sufficient to reverse hyperlipemia and is a reasonable target if the patient is not eating on their own.
    - Specially formulated diets for nasogastric tube feeding, e.g., Wellsolve Well Gel (Purina Mills, LLC, St. Louis , MO) and Enteral Immunonutrition Formula (Platinum Performance, Inc., Buellton, CA) reduce the volume and frequency required to deliver complete energy requirements.
    - Complete pelleted feeds (most often senior feed formulations) or hay pellets can be used as alternatives or additives to the above diets.
    - Recommend 4–6 L water per 1 kg feed, maximum 6–8 L volume per meal for average adult horse. Scale down for size.
  - Parenteral nutrition: Hyperlipemia is an indication for emergency use of parenteral nutrition and is a primary reason for early referral of these cases. Parenteral nutrition should be provided without lipids.
  - Feed anything the horse will eat.
- **Promote fatty acid uptake by administering insulin and IV dextrose.**
  - Regular insulin 0.1–0.5 IU/kg IM q3–6 h, 100 IU/500 kg horse. Usually used short-term until longer-acting insulin formulations below can be obtained. Start at low end of range and titrate up if needed to control hyperglycemia, or
  - Protamine zinc insulin 0.4 IU/kg IM q24 h. Titrate dose or frequency (q12–24 h) to effect, or
  - Regular insulin CRI 0.01–1.0 IU/kg/h IV. Start at low end of range and titrate up if needed to control hyperglycemia. Allow two to three hours adjustment period before increasing the rate.
  - Horses on insulin should concurrently be provided with enteral or parenteral nutrition and have serial blood glucose monitoring. CRI of IV dextrose at 1–5% solution in polyionic fluids at maintenance rate is typically sufficient to maintain blood glucose.

- **Heparin to stimulate lipoprotein lipase.** The lipase is likely already maximally activated and this might be of little benefit.
  - Unfractionated heparin 40–60 IU/kg IV/SQ q12 h, 25,000 IU/500 kg horse. Can cause coagulopathies. Low-molecular-weight heparin is preferred.
  - Low-molecular-weight heparin (enoxaparin) 0.35–0.5 mg/kg SQ q24 h.
- **Treat the underlying cause.** If a mare is pregnant, the pregnancy should be terminated unless there is an almost immediate response to medical treatments. If a mare is lactating, the foal should be weaned. Treat pars pituitary intermedia dysfunction (PPID) if present.

### Referral Decision

- Referral is preferred for horses with hyperlipemia. Intensive nutritional management and monitoring are typically required for successful treatment.
- If referral is declined, enteral feeding can be attempted on farm with multiple farm visits per day for nasogastric tube feeding. Depending on owner capabilities, an indwelling tube can be left for owner feeding.

### Prognosis and Euthanasia Decision

- Prognosis is fair to good with aggressive therapy if the underlying cause/illness can be corrected.
- Severe ventral edema indicates poor prognosis.
- Failure to regain appetite within a few days of treatment indicates poor prognosis and is a reason for euthanasia.
- Inability to correct underlying diseases can warrant euthanasia.
- Rarely, lipid accumulation in the liver is severe and can result in rupture and hemoabdomen. Prognosis is grave and euthanasia is warranted.

## Tyzzer's Disease

### Summary

***Clostridium piliforme*** **infection of the liver in 8–42 day old foals results in acute hepatic failure.** Usually only one foal on a farm is affected, although there can sometimes be multiple cases.

### Clinical Signs

- Immediate death.
- Shock.
- Hyper- or hypothermia.
- Jaundice.
- Seizures.
- Diarrhea.

### Biochemical Findings and Diagnostic Criteria

- Hepatocellular enzymes elevated, AST, SDH.
- Increased direct and indirect bilirubin.
- Hypoglycemia.
- Severe metabolic acidosis.
- Biopsy shows clostridia in liver.

### Patient Stabilization

**See section above on Patient stabilization of horses exhibiting fulminant liver failure and hepatic encephalopathy*

- Preferred antibiotics for Tyzzer's disease are:
  - **Penicillin** 44,000 IU/kg IV q6 h.

  - **Gentamicin** 6.6 mg/kg IV q24 h.
  - **Metronidazole** 15–25 mg/kg PO q6–12 h.
- Normalize blood pressure
  - Non-lactated crystalloid fluids.
  - If MAP remains low and central venous pressure rises above 11 cm $H_2O$, add **dobutamine** 5–10 μg/kg/min. **or norepinephrine** 0.1–1.0 μg/kg/min.
- Hyperimmune plasma 1–2 L IV.

### Referral Decision

- Referral is recommended for any foal showing signs of shock or severe illness.

### Prognosis and Euthanasia Decision

- Prognosis in fulminant cases is grave even with aggressive therapy.

## Starvation and Refeeding Syndrome

### Summary

**Horses can become emaciated because of underlying disease or starvation.** The prognosis and treatment will differ greatly depending on the cause. The following discussion regards horses that have been starved, with inadequate access to feed, but which have no underlying illness.

Starvation results in dysregulation of most bodily functions, resulting in weakness, poor thermoregulation, and reduced immunity. Prolonged lack of feed intake also alters the gut microbiome, making the horse less able to digest feed that is provided. If rapid increases in feed are provided, this can result in colic, diarrhea, and laminitis.

**Refeeding syndrome is a condition of electrolyte dysregulation that occurs in starved animals that are rapidly refed.** Electrolytes are depleted during starvation. When animals are fed, insulin is released and triggers movement of phosphorous, magnesium, and potassium into cells, resulting in low blood concentrations of these electrolytes. This can cause neurologic signs, and cardiac and pulmonary failure. Slow re-introduction of feed with high protein content and low glycemic index is recommended for successful treatment of the starved horse.

### Clinical Signs

- Poor body condition score (1–2/9).
- Symmetric muscle wasting.
- Weakness.
- Reduced responsiveness to stimuli.
- +/– recumbency.
- History of lack of access to feed.

### Biochemical Findings and Diagnostic Criteria

- Complete physical examination, complete blood count, serum biochemistry, fecal flotation, and thoracic and abdominal imaging are indicated to look for underlying illness as a cause of emaciation.
- In the starved horse without underlying disease, the following biochemical abnormalities can be observed:
  - Low serum magnesium.

- Normal-to-mildly low serum total calcium.
- Hypochromic anemia.

## Patient Stabilization of Starved Horses

- **Recumbent horses should be relocated to a temperature controlled, dry environment** (cool in summer, warm in winter).
- **Hydration, electrolyte abnormalities, and blood glucose should be addressed by intravenous supplementation** before attempts to make the recumbent horse stand.
- **Initial refeeding:**
  - Choose high protein, low glycemic index, high phosphorus and magnesium.
    - Alfalfa hay is recommended.
    - Complete feeds often have higher glycemic index.
    - Grass hay and low starch complete feeds have not been evaluated.
  - Gradually increase feed over the first 10 days (Table 21.3).
  - After 10 days, increase to free choice alfalfa hay. At this time you can slowly add in grass hay.
  - Offer a salt block after four to six weeks.
  - DO NOT feed grain, treats, carrots, apples, etc. until months into refeeding.
  - Add grain after the horse is near normal body weight.
- Deworming and vaccination should be addressed after two to three weeks of refeeding.
- **Avoid sedation during the initial refeeding.** If dental care is required, consider feeding a soaked pelleted diet initially until the horse is stable.

## Referral Decision

- Referral recommendation will depend on the facilities at the farm. Treatment of emaciated starved horses is often performed by rescue organizations which might have adequate facilities, staff, and experience to manage these cases in the field.
- Referral may be required if concurrent diseases require additional treatments or diagnostics, if the horse is recumbent and requires sling assistance to stand, and/or if intravenous therapy is required for resuscitation.
- For a standing, starved horse, refeeding can often be accomplished successfully in the field. This also avoids the stress and energy expenditure associated with shipping.
- Rapid refeeding can result in electrolyte derangements and colitis, typically a few days after feeding begins. Deterioration in a horse that has recently started being refed is an indication for immediate referral for intravenous management of electrolytes and colitis, although prognosis is likely poor in that situation.

## Prognosis and Euthanasia Decision

- Poor prognostic indicators:
  - Recumbent >72 h.
  - Concurrent diseases will have worse prognosis.
  - Weight loss of >50% normal body weight.
  - Neurologic, respiratory, or cardiac signs develop during refeeding. Death usually results within days.
- In successful refeeding, horses will begin to show more energy within the first few weeks, will show notable weight gain within the first month, and will achieve healthy weight within 3–10 months.
- Full assessment should be performed prior to any return to work, as there can be permanent organ dysfunction, particularly to the heart, which could limit athletic potential.

**Table 21.3** Recommended refeeding plan for the starved horse with estimated healthy weight of 450–500 kg. Alfalfa hay is preferred, if available, based on better combination of low starch, high protein, and electrolytes. Use of a scale for weighing hay is essential.

| Day | Percent DE/day | Number of meals/day | Alfalfa lbs/meal |
|---|---|---|---|
| 1–3 | 50 | 6 | 1.0 |
| 4–5 | 75 | 6 | 1.5 |
| 6–10 | 100 | 3 | 4 |
| 11+ | Free choice alfalfa | | |

DE, daily energy requirement of healthy weight.

## Case Example 21.1 Hepatic Encephalopathy

Patient: 11-Year-Old Thoroughbred Mare
History
Horse appeared normal on the morning of presentation but was found in the afternoon with her head pressed against the wall and minimal responsiveness to non-noxious stimuli. She has no recent medical issues in the last three months.

Step 1: On-Farm Assessment and Immediate Stabilization

*Perform a quick, yet focused patient assessment to evaluate the following:*

1) Systemic status: TPR, membranes.
2) Neurologic status: mentation, cranial nerves.
3) Palpate and examine head and neck for traumatic injury.

Your initial examination shows normal TPR, icteric tacky mucous membranes (Figure 21.3a) with 2 second CRT, prolonged skin tent, and slow jugular refill. The mare is standing but dull. There is intermittent menace response and sluggish PLR OU, consistent with central blindness. The mare is grade 3/5 ataxic in all 4 limbs when forced to move but returns to standing with the head pressed against the wall (Figure 21.3b).

(a) (b) (c)

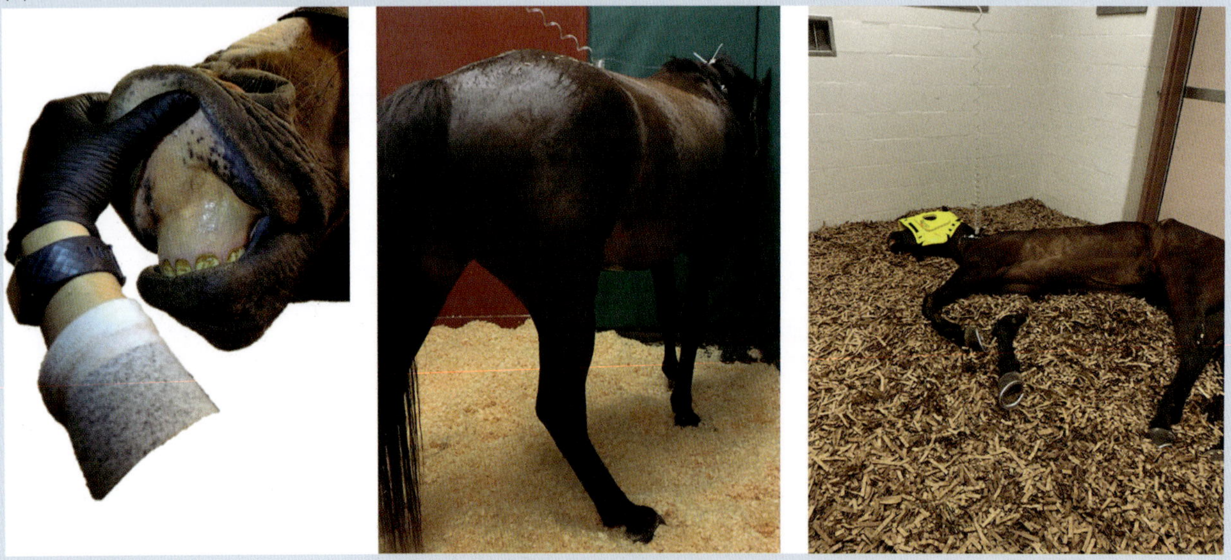

**Figure 21.3** Horse presenting with hepatic encephalopathy. (a) icteric mucous membranes. (b) Head pressing, horse in padded stall. (c) Recumbent horse with padded head protector to prevent injury. *Source:* Courtesy of Dr. Joy Tomlinson and Dr. Megan Palmisano.

*Provide immediate stabilization steps*

1) IV catheter: Based on the cortical signs with icterus, hepatic encephalopathy should be suspected. Deterioration can occur rapidly. Place an IV catheter immediately with an extension line to provide easy access for sedation if needed emergently.
2) IV fluids: Your initial examination suggests likely hypovolemia. Provide immediate resuscitation with an acetate buffered crystalloid (e.g., Plasma-Lyte). Continue with 1-2.5% dextrose and 40 mEq/L KCl at 80 mL/kg/day (~1.5× maintenance rate).
3) *Control neurologic signs*
   a) Ataxia and head pressing are significant in this case. Consider mannitol or hypertonic saline to reduce cerebral edema. You might wait on this until lab results are obtained or the horse is referred if referral is prompt.
   b) If the horse becomes manic or difficult to handle, sedate with low-dose xylazine or detomidine to effect.
   c) To prevent injury, keep the horse in a padded stall (Figure 21.3b) or place a padded head protector (Figure 21.3c).
4) Offer referral: This horse has significant forebrain disease and ataxia – always offer referral. These cases can require hospitalization for optimal diagnostics, treatment, and safe handling. Examples include on-site labs, expertise in sampling spinal fluid if required, continuous infusion of medications, immediate access to medications, and sling support if required.
   a) If hepatic encephalopathy/hyperammonemia is suspected, offer referral even if signs are mild. These horses can deteriorate rapidly.

Step 2: Formulating a Diagnostic Plan

Once stabilization is initiated, formulate a problem list, differential list, and plan if referral is declined:

*Problems*

1) *Neurologic disease with forebrain signs and ataxia in the absence of fever.*
2) *Icterus.*
3) *Hypovolemia.*

*Differentials*

1) Encephalopathy can be viral (e.g., WNV, EEE), metabolic (e.g., hepatic encephalopathy or primary hyperammonemia), other infectious (e.g., EPM), traumatic, or neoplastic.
   a) The absence of fever reduces likelihood of viral conditions.
   b) The presence of icterus and specific sign of head pressing increase likelihood of hepatic disease.
   c) EPM does not typically present as acute forebrain disease; multifocal spinal cord disease is more common.
   d) History and careful clinical examination for pain, swelling, external injuries, or hemorrhage, especially around the head or ears might reveal likelihood of traumatic injury.
   e) Primary neoplastic conditions of the CNS are rare in horses.
2) Icterus can be primary or secondary
   a) Primary icterus can be hepatic origin, which would tie into hepatic encephalopathy.
   b) Secondary icterus due to inappetence is common, but usually requires a few days of being anorexic, which is not reported in this case.
   c) Icterus from hemolysis should be accompanied by anemia.

*Diagnostic Plan*

1) Hepatic disease ties both icterus and encephalopathy and diagnostics should focus there initially.
   a) Serum biochemistry: if possible, add liver panel/specific analytes to include AST, GGT, direct and indirect bilirubin, bile acids, ammonia, and blood glucose.
      i) *Ammonia requires special handling; see lab website for specific instructions.
   b) Complete blood count, or minimally PCV/TS: this can also help rule in or out hemolysis.
   c) If the horse urinates, run a urine dipstick. Positive blood could indicate hemolysis, while positive bilirubin indicates high direct bilirubin, i.e., cholestasis.

d) Liver ultrasound
    i) Acute disease might have normal appearance or small hypoechoic liver.
    ii) Chronic disease might have increased or heteroechoic/nodular appearance.

2) Additional testing for other causes of encephalopathy could be considered after the above initial tests are completed.

*Diagnostic Results*

In-house you have PCV/TS and standard chemistry panel available for same-day results. This horse has:

PCV 65%, TS 7.0.
AST 3,071 (RI 222–489 U/L), GGT 354 U/L (RI 8–33 U/L).
BG 60 mg/dL (71–122 mg/dL).

These results confirm your suspicion of hepatic encephalopathy. Additionally, the relatively high AST compared to GGT suggests acute liver failure (e.g., parvoviral hepatitis/Theiler's disease), rather than chronic liver failure (e.g., PA toxicity). Aligned with this, your ultrasound shows normal-to-small liver and the echogenicity is unremarkable.

Counsel the client about the risk of maniacal or dangerous behavior from the horse and the possibility of sudden death. If the client declines referral, proceed with on-farm treatment.

Step 3: Emergency Treatment Guidelines
Following initial stabilization and diagnostic evaluation, further specific treatment is indicated.

- If you have not administered mannitol or hypertonic saline, do so now. Remember to follow up with isotonic crystalloids, at least a bolus if a CRI is not feasible.
- Add dextrose to IVF if using CRI or administer karo syrup orally to raise blood glucose. Once horse is stabilized, small meals can be offered.
- Reduce blood ammonia: If you have lactulose, start immediately. If you do not have it, order some and start one of the following alternatives:
  - Metronidazole.
  - Neomycin sulfate.
  - Mineral oil is a least preferred option, especially as nasogastric intubation is required, which increases risk of hemorrhage and ingestion of blood, which is digested to ammonia.
- Treat endotoxemia and bacterial translocation
  - Low-dose flunixin
  - Bactericidal, non-toxic antimicrobial – e.g., ceftiofur
- Keep the horse out of the sun and preferably in a stall with solid walls. Recommend it not be handled alone and there should be someone outside the stall to call for help in an emergency.

Step 4: Assessment and Monitoring
Serial patient monitoring is essential during emergency triage

- Routine assessment should include a physical exam including monitoring of respiratory and heart rates and mentation.
- For example, adequate treatment of hyperammonemia should improve mentation such that propulsive or maniacal behavior is reduced, responsiveness to stimuli improves, and cortical blindness resolves.
- In contrast, progression could result in a horse that is too dangerous to handle, or that becomes recumbent.
- Horses in liver failure can have polycythemia, so monitoring of PCV/TS is not a good indication of hydration. Monitor water intake, provide IVF as required (CRI at 1.5× maintenance is preferred), and monitor clinical examination/urine production/USG to aid in determining volume status.
- Liver enzymes might worsen initially, especially GGT will often continue to rise as it is associated with remodeling and response to injury. This alone is not an indication to stop treatment.

Step 5: Decision Making During Triage
Many difficult decisions face the emergency clinician working with encephalopathic patients.

- Following stabilization, referral is recommended for horses with hepatic encephalopathy. Many of the medications are not commonly stocked by field veterinarians; these horses often benefit from CRI infusion or IV medications, and the horses can easily become dangerous to handle in the field.
- Intractable behavior and lack of improvement in neurologic signs in response to treatment is the most common reason for euthanasia of these cases, although some progress to recumbency or sudden death.
- While the prognosis for a horse with hepatic encephalopathy is poor, if the process is acute and the horse survives the first few days, they can often recover fully.
  - If horses survive the immediate triage period, further diagnostics to confirm the presumptive diagnosis of acute hepatic necrosis could be pursued. These could include serum liver virus PCR and liver biopsy.

## References


Aleman, M., Nieto, J.E., Carr, E.A., and Carlson, G.P. (2005). Serum hepatitis associated with commercial plasma transfusion in horses. *JVIM* 19: 120–122.

Baird, J., Tegtmeyer, B., Arroyo, L. et al. (2020). The association of Equine parvovirus-hepatitis (EqPV-H) with cases of non-biologic-associated Theiler's disease on a farm in Ontario, Canada. *Vet. Microbiol.* 242: 108575. https://doi.org/10.1016/j.vetmic.2019.108575.

Delvescovo, B., Tomlinson, J., DeNotta, S. et al. (2021). Bile acids, direct bilirubin and gamma-glutamyltransferase as prognostic indicators for horses with liver disease in the Eastern United States: 82 cases (1997–2019). *J. Equine Vet. Sci.* 105: 103729. https://doi.org/10.1016/j.jevs.2021.103729.

Divers, T.J. (2008). Liver failure and hemolytic anemia. In: *Equine Emergencies Treatment and Procedures* (ed. J.A. Orsini and T.J. Divers), 237–258. St. Louis, MO: Saunders.

Divers, T.J. (2015). The equine liver in health and disease. *Proc. Am. Assoc. Equine Practitioners,* Las Vegas, 66–103.

Divers, T.J. and Tomlinson, J.E. (2020). Theiler's disease. *Equine Vet. Educ.* 32: 63–65. https://doi.org/10.1111/eve.13053.

Divers, T.J., Tennant, B.C., Kumar, A. et al. (2018). A new parvovirus associated with serum hepatitis in horses following inoculation of a common equine biological. *Emerg. Infect. Dis.* 24: 303–310. https://doi.org/10.3201/eid2402.171031.

Elia, G., Lanave, G., Lorusso, E. et al. (2017). Equine hepacivirus persistent infection in a horse with chronic wasting. *Transbound. Emerg. Dis.* 64: 1354–1358. https://doi.org/10.1111/tbed.12679.

Ferraro, G., Stull, C., and Madigan, J.E. (2009). Equine sanctuary and rescue facility guidelines. https://ceh.vetmed.ucdavis.edu/local_resources/pdfs/pubs-Sanctuary-bkm-sec.pdf (accessed May 202).

Hurcombe, S. (2008). Equine hepatic encephalopathy. In: *Equine Neurology* (ed. M. Furr and S. Reed), 257–268. Ames, IA: Blackwell Publishing.

Liotta, E.M., Lizza, B.D., Romanova, A.L. et al. (2016). 23.4% saline decreases brain tissue volume in severe hepatic encephalopathy as assessed by a quantitative CT marker. *Crit. Care Med.* 44: 171–179. https://doi.org/10.1097/CCM.0000000000001276.

Mendel, V.E., Witt, M.R., Gitchell, B.S. et al. (1988). Pyrrolizidine alkaloid-induced liver disease in horses: an early diagnosis. *Am. J. Vet. Res.* 49: 572–578.

Moore, B.R., Abood, S.K., and Hinchcliff, K.W. (1994). Hyperlipemia in 9 miniature horses and miniature donkeys. *J. Vet. Intern. Med.* https://doi.org/10.1111/j.1939-1676.1994.tb03253.x.

Pearson, E.G. (1991). Liver failure attributable to pyrrolizidine alkaloid toxicosis and associated with inspiratory dyspnea in ponies: three cases (1982–1988). *J. Am. Vet. Med. Assoc.* 198: 1651–1654.

Peek, S.F. (2004). Cholangiohepatitis in the mature horse. *Equine Vet. Educ.* 16: 72–75. https://doi.org/10.1111/j.2042-3292.2004.tb00270.x.

Peek, S.F. and Divers, T.J. (2000). Medical treatment of cholangiohepatitis and cholelithiasis in mature horses: 9 cases (1991–1998). *Equine Vet. J.* https://doi.org/10.2746/042516400777032156.

Peek, S.F., Divers, T.J., and Jackson, C.J. (1997). Hyperammonemia associated with encephalopathy and abdominal pain without evidence of liver disease in four mature horses. *Equine Vet. J.* 29: 70–74.

Smith, G.W., Davis, J.L., Malone, J.B. et al. (2020). Diseases of the hepatobiliary system. In: *Large Animal Internal Medicine* (ed. B.P. Smith, D.C. van Metre, and N. Pusterla), 921–955. St. Louis, MO: Elsevier.

Stegelmeier, B.L., Gardner, D.R., James, L.F., and Molyneuz, R.J. (1996). Pyrrole detection and the pathologic progression of *Cynoglossum officinale* (houndstoungue) poisoning in horses. *J. Vet. Diagn. Invest.* 8: 81–90.

Stull, C. (2012). *Nutrition for Rehabilitating the Starved Horse*. Davis: A publication of the Center for Equine Health, School of Veterinary Medicine, University of California https://ceh.vetmed.ucdavis.edu/sites/g/files/dgvnsk4536/files/local_resources/pdfs/pubs-July2012-bkm-sec.pdf (accessed May 2025).

Tegtmeyer, B., Echelmeyer, J., Pfankuche, V.M. et al. (2019). Chronic equine hepacivirus infection in an adult gelding with severe hepatopathy. *Vet. Med. Sci.* 5: 372–378. https://doi.org/10.1002/vms3.181.

Tomlinson, J. (2021). Equine hepatitis viruses. *AAEP Proc.* 67: 296–301.

Tomlinson, J., Kapoor, A., Kumar, A. et al. (2019). Viral testing of 18 consecutive cases of equine serum hepatitis: a prospective study (2014–2018). *J. Vet. Intern. Med.* 33: 251–257. https://doi.org/10.1111/jvim.15368.

Tomlinson, J.E., Tennant, B.C., Struzyna, A. et al. (2019). Viral testing of 10 cases of Theiler's disease and 37 in-contact horses in the absence of equine biologic product administration: a prospective study (2014–2018). *J. Vet. Intern. Med.* 33: 258–265. https://doi.org/10.1111/jvim.15362.

Tomlinson, J.E., Jager, M., Struzyna, A. et al. (2020). Tropism, pathology, and transmission of equine parvovirus-hepatitis. *Emerg. Microb. Infect.* 9: 651–663. https://doi.org/10.1080/22221751.2020.1741326.

Waitt, L.H. and Cebra, C.K. (2009). Characterization of hypertriglyceridemia and response to treatment with insulin in horses, ponies and donkeys: 44 cases (1995–2005). *J. Am. Vet. Med. Assoc.* 234: 915–919.

Witham, C.L. and Stull, C. (1998). Metabolic responses of chronically starved horses to refeeding with three isoenergetic diets. *J. Am. Vet. Med. Assoc.* 212: 691–696.

# 22

# Triage and Management of Injuries Associated with Fire and Flood Exposure

*Lauren Bookbinder*

*Large Animal Clinical Sciences, College of Veterinary Medicine, Michigan State University, East Lansing, MI, USA*

## Triage and Management of Injuries Associated with Fire Exposure

### Cutaneous Thermal Injury, Burn Shock, and Smoke Inhalation

Key points to remember for cutaneous thermal injury, burn shock, and smoke inhalation are provided in Box 22.1.

Equine emergencies associated with barn or wildfire exposure are uncommon but potentially devastating. Fire-related injuries can be broadly categorized into cutaneous damage and respiratory tract compromise. The triaging veterinarian must assess the extent of these injuries to provide a prognosis and plan for the owner. Importantly, serious injury related to fire exposure may progress for up to 72 hours.

Burns are the result of direct thermal injury to cutaneous structures and cause variable damage to the epidermis, dermis, adnexa, and subcutaneous tissues. Burns are categorized into degrees that are defined by the depth of tissue damage (Figure 22.1 and see below). Accurately characterizing burn degree and the percent of body surface affected provides important diagnostic and prognostic information. Burns affecting the dermis and adnexa over >10% of the body can lead to significant fluid and protein loss resulting in burn shock, a potentially life-threatening state of cardiovascular instability and systemic inflammation requiring intensive care. Consequences of burn shock, including organ failure, may develop days to weeks following initial injury. Burns affecting the germinal cells of the dermis (deep second degree or higher) will cause scarring that may be disfiguring and/or impair athletic function based on location. Importantly, the extent of burn injury may not be evident for up to 72 h after initial injury because of secondary inflammation, thrombosis, and edema developing at the burn site.

Direct thermal injury and chemical inhalation may cause respiratory disease in horses exposed to fire. Thermal injury is typically contained to the upper respiratory tract and should always be expected if burns localize to the face or muzzle but can occur without these obvious local burns. Upper respiratory tract thermal injury manifests as progressive edema over 72 h after exposure and may necessitate emergency tracheostomy to maintain an airway. Chemical inhalation of toxic gas (smoke) or carbon monoxide primarily affects the lower respiratory tract and is more likely to occur when horses are exposed to contained barn fires compared to open wildfires. Smoke inhalation causes lower airway disease through three mechanisms: immediate direct damage to the pulmonary epithelium, latent inflammatory changes including edema, cellular necrosis, mucous secretion, and hyaline membrane formation, and increased risk of secondary bacterial bronchopneumonia. Carbon monoxide poisoning results in high circulating levels of carboxyhemoglobin which impairs oxygen transportation and causes tissue hypoxemia shortly after inhalation. Importantly, acute lung injury associated with burn shock can occur in the absence of significant smoke inhalation.

### Emergency Triage Following Fire Rescue (<Six Hours After Injury)

1) Relocate the horse as needed.
2) Administer sedation and analgesia as needed for safety.
   - Xylazine: 0.5–0.75 mg/kg IV.
   - Detomidine: 5–20 μg/kg IV.
   - Butorphanol: 0.01–0.02 mg/kg IV.

*Emergency Triage of the Horse*, First Edition. Edited by Rolfe M. Radcliffe and Jamie J. Kopper.

Companion website: www.wiley.com/go/radcliffe/triage

**Box 22.1 Key Points to Remember – Cutaneous thermal injury, burn shock, and smoke inhalation**

1) Fire exposure can result in significant cutaneous damage, burn shock, and respiratory compromise. Each of these requires time, financial, and emotional investment from owners. Understanding and identifying these three consequences of fire exposure informs the decision-making triage exam.
2) Characterize burns based on degree and extent:
   - Deep second-degree (or greater) burns will scar.
   - Burn shock is likely if third- or fourth-degree burns cover >10% of the body.
   - Euthanasia should be considered if third- or fourth-degree burns cover >30–50% of the body.
3) Burn shock is a state of hypovolemia, hypoproteinemia, hypermetabolism, and systemic inflammation that results in cardiovascular instability and is a medical emergency.
4) Carefully evaluate horses surviving fire for upper respiratory thermal damage and lower respiratory tract chemical damage; both are medical emergencies.

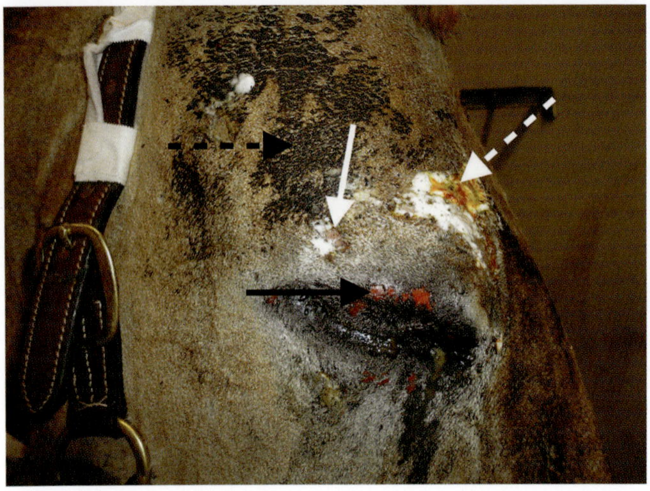

**Figure 22.1** Demonstration of various burn degrees. Superficial second degree (black solid arrow); deep second degree (black dashed arrow); third degree (white dashed arrow); fourth degree (white solid arrow). Note the various burn colors associated with each degree. First-degree burns are typically bright red; second-degree burns may have a black eschar, third-degree burns can be pink, white, or yellow based on the variable damage to the dermis and adenexa, fourth-degree burns will expose the subcutaneous tissues with reflect the color of those tissues (bone, tendon, fat, muscle, etc.). *Source:* Courtesy of Dr. Betsy Carr.

3) Limit continued cutaneous thermal injury.
   - Remove flammable material.
   - Cool tissues using *lukewarm* water (cold water potentiates local vasoconstriction).
4) Establish intravenous access.
   - Significant cutaneous edema may develop and challenge catheter placement.
5) Provide temperature and humidity control.
   - Cutaneous burns impair thermoregulation.
6) Administer anti-inflammatories.
   - Phenylbutazone: 2.2–4.4 mg/kg IV or PO q12 h.
   - Flunixin meglumine: 0.25–1.1 mg/kg IV or PO q8–12 h.
   - *Note: administration of steroids does not influence long-term prognosis and is not recommended.*
7) Manage upper airway edema if present (Figure 22.2).
   - Mild edema: intranasal phenylephrine, 5–6 cc in each nostril administered through a flexible catheter, with the head elevated for 30–60 seconds following administration.
   - Moderate/severe edema, stridor, stertor, or dyspnea: tracheostomy (see Chapter 5 for tracheostomy procedure).

## Emergency Diagnostic Evaluation Following Fire Rescue (<Six Hours After Injury)

Following immediate stabilization an initial diagnostic evaluation of the horse should be performed and is aimed at: determining the location and severity of thermal and non-thermal injury, assessing for burn shock, and estimating the degree of respiratory compromise. These evaluations will aide in clinical decision-making, including decisions for referral or euthanasia. An initial diagnostic evaluation includes a comprehensive physical examination, point-of-care bloodwork, and respiratory tract imaging.

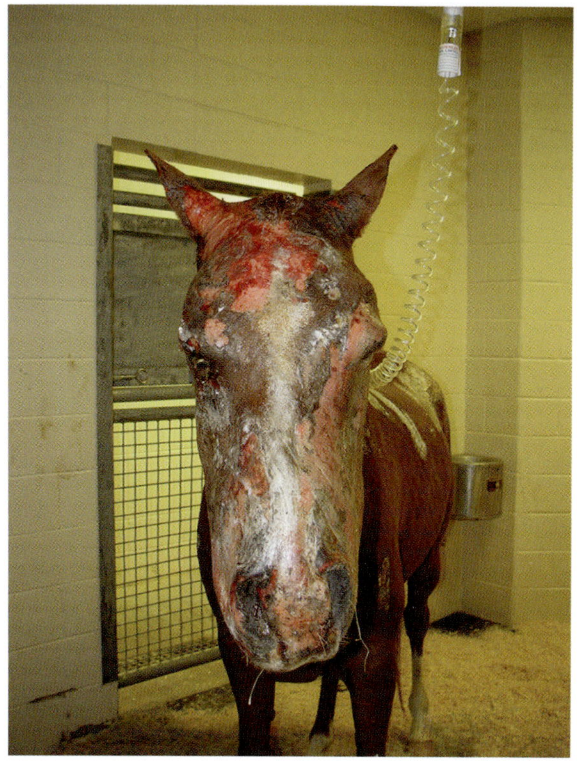

**Figure 22.2** Facial burns associated with significant facial edema. Upper respiratory tract thermal damage and lower respiratory tract smoke inhalation should be expected in cases with facial burns. *Source:* Courtesy of Dr. Jen Gold.

#### Comprehensive Physical Examination

1) Identify thermal and non-thermal injuries.
   - Pay particular attention to damage to the face, eyes, dorsum, and hooves.
   - Evaluate for traumatic wounds and lacerations.
2) Classify burn degree(s) and approximate the percent of body surface area affected (Figure 22.1).
   - *First-degree burns* are limited to the superficial layers of the epidermis. They singe the hair and are erythematous and painful, but will heal without complications or scarring in 7–14 days.
   - *Second-degree burns* variably involve deeper structures of the skin and can be categorized as superficial or deep.
     i) *Superficial second-degree* burns involve all superficial layers of the epidermis, and only a few cells of the basal (germinal) layer. As with first-degree burns, superficial second-degree burns are erythematous and painful, but will heal with minimal complication or scarring.
     ii) *Deep second-degree* burns involve all layers of the epidermis including the basal layer. These burns cause severe edema at the dermal/epidermal junction and epidermal necrosis resulting in eschar formation (blackened, sloughed epidermal layers). Healing is prolonged (three to four weeks) and occurs with the potential for significant scarring. These burns are less painful and erythematous than lesser degree burns.
   - *Third-degree burns* involve all layers of the epidermis and extend into the dermis and adnexa. These burns are minimally painful, have a white, black, or yellow appearance, and heal with significant scarring. Third-degree burns are medical emergencies (Figure 22.3).
   - *Fourth-degree burns* involve all layers of the skin and expose underlying subcutaneous tissues including fat, muscle, tendons, ligaments, or bones. Fourth-degree burns often carry a grave prognosis. These burns heal with significant scarring that may impair function of underlying structures.
   - *Note: lesser-degree burns often radiate from the primary burn site*
3) Identify clinical evidence of burn shock (Table 22.1)
   - Third- and fourth-degree burns covering >10% of body surface area may result in burn shock, a clinical state of significant systemic inflammation and fluid/protein loss that causes cardiovascular instability, electrolyte derangements, and possible organ dysfunction. Burn shock is a medical emergency.
4) Identify clinical evidence of respiratory compromise
   - Pay particular attention to respiratory rate, effort, auscultation, and any evidence of upper airway edema including stertor, stridor, or reduced nasal airflow/palpable nasal edema. Evidence of respiratory compromise is a medical emergency.

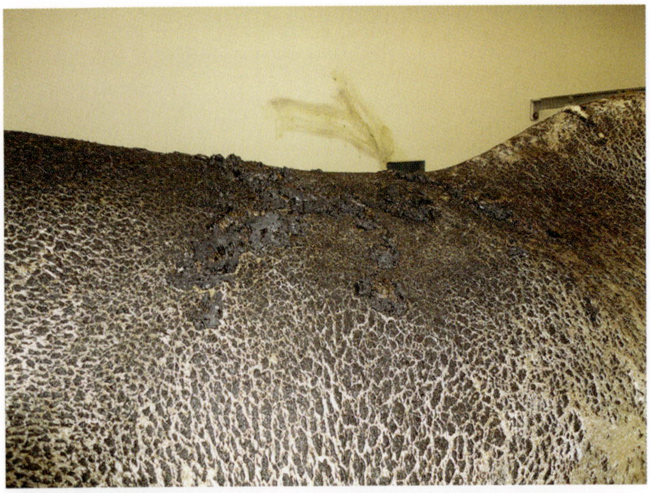

**Figure 22.3** Image of a horse with deep second- and third-degree burns of the dorsum. Falling debris caused foci of third-degree burns with radiating deep second-degree burns. *Source:* Courtesy of Dr. Betsy Carr.

**Table 22.1** Common clinical presentations of burn shock.

| **Indicators of burn shock** |
|---|
| *Clinical features* |
| • Local and systemic edema |
| • Tachycardia |
| • Dysrhythmias |
| • Tachypnea |
| • Altered mucous membrane color and capillary refill time |
| • Syncope or ataxia |
| *Clinicopathologic features* |
| • Elevated PCV |
| • Hypoproteinemia |
| • Elevated L-lactate |
| • Hypernatremia, hyperchloremia |
| • Hyperkalemia |

### Baseline Diagnostic Evaluation

1) Perform a baseline packed cell volume/total solids (PCV/TS), L-lactate, arterial blood gas, complete blood count, and biochemistry profile as able
   - Changes to these clinicopathologic variables can indicate various manifestations of burn shock (hypoproteinemia, hypovolemia, electrolyte derangements, and organ dysfunction) as well as a degree of cardiovascular compromise. Generally, the degree of fluid and protein loss parallels the extent and severity of cutaneous burns.
   - Carbon monoxide poisoning should be suspected if there is clinical evidence of hypoxemia, but arterial blood gas parameters and/or $SpO_2$ are normal. Definitive diagnosis of carbon monoxide poisoning is made by measuring serum carboxyhemoglobin levels near the time of intoxication. High $SpVO_2$ or low oxygen extraction ratios (see Appendix 2 for calculations) are also suggestive.
2) Perform baseline respiratory tract evaluation
   - Endoscopy/bronchoscopy is used to evaluate thermal injury, edema, and contamination of the lower airways (Figure 22.4). Thoracopulmonary imaging is used to evaluate the lower airways and includes transcutaneous ultrasound to identify pulmonary edema, pleural fluid, and/or superficial parenchymal disease and/or radiographs to identify parenchymal disease consistent with inflammation or infection.

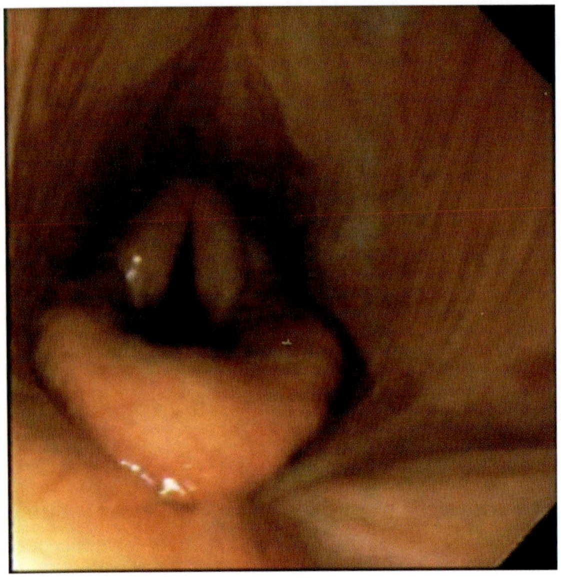

**Figure 22.4** Laryngeal edema and erythema associated with thermal damage. *Source:* Courtesy of Dr. Jen Gold.

## Decision-Making Following Initial Triage

The decision for farm management, referral management, or euthanasia should be made based on the degree of cutaneous damage and the risk of burn shock and/or significant upper or lower respiratory tract dysfunction. Cutaneous burn management is labor and cost intensive, and significant scarring is likely when burns are deep second degree or greater. Owners must be aware of this before embarking on treatment, particularly if scarring is likely to impair athletic function. Burn shock and respiratory compromise are potentially life-threatening complications associated with fire exposure, and owners must be aware of the seriousness of these conditions to make well-informed treatment choices. Remember that the full extent of fire-related injury may not be apparent for 72 hours. Close veterinary follow-up, owner compliance, and owner education are requisite before considering on-farm management. Understanding what services can be provided on the farm versus in a hospital setting can aid in this decision making.

## What Can Be Done on Farm Versus Referral Hospital

In general, first- and superficial second-degree burns can be successfully managed on the farm in the absence of respiratory compromise or unique patient co-morbidities (Figures 22.5 and 22.6). Deep second-degree or more severe burns require daily cleaning and frequent debriding, and are therefore best managed in a hospital setting. Third- or fourth-degree burns affecting >10% of the body are likely to result in burn shock. Burn shock can be stabilized in the field with anti-inflammatories and intravenous fluids, but is a highly dynamic systemic disease that is best managed with 24-hour care. Similarly, initial respiratory evaluation and stabilization can be performed in the field, however, respiratory compromise is identified or suspected, referral for intensive care including intranasal oxygen, continuous monitoring, bronchoscopic lavage, and tracheostomy management is recommended. Patients with significant upper respiratory tract edema may require tracheostomy prior to referral (see Chapter 5).

Decision tree based on cutaneous thermal damage and risk of burn shock

Consider farm management if:
1. Burns are first or superficial second degree
2. There is no clinical or clinicopathologic evidence of burn shock
3. Patient is willing and able to eat and drink

Consider referral management if:
1. Burns are deep second-degree or more severe, particularly if over >10% of the body
2. There is clinical or clinicopathologic evidence of burn shock
3. Burn damage involves the eyes or hooves
4. Patient is unwilling or unable to eat or drink
5. Criteria for farm management is met, but follow-up care is insufficient

Consider euthanasia if:
1. Third or greater degree burns cover >30–50 % of the body
2. Deep second degree burns cover >30–50% of the body with patient comorbidities (i.e. poor body condition)
3. Fourth degree burns expose critical structures
4. There is significant damage to the hoof
5. Athletic function is important and is likely to be affected by scarring
6. Criteria for referral is met, but not an option for the owner

**Figure 22.5** Management decision tree based on evaluation of cutaneous thermal damage and risk of burn shock following fire survival.

Decision tree based on respiratory compromise

Consider farm management if:
1. Open or wild fire
2. Wounds are not localized to head/neck
3. No evidence of respiratory tract dysfunction
   - *Note: dysfunction may develop over up to 72 hours*
4. Patient is willing and able to eat and drink

Consider referral management if:
1. Contained barn fire
2. Wounds are localized to head/neck
3. There is evidence of respiratory tract dysfunction
   - *Note: tracheostomy may be required prior to transport if upper airway edema is present*
4. Patient is unwilling or unable to eat or drink
5. Criteria for farm management are met, but follow-up care is insufficient

Consider euthanasia if:
1. Lower respiratory compromise is evident (i.e. cannot be managed with a tracheostomy)
2. Criteria for referral is met but is not an option for the owner

**Figure 22.6** Management decision tree based on evaluation of respiratory compromise following fire survival.

## Post-Triage Care

### Supportive Care

***Intravenous Fluids*** Intravenous fluids are required to maintain vascular volume if burns exceed 10% of total surface body area. Fluid therapy should be limited to the minimum effective volume to maintain peripheral perfusion as indicated by urine output and blood pressure. Over-hydration will potentiate burn shock and tissue edema and hasten organ failure (particularly respiratory failure). Colloid oncotic support should be considered based on evaluation of peripheral perfusion and serum albumin concentrations. Plasma administered at 2–10 L/500 kg horse is the primary colloid used in large animal practice. Hetastarch 6% (up to 10 mL/kg IV q24–48 h) may also be used, but risk of acute kidney injury and coagulopathy should be considered based on individual patient co-morbidities.

***Anti-Inflammatories and Analgesics*** Anti-inflammatories are indicated to manage pain and inflammation and include phenylbutazone (2.2–4.4 mg/kg IV or PO q12 h) or flunixin meglumine (0.25–1.1 mg/kg IV or PO q8–12 h). Additional anti-inflammatories such as pentoxifylline (7.5–10 mg/kg IV or PO q8–12 h) or DMSO (1 g/kg IV) have been reported, but their use in horses surviving fire is not evidence based. Acetaminophen (20 mg/kg PO q12) and continuous rate infusions of lidocaine (1.3 mg/kg IV bolus over 15 minutes followed by 0.02–0.05 mg/kg/min), butorphanol (0.013 mg/kg/h IV), and ketamine (0.5–0.1 mg/kg IV bolus followed by 0.006–0.02 mg/kg/min) may provide additional pain control.

***Broad-Spectrum Systemic Antimicrobials*** Bronchopneumonia is a common sequela to smoke inhalation and can occur without obvious respiratory tract damage. Concern for bronchopneumonia is the most important indication for systemic antimicrobial administration in horses surviving fires, and broad-spectrum coverage is recommended if bronchopneumonia is suspected. Trans-tracheal wash and culture should be performed if able, otherwise select empirical broad-spectrum antimicrobials. Systemic antimicrobials do not penetrate the devitalized cutaneous burns and are not indicated unless there is obvious infection of deeper structures, or other risk factors for systemic infection.

***Nutritional Support*** Burn shock causes a hypermetabolic state. The basal metabolic rate increases by 2–3 times if >30% of the body is burned. Providing enteral (preferred) or parenteral nutrition is necessary to support clinical recovery. High calorie feeds and additives such as canola oil are effective in maintaining weight in patients with adequate appetites. Preventing protein malnutrition will aid in wound healing. In patients with reduced voluntary intake, parenteral protein repletion should be provided at a minimum of 1–1.5 g/kg/day (maintenance) and forced enteral nutrition through feeding tubes should be considered.

### Cutaneous Burn Care

***Initial/Superficial Burn Care*** Once the skin is cooled, hair surrounding the wound should be clipped and the wound debrided of obvious necrotic tissue. Debride judiciously, so germinal cell layers are not inadvertently removed. Vesicles, blisters, and eschars should be left intact until they are no longer adhered to underlying structures. Lavage the wound with 0.05% sterile chlorhexidine solution and apply a water-based antibiotic ointment such as Silver Sulfadiazine or medical-grade honey liberally. In human medicine, honey is a preferred treatment for cutaneous wounds, but maintaining cleanliness and minimizing insects can be challenging in a barn setting. For first-degree and superficial deep wounds, this treatment should be repeated daily until healing occurs in 7–14 days; no additional treatment is required.

***Deep Burn Care*** For deeper burns with eschar formation there are four potential long-term wound management strategies.

1) Closed management: Eschars are debrided and the wound is covered with an occlusive dressing. These dressings are changed frequently and the wound bed is debrided and cleaned at each dressing change. This can result in significant pain and expense for large wounds, but may be manageable for small, deep burns in amenable locations.
2) Semi-open management: Eschars are left in place but covered with antimicrobial soaked dressings (usually 0.05% chlorhexidine solution). As with closed management, burn location dictates practicality.
3) Open management: Eschars are left in the open air and covered with an antimicrobial ointment at least twice daily. The eschar will slough in approximately four weeks and the resultant wound bed heals by contracture or grafting. This is the most effective, practical form of management for large burns.
4) Excision: Eschars are excised and completely grafted with allogenous or autogenous grafts. This is cost and time prohibitive for large wounds.

***Topical Wound Treatments*** There is no current consensus on the ideal topical treatment for burn wounds in human or veterinary patients. Silver sulfadiazine is the topical antimicrobial most commonly applied to burns. It has a broad spectrum of antimicrobial activity, is easy to apply, and associated with infrequent complications. Silver sulfadiazine is inactivated in the presence of exudate and must be applied at least twice daily. In human medicine, honey is preferred over silver sulfadiazine for the treatment of burn wounds, though this evidence is generally considered weak. Compared to silver sulfadiazine, honey has an improved spectrum of activity against *Staphylococcus* spp. and *Pseudomonas* spp., provides some analgesia, and may reduce scar formation and wound contracture in human medicine. However, there are practical considerations with managing open honey dressings in a barn setting. Nitrofurazone, chlorhexidine, providine-iodine, or gentamicin-sulfate ointments can also be used, but have either a narrower spectrum of antimicrobial activity, or increased risk of systemic absorption compared to silver sulfadiazine, and are only used under specific circumstances. Sterile starch copolymer can be used in conjunction with topical antimicrobials to absorb wound exudate.

***Miscellaneous Wound Treatments*** Animals with burns affecting a significant percentage of total body surface area cannot thermoregulate and require temperature and humidity control. Additionally, deep burns can be severely pruritic during the first few weeks of healing. Mechanical intervention (muzzle, cross-ties) or sedation may be required to prevent self-mutilation. (See Chapter 7 for more discussion.)

Advanced wound-healing techniques, including amniotic membrane grafts in conjunction with synthetic dermal matrix and partial thickness skin grafts, increase elasticity of healed skin, decrease healing time, and reduce wound contracture in humans. Application of platelet-rich plasma to burns may hasten healing and reduce bacterial infection in horses. Extra-corporeal shockwave of healing burns has been reported to promote resolution in one horse. These therapies may be considered to maximize likelihood of return to athletic function.

### Respiratory Therapies

***Upper Respiratory Thermal Damage*** Edema secondary to thermal damage of the upper respiratory tract may result in airway obstruction which is best managed with a temporary tracheostomy (see Chapter 11). Ancillary therapy for non-obstructive upper respiratory tract edema includes intranasal phenylephrine administration (see above), nebulization to humidify the airways, and administration of mucolytics and local antimicrobials as indicated (see below). Administration of furosemine at 1 mg/kg IV q12 h with attention to electrolyte and hydration status has been reported, but is controversial in cases of non-cardiogenic edema.

***Lower Respiratory Chemical Damage*** Therapies to support the lower airway tract following fire exposure are focused on maintaining normoxemia, minimizing inflammatory exudate and mucus production, and controlling bronchopneumonia.

1) Support normoxemia
   - Humidified intranasal oxygen insufflation:
     i) Rates of 15–20 L $O_2$/min can be achieved by oxygen infusion through either bilateral nasal cannulas or tracheostomy
   - Hyperbaric oxygen chamber therapy
     i) Significantly reduces circulating carboxyhemoglobin concentrations if performed <5 hours after inhalation.
2) Nebulization
   - N-acetylcysteine: 0.25–1 g q6–8 h
   - Albuterol: 3–5 mL 0.5% solution q4–6 h
   - Antimicrobials
     i) Gentamicin: 2.2 mg/kg of 50 mg/mL solution q24 h
     i) Amikacin: 6.6 mg/kg of 250 mg/mL solution q24
        - *Note: reduce systemic aminoglycoside therapy by 10% if aminoglycosides are concurrently nebulized*
     ii) Ceftiofur: 1 mg/kg of 25 mg/mL solution q12 h
   - Heparin: 5,000–10,000 IU q8 h
     i) *Note: this therapy is recommended in human fire victims but has not been reported in horses. Dose is extrapolated from human literature. Systemic administration of low-molecular-weight heparin (enoxaparin 0.35 mg/kg SQ Q24 for three doses) could also be considered*

3) Inhaled therapy
   - Albuterol: 720 μg inhaled q4–6 h in an adult
4) Bronchoscopic lavage
   - High-volume bronchoscopic lavage to clear soot and inflammatory debris is reported in humans and dogs. This therapy has not been reported in horses, but may be considered based on the quantity and character of lower airway debris, patient stability, and patient compliance.

### Post-Triage Continued Diagnostic Evaluation

Equine patients surviving a fire require continued close monitoring for at least the first 72 h after injury to identify latent consequences of fire exposure, particularly burn shock and respiratory tract compromise. Following an initial triage evaluation, serial physical examinations, bloodwork, and respiratory tract evaluation are recommended to maintain a comprehensive evaluation of the patient. Additional organ-specific therapies may be required based on clinical signs of organ dysfunction as a manifestation of burn shock.

## Triage and Management of Injuries Associated with Flood Exposure

Key points to remember for triage and management of injuries associated with flood exposure are summarized in Box 22.2.

### Flood Preparedness and Rescue

Horse owners are responsible for preparing for a safe evacuation of their horses prior to a significant flood. Local state animal response teams (SARTs) can provide resources for veterinarians and owners to help prepare farms for natural disasters. This preparation includes readying the animal for evacuation and securing the materials required to safely evacuate the horse. In order to be safely relocated, horses need to be haltered, easily accessible, and up to date on vaccinations, ideal with up to date microchips, Coggins tests, and health certificates (if time allows). The owner needs to secure a truck, trailer, and relocation barn and pack a basic emergency medical kit as well as three to five days' worth of hay and clean drinking water per horse. If a horse cannot be safely evacuated before a flood occurs, the horse should be let loose to seek high ground. Owners should **never** confine horses to a stall or barn during flood conditions. The owners' last name and phone number should be marked on the horse's dorsum with spray paint, permanent marker, livestock chalk, or etched with clippers.

Animal rescue teams are available in flood-prone areas, but these teams are frequently overwhelmed by animals in need during these disasters. These services do not replace owner preparation.

### Emergency Triage and Diagnostic Evaluation Following Flood Rescue

Equine flood victims are often stranded without access to shelter, food, or water for prolonged periods of time. Thus, systemic compromise and external trauma are common and a complete, systemic assessment of the patient must be performed. Common injuries and conditions associated with flood survival are outlined in Table 22.2.

1) Administer sedation as needed for safety
   - Xylazine: 0.5–0.75 mg/kg IV
   - Detomidine: 5–20 μg/kg IV
   - Butorphanol: 0.01–0.02 mg/kg IV

**Box 22.2 Key Points – Triage and management of injuries associated with flood exposure**

1) The likelihood that a horse survives a flood is heavily dependent on owner preparation. Owners should not consider emergency rescue services as an alternative to proper preparation.
2) Horses rescued from a flood are frequently affected by external trauma as well as systemic disease associated with chemical exposure and food and water deprivation. These systemic consequences may include cardiovascular shock, gastrointestinal, respiratory, or neurologic dysfunction, and require specific attention.
3) Bacterial or fungal cellulitis associated with standing water exposure can be extensive and require months to years of wound care with significant scarring.

**Table 22.2** Problems commonly associated with flood exposure.

| Traumatic injuries | Systemic diseases |
|---|---|
| *Musculoskeletal/cutaneous injuries*<br>• Wounds, lacerations, or penetrating foreign bodies of the head, neck, trunk, limbs, and hooves<br>• Dermatitis and cellulitis; bacterial or fungal<br>• Synovial or tendon sheath sepsis<br>• Fractures<br>• Thrush<br>• Laminitis<br>• Rhabdomyolysis<br>*Ophthalmic injuries*<br>• Corneal ulceration or laceration<br>• Uveitis | *Hemodynamic instability*<br>• Hypovolemia/dehydration<br>• Distributive shock/sepsis<br>• Cardiovascular arrhythmias or dysfunction associated with electrolyte derangements or toxin exposure<br>*Gastrointestinal dysfunction*<br>• Colic<br>• Colitis<br>*Respiratory diseases*<br>• Aspiration and secondary bronchopneumonia<br>• Upper and lower respiratory tract inflammation/edema<br>• Respiratory tract infections from co-mingling and immune compromise<br>*Neurologic diseases*<br>• Head and neck injuries<br>• Salt intoxication or other neurotoxin exposure<br>• Neurologic infections such as viral encephalidities, tetanus, and botulism |

- Horses that are fractious, panicked, or require emergency rescue transportation may need intravenous anesthesia, or "triple drip":
  i) Premedication: detomidine 5–20 μg/kg IV
  ii) Induction: ketamine 2 mg/kg IV +/− midazolam/diazepam 0.5–1 mg/kg IV
  iii) Triple drip protocols:
    1) 1L guaifenesin 5% with 500 mg xylazine and 1,000 mg ketamine
       - Rate of approximately 1–2 drop/second through a 15 mL drip set for a 450 kg horse (2 mg/kg/h)
    2) 1L saline bag with 25 mg midazolam (NOT diazepam) 650 mg ketamine and 325 mg xylazine
       - Rate of approximately 1 drop/second through a 15 mL drip set for a 450 kg horse (1.6 mg/kg/h)

2) Assess for signs of cardiovascular or distributive shock including tachycardia, tachypnea, arrhythmias, mucous membrane color and capillary refill time abnormalities, alterations in body temperature, altered mentation, and syncope
   - Obtain intravenous access and administer resuscitative fluids (20–30 mg/kg IV crystalloids or 4 mg/kg hypertonic saline followed by 10 L crystalloids IV) as needed.
3) Administer a tetanus booster if vaccination status is unknown
4) Perform a complete physical examination to classify injuries/diseases based on body system and severity. Specifically assess:
   - The location, depth, and contamination of wounds, paying attention to the hooves.
   - Both eyes for trauma and uveitis.
   - Neurologic, respiratory, and gastrointestinal function.
5) Perform point-of-care bloodwork as able including PCV/TS, L-lactate, complete blood count, and clinical chemistry
6) Perform point-of-care diagnostic imaging based on body system abnormalities as indicated by physical exam and point-of-care bloodwork
   - For example, radiography to identify fractures, synovial sepsis or transcutaneous thoracoabdominal ultrasound to assess respiratory and gastrointestinal dysfunction.
7) Decontaminate the skin
   - As conditions allow, horses should be bathed with a gentle shampoo to remove gross skin contamination. Clean the bottom of the hooves and assess for punctures. Deep wounds with suspected synovial involvement require sterile cleaning and lavage.
8) Administer anti-inflammatories
   - Phenylbutazone: 2.2–4.4 mg/kg IV or PO q12 h
   - Flunixin meglumine: 0.25–1.1 mg/kg IV or PO q8–12 h

Decision tree after initial evaluation of equine flood survivor

Consider farm management if:

1. Cardiovascular evaluation is normal
2. Neurologic disease is absent
3. There is no or minimal gastrointestinal or respiratory disease
4. Musculoskeletal or cutaneous trauma is minor, and fractures, synovial sepsis, or significant cellulitis/laminitis are not suspected
5. Ocular trauma is superficial without evidence of infection, uveitis is mild
6. Patient is willing and able to eat and drink

Consider referral management if:

1. Cardiovascular evaluation is abnormal
2. Neurologic disease is present
3. Gastrointestinal or respiratory diseases is moderate to severe
4. Musculoskeletal or cutaneous trauma is moderate to severe, and may include fractures, synovial sepsis, or significant cellulitis/laminitis
5. Ocular trauma is deep or with evidence of infection, uveitis is severe
6. Patient is unable or unwilling to eat or drink
7. Patient meets criteria for farm management but follow-up care is insufficient

Consider euthanasia if:

1. Musculoskeletal or cutaneous trauma is severe, and may include irreparable or open fractures, synovial sepsis, or severe cellulitis/laminitis
2. Neurologic disease makes the patient dangerous to handle or trailer
3. Patient meets criteria for referral management but this is not an option for the owner

**Figure 22.7** Management decision tree based on initial body system evaluation following flood survival.

## Important Decisions Following Initial Triage

Following initial triage the extent and severity of injury/disease associated with flood survival should be documented and categorized by body system. Under many circumstances, horses exposed to flood conditions simply need supportive care, wound management, feed, water, and shelter. However, there are several conditions which may be more appropriately managed in a referral setting. Understanding what care can be reasonably provided on the farm versus in a referral hospital can aid in this decision making. Referral should be considered for horses with signs of body system dysfunction (cardiovascular, neurologic, respiratory, gastrointestinal), or musculoskeletal injuries such as fractures, severe cellulitis/dermatitis or laminitis, or synovial sepsis. Based on the severity of these conditions and owner limitations, euthanasia may be recommended. Close veterinary follow-up, owner compliance, and owner education are requisite before considering on-farm management. Understanding what services can be provided on the farm versus in a hospital setting can aid in this decision making (Figure 22.7).

## What Can Be Done on the Farm Versus Referral Hospital

Many conditions associated with flood exposure can be successfully managed on farm including superficial injuries or lacerations, mild respiratory infections, mild gastrointestinal upset, and superficial or mild ocular disease. More serious conditions should be identified and stabilized on the farm while the decision for referral or euthanasia is made. In general, if the horse is willing and able to eat and drink, can urinate and defecate normally, and is free from neurologic disease, or significant lameness suggesting a fracture, synovial sepsis, severe cellulitis, or severe laminitis, farm management could be considered based on the specific client, veterinarian, and patient scenario.

## Post-Triage Care

Post-triage care for flood survivors can be variable and is heavily dependent on the patient's specific injuries. Many of these therapies can be initiated on farm, but continuous care necessitates referral.

### Cutaneous and Musculoskeletal Injuries

Lacerations and wounds should be evaluated for suspected chronicity, depth, degree of contamination, and location. Minor wounds and lacerations may be treated on farm with a primary closure, secondary closure, or delayed primary closure and bandaging based on the location of the wound and degree of contamination. Serial regional limb perfusions (amikacin at 250–1,000 mg daily; gentamicin at 2.2 mg/kg daily) can be performed for local antimicrobial therapy if indicated (this procedure is described in detail in Chapter 5). Systemic antimicrobials are also indicated unless the wound is superficial, fresh, and minimally contaminated - this is unlikely in flood survivors. If gentamicin is used both systemically and in a regional limb perfusion, reduce the systemic dose by 30% each day that a regional limb perfusion is performed. Wounds that are heavily contaminated, are associated with suspected synovial sepsis, or expose critical structures such as bone or tendons likely warrant referral management or euthanasia. Prior to referral the wound should be cleaned and wrapped if possible. An initial regional limb perfusion and antimicrobial administration can be performed prior to referral based on consultation with the referral center.

A primary source for any significant lameness should be identified. Horses with severe lameness should be evaluated for fractures, synovial sepsis, cellulitis, or laminitis. Identified fractures should be immediately stabilized (see Chapter 5) and referral versus euthanasia considered based on fracture location and classification. Minor lameness without wounds, evidence of infection, or palpable musculoskeletal abnormalities may be treated conservatively with rest and anti-inflammatories. Systemic conditions such as rhabdomyolysis or hoof diseases such as laminitis or severe thrush should be considered in horses with multiple limb lameness.

Severe cellulitis and dermatitis are common following flood rescue and may be caused by bacterial or fungal organisms (Figure 22.8). Cellulitis and dermatitis require prompt antimicrobial therapy to prevent infection of the deeper synovial structures (see Chapter 8). Fungal cellulitis or dermatitis should be suspected if granulomatous proliferations are present or lesions do not respond to antibiotic therapy, and is confirmed with biopsy and fungal culture. Prolonged standing water exposure often leads to skin sloughing. Sloughed wounds are managed similarly to burn wounds and may follow a similar prolonged, expensive course of treatment with significant infection and scarring (Figure 22.9).

Care should be taken to clean and dry the hooves and soles to assess for evidence of trauma, thrush, and white line diseases. Thrush medication and providine-iodine solutions can be used to treat diseased soles if punctures wounds are not suspected.

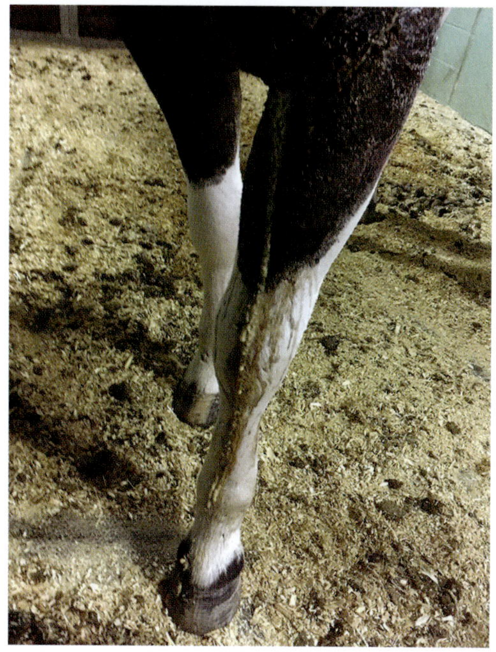

**Figure 22.8** Purulent exudate on the forelimb of horse rescued from flood conditions and standing water. Much of the skin overlying the forelimbs is necrotic and will slough over the ensuing days. *Source:* Courtesy of Dr. Caroline Burglass.

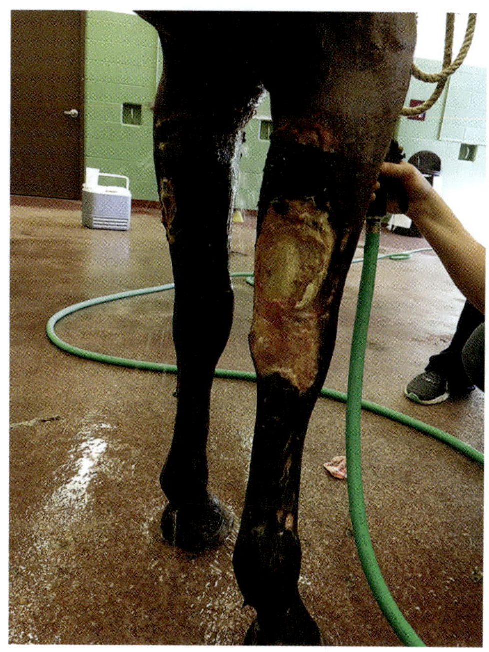

**Figure 22.9** Wounds and sloughed skin associated with standing water exposure. *Source:* Courtesy of Dr. Caroline Burglass.

### Ophthalmic Injury

Ophthalmic injuries associated with flood survival commonly include corneal abrasions and uveitis. A thorough ophthalmic examination should be performed so these injuries are not overlooked. Vision should be assessed in all horses rescued from floods, as visual deficits can exacerbate panic in already-stressed animals. Corneal abrasions, particularly with stromal loss, are likely to be infected and require aggressive treatment. Fungal keratitis should be suspected if melting corneal ulcers are present. Mild uveitis manifests as aqueous flare, blephrospasm, and miosis and should be treated to prevent progression. See Chapter 16 for detailed ophthalmic emergency protocols.

### Gastrointestinal Disease

Exposure to contaminated hay, grain, and water is common in horses surviving flood conditions and can lead to hypovolemia, colic, colitis, and endotoxemia. These conditions are identified during the triage physical exam and can be treated supportively with intravenous fluids, pain control, and anti-endotoxic therapies based on the needs of the individual animal.

Horses with evidence of moderate-to-severe colic or colitis are best managed in a referral center with continuous supportive care. Specific management of these conditions is described elsewhere (Chapter 10).

### Respiratory Disease

Bronchopneumonia associated with aspiration or contagious respiratory tract infections is common in horses surviving flood injury. The presence of these conditions can be identified at initial rescue with careful physical and diagnostic evaluation or may develop over the first few days to weeks of recovery. Specific management of these conditions is described elsewhere (Chapter 11).

### Neurologic Disease

Head and neck injuries, exposure to infectious agents, and ingestion of toxins or high salinity water are the most common neurologic consequences of flood survival. Suspected head and neck injuries resulting in proprioceptive, cranial nerve, mentation, or forebrain deficits should be emergently evaluated with diagnostic imaging (i.e., radiographs) as safety allows to identify bony instability or fractures. Referral or euthanasia should be considered based on the extent and location of damage. Seizures associated with cranial trauma can be controlled with 0.1–0.5 mg/kg diazepam or midazolam. Hypertonic saline at 1–2 mL/kg can be administered if cerebral edema is suspected and can be repeated in four hours if needed prior to referral.

Horses presenting with neurologic disease without obvious localizing signs of trauma need a complete neurologic examination to inform neurolocalization and assess of severity of the deficits. These horses should be evaluated for systemic conditions and infections that cause neurological deficits (i.e., salt toxicity). Horses with suspected salt toxicity should be managed in a referral setting since careful return to normonatremia is imperative to prevent cerebral edema. Advanced diagnostics such as CT, MRI, or CSF collection and analysis can be considered in a referral setting based on patient clinical status and suspected etiology of neurologic disease. Detailed management of neurologic emergencies is provided elsewhere (Chapter 15).

### Case Example 22.1 Barn Fire Injury

#### Case 1

A 10-year-old gelding presents three hours after surviving a barn fire. He presents with obvious pink to red burns along his muzzle, face, and dorsum. Wounds extend over approximately 15% of his body. At this time you determine an approximately even mix of first-degree and second-degree burns (few deep second-degree burns). He is agitated with a heart rate of 66 beats/min, respiratory rate of 16 breaths per minute, and temperature of 101.3 °F. Stall-side evaluation reveals the following:

PCV 48%, TS 7.2 g/dL (RR 30–40%, 6.0–7.5 g/dL)
L-lactate 3.6 mmol/L (RR < 2 mmol/L)

Question 1: What additional body systems are you most concerned about given the distribution of this horse's burns?
Answer: This horse is at high risk of respiratory complications (upper or lower respiratory tract) and ocular trauma based on the distribution of burns to the face. At the initial time of presentation, there is no obvious ocular trauma or uveitis, and he is eupneic despite his agitation. Nasal airflow is bilaterally symmetrical and appropriate.

Question 2: How might this horse's condition change over the next 72 h?
Answer: Secondary inflammation can cause progressive tissue dysfunction following a burn injury. *Specifically, over the next 72 h this horse may develop progressive:*

1) Cutaneous edema of the burned areas causing upper respiratory tract obstruction
2) Inflammation of the lower airways and secondary bacterial colonization
3) Evidence of ocular trauma
4) Cutaneous damage as the full extent of thermal damage is realized
5) Burn shock if <10% of the body is ultimately affected by deep second-degree burns.

Question 3: Define your management recommendations to the owner. Does this horse meet the criteria for attempted farm management, referral management, or euthanasia?

Answer: At the time of initial presentation, this horse clinically meets the criteria for farm management provided the client is compliant and there is the opportunity for careful veterinary follow up. If these requirements are not met, referral should be offered. An example field management plan for the owner for this patient could be:

1) *Therapeutic management/medication recommendations*
   a) Gentle cleaning of the burns and application of silver sulfadiazine or honey twice daily
   b) Anti-inflammatory and antibiotic therapy to prevent secondary bacterial bronchopneumonia
   c) Complete blood count and clinical chemistry performed at initial presentation.
2) *Monitoring*
   a) Take rectal temperature twice daily, call if >101.5 °F.
   b) Monitor for respiratory noises, such as "snoring" or coughing, and any swelling of the face or throat latch. If these signs are noticed, please call right away.
   c) Ensure the horse is eating and drinking voluntarily and in appropriate quantities. Ensure normal urination and defecation. If any concerns or signs of colic, please call right away.
   d) Perform no forced exercise, but ensure the horse can walk soundly and willingly on all four legs. Call if lameness develops.
   e) Monitor for any squinting or discharge from the eyes.
3) *Recommended follow-up*
   a) A daily veterinary visit is recommended for the next four days. At each visit the burn wounds will be assessed and a full physical examination will be performed. We will be specifically evaluating for progression of cutaneous (skin), respiratory, or ocular trauma, and development of secondary complications (i.e., impaction colic, trouble drinking).
   b) Daily PCV/TS and L-lactate will be measured for each of the four recheck days, with a repeat clinical chemistry and complete blood count performed on day 4 (sooner if clinically indicated).
   c) After day 4, weekly veterinary visits will be recommended to continue to evaluate wound healing and for secondary complications. This will likely occur for at least the next month.
   d) **At any point referral may elected and supported.**

## Further Reading

Freeman, C., Mirza, M., Pescosolido, K., and McConnico, R. (2015). Injuries and outcome of three horses hospitalised in the aftermath of Hurricane Isaac. *Equine Vet. Educ.* 27 (6): 308–315.

Hanson, R. (2005). Management of burn injuries in the horse. *Vet. Clin. North Am. Equine Pract.* 21 (1): 105–123.

Hatzfeld, A., Pasquesoone, L., Germain, N. et al. (2019). Benefits of cryopreserved human amniotic membranes in association with conventional treatments in the management of full-thickness burns. *Int. Wound J.* 16 (6): 1354–1364.

Herbert, E. (2017). Findings and strategies for treating horses injured in open range fires. *Equine Vet. Educ.* 30 (4): 177–186.

Johnson, J., McClure, S., and Liskey, C. (2010). Shockwave therapy for treatment of a burn injury in a horse. *Equine Vet. Educ.* 22 (2): 67–72.

Maciel, F., DeRossi, R., Módolo, T., Pagliosa, R., Leal, C., and Delben, A. (2012). Scanning electron microscopy and microbiological evaluation of equine burn wound repair after platelet-rich plasma gel treatment. *Burns* 38 (7): 1058–1065.

Marsh, P. (2007). Fire and smoke inhalation injury in horses. *Vet. Clin. North Am. Equine Pract.* 23 (1): 19–30.

McConnico, R. (2007). Flood injury in horses. *Vet. Clin. North Am. Equine Pract.* 23 (1): 1–17.

Miller, A., Elamin, E., and Suffredini, A. (2014). Inhaled anticoagulation regimens for the treatment of smoke inhalation-associated acute lung injury. *Crit. Care Med.* 42 (2): 413–419.

Norman, T., Chaffin, M., Johnson, M., Spangler, E., Weeks, B., and Knight, R. (2005). Intravascular hemolysis associated with severe cutaneous burn injuries in five horses. *J. Am. Vet. Med. Assoc.* 226 (12): 2039–2043.

Orsini, J., Divers, T., and Orsini, J. (2008). *Equine Emergencies*. St. Louis, MO: Saunders/Elsevier.

Osman, S., Umar, H., Hashmi, Y., Jawaid, A., and Ahmed, Z. (2022). The efficacy of honey compared to silver sulfadiazine for burn wound dressing in superficial and partial thickness burns—a systematic review and meta-analysis. *Trauma Care (Basel, Switzerland)* 2 (4): 523–534. https://doi.org/10.3390/traumacare2040043.

# 23

# Emergency Conditions of the Racehorse

*John Pigott*[1] *and Samuel D. Hurcombe*[2]

[1] *Cornell Ruffian Equine Specialists, Cornell University, Elmont, NY, USA*
[2] *Department of Clinical Studies - New Bolton Center, University of Pennsylvania School of Veterinary Medicine, Kennett Square, PA, USA*

## Specific Considerations

Emergencies in racehorses can occur at unique times at racetracks including entering a starting gate, during a race or race training, and in the post-race period. As such, track veterinarians including private practitioners and those affiliated with racing authorities should have familiarity with typical conditions commonly affecting racehorses and have a plan on how to provide emergency care. Further, attending veterinarians should understand several important considerations relevant to racehorses (Box 23.1).

Racehorses may also behave differently during periods of stress. Often the sympathoadrenal responses to racing and race training impact the physiological and behavioral responses to painful conditions. For example, a horse can still ambulate or even continue to run if they sustain a catastrophic injury during a race.

## Orthopedic Emergencies

### Emergency Triage Steps

#### History and Initial Patient Evaluation

A thorough history is important including duration of lameness, severity, and any previous treatments administered. Then, perform a thorough physical exam and quick assessment of overall patient stability. Lameness is a component of most orthopedic emergencies. Examine the horse for any obvious fractures, wounds, foreign bodies, soft-tissue swelling, joint effusion, elevated digital pulses, hoof tester sensitivity, or focal pain on palpation or limb manipulation. Assess the patient's pain level, degree of blood loss, and degree of shock that is present. Tetanus vaccine status should also be determined for any horse with a wound.

### Breakdown Injury with Disruption of the Suspensory Apparatus

1) Examination and assessment of stability: Look for instability in the fetlock region, with fetlock hyperextension typically observed during attempted weight bearing. Palpation and passive range of motion are used to assess stability and for regions of crepitus. Breakdown of the suspensory apparatus requires immediate first aid and fetlock immobilization through splinting to minimize secondary damage to the palmar/plantar vasculature and soft tissue during attempted weight bearing.
   Bandaging and initial immobilization: Any wounds are quickly cleaned with isotonic saline and a distal limb bandage placed. If fetlock or pastern instability is observed on physical exam, a Kimzey leg saver splint or similar splint is immediately placed over a light bandage until further diagnostics can be performed. Analgesics (typically phenylbutazone or flunixin meglumine) are administered after initial immobilization is achieved.

*Emergency Triage of the Horse*, First Edition. Edited by Rolfe M. Radcliffe and Jamie J. Kopper.

Companion website: www.wiley.com/go/radcliffe/triage

**Box 23.1 Important considerations for racehorse emergencies**

- Emergencies can occur in view of the general public. This requires special care and consideration when considering how to treat an emergency and the public's perception.
- Drug withdrawal times should be considered in any instance where the horse is administered certain medications and in active race training.
- Complex ownership of racehorses. It is common for a horse to be owned by a syndicate. Factors to consider include: who is the appropriate authority to make decisions? Is this a single person or must all shareholders agree on diagnostic and treatment decisions?
- Some racehorses are insured. Policies vary including major medical to mortality policies. It is essential owners and/or veterinarians (with policy holder permission) contact insurance adjusters to discuss the medical condition of the animal. Regardless, the provision of first aid and pain relief is an obligation while decisions are made.

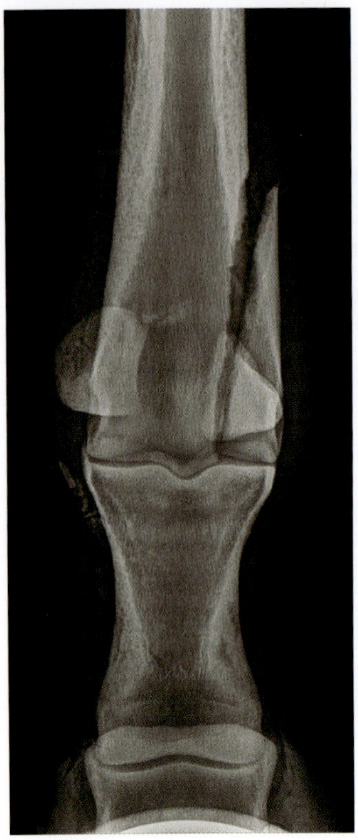

**Figure 23.1** Radiograph of a fetlock breakdown injury showing a displaced lateral condylar fracture with increased separation of the sesamoids secondary to sesamoid fracture and avulsion of the intersesamoidean ligament.

2) Imaging: Digital radiography is utilized next to characterize the injury, to provide prognostic information, and to determine if surgical repair is possible. During radiographic assessment, any metal splints will need to be removed, but the horse should not be allowed to bear full weight on the limb. A standard series of radiographs should be taken (DP, LM, DLPMO, DMPLO, Flexed DP) with any additional slight oblique projections to help further characterize the injury. Ensure the most proximal and distal extent of the injury is imaged. Some radiographic signs of suspensory apparatus breakdown include biaxial mid-body sesamoid fracture, increased medial–lateral separation of the sesamoids from axial sesamoid fracture and/or rupture of the intersesamoidean ligament, proximal displacement of the sesamoid bones from rupture of the distal sesamoidean ligaments, or distal displacement of the sesamoids seen with suspensory rupture (Figure 23.1).
3) Immobilization and transport: After imaging, any wounds are further cleaned or flushed with isotonic saline while an assistant is lightly supporting the limb. A distal limb bandage is placed followed by application of a splint to maintain the fetlock in flexion (Box 23.2). The Kimzey leg saver splint is commonly used and is acceptable for short distance transport but will not provide much medial to lateral stability. An alternative is to maintain slight fetlock flexion using a dorsal splint secured with cast material over the bandage, incorporating a heel wedge to help increase medial to lateral stability (Wright 2020). A bandage alone will not provide enough stability after suspensory apparatus disruption.
4) Referral center: Ultrasound is useful to evaluate the palmar/plantar digital vessels for flow and patency. Assessment of disruption of the suspensory and distal sesamoidean ligaments is also performed at the same time, but can be challenging due to edema, any subcutaneous gas if wounds are present, and the more typical, unweighted position of the leg.

   Foot viability: Any case considering surgical repair needs to have perfusion to the foot assessed. In addition to ultrasound assessment of blood flow, can palpate for digital pulses, check the hoof capsule for any warmth, and prick the coronary band with a needle while watching for bleeding.

**Box 23.2 Immobilization of a breakdown injury with disruption of the suspensory apparatus**

- Distal limb bandage.
- Splint to maintain the fetlock in flexion.

**Box 23.3 Immobilization of distal limb fractures not involving the suspensory apparatus**

- Distal limb compression bandage from foot to proximal metacarpus/metatarsus.
- Kimzey leg saver for comminuted P1 fractures.
- Kimzey leg saver or dorsal splint for uniaxial sesamoid fractures.
- Bandage cast extending from distal row of carpal/tarsal bones or bandage with medial and lateral splints for propagating medial or lateral condylar fractures.

Treatment: The treatment decision is typically between euthanasia or salvage with a fetlock arthrodesis as a non-athletic pasture pet or as a breeding animal. For cases with decreased blood flow to the foot, surgery is delayed (typically one to three days) with treatment initiated while monitoring blood flow to the foot. Treatment protocols vary but may involve intravenous fluids, aspirin, unfractionated or low-molecular-weight heparin, non-steroidal anti-inflammatories and/or dimethyl sulfoxide (DMSO). Systemic or local antibiotics should be administered for any open fractures or wounds in the region of the anticipated surgery site (Mudge and Bramlage 2007). If signs of compromised blood flow to the foot persists or worsens despite treatment, euthanasia is recommended.

#### Distal Limb Fractures Without Suspensory Apparatus Disruption

1) Examination: Perform a thorough physical exam and quick assessment of overall patient stability. Note any areas of swelling, pain on palpation, or crepitus. Fetlock hyperextension is not typically seen with this type of fracture.
2) Digital radiographs: A full set of radiographs are obtained including (DP, LM, DLPMO, DMPLO, Flexed DP). For lateral condylar fractures of the distal metacarpus/metatarsus, particularly if they are displaced, a 20° DMPLO view should be taken to assess the lateral sesamoid for a sagittal, axial fracture (Labbe and Pigott 2022). Examine the flexed DP views for evidence of palmar/plantar comminution along the fracture line and for pre-existing condylar disease. For propagating medial or lateral condylar fractures, a series of slightly obliqued radiographs are taken every 5–10° to characterize the orientation, while looking for additional fracture lines. CT or MRI can be very useful to characterize and to identify additional fracture lines. Imaging through the proximal extent of the metacarpus/metatarsus is important for any fracture with proximal propagation. For sagittal P1 fractures, examine for distal propagation on seemingly incomplete fractures and look for frontal plane components on lateral-medial views. All fractures should be assessed for signs of displacement or possible comminution along the fracture line.
3) Immobilization and transport: Immobilization of distal limb fractures not involving the suspensory apparatus is summarized in Box 23.3. A distal limb compression bandage that goes from the foot to the proximal metacarpus/metatarsus will be sufficient for most non-propagating condylar fractures and simple sagittal P1 fractures. The bandage can consist of a sterile or non-sterile cotton, secured on with brown gauze, Vetrap, and Elastikon. Additional layers of brown gauze and Vetrap can be added for additional compression and support. Transport of these fractures in a good bandage is typically sufficient. A Kimzey leg saver splint is frequently not necessary as this splint does not provide medial-to-lateral stability and tends to cause distal metacarpal/metatarsal condylar fracture displacement due to the flexed position. For comminuted P1 fractures, a bandage cast, cast, or compression boot is recommended, or a Kimzey leg saver for short distance transport. For uniaxial sesamoid fracture, a Kimzey leg saver or dorsal splint can be utilized. For propagating medial or lateral condylar fractures, a bandage cast that extends to the distal row of carpal/tarsal bones or a bandage with medial and lateral splints to the distal row of carpal/tarsal bones is typically sufficient (Wright 2020).

#### Carpal Fractures

Slab fractures of the third carpal bone do not typically need additional support besides a good bandage. If comminuted carpal fractures are present with associated instability in the carpus, a carpal tube cast is recommended from the distal cannon bone through the proximal antebrachium (Wright 2020).

## Cellulitis

1) Diagnostic approach: Rule out fracture or soft-tissue trauma as underlying cause for swelling. Treat the infection while monitoring response.

2) Examination: These horses can present with varying degrees of limb swelling, lameness, and fever. Examine the region of swelling for any puncture wounds, dermatitis, or other predisposing causes. Many will have no obvious external cause. In Thoroughbred racehorses, dorsal hock cellulitis is a common presentation with moderate-to-severe soreness to passive flexion and palpation. Palpate the digital pulses for any early signs of contralateral limb laminitis (see Laminitis). For pastern or distal limb swelling, examine the bottom of the foot for any punctures that could be causing ascending swelling. Palpate the swollen limb for any soft areas that could be consistent with deeper abscess formation.
3) Blood work: Frequently these horses will have elevated serum amyloid A (SAA) values, with either normal or elevated total nucleated cell count on complete blood count (CBC). More significant increases in total nucleated cell count can be observed with limb abscessation.
4) Imaging
   Ultrasound: Examine the soft tissues for any signs of abscess formation or compromise. Subcutaneous abscess formation is not uncommon and can develop anywhere along the cellulitic leg, although the medial aspect of the cannon bone adjacent to the suspensory or flexor tendons is a more typical location. Abscesses can develop inside the tendons or ligaments with the suspensory ligament, deep digital flexor tendon and distal sesamoidean ligaments as more common sites (Figure 23.2).

   Evaluate the synovial structures for any signs of sepsis (see Septic Synovial Structure). Ultrasound image quality may be decreased in the presence of severe inflammation, sometimes requiring repeat imaging in 24-48 h after starting treatment.

   Radiographs: Baseline radiographs should be taken to rule out fracture and to evaluate for signs of osteomyelitis and septic osteoarthritis on more persistent cases.
5) Treatment: Cellulitis is typically bacterial in origin with *Staphylococcus aureus* as a common cause. Any subcutaneous abscess visible on ultrasound should be drained through small stab incisions using ultrasound guidance with a culture taken of the purulent material and cytology performed. Anti-inflammatories and analgesics are administered to improve comfort. Cold hosing helps to provide analgesia and decrease swelling. Cold compression therapy is frequently not tolerated during the early phases of treatment for moderate-to-severe cases. Regional perfusion with antibiotics is effective at helping to treat the infection. This can be combined with systemic antibiotic therapy, but the risk of antibiotic-induced colitis should be assessed and considered in the management. Sweat bandages or dry compression wraps are applied to help decrease swelling. Some horses, particularly with prominent hock cellulitis, can react severely after placing a compression bandage over the painful hock. Epidural analgesia can be considered for severe hind limb cases. Foot support should be placed as part of initial management for any lame horse to try and prevent laminitis in the other feet. Cases that are not showing some clinical improvement after two to three days of treatment, should be re-assessed for possible joint or tendon sheath sepsis or abscess development.
6) Prognosis: Cellulitis in general has a good–excellent prognosis for return to racing as long as laminitis does not develop, abscesses do not develop inside the flexor tendons or ligaments, and the adjacent joints or tendon sheaths are not infected.

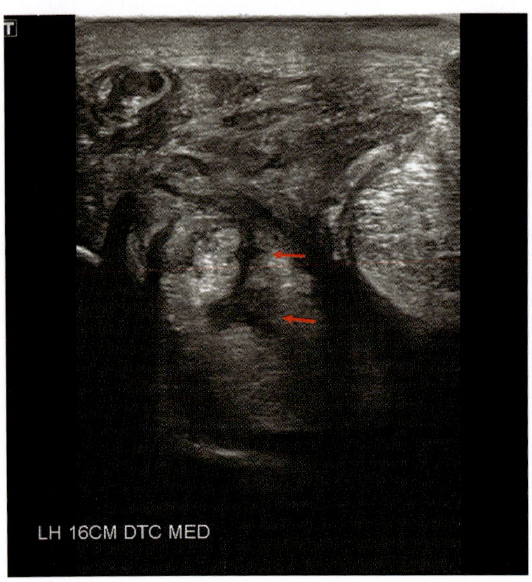


**Figure 23.2** Ultrasound of a left hind suspensory ligament viewed from the medial aspect of the limb located 16 cm distal to the chestnut. The image shows a suspensory body abscess that ruptured into the medial subcutaneous space.

## Septic Synovial Structure

1) Diagnostic approach: While diagnosis of synovial sepsis in some cases is obvious, many require multiple tools and pieces of information to arrive at the correct diagnosis.
2) Examination: Typically, lameness is present in the case of synovial infection ranging from mild to severe. Acute wounds over joints that have synovial communication without infection yet may not present with any significant lameness. Further, cases of chronic wounds with joint communication that allow egress of synovial fluid can present remarkably comfortable. Look for joint effusion or localized swelling around a joint, soreness to palpation, and passive flexion. Examine for the presence of any wounds or punctures over the synovial structure. Some will have varying degrees of cellulitis that can complicate the interpretation. A fever is not always present and is not a reliable indicator of synovial sepsis by itself.
3) Blood work: A CBC, serum chemistry, and SAA from a blood sample provides information about the degree of inflammation or infection present but is not conclusive by itself for synovial sepsis.
4) Imaging:
   Ultrasound: Ultrasound exam is another tool that provides useful information. Ultrasound findings that can be observed with synovial sepsis or synovial communication of a wound include intra-synovial fibrin, a more hyperechoic appearance to the synovial fluid, intra-synovial gas, and wound tracts that are observed to penetrate the joint capsule. In many joints, portions of the articular cartilage can be evaluated for thinning. Examination of tendons and adjacent ligaments in cases of suspected tendon sheath sepsis is important to evaluate for septic tendinitis.

   Radiographs: Digital radiographs should be performed in all cases of suspected synovial sepsis. Intra-synovial gas can be observed on some radiographs with wounds or sepsis. Chronic septic synovial structures can result in bony lysis, cartilage thinning, joint collapse, and secondary osteoarthritis.

   Magnetic resonance imaging (MRI): In cases of penetrating injuries to the foot, MRI can provide useful information about the tract location, relative to the navicular bursa, coffin joint, and digital sheath.
5) Synoviocentesis: Sampling of synovial fluid provides the most direct information regarding inflammation or infection in the structure. Sampling may be delayed one to two days in some cases if prominent cellulitis is present while the swelling is treated with regional limb perfusion, leg sweats with bandaging, and anti-inflammatories. If synovial fluid is obtained, the volume will dictate the analysis that can be performed. Gross evaluation for color, clarity, viscosity provides initial information. A CBC, total protein and cytology should be prioritized, with ancillary tests that could be considered including glucose, SAA, lactate, and pH. If minimal fluid is obtained, cytology from a smear is the recommended test (Steel 2008). With adequate volume obtained, a sample should be submitted for aerobic and anaerobic culture, with some persistent or more chronic cases submitted for fungal culture and microbial DNA sequencing in addition. Interpretation of the fluid analysis can be challenging in some cases with a large overlap area existing between primary inflammatory conditions and mild septic cases. In general, normal synovial fluid parameters include a total nucleated cell count less than 1,000 cells/μL, a total protein less than 2.0 g/dL and neutrophil percentage less than 10% (Box 23.4). Sepsis is generally presumed with a total nucleated cell count over 30,000 cells/μL, greater than 80% neutrophils, or a total protein greater than 4.0 g/dL (Steel 2008). But these numbers are not absolute cut offs with some septic synovial fluid having total nucleated cell counts under 10,000 cells/μL or a total protein less than 4.0 g/dL (Steel 2008). It is important to consider the synovial fluid analysis in combination with other clinical parameters.
6) Treatment on the farm: Standing needle lavage of the joint or tendon sheath can be considered on the farm in select scenarios, combined with antibiotic therapy. However, referral for more aggressive lavage and therapy is preferred. Standing needle lavage of a tendon sheath is frequently unrewarding due to subcutaneous fluid accumulation.

**Box 23.4 Normal synovial fluid parameters**

- Total nucleated cell count <1,000 cells/μL
- Neutrophil percentage <10%.
- Total protein <2.0 g/dL.

7) Treatment in the referral center: Arthroscopic or tenoscopic examination and debridement is preferred to allow high flow lavage, inspection of the cartilage or tendons, removal of fibrin, and debridement of any wound edges if present. A sample of synovium from surgery can be added to the culture sample to optimize the chances of a positive result. Needle lavage can be successful in some cases without significant fibrin accumulation. Small incisions with insertion of lavage cannulas can also be performed as an alternative. Placement of drains or leaving arthrotomy incisions open is an option for achieving ongoing drainage postoperatively. Local antibiotic therapy is a mainstay of treatment and can be achieved in multiple ways. Placing subpalpebral lavage tubing in the synovial structure at surgery allows for easy local antimicrobial administration postoperatively. Regional perfusion is another common antibiotic delivery mechanism for distal limb structures. Systemic antibiotics are frequently administered, but some cases can be managed with local therapy only. The risk of antibiotic-induced colitis should always be considered in the management of these cases. Judicious use of systemic non-steroidal anti-inflammatory drugs is recommended to decrease inflammation but not to mask clinical assessment of comfort.
8) Prognosis: Prognosis is variable depending on duration of sepsis, type of bacteria cultured, involvement of cartilage, bone, tendon, or ligament, and development of other complicating factors such as support limb laminitis. For more acute cases with early aggressive treatment, the prognosis is generally favorable for resolution and return to racing. More chronic cases can still have a positive outcome, but cartilage, bone, tendon, or ligament involvement can significantly lower prognosis for racing and resolution of the infection. Development of laminitis with radiographic changes secondary to chronic lameness will, in many cases, result in a poor racing prognosis depending on the severity.

## Laminitis

1) Diagnostic approach: In racehorses, laminitis tends to develop secondary to acute or chronic lameness issues causing uneven weight bearing, or secondary to systemic illness like colitis or pneumonia. Early recognition along with identifying and treating any predisposing factors is critical to help optimize outcome.
2) Examination: Laminitis can have multiple clinical presentations ranging from involvement of one to all four feet, with pain levels ranging from walking comfortably to recumbent. Evaluate digital pulses, willingness to pick up a limb and fully load the opposite limb, hoof tester response and pattern if positive. Palpate and inspect the coronary band for any separation and cleft development and the sole of the foot for any drainage, particularly near the toe. Watch the horse walk and circle in both directions looking for lameness or certain positions that exacerbate the lameness.
3) Digital radiographs: Good-quality radiographs with consistent positioning is critical to help identify laminitic changes and to follow any progression over time. Radiographs should be taken on a wooden block to allow complete visualization of the solar surface. A lateral–medial (LM) and dorsal–palmar/plantar (DP) projection should be taken of all four feet, even if the horse is initially presenting with only one lame limb. The x-ray generator is placed on the ground on a flat surface, so that sole depth can be evaluated. Placing radio-opaque paste or markers along the dorsal hoof wall to the coronary band can be considered, but subtle changes in placement can result in interpretation challenges. Measurements can be made on digital radiographs and compared to the other feet but also to published normal values for the breed. The measurements also serve to help document progression on serial radiographs.

   In general, the normal coronary extensor distance can be up to 10mm, the dorsal hoof capsule thickness up to 18 mm, and the sole depth greater than 11mm in Thoroughbreds (Sherlock and Parks 2013). In addition to measurements, evaluate to see if the dorsal margin of P3 is parallel to the dorsal hoof wall, for any roughness or irregularity in the dorsal margin of P3, particularly at the distal–dorsal tip, and for any gas in the subsolar surface or deep to the dorsal hoof wall. Ensure the dorsal hoof wall thickness is not increasing on serial radiographs, even if dorsal P3 remains parallel to the wall. On the DP view, evaluate the medial-to-lateral balance of P3 relative to the ground surface, and widening of the distance between P3 and the hoof capsule margin. Radiographic changes with laminitis can demonstrate predominately rotational changes of P3, unilateral or diffuse sinking of P3, or combinations of the two (Figure 23.3).
4) Venogram: A venogram provides additional prognostic information as well as documenting early changes in blood flow prior to the development of radiographic changes. Sedate the horse appropriately and perform an abaxial block on the limbs to be imaged. The feet to be imaged are placed on blocks. Place a tourniquet at the level of the fetlock and a 21-gauge butterfly catheter in the lateral or medial digital vein in the mid-pastern region. After placing an injection cap, inject iohexol or comparable intravenous contrast material into the vessel. Injection volume varies based on the size of the foot with most average-sized feet requiring 22–26cc. Leaving the catheter in the vessel, secure the tubing to the tourniquet with a piece of tape. Then perform a set of radiographs (LM, DP, unweighted LM) within 45 seconds of finishing the injection (Rucker 2010) (Figure 23.4).

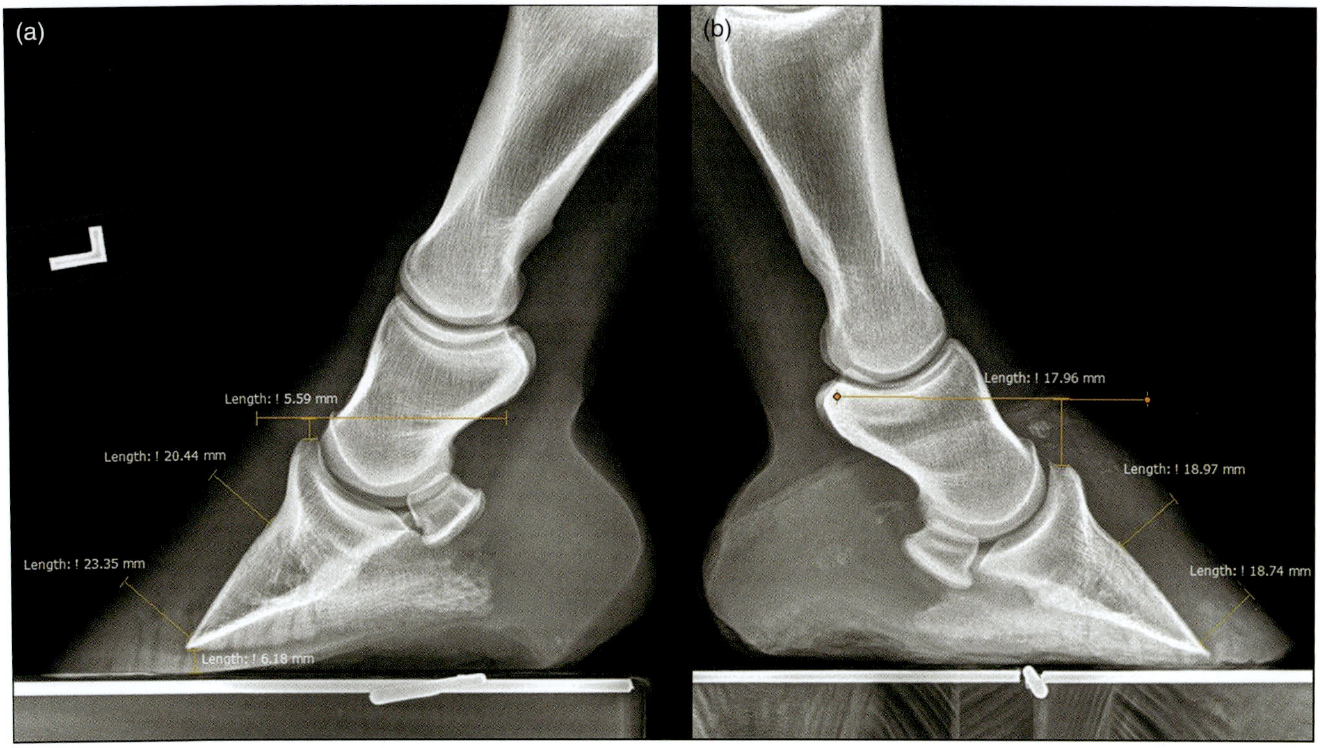


**Figure 23.3** Lateral foot radiographs from two different laminitis cases demonstrating measurements for sole depth, dorsal hoof wall thickness, and coronary extensor distance. (a) Predominately rotational laminitis observed. (b) Predominately sinking laminitis observed.

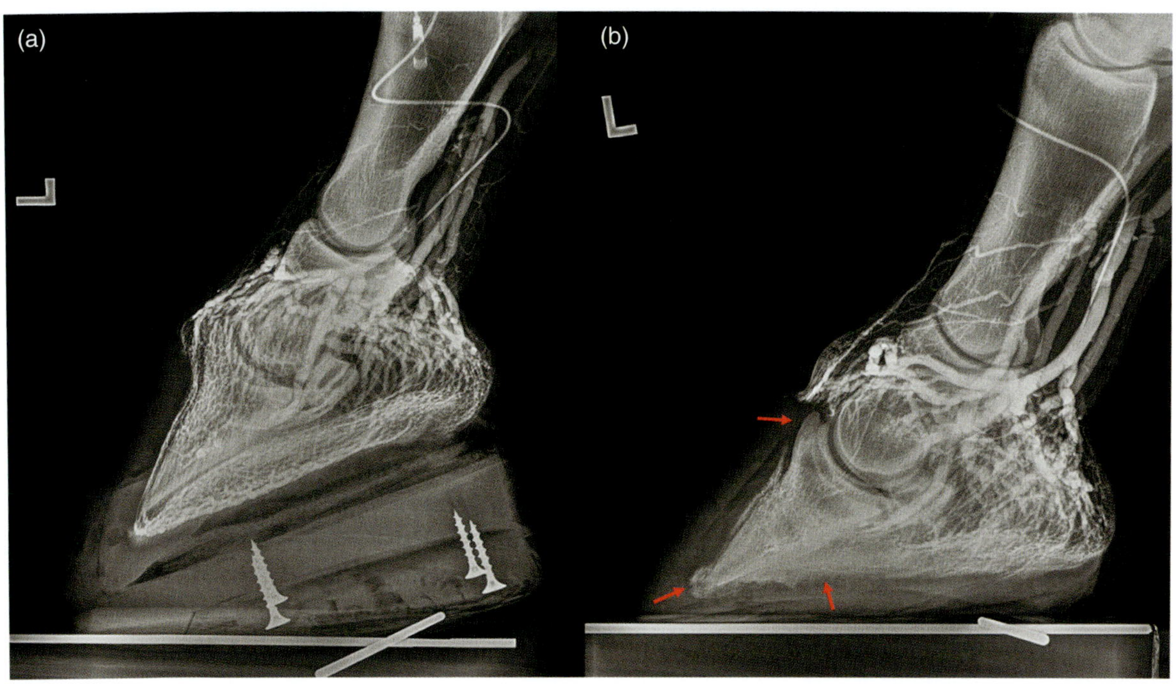


**Figure 23.4** Lateral radiograph from a venogram of the left front foot on a sinking laminitis case, 30 days apart. (a) Foot in a heel wedge with no significant changes. (b) 30 days later: foot flat on ground with reduced to absent contrast in dorsal half of coronary plexus, with displacement and distortion of the circumflex vasculature and reduced solar contrast fill along the dorsal half of P3.

5) Treatment: If there is an identified inciting cause (e.g., lameness, systemic illness), that needs to be addressed and resolved as quickly as possible. The hallmarks of laminitis treatment include foot support to help optimize mechanics while decreasing laminar stress, decreasing foot inflammation and rest to allow healing. Submerging the feet in continuous ice water decreases local inflammation and provides analgesia. Softening of the hoof capsule and sole can occur with ice water submersion for multiple days. Systemic analgesia is provided with non-steroidal anti-inflammatories, with some cases needing opioids or more involved constant rate infusions of analgesic medication. Foot support varies depending on the changes present on radiographs and the venogram with many incorporating a form of frog support in the mechanics, while trying to decrease laminar stress. Heel wedges to decrease strain on the deep digital flexor tendon are common in the acute phase, with clogs, foam support pads, or foot casts utilized for certain cases. Deep digital flexor tenotomy can be considered as a salvage procedure in severe cases with application of a P3 derotation shoe at the same time. Horses with diffuse sinking of P3 tend to be more unstable and are frequently a challenge to stabilize.
6) Prognosis: This depends on the severity, chronicity, and the degree of radiographic changes present. Racehorses that develop mild–moderate acute laminitis without radiographic changes can have a favorable chance at returning to racing if stabilized with appropriate healing. In general, Thoroughbreds with laminitis that develop mild radiographic changes have a guarded prognosis for racing. Thoroughbreds that progress to moderate or worse radiographic signs of laminitis typically have a poor prognosis for racing.

**Cardiac Emergencies – Dysrhythmia**

A cardiac event can be challenging in racehorses, particularly if a rhythm disturbance is paroxysmal or episodic in nature. A full cardiac evaluation is recommended as part of a comprehensive poor performance evaluation. Please also see Part 2, Chapter 12 for additional information on cardiovascular emergencies

1) Examination: Often there are no obvious external signs. Dysrhythmia with congestive heart disease (i.e., secondary to a congenital anomaly) or severe pleural space disease (i.e., pleuropneumonia) might have distended jugular veins with a prominent jugular pulse. Jugular fill should always be evaluated with the horse's head in a neutral upright position. If the veins are full and a jugular pulse is observed higher than the lower 2/3rds (i.e., toward the linguofacial/maxillary bifurcation), this is abnormal. Assessment in horses with low head carriage will increase venous fill and should not be overinterpreted as abnormal.

   Auscultation of the heart (and lungs) is essential: Rhythm disturbances and murmurs may be detectable. Atrioventricular (AV) blocks (second and third) can be suspected based on auscultation findings. First-degree AV block will not be detectable by auscultation.

   Atrial flutter/fibrillation (AF) is a common cause of poor performance in racehorses and can be suspected during auscultation as an irregularly irregular rhythm and no discernable S4 heart sound. Any rhythm disturbance must be qualified by an electrocardiogram before considering treatment with an antiarrhythmic medication.
2) Electrocardiogram (ECG): A simple base–apex (+ left heart; – and ground right jugular furrow) lead approximates lead II and is often all that is required to make a diagnosis of common rhythm abnormalities such as second-degree and third-degree AV block, atrial premature complexes, ventricular premature complexes, AF, sinus tachycardia, and ventricular tachycardia. Paper speed is set to 25 mm/s.
3) Blood work: Electrolyte and acid–base disturbances can create a permissive metabolic environment for the generation of some dysrhythmias (i.e., alkalosis, hypokalemia predisposing to AF). Other causes of localized or systemic inflammation can also predispose to dysrhythmia.

   Minimum database blood work should include CBC, PCV/HCT, Fibrinogen/SAA, electrolytes. A venous blood gas analysis including pH, ionized calcium, magnesium, potassium, $p_VO_2$, $p_VCO_2$, and $HCO_3^-$ (or $TCO_2$, base excess/deficit) as well as cardiac troponin I (CTnI) is also recommended when cardiac disease is suspected.
4) Referral services: Treatment for cardiac disease should be done in a hospital setting where close monitoring, continuous ECG assessment, and ability to swiftly treat potential side effects can be done efficiently.
   a) Imaging: A complete echocardiogram is recommended to assess the structure of the heart. While lone AF (without structural changes) is a common cause of poor performance in racehorses, ruling out structural changes is important before starting treatment and to better prognosticate. This can be done in the hospital setting or stall-side where available mobile ultrasonography service is available.
   b) Treatment: Treatment is based on the rhythm diagnosis and other diagnostic findings, i.e., blood work abnormalities or imaging findings. Some cases simply require treatment of a primary condition and provision of rest followed by a slow return to training. Others require the administration of antiarrhythmic medication that, while therapeutic, can have unwanted potentially life-threatening side-effects necessitating emergency treatment.

### Respiratory Emergencies

Respiratory disease is very common in racehorses and in racehorse barns. Husbandry practices including indoor housing, congregation of a large cohort of often young horses, horse handlers interacting with multiple horses, transportation stresses, and movement of horses from various locations create a perfect environment for the introduction and spread of infectious respiratory disease that can affect many horses in a barn (i.e., upper respiratory viruses, and Streptococcal disease) or individuals in a barn (pneumonia, pleuropneumonia from various causes). Racehorses are also at risk for non-infectious diseases such as inflammatory airway disease (IAD) and the various types (neutrophilic, eosinophilic, metachromatic) and exercise-induced pulmonary hemorrhage (EIPH). Additional information on respiratory emergencies can be found in Part 2, Chapter 11.

1) Examination: Perform a complete physical examination including rectal temperature, respiratory rate, and effort. Note coughing frequency and presence/absence of nasal discharge. Palpate submandibular and retropharyngeal lymph nodes for enlargement and/or pain.
   Respiration pattern/effort:
   - Rapid, shallow breathing is suggestive of pleural space disease.
     - Focus your assessment on the lower respiratory tract first.
   - A long inspiratory phase +/− stridor is suggestive of laryngeal disease.
     - Focus your assessment on the upper respiratory tract first and consider if an emergency tracheostomy is indicated (marked inspiratory stridor, swollen retropharyngeal region). When in doubt, place a tracheostomy tube. When a specific tube is not immediately available, a clean, cut off nasogastric tube placed into the proximal trachea via the nares can temporarily suffice.

   Auscultation: this is essential to perform and best done in a quiet environment out of the elements (wind, etc.) or noisy areas. Auscult all lung fields (left and right).

   Rebreathing exam: In patients with minimal distress or effort, a rebreathing examination helps to make the horse breathe deeper facilitating auscultation through rebreathing exhaled carbon dioxide ($CO_2$). A safe way to perform this is by placing a muzzle over the nose then placement of a well-fitted plastic bag over the muzzle. The muzzle aids in minimizing distress of the patient, particularly if they suck in the plastic during a deep inspiration. When the patient is visibly perturbed by the rebreathing phase, release the plastic bag and listen as the horse takes deeper breaths.

   Absence of adventitial lung sounds could indicate pleural space disease (pleural fluid or air). Muffled heart sounds can indicate pleural fluid.
2) Diagnostic testing: Minimum database should include a CBC and acute inflammatory biomarker such as fibrinogen and/or SAA.
3) Imaging:
   Endoscopy – upper airway endoscopy is indicated for cases of suspected upper airway obstruction or disease or tracheal endoscopy for cases of recent hemorrhage.

   Transthoracic ultrasound is indicated for cases of suspected pleural space disease and/or parenchymal disease. Note – marked parenchymal disease can still be present deep to the pleural surface despite a normal thoracic ultrasound.

   Thoracic radiographs are indicated for cases of suspected parenchymal disease especially when an ultrasound is unrewarding as this can show small airway disease, deep abscesses, evidence of pneumonia, and hemorrhage.
4) **Bronchoalveolar lavage (BAL)** is indicated in cases of non-infectious lower airway disease such as IAD or EIPH. Cytological assessment of BAL fluid is essential for a diagnosis.
5) Infectious disease testing:
   Upper respiratory infectious diseases: where multiple risk factors are present, or clinical findings are indicative of infectious disease, nasal swabs and blood (EDTA tube) should be collected for PCR analysis of common respiratory pathogens (EHV-1, EHV-4, ERVA, Influenza, *Streptococcus equi equi*).

   Pneumonia/pleuropneumonia: aerobic and anaerobic culture of the airway is recommended. A transtracheal wash (TTW) or endoscopically obtained guarded transtracheal aspirate (TTA) is the sample of choice. Strict aseptic technique should be employed when obtaining this sample to avoid contaminants.
6) Treatment in the field: reserved for mild cases requiring less intense treatment, i.e., once/twice a day antibiotics or anti-inflammatories.
7) Referral: Indications for referral of a respiratory patient including moderate or severe respiratory disease, need for oxygen provision, need for IV therapy (including antibiotics and fluids), need for indwelling chest tubes for drainage and pleural lavage, need for imaging or diagnostics when not available in the field (i.e., BAL, TTW, thoracic radiographs).

### Gastrointestinal Emergencies

True gastrointestinal emergencies may include acute colic (abdominal pain) or acute diarrhea syndromes and warrant immediate evaluation and treatment. Colic and diarrhea can occur in any horse; however, racehorses are at higher risk than other cohorts for certain types of colic.

The diagnostic approach to colic in the racehorse is not unique; however, the practitioner should consider factors specific to the patient including training type and schedule and diet.

Almost all racehorses have some grade of squamous gastric ulceration that is rarely an emergency to treat. However, pain after eating (post-prandial), hypersalivation, and poor performance could indicate clinically significant gastric ulcer disease. Emergency diagnostics are seldom indicated. Gastroscopy is recommended to confirm the presence and severity of ulcers in both the squamous and glandular regions.

An important factor for a practitioner to consider are the colic lookalikes such as laminitis or exertional rhabdomyolysis "tying up" which racehorses are commonly affected by.

See gastrointestinal emergencies (Part 2, Chapter 10) for more specific details on the diagnostic evaluation of colic in horses with abdominal pain.

1) Examination: As with all emergencies, the basis for developing an accurate differential list and treatment plan starts with a thorough physical examination, remembering that there are many colic lookalikes that owners will report as "colic." Additionally, some horses will have acquired co-morbidities (i.e., corneal ulceration, lacerations with the potential for synovial structure involvement) that may require concurrent treatment to ensure a positive outcome.
2) Diagnostics: Diagnostics to consider, depending on the horse and situation, include
   a) Abdominal palpation per rectum and passage of a nasogastric tube.
   b) Transcutaneous thoracic and abdominal ultrasound.
   c) Hematological evaluation including PCV/TP, blood L-lactate, CBC, and/or serum chemistry.

   The goal of these diagnostics is to evaluate the horse for evidence of systemic compromise, abnormalities that are not consistent with gastrointestinal disease and/or evidence of colic requiring surgical correction.
3) Treatment and stabilization in the field: Regardless of the cause of an acute gastrointestinal emergency, supportive care is always indicated, even before some specific diagnostics are performed. Supportive care aimed at normalizing derangements of hypohydration/dehydration and metabolic disturbances is recommended.

   Fluid provision: oral rehydration solutions (water, water and electrolytes) are recommended in horses with no enterogastric fluid accumulation (always check for reflux first) and who are mildly dehydrated (estimated <5%). Parenteral fluids using isotonic crystalloids, preferably balanced (Lactated Ringer's solution, Hartmann's solution, Plasmalyte-A, Plasmalyte-148) should be provided to horses with enterogastric reflux and/or moderate-to-severe clinical dehydration (>5%). Rates of 60–120 mL/kg/day are safe and supportive.

   For horses with severe dehydration or evidence of shock (see SIRS/Sepsis and Shock Part 3, Chapter 18), hypertonic saline solution (7.2%; HSS) can be given at 2–4 mL/kg IV as a bolus.

   Analgesia: Analgesia is important both for the welfare of the horse and the safety for those working around the horse. Part 4, Chapter 31, provides a list of medications, dosages, and side effects to consider. Remember that it is important to communicate and record all administered medications to racing authorities with consideration of drug withdrawal times. Common medications with analgesic properties used for horses with abdominal pain include:

   Flunixin meglumine (NSAID): 1.1 mg/kg IV.
   Xylazine hydrochloride (sedative): 0.5–1.0 mg/kg IV, IM.
   Butorphanol tartrate (opioid): 0.1 mg/kg IV, IM.
   *N*-butylscopolammonium bromide (spasmolytic): 0.3 mg/kg IV.
   Lidocaine continuous rate infusion (CRI): 1.3 mg/kg IV over 15 minutes, 0.05 mg/kg/min.

   Supportive care: Depending on the cause of colic consideration should be given to nutrition (i.e., holding off feed versus small volume low bulk diets) and exercise (i.e., hand walking to promote GI motility).
   For cases requiring IV fluids or those that do not respond to analgesia referral is recommended for additional diagnostics, more intensive medical therapy and/or surgical exploration.

### Ocular Emergencies

Periorbital and globe emergencies are common in racehorses. Racehorses are at risk for injury from blunt-force trauma, whip-related globe injury, and foreign body injury from flying debris (kick-back injury). Every effort should be made early to evaluate and treat an injured or infected eye to preserve vision and save the eye. Enucleation should be considered a last option in most cases. Additional information regarding ophthalmic emergencies can be found in Part 2, Chapter 16.

1) Examination: a complete ocular and periocular examination is essential in any horse showing signs of epiphora, blepharospasm, swelling, changes in corneal color and clarity, or any discharge.

   Examination may require sedation, staining techniques, and local anesthesia (blocks) to fully evaluate the globe including the nictitans gland and periorbital structures. See ophthalmology emergencies (Part 2, Chapter 16) for a review of a complete ophthalmology examination.
2) Empirical treatment:
   a) Eye lavage: commercial eye wash solutions are ideal. Never use water or antiseptic solutions.
   b) Broad-spectrum topical antibiotics: topical antibiotic ointments or solutions of medications that do not contain corticosteroid are recommended.
   c) Broad-spectrum systemic antibiotics: for more serious injury or disease, systemic therapies may be warranted such as penicillin and gentamicin.
   d) Antiprotease therapy: autologous serum or EDTA-plasma should be considered.
3) When to treat at the barn
   a) Mild injury (eye mostly open, minimal to no pain), non-progressive disease, vision intact. Fluoresceine positive, superficial lesions.
4) When to refer
   a) Injury or disease that is causing vision impairment, progressive disease, corneal changes (cloudiness, melting cornea (keratomalacia), foreign body or laceration, descemetocele), blunt trauma including head trauma. Horses that are fractious or difficult to medicate should also be referred. These cases often require placement and maintenance of a subpalpebral lavage tube to ensure effective treatment of the eye.

#### Neurologic Emergencies

Spinal ataxia is common in racehorses. Common causes of spinal ataxia including trauma, equine protozoal myelitis (EPM), and cervical vertebral stenotic myelopathy (CVSM; Wobbler syndrome) can cause subtle-to-significant gait abnormalities that represent a safety risk to the horse, rider and handler. Please see Part 2, Chapter 15, for additional information regarding neurological abnormalities in the horse.

1) Examination: Assessing a horse for possible ataxia or other neurological disease must start with a thorough physical examination and neurological assessment. After completing a physical examination, a neurological assessment includes three components:
   a) Mentation Assessment.
   b) Cranial Nerve Assessment.
   c) Gait Assessment.
2) Once an examination has been completed, this information can be used to determine a neurolocalization for the horse, as described in the neurological emergencies chapter.
3) The majority of racehorses neurolocalize to C1–C5 due to spinal cord compression (Cervical Vertebral Stenotic Malformation/CVSM/Wobblers or a traumatic injury) or Equine Protozoal Myeloencephalitis (EPM). Assuming that the horse has neurolocalized to C1–C5 the following diagnostic steps should be considered:
   a) Cervical radiographs to assess for overt signs of trauma, canal stenosis, or malalignment of the vertebrae.
   b) Assuming no abnormalities were identified on cervical radiographs, further assessment for EPM with assessment of serum immunodiagnostic testing of blood and cerebral spinal fluid (CSF).
      i) It is incredibly important to remember that in most areas of the US most horses have been exposed to EPM; thus, positive serology cannot be used to diagnose EPM. EPM is widely over-diagnosed and over-treated. A horse with negative serology for EPM most likely does not have the disease; however, repeat testing can be performed in two weeks to ensure that the horse did not seroconvert.
      ii) As described, if the horse is positive on serology for EPM, further testing should include collection of CSF for cytology and immunodiagnostics.
      iii) If EPM testing is negative, further testing would include assessing vitamin E levels and a myelogram to better assess the horse for area(s) of stenosis.
4) Treatment: Acute general treatment for cervical ataxia includes supportive care (anti-inflammatory medication, ensuring adequate hydration and nutrition) and ensuring a safe environment for the horse and those handling it, depending

on its degree of ataxia. Acutely, moderately to severely affected horses may need to be stall confined. Empirical treatment for EPM may be instituted until testing results are received to confirm or rule out a diagnosis.

5) Referral: Referral should be considered for horses that are moderately to severely ataxic and at risk for becoming recumbent or in need of intensive supportive care, or in need of a myelogram or CSF collection if it is not feasible in the field.

**Case Example 23.1 Septic Synovitis**

You are presented with a 3-year-old race filly with a non-weight bearing lameness of the left forelimb. The filly had intra-synovial injection of the right and left radiocarpal joints with triamcinolone and hyaluronic acid performed seven days prior.

1) **What are four to five differential diagnoses to consider for a horse with a non-weight bearing lameness?**
   Fracture of the limb.
   Hoof abscess.
   Cellulitis.
   Non-septic joint flair or inflammation.
   Septic synovitis.
2) **Describe a diagnostic plan to help you arrive at a definitive diagnosis for this patient.**
   Start with a thorough physical examination of the horse and specifically of the affected limb. With cellulitis there should be palpable swelling or edema, typically of the distal limb extending proximally. For a fracture, there should also be localized swelling and/or instability upon palpation if there is not obvious deformity of the limb (the exception being fracture of the third phalanx). Horses with septic synovitis often have pain and swelling of the associated joint. If the limb otherwise appears unremarkable on your examination you can consider using regional diagnostic analgesia (i.e., a palmar digital and/or abaxial) nerve block to rule out the hoof as a source of lameness.
   Examination of the left forelimb reveals radiocarpal joint effusion and pain upon palpation of the joint.
3) **Based on this finding what are your top differential diagnoses and diagnostic tests that you can consider?**
   Given the history and examination findings septic synovitis or a non-septic joint flair/inflammation are top considerations, with preference given to septic synovitis. Additional diagnostic testing that can be considered include:
   - Complete Blood Count (CBC), Serum amyloid A (SAA), and serum chemistry to look for evidence of systemic inflammation, although this is not conclusive.
   - Ultrasonographic evaluation of the radiocarpal joint to assess it for intra-synovial fibrin or thinning of the articular cartilage.
   - Radiographs should be performed to look for evidence of bony lysis, cartilage thinning, joint collapse, and secondary osteoarthritis.
   - Synoviocentesis to obtain a joint fluid sample to assess for:
     - Gross evaluation of color, clarity, viscosity.
     - Differential cell count, total protein, and cytology.
     - Culture.
     - If large enough volume fluid sample is obtained can also consider glucose, SAA, lactate, and pH.
4) **You obtain a synovial sample with the following results:**
   a) **Gross appearance: Hazy, orange with decreased viscosity.**
   b) **Differential cell count: 75,000 total cell count/μL with 95% non-degenerate neutrophils, no organisms observed, total protein of 4.5 g/dL.**

   **Based on these results, what is your diagnosis for this horse?**
   Septic synovitis likely secondary to intra-articular injection.
5) **What is your recommended treatment plan for this horse?**
   Ideally, the horse should be referred for arthroscopic examination, debridement, and high flow lavage. Post operatively the horse may receive local antimicrobial therapy, systemic antimicrobial therapy, repeat lavage and/or regional limb perfusion depending on the findings and course of treatment. If referral is not an option standing needle lavage can be attempted with local and systemic antimicrobial therapy; however, prognosis for survival and athleticism is likely decreased compared to a more aggressive approach.
6) **What are common complications associated with septic synovitis?**
   Failure to resolve the infection, osteoarthritis secondary to cartilage damage, contra-lateral limb laminitis.

## References

Labbe, K.A. and Pigott, J.H. (2022). Radiographic technique to improve diagnosis of sagittal axial sesamoid fracture in racing Thoroughbreds with lateral condylar fracture. *Equine Vet. Educ.* 34 (4): 200–206.

Mudge, M.C. and Bramlage, L.R. (2007). Field fracture management. *Vet. Clin. N. Am. Equine Pract.* 23 (1): 117–133.

Rucker, A. (2010). Equine venography and its clinical application in North America. *Vet. Clin. N. Am. Equine Pract.* 26 (1): 167–177.

Sherlock, C. and Parks, A. (2013). Radiographic and radiological assessment of laminitis. *Equine Vet. Educ.* 25 (10): 524–535.

Steel, C.M. (2008). Equine synovial fluid analysis. *Vet. Clin. N. Am. Equine Pract.* 24 (2): 437–454.

Wright, I.M. (2020). Racetrack fracture management and emergency care. In: *Equine Fracture Repair*, 2e (ed. A. Nixon), 44–82. New Jersey: Wiley Blackwell.

# 24

# Emergency Conditions of Draft Horses

Garett Pearson[1] and Eileen S. Hackett[2]

[1] Department of Clinical Studies - New Bolton Center, University of Pennsylvania School of Veterinary Medicine, Kennett Square, PA, USA
[2] Department of Clinical Sciences, College of Veterinary Medicine, Cornell University, Ithaca, NY, USA

## Introduction

Early recognition and intervention are particularly important in draft horse emergencies. Due to their size, emergency conditions requiring general anesthesia (i.e., colic surgery, dystocia) are inherently higher risk. Surgeons and anesthetists should be acutely aware of these risks (i.e., myelomalacia, myopathy) and will prioritize expedient surgery where possible, optimize oxygenation and blood pressure support as well as proactive recovery support (head, tail ropes, and/or sling assistance) routinely (Figure 24.1). Because these are such large horses, some consider draft horse medicine and husbandry a sub-specialty for veterinarians and farriers. This chapter outlines key features and pathophysiology of disease specific to draft horses.

## Defining Draft Breeds

Draft horses are large-bodied horse breeds such as Percherons, Belgians, Shires, Clydesdales, Friesians, the Suffolk Punch and Gypsy Vanners. These breeds are uniquely different to Warmblood or hot-blooded breeds due to their size (height (often >16 hands) and weight (often >600 kg)), heavy muscling, coloring, and specific phenotypic features. While some may be kept as pets, they are typically show or working animals, used for pulling machinery or carts for logging and farming activities. These factors can contribute to owner decision making and should be considered. The use of these horses has evolved which has resulted in breeding for specific characteristics including increased height, weight, and foot confirmation. In addition, hazards of their public work, such as parades and police work, can present environmental difficulties. Draft horses require appropriate equipment and facilities to accommodate their increased size. This includes stocks, headstands, halters, instrumentation, endoscopes, and fluid poles with adequate height, etc. (Figure 24.2). Additionally, the sheer size of these horses can limit diagnostic capabilities and modalities available. Draft horses present a unique challenge in the emergency setting because of these features as well as their often stoic nature. Veterinarians must rely not only on abnormalities observed during a physical examination (i.e., wound, abnormal rectal exam, etc.) but also the physiologic parameters (Figure 24.3). Veterinarians should rely less on expected behavioral changes that might be observed in other breeds. For example, a draft horse with a colonic volvulus may not present with overt signs of abdominal pain such as pawing, rolling, and striking, but rather, stand quiet and stoic with an elevated heart rate (e.g., 100 beats/min) (Figure 24.4). Prognosis should be relayed with the distinct features of the draft horse in mind.

## Pharmacology

Given the large size of draft horses and difficulty in accurately calculating drugs based on body surface area, start at the low end of standard dose rates based on body weight alone to minimize potential drug overdoses. For example, if the daily maintenance fluid rate is 40–60 mL/kg/day, start conservatively at 40 mL/kg/day, reassess the patient and

*Emergency Triage of the Horse*, First Edition. Edited by Rolfe M. Radcliffe and Jamie J. Kopper.

Companion website: www.wiley.com/go/radcliffe/triage

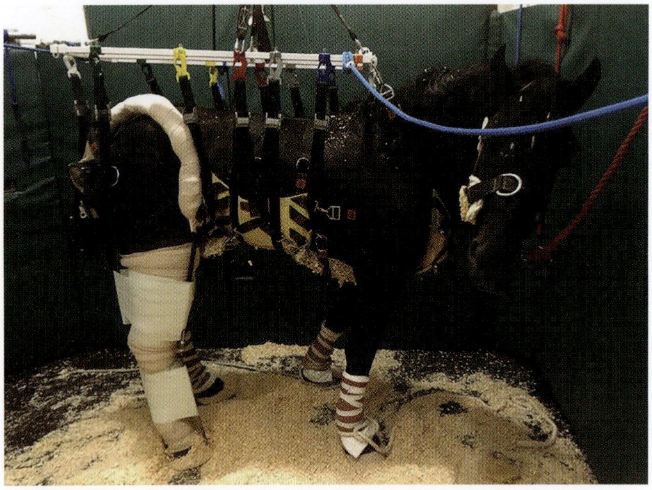

**Figure 24.1** A draft horse placed in the Anderson Sling for recovery. Because of the increased incidence of complications, such procedures may be necessary during recovery from anesthesia in the draft horse. *Source:* Courtesy of Dr. Jackie Hill.

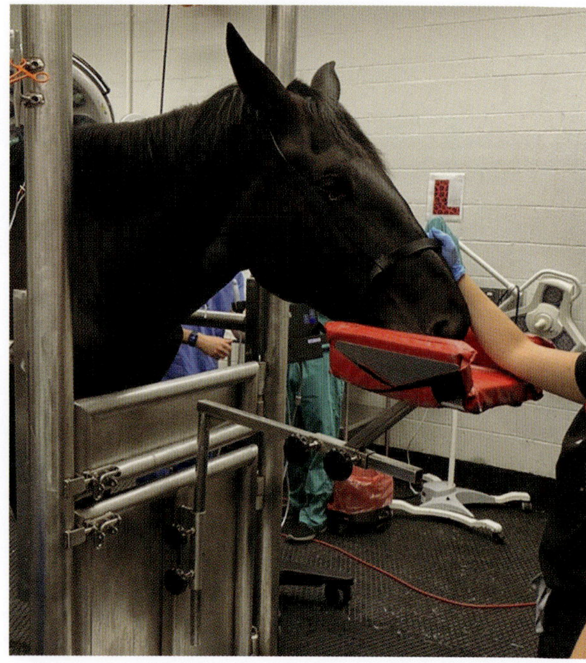

**Figure 24.2** Stocks built with ample height, adjustable head stand, and side bars to accommodate larger horses work well for draft horses.

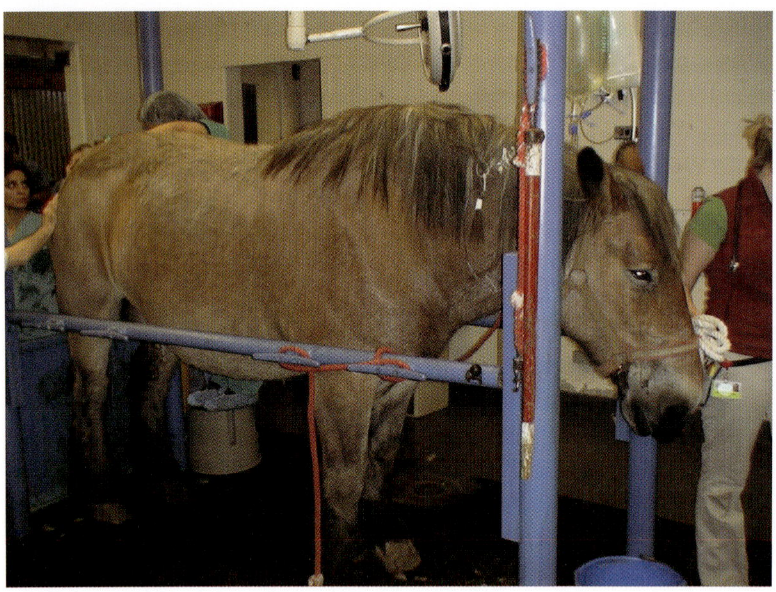

**Figure 24.3** A thorough physical examination of the sick draft horse is imperative. A concise yet thorough evaluation of body systems and recognition of the most common problems of draft horses will facilitate efficient emergency triage.

adjust the rate based on clinical examination of hydration. Desired effect can often be observed with conservative dosing, particularly in cardiovascular medications, sedatives, and anesthetic agents (Goble 2011). Sedation and anesthesia dosing in draft horses should be reduced by 10% (Branson 2011). For draft horses receiving surgery, it is reported that horses >680 kg had longer duration of anesthesia, increased incidence of postoperative morbidity, and reduced short-term survival of 60% compared to lighter horses. Additionally, the large size of draft horses often results in higher cost of treatments.

## Airway Disorders

Laryngeal disfunction is common in draft horses (Hackett and Leise 2018). Acute arytenoid cartilage collapse can be a source of life-threatening emergency. Acute airway obstruction can result in distress, collapse, and even death. Recurrent laryngeal neuropathy, which can predispose to arytenoid cartilage collapse, occurs in 35% of competition draft horses. There is a difference in incidence between Belgians (42%), Percherons (31%), and Clydesdales (17%) (Brakenhoff et al. 2006). If the animal collapses while in a harness, this can cause significant injury to both horses and handlers. In cases of upper airway obstruction, tracheostomy should be performed to restore airway patency, as described in Chapter 5. Draft horses are often transported long distances.

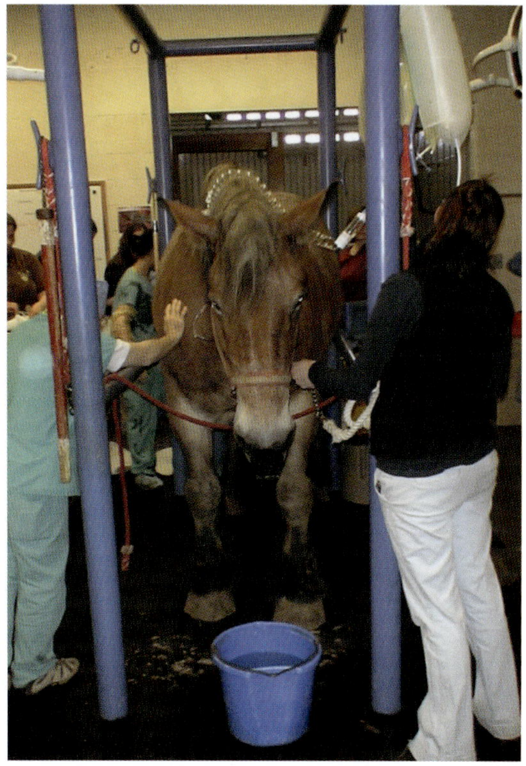

**Figure 24.4** A colicky draft horse. Overt colic signs commonly seen in light breed horses may not be evident in these animals, and clinicians must often use other available techniques to facilitate efficient triage.

## Gastrointestinal Disorders

Owners of drafts are often savvy to the unique behavioral aspects of these breeds. Any change in feeding behavior, manure output, water intake, overt signs of abdominal distension, and/or discomfort should be taken seriously. Veterinarians should observe from a distance to assess for overt clinical signs and determine whether chemical sedation or analgesia is needed immediately and to identify other abnormalities such skin abrasions secondary to trauma from being recumbent or rolling or problems such as scrotal enlargement. A thorough examination should also include heart rate, respiratory rate and effort, rectal temperature, auscultation for borborygmi, mucous membrane color, and capillary refill time. If possible, record the heart rate prior to sedation of other treatments. Given the size of most draft horses, transrectal palpation can be challenging compared to light breed horses. However, the rectal exam remains valuable in these animals and many problems can be identified similar to other horses, including small and large intestinal strangulating and non-strangulating diseases. Passing a nasogastric tube is essential. Make sure you have a tube long enough and with a large enough bore to reach the stomach and siphon fluid and thick ingesta. A net positive volume indicates a proximal obstruction, either mechanical or functional.

When available, abdominal ultrasound can provide vital information regarding the appearance of the abdominal viscera and overall condition of the abdomen. Increase in free abdominal fluid, distension or wall thickening of gastrointestinal viscera, or abnormal vessels can help identify the disease. Abdominal ultrasound is particularly important in draft horses when transrectal palpation proves challenging or unrewarding. Obtaining peritoneal fluid in the field or hospital setting can provide important information to help determine a diagnosis, treatment plan, or decision for referral. In draft horses, occasionally longer instruments (such as a long teat cannula or bitch urinary catheter) are required to collect abdominal fluid due to their larger body size. Box 24.1 outlines indications for referral in draft horses with colic.

**Box 24.1 Indications for referral in the draft horse with colic**

- Moderate-to-severe colic pain, persistent colic pain, recurrent colic pain
- Tachycardia, tachypnea, tacky mucous membranes, injected mucous membranes
- Distended small intestine on rectal palpation and/or on transabdominal ultrasound
- Markedly distended large intestine and/or tight colonic tenial bands on rectal palpation
- Abnormal peritoneal fluid including color, total nucleated cell count, protein, L-lactate
- Presence of nasogastric reflux
- Clinical evidence indicating the need for intravenous fluids and/or blood product

When evaluating a painful animal, it is important to ascertain the source of the pain. Colic is common and abdominal pain is often considered first; however, other possibilities exist such as laminitis, pleuritis, or dystocia. If the source of pain cannot be determined, or the severity of pain does not appear to match the clinical findings, consider other sources. If surgery is pursued, appropriate positioning and padding is imperative to mitigate anesthetic risks. Anesthetic complications including hypoxia, myopathy, neuropathy, musculoskeletal injury, and prolonged and complicated recovery are common in draft horses (Dupont et al. 2018; O'Donovan et al. 2023). Surgery should be performed standing when possible; when surgery under general anesthesia is necessary (e.g., most colic surgeries), draft horses should be placed in a slight dorsolateral position to help avoid some of these positional complications. The time spent in surgery, anesthesia, and recovery should be limited to as short as possible to decrease the aforementioned anesthetic complications.

## Musculoskeletal Disorders

Polysaccharide storage myopathy (PSSM) is highly prevalent in draft breeds, particularly in Belgian and Percheron horses (McCue et al. 2008). This results in an abnormal accumulation of glycogen stored within muscle, predisposing affected horses to exertional rhabdomyolysis. This may present as reluctance to move, firmness of the musculature, sweating, lameness, or muscle fasciculations. Assessment of creatine kinase and aspartate aminotransaminase, as well as creatinine and blood urea nitrogen is beneficial to quantify the extent of muscle and renal injury, respectively (Valberg 2018). Acute treatment includes sedation, analgesia, muscle relaxants, and non-steroidal anti-inflammatory drugs (Valberg 2018). With severe cases of muscle injury or where acute kidney injury is suspected, intravenous fluids using a balanced, polyionic fluid is recommended. For long-term management, it is important that affected horses are fed a diet comprising digestible energy less than 10% nonstructural carbohydrate (NSC) and greater than 20% fat (McKenzie et al. 2003).

Chronic progressive lymphedema consists of severe progressive swelling of the distal limb, scaling of the skin, dermal fibrosis, development of skinfolds and nodules, complicated by secondary infection (Brys et al. 2023). These horses may present on emergency for severe lameness, and require treatment of associated secondary infection and support of lymph drainage through hosing, massage, and bandaging.

Cerebellar Purkinje cell axonal degeneration, or shivers, has been identified in draft horses with abnormal hindlimb movement characterized by a hyperflexed, abducted, or rigidly extended hindlimb (Valentine et al. 1999; Aman et al. 2018). Underlying etiology end-terminal neuroaxonal degeneration in the deep cerebellar nuclei and a genetic predilection is suspected (Valberg et al. 2015). Lifting the limb for cleaning or trimming can also trigger this movement (Aman et al. 2018). Signs are exacerbated with prolonged standing, excitement, backing and turning, stress, or mental agitation (Valberg et al. 2015; Aman et al. 2018). Definitive antemortem diagnosis is challenging, but familiarity with breed predilection, typical abnormal movements, and exacerbating circumstances is beneficial.

Common emergency conditions of the foot including subsolar abscessation, hypertrophic pododermatitis, and laminitis can also present in draft horses. Information regarding diagnostics and treatments recommended for these conditions can be found elsewhere in Chapter 8. When evaluating the foot, draft horses often have large, flared hoof walls that displace the radiograph detector from the limb, contributing to magnification artifact (Larsen et al. 2023). The ratio of the dorsal hoof wall thickness to the length of the distal phalanx is generally greater in draft horses than light breed horses (Larsen et al. 2023). This should be taken into account, specifically when evaluating radiographs for evidence of thickening of the dorsal hoof wall in cases of laminitis, as symmetric sinking of the distal phalanx can be more challenging to identify and diagnose (Larsen et al. 2023). Draft horses have a unique lamellar architecture related to their hoof size (Senderska-Plonowska et al. 2022). This is characterized by elongated primary epidermal lamellae. Importantly, obesity is not responsible for lamellar failure (Senderska-Plonowska et al. 2022). Box 24.2 summarizes common musculoskeletal disorders of draft horses.

**Box 24.2 Common musculoskeletal disorders of draft horses**

- Polysaccharide storage myopathy (PSSM)
- Chronic progressive lymphedema
- Shivers/Cerebellar Purkinje cell axonal degeneration
- Subsolar abscessation
- Hypertrophic pododermatitis
- Laminitis

## Urogenital Disorders

Dystocia is a known issue in many draft breeds, particularly in Friesian and Belgian mares. The incidence can be as high as 10% of draft pregnancies (Sabbagh et al. 2014). The large foal desired by draft horse breeders may lead to fetal–maternal disproportion. Further uterine inertia as a result of inadequate uterine muscle tone and contractions may complicate delivery (Figure 24.5). Transverse presentation is common in draft breeds. Even with proper positioning, draft mares may require assistance delivering. Due to the size of the foal and the mare, repositioning of the foal can be complicated, and controlled vaginal delivery under general anesthesia may be indicated if initial attempts to correct the fetal malposition in the standing mare fail. Further, fetotomy and cesarean section are fraught with complications associated with prolonged uterine manipulations and the consequences of being down for extended periods of time. Retained placentas are more common in draft horses than light mares, and complications may be severe including endometritis, sepsis, and laminitis (Jaworska et al. 2020). The treatment of retained placenta in the mare is described in Chapter 14.

## Skin Disorders

Draft breeds, especially males, with feathers and large cannon bone circumference are at highest risk of pastern dermatitis (Gerber et al. 2023). Additionally, this condition is more common in the hindlimb, unpigmented skin, and animals housed in moist environments (Gerber et al. 2023). Lay terms such as scratches, mud fever, and grease heel may be used by horse owners to describe this condition. Some degree of pain and exudate may accompany disease, with lameness and loss of condition occurring in severe cases (Gerber et al. 2023). Lesions are often symmetrical. Treatment includes clipping of feathers, cleansing skin with an antiseptic, and treatment with topical antibiotics, antifungals, and steroids (Gerber et al. 2023). Systemic treatment may be indicated if there is severe lameness or the horse is febrile (Gerber et al. 2023). Prognosis is good if mild, but can decrease as disease severity increases (Gerber et al. 2023).

Squamous cell carcinoma is the most important neoplasia affecting the equine eye (Crausaz et al. 2020). This disease is caused by an inherited recessive gene in Belgian draft horses (Crausaz et al. 2020). Variably ulcerated, pink raised masses of the skin, conjunctiva, or corneal tissue (Crausaz et al. 2020). These masses grow rapidly and may cause visual impairment and destruction of the eye (Crausaz et al. 2020). Biopsy and histopathologic evaluation are required for definitive diagnosis (Crausaz et al. 2020). While excision or other treatment may not be necessary on an emergency basis, owner counselling regarding likely etiology, severity, and treatment options may be necessary (Crausaz et al. 2020).

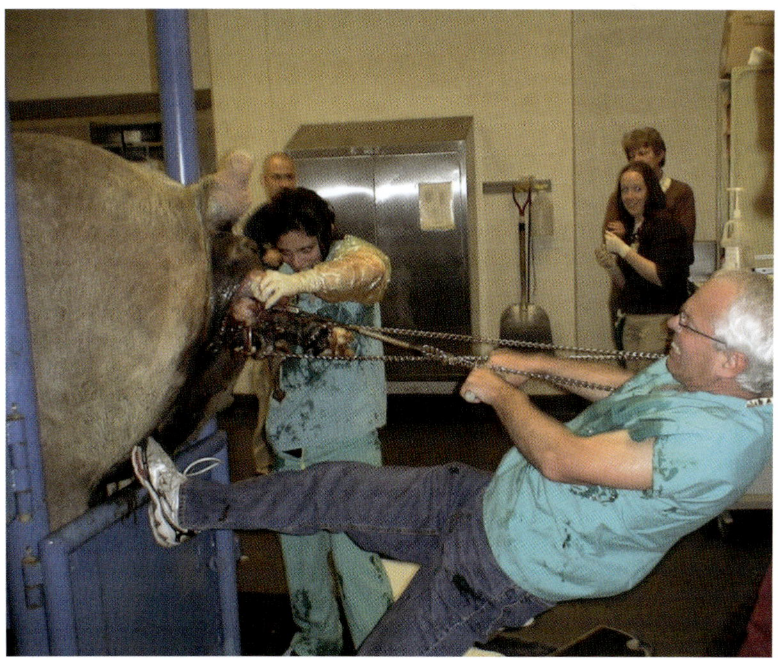

**Figure 24.5** A Percheron mare dystocia with the dead fetus is trapped in the birth canal. Controlled vaginal delivery under general anesthesia may be required for fetal extraction in the draft horse when fetal removal standing is not possible. Fetotomy or cesarean section are other options for resolving dystocia in the draft mare, but also carry with significant risks (see also Dystocia in Chapter 14).

Junctional epidermolysis bullosa (JEB) is a fatal disease causing a defect in the lamina propria that presents as a split in the dermo–epidermal junctional (Capelli et al. 2015). This disease is heritable in Belgian and other draft breeds (Capelli et al. 2015). Present at birth or shortly after, horses will develop vesicles and ulceration at the mouth and distal extremities. Subsequent effects include inability to suckle and sloughing of the affected hoof (Capelli et al. 2015). Biopsy and histopathology are required to confirm diagnosis (Capelli et al. 2015).

Box 24.3 summarizes common skin disorders of draft horses.

**Box 24.3 Common skin disorders of draft breeds**

- Pastern dermatitis
- Squamous cell carcinoma
- Junctional epidermolysis bullosa (JEB)

**Case Example 24.1 Emergency Triage of the Draft Horse**

Step 1: Patient Stabilization
*When perform an assessment of a draft horse on emergency, you should pay particular attention to what differences in clinical presentation of a painful the draft horse?*

Stoic nature
Use lower end of standard dosing ranges for sedation and stabilization therapy

*What conditions may be more prevalent in or specific to draft breeds?* , Airway disorders

Gastrointestinal disorders
Musculoskeletal disorders
Urogenital disorders
Skin disorders

Step 2: Formulating a Diagnostic Plan
Once the horse is stable, what should be taken into consideration when developing a diagnostic plan? What diagnostics are available at the location of the examination

Image quality of radiographs and ultrasonography
Restraint requirements

Step 3: Emergency Treatment Guidelines
Following initial stabilization and diagnostic evaluation, further specific treatment is indicated. Treatment will depend on the specific condition; however, what specifics regarding draft horses should be considered?

Appropriate facilities and equipment to facilitate the size of the patient
Appropriate dosing of medications and fluid therapy

Step 4: Assessment and Monitoring
Finally, when setting up a monitoring plan what considerations with staff and personnel should be taken into consideration?

Staff and personnel should be trained to monitor draft horses appropriately. Ensuring

staff are appropriately performing full physical examinations rather than relying heavily on overt signs of discomfort to monitor for pain. Personnel should also be trained in the specifics of handling draft horses to ensure safety of those involved.

## References


Aman, J.E., Valberg, S.J., Elangovan, N. et al. (2018). Abnormal locomotor muscle recruitment activity is present in horses with shivering and Purkinje cell distal axonopathy. *Equine Vet. J.* 50 (5): 636–643.

Brakenhoff, J.E., Holcombe, S.J., Hauptman, J.G. et al. (2006). The prevalence of laryngeal disease in a large population of competition draft horses. *Vet. Surg.* 35 (6): 579–583.

Branson, K.R. (2011). Sedation and anesthesia for field surgeries. *AAEP Proc.* 57: 296–298.

Brys, M., Claerebout, E., and Chiers, K. (2023). Chronic progressive lymphedema in Belgian Draft Horses: understanding and managing a challenging disease. *Vet. Sci.* 10 (5): 347.

Capelli, K., Brachelente, C., Passamonti, F. et al. (2015). First report of junctional epidermolysis bullosa (JEB) in the Italian draft horse. *BMC Vet. Res.* 11: 55.

Crausaz, M., Launois, T., Smith-Fleming, K. et al. (2020). DDB2 genetic risk factor for ocular squamous cell carcinoma identified in three additional horse breeds. *Genes (Basel)* 11 (12): 1460.

Dupont, J., Serteyn, D., and Sandersen, C. (2018). Prolonged recovery from general anesthesia possibly related to persistent hypoxemia in a draft horse. *Front. Vet. Sci.* 5: 235.

Gerber, V., Kaiser-Thom, S., and Oesch, S. (2023). Equine pastern dermatitis: a narrative review on clinical presentation, diagnosis, risk factors, preventation, and therapeutic approaches. *J. Am. Vet. Med. Assoc.* 261 (S1): S58–S65.

Goble, D.O. (2011). Lameness in draft horses. In: *Diagnosis and Management of Lameness in the Horse*, 2e (ed. M.W. Ross and S. Dyson), 1216–1228. Philadelphia: Saunders.

Hackett, E.S. and Leise, B.S. (2018). Exercising upper respiratory videoendoscopic findings of 50 competition draught horses with abnormal respiratory noise and/or poor performance. *Equine Vet. J.* 51: 370–374.

Jaworska, J., Tobolski, D., and Janowski, T. (2020). Is similarity in major histocompatibility complex (MHC) associated with the incidence of retained fetal membranes in draft mares? A cross-sectional study. *PLoS One* 15 (8): e0237765.

Larsen, C.D., Wilkinson, T.E., Roberts, G.D. et al. (2023). Radiographic analysis of the dorsal hoof wall thickness in clinically normal draft horses. *Am J Vet Res.* 85 (1) ajvr.23.06.0145. https://doi.org/10.2460/ajvr.23.06.0145: PMID: 37903451.

McCue, M.E., Valberg, S.J., Lucio, M., and Mickelson, J.R. (2008). Glycogen synthase (GYS1) mutation in diverse breeds with polysaccharide storage myopathy. *J. Vet. Intern. Med.* 22 (5): 1228–1233.

McKenzie, E.M., Valberg, S.J., and Pagan, J. (2003). *Current Therapy in Equine Medicine*, vol. 5, 727–734. Philedelphia PA: Robinson E Saunders.

O'Donovan, K.A., Aarnes, T.K., Hubbell, J.A. et al. (2023). Risk of anesthesia-related complications in draft horses: a retrospective, single-center analysis. *Vet. Anes. Analg.* 50: 157–162.

Sabbagh, M., Danvy, S., and Ricard, A. (2014). Genetic and environmental analysis of dystocia and stillbirths in draft horses. *Animal* 2: 184–191.

Senderska-Plonowska, M., Siwinska, N., Zak-Bochenek, A. et al. (2022). The difference in histoarchitecture of hoof lamellae between obese and lean draft horses. *Animals (Basel)* 12 (14): 1774.

Valberg, S.J. (2018). Muscle conditions affecting sport horses. *Vet. Clin. North Am. Equine Pract.* 34 (2): 253–276.

Valberg, S.J., Lewis, S.S., Shivers, J.L. et al. (2015). The equine movement disorder "shivers" is associated with selective cerebellar purkinje cell axonal degeneration. *Vet. Pathol.* 52 (6): 1087–1098.

Valentine, B.A., de Lahunta, A., Divers, T.J. et al. (1999). Clinical and pathologic findings in two draft horses with progressive muscle atrophy, neuromuscular weakness, and abnormal gait characteristic of shivers syndrome. *J. Am. Vet. Med. Assoc.* 215 (11): 1661–1665.

# 25

# Emergency Problems of Donkeys and Mules

*Erin L. Goodrich*[1] *and Cynthia Xue*[2]

[1] *Animal Health Diagnostic Center, College of Veterinary Medicine, Cornell University, Ithaca, NY, USA*
[2] *Department of Clinical Sciences, School of Veterinary Medicine, Ross University, Basseterre, St. Kitts, West Indies*

## Introduction

To provide the best veterinary care, it is imperative that veterinarians develop a thorough understanding of the ways in which donkeys and mules differ from horses. Behavioral, anatomic, physiologic, and metabolic differences exist among these equids and can influence the diagnostic and therapeutic approaches required in emergency situations (Mendoza et al. 2018a, b, Parts I and II).

## Clinical Assessment

### Behavior

*Donkeys, and to some extent mules and hinnies* (the reciprocal hybrid cross, a male horse and female donkey) *often express signs of pain or illness more subtly than horses* (Taylor and Matthews 2002; Burden and Thiemann 2015) (Box 25.1). This can pose a challenge to equine veterinarians. It is imperative that veterinarians have a good understanding of the ways in which donkey and mule behavior and pain responses tend to differ from horses so that emergent issues can be identified promptly and treated appropriately.

#### Observe for Subtle Signs of Pain

To diagnose pain in donkeys or mules when apparent injuries or lesions are not present, pay special attention to the tail (slight twitching), facial expression (clamped nostril, tensed muzzle, semi-closed eyes or conversely visible sclera, a "glazed" look), a fixed ear position (out to the side or back), and the donkey's orientation in the stall (standing toward the back, facing away from the entrance) or its interaction with other animals and humans (isolating itself from other donkeys, decreased or complete unresponsiveness to human handling). It is important to look at the overall, composite expression of behaviors and body cues in the determination of pain, as healthy donkeys can (and do) demonstrate these behaviors individually as part of their normal ethograms. For example, a donkey engaged in minor intra-species conflict may have backward facing ears, a tense muzzle, and tail twitching, but these transient behaviors cease once the conflict is over. These donkeys also tend to be mobile within their environment throughout the interaction despite expression of some behaviors that can be associated with pain. In contrast, truly painful donkeys are often noted to have a combination of decreased responsiveness to external stimuli (lack of ear movement, lack of herd interaction, and/or lack of positive or negative engagement with a handler) with behaviors like tail swishing and/or active facial tension, in addition to ignoring a food incentive. Thus, utilizing information from the astute owner or handler, who has a higher likelihood of detecting subtle but crucial observations in a donkey they are familiar with (McLean et al. 2019), can increase the accuracy of a clinician's eventual interpretation. See Table 25.1 for common analgesic dosages (Mendoza et al. 2019; Archer et al. 2021; Evans et al. 2021).

*Emergency Triage of the Horse*, First Edition. Edited by Rolfe M. Radcliffe and Jamie J. Kopper.

Companion website: www.wiley.com/go/radcliffe/triage

**Box 25.1 Signs of pain or illness in a sick donkey or mule**

*Reliance on a complete history and astute observations is essential; a dull donkey is an emergency! (Figure 25.1).* Obtain a detailed history from the owner, with special attention paid to any recent changes in their equid's demeanor or behavior. Realize that even severe colic in a donkey may present very differently from the same process in a horse with donkeys sometimes only displaying increased bouts of recumbency, dullness, isolation, or reduced appetite (sometimes even appearing to eat when they actually are not – sham eating) (Evans and Crane 2018). Pain-associated behavior exhibited by mules also tends to be more subtle than horses but is typically still more pronounced than in donkeys (McLean et al. 2019).

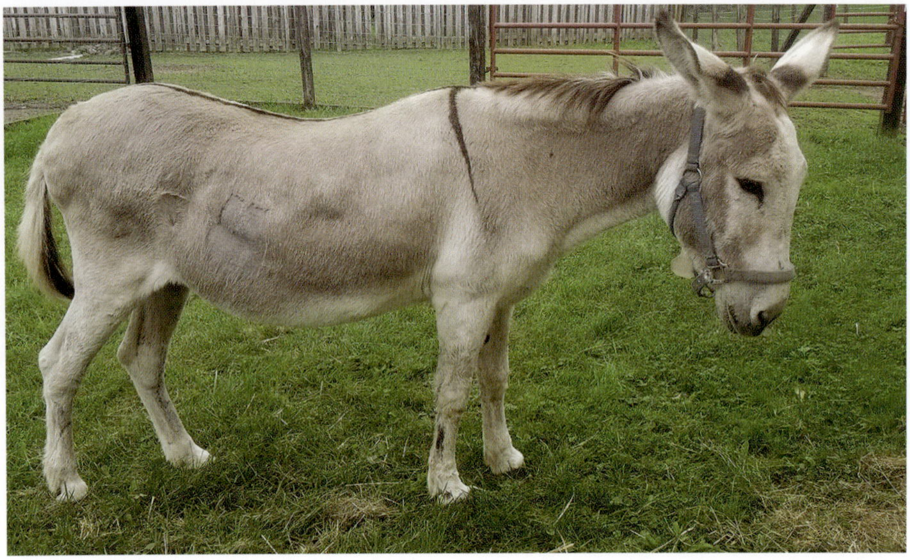

**Figure 25.1** A sick donkey showing only dull behavior. A donkey with severe hepatic failure and marked abnormalities on ultrasound exam and biochemical analysis. Note the donkey is not showing evidence of pain or recumbency, but rather is only displaying the typical dull behavior often seen with advanced disease.

**Table 25.1** Commonly used analgesic drug dosages in donkeys and mules.

| Drug | Dose (mg/kg) | Route of administration | Comments |
|---|---|---|---|
| <u>NSAID's</u> | | | |
| Phenylbutazone | 2.2–4.4 | IV, PO | Metabolized faster in donkeys and breed differences exist; consider twice daily administration in standard, and three times daily in miniature donkeys |
| Flunixin meglumine | 1.1 | IV | Conflicting information on clearance in donkeys compared to horses but fewer side effects seen with long-term use compared to long-term phenylbutazone administration in donkeys |
| Carprofen | 0.7 | IV | Metabolized more slowly in donkeys than horses |
| Firocoxib | 0.1 | PO | Much shorter half-life in donkeys than in horses; consider adjusting dosing interval; in horses 3× loading dose (0.3 mg/kg, once) is recommended but no data exists regarding the use of a loading dose in donkeys |
| Meloxicam | 0.6 | IV | Not advised for use in donkeys as half-life is very short |

## Restraint

### Establish Trust and Use Patience with Your Approach

Approach the donkey or mule at their face, rather than their neck, and use voice commands to set them at ease. Having patience when working with donkeys and mules is essential and will improve the outcome of the interaction. After successfully approaching the patient, options for securing the equid within the treatment area may include stocks, chutes, snubbing posts, or even swinging gates. Note that many equids form bonded pairs and if possible, that bonded pair animal

Table 25.2 Commonly used sedative and anesthetic drug dosages in donkeys and mules.

| Drug | Dose (mg/kg) | Route of administration | Comments |
|---|---|---|---|
| ***Sedative or Anesthetic drug*** | | | |
| Detomidine | 0.01–0.04 | IV | Alpha-2 adrenoreceptor agonists (detomidine and xylazine) may need to be given at about a 50% higher dosage in mules than in donkeys and horses. |
| | 0.04–0.08 | IM | |
| | 0.04 | PO (oral gel) | |
| Xylazine | 0.4–1.5 | IV | |
| Butorphanol | 0.02–0.05 | IV, IM | Can be given in combination with an alpha-2 agonist to enhance the sedative and hypoalgesic effects. |
| Acepromazine | 0.02–0.05 (0.03–0.1 in mules) | IV, IM, sublingual | |
| Ketamine | 2.2–2.8 | IV | Metabolized faster in donkeys (especially miniature donkeys); mules also require a shorter dosing interval than horses. |

should be present in proximity (even transported into the hospital with the affected equid if necessary) to provide a calming companion. If the equid is not part of a pair-bond, the presence of another calm donkey near the patient is advised (Taylor and Matthews 2002; Evans and Crane 2018; McLean et al. 2019). A fearful donkey tends to freeze in place or pull away, so take care to remove frightening objects from the environment, turn on lights, open doorways wide and use a companion equid for assistance, along with food incentives when possible (Evans and Crane 2018).

### Effective Restraint Can Come in Many Forms

Distractions with food rewards during procedures can help immensely. Nose twitches (not ear twitches) may be used with success when necessary in mules and hinnies, but the response seen in donkeys varies widely across individuals (Evans and Crane 2018; McLean et al. 2019). Consider the use of blindfolds or lifting a front or hind limb during short procedures. One author (CX) has also found surprising success in either rubbing the base of the pinnae or inside donkey's ears as a distraction technique for short procedures. Care must be taken to reserve this for donkeys that are not ear shy. In certain situations, trained personnel may even consider tying a front leg up with a safety knot to a non-slip loop made around the neck (McLean et al. 2019). Sedation may ultimately be necessary if all other non-chemical methods of restraint have failed. See Table 25.2 for dosages of commonly used sedatives and anesthetics (Mendoza et al. 2019; Archer et al. 2021; Evans et al. 2021).

## Physical Examination

Physical examination should proceed in a similar manner to that of the horse with considerations for anatomical and physiological differences relevant to emergency scenarios as outlined throughout this chapter. Refer to Table 25.3 for the normal temperature, pulse, and respiratory rate of horses, donkeys, and mules for comparison.

Table 25.3 Comparative horse, donkey, and mule normal temperature, heart, and respiratory rates.

| | Heart rate (beats/min) | Respiratory rate (breaths/min) | Rectal temperature (°F) | Reference |
|---|---|---|---|---|
| Horse | 28–44 | 8–15 | 99–101 | Smith (2020) |
| Mule | 29–37 | 8–16 | 98.8–100.6 | Brooke (2013) |
| Adult donkey | 31–53 | 13–31 | 97.7–99.9 | Burden and Thiemann (2015) |
| Young donkey <2 years | 40–80 | 16–48 | 97–102 | Orsini and Divers (2008) |

## Clinical Pathology

*Utilize donkey- or mule-specific reference intervals when available as their hematologic and biochemical data differs from that of horses.*

### Sample Collection

#### Venipuncture of Donkeys Can Be Challenging

While the cutaneous colli muscle of the horse is relatively small, arising from the manubrium sterni then thinning out and eventually blending into the superficial cervical fascia, this muscle is remarkably thicker and more extensive in the neck of donkeys (Burnham 2002). For this reason, it can be quite difficult to palpate or visualize the external jugular vein in donkeys. Utilizing the upper one-third of the vein for venipuncture in donkeys may improve palpation of the jugular vein, increased its visualization, and avoids inadvertent intracarotid injection. Additionally, a slightly steeper angle (but not a longer needle) may be necessary to facilitate successful venipuncture. Some donkeys may react (i.e., shoving, pushing, jerking, or shaking the head) to the act of jugular vein distention in anticipation of venipuncture. In those situations, pressing the tip of the needle flush against the skin prior to sliding it into the vein may prove more effective. This seems to decrease their responsiveness to the subsequent venipuncture in comparison to a sharp poke through the skin.

Intravenous catheterization of the donkey is similarly challenging due to their thicker skin. Thus, a stab incision made at the insertion site may be necessary to minimize drag of the catheter through the skin. In donkeys where long-term catheterization may be expected (i.e., hospitalization), an over-the-wire catheter is recommended to optimize catheter insertion and its subsequent patency.

### The Hemogram

#### Use Caution When Interpreting the Packed Cell Volume

Donkeys are very well adapted for life in the desert where their ancestors originated. For that reason, care must be taken when interpreting the packed cell volume (PCV) of donkeys. A donkey's PCV, pulse quality, and capillary refill time (CRT) are all minimally affected from fluid loss until dehydration becomes quite severe. They do not tend to hemoconcentrate until they are up to 15–20% dehydrated (Yousef et al. 1970). Therefore, clinicians unfamiliar with this difference in donkeys could misinterpret a normal PCV for lack of hypovolemia, when in fact, moderate-to-severe fluid deficits may be present. The authors are not aware of a similar issue in mules or hinnies. Further, changes in PCV should always be interpreted in light of changes with TS and TP. Splenic contraction may be a differential for a bright, clinically euhydrated and otherwise systemically stable donkey with elevations in PCV and normal TS/TP, whereas changes in PCV and TS/TP should be investigated more closely in donkeys that are quiet to depressed, inappetent, or have physical exam abnormalities consistent with dehydration and/or fluid losses.

### The Serum Biochemistry

A serum triglyceride concentration (TG) should be measured in any donkey that is experiencing pain or has any degree of appetite suppression, realizing that donkeys are also known for their ability to pretend to eat even when they are ill (i.e., "sham eat") (Box 25.2).

Importantly, the reference interval for TG in the donkey is much different from that of the horse, or the mule or hinny with the normal values in donkeys sometimes approaching 200–250 mg/dL and those of horses, mules and hinnies all fairly

**Box 25.2 Serum triglyceride and the sick donkey or mule**

*Triglyceride concentrations should be evaluated and monitored in every sick or painful donkey*: Hyperlipidemia is likely the most common disease process seen in donkeys, whether occurring as the primary problem or a secondary sequela. There is a high incidence and high mortality associated with hyperlipidemia in donkeys, especially those with concurrent disease processes, such as colic or liver disease. The visualization of opalescent serum facilitates a preliminary diagnosis, but normal-appearing serum does not exclude hyperlipidemia.

similar (~14–65 mg/dL) (Burden et al. 2016; McLean et al. 2016; Goodrich and Behling-Kelly 2019; Lagos and Tadich 2019). In addition, the TG can be utilized as a prognostic indicator and to help guide the therapeutic approach. While strong voluntary feeding encouragement coupled with glucose drenches may be enough to restore normal values in donkeys with TG concentrations of 250–700 mg/dL, more aggressive medical management is likely necessary in donkeys with hypertriglyceridemia above that concentration (see *Important considerations by body system: Hepatic Disease*). A guarded-to-poor prognosis can be expected in cases where the triglyceride concentration exceeds 1,300 mg/dL (Barrio et al. 2019).

#### Gamma Glutamyl Transferase (GGT) Reference Intervals Can Also Differ for Donkeys

GGT is an enzyme used as a marker of biliary hyperplasia, structural cholestasis, or biliary necrosis. In equids, GGT is often elevated in cases of cholangiohepatitis or sometimes with gastrointestinal disorders such as proximal enteritis, colonic displacement, or small intestinal strangulation. In healthy donkeys, it is interesting to note that the upper limit for GGT can be about twice as high (up to about 60 U/L) compared to horses (Goodrich and Behling-Kelly 2019). The same was found to be true in a study of Chilean mules; however, another study of mules and hinnies in Portugal found GGT reference intervals that corresponded more closely to those of horses (McLean et al. 2016; Lagos and Tadich 2019).

## Important Considerations by Body System

### Oral Cavity

#### Dental Problems in Geriatric Animals May Increase the Risk of Gastrointestinal Disease

Large intestinal impactions appear to be the most prevalent type of non-strangulating obstructive colic in donkeys based on an epidemiologic study from the UK Donkey Sanctuary (Cox et al. 2007). Although the association between dental disease and impaction colic needs further elucidation, this appears to align with risk factors in older horses.

#### Donkeys May Not Present with Clinical Signs of Dental Disease Despite Significant Abnormalities

Despite having significant dental problems, donkeys may not exhibit clinical signs (Rodrigues and Lilly 2019). Common dental issues in donkeys include diastemas, displaced teeth, and wave mouth (du Toit and Dixon 2012; Rodrigues and Lilly 2019). Other mechanically obstructive teeth disorders that can impair mastication and proper occlusion of the mouth include congenital conditions (brachygnathism or overbite, and less commonly prognathism or underbite), retention of deciduous teeth, and supernumerary teeth. Periodontal disease can be significant in elderly animals, and donkeys may present with considerable malodorous calculi around teeth adjacent to salivary duct openings – particularly around the incisors, canines, and occasionally premolars. Significant deposits can form sharp edges that have the potential to traumatize soft tissues (Emmett, the Donkey Sanctuary, unpublished data). Because donkeys have less sexual dimorphism when it comes to canines, both male and female donkeys may be affected by calculi accumulation around all four canines.

#### Oral Examination with a Speculum Is Recommended for Comprehensive Evaluation of the Oral Cavity in Donkeys Where There Is Concern for Dental Disease

This is because dental disorders can predispose to pain leading to inappetence, weight loss, and an increased risk of dyslipidemias (see *Important considerations by body system: Hepatic Disease*). Donkeys will tolerate an un-sedated speculum exam if the examiner takes time to establish a rapport with the patient (see *Clinical assessment: Restraint*), but sedation will facilitate the dental exam particularly if the patient has painful lesions. Ancillary diagnostics such as dental radiographs are recommended where available. Computed tomography and scintigraphy have been described in donkeys (Barakzai et al. 2006) but are not practical in a field situation.

### Gastrointestinal Tract

Anatomic variation of upper airway structures (smaller nares and a prominent pharyngeal recess) and the tendency toward fat deposition along the linea alba increase the difficulty of colic diagnostics in donkeys (Thiemann and Sullivan 2019; Wissdorf et al. 2021). Physiologic variations in gastrointestinal transit time between donkeys, mules, and horses also need to be considered to avoid overinterpretation of imaging results (see below; *gastric transit time is slower in donkeys and mules*).

### Choose a Smaller Bore Tube for Nasogastric Intubation

Donkeys have a narrower nasal meatus in comparison to a similarly sized horse. Use of smaller-diameter tubes (pony or foal sized) will decrease the risk of irritating the nasal passage and subsequent hemorrhage (Thiemann and Sullivan 2019). This consideration should also be kept in mind for diagnostics such as airway endoscopy or gastroscopy.

### Ensure the Tube Is in the Ventral Meatus

The narrower nasal meatus can increase the difficulty of maintaining the tube in the ventral meatus during advancement. Lubricating the end of the tube and guiding it ventrally with a finger placed in the nasal passage can prevent the end of the tube from slipping dorsally during nasogastric intubation. Accidental placement of the stomach tube into the dorsal meatus in horses and donkeys will cause trauma and hemorrhage to the ethmoidal labyrinth.

### Consider that the End of the Tube May Be Trapped in the Pharyngeal Recess If There Is Difficulty Advancing Into the Esophagus

Donkeys have a well-developed pharyngeal recess lying between the ostia of the guttural pouches and dorsal to the glottis (Lindsay and Clayton 1986). This membranous sac reaches depths of up to 7 cm, widths of 2–3 cm, and a height of 1 cm (Wissdorf et al. 2021). Iatrogenic trauma to the blind pouch can be induced if a practitioner continues to advance a nasogastric tube or endoscope despite resistance. Slightly extending the neck once the nasogastric tube has passed the expected location of the ethmoids seems to facilitate guiding the tip of the tube ventrally into the oropharynx and esophagus. (See supplemental video.)

### Donkeys Tend to Deposit Fat Along the Linea Alba

This thick layer of abdominal fat can confound abdominocentesis. Thus, use of a teat cannula (3.75 in.) or longer needle is recommended, even in animals that appear lean. However, care should be taken whenever using a needle for abdominal fluid collection in equids as in advertent enterocentesis is likely as the layers of the abdominal wall cannot be identified or felt during placement. Transcutaneous abdominal ultrasonography can facilitate visualization of this fat layer for preplanning of abdominocentesis and can also be used to guide placement if using the needle technique. To prevent inadvertent enterocentesis, the use of a teat cannula for abdominal fluid collection in donkeys and mules is recommended over a spinal needle even when ultrasound is available. Because of the stoic nature of donkeys and their tendency to present in advanced stages of disease, any donkey suspected of colic should have abdominocentesis performed. Sterile preparation, performing the procedure, and analysis of peritoneal effusion are similar to horses with the noted exceptions above. The predictive values of total nucleated cell count, protein, and lactate have not yet been established in donkeys for specific types of colic. Based on existing literature in healthy donkeys (Mori et al. 2003; Ibrahim and Shoieb 2020), use of normal horse reference ranges and gross color characteristics of peritoneal fluid would be appropriate for the evaluation of colic and other diseases of the abdominal cavity in donkeys.

### The Normal Donkey Abdomen May Be More Pendulous than Horses

This abdominal contour may be a normal morphologic feature of donkeys owing to their fibrous diet, decreased abdominal muscle tone, and tendency for fat deposition in the linea alba (Thiemann et al. 2017). The contour itself may not correspond with the presence of abdominal fluid (Xue and Cavanaugh 2022), and its appearance alone should not be used as positive evidence for disease.

### Gastric Transit Time Is Slower in Donkeys and Mules

Care must be taken not to overinterpret the presence of food in the stomach as indicative of a gastric impaction in the absence of other clinical signs attributable to colic (see *Clinical Assessment: Behavior*). The slower gastrointestinal transit time must also be taken into consideration when planning gastroscopy (Pearson and Merritt 1991), and when interpreting visualization of the greater curvature of the stomach (which can be normally seen at the 15th–16th intercostal space) on ultrasonography. One gastroscopy study cited a fast of at least 15 h (Sgorbini et al. 2018). In other words, there should be some consideration that the stomach has not yet undergone full emptying if it is seen to be full or if the caudal border is detected beyond the 16th intercostal space in a donkey that is bright, appetent, and has been seen to eat within the last 15 h. If gastric impaction is diagnosed, preferably with endoscopy, treatment is as with horses (Thiemann and Sullivan 2019).

**Box 25.3 Recommendations for gastrointestinal disease in donkeys and mules**

Where possible and safe, performing transrectal palpation (facilitated by liberal use of lubrication) along with abdominocentesis is recommended to rule out colic that requires surgical intervention. This is especially important in cases of colic refractory to medical management as prolonging an available surgical decision can further compromise bowel integrity and systemic health by the time a patient is brought to surgery.

#### The Large Colon Is the Most Common Site of Gastrointestinal Impaction

Risk factors include increasing dental disease with age (although the association is not well studied in donkeys), ingestion of foreign bodies, coarse dry feed, and decreased water accessibility, particularly in working animals (Cox et al. 2007; du Toit et al. 2008). Transrectal palpation is valuable in donkeys and mules when possible (Box 25.3); findings consistent with an impaction may include non-specific gas distention with or without the presence of doughy or firm ingesta (Xue, unpublished data). Based on existing epidemiologic data, clinical diagnosis of large intestinal impaction is often reached without reliance on transrectal palpation findings due to concerns of rectal tears in small donkeys.

### Cardiovascular/Hematopoietic Systems

#### Donkey Factor Is a Red Blood Cell Antigen Unique to Donkeys and Their Hybrid Offspring

This RBC antigen complicates interspecies blood donations. Ideally, when blood transfusion (as in hemorrhage) or use of blood product (as in failure of passive transfer) is indicated, a donor donkey or mule should be used. Cross-matching should occur as for horses, although this may not be necessary if the recipient has no prior exposure to blood products (Mudge 2014). Donkeys and mules should *not* be used as blood donors for horses to decrease the risk of transfusion reactions in horses. Similarly, as no information currently exists on the incidence of anti-donkey factor antibodies in horses, all blood products from horse donors (whole blood, plasma) should first be confirmed free of anti-donkey factor antibodies prior to donation to a donkey or mule (Mudge 2014; Archer et al. 2021).

Although rarely the cause of acute hemorrhage in equids, the diagnosis of coagulopathies in donkeys requires the use of donkey-specific hemostatic reference intervals. Previous studies have found prothrombin time (PT) and/or activated partial thromboplastin time (aPTT) to be significantly shorter in donkeys compared to horses (Mendoza et al. 2011; Perez-Ecija and Mendoza 2017).

### Hepatic Disease

#### Dyslipidemias (Hypertriglyceridemia, Hyperlipidemia, Hyperlipemia) Are Common in Sick Donkeys and Mules

Any systemic disease, stress, or physiologic state (pregnancy, lactation) that causes a donkey to become inappetent or go into negative energy balance can induce dyslipidemia. The authors recommend checking serum triglycerides in all donkey patients. A point-of-care triglyceride analyzer (Accutrend Plus, Diagnostics Roche) is validated in donkeys for use in the field (Pongratz et al. 2016). However, limitations include the narrow analytical range and overestimation of TG in comparison to laboratory-based methods. Specifically, the analyzer only reads TG between 0.80–6.86 mmol/L (70–600 mg/dL), and TG values tend to be higher than those obtained in the lab. Nonetheless, the benefit of early detection of hypertriglyceridemia outweighs the potential for false-positive results as prophylactic treatment of hypertriglyceridemia, especially in an overtly sick donkey, confers a better prognosis by mitigating the risk of developing hepatic lipidosis.

In donkeys with hepatic lipidosis, increases in hepatocellular and biliary enzyme activities may also be seen, but the magnitude of increase may not necessarily correlate with liver function (DeNotta and Divers 2020). Ultrasonography in those cases can be a useful adjuvant, although diagnostic imaging results are typically non-specific (e.g., increased echogenicity of the hepatic parenchyma). Definitive diagnosis of hepatic lipidosis is made based on liver biopsy results. In the absence of these ancillary diagnostics, a putative diagnosis of hepatic lipidosis in a sick, inappetent, lethargic donkey with opaque plasma (post-centrifugation or in an anticoagulant vacutainer tube left sitting upright) is often reached in the field. The authors do not recommend waiting on a definitive diagnosis of hepatic lipidosis to initiate treatment when there is strong evidence for a clinical diagnosis (Box 25.4).

**Box 25.4 Prophylactic treatment of dyslipidemias is key to improved prognosis**

Interventions include enteral (oral drenches or administration of food as a slurry via nasogastric tube) or parenteral nutrition (intravenous fluids including dextrose and potassium supplementation, or partial/total parenteral nutrition) in addition to treating the primary disorder. Treatment of the primary disorder is of utmost importance as treating dyslipidemias without addressing the inciting cause will not resolve the dyslipidemia.

In hyperglycemic patients, concomitant administration of insulin with dextrose in fluids is indicated. However, dosages of both are translated over from horses, and intervention beyond oral drenches is often not possible in the field. Heparin (40–100 IU/kg q12 SQ) may also be used to treat hyperlipemic donkeys, as heparin stimulates lipoprotein lipase activity to enhance lipogenesis and promote peripheral uptake of triglycerides. Prognosis for hepatic lipidosis is poor to guarded (up to 80% mortality) (Burden et al. 2011). Therefore, prevention of this disorder in any inappetent donkey is key. Where possible, the practitioner is encouraged to refer to an in-hospital clinic with available resources of aggressive medical management as the aforementioned interventions are logistically difficult to perform without constant nursing care.

## Respiratory System

*Donkeys have an insensitive cough reflex* compared to the horse, allowing for subtle respiratory pathologies to go unnoticed in the early stages of the disease.

*Secondary bronchopneumonia* is more common in donkeys infected with equine influenza than in horses.

Donkeys and mules can be infected with alpha (EHV-1, EHV-4) and gamma (EHV-2, EHV-5) equine herpesviruses as well as many asinine herpesviruses (AHV-2, AHV-3, AHV-4, AHV-5), all of which have been associated with a range of respiratory signs (Rickards and Thiemann 2019).

As with horses, donkeys and mules can suffer from respiratory disease associated with both *Streptococcus equi subsp. equi* and the commensal *Streptococcus equi subsp. zooepidemicus*. However, while *Streptococcus equi* subsp. *equi* is the most common causative agent of empyema and chondroid formation in the guttural pouches, there is some evidence suggesting that *Streptococcus equi* subsp. *zooepidemicus* may also lead to chondroid formation in donkeys (Evans et al. 2021).

*Tracheal collapse* due to dorsal ligament separation or structural tracheal ring abnormalities is common in aged donkeys. It can also occur secondarily to pulmonary fibrosis, or other conditions leading to increased inspiratory effort (Evans et al. 2021). Donkeys are unlikely to show clinical signs of dyspnea or stridor associated with these tracheal abnormalities unless they have a concurrent lung pathology or are subject to work (Powell et al. 2010). When clinical signs are present, an inspiratory stridor may be appreciated, as most often the extrathoracic tracheal rings are affected. However an expiratory noise may be present if the intrathoracic trachea is deformed (Boyle 2021). Diagnosis and treatment of tracheal abnormalities in the donkey is like that of the horse with a few anatomical differences that should be considered. Donkeys have narrow nasal passages, so small-bore endoscopes (see *Important Considerations by Body System: Gastrointestinal Tract*), good sedation, and restraint are necessary to avoid hemorrhage (Rickards and Thiemann 2019).

*Donkey asthma* may present as an emergency with severe expiratory dyspnea, often due to recent exacerbation of a chronic condition associated with environmental allergens (Rickards and Thiemann 2019; Archer et al. 2021).

*Pulmonary fibrosis* is also common in aged donkeys and should be considered as a differential for a donkey in respiratory distress. The underlying etiology is unknown, but the condition may be associated with asinine herpesvirus infections (AHV-4 & AHV-5), secondary bacterial infections, or acute allergen exposure (Miele et al. 2014). It can also result in secondary tracheal collapse. Reduced lung sounds coupled with characteristic ultrasonographic findings can be diagnostic. Treatment centers on supportive care and is often unrewarding in severely dyspneic patients (Archer et al. 2021).

## Musculoskeletal System

*Laminitis* (mostly endocrine in origin, though sepsis-related and supporting limb laminitis also possible) is a common cause of lameness in donkeys and mules (Figure 25.2). Donkeys may present with shifting weight, short strides, or even recumbency. As with any other pathologic process, serum triglyceride concentrations should be carefully monitored to detect hyperlipidemia as a secondary sequela. It is very important to understand important anatomical differences between donkeys and horses when attempting to diagnose laminitis. The hoof pastern axis is more upright and the distal phalanx is located more distally within the hoof capsule in the donkey compared to the horse, necessitating the use of donkey-specific radiological parameters (Collins et al. 2011; Nocera et al. 2020). In addition, the apex of the frog does not extend as far rostrally under the pedal bone in donkeys. For this reason, traditional frog supports typically used in laminitic horses may actually be contraindicated for use in donkeys as they do not provide the needed mechanical support, and may instead act as a fulcrum (Evans and Crane 2018). The hooves of mules have components of both donkeys and horses; thus, specific mechanical treatment should be tailored to the individual mule.

*White line abscesses* are another common cause of severe lameness in donkeys. Hoof testers are rarely useful for localizing an abscess in donkeys, due to the nature of their hard hoof capsules and thick soles (Evans and Crane 2018). In addition, due to the thickness of the donkey sole, pus tends to travel dorsally to the coronary band or inward to the pedal bone in more persistent cases, rather than under-running the sole (Thiemann and Rickards 2013). Paring out the sole to drain abscesses can be frustrating for this reason, and the pus may become inspissated by the time it is finally noted in the pared-out region (Figure 25.3). Medical management should be as with horses, even in the absence of obvious purulent drainage on poultice pads, until clinical resolution of lameness. Donkeys that are in severe pain should also be monitored for inappetence to avoid dyslipidemias.

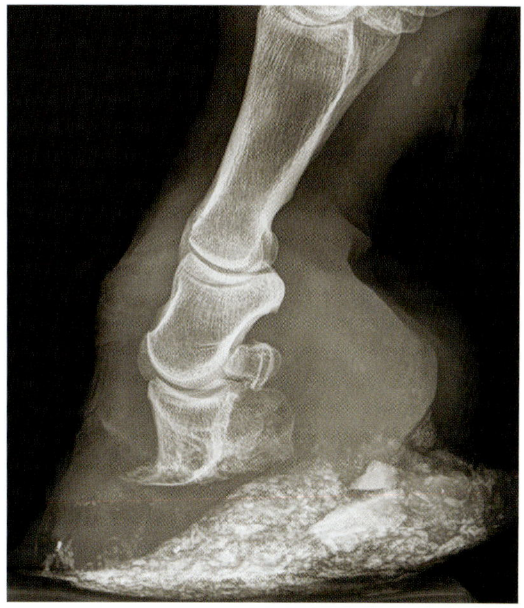

**Figure 25.2** A donkey with severe chronic laminitis. Note the flexural deformity of the distal interphalangeal joint secondary to displacement and rotation of P3 within the hoof capsule. Also, note the marked remodeling of the third phalanx associated with chronic disease. Corrective trimming and shoeing are required for such cases to help realign the pedal bone and hoof. Radiographs are valuable to establish baseline anatomic information and to monitor disease progression and response to treatment.

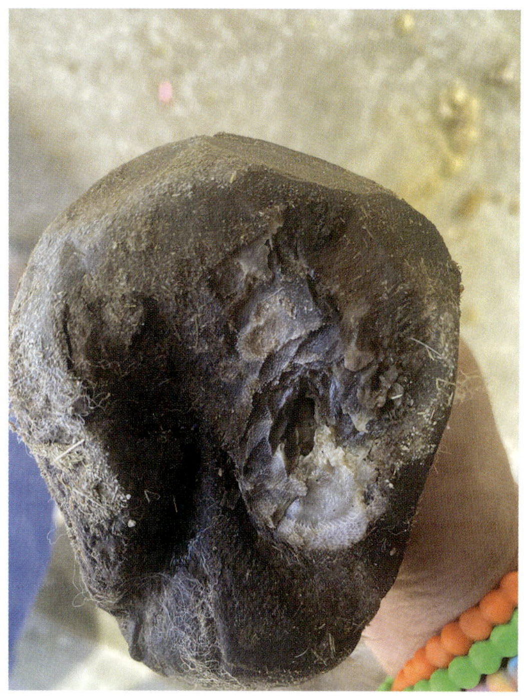

**Figure 25.3** A donkey with a sole abscess. Donkeys often suffer foot problems in captivity because of improper nutrition, poor hoof care management, and the environment. Sole abscesses may be related to overgrown hoofs, separation of the white line, secondary to laminitis, or associated with hoof trauma or other injury. Like the horse establishing ventral drainage is the first step, followed by soaking and hoof bandaging depending upon the local environment. Gravel (drainage from the coronary band) is common in donkeys because of their hard hoof structure.

**Table 25.4** Comparison of select cytologic values of equine and donkey cerebrospinal fluid.

| | Atlanto-occipital | | Lumbosacral | |
|---|---|---|---|---|
| **Parameter** | **Horse** | **Donkey**[e] | **Horse** | **Donkey**[e] |
| Specific gravity | 1.004–1.008[a] | 1.004–1.005 | 1.004–1.008[a] | 1.004–1.006 |
| Leukocytes (cells/uL) | 0–7[b] | 1.5–2.7 | 0–7[b] | 1.3–2.7 |
| Erythrocytes (cells/uL) | <50[c] | 1.5–2.7 | <50[c] | 1.3–2.7 |
| Total protein (mg/dL) | 45–61[d] | 15–30 | 55–73[d] | 10–26 |

*Source:* Modified from [a]Green et al. (1993), [b]Mayhew et al. (1977), [c]Furr and Andrews (2008), [d]Furr et al. (1997), [e]Abdelhakiem and Hussein (2021).

### Nervous System

The neurological examination in a donkey or mule is very similar to that of the horse. *Neurolocalization of lesions in and of itself is not different, but performance of the exam and response to certain tests differs.* Be aware that donkeys often do not exhibit a menace response reliably and that test should be repeated before diagnosing a donkey with a truly absent menace response (Evans et al. 2021). The dynamic component of the neurologic exam in donkeys is often complicated by their reticence to move in a new and/or stressful hospital environment, so allowing the donkey to move freely in a closed-off pen may be necessary for assessment of gait, ataxia, and weakness.

Cerebral spinal fluid can be collected from donkeys and mules as in horses. Literature exists regarding atlanto-occipital (AO) and lumbosacral (LS) CSF collection in donkeys (Abdelhakiem and Hussein 2021). One author (CX) has successfully performed an atlantoaxial (C1–C2 tap) in a donkey as described in horses. Donkey specific-reference ranges should be utilized when analyzing CSF fluid (Table 25.4). Although the normal gross appearance (clear) and cytologic components (WBC, RBC, and total protein) of CSF are similar to published horse reference ranges, the chemical constituents differ (Abdelhakiem and Hussein 2021).

Both equine herpesvirus-1 and asinine herpesvirus-3 have been associated with neurological disease in donkeys.

*Extrapolating the horse dose of anti-epileptic drugs to a seizing donkey or mule is reasonable* in the absence of established dosing regimens in donkeys and their hybrid crosses. Clinically, anti-epileptics (mainly diazepam) used in this manner has conferred successful seizure control in neurologic donkeys (Jule et al. 2023). One author (CX) has similarly successfully controlled an actively seizing donkey with diazepam (0.1 mg/kg IV) and maintained the same donkey on long-term seizure control with levetiracetam (32 mg/kg PO q12 h). More pharmacokinetic and pharmacodynamic data on these anti-seizure pharmaceuticals is not currently available and will be necessary to tailor donkey and mule-specific recommendations in the future.

## Fluid Therapy

Specific recommendations for fluid therapy do not yet exist in donkeys, but clinically donkeys seem to tolerate fluid therapies extracted from equine principles (Fielding and Magdesian 2015; Thiemann et al. 2017). As a desert-adapted species, donkeys are able to tolerate greater degrees of dehydration before hemoconcentrating or showing associated clinical sequelae (see *Clinical Pathology: The Hemogram*). Donkeys can resolve their fluid deficits faster when given the opportunity to drink, and rapid PCV/TS changes will reflect this. In general, oral, intragastric (via nasogastric tube), or rectal fluid therapy is the most practical in the field. The latter is complicated to manage without appropriate nursing care and is best achieved in a clinical setting along with intravenous fluid therapy. Because of the increased incidence of dyslipidemias in donkeys, dextrose supplementation in fluids is often recommended unless contraindicated by existing hyperglycemia.

Enteral fluids are not recommended in patients with gastric reflux and where intestinal perfusion is suspected to be compromised. Care must also be taken to consider a donkey's size in the administration of enteral fluids (no more than 3 L intragastrically for a 180 kg donkey) (Thiemann et al. 2017). Additionally, it appears that conservative fluid therapy leads to less complications (mural edema and poorer prognosis) associated with overhydrating animals with colitis (Thiemann et al. 2017). This is likely due to a similar mechanism in horses with colitis in which decreased oncotic pressure from loss of plasma proteins leads to fluid shifts from the extracellular to intracellular fluid compartments (i.e., from vasculature into interstitial spaces). When aiming to correct electrolyte and acid base derangements, the authors recommend following equine guidelines.

## Diseases of the Foal and Periparturient Jenny

### All Mule Foals (Jack × Mare) Are at Risk of Neonatal Isoerythrolysis

This is related to a unique donkey and mule erythrocyte antigen known as "donkey factor" (McClure et al. 1994). Mares carrying mule foals that develop anti-donkey factor antibodies pass these antibodies off to their offspring in colostrum, which subsequently cause immune mediated hemolysis in the mule. The incidence rate of neonatal isoerythrolysis is 10% in mules (compared to 2% in horses), but reasons behind the increased sensitization of mares to donkeys are unknown (McClure et al. 1994; Traub-Dargatz et al. 1995). Mule foals are typically normal at birth and develop clinical signs within 48–72 h after consumption of colostrum. Clinical signs and laboratory abnormalities (icterus, tachycardia, tachypnea, anemia, weakness, dark urine secondary to hemoglobinuria, and seizures if anemia and hypoxia are severe) are as with horse foals (Mair et al. 2013). Thrombocytopenia may also be seen in mule foals with neonatal isoerythrolysis, presumably from the presence of anti-platelet antibodies (Ramirez et al. 1999; Boyle et al. 2005).

A presumptive diagnosis of neonatal isoerythrolysis can be made based on clinical abnormalities, a positive Coombs test, or demonstration of anti-donkey factor antibodies in the mare's serum or colostrum to the mule foal's erythrocytes (i.e., minor cross-matching or jaundice foal agglutination test, respectively). Treatment that has been described includes administration of polymerized bovine hemoglobin, transfusion of washed erythrocytes from the dam, and provision of oxygen to the mule foal (Boyle et al. 2005). Prevention includes testing mares for anti-donkey factor antibodies 1–2 weeks prior to foaling, monitoring mule foals of multiparous mares that have previously foaled mules with neonatal isoerythrolysis, and preventing such foals from nursing their dam until gut closure (during the first 48 h postpartum) (Boyle et al. 2005; Mair et al. 2013).

To the authors' knowledge, no literature exists yet on the incidence of neonatal isoerythrolysis in the reciprocal donkey hybrid, the hinny (stallion x jenny). Thus, it seems reasonable to be overly cautious and presume the same risk in hinnies until further research elucidates otherwise.

*Hyperlipemia is more common in pregnant donkeys during the last trimester and in lactating donkeys.* This condition has a negative impact on the quality and volume of colostrum produced by the dam and therefore can increase the foal's risk for developing failure of passive transfer of immunity (FPT) (Evans et al. 2021). Diagnosis and treatment of FPT in donkey foals is as with horses.

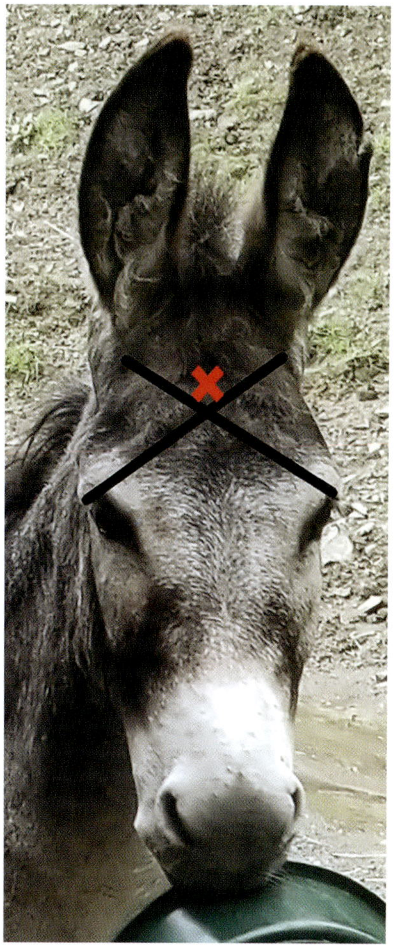

**Figure 25.4** Captive bolt placement in the donkey. A penetrating captive bolt is one method of euthanasia approved by the AAEP for euthanasia of equids. Note that placement of a captive bold or gunshot should be 1-2 cm above the intersection of two lines drawn between the lateral canthus of each eye and the base of the contralateral ear, slightly higher than the recommendation in horses.

## Euthanasia

Use of penetrating captive bolt (followed by pithing or exsanguination) or gunshot may be appropriate means of euthanasia in some instances. For donkeys, it is important to realize that the recommended site for captive bolt or gunshot entry is located about 1–2 cm above the intersection of two lines drawn between the lateral canthus of each eye and the base of the contralateral ear (Evans et al. 2021). Note that this landmark is slightly higher than that for horses and ponies (Figure 25.4).

Intrathecal lidocaine administered through the AO space is another option for euthanasia (Aleman et al. 2015). The landmarks are as described in horses. This option is useful when venipuncture is difficult in severely hypoperfused animals, or if avoidance of barbiturates is desired for environmental considerations or lack of availability. The practitioner must ensure that the animal is under a surgical plane of anesthesia to use this method.

### Case Example 25.1 Colic in a Donkey

Patient: 4-Year-Old Unknown Breed Jenny

*History:* Low body condition score, diarrhea since rescue (1 month prior), and a recent decrease in appetite (approximately two weeks). A week prior, the donkey was found to have a markedly elevated strongyle ova count (3,450 eggs per gram). Anti-helminthic therapy was initiated and a repeat fecal was planned in two weeks for a fecal egg count reduction test. However, the jenny was re-presented on emergency before the two-week recheck for refusing its evening meal and having difficulty rising after an unknown duration of being down in the field.

Step 1: Patient Stabilization
Because donkeys often present with non-specific signs of illness, the initial triage examination should always include evaluation of the following:

1) Mentation and body condition score (BCS; Figure 25.5)
2) Vital parameters (heart rate, respiratory rate, temperature)
3) Perfusion status (mucous membranes, jugular refill time, skin tent above the superior eyelid)
4) Lung and tracheal sounds
5) Gastrointestinal borborygmi
6) Hoof wall contour, sole appearance, and digital pulses

If the patient is tachycardic (>60 beats/min), it would be reasonable to treat the donkey like a colic and sedate and pass a nasogastric tube to avoid fatal gastric rupture at this point in the physical exam. Recall that donkeys are inherently stoic compared to horses and can show minimal signs of severe pain despite having a severe lesion.

If there is strong clinical evidence of severe hypoperfusion, placement of an IV catheter for IV fluids to prevent cardiovascular collapse is necessary before proceeding forward with any additional diagnostic workup.

Divergent hoof wall growth ("rings") in the absence of digital pulses does not rule out chronic laminitis. Donkeys with a high BCS are at greater risk for endocrinopathic laminitis and may remain undiagnosed due to their stoicism. Clinicians should also do their due diligence to examine the soles in amenable animals as donkeys can remain standing on their feet even if the frog has eroded from laminitis.

*Presuming that the triage examination reveals a systemically stable animal, the initial exam can also include brief evaluation of:*

7) Dentition (broken incisors, bleeding from the oral cavity)
8) Gait (weight bearing, stride length, ataxia, obvious fractures)

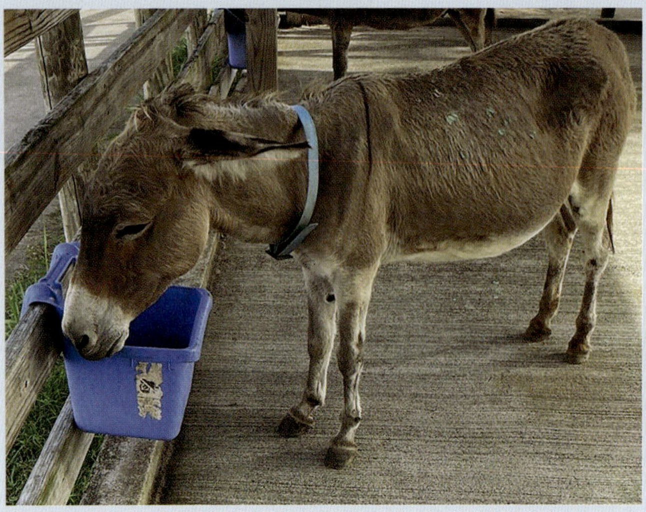

**Figure 25.5** An example of a thin donkey with a low BCS. Note the prominence of the scapular spine, tuber coxae, and lack of hamstrings. The ribs of the donkey were easily felt on palpation. *Source:* Courtesy of Dr. Claire Robinson.

These can help provide more information to guide formulation of a diagnostic plan (*Step 2*). Ideally, gait evaluation would be performed during the distance exam while the patient is walking into the examination room. If this was not possible, ask the handler to walk the donkey to ensure there are no obvious musculoskeletal issue or laminitis belying the patient's reported anorexia and difficulty rising. Unresolved dental abnormalities may also be an underlying cause of chronic pain contributing to the patient's history of progressive inappetence.

Step 2: Formulating a Diagnostic Plan

If the initial examination reveals obvious abnormalities referable to a particular organ system, the diagnostic plan should be tailored to working up that organ system. However, it is commonly very difficult to immediately determine the primary pathologic organ system causing anorexia in a donkey. In such cases, it is reasonable to work them up as a colic case. This includes:

1) Bloodwork (Figure 25.6)
2) Sedation and passage of a nasogastric tube to determine the presence of reflux
3) Rectal palpation
4) Abdominal ultrasonography (Figure 25.7)
5) Abdominocentesis

**Hematology**

**Complete Blood Count (CBC)**
(WB EDTA)

| Test | Result | Reference Range | Units |
|---|---|---|---|
| Specimen Tube Level | Adequately filled | | |
| Plasma Appearance | Turbid | | |
| Plasma Protein (PP) | **9.0 (H)** | 6.0–8.5 | g/dL |
| Packed Cell Volume (PCV) | **26 (L)** | 32–48 | % |
| Fibrinogen | 0.4 | 0.1–0.4 | g/dL |

**WBC Indices**

| Test | Result | Reference Range | Units |
|---|---|---|---|
| WBC Count | 7,120 | 5,400 – 14,320 | cells/uL |
| Segmented neutrophils | 5,700 | 3,000 – 6,000 | cells/uL |
| Lymphocytes | **520 (L)** | 1,500 – 5,000 | cells/uL |
| Monocytes | **900 (H)** | 0 – 600 | cells/uL |
| Eosinophils | 0 | 0 – 200 | cells/uL |
| Basophils | 0 | 0 – 200 | cells/uL |

**Clinical Chemistry**

| Test | Result | Reference Range | Units |
|---|---|---|---|
| Triglycerides | **>375 (H)** | 11 – 68 | g/dL |

**Mammalian Liver Profile**

| Test | Result | Reference Range | Units |
|---|---|---|---|
| ALP | **2,261 (H)** | 50 – 170 | U/L |
| ALT | **53 (H)** | 5 – 20 | U/L |
| GGT | **2,125 (H)** | 5 – 24 | U/L |
| BA | **105 (H)** | 0 – 25 | mmol/L |
| TBili | 0.8 | 0.5 – 2.3 | mg/dL |
| Albumin | 3.6 | 2.2 – 3.7 | g/dL |
| BUN | 9 | 7 – 25 | mg/dL |
| Cholesterol | **155 (H)** | 50 – 140 | mg/dL |

HEM 0, LIP 2+, ICT 0

**Figure 25.6** CBC and selected chemistry findings from this case of an anorexic donkey. Note that the plasma is turbid, which is consistent with the chemistry findings of hypertriglyceridemia and 2+ lipemia. Overall, the CBC results were interpreted as an anemia of chronic disease secondary to an unknown chronic inflammatory condition. The serum biochemistry results were consistent with a hepatopathy, either primary or secondary. Although these results were non-specific for a particular organ system, it prompted further evaluation with abdominal ultrasonography to search for possible etiologies, especially given the protracted history of low BCS and diarrhea.

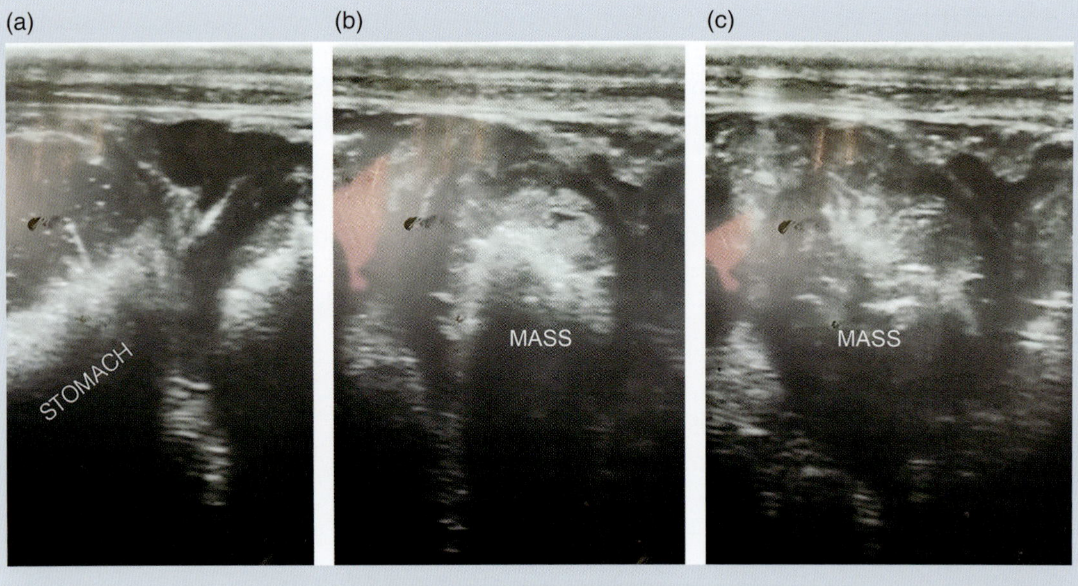


**Figure 25.7** Abdominal ultrasonography can be a useful diagnostic tool in smaller donkeys, as their size permits increased visualization of deeper structures. This is an image taken from the left 14th/15th ICS of this anorexic donkey. An ill-defined mass was detected caudal to the stomach where the spleen is usually visualized. Left is cranial, right is caudal. The spleen is not seen caudal to the stomach (a), instead being replaced by a heterogenic mass (b, c). This donkey was ultimately diagnosed with a pancreatic carcinoma on necropsy (Figure 25.9). Note that the pancreas should not normally be visualized in any equid.

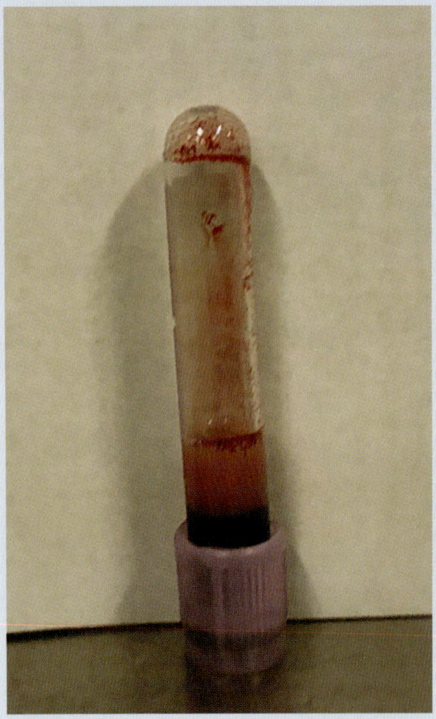

**Figure 25.8** Opaque plasma in a EDTA tube indicative of hyperlipemia. In the field, a blood tube may be set aside to allow the erythrocytes to settle out, leaving the plasma for gross evaluation. This technique can be used for subjective assessment of triglyceride concentrations if sample submission to a lab is delayed. *Source:* Courtesy of Dr. Georgia Ann Macy.

In the field, a PCV/TS, lactate, and triglycerides would be reasonable to start. Hyperlipidemia must be evaluated for in all donkeys with attributable historical factors (inappetence/anorexia) and would be supported by an increase in refractometric TS and opaque plasma even in the absence of laboratory confirmation of hypertriglyceridemia. Field practitioners can set aside a blood tube to allow erythrocytes to sediment out (Figure 25.8), which will permit quick determination of a potential dyslipidemia without interfering with the forward progression of a workup. Where available, a minimum database consisting of the above and a CBC, serum biochemistry, and triglycerides is ideal to evaluate systemic health and specific organ pathology. Note that finding abnormal liver values may simply reflect a hepatopathy secondary to the primary problem given the high risk of hyperlipidemia in this species (Figure 25.6).

Palpation per rectum is recommended in all donkeys that potentially have a gastrointestinal lesion. However, the decision to do so in a donkey that is significantly smaller than the examiner needs to be strongly weighed against the risk of rectal tears. Copious use of lube is necessary to decrease this risk in all equids regardless of size.

In patients with high BCS and those with gross hoof wall abnormalities, foot radiographs should also be considered if there is a low index of suspicion of gastrointestinal disease as acute on chronic laminitis pain can induce inappetence in a donkey. The decision to proceed with this diagnostic on an emergency basis should be weighed against a patient's systemic stability and presence of clinical findings suggestive of musculoskeletal disease.

### Step 3: Emergency Treatment Guidelines

Specific treatment in donkeys presenting for emergencies is often difficult because of the non-specific nature of their clinical signs. If a primary problem can be identified on triage, then treatment for that problem should be enacted. Additionally, all donkeys should have supportive care that addresses:

- Perfusion deficits (see *Fluid therapy* within Chapter 25)
- Inappetence
- The increased risk of hyperlipidemia (see *Hepatic disease* within Chapter 25)
- Pain control (see Table 25.1)

If donkeys are unwilling to eat on their own, the clients are unable to frequently monitor their donkey's appetite, and/or there is a concern that the disease process has been ongoing for longer than reported, parenteral nutrition (starting with dextrose added to IV fluids) is recommended. Referral at that stage is recommended as monitoring a patient on fluids with dextrose is often not logistically feasible in the field.

#### Step 4: Assessment and Monitoring

Donkeys should always have triglycerides monitored. If this is not possible, refractometric total solids can serve as a proxy for improving or worsening hypertriglyceridemia if there is a serial rise or fall, respectively, in TS over time.

Donkeys receiving IV dextrose should also have blood glucose monitored concurrently with their triglycerides. Measuring the amount of food that a donkey has eaten will also help objectively track a donkey's appetite. Monitoring fecal output will also provide an indirect assessment of gastrointestinal function.

#### Step 5: Decision Making During Triage

Referral is highly recommended for donkeys that have grossly opaque plasma as management of a hyperlipidemic animal requires supportive care that is difficult in the field (see *Hepatic Disease* within Chapter 25). Further, attempts to feed in the field by clients is often unrewarding, prolongs the duration in which the primary problem remains unresolved, exacerbates subclinical and clinical dyslipidemias, and worsens prognosis (Figure 25.9). It is important to advise owners that the financial burden of delaying referral for an inappetent/anorexic donkey is also likely to increase as more aggressive supportive care will be needed by the time of referral.

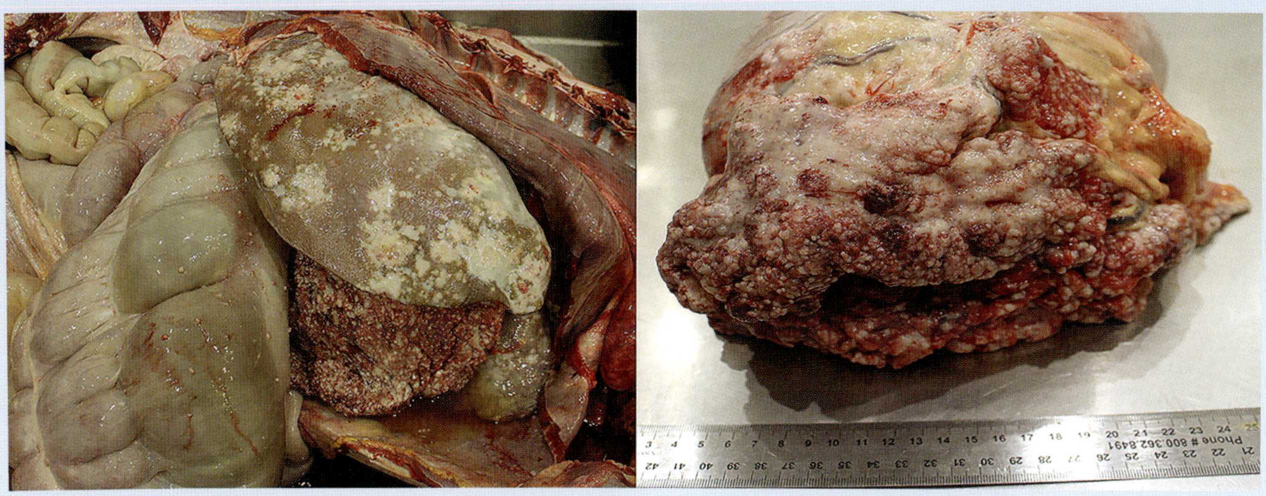

**Figure 25.9** Gross necropsy images from the same anorexic donkey with abnormal ultrasonography findings from Figure 25.6. The left image shows the relationship between the liver, mass, and right colon (cranial is right, caudal is left). The liver surface appeared mottled. Histologically, the majority of the liver sections were effaced by multifocal to coalescing regions of thick fibrosis associated with multiple islands, cords, and acini of neoplastic epithelial cells. The right image shows a close-up view of the pancreatic mass. Histologic findings included regions of coagulative necrosis present throughout the pancreas that extended into the peri-pancreatic fat; normal pancreatic tissue was rare. *Source:* Courtesy of the Pathology Laboratory, Ross University School of Veterinary Medicine.

## References


Abdelhakiem, M.A.H. and Hussein, H.A. (2021). Collection of cerebrospinal fluid in 50 adult healthy donkeys (Equus asinus): clinical complications, and cytological and biochemical constituents. *BMC Vet. Res.* 17: 302. https://doi.org/10.1186/s12917-021-03007-4.

Aleman, M., Davis, E., Williams, D. et al. (2015). Electrophysiologic study of a method of euthanasia using intrathecal lidocaine hydrochloride administered during intravenous anesthesia in horses. *J. Vet. Intern. Med.* 29: 1676–1682.

Archer, D.C., Sullivan, R.J.E., and Rickards, K. (2021). Emergency management for donkeys and mules. *Vet. Clin. North Am. Equine Pract.* 37: 495–513. https://doi.org/10.1016/j.cveq.2021.04.013.

Barakzai, S., Tremaine, H., and Dixon, P. (2006). Use of scintigraphy for diagnosis of equine paranasal sinus disorders. *Vet. Surg. VS* 35: 94–101. https://doi.org/10.1111/j.1532-950X.2005.00118.x.

Barrio, E., Rickards, K.J., and Thiemann, A.K. (2019). Clinical evaluation and preventative care in donkeys. *Vet. Clin. Equine Pract.* 35: 545–560. https://doi.org/10.1016/j.cveq.2019.08.013.

Boyle, A.G. (2021). Respiratory distress in the adult and foal. Management of emergency cases in the field. *Vet. Clin. North Am. Equine Pract.* 37: 311–325. https://doi.org/10.1016/j.cveq.2021.04.005.

Boyle, A.G., Magdesian, K.G., and Ruby, R.E. (2005). Neonatal isoerythrolysis in horse foals and a mule foal: 18 cases (1988–2003). *J. Am. Vet. Med. Assoc.* 227: 1276–1283. https://doi.org/10.2460/javma.2005.227.1276.

Brooke (2013). *The Working Equid Veterinary Manual*, 8e. Essex: Whittet Books.

Burden, F. and Thiemann, A. (2015). Donkeys are different. *J. Equine Vet. Sci.* 35: 376–382. https://doi.org/10.1016/j.jevs.2015.03.005.

Burden, F.A., Du Toit, N., Hazell-Smith, E., and Trawford, A.F. (2011). Hyperlipemia in a population of aged donkeys: description, prevalence, and potential risk factors. *J. Vet. Intern. Med.* 25: 1420–1425. https://doi.org/10.1111/j.1939-1676.2011.00798.x.

Burden, F.A., Hazell-Smith, E., Mulugeta, G. et al. (2016). Reference intervals for biochemical and haematological parameters in mature domestic donkeys (Equus asinus) in the UK. *Equine Vet. Educ.* 28: 134–139. https://doi.org/10.1111/eve.12512.

Burnham, S.L., 2002. Anatomical differences of the donkey and mule. *Proceedings of the Annual Convention of the AAEP*, Vol 48,. pp. 102–109.

Collins, S.N., Dyson, S.J., Murray, R.C. et al. (2011). Radiological anatomy of the donkey's foot: objective characterisation of the normal and laminitic donkey foot. *Equine Vet. J.* 43: 478–486. https://doi.org/10.1111/j.2042-3306.2010.00312.x.

Cox, R., Proudman, C.J., Trawford, A.F. et al. (2007). Epidemiology of impaction colic in donkeys in the UK. *BMC Vet. Res.* 3: 1. https://doi.org/10.1186/1746-6148-3-1.

DeNotta, S.L. and Divers, T.J. (2020). Clinical pathology in the adult sick horse: the gastrointestinal system and liver. *Vet. Clin. North Am. Equine Pract.* 36: 105–120. https://doi.org/10.1016/j.cveq.2019.11.004.

Evans, L. and Crane, M. (2018). *The Clinical Companion of the Donkey*, 1e. Sidmouth, Devon: Matador.

Evans, L., Crane, M., and Preston, E. (2021). *The Clinical Companion of the Donkey*, 2e. Devon: Sidmouth.

Fielding, C.L. and Magdesian, K.G. (2015). *Equine Fluid Therapy*. Iowa: Wiley.

Furr, M. and Andrews, F. (2008). Cerebrospinal fluid and the blood-brain barrier. In: *Equine Neurology* (ed. M. Furr and S. Reed), 40. Blackwell Publishing.

Furr, M., Chickering, W.R., and Robertson, J. (1997). High resolution protein electrophoresis of equine cerebrospinal fluid. *Am. J. Vet. Res.* 58: 939–941.

Goodrich, E.L. and Behling-Kelly, E. (2019). Clinical pathology of donkeys and mules. *Vet. Clin. North Am. Equine Pract.* 35: 433–455. https://doi.org/10.1016/j.cveq.2019.08.002.

Green, E., Constantinescu, G., and Kroll, R. (1993). Equine cerebrospinal fluid: analysis. *Compend. Contin. Educ. Pract. Vet.* 15: 288–301.

Ibrahim, H.M.M., Shoieb, S.M., EI-Ashker, M.R., and Abouelnasr, K.S. (2020). Sensitivity and specificity of abdominal fluid variables as a marker of intestinal ischemia in donkeys (Equus asinus). *JAPS J. Anim. Plant Sci.* 30: 1136–1144. https://doi.org/10.36899/JAPS.2020.5.0130.

Jule, C., Maxwell-Buechner, V., Southard, T., and LeCuyer, T. (2023). Listeria monocytogenes encepalitis in a donkey foal. *EVE* 36: e79–e84. https://doi.org/10.1111/eve.13915.

Lagos, J. and Tadich, T.A. (2019). Hematological and biochemical reference intervals for mules in Chile. *Front. Vet. Sci.* 6: 400.

Lindsay, F.E. and Clayton, H.M. (1986). An anatomical and endoscopic study of the nasopharynx and larynx of the donkey (Equus asinus). *J. Anat.* 144: 123–132.

Mair, T., Love, S., Schumacher, J. et al. (2013). *Equine Medicine, Surgery and Reproduction - E-Book*. Elsevier Health Sciences.

Mayhew, I.G., Whitlock, R.H., and Tasker, J.B. (1977). Equine cerebrospinal fluid: reference values of normal horses. *Am. J. Vet. Res.* 38: 1271–1274.

McClure, J.J., Koch, C., and Traub-Dargatz, J. (1994). Characterization of a red blood cell antigen in donkeys and mules associated with neonatal isoerythrolysis. *Anim. Genet.* 25: 119–120. https://doi.org/10.1111/j.1365-2052.1994.tb00091.x.

McLean, A.K., Wang, W., Navas-Gonzalez, F.J., and Rodrigues, J.B. (2016). Reference intervals for hematological and blood biochemistry reference values in healthy mules and hinnies. *Comp. Clin. Pathol.* 25: 871–878. https://doi.org/10.1007/s00580-016-2276-3.

McLean, A.K., Navas González, F.J., and Canisso, I.F. (2019). Donkey and mule behavior. *Vet. Clin. North Am. Equine Pract.* 35: 575–588. https://doi.org/10.1016/j.cveq.2019.08.010.

Mendoza, F.J., Perez-Ecija, R.A., Monreal, L., and Estepa, J.C. (2011). Coagulation profiles of healthy Andalusian donkeys are different than those of healthy horses. *J. Vet. Intern. Med.* 25: 967–970. https://doi.org/10.1111/j.1939-1676.2011.0748.x.

Mendoza, F.J., Toribio, R.E., and Perez-Ecija, A. (2018a). Donkey internal medicine-part i: metobolic, endocrine and alimentary tract disorders. *J. Equine Vet. Sci.* 65: 66–74.

Mendoza, F.J., Toribio, R.E., and Perez-Ecija, A. (2018b). Donkey internal medicine-part II: cardiovascular, respiratory, neurologic, urinary, ophthalmic, dermatology, and musculoskeletal disorders. *J. Equine Vet. Sci.* 65: 86–97.

Mendoza, F.J., Perez-Ecija, A., and Toribio, R.E. (2019). Clinical pharmacology in donkeys and mules. *Vet. Clin. North Am. Equine Pract.* 35: 589–606. https://doi.org/10.1016/j.cveq.2019.08.011.

Miele, A., Dhaliwal, K., Du Toit, N. et al. (2014). Chronic pleuropulmonary fibrosis and elastosis of aged donkeys: similarities to human pleuroparenchymal fibroelastosis. *Chest* 145: 1325–1332. https://doi.org/10.1378/chest.13-1306.

Mori, E., Fernandes, W.R., Mirandola, R.M.S. et al. (2003). Reference values on serum biochemical parameters of brazilian donkey (Equus asinus) breed. *J. Equine Vet. Sci.* 23: 358–364.

Mudge, M.C. (2014). Acute hemorrhage and blood transfusions in horses. Emergency and critical care. *Vet. Clin. North Am. Equine Pract.* 30: 427–436. https://doi.org/10.1016/j.cveq.2014.04.004.

Nocera, I., Aliboni, B., Ben David, L. et al. (2020). Radiographic and venographic appearance of healthy and laminitic feet in amiata donkeys. *Front. Vet. Sci.* 7: https://doi.org/10.3389/fvets.2020.601665.

Orsini, J.A. and Divers, T.J. (2008). *Equine Emergencies Treatment and Procedures*, 3e. St. Louis, MO: Saunders Elsevier.

Pearson, R.A. and Merritt, J.B. (1991). Intake, digestion and gastrointestinal transit time in resting donkeys and ponies and exercised donkeys given ad libitum hay and straw diets. *Equine Vet. J.* 23: 339–343. https://doi.org/10.1111/j.2042-3306.1991.tb03734.x.

Perez-Ecija, A. and Mendoza, F.J. (2017). Characterisation of clotting factors, anticoagulant protein activities and viscoelastic analysis in healthy donkeys. *Equine Vet. J.* 49: 734–738. https://doi.org/10.1111/evj.12685.

Pongratz, M.C., Junge, H.K., Riond, B., and Schwarzwald, C.C. (2016). Validation of the Accutrend Plus point-of-care triglyceride analyzer in horses, ponies, and donkeys. *J. Vet. Emerg. Crit. Care* 26: 682–690. https://doi.org/10.1111/vec.12512.

Powell, R.J., Du Toit, N., Burden, F.A., and Dixon, P.M. (2010). Morphological study of tracheal shape in donkeys with and without tracheal obstruction. *Equine Vet. J.* 42: 136–141. https://doi.org/10.2746/042516409X480412.

Ramirez, S., Gaunt, S.D., McClure, J.J., and Oliver, J. (1999). Detection and effects on platelet function of anti-platelet antibody in mule foals with experimentally induced neonatal alloimmune thrombocytopenia. *J. Vet. Intern. Med.* 13: 534–539. https://doi.org/10.1892/0891-6640(1999)013<0534:daeopf>2.3.co;2.

Rickards, K.J. and Thiemann, A.K. (2019). Respiratory disorders of the donkey. *Vet. Clin. North Am. Equine Pract.* 35: 561–573. https://doi.org/10.1016/j.cveq.2019.08.009.

Rodrigues, J.B. and Lilly, G. (2019). Dental disorders of donkeys. *Vet. Clin. North Am. Equine Pract.* 35: 529–544. https://doi.org/10.1016/j.cveq.2019.08.008.

Sgorbini, M., Bonelli, F., Papini, R. et al. (2018). Equine gastric ulcer syndrome in adult donkeys: Investigation on prevalence, anatomical distribution, and severity. *Equine Vet. Educ.* 30: 206–210. https://doi.org/10.1111/eve.12747.

Smith, B.P. (2020). *Large Animal Internal Medicine*. St. Lous, MO: Elsevier.

Taylor, T.S. and Matthews, N.S. (2002). Donkey and mule scenarios: when to stop, think, read or call. *AAEP Proc.* 48: 115–116.

Thiemann, A. and Rickards, K. (2013). Donkey hoof disorders and their treatment. *In Pract.* 35: 134–140. https://doi.org/10.1136/inp.f1074.

Thiemann, A.K. and Sullivan, R.J.E. (2019). Gastrointestinal disorders of donkeys and mules. *Vet. Clin. North Am. Equine Pract.* 35: 419–432. https://doi.org/10.1016/j.cveq.2019.08.001.

Thiemann, A.K., Rickards, K.J., Getachew, M., and Parashou, G. (2017). *The Acute Equine Abdomen*, 3e. New Jersey: Wiley.

du Toit, N. and Dixon, P.M. (2012). Common dental disorders in the donkey. *Equine Vet. Educ.* 24: 45–51. https://doi.org/10.1111/j.2042-3292.2011.00236.x.

du Toit, N., Gallagher, J., Burden, F.A., and Dixon, P.M. (2008). Post mortem survey of dental disorders in 349 donkeys from an aged population (2005–2006). Part 1: prevalence of specific dental disorders. *Equine Vet. J.* 40: 204–208. https://doi.org/10.2746/042516408X266060.

Traub-Dargatz, J.L., McClure, J.J., Koch, C., and Schlipf, J.J. (1995). Neonatal isoerythrolysis in mule foals. *J. Am. Vet. Med. Assoc.* 206: 67–70.

Wissdorf, H., Jerbi, H., and Meier-Schellersheim, M. (2021). *Anatomical Differences of the Donkey, Mule, and Horse*. utzverlag GmbH.

Xue, C. and Cavanaugh, S.M. (2022). Echocardiographic findings of a donkey (Equus asinus) Jenny with suspected mitral valve dysplasia. *J. Equine Vet. Sci.* 111: 103871. https://doi.org/10.1016/j.jevs.2022.103871.

Yousef, M.K., Dill, D.B., and Mayes, M.G. (1970). Shifts in body fluids during dehydration in the burro, Equus asinus. *J. Appl. Physiol.* 29: 345–349.

# 26

# Toxicologic Emergencies

*Megan Romano*[1] *and Karyn Bischoff*[2]

[1] *Department of Veterinary Sciences, Veterinary Diagnostic Laboratory, University of Kentucky, Lexington, KY, USA*
[2] *California Animal Health and Food Safety and Department of Molecular Biosciences, University of California Davis, Davis, CA, USA*

## Toxicologic Emergencies

Acute toxicosis is less common in equines than in other domestic species; however, when it occurs, it can be a very stressful situation for owners, patients, and practitioners alike (Caloni et al. 2018; Gwaltney-Brant 2018). Often, multiple animals are affected, especially in cases of feed or water contamination. Circumstances that should lead the practitioner to consider toxicosis are listed in Box 26.1.

If the animal is stable enough, removing the animal from the source of the toxicant is the first step in a toxicology emergency. This is immediately followed by triage and patient stabilization, which are foremost concerns in toxicant exposures just as in any other emergency; initial treatments and supportive measures necessary depend on the individual patient's status. Treatment considerations unique to toxic exposures are decontamination methods and antidotes or specific treatments. Once patients are stabilized, thorough physical examinations, history documentation, and environmental investigations are critical in diagnosis and prevention of future intoxications (Dechant 2021).

### General Stabilization

Severely affected patients require stabilization before further intervention. If possible, collect blood, serum, and urine for baseline analyses prior to administering treatments.

#### Airway

Envenomations in horses often involve the head and can cause swelling of the nasal passages. Airway maintenance is critical in these obligate nasal breathers. Nasal intubation with an endotracheal tube, nasogastric tube, or PVC pipe may be appropriate to maintain a patent airway (Landolt 2007). If swelling is too severe to permit nasal intubation, emergency tracheostomy may be necessary.

#### Breathing

Toxicants that cause severe CNS depression (e.g., amitraz) or paralysis of respiratory muscles (e.g., botulism) can impair respiration (Landolt 2007). Supplemental oxygen or endotracheal intubation and mechanical ventilation may be required in these cases. Likewise, toxicants that require anesthesia to control seizures (e.g., strychnine) will require mechanical ventilation (See Table 26.1).

#### Circulation/Cardiovascular Support

Basic cardiovascular support includes administration of intravenous fluids to restore or maintain blood volume and correct electrolyte and acid–base abnormalities. Toxicants that cause shock or hypovolemia (e.g., arsenic) may require shock doses of balanced electrolyte solutions or normal saline (Landolt 2007). Toxicants that cause severc electrolyte derangements

*Emergency Triage of the Horse*, First Edition. Edited by Rolfe M. Radcliffe and Jamie J. Kopper.

Companion website: www.wiley.com/go/radcliffe/triage

## Box 26.1 When to Suspect a Toxic Exposure

- Multiple dead or sick animals displaying similar clinical signs within a short time period
- New feed supplier, new batch or bag of feed, new batch or bale of hay
- New water source or interruption of water supply
- New medications or supplements, including over-the-counter products
- Recent management changes, e.g., movement to new or different barn or pasture
- Recent access to sheds, barns, storage areas, dump piles, burn piles, or other areas
- Recent nearby landscaping, construction, remodeling, mining, digging, drilling, or other activity
- Recent nearby use of pesticides or other agricultural chemicals
- Recent severe weather or changes in weather conditions (e.g., drought, flooding, freeze, downed limbs, uprooted trees)
- Recent conflict with neighbors or employees
- Any other recent changes

**Table 26.1** Potential toxicants, common sources, and treatments to consider. Note: many toxicants affect multiple body systems. To avoid repetition, source and treatment details are listed only once. Other listings refer the reader to the appropriate section.

| Toxicants | Sources | Treatments |
|---|---|---|
| | **Toxicants That Can Be Associated with Abdominal/Gastrointestinal Emergencies** | |
| **Colic** | | |
| **Amitraz** | • See **CNS Depression** | |
| **Arsenic** | • See **Acute Diarrhea** | |
| **Atropine** | **Medications:**<br>• Injectable solutions used to treat bradycardia, organophosphate and carbamate intoxications, and as a bronchodilator<br>• Ophthalmic preparations used in treating various ocular disorders to dilate pupils<br>**Plants:**<br>• Tropane alkaloids including atropine<br>• Most commonly:<br>– Jimsonweed (*Datura*)<br>– Some nightshades (*Solanum* spp.)<br>– Carolina horsenettle (*Solanum carolinense*)<br>– Henbane (*Hyoscyamus*) | **Impaction:**<br>• Mineral oil may be useful as a laxative to resolve mild impactions<br>• **Severe impactions** may require **surgical intervention**<br>**Analgesia:**<br>• NSAIDs<br>• α-2 agonists<br>• Opioids: **Use with caution**<br>– Can exacerbate ileus (Sellon et al. 2001)<br>AC: **Use with caution**<br>• Ileus may cause AC to release atropine, allowing further absorption<br>Hospitalize if **severe impaction** |
| **Azaleas** | • See **Rhododendron** in **Colic** | |
| **Black locust** | • See **Acute Diarrhea** | |
| **Blister beetle** | • See **Shock** | |
| **Blue-green algae** | • See **CNS Excitation** | |
| **Botulism** | • See **Respiratory Paralysis** | |
| **Cardiotoxic plants** | • See **Dysrhythmias** | |
| **Castor bean** | • See **Acute Diarrhea** | |
| **Cholinesterase inhibitors** | • See **Acute Diarrhea** | |
| **Cobalt** | • See **CNS Excitation** | |
| **Iron** | • See **Shock** | |
| **NSAIDs** | • See **Acute Diarrhea** | |

**Table 26.1** (Continued)

| Toxicants | Sources | Treatments |
|---|---|---|
| **Red maple**<br>*Acer rubrum* | • Also red maple hybrids<br>– e.g., sugar maple (*Acer saccharum*)<br>• Likely other *Acer* species | **Hemolytic anemia:** if Packed Cell Volume (PCV) is low or declining rapidly<br>• Packed red cells<br>• Whole blood<br>**IV Fluids:**<br>• **Once PCV corrected**<br>• Prevent/minimize **pigmentary nephropathy**<br>**Decontamination:**<br>• AC<br>**Oxidative stress:**<br>• **Ascorbic acid:** Extra-label<br>– 10–20 **g/horse** (NOT per kg) PO once daily (Davis and Wilkerson 2003)<br>– 30–50 mg/kg IV diluted in 5–10 L crystalloid fluids q12 h (McConnico and Brownie 1992)<br>**Analgesia:**<br>• Opioids:<br>– Butorphanol<br>– Consider transdermal fentanyl for longer use (Hovda 2022)<br>• NSAIDs: **With caution**<br>– **Correct fluid deficits** first<br>– Can exacerbate **renal effects**<br>**Hospitalization recommended** |
| **Rhododendrons**<br>*Rhododendron* spp. | • Fresh plants growing within animals' reach<br>• Clippings placed within reach after landscaping<br>• Rhododendrons are evergreen; particularly dangerous in winter when little other green forage is available | **Bloat:**<br>• Pass NG tube<br>**Decontamination:**<br>• AC<br>Hospitalize if **severe colic** |
| **Acute Diarrhea/Colitis** | | |
| **Antibiotics** | • **Any antibiotic** has some potential to cause colitis in equids (Haggett and Wilson 2008)<br>• More common with<br>– **Frequent** or **prolonged** use<br>– **High dosages**<br>– Use in **stressed** animals<br>– Macrolides (e.g., **erythromycin**)<br>○ Especially adult horses<br>○ Occasionally foals | **Hypovolemia:**<br>• **Shock dose** IV fluids<br>**Diarrhea:**<br>• **AC:**<br>– Consider repeating in 12 h if diarrhea still present<br>• Di-Tri-Octahedral smectite (BioSponge®): Per label instructions<br>• Probiotics: Per label instructions<br>Hospitalize if **severe diarrhea** |
| **Arsenic** | • See **Shock** | |
| **Azaleas** | • See **Rhododendrons** in **Colic** | |
| **Black locust**<br>*Robinia pseudoacacia* | • Bark stripped from the trees<br>• Leaves | **Hypovolemia:**<br>• **Shock dose** IV fluids<br>**Decontamination:**<br>• AC<br>**Hyperammonemia:**<br>• Lactulose: 333 mg/kg PO q8 h (Scarratt and Warnick 1998)<br>Hospitalize if **severe diarrhea** |

(*Continued*)

**Table 26.1** (Continued)

| Toxicants | Sources | Treatments |
|---|---|---|
| **Blister beetle** | • See **Shock** | |
| **Cardiotoxic plants** | • See **Arrhythmias** | |
| **Castor bean**<br>*Ricinus communis* | • Seeds are most toxic<br>• Plants growing within reach<br>• Malicious poisoning possible | **Hypovolemia:**<br>• **Shock dose** IV fluids<br>**Decontamination:**<br>• AC<br>**Hyperammonemia:**<br>• Lactulose: 333 mg/kg PO q8 h (Scarratt and Warnick 1998)<br>Hospitalize if **severe diarrhea** |
| **Cholinesterase inhibitors** | **Pesticides:**<br>• **Carbamates**<br>• **Organophosphates** | **Anticonvulsants:**<br>• Benzodiazepines<br>• Phenobarbital<br>**Tremors:**<br>• Methocarbamol<br>**Decontamination:**<br>Dermal exposure:<br>• Bathe in warm water with mild detergent<br>Ingestion:<br>• AC<br>**Antidotes:**<br>• **Atropine:**<br>– ***Test*** dosage: **0.02** mg/kg IV (Wismer and Means 2012). Monitor for mydriasis and salivation. If pupils dilate or salivation resolves, cholinesterase inhibitor intoxication is unlikely. Maximum effect may be delayed 5–10 minutes.<br>– ***Treatment*** dosage: **0.2** mg/kg (1/4 of the dose IV and remainder IM or SC) (Wismer and Means 2012). May need to repeat, typically q3–4 h.<br>– Use **extreme caution**; **severe ileus** can occur (See **Atropine**)<br>• **Pralidoxime (2-PAM)**: Extra-label<br>– 20 mg/kg (up to 35 mg/kg) slowly IV (Oehme 1987b)<br>– Reconstitute (Plumb 2018):<br>○ Add 20 mL sterile water for injection to yield 50 mg/mL solution<br>○ For IV infusion, 10–20 mg/mL in 0.9% NaCl is recommended<br>– Repeat q4–6 h as needed<br>– Note: Use is uncommon in equids<br>○ Limited availability<br>○ Expensive<br>○ Efficacy not demonstrated in horses<br>○ Carbamates bind reversibly to acetylcholine receptors; 2-PAM is of limited use in carbamate poisoning<br>**Hospitalization recommended** |

**Table 26.1** (Continued)

| Toxicants | Sources | Treatments |
|---|---|---|
| **Iron** | • See **Shock** | |
| **NSAIDs** | **Medications**:<br>• Accidental overdose (commonly paste formulations)<br>• Use of multiple products<br>• Use of steroids concurrently with NSAIDs<br>• Long-term use<br>• Use in **dehydrated animals** or animals with **underlying renal disease** | **Decontamination:**<br>• AC<br>• IV fluids to enhance renal clearance<br>**Antidote:**<br>• Misoprostol (extra-label): 5 µg/kg PO q8–12 h (Jacobson et al. 2013)<br>**Gastrointestinal protectants**:<br>• Omeprazole: 2–4 mg/kg PO q24 h (*Gastrogard*® label directions)<br>• Sucralfate (extra-label): 22 mg/kg PO q6–8 h (Videla and Andrews 2009)<br>– Administer on an empty stomach at least two hours after other oral medications (Marks et al. 2018)<br>Hospitalize if **severe diarrhea, severe colic**, or **renal compromise** |
| **Rhododendrons** | • See **Colic** | |
| | **Toxicants That Can Be Associated with Respiratory Emergencies** | |
| **Airway obstruction** | | |
| **Pit viper (Crotalid)** | • See **Shock** | |
| **Dyspnea** | | |
| **Anticoagulants** | • See **Shock** | |
| **Azaleas** | • See **Rhododendrons** in **Colic** | |
| **Blue-green algae** | • See **CNS Excitation** | |
| **Carbon monoxide** | • Smoke inhalation<br>– Barn fires<br>– Wildfires<br>• Space heaters or other equipment used in poorly ventilated areas | **Decontamination:**<br>• Move to **fresh air**<br>• Consider **supplemental oxygen**<br>Hospitalization usually **not required**<br>• Rapid death or recovery |
| **Cardiotoxic plants** | • See **Arrhythmias** | |
| **Cholinesterase inhibitors** | • See **Acute Diarrhea** | |
| **Cyanide** | **Smoke inhalation:**<br>• Barn fires<br>• Wildfires<br>**Cyanogenic forages:**<br>• Rare in monogastrics | **Decontamination:**<br>Smoke inhalation:<br>• Move to **fresh air**<br>• Consider **supplemental oxygen**<br>**Cyanogenic forages:**<br>AC **ineffective**<br>Hospitalization usually **not required**<br>• Rapid death or recovery |
| **Phosphides** | • Grain fumigants (aluminum phosphide)<br>– Treated grains<br>– Products used near animals<br>• Rodenticides (zinc phosphide) | **Anticonvulsants:**<br>• Benzodiazepines<br>• Phenobarbital<br>**Decontamination:**<br>• **Use extreme caution** passing NG tube<br>– **Phosphine gas** dangerous to personnel<br>– **Well-ventilated** area<br>– Administer liquid antacid **before** lavage<br>• Liquid antacid: Reduce liberation of phosphine gas (Regehr 2022)<br>– Aluminum hydroxide: 17–30 g/**adult horse** PO<br>– Magnesium hydroxide: 15 g/**adult horse** PO<br>– 5% Sodium bicarbonate: 10–12 g/**adult horse** PO<br>• AC **ineffective** |

(*Continued*)

**Table 26.1** (Continued)

| Toxicants | Sources | Treatments |
|---|---|---|
| | | **Tremors:**<br>• Methocarbamol<br>**Analgesia:**<br>• Flunixin (Regehr 2022)<br>**Severe acidosis:**<br>• Sodium bicarbonate IV: Dosage depends on calculated base deficit (Plumb 2018)<br>**Gastrointestinal protectants:**<br>• Omeprazole: 2–4 mg/kg PO q24 h (*Gastrogard®* label directions)<br>• Misoprostol (extra-label): 5 µg/kg PO q8–12 h (Jacobson et al. 2013)<br>• Sucralfate (extra-label): 22 mg/kg PO q6–8 h (Videla and Andrews 2009)<br>– Administer on an empty stomach at least two hours after other oral medications (Marks et al. 2018)<br>**Hospitalization recommended** |
| **Red maple** | • See **Colic** | |
| **Rhododendrons** | • See **Colic** | |
| **Respiratory Paralysis** | | |
| **Botulism** | *Clostridium botulinum* toxins<br>Ingestion of **preformed toxins**:<br>• Decaying vegetation<br>– Often round bale hay<br>• Hay contaminated with animal carcass<br>**Toxico-infectious:**<br>• "Shaker foal" syndrome<br>– Usually 2-6 weeks old<br>• Spores germinate within GI tract and produce toxin<br>**Wound botulism:**<br>• Spores germinate within a deep or penetrating wound and produce toxin | **Respiratory muscle paralysis:**<br>• Artificial ventilation<br>**Decontamination:**<br>• **Wound botulism:** clean/debride open wounds with antibacterial products<br>**Antidote:**<br>• *Clostridium botulinum* antitoxin<br>– **Does not** reverse clinical signs (Galey 2001)<br>○ Resolution can take **weeks to months**<br>**Hospitalization** recommended |
| **Poison hemlock** | • See **CNS Excitation** | |
| **Strychnine** | Rodenticides | **Anticonvulsants:**<br>• Benzodiazepines<br>• Barbiturates<br>• **General anesthesia** may be required<br>**Respiratory muscle paralysis:**<br>• Artificial ventilation<br>**Decontamination:**<br>• AC<br>**Hospitalization recommended** |

**Table 26.1** (Continued)

| Toxicants | Sources | Treatments |
|---|---|---|
| **Tetanus** | *Clostridium tetani* toxins<br>• Often introduced into **deep or puncture** wounds | **Antidotes:**<br>• Tetanus antitoxin<br>– **Does not** reverse clinical signs<br>– Prognosis is **grave** in symptomatic horses<br>**Hospitalization recommended** |
| **Toxicants That Can Be Associated with Cardiovascular/Circulatory System Emergencies** | | |
| **Shock** | | |
| **Anticoagulants** | **Rodenticides:**<br>• Active ingredients include:<br>– Brodifacoum<br>– Bromadiolone<br>– Chlorophacinone<br>– Coumachlor<br>– Difethialone<br>– Diphacinone<br>– Pindone<br>– Warfarin<br>**Moldy forages:**<br>• Dicoumarol<br>• **Moldy** sweet clover<br>• **Moldy** sweet vernal grass | **Coagulopathy/hemorrhage:**<br>• **Active clotting factors**<br>– Fresh frozen **plasma** if PCV stable<br>– **Whole blood** if **PCV is low** or rapidly falling (active bleeding)<br>• **Correct PCV** prior to administering IV fluids<br>**Antidote:**<br>• **Vitamin K1** (phytonadione):<br>– Recommended dosages vary widely<br>○ Refer to specific product label<br>– General range is 0.5–2.5 mg/kg IM or SC q24 h (Plumb 2018)<br>– PO vitamin K is well absorbed if given with a fatty meal<br>– Duration depends on product ingested; ranges from 14 to 28 days or longer<br>• Alfalfa hay provides additional vitamin K (Smit 2022)<br>AC **ineffective** once symptomatic<br>May be useful if very recent ingestion, but beginning vitamin K1 therapy is preferable to decontamination<br>Hospitalize if **coagulopathy or hemorrhage** |
| **Arsenic** | **Pesticides:**<br>• Arsenic-based **herbicides, insecticides**, and other pesticides (e.g., lead arsenate, Paris Green)<br>• Fowler's solution (potassium arsenite), a historical medication<br>• Soils in **old orchards and reclaimed strip mines** can be contaminated<br>• **Ashes** from burned pressure-treated wood may contain large amounts of chromated copper arsenate (CCA) | **Hypovolemia:**<br>• **Shock dose IV fluids**<br>• Consider **hypertonic saline**<br>**Analgesia:**<br>• Butorphanol<br>• NSAIDs: **With caution**<br>– Can exacerbate **GI and renal effects**<br>– Correct **fluid deficits** first<br>**Decontamination/Antidotes:**<br>**Chelators:**<br>• **Succimer** (2,3-Dimercaptosuccinic acid):<br>– Dosage in horses not well-established<br>– Extrapolated dosage from small animals 10 mg/kg PO q8 (Puschner and Aleman 2010)<br>• Dimercaprol (British Anti-Lewisite; BAL):<br>– Deep IM injection (Oehme 1987a):<br>○ 5 mg/kg loading dosage<br>○ 3 mg/kg q6 h for 24 h<br>○ 1 mg/kg q6 h for 2 days as needed<br>AC **ineffective**<br>Cathartics **contraindicated**<br>**Hospitalization recommended** |

(*Continued*)

Table 26.1 (Continued)

| Toxicants | Sources | Treatments |
|---|---|---|
| **Blister beetle**<br>(cantharidin) | • Alfalfa hay produced in native ranges of blister beetles (e.g., western US) | **Hypovolemia:**<br>• **Shock dose balanced** IV fluids<br>**Hypocalcemia:**<br>• Replacement:<br>– Up to 1 mL/kg 23% calcium gluconate diluted 1 : 4 in isotonic fluids administered over 30 minutes or more (Ward 2022)<br>• Maintenance/ongoing losses<br>– 250–500 mL 23% calcium gluconate/5 L (Ward 2022)<br>– Maintenance rate<br>**Hypomagnesemia:**<br>• **Note:** Use **extreme caution** calculating magnesium dosages. **Concentrations** can be reported as mEq/mL, mEq/kg, mmol/mL, mmol/kg, mg/mL, and mg/kg; *these units are **NOT equivalent**!* (Plumb 2018).<br>• Magnesium **sulfate:**<br>– 50–100 **mg/kg** IV diluted in fluids and given over 30 minutes (Toribio 2011)<br>• Magnesium **chloride:**<br>– Dosage is **NOT EQUIVALENT** to magnesium sulfate dosage<br>○ 100 mg/kg **magnesium sulfate = 9.7 mg/kg $Mg^{++}$**<br>○ 100 mg/kg **magnesium chloride = 25.5 mg/kg $Mg^{++}$**<br>○ Confusing these products can be **fatal**<br>**Analgesia:**<br>• Butorphanol<br>• Flunixin<br>**Decontamination:**<br>• AC<br>**GI protectants:**<br>• Sucralfate<br>**Hospitalization recommended** |
| **Ionophores** | **Feed/mineral additives:**<br>• Monensin best known<br>• Lasalocid<br>• Narasin<br>• Salinomycin<br>• Feeds/minerals produced for other species<br>• Horse feeds from mills that also produce medicated feeds<br>• Bulk horse feeds transported after medicated bulk feeds without sufficient flushing | **Hypovolemia:**<br>• **Shock dose balanced IV fluids**<br>• Once deficits are corrected, consider supplemental **potassium** and **phosphorus** if indicated<br>**Ventricular arrhythmia:**<br>• Lidocaine: 0.5 mg/kg slowly IV over several minutes (Boesch 2013)<br>– Repeat every 5–10 minutes prn (maximum 2 mg total)<br>– If multiple boluses needed, consider CRI<br>**Decontamination:**<br>• AC<br>• Mineral oil is contraindicated; could increase absorption (Divers 2022)<br>**Hospitalization recommended** |

**Table 26.1** (Continued)

| Toxicants | Sources | Treatments |
|---|---|---|
| **Iron** | • Oversupplementation<br>  – Often neonates<br>• Recent cases due to high-iron water sources | **Hypovolemia:**<br>• **Shock dose IV fluids**<br>• Consider **hypertonic saline**<br>**Decontamination/antidotes:**<br>Chelators:<br>• Deferoxamine mesylate:<br>  – Foals: 1 g in 5 mL SC q12 h to reduce iron overload after transfusion (Elfenbein et al. 2010)<br>• **Caution: Nephrotoxic**<br>  – **Do not use** in patients with renal disease<br>  – **Correct fluid deficits** first<br>• Rapid administration can cause **arrhythmias** and exacerbate **hypotension**<br>AC **ineffective**<br>**Hospitalization** recommended if symptomatic |
| **Pit viper (Crotalid)** envenomation | Rattlesnakes, copperheads, cottonmouth/water moccasins | **Airway:**<br>• Establish/maintain patent airway if bitten on face<br>  – Nasal intubation (NG tube, endotracheal tube, PVC pipe, etc.)<br>  – If swelling will not permit nasal intubation, consider<br>    ○ Tracheostomy<br>    ○ General anesthesia and endotracheal intubation<br>**Hypovolemia/shock:**<br>• **Shock dose** IV fluids<br>• Consider **hypertonic saline**<br>**Antidote:**<br>Several antivenom products<br>• Variable availability and efficacy<br>• Can be cost-prohibitive in horses<br>**Analgesia:**<br>• Butorphanol<br>• NSAIDs: Use **with caution**<br>  – Can exacerbate **GI and renal effects**<br>  – **Correct fluid deficits** first<br>• Corticosteroid use is controversial<br>**Hospitalization recommended** |
| Arrhythmias | | |
| **Azaleas** | • See **Rhododendrons** in **Colic** | |
| **$\beta_2$ agonists** | • See **CNS Excitation** | |
| **Blister beetle** | • See **Shock** | |

*(Continued)*

**Table 26.1** (Continued)

| Toxicants | Sources | Treatments |
|---|---|---|
| **Cardiotoxic plants** | • Death camas (*Zigadenus* spp.)<br>• Hemp dogbane (*Apocynum cannabinum)*<br>• Oleander (*Nerium oleander*)<br>• Yellow oleander (*Cascabela thevetia*)<br>• Yew (*Taxus* spp.)<br>• Plants growing within reach<br>• Clippings placed within reach after landscaping<br>• Contaminated hay | **IV Fluids**:<br>• 0.9% NaCl recommended<br>– **Avoid calcium**-containing fluids<br>– **Avoid potassium**-containing fluids if **hyperkalemia** is present<br>**Ventricular arrhythmias:**<br>• Lidocaine: 0.5 mg/kg slowly IV over several minutes (Boesch 2013)<br>– Repeat every 5–10 minutes prn (maximum 2 mg total)<br>– If multiple boluses needed, consider CRI<br>**Decontamination:**<br>• AC<br>**Antidote:**<br>Digoxin-specific FAB fragments used anecdotally in horses, but no published data is available.<br>• DigiFab<br>• Digibind<br>Hospitalize if **intractable pain** or **severe ventricular arrhythmias** |
| **Cobalt** | • See **CNS Excitation** | |
| **Ionophores** | • See **Shock** | |
| **Pit viper (Crotalid)** | • See **Shock** | |
| **Rhododendrons** | • See **Colic** | |
| **Vitamin D** | **Feeds and supplements:**<br>• Products intended for other species<br>• Feed formulation error<br>• Excessive supplementation<br>**Rodenticides**<br>• **Cholecalciferol-based** | **IV Fluids:**<br>• Enhance renal calcium excretion<br>• 0.9% NaCl recommended (Katan 2022)<br>– Avoid calcium-containing fluids<br>**Hypercalcemia:**<br>• Furosemide: 0.5-2.0 mg/kg PO or IV q 8-12 h prn (Mogg 1999)<br>– **Correct fluid deficits** first<br>• Corticosteroids: **With caution**<br>– Prednisolone: 0.05–2.0 mg/kg PO q24 h (Katan 2022)<br>– Dexamethasone: 2.5–10 mg total dose IV, IM, or PO q24 h (Katan 2022)<br>• Bisphosphonates have been used anecdotally but are **not approved** for use in Vitamin D toxicosis<br>**Decontamination:**<br>• AC<br>**Hospitalization recommended** |
| **White snakeroot** | • See **CNS Excitation** | |
| Hemolysis/Icterus | | |
| **Red maple** | • See **Colic** | |
| **Toxicants causing liver failure** | • See **Acute Liver Failure** | |

**Table 26.1** (Continued)

| Toxicants | Sources | Treatments |
|---|---|---|
| **Hemorrhage** | | |
| **Anticoagulants** | • See **Shock** | |
| **Toxicants causing liver failure** | • See **Acute Liver Failure** | |
| | **Toxicants That Can Be Associated with Renal/Urinary Tract Emergencies** | |
| **Acute Kidney Injury** | | |
| **Aminoglycosides** | **Antibiotics:**<br>• Amikacin<br>• Gentamicin | **Decontamination:**<br>• IV fluids to enhance renal clearance<br>AC **ineffective** |
| **NSAIDs** | • See **Acute Diarrhea** | |
| **Pigmenturia** | | |
| **Anticoagulants** | • See **Shock** | |
| **Box elder**<br>(*Acer negundo*) | • Winged samaras drop in autumn<br>• New sprouts in spring pastures | **IV Fluids:**<br>• Prevent/minimize **pigmentary nephropathy**<br>**Oxidative stress:**<br>• Ascorbic acid: extra-label<br>– 10–20 **g/horse** (NOT per kg) PO once daily (Davis and Wilkerson 2003)<br>– 30–50 mg/kg IV diluted in 5–10 L crystalloid fluids q12 h (McConnico and Brownie 1992)<br>• Vitamin E: Maximum 20 IU/kg PO (Finno and Valberg 2012)<br>**Analgesia:**<br>• Butorphanol<br>• NSAIDs: Use **with caution**<br>– **Correct fluid deficits** first<br>– Can exacerbate **renal effects**<br>AC **ineffective**<br>**Hospitalization recommended** |
| **Cobalt** | • See **CNS Excitation** | |
| **Red maple** | • See **Colic** | |
| **White snakeroot** | • See **Tremors** | |
| | **Toxicants That Can Be Associated with Neurologic Emergencies** | |
| **CNS Depression, Abnormal Mentation, Obtundation, or Coma** | | |
| **Amitraz** | **Pesticide:**<br>• α-2 agonist registered for use in ruminants and dogs to treat ectoparasites (ticks, mites, and lice)<br>• Toxic to **equids and cats**<br>• Various forms<br>– Sprays<br>– Dips<br>– Concentrated liquids<br>– Wettable powders | **Decontamination:**<br>Dermal:<br>• Bathe in warm water with mild detergent<br>Oral:<br>• AC: **With caution**<br>– Ileus may cause AC to release amitraz, allowing further absorption<br>**Antidote:**<br>α-2 antagonists:<br>• Atipamezole: 0.1 mg/kg IV (Dowlin 2008)<br>• Yohimbine: 0.05–0.2 mg/kg IM or slowly IV (Brosnan 2010)<br>Hospitalize if **severe CNS depression** or **severe impaction** |
| **Fumonisin** | • See **Hepatotoxins** | |

(*Continued*)

**Table 26.1** (Continued)

| Toxicants | Sources | Treatments |
|---|---|---|
| **Locoweeds** | Plants<br>• *Oxytropis* spp.<br>• *Astragalus* spp. | Handle affected animals **with caution**<br>Normally docile animals can **become aggressive** or **behave bizarrely**<br>**Anxiolytics/anticonvulsants:**<br>• Benzodiazepines<br>AC **ineffective**<br>Hospitalize if **severe CNS depression** or **mentation abnormalities** |
| **CNS Excitation, Agitation, Seizures, and/or Tremors** | | |
| **Antipsychotics** | **Medications:**<br>• Long-acting antipsychotics are often prescribed for horses on stall rest<br>– Fluphenazine<br>– Reserpine | **Agitation:**<br>• Acepromazine<br>• α-2 agonists<br>AC **ineffective**<br>**Specific treatments:**<br>Anecdotally reported to be effective (Bohannon 2022):<br>• Pentobarbital: Bolus 2 mg/kg IV or CRI 1 mg/kg/h<br>• Benztropine: 0.018 mg/kg IV or 0.035 mg/kg PO q12 h<br>• Diphenhydramine: 0.67–1.0 mg.kg IV |
| **$\beta_2$ agonists** | **Medications:**<br>• Accidental overdose or use of compounded products<br>– Clenbuterol (Ventipulmin)<br>– Albuterol<br>Feed additives intended for other species:<br>• Ractopamine (Paylean, Optaflexx, Topmax)<br>• Zilpaterol (Zilmax)<br>• Illicit use in performance horses | **Sinus tachycardia:**<br>• Lidocaine: 0.25-0.5 mg/kg IV over several minutes (Redpath and Bowen 2019)<br>– Repeat every 5–10 minutes prn (maximum 2 mg total)<br>– If multiple boluses needed, consider CRI<br>• Propranolol: 0.03–0.16 mg/kg IV q8 h (Redpath and Bowen 2019)<br>**Agitation:**<br>• α-2 antagonists<br>• Butorphanol<br>**Decontamination:**<br>• AC<br>Hospitalize if **severe cardiac dysrhythmia** |
| **Blue-green algae** | **Neurotoxic cyanobacteria:**<br>• Harmful algal blooms can develop in ponds, lakes, river, streams, and other natural water sources<br>• Toxins can be present in the water even when the bloom is not evident. | **Anticonvulsants:**<br>• Benzodiazepines<br>• Phenobarbital<br>AC **ineffective**<br>Treatment unrewarding; animals **rarely survive**<br>**Hospitalization recommended** |
| **Cholinesterase inhibitors** | • See **Acute Diarrhea** | |

**Table 26.1** (Continued)

| Toxicants | Sources | Treatments |
|---|---|---|
| **Cobalt** | **Medications:**<br>• Iatrogenic, usually injectable<br>• Products intended for other species containing cobalt salts | **Agitation:**<br>• α-2 antagonists<br>• Acepromazine<br>AC **ineffective**<br>**Tremors:**<br>• Acepromazine<br>• Methocarbamol |
| **Ionophores** | • See **Shock** | |
| **Metaldehyde** | **Pesticide:**<br>• Slug/snail bait | **Tremors:**<br>• Methocarbamol<br>**Hyperthermia:**<br>• Cool water rinse<br>• Manage tremors<br>**Decontamination:**<br>• **AC**<br>Hospitalize if **refractory tremors** or **hyperthermia** |
| **Methylxanthines** | **Caffeine, theobromine, and theophylline:**<br>• Bedding: coffee bean husks and cacao bean hulls used as bedding<br>• Foods/beverages/treats: coffee, coffee beans, tea, energy drinks and supplements, chocolate<br>• Pharmaceuticals: various products contain caffeine and/or theophylline<br>• Potential performance-enhancing stimulants | **Agitation/aggression:**<br>• Acepromazine<br>• α-2 agonists<br>  – Detomidine may be better in aggressive animals<br>• Butorphanol<br>**Sinus tachycardia:**<br>• Propranolol: 0.03–0.16 mg/kg IV q8 h (Redpath and Bowen 2019)<br>**Decontamination:**<br>• AC<br>Hospitalize if **severe arrhythmias** |
| **Phosphides** | • See **Dyspnea** | |
| **Poison hemlock**<br>*Conium maculatum* | • Fresh plants are unpalatable and rarely eaten<br>• Contaminated hay most dangerous<br>• Dried plants more palatable than fresh, but equally toxic | **Anticonvulsants:**<br>• Benzodiazepines<br>• Barbiturates<br>**Respiratory muscle paralysis:**<br>• Artificial ventilation<br>**Decontamination:**<br>• AC<br>Hospitalize if **intractable seizures** or **respiratory muscle paralysis** |
| **Tremorgenic forages** | **Mycotoxins:**<br>• Produced by **Claviceps** spp.<br>• Can infect many types of grasses, including dalllisgrass, bahia, perennial ryegrass, and corn plants | **Tremors:**<br>• Methocarbamol<br>**Decontamination:**<br>• Removing source usually sufficient<br>Hospitalization **not generally required** |

*(Continued)*

**Table 26.1** (Continued)

| Toxicants | Sources | Treatments |
|---|---|---|
| **White snakeroot**<br>*Ageratina altissima*<br><br>Rayless goldenrod<br>*Isocoma pluriflora* | • Fresh plant<br>• Hay<br>• Eliminated in milk: foals can be affected | **Tremors:**<br>• Methocarbamol<br>**IV Fluids:**<br>• Prevent/minimize **pigmentary nephropathy**<br>**Decontamination:**<br>• AC<br>**Analgesia:**<br>• Butorphanol<br>• NSAIDs: Use **with caution**<br>– **Correct fluid deficits** first<br>– Can exacerbate **renal effects**<br>Hospitalization recommended if **pigmenturia** |
| **Paresis, Paralysis, or Dysphagia** | | |
| **Botulism** | • See **Respiratory Paralysis** | |
| **Nigropallidal encephalomalacia** | • See **CNS Depression** | |
| **Tetanus** | • See **Respiratory Paralysis** | |
| **Extensor Rigidity** | | |
| **Strychnine** | • See **Respiratory Paralysis** | |
| **Tetanus** | • See **Respiratory Paralysis** | |
| | **Toxicants That Can Be Associated with Acute Liver Failure** | |
| **Acute Liver Failure** | | |
| **Alsike clover**<br>(*Trifolium hybridium*) | • The plant is widespread, but poisoning is rare (Clayton et al. 2020)<br>• Only an association between alsike clover and disease; causality unproven | **IV Fluids:**<br>• Correct fluid deficits<br>• Consider supplemental 5% dextrose and potassium (Poppenga and Sobhakumari 2022)<br>AC **ineffective**<br>**Hepatic support:**<br>• N-acetylcysteine<br>• SAM-e<br>• Silymarin<br>**Hospitalization recommended** |
| **Blue-green algae** | Hepatotoxic cyanobacteria<br>• Hepatotoxins<br>• Harmful algal blooms can be visible on ponds, lakes, rivers, streams, and other natural water sources<br>• Obvious blooms may not be evident<br>• Toxins can remain weeks after bloom collapses | Treatment **usually unrewarding**; animals often **found dead**<br>**Decontamination:**<br>• AC<br>**Hyperammonemia:**<br>• Lactulose: 333 mg/kg PO q8 h (Scarratt and Warnick 1998)<br>**Hepatic support:**<br>• N-acetylcysteine<br>• SAM-e<br>• Silymarin<br>**Hospitalization recommended** |

**Table 26.1** (Continued)

| Toxicants | Sources | Treatments |
|---|---|---|
| **Fumonisin** | **Mycotoxin:**<br>• Associated with moldy corn<br>• Equine leukoencephalomalacia (ELEM) – grave prognosis<br>• Acute liver failure<br>• ELEM and liver failure can occur separately or simultaneously | **Treatment unrewarding** with ELEM<br>• Animals with *only* liver damage may recover<br>• ELEM causes irreversible neurologic damage<br>**Hyperammonemia:**<br>• Lactulose: 333 mg/kg PO q8 h (Scarratt and Warnick 1998)<br>**Hepatic support:**<br>• N-acetylcysteine<br>• SAM-e<br>• Silymarin<br>AC **ineffective**<br>**Hospitalization recommended** |
| **Iron** | • See **Shock** | |
| | **Toxicants That Can Be Associated with Acute Laminitis** | |
| **Acute Laminitis** | | |
| **Black walnut**<br>*Juglans nigra* | • Fresh shavings made from fresh or aged black walnut wood<br>• Stripping bark from trees | **Decontamination:**<br>• Remove from source<br>Dermal exposure:<br>• Bathe in warm water with mild detergent<br>**Analgesia:**<br>• NSAIDs<br>• Butorphanol<br>Hospitalize if **intractable pain**, or if **severe sinking** or **rotation** requiring podiatrist support |
| **Hoary alyssum**<br>*Berteroa incana* | • Toxic as fresh plants and in hay up to nine months after cutting (Hovda 2022)<br>• Hay containing >30% is considered dangerous | **Hypovolemia/shock:**<br>• **Shock dose IV fluids**<br>**Decontamination:**<br>• AC<br>**Analgesia:**<br>• NSAIDs<br>• Butorphanol<br>Hospitalize if **intractable pain** or **severe sinking** or **rotation** requires podiatrist support |

(e.g., blister beetles) require electrolyte supplementation of IV fluids. Intravenous fluids can also be used to maintain thermal homeostasis and renal function. Basic supportive care for any sick horse may include administration of maintenance rates of crystalloid fluids. Intoxications requiring shock doses, special considerations as to choice of fluids or supplementation of fluids, and indications for fluid administration beyond basic maintenance needs are specified in Table 26.1.

## Specific Medications

Patients with seizures, severe muscle tremors, or severe pain including colic will need additional stabilization before other treatments are possible. Agitated or aggressive patients may require sedation to allow safe handling. Medications commonly used to treat these conditions in toxicologic emergencies are listed below. Table 26.1 lists additional medications that can be considered for a toxicosis.

#### Anticonvulsants

**Benzodiazepines** are often used for short-term seizure control (Hackett 2014). All use is extra-label; no benzodiazepine products are labeled for use in horses in the US (Plumb 2018).

- *Diazepam (Hackett 2014)*
  - Adult horses: 0.05–0.44 mg/kg IV
  - Foals: 0.1–0.2 mg/kg IV
- *Midazolam (Hackett 2014)*
  - Adult horses: 0.05–0.1 mg/kg IV
  - Foals: 0.1–0.2 mg/kg

**Barbiturates** and other long-acting drugs are often needed in the poisoned patient (Landolt 2007). All use is extra-label; no barbiturate products are labeled for use in horses in the US (Plumb 2018).

- *Phenobarbital*
  - 5–15 mg/kg slow IV (Hackett 2014)
  - Loading dosage of 16–20 mg/kg IV once, then maintenance dosage of 1–5 mg/kg PO (Knipe 2009)

*Note*: Donkeys, mules, and other equids may require higher doses or more frequent dosing of sedative and anesthetic drugs than do horses (Archer et al. 2021).

#### Muscle Tremors

- Methocarbamol: (*Robaxin*®-V package insert)
  - Moderate conditions: 4.4–22 mg/kg IV slowly to effect
  - Severe conditions: 22–55 mg/kg IV

#### Analgesia

NSAIDs: mild-to-moderate pain and inflammation

- *Flunixin*
  - 1.1 mg/kg IV or PO q12–24 h (*Banamine*® US package insert)
- *Phenylbutazone*
  - 1–2 g/454 kg horse (NOT mg/kg) slow IV once daily (*Phenylbutazone*® package insert)
  - Extra-label: 2.2–4.4 mg/kg IV or PO q12–24 h (Constable et al. 2017)
- Ketoprofen: 2.2 mg/kg IV q24 h (*Ketofen*® package insert)

Opioids: severe pain or when NSAIDs are contraindicated

- *Butorphanol*
  - 0.1 mg/kg IV q3–4 h for up to 48 h (*Torbugesic*® package insert)

α-2 agonists: sedative as well as analgesic effects.

- Xylazine: 1 mg/kg IV; 2.2 mg/kg IM (*Rompun*® package insert)
- Detomidine: 0.02–0.04 mg/kg IV (*Dormosedan*® package insert)

#### Agitation/Sedation

- Acepromazine: 0.044–0.088 mg/kg slowly IV; IM; or SC as needed (*PromAce*® package insert)
- **α-2 agonists** (see **Analgesia** above)

### Decontamination

Early decontamination involves removing contaminants from skin, mucosal surfaces such as the eyes, and the gastrointestinal tract.

- **Personal protective equipment** (gloves, masks, face shields, aprons, and goggles) is critical in protecting the animal health worker from contaminants like pesticides.

#### Dermal and Mucosal Exposures

- **Dry removal** of dry powdered or particulate material from skin can be accomplished using brushes, combs, and vacuuming (Landolt 2007).
- Copious **lavage** with tap water can be used to dilute alkaline or acidic materials. Use of a hand dish-washing detergent in addition to the tap water is helpful in removing many pesticides and oily substances, but avoid shampoos.

#### Oral Exposures

- **Gastric lavage** can be used in any recent ingestion; efficacy depends on the time since ingestion and the nature of the toxicant. For example, small pieces of recently ingested plants are easier to retrieve than loose mineral ingested hours before.
- **Activated charcoal** (AC) can adsorb and aid elimination of some toxicants. Table 26.1 indicates toxicants for which AC is potentially effective, those for which it is not effective, and other considerations regarding AC administration. Administer as soon as possible if recent ingestion of a toxicant is suspected.
  - Activated charcoal: 1–2 g/kg in a 1 g/5 mL dilution with water via NG tube (Poppenga and Puschner 2014).
- Cathartics are often added to AC and may be used, but efficacy has not been established in horses. Cathartics are contraindicated in animals with diarrhea. Additionally, adverse effects have been associated with overdose of magnesium sulfate in horses (Dawson 2011). Repeated doses of AC with sorbitol have been associated with hypernatremia and dehydration in dogs and humans (Allerton and Strom 1991; Mix et al. 2019).
- Mineral oil, often used as a laxative in equine medicine, should be avoided in most intoxications except where impactions can occur (e.g., atropine). It is not a cathartic and can interfere with the adsorptive effects of AC (Poppenga and Puscher 2014). Mineral oil also appears to increase intestinal absorption of some toxicants (Qualls et al. 2013; Divers 2022).
- **Access to potential sources** of intoxication should be limited for the patient and herd, which can mean changing the source of feed, water, or bedding or removing the horses from pasture or the contaminated environment until the diagnosis and source of exposure is confirmed.

### Antidotes and Specific Treatments

Very few true antidotes are available in veterinary medicine; most treatment for poisoning is symptomatic and supportive. More often, specific treatments are recommended to prevent or minimize effects of a toxicant. Where available, antidotes and specific treatments are provided in Table 26.1.

### Sample Collection

Thorough documentation of the case is required, including client communications; clinical signs; antemortem and postmortem examination findings; environmental observations; sources of water and feeds; and any medications, pesticides, or chemicals used, including label information from commercial products. Collection containers should be tamper-evident to maintain sample integrity from collection to analysis, and must be labeled appropriately with location of collection, time and date, collector name, owner information, and the specific contents of the sample container (e.g., "feed," "liver," "gastric contents," or "whole blood") (Gwaltney-Brandt 2016). Chain of custody tags or forms should accompany samples and will include the name, address, and contact information of the collector; the date and time of collection; sample and animal identification information; and source information including animal and property owner (Bischoff and Moiseff 2018).

***Important animal samples*** are listed in Box 26.2. Samples for toxicologic testing should be fresh, not formalin fixed. Most samples can be kept either chilled or frozen, unless otherwise indicated. Sufficient amounts of each sample should be collected to allow for multiple analyses – at least 50 g (50 mL for fluids). It is better to collect extra sample than to discover later that you didn't collect enough. Laboratory testing capabilities vary considerably; always contact the laboratory for instructions prior to sending samples. For deceased animals, the whole body can be submitted or additional tissues should be collected and saved in 10% neutral-buffered formalin for histopathology. These should include liver, kidney, heart, brain, spleen, injection sites, skin, and any gross lesions. Except for brain, fixed tissue animal samples should not exceed 1 cm in thickness.

***Important environmental samples*** can include anything unusual in the environment, such as *bait material* or *unknown containers. Water samples* can be collected by filling clean 1L glass containers. If harmful algal blooms are possible, keep the water chilled and submit it to the laboratory as quickly as possible for identification of cyanobacteria and cyanotoxins.

**Box 26.2 Important Animal Samples for Toxicologic Testing (at least 50 g or 50 mL)**

- Antemortem
  - Whole blood (*keep chilled*)
  - Serum
  - Urine
  - Gastric reflux
  - Feces
- Postmortem
  - Stomach contents
  - Intestinal contents
  - Cecal or colonic contents
  - Urine
  - Liver
  - Fat
  - Kidney
  - Brain
  - Skin (*dermal exposures*)
  - Injection sites (*parenteral exposures*)
  - Aqueous fluid (*freeze immediately in an airtight container*)

*Note:* Except for whole blood, samples can be stored frozen.

If samples from a harmful algal bloom cannot be taken directly to the laboratory, mix a subsample 1 : 1 with 10% neutral buffered formalin for organism identification. Plastic containers may be used for these samples. *Whole plants,* including leaves, flowers, roots, and seeds, can be dried and pressed for identification or frozen in plastic bags for analysis; *mushrooms* (in paper bags) can be stored in a cool dry place and should not be frozen (Poppenga and Puscher 2014). Representative sampling of *feeds* is critical. Contaminants (e.g., mycotoxins, feed additives, or toxic plants in hay) are often unevenly distributed throughout a batch or bale. Feeds should be thoroughly mixed and subsamples taken from throughout bags, bins, or other containers to fill 1 gallon plastic bags (Bischoff and Moiseff 2018). Sort hay and save weeds, unidentified plant material, mold, or carrion to submit to the laboratory. Collect multiple hay samples from different areas of separate bales and place in a large plastic garbage bag.

**Case Example 26.1 Toxicologic Emergency**

It is August in Michigan. Two days prior a bad thunderstorm caused a large amount of wind damage in the area. Today, you are being presented with three middle-aged miniature horses for lethargy, inappetence, and "red urine." They are the only three horses on the farm with no recent travel. Upon evaluation you note the following physical exam finding abnormalities for all three mares:

- Very lethargic and dull
- Very pale and icteric mucous membranes making it difficult to ascertain an accurate capillary refill time.
- Tachycardia (60–80 bpm)
- Dyspnea with a respiratory rate of 40–50 brpm
- Notably, they are afebrile
- During your examination, one mare urinates dark red urine and you collect a sample.

*You quickly spin down a sample of the blood and urine and determine the following*

- Packed Cell Volume: 5–7%, Total Solids 8.0 g/dL and the serum appears pink in color
- Urine – no change in color after centrifugation.

Given that all three miniature horses are affected, you are worried about an intoxication.

Q:What are important ante mortem animal samples to collect?

- Whole blood (kept chilled), serum, urine, feces, gastric reflux if obtained.

Q: What are important environmental samples to collect?

- Water samples in clean 1 L glass containers – kept chilled or mixed 1 : 1 with 10% neutral buffered formalin.
- Representative samples of plants found in and around the pasture (whole plants, leaves, branches)
- Representative feed samples – hay and concentrate

Q: Two primary problems for your patient include hemolysis and icterus. What are common toxicants for hemolysis and icterus in horses?

- Red maple ingestion
- Allium species ingestion (e.g., garlic and onion)

Upon walking the pasture to collect water and plant samples, you note that there are several large red maple branches in the pasture. The owner notes that they fell from a tree outside of the pen and they haven't gotten to clearing them out yet. Upon inspection, you note that many of the branches are missing leaves. Based on this, you are concerned about red maple toxicosis in these miniature horses.

Q: With concerns about red maple toxicosis, what would be your decontamination step?

- After ending exposure to maple branches administration of activated charcoal at 1–2 g/kg in 1 g/mL dilution with water via nasogastric intubation.

Q: Treatment wise, what would be your most emergent recommendation for these patients?

- Due to severity of anemia combined with clinical signs (tachycardia, dyspnea, lethargy) a whole blood transfusion is indicated.

Q: What Other Treatments are Recommended?

- *Ascorbic acid for oxidative stress. This is an extra-label recommendation. Doses recommended include*
  - 10–20 g/horse (although you may consider a dose reduction given their relatively small size) PO or 30–50 mg/kg IV in 10–20 mL/kg of crystalloid fluids
- IV fluids for renal support while the horses have pigmenturia to prevent pigmentary nephropathy
- If showing signs of colic, analgesia as needed (consider opioids over nonsteroidal anti-inflammatory drugs due to added risk of nephropathy)

## References

Allerton, J.P. and Strom, J.A. (1991). Hypernatremia due to repeated doses of charcoal-sorbitol. *Am. J. Kidney Dis.* 17 (5): 581–584.

Archer, D.C., Sullivan, R.J., and Rickards, K. (2021). Emergency management for donkeys and mules. *Vet. Clin. Am. Equine Pract.* 37 (2): 495–513.

Bischoff, K. and Moiseff, J. (2018). Equine feed contamination and toxicology. *Transl. Anim. Sci.* 2 (1): 111–118.

Boesch, J.M. (2013). Anesthesia for the horse with colic. *Vet. Clin. Equine Pract.* 29 (1): 193–214.

Bohannon, L. (2022). Antipsychotics. In: *Blackwell's Five-Minute Veterinary Consult Clinical Companion: Equine Toxicology* (ed. L.R. Hovda, D. Benson, and R.H. Poppenga), 446–450. Hoboken: Wiley.

Brosnan, R.J. (2010). Waking up is hard to do: improving anesthetic recovery in horses. *Western Veterinary Conference*, March 2010, Las Vegas NV.

Caloni, F., Berny, P., Croubels, S. et al. (2018). Epidemiology of animal poisonings in Europe. In: *Veterinary Toxicology* (ed. R. Gupta), 45–56. Cambridge: Academic Press.

Clayton, M.J., Davis, T.Z., Knoppel, E.L., and Stegelmeier, B.L. (2020). Hepatotoxic plants that poison livestock. *Vet. Clin. N. Am. Food Anim. Pract.* 36 (3): 715–723.

Constable, P.D., Hinchcliff, K.W., Done, S.H., and Grünberg, W. (2017). *Veterinary Medicine*, 11e, 2220–2231. St. Louis: WB Saunders.

Davis, E. and Wilkerson, M. (2003). Hemolytic anemia. In: *Current Therapy in Equine Medicine: 5* (ed. N. Robinson), 344–348. St. Louis: Saunders.

Dawson, D. (2011). Toxins and adverse drug reactions affecting the equine nervous system. *Vet. Clin. N. Am. Equine* 27 (3): 507–526. https://doi.org/10.1016/j.cveq.2011.08.003.

Dechant, J.E. (2021). Approach to toxicologic emergencies. *Vet. Clin. N. Am. Equine Pract.* 37 (2): 327–337.

Divers, T.J. (2022). Ionophores. In: *Blackwell's Five-Minute Veterinary Consult Clinical Companion: Equine Toxicology* (ed. L.R. Hovda, D. Benson, and R.H. Poppenga), 173–177. Hoboken: Wiley.

Dowling, P.M. (2008). Amitraz toxicosis. In: *Blackwell's Five-Minute Veterinary Consult: Equine* (ed. J.-P. Lavoie and K.V. Hinchcliff), 55. Ames: Wiley-Blackwell.

Elfenbein, J.R., Giguere, S., Meyer, S.K. et al. (2010). The effects of deferoxamine mesylate on iron elimination after blood transfusion in neonatal foals. *J. Vet. Intern. Med.* 24 (6): 1475–1482.

Finno, C.J. and Valberg, S.J. (2012). A comparative review of vitamin E and associated equine disorders. *J. Vet. Intern. Med.* 26 (6): 1251–1266.

Galey, F.D. (2001). Botulism in the horse. *Vet. Clin. N. Am. Equine Pract.* 17 (3): 579–588.

Gwaltney-Brant, S. (2016). Veterinary forensic toxicology. *Vet. Pathol.* 53 (5): 1067–1077.

Gwaltney-Brant, S. (2018). Epidemiology of animal poisonings in the United States. In: *Veterinary Toxicology*, 3e (ed. R. Gupta), 37–44. Cambridge: Academic Press.

Hackett, E.S. (2014). Appendix 6: quick reference protocols for emergency and clinical conditions. In: *Equine Emergencies: Treatment and Procedures*, 4e (ed. J.A. Orsini and T.J. Divers), 823–827. St. Louis: Elsevier.

Haggett, E.F. and Wilson, W.D. (2008). Overview of the use of antimicrobials for the treatment of bacterial infections in horses. *Equine Vet. Educ.* 20 (8): 433–448.

Hovda, L.R. (2022). Hoary alyssum. In: *Blackwell's Five-Minute Veterinary Consult Clinical Companion: Equine Toxicology* (ed. L.R. Hovda, D. Benson, and R.H. Poppenga), 294–299. Hoboken: Wiley.

Jacobson, C.C., Sertich, P.L., and McDonnell, S.M. (2013). Mid-gestation pregnancy is not disrupted by a 5-day gastrointestinal mucosal cytoprotectant oral regimen of misoprostol. *Equine Vet. J.* 45 (1): 91–93.

Katan, D. (2022). Cholecalciferol. In: *Blackwell's Five-Minute Veterinary Consult Clinical Companion: Equine Toxicology* (ed. L.R. Hovda, D. Benson, and R.H. Poppenga), 397–397. Hoboken: Wiley.

Knipe M. (2009) The short and long of seizure management. *UC Davis Veterinary Neurology Symposium*, Davis, CA, 7–8 March 2009.

Landolt, G. (2007). Management of equine poisoning and envenomation. *Vet. Clin. N. Am. Equine Pract.* 23 (1): 31–47.

Marks, S.L., Kook, P.H., Papich, M.G. et al. (2018). ACVIM consensus statement: support for rational administration of gastrointestinal protectants to dogs and cats. *J. Vet. Intern. Med.* 32 (6): 1823–1840.

McConnico, R.S. and Brownie, C.F. (1992). The use of ascorbic acid in the treatment of 2 cases of red maple (*Acer rubrum*)-poisoned horses. *Cornell Vet.* 82 (3): 293–300.

Mix, K.A., Stafford, J., and Hofmeister, E. (2019). Effects of single dose administration of activated charcoal containing sorbitol on serum sodium concentrations and hydration status in dogs. *J. Vet. Emerg. Crit. Care* 29 (6): 616–621.

Mogg, T.D. (1999). Equine cardiac disease: clinical pharmacology and therapeutics. *Vet. Clin. N. Am. Equine Pract.* 15 (3): 523–534.

Oehme, F.W. (1987a). Arsenic. In: *Current Therapy in Equine Medicine*, 2e (ed. N.E. Robinson), 668–670. Philadelphia: WB Saunders.

Oehme, F.W. (1987b). Insecticides. In: *Current Therapy in Equine Medicine*, 2e (ed. N.E. Robinson), 658–660. Philadelphia: WB Saunders.

Plumb, D.C. (ed.) (2018). *Plumb's Veterinary Drug Handbook*, 9e. Hoboken: Wiley.

Poppenga, R.H. and Puschner, B. (2014). Toxicology. In: *Equine Emergencies: Treatment and Procedures*, 4e (ed. J.A. Orsini and T.J. Divers), 580–606. St. Louis: Elsevier.

Poppenga, R.H. and Sobhakumari, A. (2022). Alsike clover. In: *Blackwell's Five-Minute Veterinary Consult Clinical Companion: Equine Toxicology* (ed. L.R. Hovda, D. Benson, and R.H. Poppenga), 261–264. Hoboken: Wiley.

Puschner, B. and Aleman, M. (2010). Lead toxicosis in the horse: A review. *Equine Vet. Educ.* 22 (10): 526–530.

Qualls, H.J., Holbrook, T.C., Gilliam, L.L. et al. (2013). Evaluation of efficacy of mineral oil, charcoal, and smectite in a rat model of equine cantharidin toxicosis. *J. Vet. Intern. Med.* 27 (5): 1179–1184.

Redpath, A. and Bowen, M. (2019). Cardiac therapeutics in horses. *Vet. Clin. Equine Pract.* 35 (1): 217–241.

Regehr, T. (2022). Phosphides. In: *Blackwell's Five-Minute Veterinary Consult Clinical Companion: Equine Toxicology* (ed. L.R. Hovda, D. Benson, and R.H. Poppenga), 398–402. Hoboken: Wiley.

Scarratt, W.K. and Warnick, L.D. (1998). Effects of oral administration of lactulose in healthy horses. *J. Equine Vet. Sci.* 18 (6): 405–408.

Sellon, D.C., Monroe, V.L., Roberts, M.C., and Papich, M.G. (2001). Pharmacokinetics and adverse effects of butorphanol administered by single intravenous injection or continuous intravenous infusion in horses. *Am. J. Vet. Res.* 62 (2): 183–189.

Smit, A. (2022). Anticoagulants. In: *Blackwell's Five-Minute Veterinary Consult Clinical Companion: Equine Toxicology* (ed. L.R. Hovda, D. Benson, and R.H. Poppenga), 383–387. Hoboken: Wiley.

Toribio, R.E. (2011). Disorders of calcium and phosphate metabolism in horses. *Vet. Clin. Equine Pract.* 27 (1): 129–147.

Videla, R. and Andrews, F.M. (2009). New perspectives in equine gastric ulcer syndrome. *Vet. Clin. N. Am. Equine Pract.* 25 (2): 283–301.

Ward, C. (2022). Blister beetles. In: *Blackwell's Five-Minute Veterinary Consult Clinical Companion: Equine Toxicology* (ed. L.R. Hovda, D. Benson, and R.H. Poppenga), 453–459. Hoboken: Wiley.

Wismer, T. and Means, C. (2012). Toxicology of newer insecticides in small animals. *Vet. Clin. North Am. Small Anim. Pract.* 42 (2): 335–347.

# Part 4

## Support of the Emergency Patient

# 27

# Monitoring Methods in Emergency Medicine

*Sally Anne L. DeNotta*

*Large Animal Internal Medicine, College of Veterinary Medicine, University of Florida, Gainesville, FL, USA*

## Physical Examination Monitoring Parameters

1) Heart rate (HR): The normal resting heart rate for an adult horse is typically between 28 and 44 beats/min (bpm). Tachycardia is commonly observed and may indicate pain, stress, endotoxemia, hypovolemia, or primary cardiac disorder, e.g., myocarditis, cardiac arrythmia.
2) Respiratory rate (RR): The healthy adult horse generally has a respiratory rate of 8–16 breaths/min. Increased respiratory rates can be observed with pain, hypoxemia, endotoxemia, and primary pulmonary disorders such as pleuropneumonia and acute respiratory distress syndrome (ARDS).
3) Temperature: Normal temperatures in adult equine patients range from 99.5 °F to 101.5 °F (37.5–38.6 °C). While hypothermia is uncommon in adult horses, fever (>101.5 °F) is common and can indicate infection, systemic inflammation, or endotoxemia. When ambient temperature and humidity is high, elevated body temperature may also reflect hyperthermia from heat stroke or secondarily to anhidrosis.
4) Oral mucous membranes: Gum color is used to assess hydration, circulatory status, and oxygenation. Oral mucous membranes should be moist and warm to the touch, and may become dry or cool in horses suffering from dehydration or hypovolemia. A normal capillary refill time (CRT) is around one to two seconds, with prolonged CRT indicating poor perfusion, usually secondary to endotoxemia, hypovolemia, or both. Pale or grayish mucous membranes signify poor perfusion or hypovolemia, while bright red or "toxic" membranes are indicative of endotoxemia, septicemia, or substantial systemic inflammation.

## Pain Assessment

Recognizing pain in hospitalized horses is challenging, and behavior-based pain ethograms have been proposed as objective, quantifiable methods for identifying pain in horses. Horses may not always show obvious signs of pain, and monitoring for subtle signs of discomfort, such as restlessness or changes in facial expression and posture can enable clinicians to initiate prompt analgesic interventions.

Various pain scales have been developed for a number of equine conditions; examples include the Horse Grimace Scale (HGS) (Dalla Costa et al. 2014) (Figure 27.1) and Behavior Pain Score (BPS), which evaluate changes in facial expression and deviations from normal equine behavior, respectively, as indicators of underlying discomfort. Individual horses may display differing degrees of pain tolerance when evaluated by a pain ethogram, and comfort trends over time are likely to be more useful than single timepoint evaluation for identifying when analgesic intervention is warranted.

*Emergency Triage of the Horse*, First Edition. Edited by Rolfe M. Radcliffe and Jamie J. Kopper.

Companion website: www.wiley.com/go/radcliffe/triage

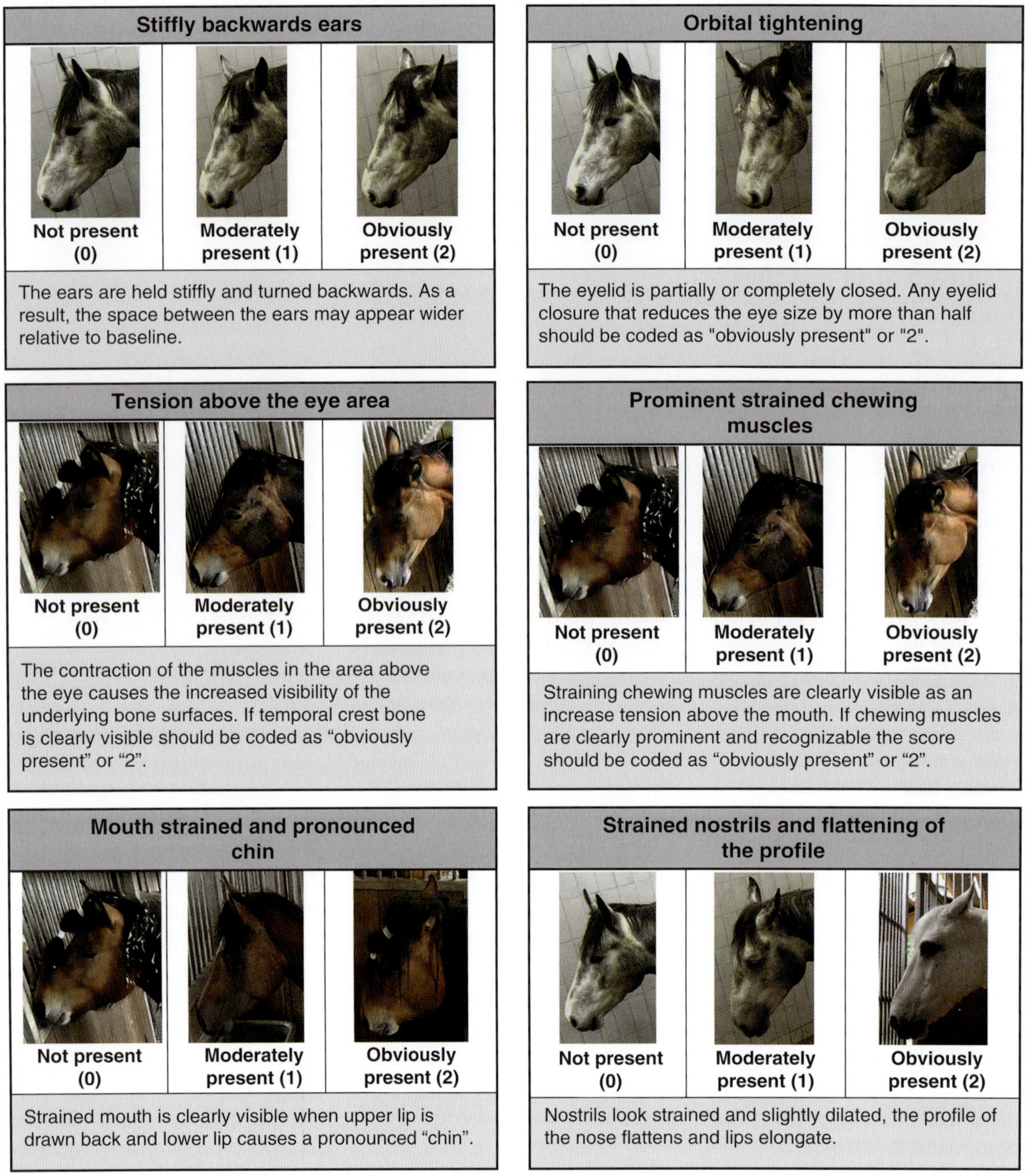


**Figure 27.1** The Horse Grimace Scale (HGS) is a pain ethogram that utilizes various aspects of facial expression to identify underlying discomfort in horses. *Source:* Dalla Costa et al. (2014)/PUBLIC LIBRARY OF SCIENCE (PLOS)/CC BY 4.0.

## Monitoring Respiratory Function

Serial monitoring of the respiratory system is helpful for determining when to intervene with supplementary oxygen or mechanical ventilation. In addition to physical parameters such as respiratory rate and quality, mucous membrane color, and thoracic auscultation, specialized monitoring tools may be utilized to assess respiratory function and determine when intervention is indicated (Pachtinger 2013) (Box 27.1).

**Box 27.1 Tools for evaluating the respiratory system**

- Pulse oximetry
- Arterial blood gas analysis

*Pulse oximetry*

- Pulse oximetry measures red blood cell (RBC) oxygen saturation percentage in the blood (Pachtinger 2013).
- Pulse oximeters are non-invasive, often portable, and also provide continuous heart rate monitoring. They can be applied to the tongue in anesthetized patients, and the ear, nostril, or vulva in standing patients. Pigmented skin frequently hinders accurate oximetry readings, and trying multiple locations and positions may be necessary to achieve accurate results.
- Pulse oximetry readings of less than 95% in standing patients are considered abnormal.
- Anemic animals may be clinically hypoxemic (due to low oxygen-carrying capacity) despite normal pulse oximetry readings

*Arterial blood gas analysis*

- Arterial blood gas analysis (ABG) is indicated in any patient demonstrating clinical signs of respiratory compromise including but not limited to tachypnea, increased respiratory effort, abnormal mucous membrane color, and/or abnormal lung sounds on auscultation (Pachtinger 2013).
- Arterial blood samples can be obtained from adult horses using the dorsal metatarsal, transverse facial, facial, or carotid arteries. Blood is collected into a heparin-coated syringe after which any air bubbles are quickly removed, the syringe is capped with a rubber stopper, and the sample is placed on ice until analysis. Collection sites should be antiseptically prepped and lidocaine either injected subcutaneously or applied as a gel.
- ABG analyzers are available as benchtop and handheld point-of-care models, all of which have been validated for horses.
- Contamination of samples with room air will artificially increase $PaO_2$, decreased $PaCO_2$, and alkalinize blood pH.
- $PaO_2$ is the partial pressure of oxygen in arterial blood and measures the amount of dissolved oxygen in an arterial blood sample. $PaO_2$ is an indicator of oxygenation capability. Unlike $SaO_2$, or arterial oxygen saturation, $PaO_2$ is independent of hemoglobin (Hb) concentrations.
- $PaO_2$ in normal standing horses at rest should be greater than 90 mmHg.
- $PaO_2$ less than 80 and 60 mmHg are indicative of moderate and severe hypoxemia, respectively.
- $PaCO_2$ is the partial pressure of carbon dioxide in blood and measures the amount of dissolved carbon dioxide in an arterial blood sample. $PaCO_2$ reflect ventilatory function and the lung's ability to remove $CO_2$ from circulation.
- Elevated $PaCO_2$ occurs with hypoventilation, impaired pulmonary diffusion, and ventilation/perfusion (V/Q) mismatch.
- $PaCO_2$ in normal standing horses at rest should be less than 45 mmHg. Venous $PCO_2$ is generally 3–6 mmHg higher than arterial $PCO_2$.
- $PaCO_2$ levels greater than 60 mmHg should prompt ventilation stimulant support (e.g., caffeine, doxapram, aminophylline), while $PaCO_2$ levels greater than 80 mmHg is an indicator for mechanical ventilation.
- As a general rule, the body will not "over-compensate" for acid–base disturbances, and disturbances outside of the guidelines below should be interpreted as mixed acid–base disorders:

*Estimations for acid–base expected compensatory responses*

1) Acute respiratory acidosis: bicarbonate concentration increases by 1 mEq/L for every 10-mmHg increase in $PCO_2$
2) Chronic respiratory acidosis: bicarbonate concentration increases by 3–4 mEq/L for every 10-mmHg increase in $PCO_2$
3) Acute respiratory alkalosis: bicarbonate concentration decreases by 1–3 mEq/L for every 10-mmHg decrease in $PCO_2$
4) Chronic respiratory alkalosis: bicarbonate concentration decreases by 5 mEq/L for every 10-mmHg decrease in $PCO_2$
5) Metabolic acidosis: $PCO_2$ decreases by 1.2 mmHg for every 1-mEq/L decrease in bicarbonate concentration
6) Metabolic alkalosis: $PCO_2$ increases by 0.6–1 mmHg for every 1-mEq/L increase in bicarbonate concentration

## Monitoring Circulation

Circulation and tissue perfusion are frequently compromised in critically ill equine patients as a result of hypovolemia, dehydration, or hypotension. Peripheral hypotension and relative hypovolemia are observed in horses with systemic inflammatory response (SIRS) or sepsis. Several monitoring tools are valuable for monitoring circulation in the emergent horse or foal (Divers and Hackett 2014) (Box 27.2).

*Arterial blood pressure*

- Arterial blood pressure (ABP) is the product of heart rate and stroke volume, and is a primary indicator of circulatory status in equine patients.
- Hypotension can occur as a result of hemorrhage, hypovolemia, sepsis, anaphylaxis, and systemic inflammatory response syndrome (SIRS).
- In adult horses, mean arterial blood pressure (MAP) must remain above 60 mmHg to maintain adequate cerebral, pulmonary, renal, and coronary circulation.
- Direct (invasive) ABP measurement: ABP may be measured in horses directly via arterial catheters and compatible continuous monitoring equipment. In adult horses, the transverse facial artery may be catheterized with 20-gauge catheter, while a similar-sized catheter in the great metatarsal artery is effective in foals. Advantages of direct ABP measurement include accuracy and ability to monitor continuously. Direct ABP in adult horses is normally between 126 and 168 mmHg systolic pressure and 85–116 mmHg diastolic pressure. Average MAP in adult horses ranges from 110 to 133 mmHg (Divers and Hackett 2014).
- Indirect (non-invasive) ABP measurement: Indirect ABP is most commonly obtained with oscillometric pressure cuffs placed on the coccygeal, dorsal metatarsal, palmar digital, or median arteries. Advantages of indirect ABP measurement include technically straightforward and non-invasive methodology, while disadvantages include frequent inaccuracy of results and single timepoint measurement. Inaccurate results are exacerbated by poorly fitting cuffs and variability in horse head position between measurements. In general, the length of the internal inflatable bladder should be approximately 80% of the appendage circumference, while the bladder width should be approximately 25% of the tail circumference or 50% of the limb circumference. In general, too narrow cuffs overestimate blood pressure, while too wide cuffs underestimate blood pressure. Horses should be standing quietly with the head in neutral position and minimal restraint, whenever possible. ABP measurements will be elevated in recumbent horses due to the relative position of the heart to the cuff placement, and monitoring trends in ABP over time may be more clinically helpful than any one single timepoint measurement. Indirect ABP in adult horses is normally between 99 and 125 mmHg systolic pressure and 54–91 mmHg diastolic pressure.

*Central venous pressure*

- Central venous pressure (CVP) is the pressure within the intrathoracic cranial vena cava and is an estimate of blood volume relative to blood vessel capacity (Divers and Hackett 2014, Magdesian 2004). It is affected by cardiac function, venous blood volume, and venomotor tone. Monitoring CVP is helpful for assessing response to fluid therapy, especially in patients with cardiac compromise. It can also be used to identify patients at risk for developing edema.
- Elevations in CVP are observed in patients with cardiac failure as well as with iatrogenic fluid overload.
- CVP is obtained with either a specialized CVP kit or 24-in. intravenous catheter placed in the jugular vein and terminating in the anterior vena cava or right atrium. The catheter is attached to a plastic hand-held manometer for single timepoint measurement or to a pressure transducer for continuous monitoring.

**Box 27.2 Tools for monitoring circulation (normal values in parentheses)**

- Arterial blood pressure (MAP ~60 mmHg)
- Central venous pressure (6–18 mmHg)
- Urine output (15–30 mL/kg/day)
- Blood L-lactate (<2 mmol/L)
- Colloid oncotic pressure (19–31 mmHg)

- CVP in standing adult horses should be less than 24 cm $H_2O$, with reported values ranging from 6 to 18 cm $H_2O$.
- CVP results are highly dependent on placement of the manometer or transducer relative to the heart, and therefore, it is imperative that the measuring device be placed in the same location relative to the horse for every measurement. The point of the shoulder or the sternum are commonly used landmarks. Furthermore, monitoring trends over time may be more clinically useful than a single timepoint measurement in any given patient.
- CVP results are also affected by respiration phase, and measurements should ideally be taken at end-expiration (when CVP is at its highest) every time. Large fluctuations in CVP are indicative of intracardiac placement and may be corrected by repositioning of the intravenous catheter.

*Urine output*

- Urine output is an indicator of renal perfusion and represents a simple and non-invasive method for assessing circulation status in both adult and neonatal equine patients (Magdesian 2004). Urine production can be measured quantitatively via urinary catheterization and collection (Figure 27.2), or qualitatively by observing micturition frequency.
- Urine output is reduced in hypovolemic patients as well as those with compromised perfusion. It is also reduced or absent in patients with oliguric or anuric renal disease, respectively.
- Urine production in adult horses is highly variable depending on ambient conditions and water, and ranges from 15 to 30 mL/kg/day. Anorexic and hyporexic horses produce less urine as a result of reduced fluid requirements, which can be as little as 16% of normal daily water intake in horses held off feed completely.
- Urinalysis is also useful for assessing hydration status in hospitalized horses. While urine-specific gravity (USG) in normal adult horses is variable, concentrated urine is indicative of dehydration or hypovolemia, while isosthenuria (1.008–1.014) may be observed in horses with renal failure.

L-*Lactate*

- L-Lactate is a metabolic product of glycolysis, and accumulates in tissues and circulation secondary to local or global hypoxia, inflammation, or decreased clearance (Magdesian 2004). As with other monitoring methods for ill equine patients, serial measurement to assess lactate trends over time is generally more clinically valuable than any one single timepoint measurement.
- L-Lactate may be measured in whole blood, plasma, and body fluids. Handheld point-of-care analyzers have been validated in horses.
- Blood L-lactate is a useful indicator of peripheral perfusion, with elevated concentrations noted in patients with hypovolemia, dehydration, and hypoxemia secondary to anemia. These patients respond rapidly to correction with fluid therapy, blood transfusion, etc., with normalization of blood lactate concentrations expected within 12–24 hours.
- Blood L-lactate concentrations may also be elevated as a result of local tissue inflammation or ischemia, especially in the intestinal tract, and hyperlactatemia that does not resolve with correction of perfusion and oxygen-carrying capacity should prompt clinicians to search for a localized source of elevated lactate production.
- L-Lactate is cleared by primarily the liver and may accumulate in circulation in horses with hepatic disease or failure. These horses should not be administered Lactated Ringer's Solution fluids, as this will exacerbate the hyperlactatemia further.

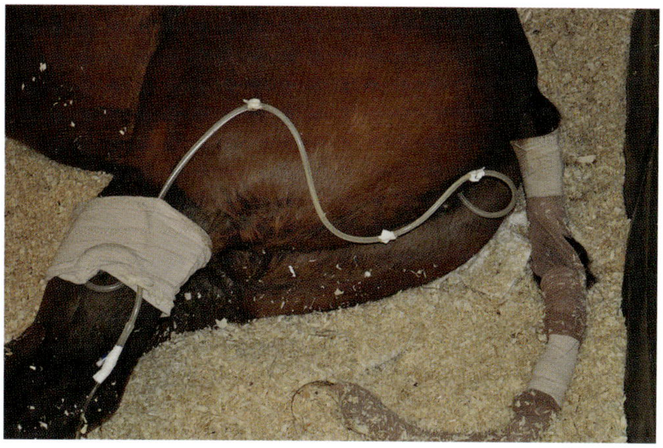

**Figure 27.2** Indwelling urinary catheter in a recumbent mare. Catheterization is helpful for both quantitative monitoring of urine output as well patient hygiene.

*Colloid oncotic pressure*

- Colloid oncotic pressure (COP) is a measurement of intravascular osmotic forces created by macromolecules, primarily albumin. These macromolecules are responsible for maintaining intravascular volume and pressure by drawing fluid from the interstitial space to the vascular space.
- COP is measured using commercial analyzers and is indicated in hypoproteinemic patients as well as those administered synthetic colloids. Normal COP in healthy adult horses and foals is reported to be 19–31 and 15-23 mmHg, respectively (Magdesian 2004).

COP is primarily determined by serum albumin concentrations. It is also affected by administration of exogenous synthetic colloids such as hetastarch. In patients that have received synthetic colloids, serum albumin and total solids as measured by refractometry will remain constant or even decrease secondary to dilution of plasma proteins. In these patients COP monitoring is helpful for assessing oncotic pressure and determining the risk of edema formation as well as the need for further oncotic therapeutic intervention.

## Conclusion

Monitoring equine patients in a hospital setting is achieved through serial physical examination complemented by clinicopathologic marker measurement and specialized monitoring equipment. The cardiovascular system is often the primary focus of homeostatic monitoring, but the function of all organ systems must be carefully monitored for changes suggestive of patient deterioration.

## References

Dalla Costa, E., Minero, M., Lebelt, D. et al. (2014). Development of the horse grimace scale (HGS) as a pain assessment tool in horses undergoing routine castration. *PLoS One* 9 (3): e92281. https://doi.org/10.1371/journal.pone.0092281.

Divers, T.J. and Hackett, E.S. (2014). Emergency and critical care monitoring. In: *Equine Emergencies* (ed. J.A. Orsini and T.J. Divers), 33–36. Elsevier.

Magdesian, K.G. (2004). Monitoring the critically ill equine patient. *Vet. Clin. North Am. Equine Pract.* 20 (1): 11–39. https://doi.org/10.1016/j.cveq.2003.12.001. PMID: 15062457.

Pachtinger, G. (2013). Monitoring of the emergent small animal patient. *Vet. Clin. North Am. Small Anim. Pract.* 43 (4): 705–720. https://doi.org/10.1016/j.cvsm.2013.03.014. Epub 2013 Apr 28. PMID: 23747256.

# 28

# Fluid Therapy for Horses and Foals

*Eric L. Schroeder*[1], *Maia R. Aitken*[2], *and Rolfe M. Radcliffe*[3]

[1] *Galbreath Equine Center, College of Veterinary Medicine, The Ohio State University, Columbus, OH, USA*
[2] *Department of Clinical Studies - New Bolton Center, University of Pennsylvania School of Veterinary Medicine, Kennett Square, PA, USA*
[3] *Department of Clinical Sciences, College of Veterinary Medicine, Cornell University, Ithaca, NY, USA*

## Introduction

Fluid therapy is a key component in treatment and supportive care of both horses and foals with a variety of conditions, especially those resulting in critical illness (Magdesian 2014a,b,c; Crabtree and Epstein 2021) (Box 28.1). Fluid and electrolyte therapy are integral to successful management of many ailments that affect horses and foals both in the hospital and in the farm setting (Schott 2006; Hollis and Corley 2007; Mudge 2014; Magdesian 2014a,b,c; Fielding 2018; Crabtree and Epstein 2021; Radcliffe et al. 2022). Despite the frequent utilization of intravenous fluids therapy, it remains challenging to make evidence-based treatment recommendations (Crabtree and Epstein 2021). Furthermore, the optimal fluid type and rate of fluid administration lacks scientific consensus and often is subject to clinician preference (Fielding 2014). Fluid therapy is considered a cornerstone to veterinary and human medicine and is constantly being studied and reevaluated to fine tune fluid resuscitation goals, optimal intravenous fluid composition, and assess the negative effects of fluid therapy and fluid physiology. As equine veterinary science has evolved, we have taken a more holistic approach to fluid therapy and physiology. While this chapter is not written to cover all facets of fluid therapy, its purpose is to serve as a primer and stepping stone to guide a practitioner on how to make and administer a fluid therapy plan.

## Body Fluid and Electrolyte Balance

Before specific aspects of fluid therapy are discussed, it is important to review normal water and electrolyte balance in the healthy horse and foal (Figure 28.1) (Forro et al. 2000; Fielding et al. 2011; Magdesian 2014a,b,c). This water balance is under tight control and is regulated by central osmole receptors within the brain resulting in hormone secretion from the posterior pituitary gland (antidiuretic hormone) resulting in dilute or ultraconcentrated urine depending on the sodium concentration of the blood. The concept of water being regulated by sodium content of the blood is referred to as water balance. Water balance is controlled by the effective osmolality (tonicity) of the plasma volume or vascular space. The tonicity is directly controlled by the sodium concentration/content of the plasma volume (Fielding 2014). Also, the water balance is under continuous tight physiological control, thus preventing large variation in total body water and total body sodium. Under mild ambient conditions (relative humidity) as would be found in most hospital settings, horses have a water requirement of about 50 mL/kg/day (maintenance fluid intake requirements) or about 25 L (or 6 gallons) per day for a typical 500 kg horse that is eating normally. In neonatal foals the daily water requirement is greater, or about 80–100 mL/kg/day (4–5 L/day for a 50 kg foal), because of their higher total body water content. With horses fed a typical hay diet, most of this water (>90%) is consumed via normal drinking habits with the remainder coming from feed (feed moisture) (Schott 2006). This water is subsequently eliminated through feces, urine, and insensible routes (via sweating and humidification of inspired and expired air). When a horse is hyporexic or anorexic, the water requirement and intake may drop by

*Emergency Triage of the Horse*, First Edition. Edited by Rolfe M. Radcliffe and Jamie J. Kopper.

Companion website: www.wiley.com/go/radcliffe/triage

**Box 28.1 Indications for fluid therapy in horses and foals**

The indications for fluid therapy in horses and foals are many; however, most commonly, fluids target emergency resuscitation, replacement of fluid deficits, maintenance support and treatment of specific problems (Crabtree and Epstein 2021). Common problems that require the administration of fluids are diseases that result in acute hypovolemia (blood loss, colitis, enteritis, and colonic volvulus) and ailments that result in whole-body dehydration and hemoconcentration (impaction colic, inability to eat/drink, electrolyte disturbance, hyponatremia) (Crabtree and Epstein 2021).

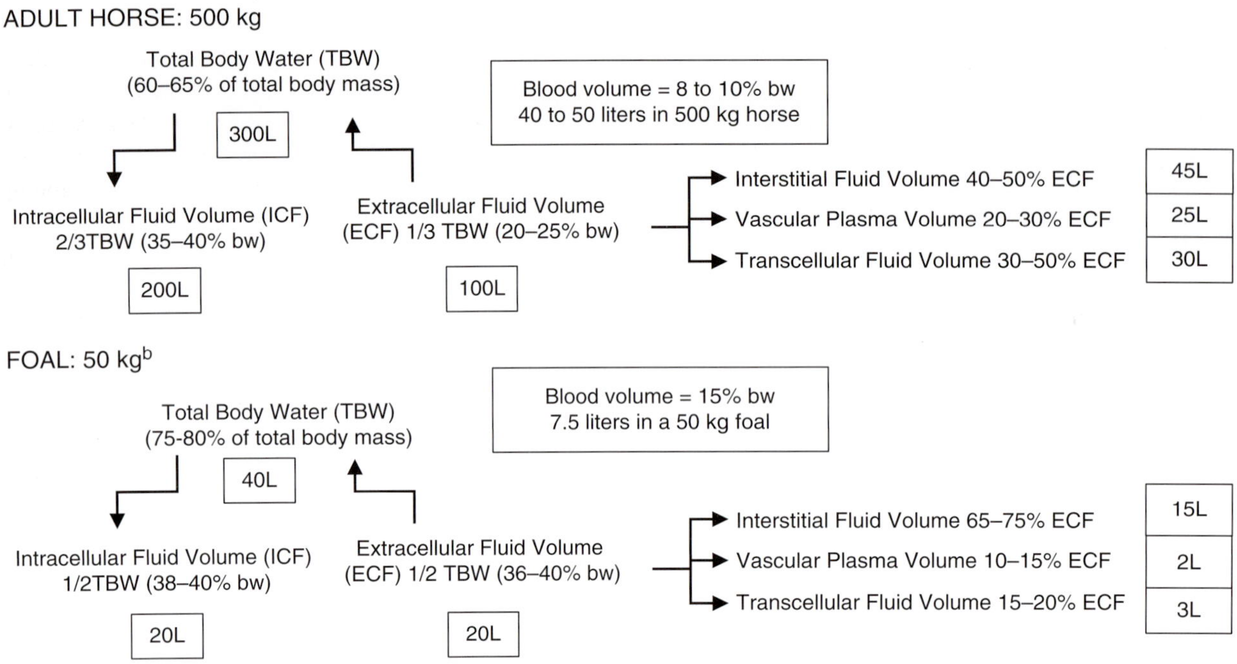


[a] Volumes and percentages estimated from literature (Fielding, 2011; Forro, 2000).
[b] Interstitial, vascular and transcellular fluid volumes are approximate in the foal and vary with age.

**Figure 28.1** A diagram illustrating the approximate water balance in liters (L) of the total body water and various compartments of the 500 kg adult horse and 50 kg foal.[a]

more than 50% without development of significant systemic and whole-body dehydration due to a similar decrease in water output in feces and urine, remembering that most of the fluid loss is via feces (Fielding 2014). Furthermore, types of feed ingested have a considerable effect on water intake with grass having a significant water component (~90%). The grazing horse will naturally drink less water (Schott 2006). More subtle dietary factors that can affect water intake include protein, calcium, and fiber content of the feed: water intake may increase mildly with increased amounts of all these factors. These dietary factors also affect water output: a diet high in protein and calcium will increase urine production and water loss by this route, while a diet high in fiber will increase fecal water output and decrease urine volume (Schott 2006).

The daily water requirement will increase significantly with the athletic performance of the horse. Horses that exercise more and have significant loss of water through sweat will require higher voluntary fluid intake. Horses are also different than small animals when it comes to body fluid stores: healthy horses have a substantial reserve of water and electrolytes in the lumen of the intestinal tract (10–12% of total body mass is gastrointestinal contents) that can initially be used to replace some types of fluid loss (e.g., sweating during prolonged exercise or transport). However, this reserve becomes useless with other problems (e.g., profuse diarrhea) and has likely already been depleted in horses that have been off feed for two to four days (Schott 2006).

Traditionally, fluid therapy has been taught with regimented standards and set fluid rates and total amounts over time which is usually calculated as an initial bolus of polyionic fluid volume and then a calculated maintenance rate. All of this is calculated for a typical 24-h day. Oral and or intravenous fluid therapy has been a "gold standard" medical therapy for decades and has been the corner stone for treatment of many medical and emergency conditions. It is important to remember however, at the simplest level, fluids are and must be considered drugs and thus have both positive intended results for both lifesaving benefits and unfortunately possibly negative life-threatening adverse effects (Crabtree and Epstein 2021).

Adult horses, like humans, are approximately 60% water, which accounts for approximately 300 L in a 500 kg horse (Schott 2006). Neonatal foals have a higher total body water content of 75–80% body weight or 38–40 L in a 50 kg foal. This fluid volume can be relatively dynamic and shift rapidly via osmosis and solvent drag among the various fluid spaces that make up total body water. As the horse ages from foal to adult the amount of total body water decreases by up to 10% and the amount of fluid located within the extracellular fluid space will decrease proportionately.

For the adult horse (500 kg), total body water (TBW, approximately 300 L) is distributed between the intracellular (ICF) (2/3, approximately 200 L) and extracellular (ECF) spaces (1/3, approximately 100 L). For comparison, in the foal (50 kg), approximate values for TBW, ICF, and ECF are 40 L, 20 L, and 20 L, respectively (Fielding 2024). The extracellular spaces include the circulating plasma volume (25–30 L, adult), interstitial space between the cells (40–45 L, adult), and the transcellular spaces (30 L, adult) (Schott 2006) including the gastrointestinal lumen, cerebrospinal fluid, pleural and peritoneal fluid, and even the synovial fluid; most of the transcellular fluid is within the lumen of the gastrointestinal tract. A 500 kg adult horse in an ambient environment requires 50 mL/kg/day or 25 L (6 gallons) of water for maintenance therapy a day most of which is acquired by voluntary water consumption and diet. Maintenance fluid requirements for the foal are higher because of the increased free body water, ranging from 80 to 100 mL/kg/day or 4–5 L/day (Fielding 2024). The greater TBW, higher basal metabolic rate, growth and increased insensible losses (sweat, respiration, urine loss, and fecal loss) results a greater water requirement to maintain hydration (Magdesian 2014c). The healthy growing foal can consume 20–30% of its body weight per day in milk with the predominant component of milk being electrolyte-rich water (89%) (Magdesian 2014c). Foals in general should have large urine production/loss 6 mL/kg/h, and the specific gravity should be hyposthenuric (<1.008) and even potentially lower (Magdesian 2014c).

If the horse is eating mostly pasture, most of its water requirement will be supplied by grass, which has very high-water content. This same horse will drink about 5 gallons (20–22 L) of water when eating hay/grain; this is due to the dry nature of the feedstuff (~12–14%). If the horse is off feed, the daily fluid requirements for maintenance needs will decrease by approximately 50% without the development of dehydration. Dehydration is prevented in this patient by having a subsequent decrease in water loss in feces as well as in urine volume. If the horse lives in a hot, humid environment, its water requirement will increase, especially during intense exercise, due to water loss through sweating. Dehydration occurs when losses are not restored by appropriate oral intake of water. Pathologic fluid losses include non-replenished sweating, diarrhea, nasogastric reflux, pleural or peritoneal effusion, hydrops, and hemorrhage.

## Patient Assessment

The initial assessment of both the adult horse and foal will require a rapid thorough physical examination (PE) including routine PE findings as well as direct assessment of cardiovascular stability of the patient (Box 28.2). Cardiovascular instability may be more prominent in the neonatal foal due to its inability to maintain cardiac output and degree if illness with septicemia resulting in significant changes in the clinical examination.

If clinical experience and technical ability allows indirect oscillometric blood pressure measurement (ideal MAP > 60–80 mmHg) will provide a more complete picture of vascular perfusion volume. Serum creatinine and urine-specific gravity can also provide significant information regarding the total fluid volume and vascular volume of the horse. There are significant cardiovascular physiologic properties that are used to maintain blood volume and perfusion in the horse; however, acute-onset clinical disease can override these fail-safe mechanisms and place the horse in a dehydrated and or hypovolemic state.

**Box 28.2 How to assess hydration status of the adult horse and foal**

Physical exam should involve assessment of pulse pressure and character (bounding vs weak and thready), jugular fill, capillary refill time (CRT), mucous membrane character (color), and warmth of the extremities (ears, limbs, nose). Skin turgor in the horse can be very misleading due the potential excessive skin; however, eye position within the orbit can give assessment of fat pad hydration. If the eyes are sunken there is likely significant dehydration. Basic lactate measurement on the farm or clinical setting and use of hematocrit concentration and total peripheral protein concentration assessment will provide the complete picture of total hydration.

Most importantly, initial patient assessment (adult and foal) is determining presence of hypovolemia (decreased vascular volume). Hypovolemia refers to loss of intravascular fluid volume either through direct blood loss or loss of plasma water. The determination of this physical state indicates clinical signs of shock, characterized by abnormalities of perfusion, dull/depressed mentation, cool-to-cold extremities, poor pulse quality, prolonged CRT, pale mucous membrane color, poor-to-absent jugular fill, and decreased to lack of urine output with subsequent increased urine-specific gravity. Heart rate can be variable depending on the primary disease process and may not provide an accurate clinical picture with regards to the severity of hypovolemia. Plasma L-lactate concentration can be used clinically to provide evidence to support the presence of hypovolemic shock. The normal plasma concentration of L-lactate is <2.0 mmol/L in the normal healthy adult horse. We often use this clinically as a marker of hydration and peripheral perfusion. However, plasma lactate concentrations must be interpreted with caution, given the various other causes of hyperlactatemia, including the euvolemic state with decreased forward cardiac output.

Dehydration (mild, moderate, severe) alone or in combination with resulting hypovolemia can be deadly. Dehydration in the broadest sense refers to global decreases in ICF and ECF, resulting in overall TBW loss and decreased body weight. The signs of dehydration in the horse include reduced skin turgor, tacky mucous membranes, and decreased corneal water content. As mentioned prior, skin turgor can be very misleading due to the overall compliance of the skin and interstitium. Clinical assessment of skin turgor should be performed over multiple areas of the body to provide a more global assessment. Urine-specific gravity may provide further proof of global dehydration by a rising USG or an USG > 1.025. In the foal, ideally the USG should never rise above isothenuria (1.008–1.012). Even better is if the USG is well below these values indicating that the foal is well hydrated. The dehydrated foal can clinically increase the USG and actively concentrate the urine.

Dehydration in the broadest sense refers to overall extravascular fluid loss not just to ECFV decrease but global decreases in ICFV, ECFV, and lastly overall TBW loss and decrease of body weight. Dehydration can be difficult to accurately assess because PCV and TP only reflect one compartment of the extracellular fluid volume and dehydration refers to more than just intravascular hemoconcentration; it also is a measurement of extravascular fluid loss (Fielding 2014). Measurement of the interstitial and intracellular fluid volumes is extremely difficult to predict. Moderate-to-severely dehydrated horses may show signs of hemoconcentration and hypovolemia including tachycardia, prolonged capillary refill time, increased packed cell volume and total solids, and prerenal azotemia. Generally, we are not able to detect dehydration <5% in horses. Horses with 10–12% dehydration will show signs of hypovolemic shock. The hospital setting allows for the ideal assessment of hydration status through body weight gain or loss (Schott 2006). Ideally patients, and especially foals, should be weighed daily to assess weight gain: most often attributed to fluid gain in a foal and in the adult potentially due to gastrointestinal fill and fluid hydration of the colon. Calculating replacement fluids to treat dehydration requires multiplying the horse's body weight in kilograms by the estimated percent dehydration. For example, a 500 kg horse with diarrhea, depression, and inappetence is assessed to be 8% dehydrated: $500 \times 0.08 = 40$-L fluid deficit. Similarly, in a 50 kg foal assessed to 8% dehydrated secondary to sepsis and diarrhea: $50 \times 0.08 = 40$-L deficit.

Dehydration assessment in the foal is more difficult to detect and quantify in the foal because most physical examination parameter findings used in the adult to assess dehydration do not work in the foal (Magdesian 2014c). Clinical understanding that the foal is not a miniature version of the adult horse is paramount. The foal can quickly die from acute rapid hypovolemia and dehydration and lead to significant cardiovascular collapse rapidly; therefore, rapid and precise clinical assessment is the most important starting point. Calculation and quantification of true dehydration of the foal is much more challenging due to ability of dynamic fluid shifts in the growing foal as well as the unpredictable nature of the foal physical examination. Such that skin turgor in the foal may provide a false/opposite direction in the true hydration status of the foal (Magdesian 2014c).

## Understanding Fluid Therapy

After clinical assessment of the patient has been performed, the next step is to decide if the patient is dehydrated (hemoconcentrated as evidenced by increased hematocrit, packed cell volume, and total peripheral protein), hypovolemic, or both (Box 28.3). This decision can influence how fluid therapy is provided to the horse: the type of fluid given (isotonic vs hypertonic), the rate of administration, the route of administration, and whether a bolus fluid therapy is required. If the horse is being resuscitated in the ambulatory medicine setting, bolus therapy will likely be used. This, however, is not the most physiologic approach, but it is the easiest to accomplish in the field. One must also consider the overreaching goals and potential consequences of fluids provided. Traditionally, fluid therapy in the horse uses polyionic isotonic crystalloid style fluids, though hypertonic fluids, synthetic colloids (starches), or natural colloids (plasma, whole blood) may also be used.

Isotonic crystalloid fluids are polyionic and balanced solutions that are like the fluid components of plasma, however, are lacking protein and clotting factors. Most of them contain multiple electrolytes and some contain energy sources dissolved in solution. These types of fluids are commonly used for both "resuscitation" and "maintenance" fluid therapy in the horse,

**Box 28.3 How to correct fluid imbalance in the horse**

Hydration status correction in cases of hypovolemia, dehydration, or hemoconcentration with fluid therapy must account for correction of volemic loss, dehydration, ongoing maintenance fluid requirements, and insensible fluid losses. Monitoring of the hydration status of the horse and the use of fluid therapy is the mainstay of supportive care in equine medicine (Fielding 2014).

and the overall goal is to provide maintenance of hydration of the ECF and ICF volumes via osmolarity-induced distribution (osmosis). Maintenance fluid therapy provides hydration to the ICF and ECF spaces; however, over time the horse will generate a relative excess of both sodium and chloride. As such, the horse must have a source of free water available. With time, the horse will become relatively sodium rich and will likely retain water in the form of interstitial edema. The excess chloride will result in a potential hyperchloremic metabolic acidosis (Fielding 2014). Isotonic fluids are indicated in the immediate resuscitation of the horse (adult and foal) for most clinical problems.

Once a particular fluid type (LRS, Plasma-Lyte 148, Normosol R) is decided upon for intravenous administration, a rate and amount of total fluid administered needs to be considered; continuous or bolus administration rates are common (Hollis and Corley 2007; Fielding 2018). Bolus administration of fluids, especially in foals, has the advantage of correcting hypovolemia and dehydration more rapidly as well as saving the clinician time. The fluid rate is highly controversial and depends directly on the patient's degree of presumed hypovolemia and overall percentage of dehydration (Fielding 2014). Care in estimation of percent dehydration needs to be realized to prevent potential overall excess interstitial fluid accumulation with excess sodium and chloride retention. The "fluid challenge" or "goal-directed" method of administration can also be used in which 10–20 mL/kg fluid boluses over 20–30 minutes are given with frequent patient reassessment (Magdesian 2014a). The initial bolus can be administered rapidly over approximately 20 minutes and each additional bolus over 45–60 minutes. Patient physical examination normalization, normalization of perfusion parameters, production of urine, and increased mental awareness are used to guide total fluid administration. Maximum administration will likely depend on the disease process and the ability to administer large volumes of fluid on the farm; this is a common reason for referral. The overarching goal of the resuscitation phase in the fluid therapy plan is to reestablish tissue perfusion (Magdesian 2014a).

Generally, all horses that show clinical evidence of dehydration are candidates to have a fluid therapy plan developed and receive fluid therapy (Schott 2006). The route of administration of the fluid and the type of fluid should be considered based on the physical examination assessment, where the most significant loss of the fluid is coming from (intracellular vs extracellular) and how rapid the loss occurred. In addition, horses that show marginal evidence of dehydration would likely also benefit from an initial period of fluid therapy, if they are azotemic (increased serum concentrations of urea nitrogen and creatinine) at admission or have a history of use of nephrotoxic medications (e.g., non-steroidal anti-inflammatory drugs or gentamicin) for several days.

Horses with moderate-to-severe dehydration (7–15%) or hypovolemia frequently require intravenous fluids due to malabsorption of enteral fluids secondary to decreased perfusion of the intestinal tract and/or urgency of vascular volume replacement (Schott 2006). With a standard intravenous catheter (14-gauge, 5¼″ length) placed in the jugular vein, intravenous isotonic crystalloid fluids can be administered at a rate of 5–7 L/h, depending on the height at which fluid bags are hung, bore of the extension set, and the type and size of IV tubing used as the fluid administration set (Schott 2006). The rate of fluid administration may be increased most effectively by increasing the catheter size (Box 28.4).

Increased rate of fluid administration can also be achieved by increasing catheter and tubing diameter, decreasing length of tubing, and increasing height of fluids from the horse to increase gravity flow. In extreme circumstances, a fluid roller pump can also be used; however, it often leads to severe endothelial damage increasing the risk of phlebitis, and or thrombophlebitis. Further, placement of catheters in both jugular veins should be approached with caution at initial presentation because venous thrombosis can be a significant complication in critically ill patients (Schott 2006).

**Box 28.4 How to increase fluid rate in horses with hypovolemic shock**

Horses in hypovolemic shock may require an increased rate of fluid administration. The most effective way to increase the rate of fluid administration is to increase the catheter size (e.g., 10 or 12 ga catheter; the rate of fluid administration is directly proportional to the radius of the catheter to the fourth power). Rarely is more than one intravenous catheter required for initial rehydration and correction of hypovolemia unless multiple types of products (e.g., crystalloid solutions and colloids) are being administered simultaneously.

Isotonic crystalloid fluids include products such as Normosol-R, lactated Ringer's solution (LRS), and Plasma-Lyte A. Saline or 0.9% sodium chloride contains a bit more sodium and equal parts sodium to chloride, resulting in intravascular acidification, but can be used as a replacement/resuscitative solution. All commercially produced 5 L bagged fluids are considered replacement or resuscitative fluids. A list of commonly used fluid products is in *Appendix 3: Emergency Medications and Fluids.* A full shock dose of isotonic fluids is equal to one blood volume or 8–10% of the body weight in kg (80–100 mL/kg in the adult horse). A shock dose of crystalloid fluids for a 500 kg horse is 80–100 mL × 500 kg = 40–50 L. This is typically given in doses of 10 L or approximately 20 mL/kg given up to four times. As with goal-directed therapy, the patient is reassessed to monitor volemic status after each 10-L bolus with particular attention to improvement/normalization of heart rate, capillary refill time, pulse pressure, jugular fill, plasma lactate values, and urine production. The improvement with isotonic crystalloid fluid boluses will be short lived, depending on the degree of debilitation and dehydration, because crystalloid fluids will distribute to the interstitium within 30–60 minutes. Generally, 25% of the fluids administered intravenously will stay within the vascular space, whereas the other 75% will move into the interstitium based on the Starling principles of fluid shift.

Shock crystalloid fluid therapy for the foal is 50–80 mL/kg = 2.5–4 L in a 50 kg foal. Like the adult horse, fluid challenges of one-quarter of the shock dose are given with continuous monitoring. Repeat one-quarter (20 mL/kg) doses or 1 L in a 50 kg foal as needed up to 80 mL/kg to achieve normal tissue perfusion and clinical improvement. This volume is quite controversial because of the severe sodium load that the foal will be receiving, and the neonatal kidney will have to excrete over time as well as lack of true evidence as to how much fluid should be bolused to the hypovolemic foal. Currently, most believe that following administration of 2 L of fluid, inotropic or vasopressor agents should be implemented if the expected results are not clinically achieved (Fielding 2024).

## Route of Administration

Several routes of administration are possible with horses and foals, including intravenous, enteral (intragastric), or rectal administration (Crabtree and Epstein 2021). The choice of fluid route will depend on the clinical problem and other co-morbidities, the goal of fluid therapy, as well as other patient and client factors. With continuous availability of 3- and 5-L intravenous fluid bags both to the general practitioner for ambulatory use and in hospital use, in combination with systems designed to hang multiple bags (e.g., 10–20 L at a time), the use of intravenous fluids in equine practice has expanded considerably over the past 10–20 years (Fielding 2018). The advantage of using large fluid bags is improved asepsis of fluid administration and better delivery of more appropriate total fluid volumes and rates. If using 1-L bags to give an appropriate fluid amount to a 500 kg horse you would need to change your lines 12–15 times while on the farm or in the hospital, greatly increasing the risk of contamination, not to mention physical labor. Accompanying this advance in treatment capability, a consequence appears to have been a decrease in the use of enteral fluid therapy. This is somewhat unfortunate because enteral fluids are rapidly absorbed across the small intestine, as long as that portion of bowel remains functional. In fact, a larger volume of fluids can often be given via this route (e.g., 8 L every 30–60 minutes via an indwelling nasogastric tube) than can be administered through a single intravenous catheter. The only real contraindications for use of enteral fluids are presence of gastric reflux when a stomach tube is passed, severe resistance by the horse to nasogastric intubation, or true hypovolemia. Clinically, gastric reflux > 4 L, evidence of ileus of the gastrointestinal tract or ultrasonographic documentation of ileus or gastric distention will alert the clinician that enteral fluid therapy may not be appropriate (Fielding 2018). Further, enteral fluid solutions can easily be made when needed without specialized equipment (e.g., 30 g of table salt, either iodized or non-iodized, or lite salt [a 1 : 1 mixture of NaCl and KCl] added to each gallon of water) (Schott 2006). All in all, enteral fluids are ideal for horses with mild-to-moderate dehydration (5–7%) if the intestinal tract is healthy and functional enough to absorb the fluids administered and there is no gastric reflux (Fielding 2018). However, as previously mentioned, if the horse is displaying signs of hypovolemia and or severe dehydration (10–12%) this horse must be treated with a bolus of 10–20 mL/kg isotonic crystalloid fluids rapidly via a large gauge intravenous catheter.

## Type of Fluid

Although sterile water is the most abundant component of commercially available fluid therapy solutions administered intravenously or via a nasogastric tube, these solutions also contain electrolytes and/or nutrients (glucose) to make the fluids balanced and isosmotic to the electrolyte concentration and osmolality of the plasma. Traditionally, fluids that are administered intravenously have an electrolyte composition and concentration like the blood, thus allowing these fluids to be given at a rapid rate. The most important electrolytes to consider are $Na^+$, $K^+$, $Cl^-$, and $Ca^{++}$. The $Cl^-$ ion is the major exchangeable anion and typically follows losses of the major cations, $Na^+$ and $K^+$.

As mentioned above, as essentially all commercially available isotonic crystalloid fluids have an electrolyte composition like plasma, they are rehydration fluids designed to replace acute losses of fluid from the ECF. As a result, most of these solutions are appropriate choices for initial treatment of dehydrated and hypovolemic horses and variation in products used between hospitals often reflects different costs and availabilities, rather than a physiological preferable solution. Realistically, there are minimal differences among all commercially available isotonic crystalloid fluids. Common crystalloid fluids used in the field include Normosol R, Lactated Ringer, Isotonic Saline, and Hypertonic Saline solutions (Fielding 2018).

## Developing a Fluid Therapy Plan

Initial rehydration plan: Once hydration and volemic status has been assessed, a fluid therapy plan can be developed. Initially, plans are made for the first 12–24 h and subsequently modified after assessing the patient's response to treatment. This may have to be reassessed frequently based on the critical nature of the patient and evaluation of ongoing losses (urine, sweat, diarrhea, effusion, and reflux). This will likely be truer in the foal due to the dynamic nature of how quickly physiologically their clinical condition may change. Consideration to the volume of fluid administered should include: (i) amount estimated to correct dehydration (5–15% sliding scale that is very subjective based on clinical assessment) and correction of hypovolemia if present; (ii) amount needed for maintenance typically for the adult horse estimated to be 40–60 mL/kg/day; and (iii) amount to replace estimated ongoing fluid losses (extremely difficult to quantify). The foal fluid therapy plan can be extremely controversial due to clinician beliefs/preferences on maintenance fluid therapy plans. It is true, however, that hypovolemia in the foal should be treated with intravenous polyionic resuscitative fluid (LRS, Plasma-Lyte 148, Normosol R) because these fluid compositions mimic those of the vascular space (Fielding 2024). The rate of "shock" dose administration in the foal is approximately 20 mL/kg over at least 20 minutes. Additional boluses become even more dependent on clinical experience, preference, and continued patient reassessment; most of the time if another bolus is warranted the rate is 20 mL/kg, however, it is given over about one hour (Fielding 2024). Assessment and prediction of ongoing losses and the inherent variability make this portion of the fluid therapy plan almost impossible to predict. However, ignorance of estimated ongoing losses will lead to failure of the fluid therapy plan and likely will result in decline of the horse. Please see the chapter case summary for examples of how to prepare a fluid plan for the adult horse and foal.

In general, selection of almost any of the commercially available crystalloid polyionic solutions would be appropriate for initial intravenous rehydration as the most important factor is to administer an appropriate volume of fluids. Fine-tuning of the fluid therapy plan is usually performed after initial laboratory data becomes available and after the response to the initial three to six hours of treatment is observed. Modifications to the initial plan may include changing the rate of fluid administration, correction of acid–base disorders, and replacement of specific or anticipated electrolyte deficits by adding electrolytes to the base fluid or supplementing needed electrolytes in enteral solutions or as oral pastes.

## Additives to the Base Fluid

At present, limitations of fluid therapy in equine patients are that commercially available intravenous rehydration solutions fail to address $K^+$ and $Ca^{++}$ deficits, $K^+$ and $Ca^{++}$ requirements, and large volume, bagged maintenance fluid solutions (for use once rehydration has been accomplished) are not currently available and likely will not be in any foreseeable future. Ideal maintenance solutions would contain less $Na^+$ and more $K^+$ and $Ca^{++}$ than rehydration solutions and would also partially supply energy needs, typically in the form of dextrose. However, due to the risk and prevalence of endocrine diseases in the adult equine population, dextrose energy sources may not be the best energy source for maintenance of polyionic, isotonic solutions. When considering additives to base fluids, consideration must be given to the type of dehydration that the horse is presenting for in the emergent setting. If the horse is primarily dehydrated and requiring fluid therapy because there has been a lack of water either due to a frozen water source or empty water trough, this style of dehydration has occurred over days. Therefore, rehydration likely will need to require fluid delivery to both the extracellular and intracellular space (true loss of total body water). While electrolyte supplementation will occur if using intravenous fluids, rapid administration is likely not required and rehydration may be possible with the use of oral fluid therapy. If the horse has lost electrolyte-rich fluid due to diarrhea or nasogastric reflux over a 12-h duration and is presenting with evidence of hypovolemic shock, this patient requires rapid intravenous administration of polyionic isosmotic crystalloid fluid. In the horse deprived of water, fluid deficits have developed more slowly, and dehydration involves a loss of both ECF ($Na^+$ rich) and ICF ($K^+$ rich) fluid. In contrast, the refluxing or enterocolitis horse produces more acute losses of fluid that are predominantly from the ECF. Thus, the water-deprived horse would have a greater depletion of body $K^+$ stores while the refluxing enterocolitis horse would have a greater depletion of body $Na^+$ stores.

It is important to emphasize that most horses have adequate body reserves of these electrolytes and energy to get them through a few days of disease. Therefore, additives to crystalloid fluids are not routinely necessary for horses receiving fluid therapy for 12–48 h for supportive treatment for impaction colic or a mild case of diarrhea. This is especially true for patients that, although depressed, continue to eat 25–50% of their daily feed ration; these patients are likely ingesting physiologically normal concentrations of electrolytes from their diet (Schott 2006). Additives to the intravenous fluids are most critical for completely anorectic patients receiving intravenous fluids for more than 48 h and in patients that are losing large amounts of fluid in the form of ongoing gastric reflux or profuse diarrhea where the loss of electrolyte-rich water is immense. In these patients, acid–base status and serum electrolyte concentrations often need to be reassessed once or twice a day, and these results are used to modify the fluid therapy plan and electrolyte supplementation. These patients then often require significant fluid additives to the intravenous base polyionic fluids that are being administered to them.

A common practice to address the anticipated $Ca^{++}$ deficit in hyporexic and anorectic horses is to add 50–125 mL of a 23% calcium borogluconate solution to each 5-L bag of polyionic intravenous fluids. This addition of calcium borogluconate provides about 1.0–2.7 g of $Ca^{++}$ in each 5-L bag that would replace about one-eighth of the exchangeable $Ca^{++}$ pool in a 500 kg horse (Schott 2006). Although hypercalcemia is rarely a problem in the supplemented horse, excess is typically excreted via the urine. Monitoring for correction of hypocalcemia and prevention of excessive $Ca^{++}$ supplementation is a further reason that follow-up measurement of serum electrolytes should be considered for horses that are receiving fluid therapy for more than 48 h, especially when initial laboratory results were outside of the reference ranges for one or more values.

Most crystalloid rehydration fluids contain relatively modest amount of $K^+$ (5 mEq/L or less for most polyionic solutions); thus, addition of supplemental $K^+$ to the base fluid may be needed due to protracted disease and the large requirements of potassium the horse requires and the large amounts that the horse continues to excrete in urine on a daily basis. Because $K^+$ is the most abundant cation in body (largely an intracellular ion) fluids, supplementation is usually not necessary unless horses have significant anorexia for several days or have been on fluid therapy for more than 48 h. In these instances, depletion of total body $K^+$ stores can be substantial, yet serum $K^+$ may still be within the normal range because <0.5% of exchangeable $K^+$ is in plasma (Schott 2006). Thus, if evaluating the urine of these horses there is typically minimal $K^+$ loss and maximal acid loss ($H^+$) making the horse have paradoxic aciduria. Again, with prolonged support (>48 h) with intravenous fluids designed for rehydration (high in sodium, low in potassium), excessive replacement of body $Na^+$ stores may increase urine output (excrete excess sodium) and further exacerbate $K^+$ depletion by increasing obligate $K^+$ loss in urine. For example, if a fluid therapy plan was to administer about 35 L of polyionic intravenous fluid over the subsequent 12 h (1 L/h for maintenance and 2 L/h for anticipated losses in diarrhea, after rehydration has been accomplished), only about 175 mEq of $K^+$ would be replaced using a typical polyionic crystalloid fluid based on the composition of the fluid without additional supplementation (Schott 2006). This would represent replacement of <1% of body $K^+$ stores while urine $K^+$ losses could result in further depletion of as much as 3–4% of body $K^+$ stores through production of 10 L of urine (~threefold increase in urine flow due to a natriuresis) with a $K^+$ concentration as low as 100 mEq/L (Schott 2006). To simply match this estimated urine $K^+$ loss, 25 mEq of additional $K^+$ would need to be added to each of the 35 L of fluid administered. Remember with potassium supplementation, that the maximum amount per hour of supplementation is 0.5 mEq/kg/h; therefore, for the 500 kg horse, a total of 250 mEq can be provided per hour of fluid administration. An alternative to adding KCl to the intravenous fluids is to administer a mixture of NaCl:KCl (Lite salt) in enteral fluids or as an oral paste. For example, to provide 1500 mEq of KCl daily (≈5% of body $K^+$ stores), 110 g of KCl (1 g of KCl provides 13.4 mEq of both $K^+$ and $Cl^-$) could be administered as four doses of 25–30 g KCl via a nasogastric tube or as an oral paste (Schott 2006).

Critically ill adult horses and foals with watery diarrhea, especially those with profuse diarrhea, commonly develop a primary metabolic acidosis that may also need to be addressed (decreased pH with a decrease in serum bicarbonate concentration, $[HCO_3^-]$). One must recognize though that these patients in this state cannot have an increase in the plasma lactate concentration. If the plasma lactate concentration is increased this is likely due to vascular hypovolemia resulting in a hyperlactatemic acidosis and this needs to first be corrected before bicarbonate supplementation is calculated and therapy initiated. This is different from a patient that is presenting with acute hypovolemic shock, hyperlactatemia, and lactic acidosis. These patients do not need intravenous bicarbonate administration; instead, they need rapid intravenous administration of polyionic intravenous fluids. Initially, rehydration with crystalloid fluids (administered intravenously and enterally) is the treatment for both dehydration and acidosis. Vascular volume expansion with polyionic crystalloid fluids alone will likely improve perfusion (decrease lactate) and correct the acidosis. However, when acidosis is severe ($pH < 7.2$ or serum $tCO_2 < 15$ mEq/L) and unresponsive to initial resuscitation rehydration, addition of intravenous $HCO_3^-$ to the base polyionic fluid may be necessary (Schott 2006). In general, supplemental $HCO_3^-$ is not needed unless serum $tCO_2$ concentration (95% of which is $HCO_3^-$) falls below 15 mEq/L (compared to a normal value of 25–30 mEq/L). To estimate the amount of $HCO_3^-$ to add to the base fluid, the base deficit (BD), a calculation made from the venous blood gas analysis that provides a measure of the decrease in $HCO_3^-$ concentration, is multiplied by body mass (kg) and a fraction representing the portion of body mass that is composed of fluid containing $HCO_3^-$. Recommendations for the latter fraction range from 0.3 to 0.6 and the authors typically use a value of 0.5 to represent the entire ECF as well as a portion of the ICF. This calculation can be used for both the adult horse and the foal. If a venous blood gas is not available a serum chemistry can be used as a surrogate.

As an example, the $HCO_3^-$ deficit in a 500 kg horse with profuse diarrhea and a BD of 14 mEq/L (serum $tCO_2$ concentration of 13 mEq/L in comparison to a normal value of 27 mEq/L) would be estimated as (assuming that $1\ kg \approx 1\ L$):

$$HCO_3^-\ \text{deficit} = 14\ \text{mEq} / \text{L}(\text{BD}) \times 500\ \text{kg} \times 0.5 = 3500\ \text{mEq}\ HCO_3^-\ \text{deficit}.$$

For immediate correction as an isotonic solution, half of this deficit can be corrected quickly over a few or over 6–12 h, by addition of $HCO_3^-$ typically provided either in the base polyionic fluid (must not contain calcium due to precipitation) or as individual boluses made up in sterile water. Lastly it can also be given enterally either as oral paste solutions or to the base intravenous fluid or by enteral administration of $HCO_3^-$ via a nasogastric tube. It is important to remember that $HCO_3^-$ must be coupled with a cation, typically $Na^+$ if given intravenously or orally; however, chemical-grade solutions of potassium hydrocarbonate are available, making it possible to add $HCO_3^-$ without also adding $Na^+$, which will decrease the risk of causing further risk of patient hypernatremia. Further, $HCO_3^-$ should not be added to fluids containing $Ca^{++}$ (i.e., LRS or Hartman's solution) because there is a slight risk of forming $CaCO_3$ crystals that could precipitate in the fluids. Sodium bicarbonate is available as either a 5% solution (1 mL = 0.6 mEq of $HCO_3^-$) or an 8.4% hypertonic solution (1 mL = 1.0 mEq of $HCO_3^-$), is generally added to a base fluid of 0.9%NaCl or Plasmalyte-A, if you are using hypertonic bicarbonate 8.4% solution, you can also add this to sterile water and have the base fluid osmolality be isosmotic, again remember that in both instances you are adding a significant amount of sodium into the vascular space and extracellular fluid volume and will likely cause a secondary natriuresis resulting in potential further potassium loss. In patients, whether a foal or adult, that are producing large amounts of gastric reflux or diarrhea there is a significant loss of $Na^+$ within each of these types of fluid; therefore, administration of fluids of high concentrations of $Na^+$ is generally safe. If additional supplementation with $NaHCO_3$ to a base fluid or as another fluid separately is instituted this should be approached cautiously in horses with an increased plasma $Na^+$ concentration or with acidosis from other causes. A more physiological approach would be to use enteral replacement therapy with $NaHCO_3$ to correct the $HCO_3^-$ deficit by administering $NaHCO_3$ as a separate enteral solution that ranges from 300 to 600 mOsm/kg in tonicity (concentration) if the small intestine is functioning normally. One gram of $NaHCO_3$ has 12 mEq of both $Na^+$ and $HCO_3^-$ (for a total of 24 mOsm), the 3500 mEq $HCO_3^-$ deficit could be addressed by administering three ≈100 g doses of $NaHCO_3$ (baking soda) in 4–8 L of water at four-hour intervals (Schott 2006). A third alternative would be to administer $NaHCO_3$ as an oral paste (by mixing 30 g of $NaHCO_3$ with water or corn oil in a 60 mL dosing syringe and administering two syringes every two hours for five treatments) (Schott 2006). One must be cautious with oral administration of $NaHCO_3$ because when mixed with water there is a tendency for the bicarbonate to produce gas and fizz, this may result in transient gas colic.

Unfortunately, the $Na^+$ load accompanying $NaHCO_3$ administration by any route (parenteral or enteral) will lead to increased urine output (and will exacerbate the obligate loss of $K^+$ in urine through naturesis. Therefore, attention to $K^+$ balance, by adding KCl to the base intravenous fluid or enteral solutions being administered or by giving KCl as an oral paste, merits consideration in horses receiving supplemental $HCO_3^-$. Finally, another alternative for oral supplementation of bicarbonate would be to use $KHCO_3$, rather than $NaHCO_3$, (Schott 2006).

When adding multiple supplements (e.g., KCl, $NaHCO_3$, and dextrose) to a polyionic fluid (typically LRS, Normosol R or Plasma-Lyte A for replacement fluids and 1/2 strength saline, Plasma-Lyte 56 or Normosol M for maintenance fluids), the tonicity of the final product should be considered (Schott 2006); in the adult horse and foal this is approximately 270–280 mmol/L. A general rule is that the total osmolality provided by electrolytes should not exceed more than twice the value of plasma osmolality. Since plasma osmolality is normally about 280 mOsm/kg, a final osmolality of about 600 mOsm/kg would be a reasonable limit. The osmotic contribution from dextrose can largely be ignored because this additive is metabolized rapidly at the cellular level into water and $CO_2$ and contributes little to the net total number of osmoles added to body fluids (Schott 2006).

Administering fluids that are hypertonic (greater osmolality than plasma) may be advantageous in some hypovolemic horses which have clinical evidence of hypovolemic shock. In the foal, it is quite controversial to use hypertonic saline; therefore, it is commonly not used even if there is evidence of acute hypovolemic shock. Rapid resuscitation is essential to help prevent further compromise of the horse and end organ perfusion deficits. Specifically, the initial fluid replacement in most dehydrated horses occurs in the form of voluntarily water drinking due to the sensed hypertonicity of the blood making up the vascular volume. Because an increase in plasma osmolality is the most potent stimulus for thirst, dilution of remaining plasma electrolytes by water drinking can abolish thirst. As a result, horses that lose considerable amounts of electrolytes with water via prolonged sweating, reflux, or diarrhea can remain moderately to severely dehydrated and yet may have little drive of thirst, therefore, do not naturally have a drive to drink and remain significantly volume depleted. Therefore, initial fluid resuscitation with hypertonic fluids, especially due to a higher $Na^+$ content and osmolality, will stimulate thirst in these horses and provide initial vascular volume resuscitation. It is also vital to consider continued polyionic fluid support to further bolster both the extracellular and intracellular fluid deficits.

Hypertonic saline (7.2% NaCl) is commonly used in equine practice, but not as a specific fluid additive to the base fluid. This solution is commonly administered intravenously to the acutely hypovolemic horse that requires rapid volume resuscitation (Crabtree and Epstein 2021). Hypertonic saline is contraindicated in foals for the treatment of hypovolemia because it causes rapid changes in plasma osmolarity that may have serious life-threatening consequences (Hollis and Corley 2007). The dose is 2–4 mL/kg or 1–2 L in a 500 kg horse, and it should only be given through an intravenous catheter due to the severe osmolality that can result in tissue necrosis if the solution is extravasated or given subcutaneously (Schott 2006). Hypertonic saline has $Na^+$ and $Cl^-$ concentrations of 1232 mEq/L or an osmolality of 2464 mOsm/kg, a value ~ninefold greater than plasma (Magdesian 2014a). Additionally, it should be followed by isotonic crystalloid fluid administration during initial rehydration because of the significant amount of sodium that the patient is receiving. Hypertonic saline increases the vascular volume by 4× the amount administered and supports cardiac output because of the rapid shift of water by osmotic forces from the endothelial glycocalyx and from the intracellular fluid space to rapidly increase the extracellular vascular space expanding the plasma volume. This treatment is ideally suited for horses experiencing rapid fluid loss from the vascular space resulting in cardiovascular, septic, and hypovolemic, shock but can also be useful in patients that have hypovolemic shock due to other types of fluid loss (acute, controlled blood loss). The intravascular expansion is relatively short-lived (30–60 minutes) but can be helpful in emergency situations. As a rule of thumb, give 10 L of balanced crystalloids/1 L of hypertonic saline to account for the significant concentration of salt (Schott 2006).

## Monitoring Response to Treatment

Identification of an appropriate response to fluid therapy is practically monitored by reassessing the patient's attitude and clinical parameters of hydration, including heart rate; moistness of oral membranes; temperature of the nose, ears, and extremities; skin tent response; PCV and TS; and lactate. There are more invasive tests including blood pressure monitoring, cardiac output monitoring, central venous pressure, and pulse pressure character (Magdesian 2014a,b). However, this is not commonly performed due to the invasive nature and the ability to get adequate assessment from the physical examination. In addition, an obvious, but easily overlooked, assessment is the frequency of urination and specific gravity of the urine; for example, is the horse's urine going from ultraconcentrated urine to more dilute, isothenuric urine? Most horses should be observed to pass substantial amounts of dilute urine within 6–12 h after onset of fluid therapy during the resuscitation phase and continue into more maintenance rate fluid administration. Once an increase in urine output is observed, the rate of fluid administration should be reassessed and likely can be reduced unless it is determined that there is still significant ongoing losses (diarrhea or nasogastric reflux). At times, improvement in other clinical parameters (e.g., heart rate, PCV, TS) is less than desired despite increased urine output. Rarely does maintenance of a high fluid administration rate correct these clinical abnormalities once urine output has increased (Schott 2006). This most often occurs due to the primary clinical disease that these patients have and the lack of clinical response (normalization of PE parameters, PCV and TS) to the provided fluid therapies may require further supportive care in the form of increasing oncotic pressure (synthetic, or natural colloid fluids), inotropic medications, or vasopressor medications.

## Discontinuation of Fluid Therapy

It is typically easier to decide when a horse needs fluid therapy, how much fluids to administer, and what type of fluid to use than when and how to implement discontinuing fluid therapy. De-escalation can be quite difficult to determine when this type of supportive care can be safely withdrawn and how this should be accomplished and how rapidly. Often, supportive fluid therapy is likely continued much longer than necessary and may result in potential more harm (subclinical edema formation) than good in many horses. While it is very uncommon for there to be negative side effects to fluid therapy, it is considered a drug; therefore, we are prudent to consider all negative consequences of parenteral and enteral fluids. Nevertheless, there are a couple of general rules that need to be followed. First, the medical or surgical problem that intravenous fluids are prescribed should be stable and or improving for at least 12–24 h before discontinuation of fluid therapy. This would include correction of dehydration and at least 6–12 h of fluid administration at a maintenance rate alone (Schott 2006). Intravenous or enteral fluid therapy does not need to be continued until all laboratory data has normalized, but consideration should be given to renal values to make sure that they are close to normal and that the electrolytes are trending back to the normal reference range. Some values may take weeks to fully normalize especially protein values and liver enzymatic activity. This is especially true for horses that are improving in response to treatment. Second, when the medical or surgical disorder has been accompanied by partial or complete anorexia, a reasonable goal is for the horse to be eating at least 50% of a normal feed ration, preferably with an increasing appetite, before fluid therapy is discontinued (Schott 2006). One exception would be a horse being treated medically for a pelvic flexure impaction colic with enteral fluids (via a nasogastric tube) will usually not be offered feed until after the last dose of enteral fluids and the horse has passed a considerable amount of feces. When the use of intravenous fluids has been exclusively used to treat gastric reflux or diarrheic foal or adult horse or in conjunction with enteral fluids, intravenous fluids are often continued at a maintenance rate for at least 24 h after feed is again offered, this is to help control the voluntary consumption of water that the patient would have to perform to maintain hydration. Lastly, when prescribing and administering nephrotoxic medications that likely have cumulative affects (e.g., gentamicin, oxytetracycline, polymyxin B, and flunixin meglumine or phenylbutazone), especially if indices of renal function (BUN and creatinine) are above the normal ranges, intravenous fluid therapy should be maintained to support renal perfusion and urine output. The main point of these guidelines is that fluids do not need to be continued until the patient is back on full feed and each patient must be critically evaluated to decide when is the ultimate time for discontinuation of fluid therapy.

The decision to discontinue fluid therapy is more difficult in patients with long-standing (>five days), ongoing fluid losses such as persistent gastric reflux with small intestinal disorders (nasogastric reflux or proximal duodenitis), or persistent diarrhea with more severe cases of enterocolitis (Schott 2006). Commonly these patients are on multimodal therapy (both fluids and often nephrotoxic medications) for treatment of their sustained disease pathophysiology requiring an increased maintenance fluid rate and other CRI medications that often result in a total intravenous fluid rate higher than traditional maintenance rate (40–60 mL/kg/h) (Schott 2006). These high intravenous fluid rate administrations are to combat the significant ongoing losses (diarrhea or nasogastric reflux) that the patient is chronically being affected by. Consideration needs to be given to the large amounts of continued $Na^+$ and $Cl^-$ administration and excessive replacement leading to greater urine output and acidosis. The excess urine output exacerbates depletion of total body $K^+$ stores (intracellular and extracellular $K^+$ depletion) and secondarily with $Na^+$ excess vascular dilution of plasma protein (albumin) resulting in edema formation. A potential approach may be to "challenge" these patients, once they are considered stable, by discontinuing fluid therapy for 12–24 h. If their clinical condition deteriorates (e.g., a decrease in appetite; greater depression; and increases in heart rate, PCV, and TS), fluid therapy can be started again (Schott 2006).

## Colloid Fluid Therapy

Colloid fluids consist of both synthetic products and natural colloids that hold water in the intravascular space by increasing the plasma oncotic pressure (Hughes and Boag 2012; van Galen and Hallowell 2019) (Box 28.5). Such blood volume expansion can occur as quickly as 30 minutes and last up to 24 h, depending on the specific product and the current disease state of the patient. This effect of volume expansion via a draw of water from the interstitial space, occurs without the addition of large amounts of sodium, unlike the administration of hypertonic saline. Synthetic colloids, including hydroxyethyl starches, dextrans, and gelatins, contain large multi-weighted carbohydrate molecules that hold water in the vascular space

**Box 28.5 How colloid fluids help restore intravascular fluid volume**

Because the colloid particles are too large to freely pass across the normal capillary endothelium, colloid fluids increase oncotic pressure and retain water in the vascular space. These fluids support the intravascular space and are useful in horses with clinical evidence of hypoproteinemia or hypoalbuminemia (Bellezzo et al. 2014). Further, much like hypertonic saline solution, synthetic colloids rapidly increase intravascular volume in cases of severe hypovolemia.

by increasing the plasma oncotic pressure (Hughes and Boag 2012). Natural colloids include plasma, albumin, and whole blood, though for this chapter, whole blood will be considered a separate fluid type as it has different properties and thus different applications to other natural colloids. Normal colloid oncotic pressure is 19.2–31.3 mmHg in adult horses and 15.0–22.6 mmHg in foals.

Colloid fluid therapy is less commonly used in equine medicine as compared with crystalloid solutions, primarily due to relative availability and cost, as well as potential side effects of colloids (van Galen and Hallowell 2019). As mentioned, the application of synthetic colloids is primarily either for resuscitation of the horse in hypovolemic shock or for the treatment of the horse with hypoproteinemia (Bellezzo et al. 2014). The osmotic effect of macromolecules is due to the large size, though the degree of increase in oncotic pressure is related to their number in solution rather than absolute size. Hydroxyethylstarches (HES) represent the most commonly used synthetic colloids and include hetastarch, pentastarch, and tetrastarch formulations. This group of synthetic colloids are produced by substituting hydroxyethyl groups onto the glucose units of amylopectin. HES products are described by their molecular weight and the degree of substitution as well as the C2/C6 hydroxylethylation ratio (van Galen and Hallowell 2019). Important to consider when selecting a specific HES is the lower the molecular weight, the higher the oncotic pressure but the faster the degradation of the product in vivo. The larger the molecular weight, the more likely to have undesired side effects. HES with a molecular weight average between 100 and 300 kDa appear to have the optimal weight for desired effects. The higher the degree of substitution (hydroxyethylation), the slower the degradation of the colloid in vivo. Two readily available products include Hextend, a 6% hetastarch 670/0.8 in a lactated electrolyte solution, and VetStarch, a 6% pentastarch 130/0.4 in 0.9% sodium chloride injection. In comparing the two products, the larger molecular weight of the Hextend means that it will have a smaller effect on oncotic pressure, but it also has a higher degree of substitution and as such, will have a more prolonged effect compared to the VetStarch. In addition, the larger molecular weight of Hextend renders it more likely to cause adverse reactions, though rare in the horse compared with humans. To provide colloidal support, HES solutions are administered as a 10 mL/kg IV bolus (up to 20 mL/kg/day). This would mean that a 500 kg horse would receive a 5-L bolus of an HES (e.g., 10–500 mL bags of VetStarch). A table of commonly used colloid products is in *Appendix 3: Emergency Medications and Fluids*. Determining response to treatment is accomplished by repeat assessment of the patient, just as with administration of crystalloid fluids, paying close attention to parameters of volemic status (HR, PCV, TS, lactate) that may not have improved with initial crystalloid resuscitation. When monitoring total protein, synthetic colloids may affect the refractive index of the plasma and, in turn, the accuracy of refractometry. As such, plasma total protein should be measured via other means (e.g., biuret or turbidometric).

It should be mentioned that large colloids may reduce tissue perfusion by increasing plasma viscosity. Many factors influence the volume and duration of intravascular expansion associated with synthetic colloids, including dose, number of hydroxyethyl substitutions (product formulation), and microvascular permeability. Synthetic colloids are heterogeneous in their size within a product and their degradation from particles of larger molecular weight to smaller, contributes to their challenging pharmacokinetics as well as some of the negative side effects associated with their use (van Galen and Hallowell 2019). Reports of renal injury and coagulopathies in human medicine, without the added benefit of improved morbidity or mortality for ICU patients with critical illness, has rendered synthetic colloids largely unpopular and even considered contraindicated in some cases in human medicine (Martin et al. 2002; Kozeck-Langenecker 2005); however, the side-effects of synthetic colloid administration have not been extensively studied in equids. Reports of acute kidney injury in horses receiving synthetic colloids have not been published. HES product administration has been shown to negatively affect coagulation testing parameters in healthy ponies, owing to a dilutional effect (Jones et al. 1997); however, none of the coagulation testing nor clot function testing that has been reported has been outside the normal reference range. Subsequent in vitro viscoelastic testing and platelet functional testing using healthy horse blood found that increasing amounts of HES solutions caused alterations in coagulation variables in vitro beyond a simple dilutional effect (Blong et al. 2013). While a large body of evidence is still lacking regarding the side effects of HES products in horses, because of the risk of altering coagulation function, synthetic colloids should be used with caution in cases of uncontrolled hemorrhage. Dextrans act similarly to HES products, though they generally have a smaller particle size (40 and 70 kDa are commonly used products) and thus exert a high oncotic pressure. However, due to their small size, they are also readily excreted or degraded and have more reported complications that HES and are not currently used.

Similar to synthetic productions, natural colloids can also provide volume expansion and be used in the management of horses with hypoproteinemia/hypoalbuminemia. The principal source of protein or oncotic pressure in plasma is albumin (69 kDa) which provides approximately 80% of the oncotic pressure of blood. Hypoalbuminemia/hypoproteinemia is the main indication for the use of plasma in horses and commonly occurs secondary to gastrointestinal disease, decreased production, or loss into the interstitial space due to increased vascular permeability. In such cases, the volume of plasma required to increase the total solids in a 500-kg horse by 1 g/dL would be approximately 4 L (see formula for transfusion volume below). It should be noted that the clinical experience suggests between 8 and 12 L of plasma is needed to increase the total solids by 1 g/dL. This difference between the theoretical and actual clinical result is likely due to ongoing losses of protein/albumin secondary to the primary disease as well as redistribution of the transfused albumin to the interstitial space across an inflamed endothelium or damaged glycocalyx. Both the cost and the availability of plasma products make synthetic colloids more desirable, practical, and useful for simply restitution of oncotic pressure.

$$\text{Plasma transfusion volume}(\text{L}) = (\text{desired TP} - \text{actual TP}) / \text{donor TP} \times \text{BW}(\text{kg}) \times 0.05$$

Unlike synthetic colloids, natural colloids have other properties that contribute to their versatility: coagulation factors, globulins, antithrombin III, and fibronectin. As such, natural colloids act not simply as a volume expander or provider of oncotic pressure, but also as component therapy for the treatment of hemorrhage or coagulopathy, or as an anti-endotoxic medication in the treatment of endotoxemia. Because of these properties, the use of natural colloids like plasma may be useful for the management of specific conditions in the horse, such as enterocolitis, as compared with synthetic colloids for their additional immunomodulatory coagulation properties (Kopper et al. 2019). For such purposes of providing component therapy, fresh frozen plasma is an excellent source of active coagulation factors, though it has comparatively reduced numbers of functioning platelets compared with fresh plasma or whole blood. A dose of 4–5 mL/kg, equating to approximately 2 L, can be effective in a 500 kg horse for component replacement therapy. It is critical that the plasma be fresh frozen (i.e., frozen within six hours of separation) and used within a year to minimize degradation of coagulation factors V and VIII. Hyperimmunized plasma against enteric pathogens (e.g., J-5 enteric plasma) may be useful in the treatment of endotoxemia using a similar dose of 4–5 mL/kg. The detriments associated with plasma administration include transfusion reactions for the horse, increased expense to the client, and added labor for the practitioner (maintaining a frozen product, timing of thawing prior to use, etc.). The majority of plasma transfusion reactions are mild and transient: signs of fever, tachycardia, tachypnea, and urticaria. However, more severe reactions can occur, and plasma transfusions should begin slowly with close attention paid to the horse's vital parameters, checking every 5 minutes for the first 15 minutes, then increasing the interval as the transfusion rate is increased. Should these signs occur, the transfusion should be stopped and a corticosteroid such as dexamethasone may be administered. For commercial products, the lot numbers should be recorded for the purposes of ideally using the same lot numbers in a patient as well as recording any adverse events associated with a particular lot number.

## Blood Transfusion

Blood transfusion is most often indicated in cases of acute, severe hemorrhage (Hurcombe et al. 2007; Hohenhaus and DiBartola 2012; Mudge 2014; Divers et al. 2022; Radcliffe et al. 2022). Whole blood is essentially a natural colloid solution with oxygen-carrying capacity. As such, it can provide all the benefits of plasma with also replacement of red blood cells and functional platelets. Blood volume represents approximately 8–10% of body weight (~40–50 L in a 500 kg horse) and 15% of body weight in the foal (7.5 L in a 50 kg foal). Clinical estimation of blood loss can be challenging depending on the rate of loss, but typically at least 15% of blood volume needs to be lost prior to the development of clinical signs (6 L in 500 kg horse). As the volume of blood lost increases, the horse will show progressively worsening tachycardia, tachypnea, prolongation of CRT, decreasing blood pressure, and decreasing urine production (Magdesian et al. 2006; Hurcombe et al. 2007; Mudge 2014). As hypovolemic shock ensues, severe tachycardia, hypotension, cold extremities, and altered mentation are seen. Due to the large reserve of red blood cells within the equine spleen, as well as a lag in fluid redistribution from the interstitial to intravascular spaces, there may be no negligible changes to a horse's PCV during acute hemorrhage. Rather, a relative hypoproteinemia and hyperlactatemia are initially seen (Magdesian et al. 2006; Hurcombe et al. 2007). In an acute situation, blood transfusion triggers include a PCV of <20%, plasma lactate of >4 mmol/L, or an oxygen extraction ratio of >40%. In a case of chronic anemia, a common transfusion trigger parameter is a PCV of <12% and a hemoglobin concentration <5–7 g/dL (Mudge 2014).

Horses have eight recognized blood groups, and the two most important in cases of blood incompatibility are the Qa and Aa blood antigens. Horses within a breed are more likely to have the same blood group (Trommershausen Bowling and Clark 1985). In an ideal world, any blood transfusion would be preceded by a cross-match between the potential donors and the recipient. This is due to decreased red blood cell survival in horses with prior cross-match incompatibility compared to those without, not because of the risk of other transfusion reactions (Tomlinson et al. 2015). In reality, horses rarely have naturally occurring anti-red blood cell antibodies, and a first time blood transfusion can be performed with minimal risk of transfusion reaction. Furthermore, in the case of acute, uncontrolled hemorrhage, a several-hour cross-match takes valuable time that is better utilized by administering blood from an ideal donor to manage the hypovolemic shock and provide essential coagulation factors, platelets, and essential oxygen-carrying capacity (Box 28.6).

For the reasons of blood groups, decreased likelihood of previous exposure to RBC antigens, and amount of blood able to be collected, ideal donors are characterized by the following: healthy, adult gelding, Standardbred, large size, negative for Aa and Qa, vaccinated, PCV > 35%, TS > 6.0 g/dL. Following a blood transfusion, a recipient will develop antibodies within the next week. Should a second blood transfusion be needed more than three days after the first, a cross-match should be completed. Prior to three days, a second transfusion may be performed without cross-match as alloantibodies have not yet been produced.

Blood transfusions are also indicated for treatment of normovolemic anemia (Divers et al. 2022; Radcliffe et al. 2022) (Box 28.7). Whole blood should always be administered via a commercial blood set with an in-line filter. Concurrent isotonic crystalloid administration can be performed; however, hypo- or hypertonic solutions need to be avoided as they may damage red blood cells. Calcium-containing fluids should also be avoided during blood transfusion as the calcium may promote undesired clot formation within the transfusate.

Like other natural colloids, blood transfusions are subject to transfusion reactions. In the case of whole blood, these include hemolytic reactions and inflammatory or allergic reactions. These reactions can range from mild elevations in vital parameters (temperature, heart rate, respiratory rate) to severe anaphylaxis. Reactions can occur acutely, during the transfusion, or be delayed as much as two weeks post transfusion. Importantly, appropriate cross-matching does not prevent transfusion reactions. As with plasma transfusions, the recipient should be monitored closely during the transfusion, especially during the first 15–20 minutes. Should an allergic reaction be suspected, the transfusion should be stopped, and a dose of corticosteroid or antihistamine administered. Should an anaphylactic reaction occur, the transfusion should be stopped, and a dose of epinephrine (0.01–0.02 mL/kg IV) should be administered. Although rare, all-natural colloid therapy, whether component or whole blood therapy, carries the risk of acute serum hepatitis (Theiler's disease) (Tomlinson et al. 2019).

**Box 28.6 How to transfuse for uncontrolled hemorrhage**

Typically, the amount of blood needed for treatment of uncontrolled hemorrhage (e.g., periparturient bleeding or hemoperitoneum) is the maximum amount that an ideal donor can provide, or 15–20% of the donor's blood volume (6–8 L in a 500 kg donor) (Divers et al. 2022). The blood transfusion can be administered at a fast rate, up to 10–40 mL/kg/h (5–20 L/h in 500 kg recipient) if emergent resuscitation is necessary.

**Box 28.7 How to transfuse for normovolemic anemia**

The volume of transfusion recommended for horses with normovolemic anemia may be calculated based on the donor and recipient PCV and the body weight of the recipient:

$$\text{Blood transfusion volume}\,(\text{L}) = (\text{desired PCV} - \text{actual PCV} / \text{donor PCV}) \times \text{BW}\,(\text{kg}) \times 0.08$$

An example transfusion would be a 450 kg horse with a PCV of 12% and a target PCV of 20% with a cross-matched donor having a PCV of 38%. The transfusion volume to be given would be (20 − 12/38) × 450 × 0.05 = 4.8 L. If the donor horse weighed 500 kg, this volume of blood to donate would represent approximately 12% of its blood volume, below the limit of 20%.

**Case Example 28.1 Fluid Therapy in the Horse and Foal**

**Case 1: Adult horse**

You are presented with a 500 kg horse afflicted with severe enterocolitis (Figure 28.2). The horse has had diarrhea for two days, is anorexic, and clinical examination findings result in an estimate of moderate (8%) dehydration.

*Emergency triage steps:*

Step 1: Patient Stabilization

a) Prepare a fluid therapy plan for this horse for the first 12 h. Include the replacement fluid needs to correct the fluid deficit, as well as the maintenance requirements and ongoing losses.
b) A plan for the initial **12 h** would be formulated as follows:

| | |
|---|---|
| i) rehydration needs: | 0.08 (estimated 8% dehydration) × 500 kg = 40 L |
| ii) maintenance needs: | 40 mL/kg/24 h × 500 kg = (20,000 mL/24 h)/2 = 10,000 mL = 10 L over 12 h |
| iii) ongoing losses: | estimated at 2 L/h × 12 h = 24 L |
| iv) TOTAL: | 40 + 10 + 24 = 74 L |

c) Thus, approximately 74 L of fluid need to be administered over the initial 12 h of treatment with multiple patient monitoring points during this time. Fluid administration could be accomplished by hanging 14–5-L bags with an infusion rate of about 6 L/h. This fluid plan would entail no use of a fluid bolus or by administering a 20–30 L fluid bolus and following with an infusion rate of 4 L/h. The disadvantage of using this route of administration is that most of the bolus would not last long in the vascular space, and it would take several hours to give a 20–30-L fluid bolus to a patient unless a roller pump was being used.

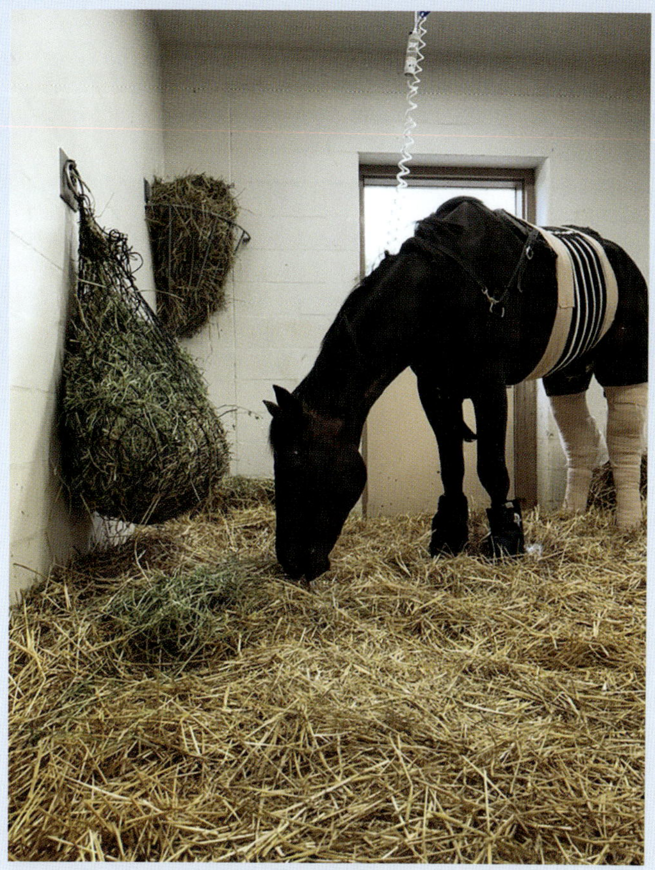

**Figure 28.2** A 12-year-old Thoroughbred horse presenting with a two-day history of diarrhea and colic. The horse had evidence of poor perfusion with purple, toxic mucous membranes, elevated heart rate, and increased gastrointestinal borborygmi. A diagnosis of enterocolitis was made based upon clinical exam, ultrasonographic evaluation, and blood work. Note fluid therapy via jugular catheterization and ice boots on forelimbs to help prevent secondary laminitis. The lateral thoracic vessel is another option for large-volume fluid therapy in the horse.

d) As an alternative, a nasogastric tube could be placed, and 10 L of fluid could be administered 7 times over the initial 12 h, provided significant gastric reflux is not present. A combination of intravenous fluids and enteral fluids is probably the most logical approach in this case to prevent phlebitis from high-volume intravenous fluid administration.
e) Most commonly, however, such horses are treated almost exclusively with intravenous fluids because most clinicians do not want to repeatedly pass a nasogastric tube in a sick, depressed horse and prefer not to place an indwelling nasogastric tube in horses that they are encouraging to eat. Also, intravenous fluids are commonly used because they are easy and convenient, the clinician can set the fluid rate and pick the type of fluids and continue with other patient evaluations. Physiologically enteral fluid therapy either alone or in combination would be very acceptable types of fluids in a fluid therapy plan.
f) From a physiological basis, however, enteral fluid therapy alone would be a completely acceptable alternative, and this point should be remembered when treating horses for which owners may not be able to afford intravenous fluid therapy (especially when the alternative may be euthanasia).

For additional information on formulating a diagnostic plan, specific treatment guidelines, monitoring, and decision making for colic in the horse, including enterocolitis, see Chapter 10, *Diseases of the abdomen*.

### Case 2: Neonatal foal

You are presented with a 24-h-old Thoroughbred foal (50 kg) that is recumbent (Figure 28.3). The mare foaled (gestation = 315 days) the previous day, and the owners reported difficulties and veterinary assistance for fetal extraction was required. Colostrum from the mare was provided to the foal following parturition; however, the foal did not stand. The foal was referred into the hospital because of progressive deterioration. On presentation, the foal has tacky mucous membranes, slow capillary refill, no urine production, tachycardia, tachypnea, sunken eyes, muddy mucous

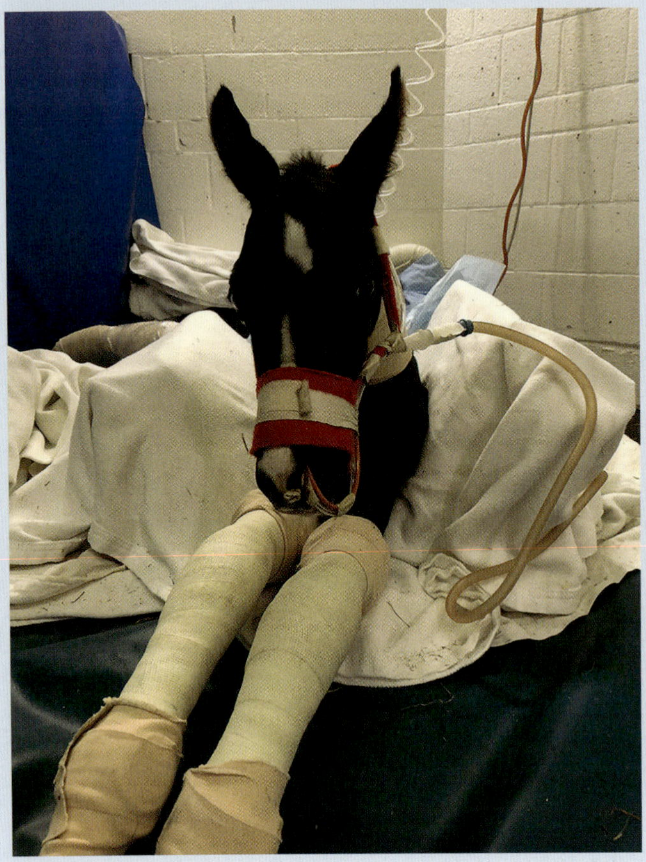

**Figure 28.3** A premature (315 days' gestation), neonatal Thoroughbred foal at 48 h of age following initial stabilization with intranasal oxygen, fluid therapy, systemic broad-spectrum antibiotics, and other supportive care. Note the intravenous fluid line, nasal oxygen supplementation line (smaller red-rubber tube entering L nostril), nasogastric feeding tube (larger clear tube entering L nostril), and the forelimb tube casts for the support of incomplete carpal bone ossification. A Bair Hugger warming device is also being used to provide thermal regulation. (3M Bair Hugger, St. Paul MN.) *Source:* Courtesy of Dr. Barbara Delvescovo.

membranes with petechial hemorrhage, poor pulse quality, and is unresponsive. Temperature of the foal is 96 °F. Emergency blood work yields a blood glucose of 37 mg/dL, systemic L-lactate of 9.7 mmol/L, and elevated PCV and TS.

*Emergency triage steps:*

Step 1: Patient Stabilization

a) Provide nasal oxygen via nasal cannula at 5–10 L/min. Place OTW catheter and begin warmed, intravenous fluid therapy. Collect blood for culture, CBC, and chemistry.
b) Estimate 15% dehydrated 50 kg foal. Fluid deficit is 50 kg × 0.15 = 7.5 L to be administered over 12 h (625 mL/h). Maintenance would be 2–4 mL/kg/h; choosing 3 mL/kg/h would be 150 mL/h + 625 mL/h = 775 mL/h after resuscitation and no ongoing losses. If on the farm, the foal may also receive 1500 mL q 2-h boluses.
c) Because the foal is hypoglycemic, begin with a 1% glucose solution (20 mL of 50% dextrose into 1-L balanced polyionic fluids) added to the resuscitation boluses at 4–8 mg/kg/min in 2 boluses and reassess in 1 h. Aim to maintain glucose concentrations from 60 to 180 mg/dL.
d) Following resuscitation, a CRI of 5% dextrose at a rate of 4 mg/kg/minute should be initiated. 50 kg foal at 4 mg/kg/minute = 50 kg × 4 mg/kg/minute × 60 minutes = 12,000 mg/hr or 12 g/h × 1000 mL/50 g = 240 mL/h of 5% dextrose in water solution. Remember glucose solutions should not be given as a bolus to prevent electrolyte derangements and further dehydration due to osmotic diuresis.
e) Positive inotrope and vasopressor therapy may be needed if intravenous fluid therapy does not improve tissue perfusion; see Chapter 29, *Pressure support in horses and foals.*
f) Warm the foal slowly using heat lamp, warm water bottles, or Bair hugger.
g) Replace any electrolyte abnormalities as required.
h) Measure IgG concentration and provide immunoglobins if value <800 mg/dL.
i) Begin parenteral nutrition as malabsorption is likely with poor perfusion. Switch to enteral nutrition once the GI tract is functioning to provide daily nutritional requirements.
j) Severe disease and evidence of sepsis (petechiae of mucous membranes) warrants broad-spectrum antibiotic therapy.
k) Radiograph carpal and tarsal cuboidal bones to grade ossification and splint if required.

For additional information on formulating a diagnostic plan, specific treatment guidelines, monitoring and decision making for foal diseases, including sepsis, see Chapter 20, *Foal emergencies.*

## References


Bellezzo, F., Kuhnmuench, T., and Hackett, E.S. (2014). The effect of colloid formulation on colloid osmotic pressure in horses with naturally occurring gastrointestinal disease. *BMC Vet. Res.* 10 (Suppl 1): S8. https://doi.org/10.1186/1746-6148-10-S1-S8.

Blong, A.E., Epstein, K.L., and Brainard, B.M. (2013). In vitro effects of three formulations of hydroxyethyl starch solutions on coagulation and platelet function in horses. *Am. J. Vet. Res.* 74 (5): 712–720. https://doi.org/10.2460/ajvr.74.5.712.

Crabtree, N.E. and Epstein, K.L. (2021). Current concepts in fluid therapy in horses. *Front. Vet. Sci.* 8: 648774.

Divers, T.J., Radcliffe, R.M., Cook, V.L. et al. (2022). Calculating and selecting fluid therapy and blood product replacements for horses with acute hemorrhage. *J. Vet. Emerg. Crit. Care (San Antonio)* 32 (S1): 97–107. https://doi.org/10.1111/vec.13127.

Fielding, L.C. (2014). Chapter 1. Body water physiology. In: *Equine Fluid Therapy*, 1e (ed. L.C. Fielding and K.G. Magdesian), 1–10. Wiley publishing.

Fielding, L.C. (2018). Practical fluid therapy and treatment modalities for field conditions for horses and foals with gastrointestinal problems. *Vet. Clin. N. Am.* 34 (1): 155–168.

Fielding, L.C. (2024). Chapter 62. Fluid therapy in the neonatal foal. In: *Equine Neonatal Medicine*, 1e (ed. D.M. Wong and P.A. Wilkins), 1344–1357. Wiley.

Fielding, L.C., Magdesian, K.G., and Edman, J.E. (2011). Determination of body water compartments in neonatal foals by use of indicator dilution techniques and multifrequency bioelectrical impedance analysis. *Am. J. Vet. Res.* 72 (10): 1390–1396.

Forro, M., Cieslar, S., Ecker, G.L. et al. (2000). Total body water and ECFV measured using bioelectrical impedance analysis and indicator dilution in horses. *J. Appl. Physiol.* 89 (2): 663–671.

van Galen, G. and Hallowell, G. (2019). Hydroxyethyl starches in equine medicine. *J. Vet. Emerg. Crit. Care (San Antonio)* 29 (4): 349–359. https://doi.org/10.1111/vec.12854.

Hohenhaus, A.E. and DiBartola, S.P. (2012). Chapter 24. Blood transfusion and blood substitutes. In: *Fluid, Electrolyte, and Acid-Base Disorders in Small Animal Practice*, 4e (ed. S.P. DiBartola), 585–604. Elsevier.

Hollis, A. and Corley, K. (2007). Practical guide to fluid therapy in neonatal foals. http://inpractice.bmj.com/. *In Pract.* 29: 130–137.

Hughes, D. and Boag, A. (2012). Chapter 27. Fluid therapy with macromolecular plasma volume expanders. In: *Fluid, Electrolyte, and Acid-Base Disorders in Small Animal Practice*, 4e (ed. S.P. DiBartola), 647–664. Elsevier.

Hurcombe, S.D., Mudge, M.C., and Hinchcliff, K.W. (2007). Clinical and clinicopathologic variables in adult horses receiving blood transfusions: 31 cases (1999-2005). *J. Am. Vet. Med. Assoc.* 231 (2): 267–274. https://doi.org/10.2460/javma.231.2.267.

Jones, P.A., Tomasic, M., and Gentry, P.A. (1997). Oncotic, hemodilutional, and hemostatic effects of isotonic saline and hydroxyethyl starch solutions in clinically normal ponies. *Am. J. Vet. Res.* 58 (5): 541–548.

Kopper, J.J., Kogan, C.J., Cook, V.L., and Schott, H.C. 2nd (2019). Outcome of horses with enterocolitis receiving oncotic fluid support with either plasma or hetastarch. *Can. Vet. J.* 60 (11): 1207–1212.

Kozek-Langenecker, S.A. (2005). Effects of hydroxyethyl starch solutions on hemostasis. *Anesthesiology* 103: 654–660.

Magdesian, K.G. (2014a). Chapter 12. Replacement fluid therapy n horses. In: *Equine Fluid Therapy*, 1e (ed. L.C. Fielding and K.G. Magdesian), 161–174. Wiley publishing.

Magdesian, K.G. (2014b). Chapter 13. Maintenance fluid therapy in horses. In: *Equine Fluid Therapy*, 1e (ed. L.C. Fielding and K.G. Magdesian), 175–189. Wiley publishing.

Magdesian, K.G. (2014c). Chapter 22. Fluid therapy for neonatal foals. In: *Equine Fluid Therapy*, 1e (ed. L.C. Fielding and K.G. Magdesian), 284–298. Wiley publishing.

Magdesian, K.G., Fielding, C.L., Rhodes, D.M., and Ruby, R.E. (2006). Changes in central venous pressure and blood lactate concentration in response to acute blood loss in horses. *J. Am. Vet. Med. Assoc.* 229 (9): 1458–1462. https://doi.org/10.2460/javma.229.9.1458.

Martin, G., Bennett-Guerrero, E., Wakeling, H. et al. (2002). A prospective, randomized comparison of thromboelastographic coagulation profile in patients receiving lactated Ringer's solution, 6% hetastarch in a balanced-saline vehicle, or 6% hetastarch in saline during major surgery. *J. Cardiothorac. Vasc. Anesth.* 16: 441–446.

Mudge, M.C. (2014). Acute hemorrhage and blood transfusions in horses. *Vet. Clin. North Am. Equine Pract.* 30 (2): 427–ix. https://doi.org/10.1016/j.cveq.2014.04.004.

Radcliffe, R.M., Bookbinder, L.C., Liu, S.Y. et al. (2022). Collection and administration of blood products in horses: Transfusion indications, materials, methods, complications, donor selection, and blood testing. *J Vet Emerg Crit Care (San Antonio).* 32 (S1): 108–122. https://doi.org/10.1111/vec.13119.

Schott, H.C. (2006). Fluid therapy: a primer for students, technicians, and veterinarians in equine practice. *Vet. Clin. N. Am.* 22 (1): 1–14.

Tomlinson, J.E., Taberner, E., Boston, R.C. et al. (2015). Survival time of cross-match incompatible red blood cells in adult horses. *J. Vet. Intern. Med.* 29 (6): 1683–1688. https://doi.org/10.1111/jvim.13627.

Tomlinson, J.E., Kapoor, A., Kumar, A. et al. (2019). Viral testing of 18 consecutive cases of equine serum hepatitis: a prospective study (2014-2018). *J. Vet. Intern. Med.* 33 (1): 251–257. https://doi.org/10.1111/jvim.15368.

Trommershausen Bowling, A. and Clark, R.S. (1985). Blood group and protein polymorphism gene frequencies for seven breeds of horses in the United States. *Anim. Blood Groups Biochem. Genet.* 16 (2): 93–108. https://doi.org/10.1111/j.1365-2052.1985.tb01458.x.

# 29

# Pressure Support in Horses and Foals

*Hope F. Douglas*[1] *and Rolfe M. Radcliffe*[2]

[1] *Department of Clinical Studies - New Bolton Center, University of Pennsylvania School of Veterinary Medicine, Kennett Square, PA, USA*
[2] *Department of Clinical Sciences, College of Veterinary Medicine, Cornell University, Ithaca, NY, USA*

## Introduction

The purpose of the circulatory system is to deliver oxygen and nutrients to the tissues and to remove metabolic waste products. Fundamental interrelated components of the circulatory system are cardiac output and blood pressure. Cardiac output is the amount of blood that is pumped into the aorta each minute, which is equal to the blood that flows through the circulation (Hall 2016). Blood pressure is defined as the force exerted by the blood against any unit area of the vessel wall (Hall 2016). *There are four primary elements that govern cardiac output and arterial blood pressure: blood volume, heart-pumping capacity, vascular compliance, and total peripheral resistance* (Guyton 1981). Based upon hydraulic principles, an analogy describing the cardiovascular system as a city water system can be effective to describe, identify, and treat circulatory disorders (Washburn and Stewart 2020). This city water pump analogy will be utilized throughout this chapter (Box 29.1).

Cardiac output (CO) is determined by heart rate and stroke volume. Heart rate is governed by the interplay between the sympathetic and parasympathetic branches of the autonomic nervous system. Stroke volume, the volume of blood ejected per cardiac contraction, is directly related to preload (the stretch of the ventricle before contraction) and contractility (the force of contraction of the ventricle). It is inversely related to afterload (the force required to achieve left ventricular outflow). Using the above-described analogy, the water (or blood) pressure in the system (or mean arterial pressure [MAP]) will be dependent upon the product of flow (cardiac output) and resistance (systemic vascular resistance [SVR]). Systemic vascular resistance is regulated systemically by the adrenergic nervous system, which can lead to alterations in the pipe dimensions (vascular tone). Systemic vascular resistance can also be regulated at the faucet, or local tissue level, by vasoactive substances including nitric oxide, histamine, prostacyclin, carbon dioxide, thrombin, thromboxane, and endothelin (Hall 2016).

The regulatory elements of the cardiovascular system mature during fetal development, with continuation during early neonatal and pediatric life. At birth, there is a pronounced transition from fetal circulation, with regression of anatomic and physiologic shunts, and there is maturation of adrenergic, neural, and endocrine regulatory pathways. The neonatal heart has altered contractility relative to the adult (Vrancken et al. 2018). Due to differences in physiology, the heart rate is particularly important for neonatal cardiac output (Driessen 2018), and higher metabolic demands require operation at near-maximum capacity. In addition, the adrenergic system is not fully mature at the time of birth, with initial dominance of the parasympathetic nervous system and later development of the sympathetic nervous system. This is particularly relevant for equine fetuses, as they have comparatively late increases in fetal cortisol relative to other species (Fowden et al. 1995; O'Connor et al., 2006; Fowden et al. 2020). Maturation of the cardiovascular system and its regulatory control continues throughout the first year of life, and the horse is considered to have adult-like heart rate and cardiovascular parameters at the time of weaning (Driessen 2018). Normal blood pressure values in awake foals and horses are summarized in Table 29.1.

*Emergency Triage of the Horse*, First Edition. Edited by Rolfe M. Radcliffe and Jamie J. Kopper.

Companion website: www.wiley.com/go/radcliffe/triage

**Box 29.1 How the cardiovascular system is like a city water system**

In this analogy, a river supplies water to the city water pump (the heart), which supplies water to a water tower (the aorta). The water tower regulates water delivery to a parallel system of homes (arteries), which subsequently each have a parallel system of pipes (arterioles) that deliver water to faucets (capillaries). The sinks (venules) collect the water and drain into a return system (venules and veins). Thus, the primary components of the system include the blood volume (the water), the heart (the pump), the vascular system (the water tower and the pipe system), and the vascular–tissue interface (water emerging from the faucet) (Swain 2000). Maximum system efficiency and tissue perfusion require each component to function normally. A problem with any component will lead affect blood (or water) delivery.

**Table 29.1** Heart rate and blood pressure values in normal, awake foals and adult horses.

| Parameter | One to three days | One week | Two weeks | Four to six weeks | Adult |
|---|---|---|---|---|---|
| Heart rate ($min^{-1}$) | 118 +/− 10 | 110 +/− 30 | 103 +/− 21 | 84 +/− 11 | 39 +/− 4 |
| SAP | 137 +/− 31 | — | — | — | 142 +/− 12 |
| DAP | 62 +/− 7 | — | — | — | 99 +/− 11 |
| MAP | 87 +/− 10 | 100 +/− 20 | 100 +/− 11 | 115 +/− 14 | 114 +/− 11 |

DAP, diastolic arterial pressure; MAP, mean arterial pressure; SAP, systolic arterial pressure.
*Source:* Adapted from Driessen 2018.

**Box 29.2 Mean arterial pressure (MAP) and tissue perfusion**

- Mean arterial pressure is an indicator of driving pressure for most tissues.
  - An exception to this is the cardiac tissue, which is reliant upon diastolic pressure for perfusion.
  - Generally, MAP should be maintained above *70 mmHg in adults and 60 mmHg in neonatal foals* to maintain organ perfusion (Hurcombe, 2018).

## Monitoring

- Tissue and organ perfusion is dependent on cardiac output and blood flow (Box 29.2).
- Because of the direct relationship between MAP, CO, and SVR, if SVR is increased, MAP may be normal or increased, but the CO will be reduced (Giguère et al. 2005; Olsen et al. 2016).
  - Thus, *blood pressure may not always directly correlate with CO and tissue perfusion.*
  - However, due to available monitoring techniques, blood pressure is often used as a surrogate (Hurcombe 2018).
- Pulse pressure is the difference between systolic arterial pressure (SAP) and diastolic arterial pressure (DAP).
- MAP can be calculated or determined graphically as the integration of the area under the pressure waveform divided by the duration of the cardiac cycle.
- Blood pressure monitoring can be performed using non-invasive or invasive techniques.
  - Non-invasive techniques include oscillometric or doppler methods.
  - Invasive blood pressure monitoring involves catheterization of a central or peripheral artery and subsequent measurement using a transducer.

*Monitoring blood pressure: what can be done on the farm*

- Non-invasive blood pressure monitoring technologies have become more portable and have been validated for use in horses and foals.
  - It is best practice to use a device that has been validated in the species and context for which you are using it.
- Multiparameter and single measurement blood pressure monitoring devices are commercially available.
- These techniques utilize the principles of oscillometric analysis.
- The selection of an *appropriately sized cuff* is critical for the accuracy of the results, and manufacturer recommendations should be followed (Figure 29.1).

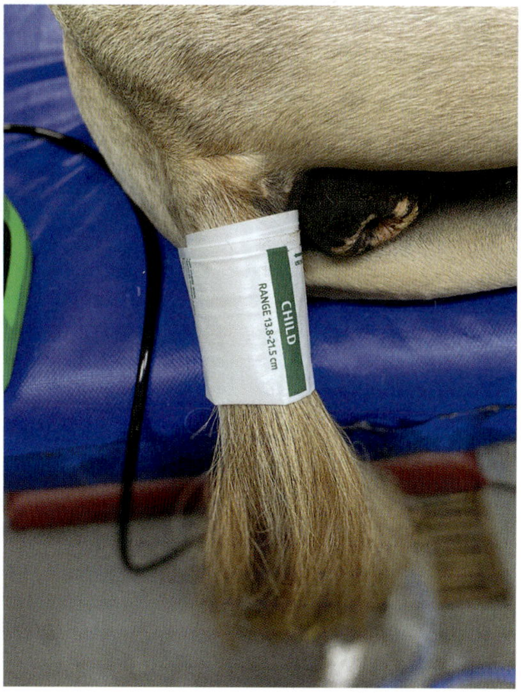


**Figure 29.1** Non-invasive blood pressure cuff placed around the tail base of a recumbent horse. Note the width of the cuff should approximate 40% of the extremity circumference; the range of acceptable extremity circumference (cm) is listed on the cuff.

  - *A cuff width-to-extremity circumference ratio of 40% is recommended* (Haskins 2015).
    - A cuff that is too large will result in incorrectly low values.
    - A cuff that is too small will yield falsely high values.
- The placement of the cuff is also important.
  - It is recommended to place a cuff around the tail base in standing adult horses centered over the middle coccygeal artery.
  - For foals, the cuff can be placed around the tail base, around the metacarpus or metatarsus, or on the antebrachium proximal to the carpus.
- Typically, measurements are obtained in triplicate, and the heart rate given by the device should agree with that measured by cardiac auscultation, pulse palpation, and ECG analysis.
- For improved accuracy in standing horses, readings can be corrected for the distance from the heart base to the base of the tail.
  - A correction factor of 0.77 mmHg/cm vertical distance from the point of the shoulder to the base of the tail can be applied (Parry et al. 1984; Heliczer et al. 2016; Olsen et al. 2016).
- Although non-invasive techniques are not considered to be as accurate as invasive techniques in equids, they are particularly useful for monitoring trends over time.
- Non-invasive monitors are more accurate in foals (Nout et al. 2002; Giguère et al. 2005).

*Monitoring blood pressure: what can be done at the referral hospital*

- Invasive blood pressure monitoring can be offered in referral settings.
  - Although catheterization of a peripheral artery can be performed on a farm, it can be logistically and technically challenging in an un-sedated or un-anesthetized patient and requires specialized equipment (e.g., pressure transducer).
  - Additionally, risks associated with arterial sepsis and thrombosis prevent routine arterial cannulation in the field.
- Invasive blood pressure monitoring is routinely performed for foals and horses undergoing general anesthesia, and it can also be utilized in critical care contexts, particularly for neonates.
- Arterial catheters can be placed in several peripheral locations in horses and foals including the facial artery, transverse facial artery, dorsal metatarsal artery, and auricular artery.
- Procedure:
  - After aseptic preparation of the site, a 22G (foals), 18G or 20G (adults) over-the-needle catheter is placed and secured in the artery.
  - Non-compliant tubing containing heparinized saline is attached to the catheter, ensuring the absence of any air bubbles.
  - A pressure transducer connected to a multiparameter monitor is then used to generate a pressure waveform and numeric values for SAP, DAP, and MAP.

- This pressure waveform not only provides data regarding blood pressure but can also provide information regarding pulse pressure variation, arrhythmias, and beat-to-beat response to therapeutic interventions.

## Disorders and Treatment: Overall Approach

- Essential to the management of blood pressure disorders is the identification of the source of the pressure problem (Boxes 29.3 and 29.4).
- Blood pressure disorders can broadly be categorized into two divisions: *hypotensive and hypertensive conditions*.
  - Hypotensive conditions (MAP < 70 mmHg in adults, <60 mmHg in foals) are more common in equine patients.
  - Hypertension can be defined as situational, secondary, or idiopathic, and in small animals has been defined as a sustained SBP >160–180 mmHg (Acierno et al. 2018). A consensus statement on equine hypertension has not been established.
  - Equine hypertension, due to pain, iatrogenic situations, pheochromocytoma, renal disease, and equine metabolic syndrome has been reported and should be considered (Navas de Solis et al. 2013; Heliczer et al. 2017; Hurcombe 2018).

### Disorders of Fluid Volume: Problems with the Source

*Fluid volume* disorders can be characterized by those resulting from a lack thereof or due to a surplus. Using the water system analogy, the river, or water source, can be low due to drought (dehydration) or uncontrolled loss (hemorrhage). Alternatively, the river can overflow due to excess input from outside sources (fluid overload). In equine patients, volume deficiencies are more common. However, fluid overload conditions can be observed particularly in neonatal foals, miniature horses, and ponies.

*Assessment: what can be done on the farm?*

1) Physical examination: A suspicion of a fluid volume disorder will become clear during the physical examination.
   a) Assessment of hydration status will govern whether the patient is suffering from volume depletion or overload.

**Box 29.3 How to diagnose blood pressure problems in horses and foals**

*Steps*

The first step of the diagnosis and management of a blood pressure disorder is the acquisition of a thorough history.

The second step is the conduction of a thorough physical examination, with a focus on the cardiovascular system.

Key elements include: These components will help to characterize the blood pressure disorder and identify treatment options.

1) Heart rate and rhythm
2) Peripheral pulse quality
3) Jugular fill
4) Capillary refill time
5) Temperature of distal extremities
6) Presence or absence of peripheral edema
7) Mental status

**Box 29.4 What is the source of the pressure problem?**

These disorders can be separated into the four primary hydraulic elements that govern cardiac output and arterial blood pressure (Guyton 1981). There can be overlap of these conditions, with multiple elements affected simultaneously.

1) *blood volume*
2) *heart-pumping capacity*
3) *vascular compliance*
4) *total peripheral resistance*

b) The following physical examination and diagnostic findings may be supportive of volume depletion:
   i) Tachycardia
   ii) Snappy/thready peripheral pulse quality
   iii) Slow capillary refill time (>two seconds)
   iv) Dry mucous membranes
   v) Slow jugular filling
   vi) Cold peripheral extremities
   vii) Elevated peripheral blood lactate (>2 mmol/L)
   viii) Hypotension
   ix) Depressed or agitated mental status
   x) Reduced/absent urination
   xi) Sweating
c) The following physical examination parameters may be supportive of volume overload:
   i) Tachypnea
   ii) Harsh bronchovesicular sounds
   iii) Foamy nasal discharge
   iv) Peripheral edema
2) Stall-side hematologic diagnostics
   a) Hand-held lactate meter
      i) Peripheral blood lactate values greater than 2.0 mmol/L suggest possible volume deficit.
   b) iSTAT
      i) Portable iSTAT results may indicate hemoconcentration.
   c) These stall-side hematologic assessments can be used during initial assessment and following response to therapy.
3) Non-invasive blood pressure analysis can be performed to obtain baseline values and to monitor trends.

*Assessment: what can be done at the referral hospital*

At the referral hospital, fluid volume status can be further assessed using diagnostic imaging and hematologic techniques.

1) Echocardiography: Echocardiography can be used to assess cardiac chamber filling and size. Echocardiographic techniques for fluid volume assessment are more commonly being employed. With continued development of advanced, portable ultrasound technologies, the use of echocardiography for the diagnosis and monitoring of volume status disorders will expand into field settings.
2) Central venous catheterization can also be used to monitor fluid volume status.
3) Serial hematologic evaluations can be performed to assess volume status and response to interventions.

*Treatment: what can be done at the farm*
*Volume deficiencies*

1) The treatment of volume deficiencies with replacement of fluid volume is the mainstay of therapeutic intervention.
2) Generally, in conditions of volume depletion, fluid therapy should be instituted early, and the response to fluid administration (goal-directed fluid therapy) should be frequently assessed.
3) In conditions of uncontrolled hemorrhage with ongoing blood loss, conservative fluid therapy may be instituted initially (permissive hypotension) until the hemorrhage has ceased to prevent clot disruption and dilution of coagulation factors.
4) Readers are referred to Chapter 28, *Fluid therapy for horses and foals*, for specific recommendations.
5) If continued or specific fluid support is required, the patient should be referred for continued care.

*Volume overload*

1) The treatment of volume overload conditions can be challenging.
2) Diuretic administration (furosemide) can be performed at the farm.
   a) Furosemide: Typically, a dose of 0.5–1 mg/kg IV of furosemide will be administered IV in acute cases of fluid overload with secondary pulmonary edema.
   b) Monitoring the response to treatment should be performed, and urination should be observed after administration of the diuretic.

*Treatment: what can be done at the referral hospital*

The treatment of blood volume disorders at the referral hospital can involve specific fluid or blood product administration based on the results of hematologic testing.

## Pump Disorder: Failure to Pump

Blood pressure issues can also be caused by *pump failure*. If the city water pump fails, water cannot reach the pipes and individual homes. Reduced cardiac contractility may be due to anatomic or functional cardiac disorders.

*Assessment: what can be done on the farm*

1) Historical information that may suggest a primary cardiac etiology leading to a secondary blood pressure disturbance include:
   a) Exercise intolerance
   b) Fatigue
   c) Vague signs of abdominal discomfort
2) Physical examination features that may indicate inefficient or inappropriate cardiac contractility include:
   a) Pronounced abnormal or new murmur
      i) It is important to remember that physiologic murmurs can be auscultated in foals. A murmur associated with a patent ductus arteriosus can be auscultated for approximately three days after birth.
   b) Abnormal cardiac rhythm
   c) Pronounced jugular pulses
   d) Bounding peripheral pulses
   e) Peripheral edema
   f) Cyanotic mucous membranes
   g) Agitation
3) Diagnostics
   a) Cardiac auscultation: A thorough cardiac auscultation should be performed. Attention should be paid to peripheral pulse quality and synchrony with heart sounds.
   b) Electrocardiography: Portable electrocardiography (ECG) technology continues to evolve.
      i) Inexpensive, portable modalities exist, and should be incorporated into field practice.
      ii) Stall-side ECG analysis should be performed anytime cardiac auscultation is abnormal or whenever a cardiac disturbance is suspected.
      iii) For continuous ECG monitoring, telemetry can be considered. Holter monitors can be rented, with ECG analysis completed by specialists.
   c) Echocardiography: Tablet or mobile ultrasonographic devices are becoming integrated into daily practice. Point-of-care ultrasound technology is useful to assess pericardial effusion, pleural effusion, and abdominal effusion, and it can be used to provide a subjective assessment of cardiac chamber size and contractility.
   d) Hematologic analysis: In cases of cardiac arrhythmia, it is useful to procure serum or plasma electrolyte values. Of particular importance to cardiac function, *potassium, calcium, and magnesium* values should be determined.

*Assessment: what can be done at the referral hospital*

Referral to an internal medicine specialist is recommended for the evaluation and treatment of complex primary cardiac conditions. At the referral hospital, further diagnostics can be offered to determine the underlying cardiac etiology.

1) Electrocardiography
   a) Multi-lead ECG analysis can be performed to further characterize a dysrhythmia.
   b) Continuous ECG analysis using telemetry is particularly important for diagnosis and monitoring response to therapeutic interventions.
2) Echocardiography
   a) A comprehensive exam can be performed to evaluate the structural cardiac components.
   b) Repeat echocardiograms can assess disease progression and response to therapy.

3) Hematologic analysis
   a) Comprehensive hematologic and serum biochemistry analyses can be repeated to monitor disease progression or response to therapy.
   b) Cardiac troponin values can also be used to evaluate and estimate prognosis for cardiac disease.

*Treatment: what can be done on the farm*

1) Identify heart rate
2) Identify arrythmia if present
   a) Is arrythmia atrial or ventricular in origin?
   b) Is there a bradyarrhythmia or tachyarrhythmia?
   c) Is the brady- or tachy-arrhythmia causing the clinical signs?
      i) If yes: proceed as described below
3) Treatment of bradyarrhythmias:
   a) Second-degree AV block is a common equine arrhythmia.
   b) Myocarditis leading to third-degree AV block has been documented in horses (Luethy et al. 2017).
   c) If the ventricular rate falls below 20 beats/min, treatment may be indicated.
      i) Ideally, obtain a blood pressure.
         - If the mean arterial blood pressure is high, bradycardia is likely reflexive and secondary to the peripheral vasoconstriction.
         - If mean arterial blood pressure is normal or low, vagal influence may be predominant.
      ii) Identify whether the bradyarrhythmia is secondary to drug administration (e.g., alpha-2 agonist administration).
         - It is counter-indicated to administer a vagolytic in the face of recent alpha-2 agonist administration. With recent administration of an alpha-2 agonist, the initial vasoconstrictive effects of the alpha-2 agonist can cause a reflex bradycardia. If a vagolytic is subsequently administered, there is increased myocardial work and oxygen demand due to the ongoing peripheral vasoconstriction.
         - Foals less than 30 days of age are particularly sensitive to the reduction in heart rate and cardiac output caused by the alpha-2 agonists. It is generally recommended to avoid alpha-2 agonist administration in foals less than 30 days of age, particularly in those that are systemically compromised.
         - If alpha-2 agonist reversal is required, an alpha-2 antagonist can be administered. Alpha-2 antagonists are typically administered intramuscularly, as rapid IV injection can cause hypotension and tachycardia.
            - Atipamezole: 0.1 mg/kg IM
            - Tolazoline: 2–4 mg/kg IM
            - Yohimbine: 0.05–0.2 mg/kg IM
      iii) Vagolytics include atropine and glycopyrrolate. In general, horses are sensitive to the vagolytic effects of antimuscarinic agents, and gastrointestinal stasis is a consequence of drug administration.
         - Atropine: 0.01–0.02 mg/kg IV
         - Glycopyrrolate: 0.001–0.005 mg/kg IV or IM
      iv) N-butylscopolamine bromide may also be considered for its vagolytic properties (Loomes 2021).
         - It is considered to have fewer negative gastrointestinal side effects relative to atropine and glycopyrrolate.
         - Dose: 0.05–0.2 mg/kg IV
4) Treatment of tachyarrhythmias
   a) Tachyarrhythmias are broadly subcategorized as supraventricular and ventricular.
   b) Supraventricular arrhythmias are most commonly due to pain, extreme physical activity, or hemodynamic disturbances. Treatment of the primary condition usually converts the rhythm.
   c) If ventricular tachycardia is identified, the following treatments can be considered:
      i) Lidocaine
         - 0.25–0.5 mg/kg slow IV bolus
         - An IV bolus can be given every 3–5 minutes for a total maximum bolus dose of 1.5 mg/kg over 15 minutes.
         - Constant rate infusion (CRI): After intravenous bolus administration, 0.05 mg/kg/min can be administered.
         - Abnormal neurologic and behavioral responses can be seen using lidocaine. If a change in mentation or ataxia is observed, the rate of administration should be slowed.

ii) Magnesium
- 40 mg/kg slowly IV given over 20–30 minutes.
- Typically administered in 1 liter of isotonic fluids.
- Can cause hypotension, particularly if administered rapidly.

5) Referral should generally be recommended in the evaluation and treatment of complex arrhythmias.

*Treatment: what can be done at the referral hospital*

Advanced therapeutic options are available for the treatment of primary cardiac disturbances in the referral hospital setting.

1) Administration of anti-arrhythmic agents
   a) With continuous ECG monitoring and after thorough diagnostic evaluation, advanced anti-arrhythmic therapy may be provided. Therapeutics offered in a referral hospital setting include, but are not limited to, amiodarone, esmolol, procainamide, diltiazem, digoxin, and quinidine.
2) Electrical cardioversion
3) Treatment of bacterial endocarditis or myocarditis
   a) Vegetative valvular lesions may require prolonged hospitalization and treatment with intravenous antimicrobials.

## Disorders of Vascular Tone: Plumbing Problems

Blood vessels are dynamic, and they constantly adjust their characteristics, *vascular tone*, to meet the demands of the tissue beds to which they are subservient. The vascular tree, with its arterial and venous arms, acts as the pipes which carry blood from the heart (the water tower) to the capillary beds (faucet). Under conditions of vasodilation, such as that which can occur with sepsis, lack of vasomotor tone prevents effective delivery of nutrients and removal of waste products. Conditions of excessive vasoconstriction can also influence oxygen delivery, leading to tissue ischemia and necrosis. Conditions of low blood pressure (hypotensive conditions) are more common in adult horses and foals than those of high blood pressure (hypertension). For neonates, particularly those that are premature and/or critically ill, reversion to fetal circulation and persistent pulmonary hypertension of the newborn must always be considered (see Chapter 20, *Foal emergencies*).

*Assessment: what can be done on the farm*

1) Physical exam: Specific elements
   a) Peripheral pulse quality
   b) Temperature of peripheral extremities (e.g., ears, distal limbs)
   c) Jugular refill time
   d) Heart rate
   e) Character of mucous membranes
      i) Are mucous membranes hyperemic and injected?
      ii) Are mucous membranes white and blanched?
2) Non-invasive blood pressure (NIBP) monitoring
   a) As described above, small, portable NIBP monitoring devices are becoming commonplace.
   b) Measurements should be repeated in triplicate, with particular note to trends over time and response to therapeutic interventions.

*Assessment: what can be done at the referral hospital*

1) Invasive blood pressure (IBP) monitoring
   a) IBP monitoring is considered to be standard-of-care for equine patients under general anesthesia.
   b) IBP monitoring is challenging in non-anesthetized horses but can be considered for recumbent, critical, neonatal foals.
2) Continuous blood pressure monitoring
   a) IBP monitoring provides continuous, beat-to-beat reporting of systolic, diastolic, and mean arterial pressure values.
   b) NIBP devices can be cycled at specific, pre-set intervals to repeat measurements over time.
   c) Sequential values should be recorded so that disease progression and response to treatment can be tracked and evaluated.

*Treatment: what can be done on the farm for hypotension*

If abnormal blood pressure has been identified, treatment can be instituted immediately to decrease end-organ damage.

1) Ensure fluid volume has been restored
   a) It is imperative to assess fluid volume status in the assessment of hypotension.
   b) The treatment of hypovolemia should be instituted immediately upon diagnosis with the placement of an intravenous catheter and initiation of fluid therapy.
   c) Hypertonic saline (7.2%) (2–4 mL/kg) can be administered rapidly and conveniently in field settings.
      i) Hypertonic saline has been demonstrated to increase SAP and MAP in anesthetized horses (Schnuelle et al. 2020).
      ii) Hypertonic saline administration should be followed by the administration of isotonic fluids.
   d) Refer to Chapter 28, Fluid therapy for horses and foals, for an in-depth discussion of fluid therapy.
2) Ephedrine
   a) Ephedrine is an indirect and direct sympathomimetic.
   b) Convenient administration by rapid IV bolus injection.
      i) The half-life and duration of action is longer than that of other vasoactive agents.
   c) Dose of Ephedrine:
      i) 0.05–0.1 mg/kg IV bolus
      ii) A second dose (0.05–0.1 mg/kg) can be administered if clinical effect not observed initially.
   d) Ephedrine demonstrates the phenomenon of tachyphylaxis.
      i) The indirect mechanism of action requires endogenous stores of norepinephrine. If reserves are depleted from repeated dosing and mobilization of supply, clinical effects may not be observed.
   e) In severely compromised animals with depletion of adrenal reserves, a clinical effect may not be observed.
      i) Catecholamine-depleted animals may not mount a clinical response to the administration of ephedrine because of the indirect mechanism of action.
   f) Caution should be employed when administering ephedrine to patients with pre-existing tachycardia.
      i) Tachycardia can worsen with ephedrine administration.
3) Parenteral calcium salts
   a) Calcium is important for effective skeletal and smooth muscle function.
   b) Conflicting results regarding the cardiovascular effects of exogenous calcium supplementation on blood pressure are reported (Schauvliege and Gasthuys 2013).
   c) Particularly in cases with low ionized plasma calcium or for cases under general anesthesia, calcium supplementation should be considered for blood pressure support.
   d) Dose:
      i) 23% calcium gluconate: 0.1–1 mL/kg diluted in fluids slowly IV
   e) Caution:
      i) Calcium gluconate can precipitate with co-administered medications. Drug incompatibility should always be assessed with co-administration.
      ii) Rapid intravenous administration can lead to hypotension, arrhythmias, and cardiac arrest.

*Treatment: what can be done at the referral hospital for hypotension*

1) Inotrope and vasopressor administration
   a) The administration of constant rate infusions (CRIs) of vasoactive agents is appropriate in referral settings.
   b) Although they can be administered as a bolus, vasoactive agents typically have a short duration of action and are best administered as a CRI for prolonged efficacy.
   c) Vasoactive agents are discussed below.
      i) Dobutamine
         - Predominant positive inotropic effects due to actions at beta-1 adrenergic receptors.
         - Dobutamine dose: 0.5–5 μg/kg/min
      ii) Phenylephrine
         - Vasopressor effects due to selective alpha-1 adrenergic agonist effects.
         - Phenylephrine dose:
           - Bolus: 0.002 mg/kg–0.004 mg/kg IV
           - CRI: 0.1–0.5 μg/kg/min

iii) Norepinephrine
- Vasopressor effects due to strong alpha-1 adrenergic receptor effects.
- Norepinephrine dose:
  - Bolus: 0.0001 mg/kg IV
  - CRI: 0.1–0.5 μg/kg/min

2) Refractory hypotension: Alternative therapies for hypotension that does not resolve with traditional modalities can be considered in referral contexts.
   a) Colloid administration
      i) In contexts requiring oncotic support, colloid administration should be considered.
      ii) The reader is referred to Chapter 28, Fluid therapy for horses and foals, for further recommendations regarding colloid administration.
   b) Vasopressin
      i) Administration typically only considered for refractory cases due to cost.
      ii) Effects due to binding of V1 and V2 receptors leading to water retention at the level of the kidney and vasoconstriction.
      iii) Vasopressin dose:
         - Bolus: 0.1–0.8 U/kg
         - CRI: 0.25–0.5 mU/kg/min

*Treatment: what can be done on the farm for hypertension*

1) Determine the cause of the hypertension.
   a) Once hypertension has been identified, the etiology should be pursued.
   b) As hypertensive disorders are less commonly identified in equine patients, its presence should trigger heightened suspicion of an underlying pathophysiology.
2) Determine if the hypertension requires specific intervention.
   a) Based on the underlying cause of the hypertension (acute pain, chronic pain, equine metabolic syndrome, renal disease), treatment of the underlying condition will contribute to management of the hypertension.
   b) Treatment of the primary condition should be considered prior to specific anti-hypertensive medication administration.
3) Acepromazine
   a) If acute intervention is required in cases of severe hypertension, the vasodilatory effects of acepromazine can be implemented.
   b) Acepromazine's vasodilatory properties are believed to be due to alpha-1 antagonist effects, with a possible central depressive contribution.
   c) Acepromazine dose: 0.01–0.05 mg/kg IV, IM
      i) Doses up to 0.1 mg/kg have been administered IV and IM.

*Treatment: what can be done at the referral hospital for hypertension*

Additional or continued intensive treatments for the underlying disease process can be offered at the referral hospital. For acute or chronic hypertensive conditions associated with pain, additional analgesic strategies can be considered. These include locoregional techniques including epidural analgesia and nerve blocks. Alternative systemic analgesics in the form of CRIs can also be considered (see Chapter 30, Anesthesia in emergency medicine). Chronic hypertension leading to hypertrophic cardiomyopathy in horses has been reported, and horses are typically euthanized due to the severity of the underlying disease (Navas de Solis et al. 2013).

## Disorders of the Vascular–Tissue Interface: Advanced Plumbing Problems

The final contributor to a blood pressure disturbance is due to a problem at the junction between the vessels and tissues, typically at the level of the capillaries – *total peripheral resistance*.

In normal vessels, the endothelium is responsible for local regulation of vascular tone (Chia et al. 2020).

1) Using our ongoing analogy, a leaky faucet will cause increased delivery of water to the sink.
2) A clogged faucet, on the other hand, will prevent effective water delivery.

Endothelial dysfunction is an emerging area of pathophysiology and treatment.

3) Increased capillary permeability, caused by disruption of the glycocalyx, is frequently observed in sepsis.
4) Thromboembolic processes and capillary microthrombi can also be observed in horses and foals leading to end-organ dysfunction.
5) The result of endothelial dysfunction leads to reduced tissue delivery of nutrients, reduced waste removal, and oxidative tissue damage.
6) Endothelial dysfunction may be a component of equine metabolic syndrome and endocrinopathic laminitis (Morgan et al. 2016; Nostell et al. 2019).
7) Endothelial dysfunction can occur simultaneously with coagulopathies.

If end-organ damage is suspected based on physical examination and diagnostic findings, treatment of the underlying disease and supportive care are indicated to treat the blood pressure disturbance.

*Assessment: what can be done on the farm*

1) Physical Exam
   a) Peripheral edema is a hallmark feature of increased capillary permeability.
2) Hematologic testing
   a) Total protein: The total protein may be reduced (<5 g/dL) due to leakage from capillary beds.
   b) Elevated renal values: Endothelial dysfunction can be seen concurrently with renal disease.
3) Indirect blood pressure monitoring: Non-invasive blood pressure monitoring can be used to indicate hypotensive or hypertensive dysfunction.

*Assessment: what can be done at the referral hospital*

1) Echocardiography
   a) Echocardiography can be used to assess ventricular remodeling, which can occur as a compensatory mechanism from chronic hypertension.
   b) Left ventricular remodeling has been documented in ponies with equine metabolic syndrome (Heliczer et al. 2016).
2) Serial blood pressure monitoring
   a) As described above, blood pressure monitoring is best performed repeatedly over time instead of one-off measurements.
   b) Hospitalization facilitates the acquisition and interpretation of serial blood pressure measurements at different timepoints in the chronology of disease and treatment.
3) Endothelial dysfunction testing
   a) Endothelial dysfunction testing has advanced in the context of atherosclerosis and coronary artery disease.
   b) Endothelial testing includes ex vivo and in vitro methods (Chia et al. 2020).
   c) Translation into the veterinary field may be available following identification and application of experimental methodologies.

*Treatment: what can be done on the farm*

The specific treatment of endovascular disorders is limited. However, drugs affecting the microvasculature have emerged, particularly in the context of microthrombi and equine metabolic syndrome.

1) Clopidogrel
   a) Clopidogrel reduces platelet aggregation.
   b) Clopidogrel can be a useful therapeutic in coagulopathic horses with hypercoagulable tendencies due to platelet activation.
   c) Clopidogrel dose:
      i) Loading dose: 4–6.5 mg/kg PO once
      ii) Maintenance: 2–4 mg/kg PO once daily
2) Pentoxifylline
   a) Pentoxifylline has been used in the treatment of a variety of allergic and immune-mediated conditions.
   b) It has been shown to reduce reactive oxygen and nitrogen species in horses with recurrent airway obstruction (Venugopal et al. 2013).
   c) Pentoxyifylline dose:
      i) 10 mg/kg PO every 12 h

*Treatment: what can be done at the referral hospital*

For cases of significant endovascular dysfunction leading to severe systemic compromise (e.g., sepsis leading to hypotension, peripheral edema, and coagulopathy), rapid referral for treatment is recommended. A multi-pronged approach will be taken to treat the underlying etiology to maximize tissue perfusion and case outcome.

**Case Example 29.1 Emergency Condition – Hypotension in the Field**

*Patient: 8-year-old Thoroughbred mare (500 kg) with her newborn foal (50 kg).*

*History: The mare foaled without complications 48 h prior to presentation when the owners found the mare recumbent with her foal in her stall in the morning* (Figure 29.2). *Both the mare and foal were observed to be acting normally the night before presentation. They were both lying quietly in lateral recumbency during the examination.*

*Emergency triage steps*

*Step 1: patient stabilization*

1) Conduct a thorough physical examination of both the mare and foal with a particular focus on:
   a) Heart rate and rhythm
   b) Peripheral pulse quality
   c) Jugular fill
   d) Capillary refill time
   e) Temperature of the distal extremities
   f) Presence or absence of peripheral edema
   g) Mental status

*Results*: Mare: Examination reveals a heart rate of 80 beats/min, with an irregular rhythm and weak pulse quality. Jugular fill and capillary refill time are prolonged, and the ears are cold. The mucous membranes are dry and pale. There is no evidence of peripheral edema. The mare has moderate abdominal distention and appears to have been rolling. Now she is anxious but does not want to stand during examination.

Foal: Examination of the foal reveals a heart rate of 200 beats/min also with poor pulse quality and cold extremities. The mucous membranes are pale white with a prolonged capillary refill time. The foal has some superficial abrasions over the left caudal abdomen and evidence of abdominal enlargement.

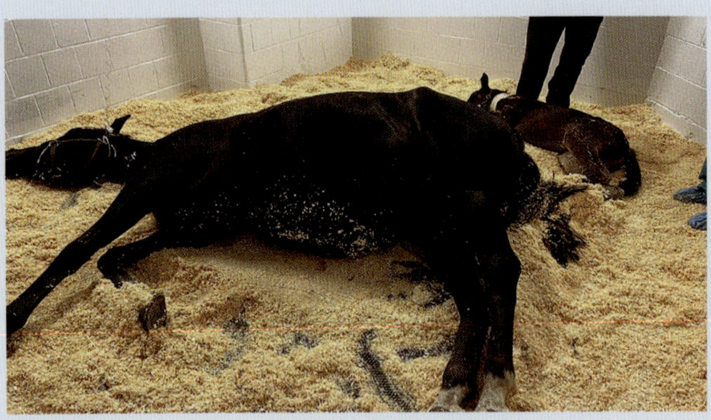

**Figure 29.2** An 8-year-old Thoroughbred mare with her newborn foal found down in her stall. The mare was anxious and depressed, weak, unable to stand, and markedly hypotensive on clinical evaluation. The foal was also hypotensive with evidence of hemorrhagic shock. Aggressive fluid resuscitation stabilized the mare and foal, allowing both to stand for referral and additional diagnostics, possible surgery, and continued supportive treatment. *Source:* Courtesy of Dr. Katharyn Mitchell.

*Step 2: formulating a diagnostic plan*

1) Point-of-care ultrasound is used to examine the thoracic and abdominal cavities of both the mare and foal.
2) A portable electrocardiogram is also performed, and a non-invasive blood pressure is determined by placing a cuff around the base of the tail. The non-invasive blood pressure measurements are repeated three times. A blood sample is obtained for point-of-care blood work, including L-lactate measurement.

*Results:* Mare: The abbreviated ultrasonographic evaluation reveals increased colon wall thickness along ventral midline and abdominal anechoic effusion. The electrocardiogram reveals a sinus tachycardia with intermittent ventricular premature complexes. The non-invasive blood pressure values yielded mean arterial pressures of 65, 68, and 64 mmHg. Peripheral venous L-lactate is 7.4 mmol/L.

Foal: Ultrasound examination of the foal reveals large amounts of swirling free hyperechoic fluid within the abdominal cavity, suggestive of hemoabdomen. The electrocardiogram reveals a sinus tachycardia, and the non-invasive mean arterial blood pressure readings are 60, 58, and 68 mmHg. The foal's PCV is 26%, TP 5.2 g/dL, creatinine 3.7 mg/dL, pH 7.21 (venous), PvO2 31, and sat vO2 46%. Peripheral venous L-lactate is 14.5 mmol/L.

*Step 3: emergency treatment guidelines*

Mare emergency triage:

The mare has evidence of hypovolemia likely secondary to gastrointestinal disease.

1) A 14G intravenous catheter is placed in the jugular vein for drug and fluid administration.
2) Two liters of 7.2% hypertonic saline solution are administered.
3) Following the administration of hypertonic saline solution, ten liters of isotonic intravenous fluids (Plasma-Lyte) are administered as a bolus during the continued evaluation.

Foal emergency triage:

The foal has evidence of hemorrhagic shock of unknown etiology.

4) A 14G over-the-wire intravenous catheter is placed in the jugular vein for drug and fluid administration.
5) One liter of isotonic crystalloid solution and 1 liter of plasma is administered prior to a whole blood transfusion of 3 liters collected from the mare.
6) Aminocaproic acid is also administered to help stabilize clot formation.

*Step 4: assessment and monitoring*

1) Frequent reassessment of the mare and foal's cardiovascular parameters and mentation is performed during your continued evaluation.
2) After the hypertonic saline and isotonic fluid therapy, the mare moves from lateral to sternal recumbency, and her attitude appears improved. The foal also improves following fluid, plasma, and whole blood resuscitation.
3) The heart rate of the mare and foal decreases to 48 and 160 beats/min, respectively. Repeated tail cuff blood pressure measurements yield mean arterial pressure values of 70, 73, and 71 mmHg and 64, 70, and 68 mmHg, for the mare and foal, respectively.
4) The etiology of the hypotension is suspected to be related to large intestinal colic in the mare and hemorrhage following renal trauma in the foal.
5) Due to the initial improvement of the mare with intravenous fluid therapy, 0.05 mg/kg ephedrine is administered intravenously as a vasoactive agent for additional blood pressure support.
6) After emergency triage and stabilization, the mare and foal stand and are transported to an equine referral hospital for further evaluation.

*Step 5: decision making during triage*

1) As the treatment of hypotension on the farm can be limited by resources, personnel, and logistics, techniques are implemented to stabilize the patient while simultaneously determining the etiology.
2) The determination of the etiology causing hypotension may not always be possible in field contexts.
3) After initial stabilization, many cases of hypotension require continued intensive supportive care.
4) Thus, after initial stabilization and assessment, referral for diagnostics and continued therapy is recommended.

*Case example outcome*:

Because of the severity of the condition of the mare and foal, both were referred for continued fluid management, further diagnostics and possible surgery. The foal required emergency surgery and left nephrectomy to prevent continued abdominal hemorrhage associated with renal trauma (the foal was likely injured by the thrashing colicky mare) (Figure 29.3). Following surgery in the foal, and because of recurrent abdominal pain unresponsive to analgesics and progressive abdominal distention, the mare also received emergency colic surgery for correction of a large colon volvulus. Both the mare and foal recovered without complications (Figure 29.4).

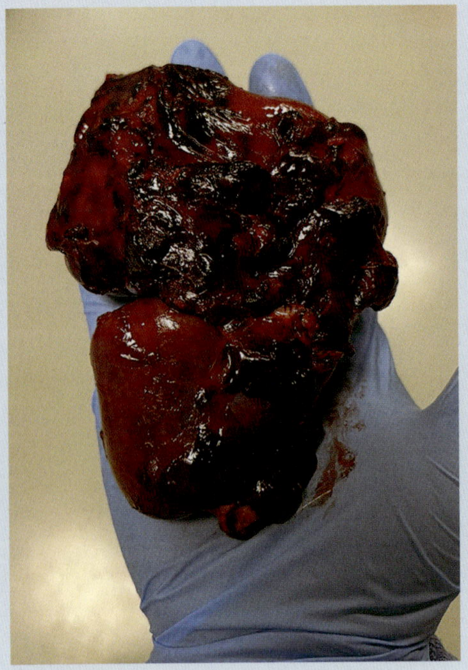

**Figure 29.3** The left kidney of the foal following nephrectomy associated with renal trauma and progressive hemorrhage likely secondary to injury from the colicky mare. *Source:* Courtesy of Dr. Katharyn Mitchell.

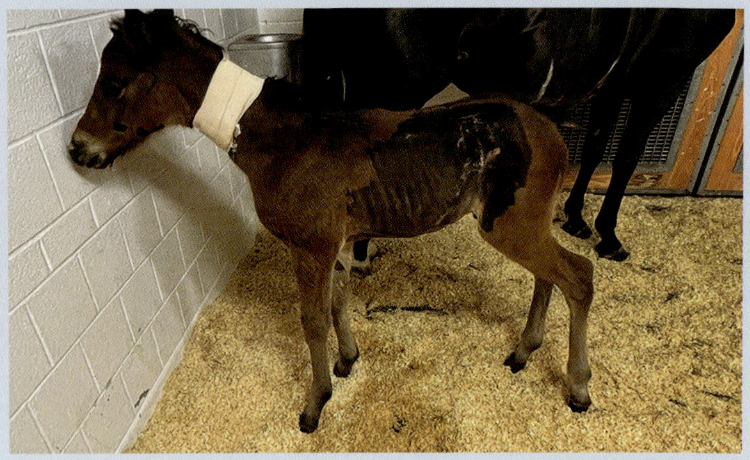

**Figure 29.4** The foal and mare following surgery for left nephrectomy and large colon volvulus, respectively. Both patients recovered following surgery and continued medical management. *Source:* Courtesy of Dr. Katharyn Mitchell.

## References


Acierno, M.J., Brown, S., Coleman, A.E. et al. (2018). ACVIM consensus statement: Guidelines for the identification, evaluation, and management of systemic hypertension in dogs and cats. *J. Vet. Intern. Med.* 32 (6): 1803–1822.

Chia, P.Y., Teo, A., and Yeo, T.W. (2020). Overview of the assessment of endothelial function in humans. *Front. Med.* 7: 542567. https://doi.org/10.3389/fmed.2020.542567.

Driessen, B. (2018). Anesthesia and analgesia for foals. In: *Equine Surgery* (ed. J. Auer, J. Stick, J. Kummerle, and T. Prange), 313–332. St. Louis, MO: Elsevier.

Fowden, A.L. and Silver, M. (1995). Comparative development of the pituitary-adrenal axis in the fetal foal and lamb. *Reprod. Domest. Anim.* 30 (4): 170–177.

Fowden, A.L., Giussani, D.A., and Forhead, A.J. (2020). Physiological development of the equine fetus during late gestation. *Equine Vet. J.* 52 (2): 165–173.

Siguère, S., Knowles, H.A., Valverde, A. et al. (2005). Accuracy of indirect measurement of blood pressure in neonatal foals. *J. Vet. Intern. Med.* 19 (4): 571–576.

Guyton, A.C. (1981). The relationship of cardiac output and arterial pressure control. *Circulation* 64 (6): 1079–1088.

Hall, J.E. (2016). *Guyton and Hall Textbook of Medical Physiology*, 13e. Philadelphia, PA: Elsevier.

Haskins, S. (2015). Monitoring anesthetized patients. In: *Veterinary Anesthesia and Analgesia* (ed. K. Grimm, L. Lamont, W. Tranquilli, et al.), 86–113. Ames, IA: Wiley.

Heliczer, N., Lorello, O., Casoni, D., and Navas de Solis, C. (2016). Accuracy and precision of noninvasive blood pressure in normo-, hyper-, and hypotensive standing and anesthetized adult horses. *J. Vet. Intern. Med.* 30 (3): 866–872.

Heliczer, N., Gerber, V., Bruckmaier, R. et al. (2017). Cardiovascular findings in ponies with equine metabolic syndrome. *J. Am. Vet. Med. Assoc.* 250 (9): 1027–1035.

Hurcombe, S.D. (2018). Chapter 4 – critical care. In: *Equine Internal Medicine*, 4e (ed. S.M. Reed, W.M. Bayly, D.C. Sellon, and W.B. Saunders), 158–190. St. Louis, MO.

Loomes, K. (2021). The use of hyoscine N-butylbromide to treat intraoperative bradycardia during isoflurane anaesthesia in three horses. *Equine Vet. Educ.* 33 (5): e113–e119.

Luethy, D., Slack, J., Kraus, M.S. et al. (2017). *Third-Degree Atrioventricular Block and Collapse Associated with Eosinophilic Myocarditis in a Horse*. Wiley.

Morgan, R.A., Keen, J.A., Walker, B.R., and Hadoke, P.W.F. (2016). *Vascular Dysfunction in Horses with Endocrinopathic Laminitis*. Public Library of Science (PLoS).

Navas de Solis, C., Slack, J., Boston, R.C., and Reef, V.B. (2013). Hypertensive cardiomyopathy in horses: 5 cases (1995-2011). *J. Am. Vet. Med. Assoc.* 243 (1): 126–130.

Nostell, K., Lindåse, S., Edberg, H., and Bröjer, J. (2019). The effect of insulin infusion on heart rate and systemic blood pressure in horses with equine metabolic syndrome. *Equine Vet. J.* 51 (6): 733–737.

Nout, Y.S., Corley, K.T.T., Donaldson, L.L., and Furr, M.O. (2002). Indirect oscillometric and direct blood pressure measurements in anesthetized and conscious neonatal foals. *J. Vet. Emerg. Crit. Care* 12 (2): 75–80.

O'Connor, S.J., Ousey, J.C., Gardner, D.S. et al. (2006). Development of baroreflex function and hind limb vascular reactivity in the horse fetus. *J. Physiol.* 572 (Pt 1): 155–164.

Olsen, E., Pedersen, T.L.S., Robinson, R., and Haubro Andersen, P. (2016). Accuracy and precision of oscillometric blood pressure in standing conscious horses. *J. Vet. Emerg. Crit. Care* 26 (1): 85–92.

Parry, B.W., McCarthy, M.A., and Anderson, G.A. (1984). Survey of resting blood pressure values in clinically normal horses. *Equine Vet. J.* 16 (1): 53–58.

Schauvliege, S. and Gasthuys, F. (2013). "Drugs for cardiovascular support in anesthetized horses", *The Veterinary Clinics of North America. Equine Pract.* 29 (1): 19–49.

Schnuelle, M., Hopster, K., and Hurcombe, S. (2020). Effects of intravenous administration of 7.2% hypertonic saline on cardiovascular parameters in healthy, anesthetized horses. *Vet. Anaesth. Analg.* 47 (6): 855.e9.

Swain, D.P. (2000). The water-tower analogy of the cardiovascular system. *Adv. Physiol. Educ.* 24 (1): 43–50.

Venugopal, C., Mariappan, N., Holmes, E. et al. (2013). Effect of potential therapeutic agents in reducing oxidative stress in pulmonary tissues of recurrent airway obstruction-affected and clinically healthy horses. *EVJ* 45: 80–84.

Vrancken, S.L., Heijst, A.F.V., and Boode, W.P.D. (2018). Neonatal hemodynamics: from developmental physiology to comprehensive monitoring. *Front. Pediatr.* 6: 87.

Washburn, S.E. and Stewart, R.H. (2020). A plumber's guide to the cardiovascular system. *Adv. Physiol. Educ.* 44 (2): 163–168.

# 30

# Anesthesia in Emergency Medicine

*Klaus Hopster*

*Department of Clinical Studies - New Bolton Center, University of Pennsylvania School of Veterinary Medicine, Kennett Square, PA, USA*

Field anesthesia for emergency situations combines two nightmare situations for the anesthesiologist: anesthetizing a possibly critically ill patient with compromised cardiovascular and/or respiratory function under non-ideal conditions with limited resources and equipment available.

Therefore, good planning, preparation, and willingness to improvise when necessary are key components for success.

The following chapter will lead through a field anesthetic emergency event and emphasis important points and consideration that will hopefully help the reader to improve outcome.

There are many indications for emergent anesthetizing horses in the field, a few of which include:

- Saving the animal from a compromising situation such as being caught in a fence
- Providing treatment to a highly uncooperative patient
- Safely transporting a severely injured or down animal

Therefore, the horse to be anesthetized in the field might be in a condition that is less than ideal for undergoing general anesthesia. It might either be cardiovascularly compromised and/or in shock or very excited, stressed, and/or painful.

## Preparation

"It is always good to be well prepared." This statement has never been truer, particularly for field anesthetic events. And while it might seem that anesthesiologists are sometimes "over-prepared" it is this 1 out 1,000 situations where this "over"-preparedness will make the difference.

Checklists are very helpful to ensure that nothing essential is forgotten, and often small things can make a difference with regards to outcome. Depending on the setting and the number of emergencies seen on a regular basis an emergency anesthesia kit can be either pre-prepared and packed or – which is the case in our hospital – needs to be packed together in emergent field situations where a horse needs to be anesthetized.

The checklist should include (but not limited to) that listed in Box 30.1.

## Assessment

Particularly under emergency situations assessment of the horse and physical examination might be brief but are still essential to optimize outcome and preparedness.

*Emergency Triage of the Horse*, First Edition. Edited by Rolfe M. Radcliffe and Jamie J. Kopper.

Companion website: www.wiley.com/go/radcliffe/triage

**Box 30.1 Emergency anesthesia kit check list**

- Stethoscope
- Pulse oximeter
- Endotracheal tube (different sizes)
  - Typical tube size for 500 kg bwt adult horse 25 mm ID for oral intubation
  - Typical tube size for 250 kg bwt pony 16 mm ID for oral intubation
  - Typical size for 50 kg bwt foal 10 mm ID for oral intubation
  - Mouth gag/ speculum
- Oxygen source
- Intravenous catheter equipment (Part 1, Chapter 4)
  - Scrub material and disinfectant for catheterization site
- Drugs – emergency drugs and anesthetics (Table 30.1 and Appendix 3)

**Table 30.1** Dosage recommendations for sedatives and anesthetics used under emergency field conditions.

| Drug | Typical dose per kg bwt | Total dose per 500 kg bwt Horse severely stressed and nervous | Total dose per 500 kg bwt Horse in cardiovascular shock |
|---|---|---|---|
| Xylazine | 0.4–0.7 mg/kg | up to 500 mg IV | 200 mg IV |
| Detomidine | 4–7 mcg/kg | up to 10 mg IV | 3 mg IV |
| Butorphanol | 0.05–0.1 mg/kg | 50 mg IV | 50 mg IV |
| Morphine | 0.1–0.2 mg/kg | 100 mg IV | 100 mg IV |
| Midazolam[a] | 0.05–0.1 mg/kg | 25 mg IV | 50 mg IV |
| Diazepam[a] | 0.05–0.1 mg/kg | 25 mg IV | 50 mg IV |
| Guaifenesin[a] | 50–75 mg/kg | 25 g IV | 50 g IV |
| Ketamine | 2–3 mg/kg | 1.5 g IV | 1 g IV |
| Tiletamine | 1–1.5 mg/kg | 750 mg IV | 500 mg IV |

[a] in combination with the induction agent.

**Table 30.2** Clinical findings associated with dehydration.

| % | Mentation | Heart rate (bpm) | Mucous membranes | CRT (seconds) | PCV/TPP (%/g/dL) |
|---|---|---|---|---|---|
| <5 | BAR | <44 | WNL | <2 | WNL |
| 6 | BAR | 44–60 | Tachy | 2 | 40/7 |
| 8 | Quiet | 60–80 | Tachy to dry | 3 | 45/7.5 |
| 10 | Dull | 80–100 | Dry | 4 | 50/8 |
| 12 | Moribund | >100 | Dry | >4 | >50/>8 |

BAR, bright, alert, and responsive; bpm, beats per minute; WNL, within normal limits.
*Source:* Modified from Hardy (2009).

The focus needs to be on the cardiovascular status of the horse. The patient should be checked for signs of

- Dehydration, hypovolemia and/or hypotension (Table 30.2)
  - Weak palpable pulse.
  - Prolonged capillary filling.
  - Tachycardia as a response to hypotension and hypovolemia.
- Anemia
  - Pale mucous membranes.
  - Tachycardia in response to reduced oxygen delivery to the periphery.

- Hypoxemia
  - May be difficult to appreciate in an anesthetized horse.
  - Cyanosis may be present.
  - Tachycardia and hypertension due to hypoxia-induced catecholamine release.
  - The horse may be tachypneic or gasping.

## Intravenous (IV) Catheter

Not many things are more important for a safe anesthetic event than reliable venous access.

Therefore, IV catheter placement needs to be high on the list of things to do in preparation for an emergent anesthetic event. In rare cases when the horse is uncooperative or struggling it can be necessary to induce general anesthesia prior to catheter placement, but ideally the order should be opposite.

Intravenous catheters are needed for fluid resuscitation, stabilization as well as the safe and reliable administration of drugs and anesthetics in case of emergent events.

Supplies needed for intravenous catheter placement as described in Box 30.2.

## Stabilization

Induction of general anesthesia results in a decrease in cardiac output, blood pressure, and ventilatory drive. In compromised horses this can increase the risk of fatal complications. Therefore, it is important to (at least attempt) cardiovascular and respiratory stabilization prior to inducing anesthesia.

- Preoxygenation with flow by oxygen
- Intravenous fluids (Table 30.3)
  - Isotonic electrolyte solution
  - Hypertonic saline
- Analgesia: these horses are sometimes uncooperative because of pain; providing good and reliable analgesia will improve outcome.

**Box 30.2 Supplies needed for placement of an intravenous catheter**

- Different size and length catheters
- Extension for safe access
- Injection port
- Suture material and/or super glue to secure the catheter
- Iodine scrub and alcohol
- Heparinized saline flush

**Table 30.3** Fluid therapy to stabilize a patient in shock.

| Fluid type | Volume per kg bwt | Volume per 500 kg bwt |
|---|---|---|
| Isotonic crystalloids, e.g., Lactated Ringer | 20 (−40) mL/kg bwt | 10 (−20) L |
| Hypertonic solutions, e.g., 7.5% NaCl | 3–4 mL/kg bwt | 2 L |
| Colloidal solutions, e.g., Hetastarch | 4–8[a] mL/kg bwt | 2 – 4[a] L |

[a] Daily maximum.

**Box 30.3 Premedication and sedation key points**

- Stabilization of the cardiovascular system with a fluid bolus if possible
- Pre-oxygenation if required (e.g., horse in respiratory distress)
- Avoid acepromazine as it can cause long lasting cardiovascular compromise
- Alpha-2-agonists
  - Detomidine
  - Xylazine

*Induction options*

- Muscle relaxation (e.g., with one these options)
  - Guaifenesin to effect, 50–100 mg/kg IV (Ketelaars et al. 1979; Hubbel et al. 1980; Matthews et al. 1997)
  - Midazolam 0.05–0.1 mg/kg IV
  - Diazepam 0.05–0.1 mg/kg IV
- Induction
  - Ketamine 2–3 mg/kg IV, if cardiovascularly stable
  - Ketamine "to effects," 1–2 mg/kg IV, if in shock (Lin et al. 2015)

## Sedation and Induction

Induction of anesthesia in the field should be safe and rapid. If the plan is to anesthetize the horse for a procedure and recover it afterwards in the field the recovery phase needs to be considered with regards to location and conditions. Ideally it should be of sufficient size, clean, and even flat ground allowing for good control of the horse. Box 30.3 provides premedication and sedation key points.

Provided there is good sedation from xylazine, the combination of xylazine and ketamine hydrochloride as a short-term intravenous anesthetic technique in the horse appears safe and acceptable providing reasonably stable cardiopulmonary function (Muir et al. 1977). But in cardiovascular unstable horses that are catecholamine depleted ketamine has shown to have negative cardiovascular effects (Lin et al. 2015). In these cases, particularly if the horse is weak or recumbent, the authors recommend administration of guaifenesin at a dose of at least 75–100 mg/kg IV prior to induction of anesthesia (Ketelaars et al. 1979; Hubbel et al. 1980; Matthews et al. 1997). The muscle relaxation and central dampening from the guaifenesin allows for using lower and therefore safer dosages of ketamine (Morris et al. 2009).

## Maintenance of Anesthesia

Under field conditions maintenance of anesthesia is most practical using total intravenous anesthesia (TIVA) protocols.

*Advantages to TIVA*

- Easy to use
- Safe
- No anesthesia equipment necessary

*Disadvantages to TIVA*

- Limited controllability
- Prolonged recovery after long anesthetic events

*Example "recipe" for a triple-drip*

| | | |
|---|---|---|
| Xylazine | 500 mg | 10% formulation = **5 mL** |
| Ketamine | 2,000 mg | 10% formulation = **20 mL** |
| Guaifenesin | 25 g | 5% formulation = **500 mL** |

*For a "normal size" horse (approx. 500 kg) should last for 45–60 minutes*

*Example "recipe" for a triple-drip*

| | | |
|---|---|---|
| Detomidine | 10 mg | 10% formulation = **1 mL** |
| Ketamine | 2,000 mg | 10% formulation = **20 mL** |
| Midazolam | 50 mg | 0.5% formulation = **50 mL** |

*Mixed together in a 500 mL Saline bag*
*For a "normal size" horse (approx. 500 kg) should last for 45–60 minutes*

## Pharmacokinetics and Pharmacodynamics in Shocked Patients

Intravenous anesthetics – as almost exclusively used under emergent field conditions – are presumed to exert their ultimate effects by action at some unknown central nervous system site. The speed with which they act here highly depends on the dose/concentration of the drugs administered and perfusion of the effector site (Voss et al. 2007). Theoretically, any drug will work quickly if a large enough bolus dose is administered but the larger the induction bolus dose, the greater the incidence and magnitude of any adverse (hemodynamic) effects.

Thus, rapid onset of action of sedation and induction drugs cannot always be safely achieved. In general, shocked patients manifest a greater hemodynamic and nervous system sensitivity to anesthetic agents. While many clinicians intuitively reduce induction agent doses in shock to reduce adverse effects, induction time and quality can be altered, often as a consequence of dose reduction. However, a "blood–brain circuit" often exists in shocked patients which paradoxically delivers the required concentration. Furthermore, many anesthetic agents exhibit high protein binding and in severe hypovolemic shock, especially after fluid resuscitation, the non-protein bound, free fraction of drug is increased which achieves high, effective concentrations despite reduced dose and increases adverse hemodynamic effects of the drug even more. Therefore, in hemodynamically compromised patients there are complex pharmacokinetic and dynamic interactions, which can increase or decrease the efficacy and adverse effects of intravenous anesthetic agents. Predicting the response (i.e., underdosing and awareness vs hemodynamic collapse) in any one patient is challenging, which favors agents being administered to effect at a minimal dose possible.

## Airway/Intubation

A safe and secure airway is essential for the anesthetic outcome. Tracheal intubation might not always be required particularly for short events under injectable anesthesia but – as mentioned earlier – being prepared will save you from most adverse events.

When intubating a horse under hectic and non-ideal situations rapid protection of the airway is more important than a large inner diameter of the tracheal tube. Further, it is often easier and faster to place a naso-tracheal tube as it does not require a rinsing and cleaning of the mouth (to prevent tracheal contamination) nor a mouth gag or other device to keep the mouth open.

- Nasal vs oral intubation – nasal often easier, faster, and safer
- Smaller inner diameter makes intubation easier
- Secure the tube to the halter to prevent displacement

## Ventilation

Ventilation can be challenging under field conditions but becomes necessary in emergency situations particularly in horses with reduced respiratory function.

A reliable way to ensure ventilation of horses is using an Equine Demand Valve, a compact oxygen demand valve for equine applications. The valve is connected to an oxygen tank and provides fast and easy emergency oxygen delivery. It uses a standard 50 PSI oxygen source to provide 160 L/min oxygen flow at the push of a button or at the demand of the horse. A simpler and easier alternative is the Vienna Equine Field Ventilator. Anesthesiologists at the University of Veterinary Medicine, Vienna, have developed an inexpensive device for the ventilation of large animals. They modified a commercial

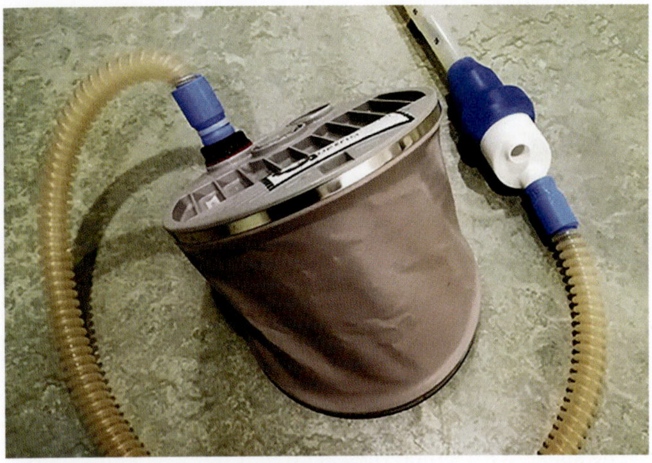

**Figure 30.1** Vienna equine field ventilator. An inexpensive 2.5 L foot pump (developed by anesthesiologists at the University of Veterinary Medicine, Vienna) enables the practitioner to provide intermittent positive pressure ventilation (IPPV) to large animals in emergency situations. *Source:* Courtesy of Dr. Schrammel.

**Box 30.4 Ventilation key points**

- Intubation is necessary
- An Oxygen source is required
- Ventilator needed
- Tidal volume ideally between 8 and 10 mL/kg bwt
- A Respiratory rate should be provided of 2–4 breaths/min

foot pump for emergency ventilation of horses. This 2.5 L foot pump, initially intended for the inflation of recreational items, enables the practitioner to provide intermittent positive pressure ventilation (IPPV) to large animals in emergency situations (Figure 30.1). Box 30.4 provides ventilation key points.

## Recovery

Recovery should be performed in an environment safe for both personnel and the horse.

Depending on the condition of the horse deep sedation and good analgesia may be required.

For example, a horse that got caught in a fence or injured during exercise will require significantly more sedation to overcome the high stress levels, whereas a horse that was exhausted and cardiovascularly compromised prior to general anesthesia might not need any further sedation.

Overall, assisted recovery might be beneficial. The most common form of assistance during recovery is head and tail rope assistance or head rope assistance alone. Head and tail rope assistance endeavors to provide stability and direction to a horse during attempts to stand. One rope attaches to the halter and aims to control the direction of the horse's attempts to stand, while the second rope attached to the tail aims to assist and stabilize the horse during rising. Currently there is conflicting evidence to clarify if the use of head tail rope assistance method leads to fewer complications when compared to unassisted recovery in horses recovering from anesthesia, but a recent study showed that it leads to lesser attempts of the horse to stand up (Arndt et al. 2020).

*Drugs that might be needed for recovery*

- Reversal drugs
  - Atipamezole 0.1 mg/kg IM (to reverse alpha-2 agonists) (Ramseyer et al. 1998)
  - Tolazoline 2–4 mg/kg IM (to reverse alpha-2 agonists) (Kollias-Baker et al. 1993)

- Flumazenil 0.02 mg/kg IV (to reverse benzodiazepines) (Douglas et al. 2021)
- Ephedrine 0.1 mg/kg IV in case of cardiovascular compromise and weakness during recovery (Fantoni et al. 2013)

## Complications

The main complications during general anesthesia involve either the respiratory or the cardiovascular system. Table 30.4 provides drugs and dosages that may be indicated for these patients. The key is to detect and immediate treat and/or prevent these complications:

- Hypoxemia
  - Defined as $PaO_2 < 65$ mmHg and or $SaO_2 < 90\%$
  - Treatment options in the field are limited, and include administration/flow by of oxygen and ventilation
- Hypotension
  - Mean arterial blood pressure lesser 65 mmHg
  - Difficult to measure in the field
  - Alternative indicators for impaired perfusion
    - Clinical assessment
      During circulatory failure cutaneous circulation is deprived of autoregulation, and the sympathetic neurohumoral response predominates, resulting in a decrease in skin perfusion and temperature in these conditions.
    - Capillary refill time (CRT)
      CRT has been validated as a measure of peripheral perfusion with significant variation. Several clinical studies have reported a poor correlation between CRT, heart rate, blood pressure, and cardiac output. However, prolonged CRT has been found to be a good predictor of dehydration and increased blood lactate levels.
    - Skin temperature
      Distal extremity skin temperature has also been related to the adequacy of the circulation. Patients with cold periphery (including septic patients) had lower cardiac output and higher blood lactate levels as a marker of more severe tissue hypoxia. In another the presence of a cold and clammy skin was a predictor of 30-day mortality in patients with cardiogenic shock complicating acute myocardial infarction.
  - Treatment
    - Fluid resuscitation
    - Catecholamines such as ephedrine, 0.1 mg/kg IV as a bolus (Fantoni et al. 2013)
- Bradycardia
  - It is recommended that bradycardia (HR <20 beats/min) in association with hypotension warrants treatment
  - Atropine 0.01 mg/kg IV bolus (Pimenta et al. 2011)
  - Glycopyrrolate 0.005 mg/kg IV bolus
  - Butylscopolamine/ butylbromide, 0.05–0.1 mg/kg IV bolus (Pimenta et al. 2011)

**Table 30.4** Dosage recommendations for rescue drugs used as single bolus under emergency field conditions.

| Drug | Indication | Dosage | Total dose per 500 kg bwt |
|---|---|---|---|
| Atropine | Bradycardia | 0.01 mg/kg IV | 5 mg IV |
| Butylscopolamine | Bradycardia | 0.05–0.1 mg/kg IV | 25 mg IV |
| Ephedrine | Hypotension | 0.1 mg/kg IV | 50 mg IV |
| Epinephrine | Severe hypotension/cardiac arrest | 0.01 mg/kg IV | 5–10 mg IV |
| Atipamezole | Reversal of alpha-2 sedation | 0.1 mg/kg IM | 50 mg IM |
| Tolazoline | Reversal of alpha-2 sedation | 2–4 mg/kg IM | 1 g IM |
| Flumazenil | Reversal of benzodiazepine muscle relaxation | 0.02 mg/kg IV | 5 mg IV |

**Case Example 30.1 Emergency Field Anesthesia**

*Field anesthesia for emergency problems*

You get called to a six-year-old and approx. 550 kg gelding which was found down in the field this morning. The horse has several distal limb abrasions and a suspect left hind open P1 fracture.

The owner wants further diagnostic and is entertaining the idea of fracture repair if prognosis is good. You decide to transport the horse to the hospital for radiographic evaluation.

Transportation is available and the transport will take approx. 45 minutes.

To reduce the risk for further worsening of the fracture you decide to transport this horse under general anesthesia.

a) What do you do before anesthesia to prepare and stabilize your patient?
- IV catheter placement
- Hypertonic saline, 2 L
- Analgesia, flunixin, or phenylbutazone
- Sedation with xylazine or detomidine
- Remember: Horses that are injured are often exhausted, stressed, excited, and painful

b) What anesthesia protocol do you want to use to keep the horse safely anesthetized for approx. 45–60 minutes?
- Muscle relaxation using infusion of Guaifenesin to effect, approx. 50–100 mg/kg IV
- Induction with Ketamine, 1.5–2 mg/kg IV
- Maintenance using Triple Drip:

| | | |
|---|---|---|
| • Xylazine | • 500 mg | • 10% formulation = **5 mL** |
| • Ketamine | • 2 g | • 10% formulation = **20 mL** |
| • Guaifenesin | • 25 g | • 5% formulation = **500 mL** |
| • This combination should last for 45–60 minutes | | |

- Monitoring
  - Heart rate and respiratory rate
  - Oxygen insufflation during the transport (if available)

## References


Arndt, S., Hopster, K., Sill, V. et al. (2020). Comparison between head-tail-rope assisted and unassisted recoveries in healthy horses undergoing general anesthesia for elective surgeries. *Vet. Surg.* 49 (2): 329–338.

Douglas, H., Hopster, K., Cerullo, M. et al. (2021). The effects of flumazenil on ventilatory and recovery characteristics in horses following midazolam-ketamine induction and isoflurane anaesthesia. *Equine Vet. J.* 53 (6): 1257–1267.

Fantoni, D.T., Marchioni, G.G., Ida, K.K. et al. (2013). Effect of ephedrine and phenylephrine on cardiopulmonary parameters in horses undergoing elective surgery. *Vet. Anaesth. Analg.* 40 (4): 367–374.

Equine AnesthesiaHardy, J. (2009). Chapter 7 - Venous and arterial catheterization and fluid therapy. In: , 2ede (ed. W.W. Muir and J.A.E. Hubbell), 131–148. W.B. Saunders https://doi.org/10.1016/B978-1-4160-2326-5.00007-9.

Hubbell, J.A., Muir, W.W., and Sams, R.A. (1980). Guaifenesin: cardiopulmonary effects and plasma concentrations in horses. *Am. J. Vet. Res.* 41 (11): 1751–1755.

Ketelaars, H.C.J., Van Dieten, J.S.M.M., and Lagerweij, E. (1979). Untersuchung von Guajakolglyzerinather bei Pferden und Ponys. 1. Pharmakokinetik nach einmaliger iv Injektion. Berliner und Munchener tierarztliche Wochenschrift. *Berl. Munch. Tierarztl. Wochenschr.* 92: 211–214.

Kollias-Baker, C.A., Court, M.H., and Williams, L.L. (1993). Influence of yohimbine and tolazoline on the cardiovascular, respiratory, and sedative effects of xylazine in the horse. *J. Vet. Pharmacol. Ther.* 16 (3): 350–358.

Lin, H.C., Passler, T., Wilborn, R.R. et al. (2015). A review of the general pharmacology of ketamine and its clinical use for injectable anaesthesia in horses. *Equine Vet. Educ.* 27 (3): 146–155.

Matthews, N.S., Peck, K.E., Mealey, K.L. et al. (1997). Pharmacokinetics and cardiopulmonary effects of guaifenesin in donkeys. *J. Vet. Pharmacol. Ther.* 20 (6): 442–446.

Morris, C., Perris, A., Klein, J., and Mahoney, P. (2009). Anaesthesia in haemodynamically compromised emergency patients: does ketamine represent the best choice of induction agent? *Anaesthesia 64* (5): 532–539.

Muir, W.W., Skarda, R.T., and Milne, D.W. (1977). Evaluation of xylazine and ketamine hydrochloride for anesthesia in horses. *Am. J. Vet. Res.* 38 (2): 195–201.

Pimenta, E.L.M., Teixeira Neto, F.J., Sá, P.A. et al. (2011). Comparative study between atropine and hyoscine-N-butylbromide for reversal of detomidine induced bradycardia in horses. *Equine Vet. J.* 43 (3): 332–340.

Ramseyer, B., Schmucker, N., Schatzmann, U. et al. (1998). Antagonism of detomidine sedation with atipamezole in horses. *J. Vet. Anaesth.* 25 (1): 47–51;Voss, L.J., Ludbrook, G., Grant, C. et al. (2007). A comparison of pharmacokinetic/ pharmacodynamic versus mass-balance measurement of brain concentrations of intravenous anesthetics in sheep. *Anesth. Analg.* 104: 1440–1446.

# 31

# Antimicrobial Therapy and Anti-inflammatory Medications

*K. Gary Magdesian[1] and Jamie Kopper[2]*

[1] *School of Veterinary Medicine, Department of Medicine and Epidemiology, University of California, Davis, CA, USA*
[2] *Department of Veterinary Clinical Sciences, College of Veterinary Medicine, Iowa State University, Ames, IA, USA*

## Antimicrobial Therapy

Sepsis and endotoxemia are leading causes of critical illness in horses and foals. Sepsis is a state of organ dysfunction, often coupled with hypotension, as a consequence of a dysregulated immune response to infection (Fielding and Magdesian 2015; Barrier 2016). With progression, sepsis or endotoxemia can lead to septic or endotoxic shock, which is defined in human medicine as a state of profound circulatory, cellular and metabolic derangements, with a higher mortality than sepsis (Barrier 2016). Foals with sepsis can develop life-threatening complications, including osteomyelitis, septic physitis or arthritis, and meningitis. Adult horses can develop hypercoagulation with thromboemboli, as well as complications such as laminitis.

Emergency patient stabilization: Sepsis in foals and horses should be treated with a triad of early antimicrobials, hemodynamic support including intravenous fluids, and critical nursing care including nutrition, recumbency care, and oxygen as needed (Fielding and Magdesian 2015; Magdesian 2017). In humans, early antimicrobial administration has been associated with improved outcome in septic patients, and there is a suggestion this may be true in septic foals (Barrier 2016; Theelen et al. 2019).

The initial antimicrobial plan for critically ill horses and foals suspected of sepsis should include bactericidal antimicrobials rather than static drugs, because affected horses are often neutropenic. The intravenous (IV) route is optimal in such patients, in order to bypass muscle (IM) or gut (PO) absorption as peripheral perfusion may be reduced to those tissues, impairing drug absorption. The initiating antimicrobials should be broad spectrum, because both Gram-negative and -positive microbes have commonly been associated with equine sepsis. Table 31.1 lists recommendations for initial, empirical antimicrobials for a variety of critical or serious illnesses and emergency situations in equine practice, when cultures are either not available or are pending.

Prior to the first dose of antimicrobials, a culture should be obtained aseptically whenever possible from the site of suspected sepsis (e.g., blood culture in septic foals, abdominal fluid culture with peritonitis or internal abscess). However, antimicrobials should be administered as early in the course of treatment as possible, and they should not be delayed for the sake of sampling for blood cultures; such delays can lead to adverse consequences such as progression of shock or joint infections (Magdesian 2017). In human medicine the early use of antimicrobials has been associated with increased survival in patients with sepsis, and standard of care now includes early treatment with IV antimicrobials (Puskarich et al. 2011; Magdesian 2017; Barrier 2016).

Pharmacologic considerations for critical care: During critical illness, the core pharmacologic principles of absorption, volume of distribution, clearance, and elimination may be altered. In addition, hypoalbuminemia, liver and kidney dysfunction, and drug interactions are additional considerations for critically ill patients. Hypoproteinemia results in reduced percentage of bound drug to albumin, with a resultant increased free or unbound drug; this free drug is the active form of the antimicrobial. This can result in increased potential for toxicity in the short term, especially for drugs

*Emergency Triage of the Horse*, First Edition. Edited by Rolfe M. Radcliffe and Jamie J. Kopper.

Companion website: www.wiley.com/go/radcliffe/triage

**Table 31.1** Guide to selection of <u>initial</u> antimicrobials for treating specific conditions while awaiting results of culture and susceptibility testing, or when no culture is available.

| Condition | Initial antimicrobial suggestions | Other options | Notes |
|---|---|---|---|
| Neonatal sepsis | Amikacin and ampicillin | • Amikacin and penicillin<br>• Amikacin and ceftiofur<br>• Ceftiofur | *Renal function and urine output should be normal with aminoglycoside use |
| Foal pneumonia | R. equi not suspected<br>Mild: penicillin, ceftiofur or TMS<br>Mod to severe:<br>• Penicillin + ampicillin<br>• Penicillin + penicillin | | |
| | R. equi suspected<br>• Clarithromycin + rifampin<br>• Azithromycin + rifampin | Macrolide Resistant Strains<br>• Doxycycline<br>• Minocycline<br>• Minocycline + Rifampin | Doxycycline and rifampin should not be used together due to risks of hemolysis or liver disease |
| Pneumonia or pleuropneumonia in adult | • Penicillin + gentamicin<br>• Ampicillin + gentamicin +Metronidazole if pleuropneumonia present | Enrofloxacin can replace gentamicin, paired with penicillin or ampicillin, if azotemia present<br>Ceftiofur + metronidazole | Inhalational therapy can be used as adjunctive treatment, using ceftiofur, gentamicin, or enrofloxacin depending on culture and susceptibility results |
| Septic peritonitis-primary | • Penicillin + gentamicin<br>• Ampicillin + gentamicin<br>• Ceftiofur | • Enrofloxacin can replace gentamicin along with penicillin or ampicillin, especially if azotemia present or when *Corynebacterium* suspected | *Actinobacillus, Streptococcal, Corynebacterium pseudotuberculosis* |
| Septic peritonitis-secondary | Same as primary, but metronidazole added | | Secondary to GI breach, foreign body, GI surgery, uterine compromise |
| Intra-abdominal abscess, primary | • Penicillin + rifampin<br>• Ampicillin + rifampin<br>• TMS + rifampin if stable<br>• (Enrofloxacin ± rifampin or TMS + rifampin, if *Corynebacterium* suspected) | • Penicillin + gentamicin<br>• Doxycycline or minocycline pending culture or titers | *Streptococcus equi ss equi*<br>*Streptococcus equi ss zooepidemicus*<br>*Actinobacillus*<br>*Corynebacterium* |
| Intra-abdominal abscess, secondary | Same as secondary septic peritonitis | | Secondary to GI breach, foreign body, GI surgery, uterine compromise |
| Cholangiohepatitis | • Enrofloxacin + penicillin<br>• Enrofloxacin + ampicillin<br>• Ceftiofur<br>• TMS + metronidazole | • Penicillin + gentamicin<br>• Ampicillin + gentamicin | • Metronidazole if gas present on ultrasound or if poor initial response |
| Septic arthritis/ osteomyelitis: foal | Neonate: As for neonatal sepsis above<br>Three weeks and older:<br>Consider *R. equi* or *Streptococcus* | | |
| Septic arthritis/ osteomyelitis: adult | • Penicillin + gentamicin<br>• Ampicillin + gentamicin<br>• Penicillin + enrofloxacin<br>• Ampicillin + enrofloxacin<br>• Ceftiofur + gentamicin | • Amikacin can replace gentamicin for serious infections or when *Staphylococcus* or enteric microbes (*Enterobacterales*) are suspected | |

**Table 31.1** (Continued)

| Condition | Initial antimicrobial suggestions | Other options | Notes |
|---|---|---|---|
| Cellulitis / Lymphangitis | • Penicillin + gentamicin<br>• Penicillin + amikacin<br>• Penicillin + enrofloxacin<br>• *Can substitute ampicillin or ceftiofur for penicillin | • TMS, doxycycline, minocycline for mild cases<br>• TMS + rifampin | |
| Colitis/ Enterocolitis: Foal | Broad-spectrum coverage as for neonatal sepsis (above) to prevent bacteremia.<br>Metronidazole is clostridial enteritis is suspected. | | |
| Colitis/ Enterocolitis: Adult; general | In general, systemic antimicrobials should be avoided unless the patient is neutropenic, persistently febrile, or immunocompromised.<br>---------------------------------<br>For clostridial enterocolitis, metronidazole should be used | | |
| *Neorickettsia risticii* or *findlayensis* enterocolitis | Oxytetracycline IV;<br>Followed by oral doxycycline or minocycline as the horse improves | | Monitor renal function when oxytetracycline is used. |
| *Lawsonia intracellularis* in foals to young horses | • Oxytetracycline IV for three to five days<br>• Doxycycline<br>• Minocycline<br>• +/− rifampin | • Azithromycin +/− rifampin can be used, but has a higher risk of antibiotic associated colitis<br>• Chloramphenicol can be used | Monitor renal function when oxytetracycline is used. |

with a narrow therapeutic index. However, with hypoalbuminemia, the free drug concentrations decrease over time because of increases in volume of distribution and drug clearance; simply put, there is more free drug available to be distributed outside of the vascular space, and also more readily available for clearance. Alterations in dosing for hypoproteinemia are only clinically indicated if: (i) the antimicrobial is highly protein bound (>70%) and (ii) the antimicrobial has a narrow therapeutic index. Fortunately, for antimicrobial therapy, there are not many drugs that fulfill these two criteria. Renal injury is a potential adverse effect of aminoglycosides; however, they are minimally protein bound. Metronidazole is another antimicrobial with potential for toxicity (anorexia, hepatotoxicity, neurotoxicity); however, it is also minimally protein bound. In contrast, many nonsteroidal anti-inflammatory drugs are highly protein bound, and severe hypoproteinemia should be a consideration for dose selection.

Some critically ill patients have increased volume of distribution for hydrophilic antimicrobials, because of increased interstitial fluid due to capillary leak syndrome associated with cytokine storms. This is a consideration for hydrophilic or water-soluble antimicrobials such as the aminoglycosides amikacin and gentamicin, as well as many beta lactam antimicrobials. In these cases, doses may need to be increased because of the increased volume of distribution (Vd) caused by the expansion of the extracellular fluid compartment. Aminoglycoside concentrations can be monitored with therapeutic drug monitoring, in order to ensure high enough peak concentrations during critical illness (see section on aminoglycosides). Beta lactam antimicrobials should be used at the higher end of the recommended doses to account for the increased Vd. Lipophilic drugs, such as macrolides, metronidazole, tetracyclines and trimethoprim-sulfa, would not be affected to the same extent as hydrophilic drugs, because the body fat content does not change acutely.

Many critically ill horses have organ dysfunction, with liver and kidney function being important to metabolism, clearance, and elimination of drugs. With severe liver dysfunction (functional failure), dosing for liver-metabolized and eliminated drugs may need to be modified. This applies primarily to drugs with narrow therapeutic indices, such as metronidazole. In horses with liver failure, an increase in the dosing interval may be required, while keeping the dose the same to allow for more time for hepatic metabolism and elimination. For example, metronidazole could be administered every 8–12 h as opposed to every 6–8 h under normal circumstances. Many of the other liver-metabolized drugs, for example doxycycline, minocycline, chloramphenicol, and enrofloxacin, do not warrant significant dose alterations during liver failure due to a wider therapeutic index. For horses with renal injury, thought should be given to renally excreted drugs. Aminoglycosides, which are renally eliminated, are not recommended for horses with kidney injury. Other renally eliminated drugs, such as penicillin or ampicillin, do not have a narrow therapeutic index and likely do not need to be altered in terms of dosing regimen. Cephalosporins could accumulate with oliguric renal failure in foals or horses, and therefore should be administered at longer intervals and lower doses to account for the reduced elimination; there has been some question about renal tubular effects in human patients with very high concentrations of the drugs. Cephalosporins are thought to be potentially nephrotoxic at high concentrations (Quin 1989).

## Antimicrobial Classes

The following section will review the commonly prescribed antimicrobials in horses and foals, with an emphasis on those used for critically ill or emergent patients. They are organized by their mechanism of action: (i) cell wall inhibition, (ii) protein synthesis inhibition, and (iii) nucleic acid dysregulation.

### Cell Wall Inhibitors

This group of antimicrobials act by binding to penicillin-binding proteins, which results in inhibition of bacterial cell wall formation through prevention of peptidoglycan binding. This is the largest group of antimicrobials and includes the beta lactam antimicrobials, which include the penicillins and cephalosporins, as well as higher-spectrum antimicrobials such as piperacillin and carbapenems.

1) Beta-Lactam antimicrobials
   Beta lactam antimicrobials are bactericidal and act through inhibition of bacterial cell wall synthesis. Suggested drug dosages are listed for foals and adult horses are listed in Tables 31.2 and 31.3, respectively. They bind to penicillin-binding proteins (PBPs), and in doing so inhibit the cross-linking of peptidoglycan strands; this is a necessary step in creation of the bacterial cell wall. Beta-lactams are time dependent; this means that the duration of time (T) plasma concentrations are above the minimum inhibitory concentration (MIC) of the cultured bacterial isolate is highly important in determining efficacy (T > MIC). Optimally, they would remain above four to eight times the MIC of the offending organism throughout the dosing interval because of this time-dependent activity. As a minimum, beta-lactam concentrations should stay above onefold the MIC of the cultured microbe for ≥50% of the time of the dosing interval for Gram-positive infections. This time should be ≥80% of the dosing interval for Gram-negative infections (Magdesian 2017). As a clinical example, the dosing interval for intravenous penicillin is every six hours; therefore, the goal of therapy should be for plasma penicillin concentrations to remain >MIC of the cultured isolate for at least 3 (50% of dosing interval) and 5 (80% of dosing interval) hours for susceptible Gram-positive and Gram-negative bacteria, respectively (Magdesian 2017).
   A) Penicillin: The classic beta-lactam antibiotics are penicillins; these include penicillin G (benzyl penicillin), ampicillin, and amoxicillin as the foundational penicillin drugs (Magdesian 2017). Penicillin G is the original beta lactam and still in heavy use. These drugs have a Gram-positive spectrum, especially for beta-hemolytic streptococci; it is important to note that many staphylococci have developed resistance to penicillin antibiotics over time (Magdesian 2017). Penicillin G has high efficacy against many Gram-positive bacteria, especially beta hemolytic streptococci, non-beta lactamase producing staphylococci, as well as most anaerobes, except for *Bacteroides fragilis* and other beta lactamase-producing anaerobic bacteria (e.g., many isolates of *Prevotella* and *Porphyromonas*). Penicillin drugs are effective against some Gram-negative non-enteric microbes, for example some isolates of *Pasteurella* and *Actinobacillus* (Magdesian 2017); However, these bacteria require antimicrobial susceptibility testing, because their sensitivity to penicillin is difficult to predict. Penicillin has lost much of its Gram-negative activity over time, but remains an excellent Gram-positive antimicrobial. Penicillin should be administered either intramuscularly (IM) or slowly IV. The IM formulation that is widely available is procaine penicillin G, whereas the IV formulations are available as potassium or sodium salts. Horses can develop reactions such as cramps and loose stool when IV potassium penicillin is administered rapidly, and therefore it should be administered diluted and slowly (Cole 2015; Magdesian 2017). There have also been anecdotal concerns over low blood pressure with the fast administration of the sodium salt of penicillin (Cole 2015; Magdesian 2017). Procaine penicillin G (PPG) can occasionally to rarely cause reactions to procaine, which can result in hyperexcitability and hyperactivity, and can present some risk to horse or handler (Olsen et al. 2017).

**Table 31.2** Suggested dosages for beta lactam antimicrobials in foals.

| Drug | Dosage | Comment |
|---|---|---|
| **Penicillins** | | |
| Ampicillin | Foal: 20–40 mg/kg IV or PO, q6–8 h | Higher IV doses target *Enterococcus*. Oral pivampicillin 19.9 mg/kg q8–12 h for bacteria with MIC ≤0.25 μg/mL. Oral for neonates only. |
| Amoxicillin | 13–30 mg/kg PO, q8 h | For neonates only |
| Penicillin, potassium, or sodium | 22,000–44,000 IU/kg IV, q6 h | Always infuse slowly |
| Ticarcillin-clavulanic acid | 50 mg/kg IV, q6 h | (Dose based on the ticarcillin) |
| Imipenem (with cilastatin) | 15–20 mg/kg IV, q6–8 h | Slow and dilute infusion<br>Use only when dictated by culture |
| Meropenem | 15–20 mg/kg IV, q6 h | Use only when dictated by culture |
| **First-generation cephalosporins** | | |
| Cefazolin | 11–22 mg/kg IV, q6–8 h | |
| Cephalothin | 10–20 mg/kg IV, q6 h | |
| Cefadroxil | 20–40 mg/kg PO, q8–12 h | Oral for neonates only |
| Cefalexin | 25 mg/kg PO, q6, or 30 mg/kg PO q8 h | Oral for neonates |
| **Second-generation cephalosporins** | | |
| Cefuroxime Na | 16–33 mg/kg IV, q8 h | |
| Cefoxitin | 20 mg/kg IV, q6 h | |
| **Third-generation cephalosporins** | | |
| Ceftazidime | 25–50 mg/kg IV, q6–8 h, slow infusion | Crosses the blood–brain barrier (BBB) |
| Cefotaxime | 40–50 mg/kg IV, q6 h, slow infusion | Crosses the BBB |
| Cefotaxime continuous infusion | 40 mg/kg loading dose, then 6.7 mg/kg/h IV; | Can go up to 8.3 mg/kg/h |
| Ceftizoxime | 20–50 mg/kg IV, q6 h, slow infusion | |
| Cefoperazone | 30 mg/kg IV, q8 h, slow infusion | |
| Cefpodoxime proxetil | 10 mg/kg PO, q6–8 h | |
| Ceftriaxone | 25–50 mg/kg IV, q12 h | Excellent for meningitis |
| Ceftiofur | 5–10 mg/kg IV, SC, IM q6–12 h | Author most often uses 5–10 mg/kg IV, q12; |
| Ceftiofur continuous infusion | 5 mg/kg loading dose, then 0.42 mg/kg/h | Can double the loading and infusion dose depending on MIC or targe |
| **Fourth-generation cephalosporins** | | |
| Cefepime | 11 mg/kg IV, q8 h | |
| Cefquinome | 1 mg/kg IM or IV q12 h | Has been used up to 2.5 mg/kg q6–8 h |

B) Aminopenicillins: These are semisynthetic penicillins and include ampicillin and amoxicillin (Magdesian 2017). Like penicillin G, the aminopenicillins have excellent Gram-positive activity, but have additional activity against some Gram-negative bacteria, and greater activity against *Enterococcus* sp (Magdesian 2017). However, the Gram-negative activity has waned over decades of use. Ampicillin has sodium ampicillin and ampicillin trihydrate forms for IV or IM use, respectively (IV use is most common) (Magdesian 2017). Amoxicillin trihydrate is an aminopenicillin that can be administered *per os* to foals, as can ampicillin trihydrate, but these should not be administered to older horses because of low bioavailability after oral administration and concerns over induction of antibiotic-associated

**Table 31.3** Suggested dosages for beta lactam antimicrobials in adult horses.

| Drug | Dosage | Comment |
|---|---|---|
| **Penicillins** | | |
| Ampicillin | 15–20 mg/kg IV q6–8 h | |
| Penicillin, potassium, or sodium | 22,000–44,000 IU/kg IV, q6 h | Always infuse slowly |
| **First-generation cephalosporins** | | |
| Cefazolin | 11 mg/kg IV, q6–8 h | |
| **Third-generation cephalosporins** | | |
| Cefotaxime | 25 mg/kg IV, q6 h, slow infusion | Crosses the BBB; watch closely for colitis |
| Ceftiofur | 2.2 mg/kg IV, IM q12–24 h | |

enterocolitis (Brown et al. 1984; Baggot et al. 1988; Horspool et al. 1992; Magdesian 2017) (Table 31.2). Ampicillin can be used orally in newborn foals up to three days of age, and amoxicillin can be administered to foals up to seven days of age (Brown et al. 1984; Baggot et al. 1988; Horspool et al. 1992; Magdesian 2017).

An advantage of ampicillin over penicillin in horses is better activity against *Enterococcus* isolates, including *Enterococcus faecalis* and *E. faecium* (Magdesian 2017; Willis et al. 2019). In a study of foal isolates, ampicillin was highly effective against *E. faecalis*, and one of the best drugs with activity against *E. faecium* (59% susceptible) (Willis et al. 2019).

The antimicrobial duo of ampicillin and amikacin has very high activity against bacteria isolated from foals with sepsis through blood cultures (Magdesian 2017; Theelen et al. 2019). A recent study of 306 bacterial isolates obtained from septic foals showed that 91.5% were susceptible to this combination (Theelen et al. 2019). This combination of amikacin and ampicillin can be used as a front-line antimicrobial combination in foals, prior to culture and susceptibility results, when kidney injury does not preclude the use of amikacin. When kidney disease is present, alternatives such as ceftiofur should be used (see Cephalosporins below). The lower activity of penicillin against enterococci noted above results in a slightly lower overall predictability for the use of penicillin and amikacin as a front-line combination (Magdesian 2017; Theelen et al. 2019).

C) Extended-spectrum penicillins

Carbenicillin, piperacillin, and ticarcillin are extended-spectrum penicillins with high activity against *Pseudomonas aeruginosa* and *Proteus* isolates, developed because these bacteria are often multidrug resistant, including to other penicillins. However, their activity does not include many Enterobacterales; most cultured isolates of *Klebsiella, Citrobacter, Serratia,* and *Enterobacter* are resistant to these extended-spectrum penicillins (*Klebsiella* isolates are still often susceptible to piperacillin) (Magdesian 2017). These drugs are broad spectrum, so they continue to be active against Gram-positive bacteria. The extended-spectrum penicillins are more often effective than penicillin or ampicillin for use with resistant anaerobic infections, including *Bacteroides fragilis* (Magdesian 2017). The extended-spectrum penicillin antibiotics are not used very much in horses, with the exception of intra-uterine administration for uterine infections, and in foals with *Pseudomonas* infections (Magdesian 2017).

D) Carbapenems

The carbapenem subclass of beta lactam antibiotics includes imipenem, meropenem, and doripenem (Magdesian 2017). These antimicrobials have some of the highest efficacy against bacteria and are very broad in spectrum (Magdesian 2017). The only drug in this class which has been studied for systemic use in horses is imipenem (Orsini et al. 2005; Magdesian 2017), Imipenem is effective against bacteria with multidrug resistance, including many *Enterococcus* and *Pseudomonas* isolates, and their activity against anaerobic bacteria is high (Orsini et al. 2005; Magdesian 2017). Meropenem has been studied for regional limb perfusion, but concentrations were inadequate as administered (Fontenot et al. 2018). The shortcomings of carbapenem antimicrobials in terms of antimicrobial spectrum include methicillin-resistant *Staphylococcus aureus* (MRSA), and the susceptibility of *Enterobacter, Pseudomonas,* and *Enterococcus faecium* isolates is unpredictable and variable (Magdesian 2017). Imipenem is highly susceptible to degradation by renal dehydropeptidases, resulting in a very short elimination half-life of the drug. To get around this, it is formulated with cilastatin, which inhibits the renal dehydropeptidases. In a study evaluating imipenem-cilastatin in adult horses, it was well tolerated and there were no significant adverse events (Orsini et al. 2005). Possible side effects of the use of imipenem in the foal noted by the author include diarrhea and thrombophlebitis if administered without proper dilution (Magdesian 2017). Seizures have been noted in other species, and therefore imipenem should be used with caution in foals with seizure activity (Magdesian 2017). Dysbiosis would be a strong concern in adult horses.

Because of antimicrobial stewardship concerns and increasing development of antimicrobial resistance, carbapenems should not be front-line antimicrobials in equine practice.

2) Cephalosporins

Cephalosporins comprise the other major group of beta lactam drugs (Magdesian 2017). Like penicillins, cephalosporins have time-dependent bactericidal activity, and penetrate into extracellular fluid more so than penicillin and ampicillin, but not very well into intracellular fluid (Magdesian 2017). This penetration into extracellular fluids is enhanced by inflammation. In horses and foals with significant renal dysfunction and reduced glomerular filtration rate (GFR), especially in those with oliguria, the dose or administration frequency may need to be decreased, due to reduced clearance (Magdesian 2017). This will avoid accumulation of cephalosporins to very high concentrations. There is some suggestion that high concentrations of cephalosporins could have effects on the kidneys (Quin 1989).

Most penicillins are renally excreted; cephalosporins are also primarily excreted into urine, with some secondary biliary excretion. Specific cephalosporins, such as the third-generation drugs cefoperazone and ceftriaxone, have significant biliary excretion.

It should be noted that enterococci have intrinsic resistance to cephalosporins. With a few exceptions, cephalosporins as a group have poor anaerobic coverage. Exceptions include cefotetan and cefoxitin, $2^{nd}$-generation cephalosporins, and cefotaxime, a third-generation drug, which have excellent anaerobe activity. Ceftiofur is effective against a few anaerobes, notably *Peptostreptococcus* and *Fusobacterium* (Samitz et al. 1996).

There are five categories or "generations" of cephalosporins, first through fifth (Magdesian 2017). The first-generation cephalosporins are mainly Gram-positive in spectrum, and Gram-negative activity increases as the generation number increases (Magdesian 2017); Fifth-generation cephalosporins are primarily aimed at targeting MRSA, but their use in horses should be limited.

i) First-generation cephalosporins:

First-generation cephalosporins have activity similar to ampicillin, with the exception of lacking anaerobe and enterococcal coverage (Magdesian 2017). They have excellent streptococcal and non-beta lactamase producing staphylococcal coverage; they also some Gram-negative, non-enteric activity (e.g., *Actinobacillus*). Cephalexin and cefadroxil can be administered to neonatal foals orally, whereas they should not be given through this route to adult horses due to risks of dysbiosis and colitis, and poor oral bioavailability (Table 31.2). Cefadroxil had close to 100% bioavailability in two-week-old foals (Duffee et al. 1997).

ii) Second-generation cephalosporins:

Second-generation cephalosporins have increased activity against Gram-negative bacteria compared to the first category of cephalosporins and are relatively broad spectrum (Magdesian 2017). Examples of second-generation drugs include cefoxitin, cefotetan, and cefuroxime. While most cephalosporins have little to no anaerobic activity, cefoxitin and cefotetan have excellent anaerobe activity.

iii) Third-generation cephalosporins:

Third-generation cephalosporins have broad activity, including many Gram-positive and Gram-negative bacteria (Magdesian 2017). When renal dysfunction or acute kidney injury precludes the use of aminoglycosides, the third- and fourth-generation cephalosporins are excellent alternatives to amikacin and ampicillin in treating septic foals (Magdesian 2017). Because they penetrate the blood brain barrier well, they are excellent choices to treat meningitis in neonatal foals. Ceftiofur is a commercially available third-generation cephalosporin for horses; it is labeled for use in horses and available in sodium salt (Naxcel; Zoetis, Parsippany NJ 07054) and crystalline-free acid (Excede; Zoetis, Parsippany NJ 07054) forms (Magdesian 2017). The anaerobic spectrum of ceftiofur is limited, being effective against *Fusobacterium necrophorum* and *Peptostreptococcus anaerobius* (these have low MIC values of ≤0.0625 and 0.125 μg/mL, respectively) (Magdesian 2017). More resistant anaerobes, such as *Bacteroides* and *Prevotella,* have higher MIC values for ceftiofur and are resistant (Samitz et al. 1996; Magdesian 2017). Cefotaxime has broad anaerobe coverage, whereas the majority of third-generation cephalosporins do not.

The literature suggests that up to 30% of the cultured isolates from septic foals are resistant to ceftiofur (Brewer and Koterba 1990; Henson and Barton 2001; Marsh and Palmer 2001; Sanchez et al. 2008; Magdesian 2017). The susceptibility patterns likely vary with geography and the antimicrobial break points used to define resistant in each study; this highlights the importance of attempting blood cultures and basing the decision to use ceftiofur on culture and susceptibility testing results. If blood cultures are negative, then hospital historical and regional antimicrobial susceptibility data would be helpful. This warrants keeping track of susceptibility results over time. Ceftiofur is labeled at a dose of 2.2–4.4 mg/kg administered once daily for therapy of equine respiratory sepsis caused by *Streptococcus zooepidemicus* (Magdesian 2017). Beta hemolytic streptococci are exquisitely susceptible to ceftiofur (MIC of ≤0.25 μg/mL) (Magdesian 2017). In foals, the dose of ceftiofur used is often higher than the labeled doses, up to 5–10 mg/kg q6–12 h; the reason for this is the high prevalence of Gram-negative bacteria cultured from septic foals and their higher MICs (Magdesian 2017). *Actinobacillus* and *Pasteurella* isolates, both Gram-negative non-enteric microbes, are usually highly susceptible to ceftiofur at MIC values similar to beta hemolytic streptococci (Magdesian 2017).

The results of one study on blood cultures from septic foals predicted that ceftiofur administered at a dose of 5 mg/kg every 12 h would be effective against 90% of *E coli, Pasteurella, Klebsiella*, and *Streptococcus* isolates ($MIC_{90}$ ≤0.5 μg/mL) (Meyer et al. 2009; Magdesian 2017). However, results have been mixed, as another study showed that 23% of bacterial isolates from foals were resistant to ceftiofur (Sanchez et al. 2008; Magdesian 2017). Again, these differences warrant assessment of local and regional trends in antimicrobial susceptibility patterns, and the breakpoints used by local microbiology labs. Even though ceftiofur is labeled for IM use in horses, the IV and SC routes are preferable for foals; it is best administered IV to treat sepsis in foals whenever possible, due to malperfusion of tissues that is often associated with shock (Slovis et al. 2006; Magdesian). The author does not exceed 2.2 mg/kg of ceftiofur every 12 h (preferably every 24 h) in adult horses, due to the risk of antimicrobial induced dysbiosis and enterocolitis. As such, it is primarily targeting streptococci and Gram-negative non-enteric bacteria for adult horses.

A crystalline-free acid formulation of ceftiofur is labeled for treating streptococcal infections in horses (MIC ≤0.25 μg/mL) (Pusterla et al. 2016; Magdesian 2017). An extra label dose of 13.2 mg/kg SC administered every 48–72 h of crystalline-free acid ceftiofur has been recommended for use in neonatal foals, to be effective against bacteria with higher MIC values, for example up to 2 μg/mL (Pusterla et al. 2016; Magdesian 2017). The recommendation is to administer the second dose at 48 h, with subsequent doses administered at intervals of 72 h (Pusterla et al. 2016; Magdesian 2017). This high dose administered subcutaneously appears to be safe for use in foals, with exception of occasional swellings at injections sites (Magdesian 2017). This extra-label dose of crystalline-free acid formulation should not be used in adult horses due to risks of dysbiosis. In adult horses, the drug is administered intramuscularly; swellings can be minimized by not injecting more than 20 cc volume per site.

It takes an average of six hours for ceftiofur-free acid equivalents to reach 2 μg/mL concentrations in plasma when the crystalline-free acid formulation is used (Magdesian 2017). This several hour delay is not optimal in foals that are already septic or have an infection; in order to work around this, an initial IV dose of ceftiofur sodium (Naxcel) can be administered to cover the time gap (Magdesian 2017).

Several additional third-generation cephalosporins are used in human medicine, including cefotaxime, ceftizoxime, cefpodoxime, and ceftizoxime. They have better Gram-negative potency than ceftiofur, and ceftriaxone, cefotaxime, and ceftazidime specifically distribute into the central nervous system (CNS) quite well, making them important to treat meningitis (especially ceftriaxone). Because they are used to treat serious infections in humans, these third-generation cephalosporins should be used sparingly and only when clearly indicated, as in foals with meningitis. Each of these third-generation drugs has unique properties; cefotaxime is the third-generation cephalosporin with the best anaerobe spectrum, whereas ceftazidime and cefoperazone are the optimal cephalosporins to treat *Pseudomonas* infections (Magdesian 2017). Cefpodoxime has been studied in horses and is an oral option for foals (Carrillo et al. 2005).

iv) Fourth-generation cephalosporins:

The pharmacokinetics of cefquinome and cefepime, fourth-generation cephalosporins, have been reported in horses and foals (Tables 31.2 and 31.3) (Gardner and Papich 2001; Rohdich et al. 2009). This generation has the widest spectrum of antibacterial activity, with similar Gram-positive and even greater Gram-negative activity than the third-generation cephalosporins; this even better enteric (Enterobacterales) activity is because the fourth-generation drugs can better resist beta-lactamase enzymes produced by bacteria (Magdesian 2017).

This generation of cephalosporins can also distribute across the blood brain barrier well, similar to the third-generation drugs (Magdesian 2017).

v) Fifth-generation cephalosporins:
Relatively new, the fifth-generation cephalosporins were developed for use in humans in large part against MRSA, but they retain the broad-spectrum coverage of the third- and fourth-generation cephalosporins (Magdesian 2017). The use of ceftaroline, a fifth-generation drug, should be restricted due to its specific indication for MRSA in human patients. Drugs in this generation have not been studied in horses.

E) Continuous infusion of beta lactam antimicrobials
Continuous rate infusion (CRI) of beta lactam antimicrobials has been studied in human medicine in the last several years. Because they are time dependent, cell wall inhibitors like penicillin, ampicillin, and cephalosporins are well suited to continuous infusions (Magdesian 2017). With antimicrobials that are dependent on time above MIC, optimal dosing includes maintaining free plasma drug concentrations at four to six times the MIC of the offending microbe for the totality of the dosing interval (Magdesian 2017). Recently, a group of international and interprofessional collaborators developed consensus guidelines on the use of prolonged infusions, including CRI, of beta lactam agents (Hong et al. 2023). Early clinical studies have been conflicting, but some have shown survival benefits in human patients receiving continuous infusions, in comparison to those being treated with boluses or short infusions of beta lactam antimicrobials (Osthoff et al. 2016). When CRI dosing is used, a loading dose is required to achieve immediate therapeutic concentrations.

Continuous infusion of ceftiofur has been studied in newborn and neonatal foals (Wearn et al. 2012; Magdesian 2017). The recommendations from that study included a loading dose of 1.26 mg/kg administered as a bolus, with subsequent continuous infusion rates of 2.86 μg/kg/min in order to keep plasma concentrations of desfuroylceftiofur (DCA), the active metabolite of ceftiofur, >2 μg/mL continuously (Wearn et al. 2012; Magdesian 2017). The goal is to maintain free drug concentrations >MIC for 100% of the dosing interval for bacteria with an MIC ≤2 μg/mL. The accumulated total daily dose of ceftiofur with this CRI rate is 5.4 mg/kg/day (Wearn et al. 2012; Magdesian 2017). An even higher continuous infusion rate would be necessary to target bacteria with MIC values >2 μg/mL, and even more to maintain concentrations four to six times the MIC of 2 μg/mL, which is currently believed to be the optimal concentration for maximum beta lactam efficacy and for minimizing the development of resistance (Magdesian 2017; Hong et al. 2023).

Cefotaxime has also reported as a continuous infusion for neonatal pony foals (Hewson et al. 2013; Magdesian 2017). The total daily dose was kept the same, comparing the traditional bolus dose protocol of 40 mg/kg IV q6 h to the CRI rate of 160 mg/kg/day (6.7 mg/kg/h, after an initial loading bolus dose of 40 mg/kg) (Magdesian 2017). Cefotaxime levels were 16.10 μg/mL throughout the administration period, which is above the MIC value of many bacteria associated with sepsis in foals (Hewson et al. 2013; Magdesian 2017). In contrast, plasma concentrations of cefotaxime fell to 0.78 μg/mL six hours after administration of standard intermittent dosing (Hewson et al. 2013; Magdesian 2017). Being very relevant to neonatal foal sepsis, synovial fluid cefotaxime concentrations were higher with the continuous infusion protocol (5.02 μg/mL) than those achieved with intermittent dosing (0.78 μg/mL) and were above the MIC of common pathogens in the joint fluid only with CRI dosing (Hewson et al. 2013; Magdesian 2017).

The practical and accurate administration of beta lactam antimicrobials as a continuous infusion includes the use of automated fluid or syringe pumps. The reconstituted or diluted antimicrobial being considered for CRI should be assessed in terms of stability at room temperature (Magdesian 2017). Ceftazidime, cefotaxime, sodium and potassium penicillin, and cefazolin are stable for 24 h at room temperature once diluted (Magdesian 2017). Ampicillin's stability depends on the dilution used and should be confirmed with the instructions on the label. Once reconstituted, ceftiofur is stable for up to 12 h at room temperature but is light sensitive and needs to be protected from light (Magdesian 2017).

## Protein Synthesis Inhibitors

1) Aminoglycosides
Aminoglycosides studied in horses and foals includes amikacin, gentamicin, and netilmicin (Magdesian et al. 2004; Burton et al. 2015; Green and Conlon 1993). Suggested doses for foals and adult horses are listed in Tables 31.4 and 31.5, respectively. They have excellent activity against Gram-negative aerobic bacteria, including enteric bacteria. Amikacin has more predictable antimicrobial coverage against enteric bacteria. The aminoglycosides are bactericidal, with a

**Table 31.4** Aminoglycoside dosing for foals.

| Drug | Dosage | Comment |
|---|---|---|
| **Antimicrobial agents** | | |
| Aminoglycosides: Amikacin | 25 mg/kg IV, q24 h for neonates | TDM[a] recommended. Monitor creatinine + UA |
| Gentamicin | 8–16 mg/kg IV, q24 h for neonates | TDM recommended. Monitor creatinine + UA |

[a] TDM, therapeutic drug monitoring (see Table 31.6).

**Table 31.5** Aminoglycoside dosing for adult horses.

| Drug | Dosage | Comment |
|---|---|---|
| **Antimicrobial agents** | | |
| **Aminoglycosides** | | |
| Amikacin | 10–20 mg/kg IV, q24 h (start with 15 mg/kg) | TDM[a] recommended Monitor creatinine + UA |
| Gentamicin | 6.6–8.8 mg/kg IV, q24 h | TDM recommended Monitor creatinine + UA |

[a] TDM, therapeutic drug monitoring (see Table 31.6).

mechanism of action of binding to the 30S ribosome, inhibiting the interaction of mRNA and tRNA, and thereby inhibiting bacterial protein synthesis. They are concentration dependent, meaning the rate and extent of bactericidal efficacy increases with increasing peak plasma concentrations rather than T > MIC (Magdesian 2017). They are polar drugs, resulting in their Vd being limited to the extracellular fluid volume primarily (Magdesian 2017). Whereas gentamicin is the most commonly used aminoglycoside for adult horses, amikacin is the primary aminoglycoside recommended for foals with sepsis, to be paired with a beta lactam drug for initial broad-spectrum coverage (Magdesian 2017). This is because it is the most potent aminoglycoside against Gram-negative Enterobacterales (Magdesian 2017). It is also highly effective against *Staphylococcus* isolates, including a high percentage of MRSA. In adult horses, gentamicin is the first-line aminoglycoside used because of the high costs of amikacin, as well as out of judicious use of amikacin.

The primary safety concern with aminoglycosides is the potential for renal and otovestibular injury, most often when preexisting risk factors are present. Foals with sepsis and hypoxic-ischemic injury (neonatal maladjustment syndrome or neonatal encephalopathy), and premature foals, as well as dehydrated horses or those on concurrent potentially nephrotoxic drugs (e.g., NSAIDS) are at greatest risk of kidney injury from aminoglycosides (Magdesian 2017). Such critically ill foals commonly have concurrent dehydration, hypoperfusion, and reduced oxygen delivery, as well as inflammatory mediators which all increase the risks off acute kidney injury (Green et al. 1992; Green et al. 1992; Magdesian 2017). Ototoxicity is another potential side effect of aminoglycoside therapy in horses, although it is much less commonly recognized in animals as compared to human patients, and as compared to renal injury (Magdesian 2017). Neuromuscular blockage is another theoretical concern, primarily for foals with neuromuscular disorders (e.g., -botulism) (Magdesian 2017).

Marked caution is advised when administering aminoglycosides to azotemic foals or horses (Magdesian 2017). Other options should be considered, including third- or fourth-generation cephalosporins. Therapeutic drug monitoring (Table 31.6) is a means of ensuring that plasma aminoglycoside concentrations are consistent with a potential for efficacy and a low risk of adverse effects. Because aminoglycosides are concentration dependent, the goal is to attain peak plasma concentrations 8–10 fold that of the MIC of the offending bacteria. The peak concentration is measured after some time has elapsed for distribution of the drug throughout the extracellular fluid. This is usually obtained 30–60 minutes after administration. The trough concentration is obtained before the next dose, usually between 20 and 23 h after administration. As an example, if an *E coli* isolate has an MIC of 1 μg/mL for gentamicin,

**Table 31.6** Therapeutic drug monitoring of aminoglycosides.

| Drug | Peak | 8 hour level | Trough |
|---|---|---|---|
| Amikacin | 30 minutes: 53–60 μg/mL<br>60 minutes: 40 μg/mL | 15–20 μg/mL | 20 h: <2 μg/mL<br>24 h: <1 μg/mL |
| Gentamicin | 30 minutes: 30–40 μg/mL<br>60 minutes: 20 μg/mL | 3–5 μg/mL | 20 h: < 1 μg/mL |

the desired peak serum gentamicin concentration would be 8–10 μg/mL (8–10× MIC) (Magdesian 2017). Because many patients with sepsis have negative cultures, empirical targets are used to cover bacteria which are considered susceptible under achievable plasma concentrations. For example, many Gram-negative bacteria frequently isolated from infections in foals and horses have MIC values ≤4 μg/mL for amikacin and ≤2 μg/mL for gentamicin (Adamson et al. 1985; Orsini et al. 1985; Jacks et al. 2003; Bucki et al. 2004; Magdesian 2017). Therefore, a peak serum concentration obtained one hour post administration optimally should be 40 μg/mL for amikacin, and 20 μg/mL for gentamicin (Table 31.6) (Magdesian 2017).

Some clinicians prefer to use a 30-minute peak for therapeutic drug monitoring of amikacin in foals (Table 31.6); for the 30-minute sample, the concentration should be ≥53–60 μg/mL, in order to result in a one-hour concentration of 40 μg/mL (Magdesian 2017). Recommendations for gentamicin, as well as goals for trough concentrations, are listed in Table 31.6.

Serial monitoring of serum creatinine and SDMA concentrations should be part of monitoring foals and horses being treated with aminoglycosides, for early detection of acute kidney injury (Magdesian 2017). The assessment of creatinine values in critically ill patients should go beyond detecting concentrations rising outside of the reference range. Instead, creatinine should be monitored for trends, as increasing values over time should raise concern, even when still within the reference range; a 0.3 mg/dL rise in creatinine within a 48-h period is considered acute kidney injury in hospitalized human patients (Magdesian 2017). Symmetric dimethylarginine (SDMA) can be monitored serially in adult horses as a means of monitoring renal function. Measurement of SDMA in foals can be complicated to interpret as their values are much higher as compared to adult horses, but trends over time may be useful. Urine output and urinalysis findings are additional tools to minimize nephrotoxicity, Aminoglycosides should not be used in foals or horses with reduced urine output.

The pairing of amikacin and ampicillin has been reported to be effective in terms of susceptibility of 91.5% of bacteria isolated from foals with sepsis (Theelen et al. 2019). Other antimicrobials or combinations with high activity were ceftizoxime (89.7% susceptible), ceftiofur + amikacin (89.6% susceptible), and amikacin + penicillin (88.6% susceptible). Ceftiofur as monotherapy was considered effective against 86.3% of isolates in vitro; gentamicin + ampicillin had 83.6% susceptible bacteria, and gentamicin + penicillin had 82% susceptible (Theelen et al. 2019). Imipenem, a carbapenem described earlier, had the highest % in vitro susceptibility in the study (92.6%); however, carbapenems should be limited to infections with culture and susceptibility results indicating no other antimicrobial choice, or for foals with clinical deterioration or lack of improvement in the face of other appropriate antimicrobials (Theelen et al. 2019). In adult horses, gentamicin is most commonly paired with a beta lactam (e.g., penicillin and gentamicin or ampicillin and gentamicin) for initial IV, bactericidal, and broad-spectrum coverage. Suggested dosages for aminoglycosides are listed in Tables 31.4 and 31.5.

2) Tetracycline, doxycycline, and minocycline:
The tetracycline class of antimicrobials is relatively broad spectrum, with excellent activity against Gram-positive aerobes and Gram-negative non-enteric microbes (Tables 31.7 and 31.8) (Magdesian 2017). They are effective against specific anaerobic bacteria, including Fusobacterium, Peptostreptococcus, and certain clostridial strains, but not uniformly so (Magdesian 2017). The primary group of bacteria with widespread resistance to the tetracyclines is the order Enterobacterales, with few exceptions. They would be considered effective against a greater % of Gram-negative enteric microbes in foals as compared to adult horses, because the bioavailability of doxycycline and minocycline is quite low in adult horses. The tetracyclines are also excellent drugs for rickettsial organisms, including *Anaplasma phagocytophilum, Neorickettsia risticii,* and *N. findlayensis*, the latter two being the agents of Potomac Horse Fever. They are also effective against the agent of Lyme disease, *Borrelia burgdorferi*, as well as *Lawsonia intracellularis*, which causes proliferative enteropathy in foals.

**Table 31.7** Other antimicrobials available for use in foals.

| Drug | Dosage | Comment |
|---|---|---|
| Azithromycin | 10 mg/kg PO, q24 h; q48 h after 5 days | Can induce anhidrosis: Keep foal out of sunlight/heat |
| Clarithromycin | 7.5 mg/kg PO, q12 h | Can induce anhidrosis: Keep foal out of sunlight/heat |
| Chloramphenicol+ | 40–50 mg/kg PO, q12 h on d 1–2 of age;<br>Dose interval: q8 h on d 3–5 of age | Handlers should wear gloves.<br>Should be used with caution in first few days of life- although not reported in foals, gray baby syndrome is a risk in human infants. |
| Doxycycline | 10 mg/kg PO, q12 h | May cause tendon laxity |
| Minocycline | 4 mg/kg PO q12 h | May cause tendon laxity |
| Rifampin | 5 mg/kg PO, q12 h | Stains urine and mucous membranes pink |
| Metronidazole for enteric clostridiosis: | 10 mg/kg PO, IV q8–12 h for 1st 2 weeks | |
| Trimethoprim-sulfonamide | 24–30 mg/kg PO, q12 h | |

**Table 31.8** Other antimicrobials available for use in adult horses.

| Drug | Dosage | Comment |
|---|---|---|
| Chloramphenicol[a] | 50 mg/kg PO q6 h | Handlers should wear gloves |
| Doxycycline | 10 mg/kg PO, q12 h | |
| Minocycline | 4 mg/kg PO q12 h | |
| Rifampin | 5 mg/kg PO, q12 h | Stains urine and mucous membranes pink |
| Enrofloxacin | 5.5 mg/kg IV, q24 h; 7.5 mg/kg PO, q24 h | Horses should not be worked or ridden while being treated |
| Metronidazole | 15 mg/kg PO,IV q8 h; 20 mg/kg per rectum q6–8 h | |
| Trimethoprim-sulfonamide | 24–30 mg/kg PO, q12 h | Commercial formulation with sulfadiazine has a dose of 24 mg/kg; tablets containing sulfamethoxazole have a dose of 30 mg/kg |

[a] Please see text regarding relatively low oral bioavailability of chloramphenicol in horses, limiting its use to select infections.

Oxytetracycline and tetracycline are similar in their spectrum, being older drugs in this class (Magdesian 2017). Doxycycline and minocycline have expanded spectrums as compared to tetracyclines, with improved activity against Gram-positive and Gram-negative non-enteric (e.g., *Actinobacillus*) microbes (Magdesian 2017). Doxycycline and minocycline may have efficacy against some isolates of enteric microbes in foals (e.g., *E coli, Klebsiella*), because they have significantly greater bioavailability in foals as compared to in adult horses. In adult horses, only bacteria with an MIC $\leq$0.25 μg/mL, and preferably $\leq$0.12 μg/mL, should be targeted because of poor oral bioavailability. This includes primarily *Streptococcus* and Gram-negative non-enteric microbes, with variable susceptibility in terms of *Staphylococcus* isolates. In contrast, the oral absorption of doxycycline in foals (four to eight week of age) is such that bacteria with an MIC $\leq$2 μg/mL can be targeted in this age group of foals and younger (Magdesian 2017). Bacteria that would be considered susceptible with MIC $\leq$2 μg/mL include a high proportion of isolates of *Actinobacillus*, *Pasteurella*, *Staphylococcus* (non-MRSA), *Streptococcus*, and *Rhodococcus equi* in horses (Womble et al. 2007; Magdesian 2017). Variably, a proportion of *E coli* and *Klebsiella* isolates are also expected to be susceptible to doxycycline at this concentration, if their MIC is $\leq$2 μg/mL, and can be targeted in foals with susceptibility data (i.e., isolate MIC values) available (Magdesian 2017). Minocycline also has a higher oral bioavailability (57.8 $\pm$ 19.3%) in foals aged six to nine weeks as compared to adult horses (32.0 $\pm$ 18.0%). This difference allows bacteria with MIC values $\leq$1.0 μg/mL to be targeted with minocycline in foals, as opposed to only those with MIC values ≤0.12–0.25 μg/mL in adult horses (Giguere et al. 2016; Magdesian 2017). This MIC target of 1 or below includes most equine isolates of *Actinobacillus*, *Staphylococcus*, *Rhodococcus equi*, and *Streptococcus equi ss. zooepidemicus* and *Streptococcus equi ss. equi* (Magdesian 2017). As with doxycycline, variably, specific isolates of *E coli* would also be considered susceptible, as long as their MIC values were ≤1.0 μg/mL (Giguere et al. 2016).

Oxytetracycline, doxycycline, and minocycline are bacteriostatic in activity, have a high degree of lipophilicity, and share both time- and concentration-dependent efficacy (Magdesian 2017). They have excellent intracellular penetration, and minocycline and doxycycline are able to cross the blood brain barrier, with minocycline having the highest extent of penetration into the CNS (Magdesian 2017). Their mechanism of action is through bacterial protein synthesis inhibition by binding the 30S ribosomal subunit. Oxytetracycline and tetracycline are renally excreted, whereas doxycycline and minocycline have both kidney and hepatic elimination (Magdesian 2017). Doxycycline has an additional means of elimination, that being directly into the gastrointestinal tract (Magdesian 2017).

The tetracycline antimicrobials can discolor the enamel of teeth in young animals (especially oxytetracycline), due to being incorporated into developing bone and enamel tissues (Magdesian 2017). In young humans, these antimicrobials can also affect bone growth. Such effects in the enamel and bone of foals have not been reported thus far (Womble et al. 2007; Giguere et al. 2016; Magdesian 2017). Diarrhea and antimicrobial associated colitis are additional potential side effects of these drugs (Magdesian 2017). Oxytetracycline and tetracycline are also potentially nephrotoxicity, especially if the horse is dehydrated or has other risk factors for nephrotoxicity (Magdesian 2017). In contrast, doxycycline and minocycline are considered safe for use in patients with kidney injury or disease (Magdesian 2017). The author has experienced laxity of forelimbs in weanlings that were on long-term doxycycline or minocycline therapy, similar to the response of contracted neonatal foals to high-dose oxytetracycline. This laxity has primarily been noted in weanlings that were debilitated due to their underlying disease, such as foals with *Lawsonia intracellularis* and *Rhodococcus equi*. Minocycline and rifampin can be used to treat macrolide-resistant *R. equi* infections; however, doxycycline and rifampin should not be used together due to a suggestion for concern over liver disease and hemolysis (Venner et al. 2013). For rifampin-resistant *R. equi* infections, doxycycline plus azithromycin can be used (Wetzig et al. 2020).

Oxytetracycline is also used to treat limb contractures in foals, at high doses (above the antimicrobial doses) along with bandages and/or splints. When oxytetracycline is used for this purpose and at these doses, it should be diluted in fluids to minimize the chances of renal injury, and pre- and post-administration creatinine should be monitored (Magdesian 2017). The IV formulations of oxytetracycline are best to be used in young foals under these circumstances whenever possible, because the IM formulations often include propylene glycol, which may increase risks of renal injury in the author's experience (Magdesian 2017). Plasma or serum creatinine levels and the foals' urine output should be monitored closely (Vivrette et al. 1993; Magdesian 2017). The intravenous use of doxycycline should be avoided in horses and foals, due to a potential for supraventricular tachycardia, hypertension, collapse, and possibly death (Riond et al. 1992; Magdesian 2017).

3) Macrolides and azalides

Macrolides are primarily used in foals, as they can cause severe colitis in adult horses (Table 31.7). Clarithromycin is the most commonly used macrolide in foals, and azithromycin is an azalide. Azalides are macrolide derivatives, with insertion of a methyl-substituted nitrogen in place of a carbonyl group within an aglycone ring. This change in structure makes azalides more stable under acid conditions, have a longer half-life, improved Gram-negative activity, and better tissue penetration. Macrolides and azalides have excellent activity against Gram-positive bacteria, with azithromycin being better against Gram-negative bacteria; the Gram-negative coverage of azithromycin is primarily against non-enterics, such as *Actinobacillus*. Their primary use is in the treatment of *Rhodococcus equi*, usually in combination with rifampin. They can also be used to treat Gram-positive infections in foals, including those caused by *Streptococcus* or some *Staphylococcus* isolates. The mechanism of action is through inhibition of bacterial protein synthesis from inhibition of the 50s ribosomal subunit. They have the advantage of being highly lipophilic and concentrating to a high extent intracellularly, which is an advantage for treating intracellular pathogens such as *R. equi*. The reader is referred to other resources for more comprehensive review of the treatment options for *Rhodococcus equi* infections. Select infections, such as umbilical, bone or joint, or pneumonia in foals may be treated with macrolides owing to their penetrability, depending on culture and susceptibility results. The latter cannot be emphasized enough as macrolides are not broad spectrum enough to be used as monotherapy empirically.

It is important to note that the dams of foals being administered macrolides or azalides could be at risk for ingesting small amounts of azithromycin or clarithromycin and developing severe colitis. Water and feed buckets should be cleaned out after treating foals, and the lips and muzzle of the foal should be wiped clean of any residual medication in order to reduce the exposure to the dams. In addition, the foal feces should be picked up daily to reduce potential exposure from that route. Another potential adverse effect of macrolides and azalides on the foals themselves includes transient hypohidrosis or anhidrosis, which can lead to impaired ability to thermoregulate and subsequent hyperthermia (Stieler Stewart et al. 2016; Magdesian 2017). Therefore, such foals being treated with these medications should be kept out of direct sunlight and as cool as possible, with shade and fans as necessary (Magdesian 2017). Finally, rifampin and macrolides should be staggered by four to six hours in terms of administration, because rifampin can reduce the oral bioavailability of macrolides and azalides (Berlin et al. 2016). For example, clarithromycin can be administered at 6 am and 6 pm, with rifampin being administered at 10 am and 10 pm.

4) Chloramphenicol

Chloramphenicol is an amphenicol class of antibiotic; it is broad spectrum in antibacterial activity, though less so in horses as compared to humans due to the reduced oral bioavailability. It is bacteriostatic, highly lipophilic, and a time-dependent antimicrobial (Tables 31.7 and 31.8) (Magdesian 2017). The mechanism of action of chloramphenicol is through inhibition of microbial protein synthesis through binding receptors on bacterial 50S ribosomal subunit (Magdesian 2017) Chloramphenicol distributes into the intracellular fluids, bone, and CNS well, owing in large part to its lipophilicity (Magdesian 2017). Chloramphenicol has several characteristics which limit its utility for horses and foals with serious infections: it is bacteriostatic, only available in oral formulations, and has a limited spectrum in horses due to limited bioavailability and a very short half-life (Magdesian 2017). Its primary use may be as an oral antimicrobial after an initial antimicrobial course with IV and bactericidal antimicrobials and based on microbial culture and susceptibility results (Magdesian 2017). Because of the poor absorption and variable serum concentrations obtained with oral dosing, chloramphenicol should only be used when the predicted or confirmed MIC of the offending bacterial isolate is ≤1–2 μg/kg.

Unfortunately, chloramphenicol is not absorbed well in adult horses (Estell et al. 2020). It has low bioavailability in horses such that it has lost a significant amount of spectrum as compared to that in humans. In adult horses, chloramphenicol should only be used to target bacteria with an MIC of 1–2 μg/mL or less (Estell et al. 2020). This includes *Streptococcus equi ss zooepidemicus* and *Streptococcus equi ss equi*, some Staphylococcus isolates, non-enteric Gram-negative microbes (some isolates of *Actinobacillus equuli)*, and a few anaerobes, including *Porphryomonas spp.*, *Prevotella spp.*, and *Peptostreptococcus spp.* It can be effective against enterococci as well, but only those isolates with 1 μg/mL or less. It is also effective against special bacteria, including *Chlamydia* and *Mycoplasma*. In contrast to adult horses, foals (one to nine days of age) absorb chloramphenicol with a high oral bioavailability (83%), so it would be expected to have a broader spectrum of activity in foals; however, potential for side effects should be considered (Brumbaugh et al. 1983; Magdesian 2017).

A problematic aspect of the use of chloramphenicol is the potential for human toxicity in susceptible individuals (Magdesian, 2017). The main concern in humans is bone marrow suppression, which can be a rare dose-independent aplastic anemia (1 in every 25,000–60,000 people), or a dose-dependent anemia. Topical contact exposure with skin, eyes, or mucus membranes can also lead to toxicity in rare, susceptible individuals (Magdesian 2017). Therefore, clients and veterinary staff should be aware of this risk, and handlers should wear gloves, and possibly face masks if risk of exposure is there, whenever handling chloramphenicol. Tablets should not be crushed in order to avoid inhalation of dust. Chloramphenicol is liver metabolized, and is a hepatic microsomal enzyme inhibitor, which will delay clearance of other liver metabolized drugs.

A "gray baby syndrome" can occur in human infants due to glucuronic acid conjugation deficiency in infants, which leads to chloramphenicol accumulation and a dose-dependent anemia and hemodynamic events. With this syndrome, hypotension and cyanosis can develop, as well as death of the infant. Gray baby syndrome has not been described in foals; however, it warrants cautious use and even avoidance in premature foals (Magdesian 2017). Based on the age-dependent pharmacokinetics described in term foals, the drug should be administered twice daily for the first one to two days of life, then q8 h after that (Table 31.7) (Adamson et al. 1991). These potential drawbacks significantly limit the use of chloramphenicol in horses and foals with critical illness. (Magdesian 2017).

## Nucleic Acid Inhibitors

1) Potentiated sulfonamides

This is a combination of antimicrobials, trimethoprim, and either sulfamethoxazole or sulfadiazine (Tables 31.7 and 31.8). Trimethoprim and sulfonamides (TMS) individually are bacteriostatic, but together they are bactericidal (Magdesian 2017). Trimethoprim-sulfonamide (TMS) is a time-dependent combination (Magdesian 2017). The mechanism of action is through synergistic inhibition of bacterial folate synthesis (Magdesian 2017). The mechanism of action of trimethoprim is through inhibition of dihydrofolate reductase; this enzyme is what produces tetrahydrofolic acid, a metabolically active form of folates. Sulfonamides are para-aminobenzoic acid (PABA) analogues competing with binding sites for bacterial PABA, thereby providing a second means of inhibiting the pathway to folate synthesis. Potentiated sulfonamides penetrate tissue well; however, it is important to note that the activity of TMS is suboptimal in the presence of exudate due to the availability of free PABA or thymidine in pus that can be utilized by bacteria (Magdesian 2017). When treating purulent abscesses, such as those with *Streptococcus equi* ss *equi* or *Corynebacterium pseudotuberculosis*, TMS is not the optimal monotherapy initially when the abscesses are quite exudative. Alternatives should be used when possible, or TMS can be combined with another effective drug such as rifampin.

Potentiated sulfonamides have a moderately broad spectrum; they target beta hemolytic streptococci and Gram-negative non-enteric bacteria, such as *Actinobacillus*, very well. Trimethoprim-sulfonamides do not target enterococci due to intrinsic resistance. Many Gram-negative enteric bacteria are resistant to TMS and TMS has poor anaerobic coverage (Magdesian 2017). Therefore, TMS should not be considered a first-line antimicrobial for treatment of sepsis in foals (Magdesian 2017). Only 60% of foals had all cultured isolates susceptible to TMS in a recent study (Theelen et al. 2019) The place for TMS in the treatment of foal sepsis, or critical illness in horses, is not in the acute stage of the disease, but rather in the convalescent period once culture and susceptibility results have been obtained to ensure susceptibility of the isolate and when the infection is under control but requires continued antimicrobial therapy (Magdesian 2017).

For older foals and adult horses, they are fairly broad spectrum for use in hemodynamically stable animals. They are indicated for mild pneumonia associated with *Streptococcus equi ss zooepidemicus*, wounds, umbilical infections that are localized and not causing serious systemic inflammatory response, and as a front line for many other non-life threatening infections. Trimethoprim-sulfonamides are highly effective against *Pneumocystis jirovecii*; this is a yeast-like fungal infection that has been associated with acute bronchointerstitial pneumonia and acute respiratory distress syndrome in foals (Magdesian 2017).

Potential side effects of TMS in horses include diarrhea and elevations in liver enzymes. Bone marrow suppression is possible with long-term use. Other reported rare side effects include hemolytic anemia, hypermetria, and agitation, Stevens-Johnson like syndrome (uveitis, skin reactions), and erythema multiforme. Intravenous formulations of TMS are available for horses; however, they should not be used concurrent to alpha-2 agonists (xylazine, romifidine, detomidine) because of concerns over hemodynamic instability and collapse when the two are administered in close temporal proximity (Corley and Hollis 2009). Experimental studies have demonstrated prolongation of the QT interval in horses receiving IV detomidine and TMS (Trachsel et al. 2021). Pregnant mares on TMS should optimally receive natural forms of folate, such as through fresh grass or alfalfa.

2) Rifampin

Rifampin is a rifamycin antimicrobial and acts through inhibition of bacterial DNA-dependent RNA polymerase (Tables 31.7 and 31.8) (Magdesian 2017). This ultimately prevents bacterial transcription and protein synthesis. Rifampin is primarily a Gram-positive drug, often effective against *Staphylococcus, Corynebacterium pseudotuberculosis,* and *Rhodococcus equi* isolates (Cole 2015). Rifampin also has selective activity against a small number of Gram-negative microbes, primarily *Actinobacillus* and other non-enteric microbes, and has reasonably good anaerobic coverage (Magdesian 2017). It is a highly lipophilic drug, which allows it to penetrate the CNS and concentrate intracellularly very well (Magdesian 2017). Rifampin is time-dependent and can be either bactericidal or bacteriostatic depending on the type of bacteria involved with the infection (Magdesian 2017). Rifampin undergoes hepatic metabolism and elimination through the bile into the gastrointestinal tract (Burrows et al. 1992). Rifampin induces hepatic microsomal enzymes, particularly cytochrome P450 enzymes, and therefore may increase the elimination of other liver metabolized drugs (Magdesian 2017). Adverse effects of rifampin include soft feces and occasionally antimicrobial-associated diarrhea (Magdesian 2017). It can make urine and other body fluids turn pink or orange-red in color (Magdesian 2017). Rifampin should not be administered IV to horses; a report of IV injection described weakness, hyperhidrosis, excessive defection, and behavioral distress during injection, even when administered slowly IV over 10 minutes (Burrows et al. 1992; Magdesian 2017).

Because bacteria can develop resistance to rifampin quickly when used alone, it should only be used in combination with other antimicrobials. One of the most common uses of rifampin is when paired with macrolides or azalides in the treatment of *Rhodococcus equi* pneumonia in foals (Magdesian 2017). It is also used in combination with other antimicrobials to treat infections that require good penetration, such as umbilical abscesses with susceptible bacteria in foals, and internal abscesses caused by *Streptococcus* or *Corynebacterium pseudotuberculosis* in adult horses (Magdesian 2017). For example, internal *Corynebacterium pseudotuberculosis* infections are often treated with TMS and rifampin, or enrofloxacin and rifampin.

3) Fluoroquinolones

Fluoroquinolones used in horses include enrofloxacin and marbofloxacin. The mechanism of action of fluoroquinolones is through inhibition of bacterial DNA gyrase, also called topoisomerase II (Magdesian 2017). The result of inhibiting DNA gyrase is inhibition of DNA repair, replication, and transcription. Topoisomerase IV is another target of fluoroquinolone inhibition; this enzyme mediates unlinking and relaxation of DNA after replication has occurred.

Fluoroquinolones have an antimicrobial spectrum similar to aminoglycosides, in that they have excellent activity against Gram-negative bacteria and many *Staphylococcus* isolates but have poor anaerobic activity (Table 31.8) (Magdesian 2017). Fluoroquinolones are also effective against *Brucella*, *Chlamydia*, and *Leptospira*. Most isolates of *Corynebacterium pseudotuberculosis* are susceptible to fluoroquinolones, and the penetrability is advantageous for internal abscesses. Fluoroquinolones are not very effective against *Streptococcus* isolates, even when in vitro MIC results suggest the isolates are susceptible (Magdesian 2017).

Fluoroquinolones are bactericidal and penetrate intracellularly well, consistent with their lipophilicity. Like aminoglycosides, they are concentration dependent in their antibacterial action (Magdesian 2017). Consistent with aminoglycosides, peak concentrations ≥8–10 fold the MIC of the offending microbe are desired (Magdesian 2017). As or more important to effectiveness of fluoroquinolones than the ratio of peak to MIC is the ratio of the area-under-the-curve to MIC, with the goal being ≥ 125 (Magdesian 2017).

Fluoroquinolones should not be used routinely in foals, because of potential for chondrotoxicity and subsequent arthropathy (Magdesian 2015). A study in neonatal foals administered enrofloxacin (10 mg/kg daily) for 8 days, starting at 14 days of age, showed consistent chondrotoxicity, joint effusion, and associated lameness (Davenport et al. 2001; Vivrette et al. 2001; Magdesian 2017). The author and other clinicians have used marbofloxacin in foals without obvious joint complications, but the risks are still a theoretical concern until further studies are conducted (Corley and Hollis 2009; Magdesian 2017).

In adult horses, enrofloxacin is commonly utilized as a Gram-negative antimicrobial, often coupled with beta lactams for broad-spectrum coverage of serious infections such as peritonitis or pleuropneumonia. It is also commonly utilized against *Staphylococcus* infections, especially limb cellulitis. With rapid IV administration of enrofloxacin, neurological signs are possible; therefore, it should be diluted and administered slowly. The author also advises owners of horses being treated with enrofloxacin to avoid forced exercise while on the medication. This is because of potential tendon and ligament effects in humans treated with fluoroquinolones, though this has not been well documented in horses.

4) Metronidazole

Metronidazole is a nitro-imidazole antimicrobial that has excellent anaerobic activity (Tables 31.7 and 31.8). It also has antiprotozoal activity against *Giardia*. It has no activity against aerobic bacteria. Metronidazole is bactericidal and highly lipophilic (Magdesian 2017). It has both concentration- and time-dependent efficacy as an antimicrobial (Magdesian 2017). Notably, metronidazole is highly effective against beta-lactamase producing anaerobes, including *Bacteroides fragilis* (Magdesian 2017). Metronidazole works through causing oxidant damage to bacterial DNA; anaerobic bacteria metabolize metronidazole to free radicals.

Possible adverse effects of metronidazole in horses include anorexia as the most common adverse effect; others include diarrhea, neurotoxicity, and subclinical hepatopathy (Magdesian 2017). Anorexia can be minimized through administration of metronidazole per rectum. Metronidazole is metabolized by the liver and is eliminated primarily through biliary excretion; secondary excretion of metronidazole metabolites occurs into urine (Magdesian 2017).

Metronidazole can be administered through the intravenous or oral routes, as well as per rectum (Steinman et al. 2000; Magdesian 2017). It has >90% oral bioavailability; the rectal bioavailability is variable, ranging from 30 to 86.7% in various studies, with a high degree of inter-individual variation reported (Steinman et al. 2000; Magdesian 2017; Stein et al. 2018). Evacuation of the rectum is not required prior to rectal administration (Stein et al. 2018). In adult horses, the author recommends 15 mg/kg PO or 20 mg/kg PR q8 h administration for routine use.

Metronidazole is administered to foals through the oral or IV route. Anorexia is apparently less of a concern in neonatal foals (Magdesian 2017). Recommendations for dosing of metronidazole in foals include lower doses and frequency of administration due to high oral bioavailability and a longer half-life in foals as compared to adult horses (Swain et al. 2014; Magdesian 2017). The author recommends metronidazole be used at a dose of 10 mg/kg PO or IV q12 h during the first two weeks of life (Swain et al. 2014; Magdesian 2017).

Metronidazole is used to treat anaerobic infections, including those caused by clostridial bacteria, including clostridial enteritis in foals and horses, both *Clostridium perfringens* and *C. difficile* enteritis/enterocolitis. Tetanus (*Clostridium tetani*) is usually treated with both penicillin and metronidazole.

## Summary of Clinical Use of Antimicrobials in Critically Ill Patients

Sepsis and infections causing critical illness are often best treated with broad-spectrum, intravenous, and bactericidal drugs until culture results are available, when spectrum can be narrowed. Often, once the patient is stabilized, antimicrobials can be changed to the oral route, as opposed to intravenous. Combinations of beta-lactam and aminoglycoside are often the broadest in spectrum. These can include combinations such as gentamicin and penicillin, gentamicin and ampicillin, gentamicin and a first-generation cephalosporin, or gentamicin and ceftiofur for adult horses. In this setting, ceftiofur can be used at low labeled doses (2.2 mg/kg every 24 h) as a drug with Gram-positive spectrum, because it is paired with gentamicin for Gram-negative coverage. For foals, amikacin is often paired with the same beta-lactams, ampicillin, penicillin, or ceftiofur. Amikacin has better Gram-negative and *Staphylococcus* coverage than gentamicin. The most active of these beta-lactam drugs against *Enterococcus* isolates is ampicillin, and because this is an emerging pathogen in foal sepsis, ampicillin has advantages over penicillin and cephalosporins in this regard (Magdesian 2017). Cephalosporins have no activity against enterococci. When enterococci are cultured, then ampicillin should be administered pending susceptibility results. Otherwise, the combination of ceftiofur and gentamicin, or ceftiofur and amikacin, is another option for broad coverage, though this combination provides no enterococcal coverage and only limited anaerobic coverage as compared to ampicillin and amikacin.

When patients are azotemic or oliguric, aminoglycosides should not be administered. For adult horses, enrofloxacin can be used instead of aminoglycosides, providing a similar spectrum. For foals with kidney disease, ceftiofur or other third-generation cephalosporins, such as cefotaxime or ceftazidime, can be used to treat serious Gram-negative infections (Magdesian 2017).

Once foals or horses with critical infections have been stabilized after five to seven days (and as clinically indicated; foals and horses with more severe illness, such as septic arthritis and osteomyelitis often need intravenous antimicrobials for longer periods of time) of the above broad-spectrum IV antimicrobials, an alternative route of administration conducive to treatment at home or on the farm can be considered if the patient is doing well. These can also be the initial antimicrobials for horses with less critical illness. This can include subcutaneous, intramuscular, or oral medications to prolong the course of antimicrobials. Ideally, the choice of antimicrobial would be based on culture and susceptibility data, but if unavailable, there are several choices listed in Tables 31.1–31.5 (Magdesian 2017). For neonatal foals, these options include oral cephalosporins such as cefpodoxime, or ceftiofur which can be administered SC or IM. Other oral choices for foals, with narrower spectrums, include TMS, minocycline/doxycycline, azithromycin, chloramphenicol, and rifampin (Magdesian 2017). In the study by Theelen et al., chloramphenicol was effective in vitro against 81.6% of cultured isolates from septic foals, whereas TMS was effective against 59.6% (Theelen et al. 2019).

After initial IV therapy, critically ill adult horses can be treated with TMS, minocycline/doxycycline, chloramphenicol, enrofloxacin, and/or rifampin depending on the disease process and suspected or confirmed bacterial agents. Ideally the decision should be based on culture whenever possible, but when not available they should be based on the most likely offending bacteria (Table 31.1).

## Anti-inflammatory Medications

### Non-steroidal Anti-inflammatory Drugs (NSAIDs) and Cyclooxygenase (COX) Selectivity

Non-steroidal anti-inflammatory drugs (NSAIDs) primarily work by inhibition of cyclooxygenase (COX) enzyme(s). COX-1 is constitutively expressed in most tissues. Inhibition of the COX-1 isoform is associated with many of the adverse effects noted with the use of NSAIDs including gastrointestinal (GI) ulceration and renal papillary necrosis. Generally, COX-2 is an inducible COX enzyme and associated with pain and inflammation. To maximize anti-inflammatory and analgesic properties while minimizing adverse effects COX-2-selective NSAIDs have been evaluated. Unfortunately, the use of COX-2-selective NSAIDS does not completely mitigate all NSAID-associated risks, as even COX-2 is constitutively expressed in some tissues, such as the kidney. COX-2: COX-1 selectivity ratios are an expression of the COX-2 to COX-1 activity of an NSAID, with higher ratios (>1:1) associated with increased COX-2 specificity. It is important to remember that these ratios are only applicable when the drug is given at the recommended dose – if a COX-2-selective drug is overdosed the selectivity is negatively affected and increased COX-1 binding occurs. Likewise, co-administration of COX-2-selective NSAIDs with non-COX-2-selective NSAIDs eliminates the COX-2 selectivity and increases the likelihood of adverse effects (Foreman and Ruemmler 2011; Kivett et al. 2014; Ziegler et al. 2017). Table 31.9 summarizes commonly used NSAIDs in equine patients.

**Table 31.9** Acetaminophen and non-steroidal anti-inflammatory drugs (NSAIDs).

| Drug | Dose<br>Adults (A)<br>Neonates (N) | Route | Mechanism of action<br>(COX2:COX1<br>selectivity ratio) | Adverse effects | Notes |
|---|---|---|---|---|---|
| Acetaminophen (paracetamol) | A: 20 mg/kg q12 h (Mercer et al. 2020)<br>N: 40 mg/kg PO q12 h, 60 mg/kg PO q24 h | PO | Weak prostaglandin inhibitor; centrally mediated effects (Graham et al. 2013) | Hepatotoxicity in humans | N dosing is based on a pharmacokinetic study (Faivre et al. 2023). Clinical efficacy studies are still lacking. |
| Diclofenac sodium | A: 5-in. strip q12 h<br>N: 1.27 cm strip (7.3 mg) q12 h (Barnett et al. 2017) | Topical | Non-selective NSAID (1 : 1) (Gan 2010) | | Minimal systemic absorption occurs in neonates (Barnett et al. 2017). |
| Dipyrone (metamizole) | A: 30 mg/kg q8 h | IV, IM | Suspected inhibition of central COX-3 (Jasiecka et al. 2014).<br>Inhibition of prostaglandin-dependent and -independent pathways (Jasiecka et al. 2014). | Leukopenia, agranulocytosis and aplastic anemia has been reported in humans (Giorgi et al. 2017). | |
| Firocoxib | A: 0.3 mg/kg loading dose; 0.1 mg/kg q24 h thereafter<br>N: 0.2 mg/kg q24 h* (Davis et al. 2017). | IV, PO | COX-2 selective (200 : 1) (Ziegler et al. 2017) | Gastrointestinal and renal | IV formulation turns catheter extension plastic white (Ziegler et al. 2017)<br>*This is a proposed dose based on a pharmacokinetic study (Davis et al. 2017); safety and efficacy of this dose has not been evaluated in neonates. |
| Flunixin meglumine | A: 0.25–1.1 mg/kg q12 (Semrad et al. 1987).<br>(no more than 2.2 mg/kg/24 h)<br>N: 1.8 mg/kg IV q24 h (Crisman et al. 1996).<br>Donkeys likely have altered PK and require a shorter dosing interval than horses and mules (Coakley et al. 1999). | IV, PO, Transdermal (Knych et al. 2021) | Non-selective NSAID (1 : 1) (Ziegler et al. 2017) | Gastrointestinal and renal (Macallister et al. 1993) | Injectable formulations achieve mean bioavailability of 72% when given PO (Pellegrini-Masini et al. 2004).<br>Flunixin meglumine is licensed for IM use but believed to be associated with increased risk of Clostridial myonecrosis (Peek et al. 2003). |
| Ketoprofen | A: 2.2 mg/kg q24 h<br>N: 3.3 mg/kg* (Wilcke et al. 1998) | IV | COX-1 selective NSAID (0.88 : 1) (Landoni and Lees 1995a, b) | No noted GI and renal adverse effects when administered q8 h for 12 days (Macallister et al. 1993). | Ketoprofen has not demonstrated oral bioavailability in the horse (Landoni and Lees 1995a, b).<br>*Prolonged dosing intervals may be necessary but have not been evaluated in the neonate (Wilcke et al. 1998). |

**Table 31.9** (Continued)

| Drug | Dose<br>Adults (A)<br>Neonates (N) | Route | Mechanism of action<br>(COX2:COX1 selectivity ratio) | Adverse effects | Notes |
|---|---|---|---|---|---|
| Meloxicam | A: 0.6 mg/kg q24 h<br>N: 0.6 mg/kg q 12 hours (Raidal et al. 2013).<br>There are significant differences in pharmacokinetic variables of meloxicam in donkeys vs horses (Sinclair et al. 2006). | IV, PO | COX-2 preferential (3–4 : 1) (Berreta et al. 2005) | Gastrointestinal and renal | Use of meloxicam is extra-label for horses in the United States. |
| Phenylbutazone | A: 2.2–4.4 mg/kg q12–24 h<br>N: 2.2 mg/kg* (Wilcke et al. 1993) | IV, PO | Non-selective NSAID (1 : 1) (Berreta et al. 2005) | Gastrointestinal and renal (Macallister et al. 1993) | *Repeat dosing was not evaluated, but given a reduced ability to eliminate phenylbutazone longer dosing intervals than adults may be warranted (Wilcke et al. 1993). |

## Non-NSAIDs with Anti-inflammatory Effects

Opioids: In addition to centrally mediated analgesic effects, work in non-equine patients supports anti-inflammatory effects of opioids in peripheral tissues (Iwaszkiewicz et al. 2013). Thus, in addition to providing centrally mediated analgesia, opioids may also decrease peripheral inflammation through several mechanisms. Table 31.10 summarizes commonly used opioids in equine patients.

Gabapentin: Gabapentin, a structural analog of $\gamma$-amino butyric acid (GABA), targets the $\alpha_2\delta_1$ subunit of voltage-sensitive calcium channels. In veterinary medicine, gabapentin is frequently used to treat neuropathic pain, provide sedation, and for its anti-epileptic effects. However, gabapentin has also demonstrated anti-inflammatory properties by reduction of pro-inflammatory mediators and upregulation of anti-inflammatory cytokines in several pain models. Current information regarding the use of gabapentin in horses is summarized in Table 31.10.

Lidocaine: The use of lidocaine, as a continuous rate infusion, may help mitigate some of the adverse effects reported with the use of flunixin meglumine on small intestinal healing after ischemic injury, which may in part be due to decreased neutrophil migration into the intestinal tissues (Cook et al. 2009). However, these potential beneficial effects of lidocaine on inflammation in the equine jejunum have been debated (Bauck et al. 2017). Lidocaine, as a continuous rate infusion, is included in Table 31.10

## Immunomodulators

Glucocorticoids (i.e., dexamethasone, prednisolone) and azathioprine are immunomodulators used in veterinary medicine for anti-inflammatory and/or immunosuppressive effects. Glucocorticoids are a class of corticosteroids which can have anti-inflammatory and/or immunosuppressive effects depending on the dose employed (i.e., immunosuppressive effects at higher doses). Commonly used doses for these immunomodulators are provided in Table 31.11.

## Neonatal Dosing

Neonates have several key differences in drug metabolism including alterations in drug-metabolizing enzymes, glomerular filtration rate, renal tubular secretory mechanisms, relative total body water, and differences in plasma protein concentrations (Warner, 1986). Unfortunately, this means that doses (dose, route, and dosing interval) established for adult horses may not be appropriate for neonates. When available, in Tables 31.9 and 31.10, information regarding neonatal doses is provided.

**Table 31.10** Gabapentin, lidocaine, and opioids.

| Drug | Dose and route Adults (A) Neonates (N) | Mechanism of action | Adverse effects | Notes |
|---|---|---|---|---|
| Buprenorphine | A: 0.01 mg/kg IV q8–12 h (Love et al. 2015) 0.005 mg/kg IV, IM q12 h (Davis et al. 2012)<br>N: 10 μg/kg IM* (Risberg et al. 2015) 0.01–0.02 mg/kg IV (Grubb et al. 2019) | Partial μ-receptor agonist | Increased locomotor activity (Love et al. 2015), decreased gastrointestinal motility (Davis et al. 2012), excitation (Davis et al. 2012) | In foals, sublingual administration did not reliably achieve sustained concentrations presumed to provide analgesia in other species (Grubb et al. 2019).<br>*Pharmacokinetics were not performed in this study to suggest a dosing interval. Pharmacokinetics in a separate study (Grubb et al. 2019), suggest a shortened dosing interval compared to adults. |
| Butorphanol | A: 0.1 mg/kg IV (Sellon et al. 2001)<br>17.8 μg/kg, IV followed by 24 μg/kg/h (Sellon et al. 2001) 0.08 mg/kg IM q3 h (Sellon et al. 2009)<br>N: 0.1 mg/kg IV* (McGowan et al. 2013)<br>0.05 mg/kg IV, IM (Arguedas et al. 2008) | μ-receptor agonist κ-receptor antagonist | Single IV injection was associated with ataxia, decreased borborygmi, and defecation (Sellon et al. 2001)<br>In neonates, decreased GI motility, sedation, and increased nursing with no increase in locomotor activity (Arguedas et al. 2008). | *Anti-nociceptor effects were observed at 0.1 mg/kg but not 0.05 mg/kg doses (McGowan et al. 2013). This study did not provide dosing interval information. |
| Fentanyl | A: Transdermal: 2–3 100 μg/h patches (Maxwell et al. 2003; Driessen et al. 2010)<br>N: 2–32 μg/kg IV (Knych et al. 2015) | Full μ-receptor agonist | Adverse effects have not been noted with the use of transdermal fentanyl patches in adult horses.<br>In foals, adverse effects including sedation, muscle rigidity, and head pressing were dose dependent, with increasing side effects occurring at doses ≥8 μg/kg (Knych et al. 2015). | Using matrix fentanyl patches, no difference was found when applied to the abdomen, ventral tail base and metacarpus (Maxwell et al. 2003).<br>An ex vivo study resulted in decreased fentanyl absorption from metacarpal vs thorax or groin skin (Mills and Cross 2007). |
| Gabapentin | 10–120 mg/kg PO q8–12 h (Gold et al. 2020). | Inhibition of excitatory neurotransmitters. | Sedation is possible at high doses (Gold et al. 2020).<br>Hepatocellular injury and chronic kidney disease have been reported in humans. | Analgesic plasma concentrations have not been described in horses. |
| Hydromorphone | A: Epidural: 0.04 mg/kg q4 h (Natalini and Linardi 2006)<br>IV: 0.025–0.08 mg/kg IV q12 h (Reed et al. 2019) | Full μ-receptor agonist | Elevation in heart rate (Reed et al. 2019; Martins et al. 2020) and hypertension (Martins et al. 2020)<br>Increased locomotion, vocalization, and rectal temperature (Reed et al. 2019). | |
| Lidocaine | A: 1.3 mg/kg IV bolus over 15 minutes followed by 0.05 mg/kg/min (IV) | Voltage gaited sodium channel blocker | Lidocaine toxicity, due to inadvertent overdose, can result in collapse, seizures, and death. | Decreased neutrophil migration in ischemic injured small intestine (Cook et al. 2009). |

**Table 31.10** (Continued)

| Drug | Dose and route<br>Adults (A)<br>Neonates (N) | Mechanism of action | Adverse effects | Notes |
|---|---|---|---|---|
| Morphine | A: 0.05–0.5 mg/kg IV q4–6 h (Driessen et al. 2010; Knych et al. 2014)<br>Cervical epidural: 0.1 mg/kg q24 0.05 mg/kg q12 h (Watkins et al. 2021)<br>Caudal epidural: 0.2 mg/kg q24 h (San et al. 2011)<br>0.1 mg/kg q8 h (Mirra et al. 2020) | Full μ-receptor agonist | Decreased GI activity, increased locomotion | |

**Table 31.11** Immunomodulators.

| Drug | Dose and route<br>Adults (A)<br>Neonates (N) | Mechanism of action | Adverse effects | Notes |
|---|---|---|---|---|
| Dexamethasone | 0.05–0.1 mg/kg IV, IM, PO q24 h | Glucocorticoid | Immunosuppression, hepatopathy, muscle wasting<br>Dexamethasone is frequently believed to be associated with the development of laminitis, but this has been questioned by several studies (McGowan et al. 2016; Potter et al. 2019). | Ideally, administer in the morning to coincide with circadian rise and fall of endogenous glucocorticoids |
| Prednisolone | 1–2 mg/kg PO q24 h | Glucocorticoid | Immunosuppression, hepatopathy, muscle wasting<br>Prednisolone is frequently believed to be associated with laminitis, but this has been questioned (Jordan et al. 2017). | Horses are unable to convert prednisone to prednisolone (the active metabolite), thus require administration of prednisolone. |
| Azathioprine | 1.5 mg/kg IV (White et al. 2005)<br>3 mg/kg PO q24 h (White et al. 2005) | Purine synthesis inhibitor | Possible immunosuppression with long-term use (White et al. 2005). | Low oral bioavailability of 1–7% (White et al. 2005). |

## Donkeys and Mules

In comparison to horses, donkeys and mules have several key differences including a higher metabolic rate and cellular water content that can impact the pharmacokinetic and pharmacodynamic properties of drugs (Mendoza et al. 2019). Unfortunately, extrapolation of horse doses to donkey or mule patients can result in either underdosing or overdosing the patient. In general, donkeys and mules tend to require higher doses and/or shorter dosing intervals compared to those established for horses. When available, donkey and mule studies are referenced in Table 31.9. To the author's knowledge, donkey- and mule-specific studies are not available for opioids and gabapentin. The reader is also referred to Chapter 25 for more in-depth information including pharmacology, specific to donkeys and mules.

## References


Adamson, P.J., Wilson, W.D., Hirsh, D.C. et al. (1985). Susceptibility of equine bacterial isolates to antimicrobial agents. |*Am. J. Vet. Res.* 46: 447–450.

Adamson, P.J.W., Wilson, W.D., Baggot, J.D. et al. (1991). Influence of age on the disposition kinetics of chloramphenicol in equine neonates. *Am. J. Vet. Res.* 52: 426–431.

Arguedas, M.G., Hines, M.T., Papich, M.T. et al. (2008). Pharmacokinetics of butorphanol and evaluation of physiologic and behavioral effects after intravenous and intramuscular administration to neonatal foals. *J. Vet. Intern. Med.* 22 (6): 1417–1426.

Baggot, J.D., Love, D.N., Steward, J., and Raus, J. (1988). Bioavailability and disposition kinetics of amoxicillin in neonatal foals. *Equine Vet. J. 120*: 125–127.

Barnett, S.E., Sellon, D.C., Hines, M.T. et al. (2017). Randomized, controlled clinical trial of safety and plasma concentrations of diclofenac in healthy neonatal foals after repeated topical application of 1% diclofenac sodium cream. *Am. J. Vet. Res.* 78 (4): 405–411.

Barrier, K.M.(2016). International surviving sepsis campaign. A clinician's guide (2018). *Crit. Care Nurs. Clin. Noth. Am.* 30: 311–321.

Bauck, A.G., Grosche, A., Morton, A.J. et al. (2017). Effect of lidocaine on inflammation in equine jejunum subjected to manipulation only and remote to intestinal segments subjected to ischemia. *Am. J. Vet. Res.* 78 (8): 977–989.

Berlin, S., Spieckermann, L., Oswald, S. et al. (2016). Pharmacokinetics and pulmonary distribution of clarithromycin and rifampicin after concomitant and consecutive administration in foals. *Mol. Pharm.* 13: 1089–1099.

Berreta, C., Garavaglia, G., and Cavalli, M. (2005). COX-1 and COX-2 inhibition in horse blood by phenylbutazone, flunixin, carprofen and meloxicam: an in vitro analysis. *Pharmacol. Res.* 52 (4): 302–306.

Brewer, B. and Koterba, A. (1990). Bacterial isolates and susceptibility patterns in foals in a neonatal intensive care unit. *Comp. Cont. Ed Pract. Vet.* 12: 1773–1781.

Brown, M.P., Gronwall, R., Kroll, W.R., and Beal, C. (1984). Ampicillin trihydrate in foals: serum concentrations and clearance after a single oral dose. *Equine Vet. J.* 16: 371–373.

Brumbaugh, G.W., Martens, R.J., Knight, H.D., and Martin, M.T. (1983). Pharmacokinetics of chloramphenicol in the neonatal horse. *J. Vet. Pharmacol. Ther.* 6: 219–227.

Bucki, E.P., Giguere, S., Macpherson, M., and Davis, R. (2004). Pharmacokinetics of once-daily amikacin in healthy foals and therapeutic drug monitoring in hospitalized equine neonates. *J. Vet. Intern. Med.* 18: 728–733.

Burrows, G.E., MacAllister, C.G., Ewing, P., Stair, E., and Burrows, S.L. (1992). Rifampin disposition in the horse: effects of repeated dosage of rifampin or phenylbutazone. *J. Vet. Pharmacol. Ther.* 15 (3): 305–308. https://doi.org/10.1111/j.1365-2885.1992.tb01021.x.

Burton, J.A., Giguere, S., and Arnold, R.D. (2015). Pharmacokinetics, pulmonary disposition and tolerability of liposomal gentamicin and free gentamicin in foals. *Eq. Vet. J.* 47: 467–472.

Carrillo, N.A., Giguere, S., Gronwall, R.R. et al. (2005). Disposition of orally administered cefpodoxime proxetil in foals and adult horses and minimum inhibitory concentration of the drug against common bacterial pathogens of horses. *Am. J. Vet. Res.* 66: 30–35.

Coakley, M., Peck, K.E., Taylor, T.S. et al. (1999). Pharmacokinetics of flunixin meglumine in donkeys, mules and horses. *Am. J. Vet. Res.* 11: 1441–1444.

Cole, C. (2015). Basics of antimicrobial therapy for the horse. In: *Equine Pharmacology* (ed. C. Cole, B. Bentz, and L. Maxwell), 16–43. Wiley Blackwell.

Cook, V.L., Shults, J.J., McDowell, M.R. et al. (2009). Anti-inflammatory effects of intravenously administered lidocaine hydrochloride on ischemia-injured jejunum in horses. *Am. J. Vet. Res.* 70 (10): 1259–1268.

Corley, K.T.T. and Hollis, A.R. (2009). Antimicrobial therapy in neonatal foals. *Eq. Vet. Educ.* 21: 436–448.

Crisman, M.V., Wilcke, J.R., and Sams, R.A. (1996). Pharmacokinetics of flunixin meglumine in healthy foals less than twenty-four hours old. *Am. J. Vet. Res.* 57 (12): 1759–1761.

Davenport, C.L., Boston, R.C., and Richardson, D.W. (2001). Effects of enrofloxacin and magnesium deficiency on matrix metabolism in equine articular cartilage. *Am. J. Vet. Res.* 62: 160–166.

Davis, J.L., Messenger, K.M., LaFevers, D.H. et al. (2012). Pharmacokinetics of intravenous and intramuscular buprenorphine in horses. *J. Vet. Pharmacol. Ther.* 25 (1): 52–58.

Davis, J.L., Crisman, M.V., Kvaternick, V. et al. (2017). Pharmacokinetics of firocoxib after intravenous administration of multiple consecutive doses in neonatal foals. *J. Vet. Pharmacol. Ther.* 40: e23–w29.

Driessen, B., Bauquier, S.H., and Zarucco, L. (2010). Neuropathic pain management in chronic laminitis. *Vet. Clin. North Am. Eq. Pract.* 26 (2): 315–337.

Duffee, N.E., Stang, B.E., and Schaeffer, D.J. (1997). The pharmacokinetics of cefadroxil over a range of oral doses and animal ages in the foal. *J. Vet. Pharmacol. Ther.* 20: 427–433.

Estell, K., Knych, H.K., Patel, T. et al. (2020). Pharmacokinetics of multiple doses of chloramphenicol in fed adult horses. *Vet. J.* 257: 105446. https://doi.org/10.1016/j.tvjl.2020.105446. Epub 2020 Feb 21. PMID: 32546355.

Faivre, C., Wong, D.M., Villarino, N.F. et al. (2023). Pharmacokinetics of multiple oral doses of acetaminophen in equine neonates. *Am. J. Vet. Res.* 84 (9): ajvr.23.04.0079.

Fielding, C.L. and Magdesian, K.G. (2015). Sepsis and septic shock in the equine neonate. *Vet. Clin. Equine Pract.* 31: 483–496.

Fontenot, R.L., Langston, V.C., Zimmerman, J.A. et al. (2018). Meropenem synovial fluid concentrations after intravenous regional limb perfusion in horses. *Vet. Surg.* 47: 852–860.

Foreman, J.H. and Ruemmler, R. (2011). Phenylbutazone and flunixin meglumine used singly or in combination in experimental lameness in horses. *Equine Vet. J. Suppl.* 40: 12–17.

Gan, T.J. (2010). Diclofenac: an update on its mechanism of action and safety profile. *Curr. Med. Res. Opin.* 26 (7): 1715–1731.

Gardner, S.Y. and Papich, M.G. (2001). Comparison of cefepime pharmacokinetics in neonatal foals and adult dogs. *J. Vet. Pharmacol. Ther.* 24: 187–192.

Giguere, S., Burton, A.J., Berghaus, L.J., and Haspel, A.D. (2016). Comparative pharmacokinetics of minocycline in foals and adult horses. *J. Vet. Pharmacol. Ther.* 40: 335–341.

Giorgi, M., Aupanun, S., Lee, H.K. et al. (2017). Pharmacokinetic profiles of the active metamizole metabolites in healthy horses. *J. Vet. Pharmacol. Ther.* 40 (2): 165–171.

Gold, J.R., Grubb, T.L., Green, S. et al. (2020). Plasma disposition of gabapentin after the intragastric administration of escalating doses to adult horses. *J. Vet. Intern. Med.* 34 (2): 933–940.

Graham, G.G., Davies, M.J., Day, R.O. et al. (2013). The model pharmacology of paracetamol: therapeutic actions, mechanisms of action, metabolism, toxicity and recent pharmacological. *Inflammopharmacology* 21: 201–232.

Green, S.L. and Conlon, P.D. (1993). Clinical pharmacokinetics of amikacin in hypoxic premature foals. *Eq. Vet. J.* 25: 276–280.

Green, S.L., Conlon, P.D., and Mama, K. (1992). Effects of hypoxia and azotaemia on the pharmacokinetics of amikacin in neonatal foals. *Eq. Vet. J.* 24: 475–479.

Grubb, T.L., Kurkowski, D., Sellon, D.C. et al. (2019). Pharmacokinetics and physiologic/behavioral effects of buprenorphine administered sublingually and intravenously to neonatal foals. *J. Vet. Pharmacol. Ther.* 41 (1): 26–36.

Henson, S. and Barton, M. (2001). Bacterial isolates and antibiotic susceptibility patterns from septicemic neonatal foals: one 15 year retrospective study (1986–2000). In: *Proceedings of the Dorothy Havemeyer Foundation Neonatal Septicemia Workshop*, vol. 3, 350–352. 2001.

Hewson, J., Johnson, R., Arroyo, L.G. et al. (2013). Comparison of continuous infusion with intermittent bolus administration of cefotaxime on blood and cavity fluid drug concentrations in neonatal foals. *J. Vet. Pharmacol. Ther.* 36: 68–77.

Hong, L.T., Downes, K.J., FakhriRavari, A. et al. (2023). International consensus recommendations for the use of prolonged-infusion beta-lactam antibiotics: endorsed by the American college of clinical pharmacy, British society for antimicrobial chemotherapy, cystic fibrosis foundation, European society of clinical microbiology and infectious diseases, infectious diseases society of America, society of critical care medicine, and society of infectious diseases pharmacists: an executive summary. *Pharmacotherapy* 43: 736–739.

Horspool, L.J., Sarasola, P., and McKellar. (1992). Disposition of ampicillin sodium in horses, ponies and donkeys after intravenous administration. *Equine Vet. J.* 11: 59–61.

Iwaszkiewicz, K.S., Schneider, J.J., and Hua, S. (2013). Targeting peripheral opioid receptors to promote analgesic and anti-inflammatory actions. *Front. Pharmacol.* 4: 132.

Jacks, S.S., Giguere, S., and Nguyen, A. (2003). In vitro susceptibilities of *Rhodococcus equi* and other common equine pathogens to azithromycin, clarithromycin, and 20 other antimicrobials. *Antimicrob. Agents Chemother.* 47: 1742–1745.

Jasiecka, A., Maslanka, T., and Jaraszewski, J.J. (2014). Pharmacological characteristics of metamizole. *Pol. J. Vet. Sci.* 17 (1): 207–214.

Jordan, V.J., Ireland, J.L., and Rendle, D.I. (2017). Dose oral prednisolone treatment increase the incidence of acute laminitis? *Equine Vet. J.* 49 (1): 19–25.

Kivett, L., Taintor, J., and Wright, J. (2014). Evaluation of the safety of a combination of oral administration of phenylbutazone and firocoxib in horses. *J. Vet. Pharmacol. Ther.* 37 (4): 413–416.

Knych, H.K., Steffey, E.P., and McKemie, D.S. (2014). Preliminary pharmacokinetics of morphine and its major metabolites following intravenous administration of four doses to horses. *J. Vet. Pharmacol. Ther.* 37 (4): 374–381.

Knych, H.K., Steffey, E.P., Casbeer, H.C., and Mitchell, M.M. (2015). Disposition, behavioural and physiological effects of escalating doses of intravenously administered fentanyl to young horses. *Equine Vet. J.* 47 (5): 592–598.

Knych, H.K., Arthur, R.M., Gretler, S.R. et al. (2021). Pharmacokinetics of transdermal flunixin meglumine and effects on biomarkers of inflammation in horses. *J. Vet. Pharmacol. Ther.* 44 (5): 745–753.

Landoni, M.F. and Lees, P. (1995a). Comparison of the anti-inflammatory actions of flunixin and ketoprofen in horses applying PK/PD modelling. *Equine Vet. J.* 27: 247–256.

Landoni, M.F. and Lees, P. (1995b). Influence of formulation on the pharmacokinetics and bioavailability of racemic ketoprofen in horses. *J. Vet. Pharmacol. Ther.* 18: 446–450.

Love, E., Pelligand, L., Taylor, P.M. et al. (2015). Pharmacokinetic-pharmacodynamic modelling of intravenous buprenorphine in conscious horses. *Vet. Anesth. Analg.* 42: 17–29.

Macallister, C.G., Morgan, S.J., Borne, A.T., and Pollet, R.A. (1993). Comparison of adverse effects of PBZ, flunixin meglumine and ketoprofen in horses. *J. Am. Vet. Med. Assoc.* 202: 71–77.

Magdesian, K.G. (2015). Foals are not just mini horses. In: *Equine Pharmacology* (ed. C. Cole, B. Bentz, and L. Maxwell), 99–117. Wiley Blackwell.

Magdesian, K.G. (2017). Antimicrobial pharmacology for the neonatal foal. *Vet. Clin. North Am. Equine Pract.* 33: 47–65.

Magdesian, K.G., Wilson, W.D., and Mihalyi, J. (2004). Pharmacokinetics of a high dose of amikacin administered at extended intervals to neonatal foals. *Am. J. Vet. Res.* 65: 473–479.

Marsh, P.S. and Palmer, J.E. (2001). Bacterial isolates from blood and their susceptibility patterns in critically ill foals: 543 cases (1991-1998). *J. Am. Vet. Med. Assoc.* 218: 1608–1610.

Martins, F.C., Keating, S.C.J., Clark-Price, S.C. et al. (2020). Pharmacokinetics and pharmacodynamics or hydromorphone hydrochloride in healthy horses. *Vet. Anaesth. Analg.* 47 (4): 509–517.

Maxwell, L.K., Thomasy, S.M., Slovis, N., and Kollias-Baker, C. (2003). Pharmacokinetics of fentanyl following intravenous and transdermal administration in horses. *Equine Vet. J.* 35 (5): 484–490.

McGowan, K.T., Elfenbein, J.R., Robertson, S.A., and Sanchez, L.C. (2013). Effect of butorphanol on thermal nociceptive threshold in healthy pony foals. *Equine Vet. J.* 45: 503–506.

McGowan, C., Cooper, D., and Ireland, J. (2016). No evidence that therapeutic systemic corticosteroid administration is associated with laminitis in adult horses without underlying endocrine or severe systemic disease. *Vet Evidence* 1.

Mendoza, F.J., Perez-Ecija, A., and Toribio, R.E. (2019). Clinical pharmacology in donkeys and mules. *Vet. Clin. North Am. Equine Pract.* 35 (3): 589–606.

Mercer, M.A., McKenzie, H.C., Davis, J.L. et al. (2020). Pharmacokinetics and safety of repeated oral dosing of acetaminophen in adult horses. *Equine Vet. J.* 52 (1): 120–125.

Meyer, S., Giguere, S., Rodriquez, R. et al. (2009). Pharmacokinetics of intravenous ceftiofur sodium and concentration in body fluids of foals. *J. Vet. Pharmacol. Ther.* 32: 309–316.

Mills, P.C. and Cross, S.E. (2007). Regional differences in transdermal penetration of fentanyl through equine skin. *Res. Vet. Sci.* 82 (2): 252–256.

Mirra, A., Birras, J., Diez, B.S., and Spadavecchia, C. (2020). Morphine plasmatic concentration in a pregnant mare and its foal after long term epidural administration. *BMC Vet. Res.* 16 (1): 19.

Natalini, C.C. and Linardi, R.L. (2006). Analgesic effects of epidural administration of hydromorphone in horses. *Am. J. Vet. Res.* 67: 11–15.

Olsen, L., Ingvast-Larsson, C., Brostrom, H. et al. (2017). Clinical signs and etiology of adverse reactions to procaine benzylpenicillin and sodium/potassium benzylpenicillin in horses. *J. Vet. Pharmacol. Ther.* 30: 201–207.

Orsini, J.A., Soma, L.R., Rourke, J.E., and Park, M. (1985). Pharmacokinetics of amikacin in the horse following intravenous and intramuscular administration. *J. Vet. Pharmacol. Ther.* 8: 194–201.

Orsini, J.A., Moate, P.J., Boston, R.C. et al. (2005). Pharmacokinetics of imipenem-cilastatin following intravenous administration to healthy adult horses. *J. Vet. Pharmacol. Ther.* 28: 3550361.

Osthoff, M., Siegemund, M., Gianmarco, B. et al. (2016). Prolonged administration of β-lactam antibiotics – a comprehensive review and critical appraisal. *Swiss Med. Wkly.* 146: w14368.

Peek, S.F., Semrad, S.D., and Perkins, G.A. (2003). Clostridial myonecrosis in horses (37 cases 1985-2000). *Equine Vet. J.* 35 (1): 86–92.

Pellegrini-Masini, A., Poppenga, R.H., and Sweeney, R.W. (2004). Disposition of flunixin meglumine injectable preparation administered orally to healthy horses. *J. Vet. Pharmacol. Ther.* 27: 183–186.

Potter, K., Stevens, K., and Menzies-Gow, N. (2019). Prevalence of risk factors for acute laminitis in horses treated with corticosteroids. *Vet. Rec.* 185 (3): 82.

Puskarich, M.A., Trzeciak, S., Shapiro, N.I. et al. (2011). Association between timing of antibiotic administration and mortality from septic shock in patients treated with a quantitative resuscitation protocol. *Crit. Care Med.* 39: 2066–2071.

Pusterla, N., Hall, T.L., Wetzlich, S.E. et al. (2016). Pharmacokinetic parameters for single- and multi-dose regiments for subcutaneous administration of a high-dose ceftiofur crystalline-free acid to neonatal foals. *J. Vet. Pharmacol. Ther.* 40: 88–91.

Quin, J.D. (1989). The nephrotoxicity of cephalosporins. *Adverse Drug React. Acute Poisoning Rev.* 8: 63–72.

Raidal, S.L., Edwards, S., Pippia, J. et al. (2013). Pharmacokinetics and safety of oral administration of meloxicam to foals. *J. Vet. Intern. Med.* 27: 300–307.

Reed, R., Barletta, M., Mitchell, K. et al. (2019). The pharmacokinetic and pharmacodynamics of intravenous hydromorphone in horses. *Vet. Anaesth. Analg.* 46 (3): 395–404.

Riond, J.L., Riviere, J.E., Duckett, W.M. et al. (1992). Cardiovascular effect and fatalities associated with intravenous administration of doxycycline to horses and ponies. *Equine Vet. J.* 24: 41–45.

Risberg, A.I., Spadavecchia, C., Ranheim, B. et al. (2015). Antinociceptive effect of buprenorphine and evaluation of the nociceptive withdrawal reflex in foals. *Vet. Anaesth. Analg.* 42 (3): 329–338.

Rohdich, N., Zschiesche, E., Heckeroth, A. et al. (2009). Treatment of septicaemia and severe bacterial infections in foals with a new cefquinome formulation: a field study. *Dtsch. Tierarztl. Wochenschr.* 116: 316–320.

Samitz, E.M., Jang, S.S., and Hirsh, D.C. (1996). In vitro susceptibilities of selected obligate anaerobic bacteria obtained from bovine and equine sources. *J. Vet. Diagn. Invest.* 8: 121–123.

San, H., Martin-Flores, M., Sants, L.C.P. et al. (2011). Effects of epidural morphine on gastrointestinal transit in unmedicated horses. *Vet. Anaesth. Analg.* 38 (2): 121–126.

Sanchez, L.C., Giguere, S., and Lester, G.D. (2008). Factors associated with survival of neonatal foals with bacteremia and racing performance of surviving thoroughbreds: 423 cases (1982-2007). *J. Am. Vet. Med. Assoc.* 233: 1446–1452.

Sellon, D.C., Monroe, V.L., Roberts, M.C., and Papich, M.G. (2001). Pharmacokinetics and adverse effects of butorphanol administered by single intravenous injection or continuous intravenous infusion in horses. *Am. J. Vet. Res.* 62 (2): 183–189.

Sellon, D.C., Papich, M.G., Palmer, L., and Remund, B. (2009). Pharmacokinetics of butorphanol in horses after intramuscular injection. *J. Vet. Pharmacol. Ther.* 32 (1): 62–65.

Semrad, S.D., Hardee, G.E., Hardee, M.M., and Moore, J.N. (1987). Low dose flunixin meglumine: effects on eicosanoid production and clinical signs induced by experimental endotoxaemia in horses. *Equine Vet. J.* 19 (3): 201–206.

Sinclair, M.D., Mealey, K.L., Mathews, N.S. et al. (2006). Comparative pharmacokinetics of meloxicam in clinically normal horses and donkeys. *Pharmacology* 67 (6): 1082–1085.

Slovis, N.M., Wilson, W.D., Stanley, S.D. et al. (2006). Comparative pharmacokinetics and bioavailability of ceftiofur in horses after intravenous, intramuscular, and subcutaneous administration. *Proc. Am. Assoc. Equine Pract.* 52: 329–330.

Stein, F., Gilliam, L., Davis, J., and Taylor, J. (2018). Rectal administration of metronidazole with and without rectal evacuation prior to use in horses. *J. Vet. Pharmacol. Ther.* 41: 838–842.

Steinman, A., Gips, M., Lavy, E. et al. (2000). Pharmacokinetics of metronidazole in horses after intravenous, rectal and oral administration. *J. Vet. Pharmacol. Ther.* 23: 353–357.

Stieler Stewart, A.L., Sanchez, L.C., and Mallicote, M.F. (2016). Macrolide-induced hyperthermia in foals: role of impaired sweat responses. *Eq. Vet. J.* 48: 590–594.

Swain, E.A., Magdesian, K.G., Kass, P.H. et al. (2014). Pharmacokinetics of metronidazole in foals: influence of age within the neonatal period. *J. Vet. Pharmacol. Ther.* 38: 227–234.

Theelen, M.J.P., Wilson, W.D., Byrne, B.A. et al. (2019). Initial antimicrobial treatment of foals with sepsis: do our choices make a difference? *Vet. J.* 243: 74–76.

Trachsel, D.S., Calloe, K., Rgensen, E.J. et al. (2021). Evaluation of electrocardiographic repolarization parameters after administration of trimethoprim-sulfadiazine, detomidine, or their combination in horses. *Am. J. Vet. Res.* 82: 207–217.

Venner, M., Astheimer, K., Lammer, M., and Giguere, S. (2013). Efficacy of mass antimicrobial treatment of foals with subclinical pulmonary abscesses associated with Rhodococcus equi. *J. Vet. Intern. Med.* 27: 171–176.

Vivrette, S., Cowgill, L.D., Pascoe, J. et al. (1993). Hemodialysis for treatment of ox tetracycline-induced acute renal failure in a neonatal foal. *J. Am. Vet. Med. Assoc.* 203: 105–107.

Vivrette, S.L., Bostian, A., Bermingham, E., and Papich, M.G. (2001). Quinolone-induced arthropathy in neonatal foals. *Proceedings of the 47th Annual Convention of the American Association of Equine Practitioners*, Denver CO, 24–28 November 2001, pp.376–377.

Warner, A. (1986). Drug use in the neonate: interrelationships of pharmacokinetics, toxicity and biochemical maturity. *Clin. Chem.* 32: 721–727.

Watkins, A.R., Hopster, K., Levin, D., and Hurcombe, S.D. (2021). Cervical epidural spinal analgesia for acute management of severe unilateral forelimb lameness: case report. *Front. Vet. Sci.* 8: 749713.

Wearn, J.M.G., Davis, J.L., Hodgson, D.R. et al. (2012). Pharmacokinetics of a continuous rate infusion of ceftiofur sodium in normal foals. *J. Vet. Pharmacol. Ther.* https://doi.org/10.1111/j. 1365-2885.2012.01403.x.

Wetzig, M., Venner, M., and Giguere, S. (2020). Efficacy of the combination of doxycycline and azithromycin for the treatment of foals with mild to moderate bronchopneumonia. *Equine Vet. J.* 52: 613–619.

White, S.D., Maxwell, L.K., Szabo, N.J. et al. (2005). Pharmacokinetics of azathioprine following single-dose intravenous and oral administration and effects of azathioprine following chronic oral administration in horses. *Am. J. Vet. Res.* 66 (9): 1578–1583.

Wilcke, J.R., Crisman, M.V., Sams, R.A., and Gerken, D.F. (1993). Pharmacokinetics of phenylbutazone in neonatal foals. *Am. J. Vet. Res.* 54 (12): 2064–2067.

Wilcke, J.R., Crisman, M.V., Scarratt, W.K., and Sams, R.A. (1998). Pharmacokinetics of ketoprofen in healthy foals less than twenty-four hours old. *Am. J. Vet. Res.* 59: 290–292.

Willis, A.T., Magdesian, K.G., Byrne, B.A., and Edman, J.M. (2019). Enterococcus infections in foals. *Vet. J.* 248: 42–47.

Womble, A., Giguere, S., and Lee, E.A. (2007). Pharmacokinetics of oral doxycycline and concentrations in body fluids and bronchoalveolar cells of foals. *J. Vet. Pharmacol. Ther.* 30: 187–193.

Ziegler, A., Fogle, C., and Blikslager, A. (2017). Update on the use of cyclooxygenase 2-selective nonsteroidal anti-inflammatory drugs in horses. *J. Am. Vet. Med. Assoc.* 250 (11): 1271–1274.

# 32

# Nutritional Support for the Emergent Patient

*Meri Stratton*[1,2]

[1] *Clinical Veterinary Nutritionist and President, All Creatures Veterinary Nutrition Consulting, Inc., Fairfield, CA, USA*
[2] *Large Animal Medicine, College of Veterinary Medicine, University of Georgia, Athens, GA, USA*

## Nutritional Support of Adult Horses

*Nutritional support should be provided to equine patients* that are unwilling or unable to consume enough feed to meet *50% of their resting energy ($DE_{rest}$) and/or 50% of their maintenance protein requirements ($CP_{maint}$) for more than two days* (Table 32.1). The type of treatment will depend upon several factors (Box 32.1).

The *type of dietary treatment* depends on where the horse is being managed (field or hospital), whether or not the horse can tolerate enteral feeding, the severity of a horse's malnourishment (determined with an assessment of body weight [BW] and body condition score [BCS]), and the expected duration that nutritional support will be needed (days to a week or more).

Currently there are no standard protocols for refeeding an equine patient in the post-operative period, regardless of the type of surgery. *Clinicians and surgeons differ in their refeeding protocols (duration after surgery, type and volume of feed offered) for post-operative colic patients based on the type of surgery, the location of the intestinal lesion, and other patient-related factors* (Lawson et al. 2021). Most post-operative colic patients will benefit from some nutritional support provided in dextrose-supplemented IV fluids especially during the time when the horse is maintained on a nothing per os (NPO) or a no-food order. Horses recovering from colic surgery that cannot be refed even small volumes (two to four pounds) of feed (hay pellets, hay chop, alfalfa leaves, low non-structural carbohydrate (NSC) complete feed pellets) within two days after colic surgery may benefit from parenteral nutrition (PN).

*Few cases require emergent nutritional treatment.* Supportive therapy with nutrition can be started on a patient at any time, but initiation of treatment is usually reserved until after a patient has been stabilized with medical or surgical care.

## Patient Assessment

*The first step in selecting a nutrition plan begins with a patient assessment.* This often is done during the initial case work up with diagnostic tests, development of a problem list, and determining a diagnosis. Cases with acute trauma, medical emergencies, and horses requiring surgical intervention should be managed with appropriate medical or surgical care prior to initiating nutritional therapy. *After patient stabilization, a plan for dietary support can be integrated into the horse's treatment plan.*

*Patient factors to evaluate before starting nutritional therapy*

1) Body weight (BW)
   a) A weigh scale should be used if available, but weight can be estimated with a weight tape or with morphometric measurements
   b) Nutrient requirements are calculated based on BW

*Emergency Triage of the Horse*, First Edition. Edited by Rolfe M. Radcliffe and Jamie J. Kopper.

Companion website: www.wiley.com/go/radcliffe/triage

**Table 32.1** Recommended energy ranges and daily protein intake for supplemental nutrition in adult horses.

| Horse weight (pounds) | Horse weight (kg) | $DE_{rest}$ (kcal/day)[a] *minimum* suggested daily energy intake | $DE_{maint}$ (kcal/day)[b] *maximum* suggested daily energy intake | Protein ($CP_{maint}$) (grams/day)[c] |
|---|---|---|---|---|
| 440 | 200 | 5,175 | 6,660 | 252 |
| 495 | 225 | 5,700 | 7,493 | 284 |
| 550 | 250 | 6,225 | 8,325 | 315 |
| 605 | 275 | 6,750 | 9,158 | 347 |
| 660 | 300 | 7,275 | 9,990 | 378 |
| 715 | 325 | 7,800 | 10,823 | 410 |
| 770 | 350 | 8,325 | 11,655 | 441 |
| 825 | 375 | 8,850 | 12,488 | 473 |
| 880 | 400 | 9,375 | 13,320 | 504 |
| 935 | 425 | 9,900 | 14,153 | 536 |
| 990 | 450 | 10,425 | 14,985 | 567 |
| 1,045 | 475 | 10,950 | 15,818 | 599 |
| 1,100 | 500 | 11,475 | 16,650 | 630 |
| 1,155 | 525 | 12,000 | 17,483 | 662 |
| 1,210 | 550 | 12,525 | 18,315 | 693 |
| 1,265 | 575 | 13,050 | 19,148 | 725 |
| 1,320 | 600 | 13,575 | 19,980 | 756 |
| 1,375 | 625 | 14,100 | 20,813 | 788 |
| 1,430 | 650 | 14,625 | 21,645 | 819 |

[a] $DE_{rest}$ (kcal/day) = 975 + 21 (BW in kg) For horses that weigh 125–856 kg
[b] $DE_{maint}$ (kcal/day) = 33.3 × (BW in kg) For horses that weigh 200–900 kg
[c] Crude Protein ($CP_{maint}$) (grams/day) = 1.26 × (BW in kg)
*Source:* National Research Council (2007).

**Box 32.1 Nutritional Support for the Equine Patient**

1) The type of dietary treatment depends on *where the horse is being managed* (field or hospital)
2) Whether or not the horse can *tolerate enteral feeding*
3) The *severity of a horse's malnourishment* (determined with an assessment of body weight [BW] and body condition score [BCS])
4) The expected *duration that nutritional support* will be needed (days to a week or more).

2) Body condition score (BCS)
   a) An important factor to guide the need for supplemental nutritional support
   b) Based on a 1–9/9 scale with 1 being emaciated and 9 being obese
      i) *Horses with a BCS of 1–3* have minimal endogenous protein and fat stores and require nutritional support early in their disease management
         - Severely malnourished horses may be at risk of developing refeeding syndrome and must be managed with a gradual refeeding protocol (see section on Refeeding Starved Horses)
         - BCS appears to be associated with survival in the 100-day period after refeeding with horses with a BCS of 1 and 1.5 less likely to survive (Schneider et al. 2021) (see Section on refeeding starved horses)
         - Energy calculations for malnourished horses should be made using the $DE_{rest}$ equation with a goal of providing 50% of the calculated daily $DE_{rest}$ at the horse's current BW
           - Adjust calorie intake during the recovery period as the horse gains weight

- Protein calculations can be made using the $CP_{maint}$ equation with a goal of providing 50% of the daily protein requirement at the horse's current BW
  - Increase dietary protein to 75–100% $CP_{maint}$ to promote recovery of organs and muscle mass gain during the recovery period

ii) *Horses with a BCS of 4–6* have an ideal BCS and supplemental nutrition can be delayed for 24–36 h after disease onset
- Calculate energy requirements between $DE_{rest}$ and $DE_{maint}$
- Calculate protein requirements using $CP_{maint}$ as long as there are no contraindications to dietary protein intake (renal or hepatic disease)
- Adjust calorie intake to $DE_{maint}$ once the horse's condition is stabilized if supplemental nutritional support is still required

iii) *Horses with a BCS of 7–9* have an elevated BCS, excess lipid deposits, and may be affected by insulin dysregulation
- Increased risk of dyslipidemia if nutritional therapy is delayed
- Calculate energy requirements between $DE_{rest}$ and $DE_{maint}$
- Calculate protein requirements using $CP_{maint}$ as long as there are no contraindications to dietary protein intake (renal or hepatic disease)

3) Ability and willingness of the horse to eat
   a) Dental disease may prevent adequate feed intake
   b) Pain from a jaw fracture, oral foreign body, tooth root abscess, or other facial trauma may decrease voluntary feed intake
   c) Neurologic disease may make food prehension, chewing, or swallowing difficult or impossible
   d) Systemic disease may result in the production of inflammatory mediators that decrease appetite and should be considered as a cause of inappetence
4) Intestinal tract function
   a) Influences the type of nutritional support
      i) Horses with choke, reflux, intestinal ileus, an impaction, or another complication that prevents oral food intake should be treated with intravenous (IV) nutrition with dextrose-supplemented fluids or PN
   b) Is the horse displaying active signs of colic?
      i) If immediate nutritional support is necessary, consider dextrose-supplemented fluids while establishing a treatment plan
   c) Is the horse recovering from abdominal surgery?
      i) Time of refeeding in the post-operative period is largely clinician dependent based on the type of surgery and the severity of intestinal lesions (Lawson et al. 2021)
      ii) Nutrition support in the early post-operative period can be provided with dextrose-supplemented fluids
5) Laboratory analyses
   a) Unless a horse is severely malnourished, most biochemical test results will remain within normal ranges
      i) Serum triglyceride (TG) should be measured before starting PN therapy
      ii) Serum TG may increase to concentrations up to 500 mg/dL in otherwise healthy horses that are deprived of feed
      iii) Serum TG concentrations >500 mg/dL may be measured in horses with prolonged feed deprivation, horses with increased energy requirements (pregnant, lactating mares) that do not eat for >48 h, or horses with excess fat deposition that do not eat for >24 h
      iv) Refeeding with supplemental nutrition often results in a normalization of elevated serum TGs
   b) Electrolyte abnormalities can be managed in IV fluids or using enteral fluids

## Choices for Nutritional Support

There are *four options for nutritional support of the adult horse* (Box 32.2). They are listed below along with a notation about whether they can be administered to patients in the field (F) or hospital (H).

Cost is always a consideration in managing patients with supplemental nutrition; however, this factor should not limit patient care or treatment decisions. Offering even a portion of a horse's daily calorie needs using one of the four options listed above will limit protein calorie malnutrition and muscle catabolism and will promote recovery.

**Box 32.2 Options for Nutritional Support of the Adult Horse**

1) *Offer highly digestible palatable feed*
   a) Should have a low concentration (≤20%) of non-structural carbohydrates (NSC as sugar and starch) (F, H)
      i) Ex: Hay pellets, hay chop, commercial low NSC complete feeds, and many complete "senior" feeds that have a concentration of NSC <20% (ideally <15% NSC)
2) *Provide dextrose-supplemented intravenous fluids* (F if a catheter can be safely maintained and monitored, H)
3) *Treat with assisted enteral feeding* (AEF) using a liquid enteral diet or feed slurry (F, H)
4) *Administer IV PN as partial parenteral nutrition* (PPN) or total parenteral nutrition (TPN) (H only)

## Offer Highly Digestible Palatable Feed

If a horse is willing and able to eat, nutritional therapy can be provided with a low NSC feed that is also highly digestible. A "cafeteria-style" approach to offering a variety of palatable feeds can be used, but the volume of all feeds offered should be weighed, so feed intake can be monitored. Wet pellet mashes can also be offered, but soaked feed becomes spoiled and rancid quickly and should not be left in a stall for more than two hours.

Cafeteria feeding is a reasonable option for horses that have a 4–6/9 BCS and are expected to start eating in one to two days. If a horse does not consume enough feed to meet 50% of their $DE_{rest}$ or $CP_{maint}$ requirements during that one-to-two-day trial period, then another form of nutritional support should be initiated.

*How to feed*

1) Select a hay pellet, hay chop or commercial complete feed that has a low-to-moderate concentration (≤20%) of NSC
   a) Three to four types of feed can be offered at a time
2) Weigh the feed (0.25–1 pound volume of each feed)
3) Offer the feed every four to six hours
   a) Remove the feed after the allotted time and weigh the feed
   b) Record the volume of feed that was consumed so you can calculate the horse's energy intake
   c) Calculate a daily energy intake for the horse and compare that number with the daily energy requirements ($DE_{rest}$, $DE_{maint}$) listed in Table 32.1 for the horse's current BW
   d) If the energy intake is <50% of the horse's daily $DE_{rest}$ for more than two days, choose another form of nutritional support
4) If the horse eats enough feed to meet ≥50% $DE_{rest}$ gradually increase the volume of feed offered during each feeding over the next three to four days (continue to offer feed every four to six hours)
5) Once the horse has recovered, gradually return the horse to their regular ration over a period of 7–14 days

## Provide Dextrose-Supplemented Intravenous Fluids

If an equine patient has an IV catheter or if a catheter can be placed and maintained safely, and if the patient is a candidate for IV fluid therapy, then dextrose can be added to the patient's fluids to provide a supplemental source of energy.

Dextrose-supplemented fluids are a reasonable option for horses that would benefit from some caloric support as an interim therapy before they are offered feed (like a post-operative colic patient) or before more substantial nutritional therapy is started with PN or a liquid enteral diet. Dextrose provides a percentage of a horse's daily $DE_{rest}$ (see case example below) but does not provide protein, electrolytes, or other essential nutrients, resulting in a patient that will be protein and nutrient malnourished.

A final dextrose solution that ranges in concentration from 2.5 to 5.0% is recommended to decrease complications from hyperglycemia. Horses with insulin dysregulation and/or hyperglycemia may be able to tolerate a 2.5% dextrose solution, but in these patients, frequent monitoring of serum glucose and insulin is recommended, making treatment of these patients in the field more complicated. Electrolytes can be added to the IV fluids, but appropriate concentrations should be determined by monitoring and adjusting the patient's electrolyte supplementation during the treatment period. Fluid infusion should be managed as a continuous rate infusion (CRI), but dextrose-supplemented fluids can also be administered in smaller volumes as a fluid bolus.

*Calories provided in dextrose solutions of different concentrations*

2.5% dextrose = 0.085 kcal/mL
5% dextrose = 0.17 kcal/mL
10% dextrose = 0.34 kcal/mL
*50% dextrose = 1.7 kcal/mL
*50% dextrose is too concentrated to use in an IV infusion without further dilution

*How to administer*
*Equipment needed for dextrose-supplemented IV fluids*

1) Intravenous catheter
2) Fluid infusion line
3) System to hang and administer the IV fluids
4) Fluids
5) Dextrose
6) Syringe and needle (if needed to transfer the dextrose into the IV fluid bag)

*Formulating A dextrose-supplemented IV fluid treatment plan* (Box 32.3)

1) Determine the concentration of dextrose you want for your patient
   a) A conservative approach is to begin with a 2.5% dextrose solution to provide calories while monitoring the patient to evaluate tolerance of the dextrose
      i) Goal:
         - Make a 2.5% dextrose solution in a 5 L (5,000 mL) bag of fluids using 50% dextrose
      ii) How to Formulate:
         - Calculate the volume of 50% dextrose to add to a bag of fluids to create the desired final dextrose solution concentration using the equation: C1V1 = C2V2
         - C1 = 50%; C2 = 2.5%; V2 = 5,000 mL
         - Solve for V1 (the volume of 50% dextrose you need to add to the 5,000 mL fluid bag)

$$V1 = \frac{C2 * V2}{C1} = \frac{(2.5)*(5{,}000)}{50} = 250 \text{ mL of } 50\% \text{ dextrose}$$

2) Make the 2.5% dextrose solution and infuse the fluids at the desired infusion rate (CRI is recommended)
   a) Monitor daily caloric intake from dextrose using the $DE_{rest}$ calculation (Table 32.1)
   b) Monitor daily fluid therapy rate
3) Patient monitoring
   a) PE/TPR
   b) Catheter site

| **Box 32.3 Case Example: Dextrose Supplementation** |
|---|
| 450 kg horse<br>IV fluid rate of 50 mL/kg/day (22.5 L/day)<br><br>Treat with IV fluids that contain 2.5% dextrose (see calculation above)<br>0.085 kcal dextrose/mL × 22,500 mL = 1,913 kcal<br><br>Total kcal administered = 1,913 kcal<br>Daily resting energy requirement (Table 32.1):<br><br>$DE_{rest}$ (kcal/day) = 975 + 21 (BW in kg) = 10,425 kcal<br><br>$DE_{rest}$ from dextrose = 1,913 kcal/10,425 kcal = 18% |

    c) Blood glucose
        i) Adjust the concentration of dextrose as needed to prevent hyperglycemia
    d) Hydration
4) Potential complications
    a) Catheter site infection
        i) Monitor for signs of infection (swelling, pain, erythema, discharge)
            - If catheter site sepsis develops, remove the catheter (submit tip for culture/sensitivity testing) and place another catheter in a different location (lateral thoracic, cephalic) to resume treatment if necessary
    b) Hyperglycemia
        i) Decrease dextrose concentration in IV fluids or discontinue treatment
    c) Overhydration
        i) Manage fluid balance as necessary
5) Returning the horse to a regular ration
    a) Attempts can be made to offer highly digestible, low NSC (≤20%) feed throughout dextrose-supplemented IV fluid treatment
    b) See guidelines for "How to Feed" under "Offer Highly Digestible Palatable Feed"
        i) If the horse consumes less than 50% of their $DE_{rest}$ or $CP_{maint}$ for more than two days consider offering a liquid enteral diet with AEF or IV nutrition as PPN or TPN

## Treat with Assisted Enteral Feeding (AEF) Using a Liquid Enteral Diet or Feed Slurry

*Candidates for AEF can tolerate the placement of an NG tube, and they do not have any gastrointestinal tract disease that would prevent enteral feeding.* Equine patients with gastric reflux, intestinal ileus or obstruction, nasal, esophageal or pharyngeal disease, or that are recumbent are not good candidates for AEF, and for these patients nutritional support should instead be started with either dextrose-supplemented fluids or PN.

AEF can be used to provide part or all of a horse's daily $DE_{rest}$, $DE_{maint}$, and $CP_{maint}$ and can be administered to horses of any BW and BCS as long as NG tube placement and enteral feeding is not contraindicated. If a horse tolerates AEF, this form of nutritional therapy can be provided for days to weeks at a time. Prolonged therapy with AEF ideally is managed with a small-diameter NG tube and a minimally viscous liquid slurry.

*Commercial equine enteral diets designed for NG tube administration* like WellSolve® W/G Well-Gel® (Purina Mills) or Enteral Immunonutrition Formula (Platinum Performance) are single-formulation treatment options. If these products are not available, then a pelleted feed that has a low concentration of NSC (≤20%) should be used. Hay pellets (grass, alfalfa, or a blend of the two) are easily acquired, are low in NSC, and can be fed alone or can be combined with vitamins, minerals, and other ingredients to provide more of a complete ration if they will be fed for more than a week. Commercial equine pelleted feeds are appropriate if they are complete feeds, which means that they do not need to be fed with any additional forage (grass or hay). Most senior feeds are complete feeds and can be used for AEF, but not all equine senior feeds have a low concentration of NSC. Some equine feed options for AEF are listed in Table 32.2.

*When can AEF be used?*

1) Horses that can tolerate NG tube feedings that do not have oral, pharyngeal, esophageal, or gastric disease that would prevent NG tube placement
2) Horses that are standing or that can maintain sternal recumbency
3) Horses that do not have contraindications for gastric feeding and can be fed enterally

*When should AEF not be used?*

1) Horses that cannot tolerate placement of an NG tube
2) Horses with gastric reflux, intestinal ileus, or when enteral feeding is contraindicated
3) Horses that are recumbent

*How to administer*

*Equipment needed for enteral diet administration*

1) Feed (commercial equine enteral diet, hay pellet, equine commercial complete pelleted feed)
2) Water

**Table 32.2** Equine feeds suitable for use in a liquid enteral diet.

| Feed | Digestible energy (kcal/pound) | Crude protein (%) | Crude protein (grams/pound) | Crude fat (%) | NSC (%) | Amount in pounds to meet $DE_{rest}$ for a 990 pound horse | Amount in pounds to meet $DE_{maint}$ for a 990 pound horse |
|---|---|---|---|---|---|---|---|
| Equine Senior®[a, c] | 1,225 | 14 | 64 | 5.5 | 19 | 8.5 | 12.2 |
| Triple Crown Senior[a, d] | 1,546 | 14 | 64 | 10 | 14.7 | 6.7 | 9.7 |
| LMF Senior Low Carb[a, e] | 1,400 | 13 | 59 | 7 | 10 | 7.4 | 10.7 |
| Nutrena SafeChoice® Senior[a, f] | 1,275 | 14 | 64 | 8 | 20 | 8.2 | 11.8 |
| Alfalfa Hay Pellets[b] | 1,089 | 15 | 68 | 2.4 | 10.4 | 9.6 | 13.8 |
| Grass Hay Pellets[b] | 1,011 | 10 | 45 | 2.9 | 13.1 | 10.3 | 14.8 |

[a] As fed, Manufacturer Analysis.
[b] As fed, Estimated Values.
[c] Purina Mills, St. Louis, MO, USA.
[d] Triple Crown Nutrition, Wayzata, MN, USA.
[e] LMF Feeds, Inc., Weiser, ID, USA.
[f] Nutrena (Cargill, Inc.), Wayzata, MD, USA.

3) NG tube (small diameter for long-term administration ≥ seven days)
   a) Mila 18 Fr, 250 cm feeding tube
4) Fluid pump for oral fluid administration
5) Bucket
6) Muzzle (if the NG tube will remain in place between feedings)
7) Blender (if needed to liquefy the diet)
8) Carboy or infusion container if the liquid diet will be administered using slow gravity flow

*Formulating the enteral feeding plan* (Figure 32.1)

1) Select a feed (Table 32.2)
   a) Equine commercial enteral feed
   b) Plain hay pellets
   c) Equine commercial complete feed with ≤20% NSC
   d) Horses with insulin dysregulation or laminitis
      i) Select a very low NSC feed (≤15%)
2) Determine the amount of feed that should be provided daily using the $DE_{rest}$ and $DE_{maint}$ equations (Table 32.1)
   a) Feed at the $DE_{rest}$ for malnourished or undernourished horses to reduce possible metabolic complications during the initial refeeding period
      i) $DE_{rest}$ (kcal/day) = 975 + 21 (BW in kg)
   b) Calculate the volume of feed that should be administered daily
      i) See Table 32.2 for calorie and protein content of common feeds
   c) After meeting energy requirements calculate the amount of protein in the diet and compare to the horse's $CP_{maint}$ (Table 32.1)
      i) Protein intake can be above requirements in most horses
      ii) Do not feed excess protein to horses with renal or hepatic disease
         - A grass hay pellet may be the option with the lowest concentration of protein
   d) Divide the total amount of daily feed volume by the number of meals to determine the volume of feed in each meal
      i) Smaller meal volumes administered multiple times throughout the day is ideal
      ii) If the diet can only be administered one to two times a day, decrease the daily volume of feed by 30–50%, so the meal size is appropriate for the horse

1. Initial body weight (kg) ________ kg
2. Stall resting energy requirement: $DE_{rest}$ (kcal/day) = 975 + 21 (BW in kg) ________ kcal
3. Maintenance energy requirement: $DE_{maint}$ (kcal/day) = 33.3 (BW in kg) ________ kcal
4. Protein requirement: Crude Protein ($CP_{maint}$) (grams/day) = 1.26 (BW in kg) ________ g
5. Fluid requirements for maintenance: 60 mL/kg/day ________ mL
6. Total kcal required/day (estimate between **2** and **3** calculated above) ________ kcal
7. Select a product for use (see Table 2 or other feed)
8. Calculate the daily volume of feed needed based on calculations from 2 and 3 above

**Example:** 450 kg horse

1. Initial body weight (kg) 450 kg
2. Stall resting energy requirement: $DE_{rest}$ (kcal/day) = 975 + 21 (BW in kg) 10,425 kcal
3. Minimum Maintenance energy requirement: $DE_{maint}$ (kcal/day) = 33.3 (BW in kg) 14,985 kcal
4. Protein requirement: Crude Protein ($CP_{maint}$) (g/day) = 1.26 (BW in kg) 567 g
5. Fluid requirements for maintenance: 60 mL/kg/day 27,000 mL
6. Total kcal required/day (estimate between **2** and **3** calculated above) 12,000 kcal

A. Meet Energy Requirements
   a. Grass pellets (1011 kcal/pound from Table 2)
   b. 12,000 kcal × 1 pound/1011 kcal = 11.86 rounded to 12 pounds of grass pellets/day

B. Calculate Protein Intake
   a. Grass pellets (10% crude protein, 45 grams of protein/pound from Table 2)
   b. 12 pounds grass pellets × 45 grams crude protein/pound grass pellets = 540 grams crude protein
   c. Slightly less protein in the diet than is required
      i. May result in slight protein malnutrition
      ii. Could supplement the diet with additional protein using 1–1.5 pounds of alfalfa pellets or plain unflavored whey protein isolate

C. How to Feed
   a. Divide the12 pounds of grass hay pellets into 4–6 meals daily
      i. 12 pounds grass pellets/4 meals = 3 pounds grass pellets/feeding
   b. Determine the volume of water to add to the pellets for soaking
      i. Daily fluid requirements can often be met with the liquid diet slurry
      For example, use 6 liters of water to soak the pellets for each meal (6 L x 4 meals = 24 L of water in the enteral diet)
      ii. An additional 0.5–1 liter of water will be needed to flush and clear the NG tube after diet infusion (0.5 L x 4 = 2 L of flush water)
   c. Soak the pellets in water for 30-60 minutes
      i. Do not soak for more than 60 minutes because the pellets may spoil and become rancid.
   d. If necessary, blend the pellets in a heavy duty blender to make a feed slurry that can be administered through the NG tube
   e. Follow diet administration instructions
   f. Diet total summary:
      Total water administered with the diet/day = 26 L/day
      Total kcal/day = 12,000 kcal
      Total grams of protein/day = 540 grams/day

Electrolytes, trace minerals and vitamins can be supplemented in the diet if plain hay pellets are used if the diet will be fed for more than 1 week. Additional nutrients are not necessary if a commercial complete equine feed is used for the liquid enteral diet.

**Figure 32.1** Assisted enteral feeding worksheet for adult horses.

e) Note: The diet should be introduced, and the volume increased slowly over two to three days
   i) Gradually introduce the volume of the diet to the horse
      - Day 1: Feed 1/4–1/3 of the total daily diet volume
      - Day 2: Feed 1/2–2/3 of the total daily diet volume
      - Day 3+: Feed the total daily diet volume

3) Prepare the meal
   a) Add 1–2 L of warm or cool water to the feed pellets
      i) Measure the volume of water that you add to each meal and include this water volume in the total daily fluid intake volume for your patient
   b) Soak the pellets until the mixture becomes a liquid slurry
      i) If needed, use a durable commercial home-use blender (Vitamix, Blendtec) to liquefy the pellets
      ii) Add more water to achieve a diet consistency that you can pump into the NG tube used for diet infusion
         - Ensure that the total volume of the meal is within an appropriate volume for the horse
   c) Test the diet slurry with the NG tube and fluid pump before placing the NG tube in the horse to make sure the diet will flow easily through the tube
4) Administer the meal
   a) Place the NG tube and ensure proper placement in the stomach
   b) Check for gastric reflux
      i) If >2 L gastric reflux, delay feeding for one hour then check again for reflux
         - If the horse has persistent gastric reflux consider an alternate form of nutritional support with either dextrose-supplemented IV fluids, or PN
   c) Pump in the diet slowly or allow the diet to flow in by gravity feed
      i) Continually stir or mix the diet to prevent separation of the feed from the water
   d) Flush with 0.25–0.5L of water after the diet has been administered
      i) Include this volume of flush water in the patient's daily total fluid intake
   e) Clear the tube of water, then cap off and remove the tube. If the tube is suitable for continuous placement, cap off the tube, and secure it on a safe halter.
      i) A muzzle like the Best Friend Deluxe Grazing Muzzle (Intrepid Internation, New Holland, PA) can be placed on the horse to help prevent them from removing the NG tube
5) Monitor for complications
   a) PE/TPR
      i) Should remain within normal limits
   b) BW/BCS
      i) Stabilization is seen as a treatment success
   c) Nasal discharge
      i) An abrupt increase in nasal discharge is abnormal
         - If observed, workup as necessary for respiratory disease
         - Perform an upper airway endoscopy to evaluate the integrity of the nasopharynx
   d) Digital pulses
      i) Laminitis is not an expected complication
      ii) Workup as necessary
   e) Fecal production
      i) Self-limiting diarrhea frequently develops
      ii) Monitor for signs of worsening diarrhea and dehydration
      iii) Workup as necessary
   f) PCV/TS
      i) Monitor the total volume of water infused with the diet and flush volume
      ii) Overhydration is usually not a complication
   g) Serum electrolytes
      i) Ensure that the horse does not develop complications from refeeding syndrome
      ii) Supplement with electrolytes in the diet and/or in intravenous fluids, if necessary
6) Returning the horse to a regular ration
   a) Provide a small volume (0.25–0.33 pounds) of a highly digestible, highly palatable feed that is low in NSC (≤20%) before the liquid meal is administered
      i) If the horse shows interest in eating, skip one meal treatment and measure the volume of feed the horse consumes voluntarily

- If voluntary feed intake is estimated to be close to 50% of their $DE_{rest}$ over a 24-h period, discontinue half of the scheduled meals on day one of voluntary feed intake and offer a weighed volume of feed instead. If voluntary feed intake continues then on day two, discontinue AEF administration and feed measured volumes of appropriate feed
- If the horse consumes less than 50% of their $DE_{rest}$ or $CP_{maint}$ for more than two days consider alternate forms of nutritional support including
  - Dextrose-supplemented IV fluids
  - Returning the horse to the liquid enteral diet
  - IV nutrition with PPN or TPN

## Administer Parenteral Nutrition as PPN or TPN

PN includes both *PPN* which is a mixture of amino acids and dextrose, and *TPN* which includes amino acids, dextrose, lipids, and often vitamins and minerals.

*Candidates for PN are horses that are hospitalized* and that either cannot tolerate enteral nutrition, or that require additional nutritional support beyond what is achieved by treatment with dextrose-supplemented IV fluids. This includes horses with gastrointestinal ileus, post-op surgical cases that will be withheld from enteral nutrition for a period of time (>three days), and horses that cannot tolerate placement of an NG tube (oral, nasal, pharyngeal, esophageal disease). Because PN infusion requires a dedicated fluid line and administration with a CRI, treatment of horses in any field setting is impractical and contraindicated. It is rare to refer an equine patient solely for PN therapy, but if a patient cannot consume 50% of their daily $DE_{rest}$ or $CP_{maint}$, and there is a desire from an owner to support the horse with nutrition therapy, then referral to a clinic that has the resources to administer PN should be considered.

The cost of PN therapy is often thought to be prohibitive; however, a hospitalized horse that is treated with even a portion of their daily caloric and protein requirements in a PPN or TPN solution will benefit from the nutritional support during the recovery and convalescent period.

*When can PN be used?*

1) Horses that cannot be treated with enteral nutrition due to a disease process (cannot tolerate NG tube placement, intestinal ileus, post-operative colic)
2) Horses that are underconditioned (BCS $\leq$ 3) where there is an expected three to five day delay in refeeding that would benefit from nutritional support
3) Horses that are overconditioned and when nutritional support is required to reduce complications from hyperlipemia and hepatic lipidosis (lipid-free PN formula)
4) Horses that are hospitalized

*When should PN not be used?*

1) Horses managed in a field or farm setting
2) Horses that cannot tolerate placement of an IV catheter

*How to formulate and administer a PN feeding plan* (Figure 32.2)
*Equipment needed for parenteral diet administration*

1) Intravenous catheter (long term, double or triple lumen strongly recommended to maintain a dedicated PN infusion port)
2) IV fluid line with extension sets
3) Fluid infusion pump
4) PN formulation
   a) Commercial pre-made PN formulation (CLINIMIX, CLINIMIX E (Baxter))
      i) 2.75–6% Amino Acid without or with Electrolytes in 5% Dextrose
   b) If making the PN formulation on-site
      i) PN admixture bag
         a) Not recommended but a sterile glass administration bottle or sterile carboy can be used
      ii) Amino Acids (Travasol 10% (Baxter), TrophAmine® 10% (BBraun))

*Patient Information*

1. Initial body weight (kg) ______________ kg
2. Stall resting energy requirement: $DE_{rest}$ (kcal/day) = 975 + 21 (BW in kg) ______________ kcal
3. Maintenance energy requirement: $DE_{maint}$ (kcal/day) = 33.3 (BW in kg) ______________ kcal
4. Protein requirement: Crude protein ($CP_{maint}$) (grams/day) = 1.26 (BW in kg) ______________ g
5. Fluid requirements for maintenance: 60 mL/kg/day ______________ mL

**Parenteral Nutrition Formulation**

6. Total kcal required/day (estimate between **2** and **3** calculated above) ______________ kcal
7. Calculate volume of 10% amino acids required to meet protein requirement (from **4**)
   Protein (grams) × 1 mL/0.1 grams protein for a 10% amino acid solution ______________ mL
8. Calorie contribution from 10% amino acid solution (from **7**)
   4 kcal/g protein × grams of protein in solution ______________ kcal
9. Total kcal required/day (from **6**) minus total kcal provided by AA (from **8**) ______________ kcal
   * *The caloric contribution from protein can be omitted from the following calculations, if desired*
10. Determine amount of lipid required to meet 20–70% of the remaining energy requirements
    10% lipid solution contains 1 kcal/mL; 20% lipid solution contains 2 kcal/mL
    Ex: If providing 50% of remaining energy requirements with 10% lipid:
    (kcal (from **9**) × 0.5) × 1 mL/1 kcal (substitute 0.5 mL/1 kcal if using 20% lipid) ______________ mL
11. Calculate remaining energy requirements to be provided by 50% dextrose
    Ex: Providing 50% of calories with dextrose: (kcal (from **9**) × 0.5) × 1 mL/1.7 kcal ______________ mL
12. Add 1–2 mL of B vitamin complex/L ______________ mL
13. Add up to 5 mL of trace minerals/day ______________ mL
14. Determine the total volume of the PN solution (**7+ 10 + 11 + 12 + 13**) ______________ mL
15. Determine the rate of PN infusion for a 24-hour period: mL (from **14**)/24 ________ mL/hour
16. Calculate the calorie:nitrogen ratio for the PN solution
    Total kcal from PN solution (from **6**)/(total g of protein/6.25) ______________
17. Calculate osmolarity of the solution

| | | | | |
|---|---|---|---|---|
| 10% Amino acid | ________ mL | (from **7**) | × 0.840 mOsm/mL = | ________ mOsm |
| 10% Lipid | ________ mL | (from **10**) | × 0.276 mOsm/mL = | ________ mOsm |
| 50% dextrose | ________ mL | (from **11**) | × 2.550 mOsm/mL = | ________ mOsm |
| | ________ Total mL | | + | ________ Total mOsm |

PN solution mOsm/L = Total mOsm/Total mL × 1000 mL/L ______________ mOsm/L

* An 8.5% amino acid solution with electrolytes contains 0.85 g protein/mL and 1.045–1.444 mOsm/mL

**Figure 32.2** Parenteral nutrition worksheet for adult horses.

- 0.4 kcal/mL for 10% amino acid solution
  - 0.1 g protein/mL of solution for 10% amino acid solution
- 0.34 kcal/mL for 8.5% amino acid solution
  - 0.085 g protein/mL of solution for 8.5% amino acid solution

iii) Dextrose
- 1.7 kcal/mL for 50% dextrose
- Limit the volume of dextrose in solutions for horses with insulin dysregulation or horses with hyperglycemia

iv) Lipid (20% CLINOLIPID (Baxter), Nutrilipid® 20% (BBraun))
- 1 kcal/mL (10% lipid); 2 kcal/mL (20% lipid)
- Limit lipid to ≤60% of the non-protein calories in the formulation
- Measure serum TGs prior to lipid use in TPN
  - Reduce or eliminate lipid from the TPN formulation in horses with TG > 500 mg/dL

- v) Vitamins (INFUVITE (Baxter))
  - Consider vitamin use if the PN will be administered for more than five days
- c) Fluid transfer sets or sterile syringes and needles
  - i) EXACTAMIX compounding bag and Three Lead Parenteral Nutrition Transfer Set (Baxter)
  - ii) EVA Gravity Mixing Container, three-lead Vented Transfer Set (B. Braun)
- d) Laminar flow hood, clean surgical suite or other clean area

*Preparing the solution*

1) Compounding agencies to make the PN formula
   - a) Human hospital pharmacies
   - b) Central Admixture Pharmacy Services (CAPS®) (www.capspharmacy.com)
   - c) Coram® CVS Specialty® Infusion Services
2) In-house
   - a) Mix aseptically (laminar flow hood, sterile prep area; wear gloves, gown, mask)
   - b) Prepare admixture bag, glass vial, or other PN compounding container
   - c) Prepare all ingredients by wiping the top of each bottle with a sterile alcohol pad
   - d) Use a separate infusion line for all ingredients
   - e) Add the dextrose and protein solutions first
   - f) Gently mix the ingredients as they flow into the bag
   - g) *Add the lipid solution last*
   - h) Add any supplemental nutrients (vitamins, minerals) to the solution after all macronutrients have been added and mixed together
   - i) Check for compatibility of all additives before adding and mixing
3) The base formula of dextrose, amino acids, and lipids can be stored in the refrigerator for 24 h, and at room temperature for 24 h
4) Electrolyte supplementation should be made in maintenance IV fluids to prevent unwanted loss of the PN formulation if abrupt changes need to be made based on serum electrolyte concentrations
5) Check for incompatibilities of the PN ingredients with medications and IV fluid additives especially when the PN is not administered through a dedicated catheter port

*PN administration guidelines*

1) All PN formulations (PPN and TPN) must be gradually introduced and gradually discontinued after a steady rate of infusion has been reached
2) A new PN infusion line should be used each time a new bag or new PN container is used
3) The PN infusion line (running from the bag to the IV infusion port) is a closed system and *cannot be broken*. If there is a break in the line a new bag or container must be used to maintain sterility of the PN formulation and reduce the risk of PN-related sepsis
   - a) Day 1: Administer 25–33% of the total PPN or TPN volume
     - i) Monitoring
       - HCT/TP, blood glucose, hydration status and PE parameters
       - If the patient is stable after 8–12 h, increase the rate by 1–3 mL/h based on body size
   - b) Day 2: Administer 50–66% of the total PPN or TPN volume
     - i) Monitoring
       - HCT/TP, blood glucose, hydration status, and PE parameters
       - If the patient is stable after day 2, increase the rate by 1–3 mL/h
   - c) Day 3: Administer 75–100% of the total PPN or TPN volume
     - i) Monitoring
       - HCT/TP, blood glucose, hydration status and PE parameters
       - If the patient is stable after day three and they are at 75% of their total daily infusion rate, increase the rate by 1–3 mL/h to 100% of the daily infusion rate on day four
   - d) *Maintenance IV fluid therapy should be adjusted to account for additional fluid infused with the PPN or TPN to prevent overhydration*

*Monitor for complications*

1) Follow the monitoring guidelines under AEF but note the following differences
   a) Catheter site
      i) Evaluate for signs of infection (swelling, pain, erythema, discharge)
         - If catheter site sepsis develops, remove the catheter (submit tip for culture/sensitivity testing) and place another catheter in a different location (lateral thoracic, cephalic) to resume treatment
   b) Nasal discharge
      i) No increase in nasal discharge or increase in respiratory rate is expected
      ii) If observed, workup as necessary for respiratory disease and rule out pulmonary edema
   c) Fecal production
      i) Self-limiting diarrhea frequently develops
      ii) Scant manure production is not uncommon
      iii) Monitor for signs of worsening diarrhea and dehydration
      iv) Workup as necessary
   d) PCV/TS
      i) Monitor every 12–24 h until stabilized
         - Adjust IV fluid therapy to prevent overhydration
   e) Serum electrolytes
      i) Ensure that the horse does not develop complications from refeeding syndrome
      ii) Supplement with electrolytes in IV fluids as necessary
   f) Blood glucose/urine glucose
      i) Monitor every 12–24 h until stabilized
      ii) If hyperglycemia develops, decrease infusion rate by 30%
         - If hyperglycemia persists, reformulate the PN solution with a lower concentration of dextrose
   g) Serum TGs
      i) Monitor every 12–24 h until stabilized
      ii) Discontinue TPN infusion for 20 minutes prior to sampling to allow time for the lipid to clear from the blood
      iii) If hypertriglyceridemia develops, decrease infusion rate by 30%
      iv) If hypertriglyceridemia persists, reformulate the PN solution with a lower concentration of lipids or omit the lipid ingredient from the TPN recipe
2) Returning the horse to a regular ration
   a) Once the horse can be offered feed, provide a small volume (0.25–0.33 pounds) of a highly digestible, highly palatable feed that is low in NSC ($\leq$20%)
      i) If the horse shows interest in eating, and if there are no gastrointestinal complications that develop (e.g., ileus, reflux, colic) then offer another small meal (0.25–0.33 pounds) in six to eight hours
      ii) If voluntary feed intake continues without complications over a 24-h period, then on day two increase the volume of feed offered to 0.33–0.5 pounds every 6–8 h
      iii) Once the horse is consuming close to 50% of their $DE_{rest}$ over a two-day period, gradually decrease the rate of PN infusion by 1–3 mL/h
         - PN infusion can be discontinued once it has been decreased to 25–33% of the total PN volume
      iv) If the horse cannot tolerate enteral nutrition or if they consume less than 50% of their $DE_{rest}$ or $CP_{maint}$ for more than two days continue the PN solution and manage the complicating factors that limit enteral feed intake
      v) Horses can be transitioned to AEN while they are being treated with PN

## Special Cases: Feeding the Starved Horse

Equine starvation cases are some of the most challenging cases that practitioners encounter, both from an emotional standpoint and from a medical management perspective. Malnutrition resulting in an excessively low BW and BCS can develop from a systemic disease that may not have been diagnosed at an initial examination (chronic renal or hepatic failure, internal abscessation, parasitism, severe dental disease), or it can be the result of inadequate calorie, protein, and essential nutrient intake due to poor feed quality, and/or an inadequate intake of feed.

## Evaluation

Initial diagnostic tests for a malnourished horse include a complete physical examination (including an examination for dental disease), blood work (complete blood count and serum biochemistry panel), and fecal parasite testing (Main et al. 2022). Dental disease may limit forage intake due to pain or mechanical complications with chewing. Joint disease may limit a horse's ability to graze or to access feed and water. The BCS of the horse can be used to help guide the prognosis for recovery with extreme emaciation (BCS 1 or 1.5) being associated with a lower likelihood of survival (Schneider et al. 2021).

A complete diet history is essential. Document the types and volumes of all feed and supplements that are offered. Include nutrient testing of all forages (pasture and hay), grains, and commercial feeds. Analyze the water source(s) to identify contaminants. Review the feeding protocols for the horse and/or herd feeding management. Herd dominance dynamics may result in one or a few horses losing access to adequate feed volumes.

## Dietary Management

Malnourished horses, like many other species, can experience the effects of refeeding syndrome when feed is first reintroduced (Witham and Stull 1998). Metabolic abnormalities including hypokalemia, hypomagnesemia, hypophosphatemia, and glucose dysregulation can develop along with alterations in cardiac and neurologic function if feed or high concentrations of dietary sugar and starch are introduced too quickly. This may result in a worsening of the horse's condition, and in severe cases, death. Blood work and clinical status can be monitored if diagnostics are available, but many rescue organizations may not be able to afford additional diagnostic tests during the first few days to weeks of refeeding.

The following refeeding protocol can be used by rescue groups and clinics to help guide nutritional care for a malnourished horse during the first one to two months of therapy (Box 32.4). Good-quality forage (alfalfa or grass hay) should be fed, although alfalfa hay is preferred. Water should be offered free choice. Hay volumes should be adjusted based on the size of the horse. Appropriate nursing care (adequate shelter, deep bedding, blankets, etc.) is also an essential part of case management.

### Box 32.4 Case Example: Malnourished Horse Refeeding Plan

Adult horse, BW = 345 kg, BCS = 2/9

1) Days 1–3
   a) 1–1.5 pounds alfalfa or grass hay six times/day
2) Days 4–7
   a) 2–2.5 pounds alfalfa or grass hay six times/day
3) Days 8–11
   a) 3–3.5 pounds alfalfa or grass hay four to six times/day
4) Days 12–15
   a) 4–4.5 pounds alfalfa or grass hay four to six times/day
5) Day 16 and beyond
   a) Free choice alfalfa or grass hay
   b) If enterolithiasis is regionally present, do not feed more than 50% alfalfa hay in the total ration volume

A plain salt block can be offered after three to four weeks.

A plain vitamin and mineral supplement can be added after three to four weeks.

Grain, concentrate feeds, and feeds with >20% NSC should not be fed for two months after refeeding.

A commercial complete feed can be offered after 30 days, but the product should be low in NSC (≤20%). Additional mineral and vitamin supplements may not be necessary if a complete feed is used.

### Prosecuting Starvation Cases: The Veterinarian's Role

When horses have been denied adequate nutrition, owners may be prosecuted for animal cruelty and veterinarians are often involved in the legal process providing evidence about the physical condition of the horses and about the nutritional management on the property (see Chapter 35). Physical examination findings, blood work analyses, necessary diagnostic tests, and feed and water samples form the basis of evidence collection. It is essential to maintain accurate documentation with objective measurements and photos (as allowed), to support case prosecution if necessary. Veterinarians are encouraged to access resources to mentally and emotionally process these cases.

## Nutritional Support of Foals

Supplemental nutrition complements the medical or surgical management of a sick foal. Foals that are unable to nurse or that cannot tolerate enteral feeding develop protein calorie malnutrition rapidly and should be treated with supplemental nutrition within 6–12 h after their feed intake is compromised. With such foals, dextrose-supplemented intravenous fluid alone does not provide adequate calories, protein, or other nutrients to support a sick foal, and should not be used without additional nutritional support (Paradis 2001).

Assessment of the neonatal foal is reviewed in Chapter 20. Along with the routine foal physical examination and appropriate laboratory tests for neonates or older foals, it is important to run a serum TG to help evaluate the safety of supplemental nutrition especially when a PN formulation will be used (Myers et al. 2009).

## Foals That Require Nutritional Support

*Three groups of foals may require supplemental nutrition* (Box 32.5). The choice of treatment depends on the health of the foal and where the foal is managed, either in the *field* (*F*) or in a *hospital* (*H*).

### The Healthy Neonatal Foal That Cannot Consume Enough Milk Because of Complications with the Mare

Foals that have a strong suckle reflex and that can tolerate enteral feeds but that cannot nurse directly from a mare require supplemental nutrition that can be provided by a veterinarian, owner, or caretaker. Mare's milk is the best option for supplemental nutrition but may not be available. A commercial foal milk replacer is a good substitution for mare's milk and can be used to support the growth of a foal until weaning. Multi-species milk replacers do not provide adequate long-term nutrition for a foal but can be used for a limited time (three to five days). Goat's milk can also be used as a substitute for mare's milk for one to three days; however, the nutrient profile is not the same as mare's milk, and some foals will develop constipation while consuming goat's milk. In an emergency when no other milk replacer is available, 2% cow's milk supplemented with 20 g dextrose per liter of milk can also be used but is only suitable for a few days until a foal milk replacer is available.

**Box 32.5 Indications for Nutritional Support in the Foal**

1) *The healthy neonatal foal that cannot consume enough milk because of complications with the mare* (e.g., death, illness, inadequate milk production, foal rejection). *(F, H)*
   a) Mare's milk or a foal milk replacer offered through a bottle or pan is appropriate unless a foal does not consume enough milk to meet at least 10% of their BW (see group 2)
2) *The foal that is unable to voluntarily or safely consume enough milk to meet nutrient requirements but can tolerate enteral feeds. (F, H)*
   a) Placement of an NG tube and AEF with mare's milk or a foal milk replacer is appropriate if the foal can tolerate enteral nutrition
3) *The critically ill foal that cannot nurse or tolerate enteral feeds for >24 h due to systemic complications from respiratory, GI, neurologic, or other disease. (H only)*
   a) PN is required to provide calories, protein, and other essential nutrients until the foal can be fed enterally

It is ideal to gradually transition a foal on to a new diet. Begin by feeding at 10% of the foal's BW in milk daily (a 50 kg foal would be fed a total of 5 L of milk daily, divided into multiple meals). If the milk is tolerated, gradually increase the volume of milk over two to four days until the foal is consuming 20% BW daily.

When a foal is first offered a milk replacer, it is best to use a bottle because the foal will be familiar with nursing from the mare's udder. Long-term bottle feeding should be avoided because it can result in poor behavior as the foal grows, and because bottle feeding is labor intensive. Training a foal to drink from a bucket or pan is ideal for orphan foals; however, it can take some foals up to one to two weeks to adapt to drinking from a pan. Never skip or withhold a meal from a foal when trying to train the foal to drink from a bucket or pan. Instead, train the foal by offering a bucket or pan for a few minutes before a scheduled meal is provided from a bottle.

***Never syringe feed a foal***

*How to feed*

1) *Evaluate the foal's suckle reflex*
   a) Only foals with a strong suckle reflex can be fed from a bottle (an 8-ounce infant bottle can be used for neonatal foals)
      i) Bottle feeding is a short-term option until a foal can be trained to drink from a bucket or a pan, or is fostered to a nurse mare
   b) A foal that has a weak or questionable suckle, a foal that cannot hold up its head, a foal that has an abnormal neurologic status, or a foal that cannot consume an adequate volume of milk voluntarily should be fed through an NG tube (see group 2)
2) *Select the diet* (listed in order of preference)
   a) Graft a foal onto a nurse mare if one is available
   b) Feed with a commercial foal milk replacer
      i) Purina® or Land O' Lakes Mare's Match® (Land O' Lakes)
      ii) Mare's Milk Plus® (MARS Horsecare)
   c) Feed with a multi-species livestock milk replacer (option for three to five days)
      i) Land O Lakes® ProNurse® Multi-Species Milk Replacer
   d) Feed pasteurized goat's milk (option for one to three days)
   e) Feed pasteurized 2% cow's milk (option for one to two days)
      i) When feeding cow's milk ONLY feed 2% milk
      ii) Prepare the milk by adding 20 g of dextrose to each liter of 2% cow's milk to provide a carbohydrate concentration that is closer to mare's milk
      iii) Do NOT add other carbohydrates (sugar, honey) because they are not digestible by foals
3) Determine the *volume of milk* to feed daily
   a) Day 1
      i) Start by feeding the foal at 10% BW daily
         - For growth and weight gain, a higher daily volume of milk is needed
      ii) A sick foal or a foal with reduced GI motility can be started at a lower volume of milk (2.5–7.5% BW)
   b) Day 2
      i) If the foal tolerates milk at a volume of 10% BW then increase the volume to 15% BW daily
   c) Day 3
      i) If the foal tolerates milk at a volume of 15% BW then increase the volume to 20% BW daily
      ii) Most foals will grow at an appropriate weight when they consume a foal milk replacer at 20% BW daily
         - If a foal grows too quickly at the 20% BW/day volume, decrease the daily volume to 15–17% BW and recheck the foal's weight and growth over two to four weeks
         - A growth chart can be made using the 2007 Horse NRC guidelines for weight gain for growing foals (https://webassets.nationalacademies.org/nrh/)
4) Decide on a *feeding schedule*
   a) Neonatal foals (within the first week of life) should be fed every hour if possible
   b) Foals between one and six weeks of age should be fed every two hours
   c) Foals >six weeks of age can be fed every three to six hours gradually decreasing the frequency of meals as the foal grows

  d) Calculate the volume of milk that will be provided at each feeding to make sure the volume is not too much for the foal
    i) For example: A 65 kg foal that is fed at 20% BW will be fed
       $65\,kg \times 0.2 = 13\,L$ of milk daily
       If the feeds are provided every two hours, for a total of 12 meals daily, the foal will be fed
       13 L/12 meals = 1.08 L, or 1,080 mL/meal which is an appropriate volume
       If the feeds were provided every eight hours, for a total of 3 meals daily, the foal will be fed
       13 L/3 meals = 4.3 L, or 4,300 mL/meal which is too much volume at a single meal for a 65 kg foal
5) *Prepare the food* and feed the foal
  a) Always follow the label instructions for mixing a milk replacer. Never overconcentrate or overdilute the formula. Adjustments in calories fed are made by changing the total daily volume of formula that is offered to the foal
  b) Water can be offered to a foal, but intake should be monitored to prevent excess water consumption

## The Foal That Is Unable to Voluntarily or Safely Consume Enough Milk to Meet Nutrient Requirements But Can Tolerate Enteral Feeds

AEF is often required for a neonatal foal and in many cases can be managed in a field setting. AEF is an appropriate choice for nutritional supplementation if a foal does not have a strong suckle reflex, if they have complications swallowing, if they have an anatomic abnormality that prevents milk consumption, if they are obtunded, or if they are unable to nurse voluntarily. Foals can be managed with NG tube feeding for prolonged periods of time (weeks to months).

The same general guidelines listed for group 1 foals above should be followed when feeding through an NG tube. Foals fed through an NG tube should be checked for gastric reflux before a meal and should have their NG tube flushed with water after a meal. All water administered through an NG tube should be added to the foal's total daily fluid intake to help maintain hydration and to prevent complications from overhydration.

Once a foal develops a strong suckle reflex and can safely drink from a bottle or pan independently, the NG tube can be removed.

*How to feed*

1) If the dam is producing milk, feed the foal using her milk
  a) Use a commercially available milker
    i) Udderly EZ™ Mare Milker
  b) Milk the mare by hand
    i) Wear gloves and ensure clean protocols are followed to prevent iatrogenic mastitis
2) If the dam is not available for milk, follow steps 2–5 outlined above for group 1 foals
  a) Note: Critically ill neonatal foals may need to be started at a lower volume of milk (2.5–5% BW/day) for the first few days of nutritional therapy to ensure dietary tolerance before milk volume is gradually increased. Concurrent treatment with dextrose-supplemented fluids may be necessary to help maintain blood glucose concentrations when very low volumes of milk are fed.
3) Ensure proper placement of the NG tube
4) Check the NG tube for residual gastric fluid
  a) Apply gentle suction on the NG tube
     OR
  b) Allow for any residual fluid to flow from the tube using gravity flow like a siphon
     OR
  c) Use a gastric decompression bag (Farrell Valve) to collect residual fluid by gravity flow
  d) Note: Some foals will develop intestinal ileus with residual gastric fluid as an early sign of illness and these foals will require supplemental IV nutrition (group 3 foals)
5) If the foal has <20 mL of residual gastric fluid (appropriate volume for a 50 kg foal) offer the meal
6) If the foal has >20 mL of residual gastric fluid (appropriate for a 50 kg foal; adjust volume based on foal weight), replace the residual fluid, flush the NG tube with 10 mL warm water, delay feeding the foal for one hour and check for residual fluid again

   a) If the foal still has >20 mL of residual gastric fluid over the next two hours, supplemental nutrition with PPN should be initiated (group 3 foals)
   b) A neonatal foal should not go without food for more than six to eight hours
7) Position the foal in sternal recumbency and administer half of the meal volume by gravity flow through the NG tube. Pause feeding to ensure that the foal is tolerating the meal, then administer the remainder of the meal.
   a) Use a 60cc catheter tipped syringe as a funnel for feeding
   b) Use a commercial enteral feeding bag
8) Flush the NG tube with 15–20 mL of warm water
   a) Add the water flush to the foal's daily fluid intake volume
9) Close or cap off the NG tube
10) Maintain the foal in sternal recumbency for an additional 10–15 minutes after the meal

## The Critically Ill Foal That Cannot Nurse or Tolerate Enteral Feeds for >24 Hours Due to Systemic Complications from Respiratory, GI, Neurologic, or Other Disease

PN as either PPN (amino acids and dextrose) or TPN (amino acids, dextrose, lipid) is administered to foals following the same guidelines as were outlined for adult horses. A serum TG concentration should be measured on every foal before a PN solution is formulated. A Parenteral Nutrition Worksheet for Foals is provided (Figure 32.3). Administration should be done through a multi-lumen catheter using a fluid pump in a hospital setting. In foals, a multi-lumen catheter is often placed as a central catheter line. A PN infusion port can be reserved for administration.

A unique aspect of using PN in foals is that often it is helpful to provide a very small volume (5–10 mL/h) of mare's milk or a milk replacer through an NG tube to help provide nutrients directly to the enterocytes while the foal is being treated

Patient history: 3-day-old Thoroughbred colt, BCS 3/9 with a diagnosis of failure of passive transfer and sepsis along with intestinal ileus. Requires nutritional support with PN.

**Patient Information:**

| | |
|---|---|
| 1. Body weight (kg) | 55 kg |
| 2. RER (Mcal/day)[1] (45–50 kcal/BW kg/d): 55 kg × 50 kcal | 2750 kcal |
| 3. Protein requirement (2–5 g/kg/d): 55 kg × 3 g/kg | 165 g |
| 4. Fluid requirement = 5 mL/kg/h × 24 hours: 5 mL × 55 kg × 24 h | 6600 mL |
| 5. Decided on 60:40 dextrose: lipid calorie source | |

**Parenteral Nutrition Formulation**

| | |
|---|---|
| ▪ Volume of 50% dextrose solution (1.7 kcal/mL) providing 60% of calories | |
| 60% of 2750 kcal = 1650 kcal / 1.7 kcal/mL | 970 mL |
| ▪ Volume of 20% lipid solution (2 kcal/mL) providing 40% of calories | |
| 40% of 2750 kcal = 1100 kcal / 2 kcal/mL | 550 mL |
| ▪ Volume of 10% amino acids (0.10 g/mL) to meet protein requirement | |
| 165 g protein /0.10 g/mL | 1650 mL |
| ▪ Total volume of macronutrient solutions: | 3170 mL |
| Add 1–2 mL of B complex vitamins/L of PN | 2 mL |
| Add 1 mL of trace minerals/day | 1 mL |
| ▪ Volume of polyionic fluids required to meet fluid requirement | |
| Fluid requirement minus PN solution 6600 mL – 3173 mL | 3427 mL |
| ▪ Osmolarity of final solution | |
| Dextrose: 970 mL × 2.550 mOsm/mL = 2474 | |
| Lipid: 550 mL × 0.260 mOsm/mL = 143 | |
| Amino acids: 1650 mL × 0.998 mOsm/mL = 1647 | |
| Polyionic fluid: 3427 mL × 0.273 mOsm/mL = 936 | |
| Total mOsm / total fluid volume = 5200 mOsm/6.6 L | 788 mOsm/L |
| ▪ Calorie to Nitrogen ratio: 2,750 kcal to 26.4 g nitrogen[2] = | 104 |

Feeding orders: administer PN solution at 275 mL/hr or 4.6 mL/min via jugular catheter.

[1] 70–100 kcal/BW kg/d for foals older than 2 months of age
[2] Protein contains on average 16% nitrogen [165 g protein × 16% = 26.4 g N]

**Figure 32.3** Parenteral nutrition worksheet for foals.

with PN. As the foal becomes more tolerant of enteral feeds, the PN can gradually be discontinued and the foal can be transitioned over to an enteral diet.

*How to feed*

1) Ensure placement of a multi-lumen catheter and gather all equipment needed for PN administration (see adult section)
2) Select the PN formulation
   a) A commercial pre-made PN formulation can be used (CLINIMIX, CLINIMIX E (Baxter))
      i) 2.75–6% amino acid solutions are available without or with electrolytes in 5% dextrose. Higher concentrations of dextrose may result in hyperglycemia
   b) If making the PN formulation on-site, see the adult section for needed ingredients and use the following guidelines to calculate the PN recipe for a foal. See the foal Parenteral Nutrition Worksheet (Figure 32.3)
      i) Daily calorie intake for a sick neonatal foal
         - 45–50 kcal/kg BW/day
      ii) Daily calorie intake for a sick older foal (>one month of age)
         - 75–100 kcal/kg BW/day
      iii) Amino acids
         - 2–5 g/kg BW/day
           - Use 2–3 g/kg BW/day if the foal has renal or hepatic disease
           - Higher protein intake (6–6.5 g/kg BW/day) may be beneficial if PN is administered for >five to seven days
      iv) Calories from lipid (if included in the PN formulation)
         - 1–2 g/kg BW/day
           - Should be <50% of the total calories in the PN formulation
           - Note: A serum TG should be measured before the PN is formulated. If a foal has hypertriglyceridemia (TG >200 mg/dL), do not add lipid to the PN formulation
      v) Divide total PN calories between dextrose and lipid (if included), then calculate the amount of amino acids needed for the solution
      vi) Adjust the osmolarity of the PN solution using sterile water if necessary
      vii) Vitamins and Minerals
         - If PN is administered for >three days, consider adding
           - 1 mL B vitamins/liter PN
           - Add up to 1 mL trace minerals/day
3) Administer the PN formula
   a) Discontinue IV fluids that contain dextrose before starting the PN formulation
   b) Decrease the foal's IV fluid rate to account for fluids infused with the PN (50% free water)
   c) Provide supplemental electrolytes in maintenance IV fluids, so concentrations can be easily adjusted
   d) Start the foal at 25% of the total PPN or TPN volume
   e) Advance PN feeds as tolerated (follow adult horse guidelines)
4) Monitor the foal's clinical response to PN and check for complications (follow general guidelines for adult horses)
   a) The total daily fluid intake from all sources (IV, enteral, parenteral) should be measured and closely monitored, while a foal is on PN to prevent serious complications from overhydration
   b) Enteral feeding
      i) Trickle feed small volumes of milk through an NG tube as tolerated (5–10 mL/h) to provide nutrients directly to the enterocytes
      ii) Monitor intestinal motility and tolerance of enteral feed and when possible gradually increase the volume of milk (see 6 below)
5) Adjust the PN formula if needed based on the foal's response
   a) If the foal develops hyperglycemia
      i) Decrease the concentration of dextrose in the formulation by 50% OR decrease the PN infusion rate by 25–30%
      ii) If hyperglycemia persists, consider insulin therapy
         - CRI of insulin (Humulin® R)
           - 0.01 IU/kg BW/hr adjusted to maintain blood glucose

- Intermittent insulin
  - 0.1–0.5 IU regular insulin SQ q12 h
- Whenever insulin is administered closely monitor blood glucose (every hour to start) to prevent complications from hypoglycemia.

b) If the foal develops hypertriglyceridemia (confirmed serum TG > 200 mg/dL after the PN has been turned off for 20 minutes)
   i) Remove the lipid from the PN formula
c) If the foal requires PN for >seven days, reformulate the solution based on any growth or positive weight gain

6) Offer milk through an NG tube as tolerated (include milk volume in total daily fluid intake)
   a) Begin with 2.5% BW/day fed every two hours
      i) If tolerated, increase milk volume by 10–20 mL/feeding until 5% BW/day is reached
      ii) Follow guidelines above (group 2 foals) about how to monitor for gastric reflux before feeding
   b) Once the foal is tolerating 5% BW/day fed every two hours
      i) Monitor the foal for 8–12 h to ensure continued tolerance of milk
      ii) Once this volume of milk is tolerated, gradually decrease the PN infusion rate by 1–2 mL/h until you reach 30% of the foal's total PN infusion volume.
      iii) Continue to increase milk volume by 10–20 mL/feeding until 10% BW/day is reached
   c) Once the foal is tolerating 10% BW/day fed every two hours
      i) Monitor the foal for 8–12 h to ensure continued tolerance of milk
      ii) If the milk is tolerated for one to two days discontinue the PN
7) Discontinue the PN once the foal is treated with 25–33% of the total PN volume

## 32.A Nutrition Resources

1) Assisted Enteral Feeding
   a) WellSolve® W/G Well-Gel® (Purina Animal Nutrition LLC, Shoreview, MN)
   b) Enteral Immunonutrition Formula (Platinum Performance, Buellton, CA)
   c) Mila 18-Fr, 250 cm feeding tube (Mila NG18100, Mila International, Inc., Florence, KY)
   d) Vitamix (Vitamix, Cleveland, OH)
   e) Blendtec (Blendtec, Orem, UT)
   f) Best Friend Deluxe Grazing Muzzle (Best Friend Equine, Supply, Inc., Fairfield Glade, TN)
2) Parenteral Nutrition
   a) CLINIMIX, CLINIMIX E (with electrolytes) (Baxter Healthcare Corporation, Deerfield, IL)
   b) Travasol 10% (Baxter Healthcare Corporation, Deerfield, IL)
   c) TrophAmine® 10% (B. Braun Medical Inc., Bethlehem, PA)
   d) 20% CLINOLIPID (Baxter Healthcare Corporation, Deerfield, IL)
   e) Nutrilipid® 20% (B. Braun Medical Inc., Bethlehem, PA)
   f) INFUVITE Multiple Vitamins for Infusion (Baxter Healthcare Corporation, Deerfield, IL)
   g) EXACTAMIX and Three Lead Parenteral Nutrition Transfer Set (Baxter Healthcare Corporation, Deerfield, IL)
   h) EVA Gravity Mixing Container, 3-lead Vented Transfer Set (B. Braun Medical Inc., Bethlehem, PA)
   i) CAPS®, Central Admixture Pharmacy Services, Inc., a B. Braun Group of Companies, Bethlehem, PA
   j) Coram® CVS Specialty® Infusion Services, Northbrook, IL
3) Foal Nutrition
   a) Mare's Match® Purina or Land O Lakes®, Arden Hills, MN
   b) Mare's Milk Plus® MARS Horsecare, Dalton, OH
   c) Udderly EZ™ Mare Milker, Humboldt, IA
   d) Farrell Valve Closed Enteral Decompression System, Avanos Medical, Alpharetta, GA
   e) Humulin R, Eli-Lilly, Indianapolis, IN

## References


Lawson, A., Sherlock, C., Ireland, J., and Mair, T. (2021). Equine nutrition in the post-operative colic: survey of diplomates of the American colleges of veterinary internal medicine and veterinary surgeons, and European colleges of equine internal medicine and veterinary surgeons. *Equine Vet. J.* 53: 1015–1024.

Main, S., Brown, L., Melvin, K. et al. (2022). Metabolomic profiles in starved light breed horses during the refeeding process. *Animals* 12 (19): 2527.

Myers, C., Magdesian, G., Kass, P. et al. (2009). Parenteral nutrition in neonatal foals: Clinical description, complications and outcome in 53 foals (1995-2005). *Vet. J.* 181: 137–144.

National Research Council (2007). *Nutrient Requirements of Horses*, 6e. Washington, DC: National Academy Press.

Paradis, M. (2001). Caloric needs of the sick foal: determined by the use of indirect calorimetry. *Proceedings of the 3rd Dorothy Havemeyer Foundation Neonatal Septicemia Workshop, Talliores, France*. Talloires, France. pp. 13–16.

Schneider, L., Self, A., Hines, M., and Ivey, J. (2021). Clinical factors associated with survival outcomes in starved equids: a retrospective case series. *J. Eq. Vet. Sci.* 101: 103370.

Witham, C. and Stull, C. (1998). Metabolic responses of chronically starved horses to refeeding with three isoenergetic diets. *J. Am. Vet. Med. Assoc.* 212 (5): 691–696.

# 33

# Resuscitation in the Foal and Adult Horse

*Maia R. Aitken*

*Department of Clinical Studies - New Bolton Center, University of Pennsylvania School of Veterinary Medicine, Kennett Square, PA, USA*

## Introduction

Cardiopulmonary resuscitation (CPR), also referred to as "resuscitation," is a lifesaving procedure to reverse the effects of cardiac and/or respiratory arrest before irreversible interruption of cardiac output, ventilation, or tissue perfusion occurs. Resuscitation in the horse is most commonly performed in the neonate immediately following birth (Palmer 2007). In cases of neonatal cardiopulmonary arrest (CPA), respiratory arrest almost always precedes cardiac arrest (Jokisalo and Corley 2014). The most common reason for asphyxia or respiratory arrest in the neonate includes prolonged dystocia, premature placental separation, airway obstruction by fetal membranes, or umbilical cord torsion (Jokisalo and Corley 2014). In some cases, neonates require resuscitation without having an associated dystocia or issues related to foaling. Immediately following birth, a foal should be assessed for signs of respiratory depression or arrest to determine the need for intervention. Outside of the foaling period, neonates are susceptible to CPA secondary to other systemic conditions such as sepsis, pulmonary pathology, neonatal ischemic encephalopathy/ neonatal maladjustment syndrome, hypoglycemia, metabolic acidosis, botulism, or other causes of respiratory failure. It is essential for the veterinarian to anticipate when resuscitation is needed in foals as early recognition of signs of CPA greatly improves the success rate of resuscitative efforts. Immediately after birth, such signs include dyspnea, open-mouth breathing, abdominal effort to breathing, bradycardia of less than 50 beats/min, gasping for longer than 30 seconds, apnea, or asystole (Jokisalo and Corley 2014). In the hospitalized foal, signs of CPA include decreases in venous oxygen saturation or end-tidal $CO_2$, bradycardia less than 50 beats/min, and apnea (Jokisalo and Corley 2014).

Resuscitation of the adult horse is a rarely performed procedure outside of the operating room, where there is a less than 1% reported mortality rate in non-colic cases and approximately one-third of these mortalities involve cardiac arrest (Bidwell et al. 2007). When CPA occurs unrelated to anesthetic events, it may be caused by a number of other factors, including drug reactions, airway obstruction, pulmonary disease, cardiac disease, respiratory arrest secondary to severe abdominal distention, sepsis or endotoxic shock, intracarotid injection, severe acid–base disturbances, and lightning strike. Due to the mass of an adult horse resuscitative efforts limited to basic life support can be challenging (Hubbell et al. 1993) and often unsuccessful. However, successful CPR in adult horses has been documented (De Moor et al. 1972; Kellaghar and Watney 1986, McGoldrick and Clarke 1998; Conde-Ruiz and Junot 2018; Duggan et al. 2022). Regardless of age or size, the following list (Box 33.1) offers signs of CPA requiring immediate intervention and resuscitative efforts:

*Emergency Triage of the Horse*, First Edition. Edited by Rolfe M. Radcliffe and Jamie J. Kopper.

Companion website: www.wiley.com/go/radcliffe/triage

**Box 33.1 Signs of cardiopulmonary arrest**

- Apnea (respiratory arrest is often first sign in horses, especially foals)
- Lack of palpable pulse
- Severe bradycardia (<50–60 beats/min in foals)
- Cardiac dysrhythmias – fibrillation, asystole
- Low venous oxygen saturation
- Low end-tidal $CO_2$
- Severe hypoventilation

## Basic Life Support

Basic life support (BLS) firstly involves the recognition of CPA, followed by the initiation of chest compressions and ventilation of the patient (Figure 33.1) (Fletcher et al. 2012; Hopper et al. 2012). A full cycle of BLS is two to three minutes of chest compressions (Fletcher et al. 2012; Hopper et al. 2012). The chest compressions may provide direct compression of the heart itself, as in the case of neonates (Javsicas and Giguere 2008), or rather utilized the thoracic pump mechanism (Haas et al. 2003), as in the case of adult horses (Muir and Hubbell 2009). Just as with human first-aid, the ABCs of CPR apply to equine patients (Box 33.2).

Establishing an airway typically involves endotracheal intubation, whether oro- or naso-tracheal, or in some cases of obstruction, tracheostomy. Initiating ventilation includes using a re-breathing bag or mechanically ventilating with an anesthesia machine or ventilator. A goal of 10 breaths/min with a tidal volume of 10 mL/kg is recommended. The ventilation rate can also be targeted to establishing normocapnia and normoxemia. Ventilating with room air instead of 100% oxygen decreases the risk of hyperoxemia and subsequent reactive oxygen species and neurologic injury. Re-establishing circulation involves performing chest compressions to increase intra-thoracic pressure, compress vascular structures, and circulate blood. Performing chest compressions will also help to disperse any medications administered during CPR. The goal of chest compressions for both neonate and adult is to compress the thorax to one-third to one-half the width of the thorax. This is most effective with the patient in lateral recumbency on a hard surface. The person performing compressions should be switched out every two to three minutes to decrease fatigue and ensure effective compression. For neonatal patients, the operator should position themselves at the foal's back, with their knees against the foal's spine and hands clasped to compress directly over the heart. If the foal has rib fractures, the foal should be positioned with the fractures most dependent, against the floor or table. An appropriate rate of compression for neonates is 100 compressions per minute (Javsicas and Giguere 2008). For adult horses, compressions can be performed by forcefully thrusting the operator's knees into the horse's chest just caudal to the point of the elbow. An acceptable rate of compression for adult horses is 30–80 compressions per minute (Hubbell et al. 1993). Chest compressions may result in rib fractures; however, this undesirable sequela is preferable to a dead patient.

### Important Considerations for Resuscitation at Birth

CPR has a better prognosis in foals immediately after birth than older foals and adults, though rapid recognition and intervention is essential. Box 33.3 provides essential steps for neonatal resuscitation.

## Advanced Life Support

Advanced life support (ALS) includes the addition of medications to BLS (Table 33.1, Figure 33.1), correction of electrolyte disturbances or volume deficits, and defibrillation if indicated (Rozanski et al. 2012). The medications utilized in ALS include vasopressors, positive inotropes, and anticholinergics. The medication of choice for ALS continues to be epinephrine. While BLS is considered a separate entity to ASL, the goal is to provide, if possible, both BLS and ALS concurrently. Or in the majority of cases, BLS is initiated immediately following diagnosis of CPA and then ALS and monitoring begin as soon as possible.

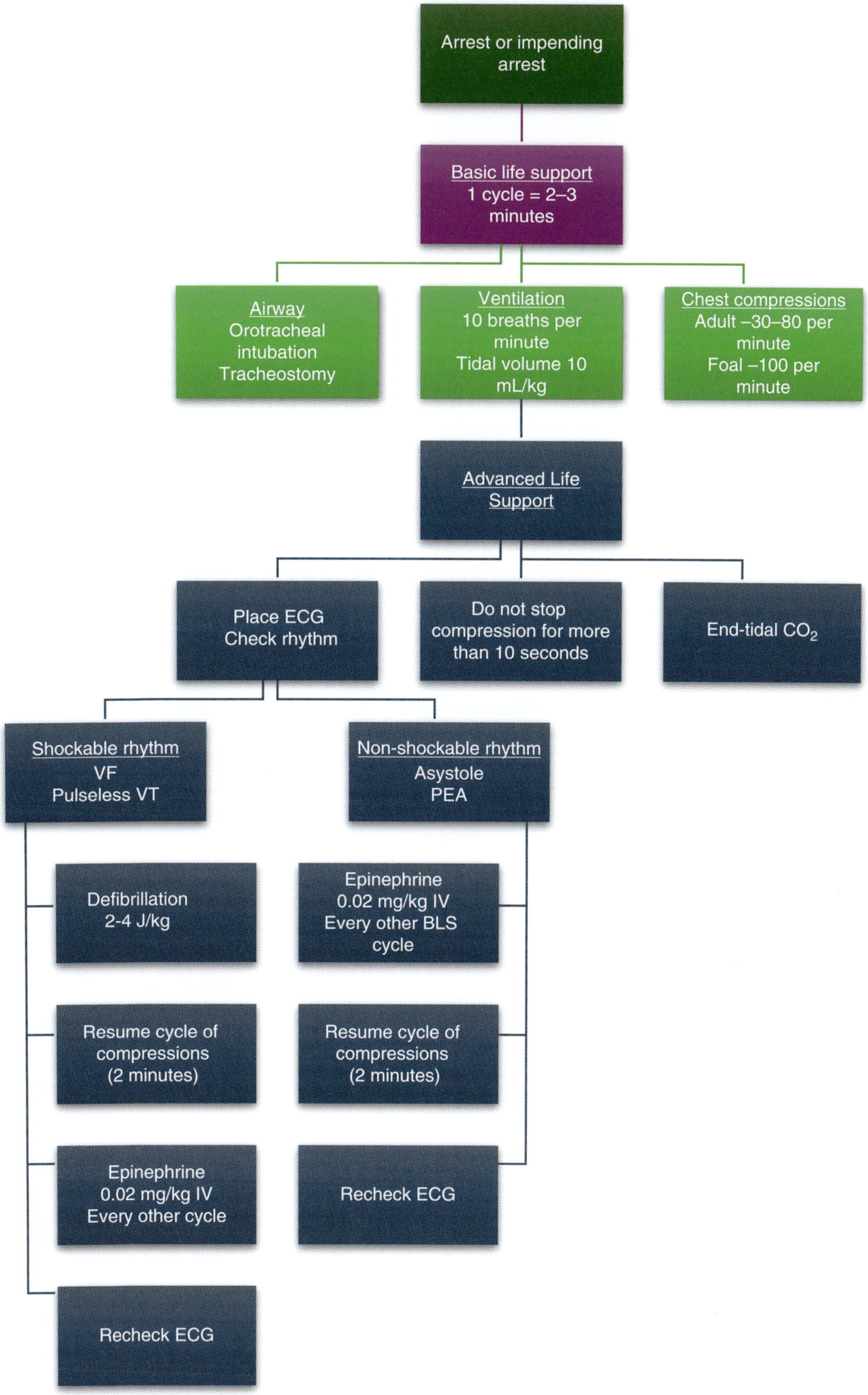


**Figure 33.1** Steps for addressing arrest or impending arrest of a patient. ECG, electrocardiogram, PEA, Pulseless electrical activity, VF, ventricular fibrillation, VT, ventricular tachycardia.

**Box 33.2 ABCs of CPR**

A – Airway: establish an airway
B – Breathing: initiate ventilation
C – Circulation: palpate for pulse, start compressions

**Box 33.3 Neonatal resuscitation**

- Quickly clean nares of mucus, suction if necessary and if meconium stained
- Vigorously towel clean to stimulate breathing
- Assess breathing (normal 60–80 brpm)
- Assess heart rate (normal 60–70 bpm)
- If apneic or gasping, intubate
  - Nasotracheal intubation with a size 9–10 internal diameter 55 cm long endotracheal (ET tube (for ~50 kg foal)
  - Intubate with head in extension, gentle pressure at cranial esophagus to prevent esophageal intubation
- If heart rate <50 bpm, intubate and ventilate
  - If heart rate <40 bpm, ventilate and start compressions
  - Administer epinephrine

**Table 33.1** Medications for ALS.

| Medication | Indications | Concentration | Dose | IV dose (mL) for 50 kg foal | IV dose (mL) for 500 kg horse |
|---|---|---|---|---|---|
| Epinephrine | Asystole, PEA, VT, VF refractory to shock | 1 mg/mL | 0.02 mg/kg<br>0.2 mg/kg Intratracheal | 1<br>10 Inratracheal | 10 |
| Vasopressin | Asystole | 20 U/mL | 0.8 U/kg | 2 | 20 |
| Lidocaine | VT, VF refractory to shock | 20 mg/mL | 1 mg/kg | 2.5 | 25 |
| Amiodarone | VT, VF refractory to shock | 50 mg/mL | 5 mg/kg | 5 | 50 |
| Atropine[a] | Vagally mediated bradycardia (rare) | 0.4 mg/mL | 0.02 mg/kg | 2.5 | [a] |
| $CaCl_2$ | Severe hyperkalemia<br>Severe hypocalcemia | 100 mg/mL | 20 mg/kg | 10<br>Diluted in 100 mL NaCl over 10 minutes | 100<br>Diluted in 1 L NaCl over 10 minutes |
| $MgSO_4$ | Refractory ventricular arrhythmias | 4.06 mEq/mL | 0.02 mEq/kg | 10<br>Diluted in 100 mL NaCl over 10 minutes | 100<br>Diluted in 1 L NaCl over 10 minutes |

PEA, pulseless electrical activity; VF, ventricular fibrillation; VT, ventricular tachycardia.
[a] Atropine has been shown to have no benefit in ALS, may cause ileus; thus, its use is not recommended.

Defibrillation can be effective in patients with shockable rhythms: cases of ventricular fibrillation or pulseless ventricular tachycardia. These are uncommon arrythmias in neonatal CPA. However, should one of these rhythms be diagnosed where abnormal pacing of groups of ventricular myocardial cells occurs, it can be depolarized by a shock. The goal is to drive these cells into their refractory period, stopping the uncoordinated electrical and mechanical activity, and allow the pacemaker cells to drive the myocardial cell. However, asystole can also occur as a result of such defibrillation. Biphasic defibrillators are recommended over monophasic, shocking at a dose of 2–4 J/kg. The amount of energy may be increased by 50–100% if the first shock is unsuccessful. Defibrillation should not be used in non-shockable rhythms: asystole or pulseless electrical activity (PEA) (Rozanski et al. 2012). It is critical that the defibrillator paddles are placed on opposite sides of the thorax and directly over the heart. Defibrillator gel should be applied to the paddles, or defibrillator patches can be used (hair must be clipped). The defibrillator operator must be aware that no one is in contact with the patient or the table prior to discharging the defibrillator. The timing of defibrillation is ideally within four minutes of CPA for patients with shockable rhythms. After an initial shock is given, a full cycle of CPR should be performed before reassessing the ECG and administering further defibrillations (two to three minute cycle). As mentioned, the energy may be increased by 50–100% once for subsequent defibrillations.

Fluid therapy is an important component of ALS. Isotonic crystalloids can be administered at a rate of 10–40 mL/kg/h to correct hypovolemia, dehydration, acidosis, or shock. Caution should be observed with respect to supplementation with calcium as increased morbidity has been reported in other species. Despite CPA causing a sometimes severe metabolic acidosis, the administration of sodium bicarbonate has also been associated with increased morbidity and mortality. Care should be taken with respect to fluid administration cases of cardiogenic shock, to avoid fluid overload.

With respect to drug interventions and ALS, by and large the most effective medication across species is low-dose epinephrine at a dose of 0.01–0.02 mg/kg IV. Vasopressin has been utilized in human and veterinary species successfully and most often, in combination with epinephrine. These drugs are often alternated in between cycles of BLS compressions (every two to three minutes). Other medications that may play an important role in ALS, depending on the specific clinical scenario, include reversal agents for sedatives, opioids, or anesthetic agents.

In neonatal foals born to a mare under general anesthesia (i.e., born via controlled vaginal delivery or cesarean section) that are not responding to initial resuscitative efforts, reversals may be administered to the foal for medications administered to the mare prior to parturition (i.e., flumazenil for diazepam, naloxone for opioids, and yohimbine for alpha-2 antagonists).

### Monitoring

Monitoring throughout the administration of CPR is critical to the success of the procedure. Using ECG and end-tidal $CO_2$ early during any CPR attempt allows verification of placement of an endotracheal tube and monitoring for shockable rhythms. While ECG monitoring can diagnose a shockable rhythm and thus change the course of CPR, it is critical that breaks of chest compressions be no longer than 10 seconds. End-tidal $CO_2$ monitoring can confirm successful placement of endotracheal tubes, confirmed by a high level of $CO_2$, as there are relatively low levels within the esophagus. However, a limitation to this method of verification can occur in patients with a longer amount of time in CPA, where low levels of end-tidal $CO_2$ can occur with correct intubation of the patient. In addition, in neonates, fluid from the lungs can also interfere with end-tidal $CO_2$ monitoring equipment.

Monitoring can also indicate the return of spontaneous circulation (ROSC), the ultimate sign of a successful resuscitation. Signs of ROSC include a palpable pulse, thoracic wall or diaphragmatic movement, present corneal/palpebral reflexes, changes in eye position, presence of a pupillary light reflex, or increased consciousness. Throughout CPR, end-tidal $CO_2$ of greater than 15 mmHg indicates perfusion and a higher chance of successful ROSC.

### Stopping Resuscitation

Equally important as performing CPR is knowing when to stop interventions. Ventilation can be stopped when spontaneous breathing has been established and the heart rate is greater than 60 beats/min in foals. Ventilation can be paused for 30 seconds to "test" the patient's response prior to complete cessation of ventilation, during which a short lag between support and the onset of regular breathing may occur. For chest compressions, there should be no pause between the cessation of compressions and the continued heartbeat of the patient. Chest compressions can be stopped when the heart rate is maintained at greater than 60 beats/min in foals. When assessing whether compressions can be stopped, a pause of less than or equal to 10 seconds can be safely allowed. Though there is no agreement on the duration of CPR, based on clinical reports the likelihood of survival is low if ROSC has not occurred within 10 minutes of initiating resuscitation.

## Conclusions

Resuscitation in equine neonates and adults is an essential procedure to treat CPA, the absence of systole or failure of ventricular contraction and cardiac output. Sustained lack of cardiac output, ventilation, and subsequent tissue perfusion will cause irreversible CPA. Early intervention using both BLS and ALS will increase the likelihood of achieving ROSC. Despite shockable rhythms being rare in neonatal CPA, these rhythms do occur, and ECG monitoring and defibrillation should be used accordingly. Ideally, a flow chart and drug doses for different weight horses will be displayed in key areas of clinical activity.

**Case Example 33.1 Basic and Advanced Life Support**

You have been called in for an equine dystocia (500 kg Thoroughbred mare) and are in charge of neonatal resuscitation if needed. While you are waiting for the mare to arrive you quickly prepare your area for potential basic and advanced life support. What should supplies should you have prepared and waiting?

*Answer*

Basic Life Support

- Endotracheal tube – 9–10 ID, 55 cm long
- Rebreathing bag
- Time keeper/three minute stop watch

Advanced Life Support

- Epinephrine – 1 mL for IV administration
- Reversals depending on the mare's potential anesthetic protocol
  - Examples: Flumazenil, Naloxone
- ECG
- End tidal $CO_2$ monitor
- Defibrillator

Upon birth via controlled vaginal delivery the foal is non-responsive to stimuli, apneic, and has a heart rate of 30 bpm. What should you do next?

*Answer*

1) Start BLS and ALS:
   a) Intubate the foal – provide respiratory support at 10 brpm, 10 mL/kg tidal volume (estimate 0.5 L)
   b) Initiate chest compressions at 100 bpm
   c) Obtain venous access
   d) Administer 1 mg (1 mL) of epinephrine IV
   e) Reassess patient every two to three minutes for <10 seconds to determine if additional rounds of BLS/ALS are indicated

You have the foal intubated and are providing ventilatory support at a rate of 10 brpm. What end-tidal $CO_2$ reading would indicate that the foal is receiving perfusion and you have a higher chance of achieving return to spontaneous circulation?

Answer: Greater than 15 mmHg

What are indications that you have successfully achieved return to spontaneous circulation and can stop resuscitation efforts?

*Answer*

1) Heart rate maintained >60 bpm
2) Ventilation maintained at >10 brpm
3) Palpable pulse
4) Present corneal/palpebral reflex
5) Presence of a pupillary light response
6) Increased consciousness or spontaneous movement

## References


Bidwell, L.A., Bramlage, L.R., and Rood, W.A. (2007). Equine perioperative fatalities associated with general anaesthesia at a private practice – a retrospective case series. *Vet. Anaesth. Analg.* 34: 23–30.

Conde-Ruiz, C. and Junot, S. (2018). Successful cardiopulmonary resuscitation in a sevoflurane anaesthetized horse that suffered cardiac arrest at recovery. *Front. Vet. Sci.* 5: 1–5.

De Moor, A., Verschooten, F., Desmet, P. et al. (1972). Intrathoracic cardiac resuscitation in the horse. *Equine Vet. J.* 4: 31–33.

Duggan, M., Schofield, W., and Vermedal, H. (2022). Successful cardiopulmonary resuscitation in an adult horse following cardiovascular collapse on recovery from general anaesthesia in the Trendelenburg position. *Equine Vet. Educ.* 34 (3): e98–e105.

Fletcher, D.J., Boller, M., Brainard, B.M. et al. (2012). RECOVER evidence and knowledge gap analysis on veterinary CPR. Part 7: clinical guidelines. *J. Vet. Emerg. Crit. Care (San Antonio)* 22 (Suppl 1): S102–S131.

Haas, T., Voelckel, W.G., Wenzel, V. et al. (2003). Revisiting the cardiac versus thoracic pump mechanism during cardiopulmonary resuscitation. *Resuscitation* 58: 113–116.

Hopper, K., Epstein, S.E., Fletcher, D.J. et al. (2012). RECOVER evidence and knowledge gap analysis on veterinary CPR. Part 3: Basic life support. *J. Vet. Emerg. Crit. Care (San Antonio)* 22 (Suppl 1): S26–S43.

Hubbell, J.A.E., Muir, W.W., and Gaynor, J.S. (1993). Cardiovascular effects of thoracic compression in horses subjected to euthanasia. *Equine Vet. J.* 25: 282–284.

Javsicas, L.H. and Giguere, S. (2008). How to perform cardiopulmonary resuscitation in neonatal foals. *AAEP Proceedings* 54: 513–519.

Jokisalo, J.M. and Corley, K.T. (2014). CPR in the neonatal foal: has RECOVER changed our approach? *Vet. Clin. North Am. Equine Pract.* 30 (2): 301–316.

Kellagher, R.E. and Watney, G.C. (1986). Cardiac arrest during anaesthesia in two horses. *Vet. Rec.* 119: 347–349.

McGoldrick, T.M., Bowen, I.M., and Clarke, K.W. (1998). Sudden cardiac arrest in an anaesthetised horse associated with low venous oxygen tensions. *Vet. Rec.* 142: 610–611.

Muir, W.W. and Hubbelll, J.A.E. (2009). Cardiopulmonary resuscitation. In: *Equine Anesthesia: Monitoring and Emergence Therapy*, 2e (ed. W.W. Muir and J.A.E. Hubbell), 418–429. St Louis, MO: Elsevier.

Palmer, J.E. (2007). Neonatal foal resuscitation. *Vet. Clin. N. Am. Equine Pract.* 23: 159–182.

Rozanski, E.A., Rush, J.E., Buckley, G.J. et al. (2012). RECOVER evidence and knowledge gap analysis on veterinary CPR. Part 4: advanced life support. *J. Vet. Emerg. Crit. Care (San Antonio)* 22 (Suppl 1): S44–S64.

# 34

# Large Animal Rescue Techniques for Emergency Incidents

*Rebecca (Gimenez) Husted*

*Technical Large Animal Emergency Rescue (TLAER), Macon, GA, USA*

## Introduction

Large animal rescue (LAR) is considered a technical specialty in the fire/rescue world (Gimenez et al. 2008a). Incidents vary in frequency and duration, but are inherently dangerous to practitioner, responders, and animals (Thompson et al. 2015). These events vary over a wide continuum – one horse slides into a muddy ravine and requires a forward assist with webbing to get to safety (Figure 34.1), another needs a vertical sling lift from a septic tank (Gimenez et al. 2012). Similarly, the number of resources to conduct a rescue across this continuum varies as well from pieces of webbing and a few bystanders to special mechanical equipment and involvement of fire/rescue responders. As complexity increases, so do the potential hazards. Straightforward techniques for LAR place emphasis on simple tools and webbing, standard manipulations, LAR specific equipment, and proper positioning of personnel to minimize iatrogenic injury and achieve effective results when moving or extricating animals in various daily clinical situations (Gimenez et al. 2002; Gimenez et al. 2004) (Box 34.1).

*Equines get entrapped in an amazing variety of scenarios* (Gimenez 2015) *and unusual types of recumbency* (Box 34.2 and Table 34.1). Practitioners will frequently deal with these incidents over their careers – requiring immediate response, usually they can be resolved within several hours, and seldom exhaust the local community emergency resources (although they may exhaust your personal resources of personnel, drugs, and equipment). Some communities experience LAR scenarios less than once a year, in others the incidence rate exceeds twice per month. Some communities have an organized team of responders for LAR through fire department or private rescue organization.

The old assumption was that horses are large, tough, and strong. *Old LAR methods (rope it by the neck and pull them out with a tractor, etc.) were based on predatory human instincts to solve the problem but caused iatrogenic injury* (traumatic amputations, lacerations, asphyxiation, corneal damage, myopathy, neurologic and soft tissue injury, etc.) In vast numbers of cases, several hours to days after a seemingly "successful" rescue, equine victims died. Retrospectively, veterinarians realized that stress, ischemic reperfusion syndrome, accidental hypothermia, and/or complications of shock caused these losses. Equine medical fragility is now better understood; utilize the "golden hours" concept from military medicine to prompt response to their rapidly deteriorating condition (Gimenez 2012).

## Large Animal Rescue Preparation in the Community

*Veterinarians are not required by law to attend a scene – however, the veterinarian is an essential part of a team response* (Box 34.3) *and prior coordination with 911 emergency services is recommended.* There are serious legal, ethical, and financial considerations for practitioners requested to respond to LAR scenes. Educate local responders that LAR can occur in your community, coordinate with local 911 communications centers how to best assist. Most fire departments do not have expertise nor recognize special hazards of animals, but they can provide power and lighting, heavy rescue rigging expertise,

*Emergency Triage of the Horse*, First Edition. Edited by Rolfe M. Radcliffe and Jamie J. Kopper.

Companion website: www.wiley.com/go/radcliffe/triage

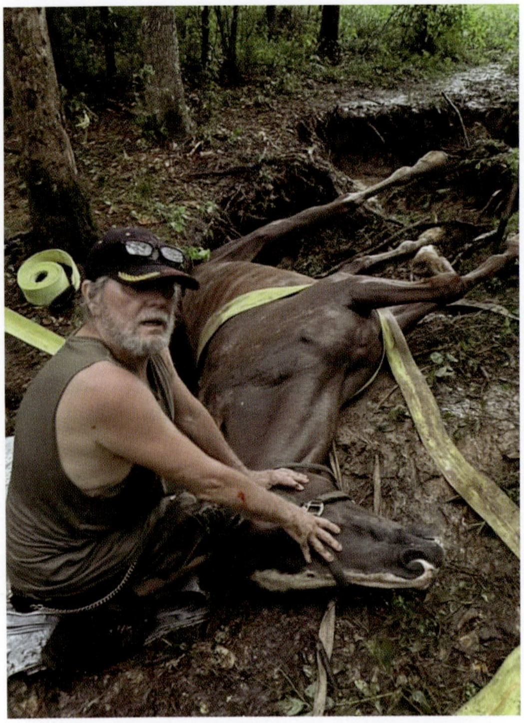

**Figure 34.1** Aged horse cast in a ravine, suffering from cold and exhaustion, was moved to solid ground with a forward assist technique using webbing. The horse was then stabilized medically, with appropriate fluid therapy and rewarming, and made a full recovery. Head protection for the horse and helmets for all personnel are recommended. *Source:* Photo by Dr. Rebecca McConnico.

**Box 34.1 Large animal rescue methods and planning**

*Overall Goal: keep technique as simple as possible to make responders safe, conduct effective triage and field treatment for the horse victim,* conduct risk assessment and extrication planning, contact equipment and fire/rescue resources earlier not later – adding to efficiency and professionalism of LAR efforts.

**Box 34.2 LAR examples**

Draft horse stuck in mud at the bottom of a steep ravine, has been there for 12 h, owner is very upset.

Horse has fallen into a well and only the front legs, head and neck are sticking out. However, he is eating hay and looks okay.

Six horses have survived a horrific trailer rollover on the interstate, three are tied and lying down between and under trailer dividers, one is loose and two are injured but removed from the trailer. 911 dispatch has asked you to respond.

A barn fire has affected 10 valuable performance horses with toxic smoke from a smoking charred tractor block heater, their barn was closed for the cold night temperatures.

**Table 34.1** Types of LAR recumbency and examples.

| |
|---|
| Anterior: Common in trailers nose down into embankments where horses are not able to rise, where heads are well below the rest of their bodies in a hole, etc. Often the neck is at strange angles which impacts breathing, and sheer weight of abdominal contents constricts lungs. Rarely survivable scenario unless attended efficiently. |
| Posterior: Common in animals that fall into a small opening but deep obstacles and holes, wells, or through bridges where the rump is well below the body. Often only the front legs and head/neck can be seen. |
| Dorsal: Horses that fall or are thrust into a tight space and end up on their backs with their hooves pointed upward – water tanks, feed bunk, horse trailer wreck, or ditch obstacles are common. Victim becomes medically fragile within short time in this position. |
| Lateral: Most common position for "downed" animals, various geriatric or debilitated as inability to get up, or injured, to technical rescue scenarios. The sheer weight of the animal contributes over time to compartment/crush syndromes, myopathies, neuropathies, and ventilation issues including collapse of the downside lung. These necessitate that the animal be attended to quickly – within four hours of being down for the best opportunity at recovery. |
| Sternal: The animal is laying on its ventral surface with legs either trapped in a downward position or folded and resting upon them. Resting on folded legs is a desired position for completing technical rescue scenarios and is considered the preferred "recovery position" for downed equines. |

**Box 34.3 A veterinarian's role in disaster and emergency response planning**

*Veterinarians are ideal leaders in animal emergency and disaster planning for their community* and can organize their practices around routine clinical emergencies, expandable to all levels of disaster preparedness using an ALL-HAZARDS approach. You are the local expert when evacuation and shelter-in-place questions come up for emergencies and disasters in your community.

and numerous response options civilians will not be aware of. Example: Practitioner is an hour from the scene – 911 dispatch might provide a law enforcement escort to scene to get around traffic. Within emergencies involving professional response personnel (fire/rescue, law enforcement, and animal control/welfare), the practitioner works as part of a team under the Incident Command System (ICS) (Emergency Management Institute 2021).

*Many useful items are simple to make or to convert from human rescue systems.* An investment of less than $7,000 can outfit a team with both basic and many advanced technical LAR items for a local cache. More expensive equipment needs for a community should be purchased and used under the direction of a veterinarian skilled in large-animal rescue techniques and maintained with local fire/rescue equipment; or privately funded and coordinated under non-profit designation.

Specialized LAR equipment (Large Animal Relocator Sked System,[1] Häst Nicopolous Needle,[2] Häst Mud Lances,[3] Häst Becker Sling,[4] LARGE Rescue Glide,[5] Häst Head Protector,[6] CDA Anderson Sling,[7] LOOPS Rescue System,[8] etc.) is commercially available.

*Routinely practice handling, manipulation, and triage skills plus remain proficient in techniques and use of LAR equipment that will result in an efficient, safe rescue.* Animals can be injured by untrained persons attempting to improvise a rescue harness, or when incorrectly attaching commercial systems. Slides, drags, vertical lifts, and manipulations are basic to LAR and often require proper use of chemical restraint – but are intimately tied to the veterinary practitioner's expertise – thus the art and science of veterinary medicine.

Note: *Natural and technological disasters* (Gimenez and McConnico 2018) *(hurricane, floods, tornado, blizzard, wildfire, earthquake, nuclear, electrical) require detailed evacuation or shelter in place planning, mitigation, and response not covered in this chapter.*

## A LAR Call Comes In

Traditionally, first contact between the owner and the veterinarian is initiated via the clinic's phone number. Practitioners should consider involvement of 911 emergency services personnel in many field scenarios, because it speeds up the overall efficiency of the LAR response and increases your safety. If emergency 911 service dispatch requests your attendance – what are your protocols or plan? How will you prepare for a call? What questions should you ask? (Box 34.4) Follow some general LAR rules to stay safe (Table 34.2).

**Box 34.4 What questions should you ask?**

*GO ENROUTE: Ask for a short video or photograph to assist with understanding of what is needed to bring or call to the scene.* Ask questions relevant to signalment and history, resources, equipment, and if the owner is available. Bring appropriate LAR equipment in addition to your medical treatment resources.

1 Large Animal Relocator Sked System, 4Hooves LA Services, LLC, Biscoe, NC. https://4hoovessmart.com/online-store/ols/categories/large-animal-skid-relocation-system 910-494-8210.
2 Nicopolous Needle, Häst, PSC, Floyd, VA. http://rescue.hastpsc.com/products/water/nicopolous/needle.html 804-286-0832.
3 Häst Mud Lance, Häst, PSC, Floyd, VA. http://rescue.hastpsc.com/products/water/lances/lances.html 804-286-0832.
4 Häst Becker Sling, Häst, PSC, Floyd, VA. http://rescue.hastpsc.com/ 804-286-0832.
5 Rescue Glide, LARGE, Inc. Inman, SC. http://www.rescueglides.com/ 864-270-1344.
6 Häst Head Protector, Häst, PSC, Floyd, VA. http://rescue.hastpsc.com/ 804-286-0832.
7 Anderson Sling, CDA Products, Porter Valley, CA https://www.andersonsling.com/andersonsling.
8 LOOPS Rescue System, Loop Lift LLC, Davis, CA https://loopsrescue.com.

**Table 34.2** General rules for large animal rescue.

| |
|---|
| Use Personal Protective Equipment (PPE) appropriate to the scenario: Firefighters will always show up with boots, gloves, reflective vest, and a helmet – follow their example especially on active roadways. |
| Do not attach anything to the head, neck, or legs and pull: A halter and lead rope are not intended for pulling – but guidance only. Head or legs are not handles or attachment points – due to opposition reflex, the animal will spend more time fighting the pressure and less time moving in the desired direction. |
| Approach from the dorsal side where possible and stay on dorsal side out of the kill zone – never get between the legs or between the legs and head: Also, remember the head of a horse can be dangerous, especially with horses that are struggling to stand. Whenever working near the head, keep one hand or your knee onto the neck to control thrashing and to feel when the horse is moving. |
| Prioritize LAR techniques – simple, low-tech, and low-risk methods should be attempted before more difficult higher tech and complicated methods are implemented: If a sideways drag out of a deep trench will work, why call in a vertical lifting sling and helicopter? |
| Perform a concise, but thorough physical exam prior to initiating a rescue: It is better to euthanize the horse in situ than to work for hours to rescue it, only to discover a life-ending injury (e.g., open tibial fracture) or have the animal die or require euthanasia immediately after extrication. |
| Use webbing with looped ends or fire hose (instead of ropes) for any type of manipulation: The greater surface area and flat surface of the webbing will minimize injury to the skin and underlying structures. Use padding to protect soft tissue if rope is the only option. |
| Use the pectoral and pelvic girdles as the slinging points for any lifting or manipulations: The muscle and bone structures here will protect the delicate soft structures (nerve, blood vessels, tendons, and ligaments) beneath. |
| Do not use the tail as an attachment point for any mechanical manipulations: only use the tail for careful manual movement of the recumbent horse by no more than 2 people. Tails can be broken, injured, or traumatically amputated by application of excessive force. |
| *Use a blindfold or head protector while horses are recumbent* (Gardner 2012; Gimenez and Smith 2017), to protect the downside eye and relax the animal. Horses use their head and neck as a lever to rise and when struggling may cause serious injury to an unprotected eye. Ensure blindfolds are easily removable – they should fall off if handler loses control. Panicked horses that stand and run with a blindfold will go until hitting a solid object or falling. |
| Always try to facilitate self-rescue: the legs, head, and neck should have free movement so that the animal can balance, stand, and move out of the entrapment. Many animals, when extricated or manipulated out of entrapment or rolled to sternal, will eventually rise and stand on their own. |
| Call for resources you may need earlier, not later: Call 911 for lighting, power, and cutting equipment, mechanical equipment, or escort to the scene; call for another Trailer for transport, LAR equipment, etc. |
| *Severely injured horses should not be transported without appropriate methods for medical support; in these situations, veterinary support or consultation is appropriate* (i.e., an animal with fracture should not be loaded on a trailer without a splint, pain treatment, and combating shock). |
| Always treat live and even dead animals with respect and professional methods – you never know who is watching or taking a video. |

## Arrival and Scene Control

- Put on personal protective equipment (PPE) appropriate to the scenario: Minimum PPE recommendations always include gloves, boots, helmet with chin strap for any LAR scene; with bright reflective vest for any on-road incident. LAR scenes have common injury hazards to personnel (Table 34.3).
- Take charge of the scene by establishing scene control zones: designate the HOT zone (area immediately around the horse) restricted to personnel immediately involved in the rescue tasks of triage, stabilization, and extrication. The WARM zone should be limited access, with only personnel providing direct support to the immediate rescue and extrication tasks. The COLD Zone is for support and logistics, bystanders, etc.
- Take a few seconds to look around the entire scene for situational awareness and size up critical factors: Identify what types of animal(s) are involved (i.e., rodeo broncs, breeding stock, racehorses). Interview knowledgeable witnesses for valuable information on mechanism and extent of injury, or locations of life safety hazards that may be present. Example: Trailer wreck may have several horses trapped, with a guard dog in the towing vehicle that is leaking fuel. Assess arrangement of obstacles and safest access to and egress for horse(s), then make an estimate of number of horses involved in the scenario (i.e., count doors and windows on horse trailers, estimate number of barn stalls, etc.)

**Table 34.3** General LAR hazards to personnel include.

- Injured by animal: bitten, kicked, crushed, knocked into, stepped on, etc.
- Injured by rescue gear: overhead hazards, rope burn, hurt lifting heavy items, hands caught in loop of webbing, crushed by heavy machinery, etc.
- Injured by environment: cut by metal on trailer, dehydration, trip over equipment, accidental hypothermia, step on a nail, etc.
- Secondary incidents: rubbernecking drivers slam into people directing traffic, horse gets loose and runs over rescuers, etc.

## Establish Control of Animal

*Assign a handler* (Husted et al. 2020) *to approach and gain control of the animal's head (if possible) with a halter or emergency rope halter* (Figure 34.2). The Handler's primary responsibility is to tend to the animal, direct and orient its movement and reactions to incident chaos. They should alert team members to potential problems, behavior, vital signs, etc. Team should alert the handler before touching, injecting, putting equipment around the animal – or when loud tools are started that may frighten the animal. The Handler is a crucial addition to the team and often directly responsible for success or failure of the rescue attempt. If loose animals cannot be caught, then secondary containment must be coordinated.

Note: Owners are rarely the best choice for handler – their priority is not consistent with maintaining safety for responders.

*Generally, humans should not enter the rescue environment with a horse (confined space, overturned trailer, floodwater, mud, etc.).* If the horse is still trapped when you arrive on scene – either self-rescue was unsuccessful, or there is a medical issue. Providing simple egress (removing obstacles, rolling it over, or making a ramp) may allow the animal to self-rescue. If those strategies don't work – technical rescue assistance from the local fire department should be called for sooner than later. Specialized resources and equipment anticipated for animal extrication are based on incident type (vertical lift sling, containment fencing, carcass disposal, transport from scene, etc.). Call for unusual resources early as response times may be long. Ask Fire Department to provide lighting (power generator/extension cords) or provide water or LAR equipment or ventilation (cooling/heating).

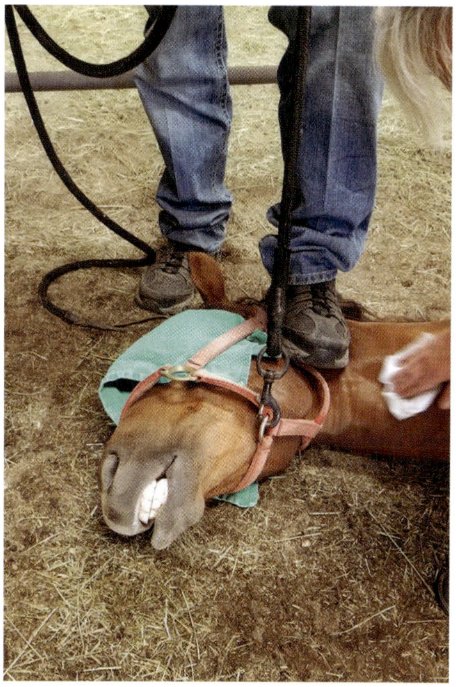

**Figure 34.2** Laterally recumbent horse with blindfold to protect the downside eye. Horse is being held down by the more ergonomic standing method (foot on the atlanto-occipital area, tip the nose up with the halter) than traditional "knee on neck" method. Note, care must be taken with the standing technique to avoid compression of the trachea and interference with normal ventilation.

## Veterinary Responsibilities

*The veterinarian has critical responsibilities as part of a team* (Box 34.5). *However, it differs from clinical practice – there are many dangers on roadways or even field extrications where the veterinarian is NOT the authority having jurisdiction (AHJ) over the scene.* The AHJ will be the firefighter or police officer that arrived first, and the practitioner is expected to fit into the working model of Incident Command System (ICS) on scene. The Incident Commander (IC) is ethically and legally responsible for the safety and lives of all personnel on his/her scene.

## Dual Planning

*A plan for triage, assessment, and treatment should occur simultaneously with the extrication planning effort, and before applying webbing or slings for lift or extrication.* If sedation, anesthesia or field euthanasia is needed – make decisions early (AVMA Policy on Euthanasia 2020; Shearer and Ramirez 2021). Plan the route of extrication to minimize obstacles and wasted time.

Assess transport and extrication resources. Veterinarians get training to remain calm, make rational decisions, and handle situations by close coordination with the owner which can ensure better outcomes based on good diagnosis and early treatment options, or in euthanasia being selected for induction at an early or rational point (Box 34.6). For example: if animal is significantly injured five miles into the wilderness, will it survive the response time, rescue effort, and subsequent walk out to transportation, be helicopter sling-lifted out, or be euthanized on scene?

Note: Recognize the limits of your knowledge, training, and experience. If the extent of the emergency is beyond your scope and resources, the animal might not be able to be rescued alive. If it cannot be safely approached and extricated, a euthanasia plan should be considered with the owner or animal control/welfare officer on scene.

## Common LAR Scene Issues

Long-term response factors: rural environments, the tendency of owners not to call for help until attempting to rescue the animal themselves, long entrapment times (hours to days) before discovery of the animal and can limit chances of success.

Ensure animal's medical status matches the rescue plan: if an animal is exhausted or dehydrated, if baseline vitals are poor, or when recumbence scenarios occur in wet or muddy environments, a sedated horse could drown or cause physiologic thermal maintenance issues. Animal may need to be aggressively treated or euthanized based on the extent of their internal or external injuries.

Triage efficiently in multiple casualty situations (Riley et al. 2016): resources should be conserved for animals more likely to survive. Primary triage should be conducted in an efficient manner on scene to effect extrication, then transport where secondary triage may be conducted at the clinic or off-site field hospital for mass casualty incidents. Veterinarian, Owner, Animal Control/Welfare Officer, and Incident Command should coordinate closely on euthanasia decisions and inform the media professionally – these are emotional events for people (Box 34.7).

**Box 34.5 Veterinary responsibilities during animal rescue**

*The veterinarian should assess the patient's condition, direct medical stabilization, and evaluate the risk/benefit of various strategies for extrication.* Let emergency responders do their job – by using a hands-off approach for extrication the practitioner can plan medical management and treatment options; advise the IC, owner, and Animal Control/Welfare officer; and prevent injury to themselves by staying out of the HOT zone.

**Box 34.6 How to triage rescue animals efficiently**

*Medically stabilizing the animal prior to and during the extrication is a dangerous task. Avoid tunnel vision: don't lose sight of hazards around you while evaluating horse(s).* If the horse is able, lead to a safer quiet spot for secondary triage. Examine animal more closely for internal injuries and provide initial treatment; once stable, transport immediately to definitive care at veterinary facilities.

**Box 34.7 How to handle people during animal rescue**

*Other responders and bystanders are not aware that recumbent or sedated animals can still be dangerous*, nor do they understand horse reactions while recovering from anesthesia. Understanding how large and fast a horse can potentially move is crucial for everyone's safety. The tendency to anthropomorphize horses with human emotions and cognition may make humans complacent.

*Animal incidents are remarkable in their ability to attract media* and tend to generate great public interest. Since they typically last longer than people extrications, the media will have time to arrive – dealing with news crews may be challenging while triaging and treating your victims.

## How to Use LAR Manipulations

### Cast Horse Rolls

This procedure assumes entrapment of head and legs are dealt with, handler has attached a halter and head protector to the animal for guidance and control, and rescuers have a pre-defined escape route – since the horse will often frantically attempt to stand after rolled.

*Simple one leg*: Because the pelvis of the horse is fixed, attaching girth hitch of rope or 4-in. webbing or rescue straps[9] to the downside hind leg at the pastern, then rolling the animal over the dorsal aspect at a 45° angle over the shoulder will ensure that the rest of the horse easily rolls over when leg is pulled.

*Simple two leg*: Attach girth hitch of rope or webbing to the downside legs (front and rear) from a safe position at the dorsum – position it around the pasterns, then pull both pieces of the webbing toward the dorsal aspect so that it rolls over the dorsum will often free the animal.

### Forward Assist

THREE configurations: SIMPLE/BASIC; CINCH/LARKSFOOT; and WIDENER/SWISS SEAT used to assist animal forward out of a ditch, edge of a muddy pond, or confined space where only the head, neck, and forelegs are reachable. The handler attaches a halter and head protector to the animal for guidance and control, uses their standing body position to hold the horse down (if laterally recumbent – uses a Rescue Glide or tarp to protect the downside skin), and ensures egress routes are clear with plenty of room for animal to move forward.

*Simple/basic forward assist*: This configuration is simplest to attach, remove, and easiest to learn to use. A 10 m piece of webbing or firehose is laid over the animal's withers at the halfway point, then each end of the webbing is wrapped under or over the chest at the sternum and pulled anteriorly between the legs, then attached with a carabiner to a long rope for manual pulling.

*Cinch/larks foot forward assist*: This configuration cinches down around the animal's chest, minimizing slippage. One 10 m piece of webbing with loops at each end is wrapped around the animal's chest at the withers, one end of the webbing is fed through the other looped end, fed anteriorly between the front legs, lastly webbing loop is attached with a carabiner to a long rope for manual pulling.

*Widener/swiss seat forward assist*: This configuration cinches around the animal's entire forequarters and pectoral girdle, effectively doubling the surface area of the webbing on the animal's skin – reducing slippage and the chance of injury from pressure used to pull or lift the animal out of entrapment. Highly recommended for posterior recumbency vertical lifts (Figure 34.3) this configuration does not come off the animal if properly emplaced and tightened before pulling or lifting.

One 10 m piece of webbing is held at the animal's chest below the thoracic inlet at the halfway point, then each end of the webbing is wrapped over the withers, around each side of the animal, down then under the chest at the sternum, then pulled anteriorly between the front legs; lastly it is fed up through the existing webbing at the thoracic inlet; then both looped ends attached with a carabiner to a long rope for manual pulling. If lifting from posterior recumbency, ensure head and neck have separate support to overhead lifting equipment.

9 Häst Rescue Straps, Häst, PSC, Floyd, VA https://rescue.hastpsc.com/products/accessories/straps/straps.html 804-286-0832.

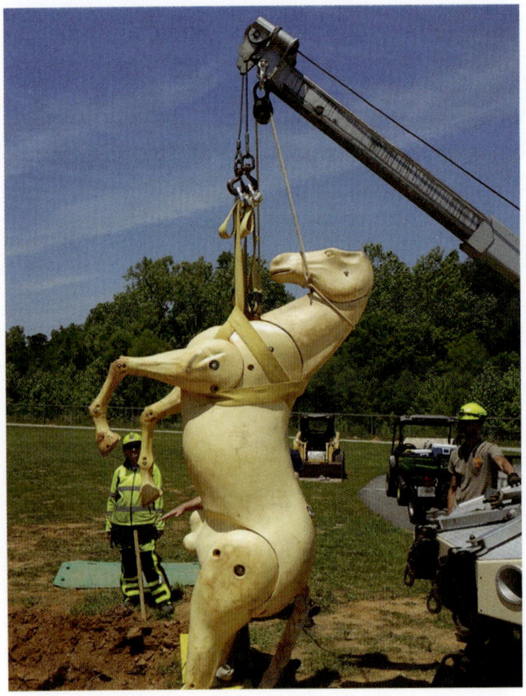

**Figure 34.3** Horse mannequin in simulated posterior recumbency. Webbing has been placed in the Widener/Swiss Seat configuration around chest and pectoral girdle to double the surface area and provide better support for a vertical lift maneuver. Note – the animal's head MUST BE SUPPORTED with rope from halter to an overhead attachment point, or it will fall to one side and injure the animal.

## Sideways Slide/Drag

This manipulation method requires two (2) pieces of 5 m long, 10 cm wide webbing or firehose (10 m length for draft horses.) The head is controlled by handler to reduce possible injury to the eye, or facial paralysis, and a Rescue Glide or tarp is used to minimize damage to the downside skin. For a standing animal (e.g., in a ditch) – two (2) pieces of webbing are separately flossed under the animal into position (front position) around the abdomen directly behind the front legs, and (back position) around the abdomen directly in front of the back legs. In a laterally recumbent animal, the webbing is passed over the down legs (front webbing passed over front leg; back webbing passed over back leg), and then back under the animal. Because of the placement of the webbing under the animal and over the down leg, the sideways slide allows both lifting and pulling from the animal's center of gravity. Following placement of the webbing, manual pulling systems are employed.

The sheer weight of the animals' body is used to keep it recumbent; this method increases the surface area of the animal on unstable ground surface (mud, slippery surface, etc.) while being moved to solid ground. Pull the animal sideways over mud or ground (Figure 34.4) or upwards over the edge of pool or ravine; or pull to roll and maneuver the animal into different positions or around obstacles on the ground. Continuous pressure will usually keep the animal from struggling.

## Backwards Slide/Drag

Horse is recumbent and safe access is to the rear end/posterior of the animal (recumbent in a trailer, culvert, stall, etc.) The head is controlled by handler to reduce possible injury to the eye, or facial paralysis, and a Rescue Glide or tarp is used to minimize damage to the downside skin. A 10 m piece of webbing is encircled around the animal's pelvis with the center of the webbing at the dorsum above the spine, at the loin. (Figure 34.5) The pieces of webbing with loops on the end are fed toward the abdomen, then are pushed between the back legs meeting at a carabiner which can be attached to a manual pulling system.

## Vertical Lift

This option involves heavy equipment, specialty slings, greater coordination between responders with increasing level of danger, and expense. Heavy sedation with close coordination between equipment operator and handler is required. However, when used with appropriate lifting equipment and attention to safety issues, Simple Vertical Lift Slings (Madigan 1993, Gimenez et al. 2004; Madigan et al. 2019a, b) provide a suitable means of short-term vertical lift of horses out of holes and obstacles, from entrapments, or from recumbency.

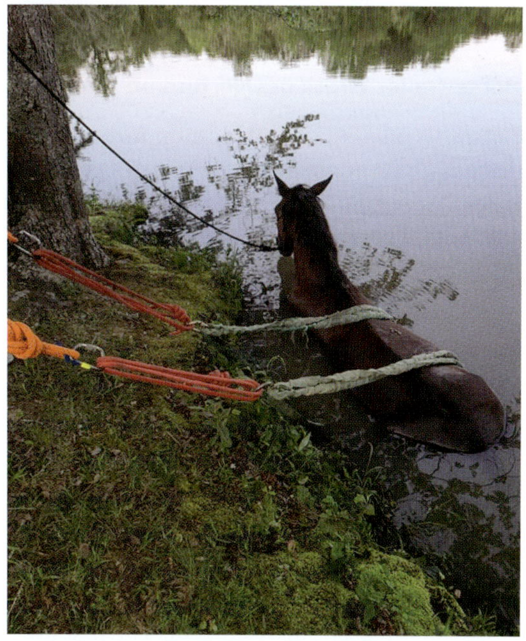

**Figure 34.4** Aged horse was stuck in mud next to the riverbank; removal was facilitated by use of the sideways drag technique. The horse was cold and exhausted, but efficient removal contributed to her stable treatment and successful outcome. Continuous loop slings from a tow truck, with carabiners and prussiks attached to a pulling rope are being used for the sideways drag.

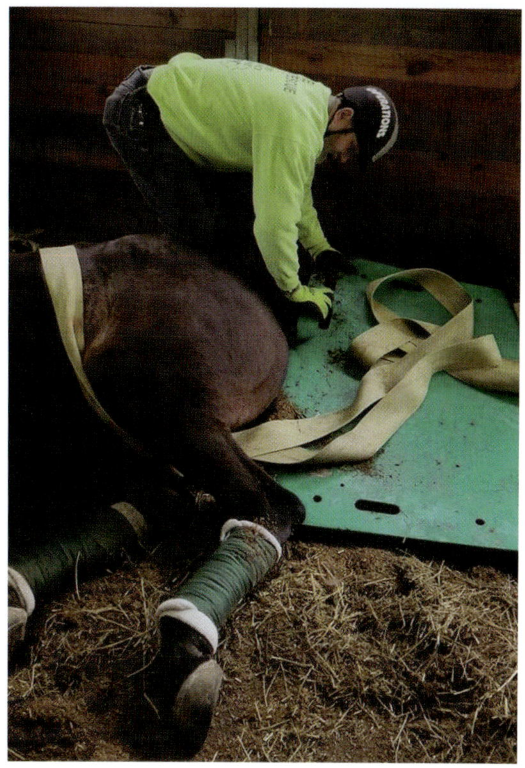

**Figure 34.5** Horse was found down in a stall with neurologic issues, necessitating transport to a veterinary school for diagnosis and treatment. Here, the backward drag configuration of webbing has been applied and the horse was pulled onto the Rescue Glide. The webbing is placed around the lumbar region and passed back through the hindlegs. Note the use of helmets, gloves, and boots for PPE on personnel. *Source:* Courtesy of Missouri Equine Response Service (MERS), MO.

## Rescue Glide Systems

Horses are notoriously difficult to move or transport when laterally recumbent. Rescue Glides or Large Animal Skeds (Gimenez 2011) provide practical means of moving a non-ambulatory horse. These skeds are modified from the human version at 2 or 2.5 m and use a restraint system to keep the horse on the equipment. Horses must usually be sedated during transport on a Glide/Sked to prevent further injury to itself or personnel. Horses with serious injuries, debilitation, or neurological symptoms can be easily relocated from a stall, removed from public view at an event/race/show, or even drawn along a wilderness trail to a trailer for transport to definitive veterinary care. This is one of the most useful LAR pieces of equipment for regular clinical use.

## Types of LAR Calls

### Horse Trailer Wreck or Overturn on the Roadway

Ensure traffic is controlled, minimize noise, assess from the outside through obvious openings (number of animals, orientation in trailer, obvious injuries or losses, location of probable exits, loose animals). Panicked horses will attempt egress through small openings (windows, etc.) If horse can stand, it will do so immediately – if recumbent, there is a reason. Slick floors, obstacles, hoof or leg trapped, and lack of leverage or space may contribute to failure to rise as much as injury or exhaustion. Hay can be given to quiet and calm horses while waiting for help.

Working with fire/rescue, prevent unintentional exit until secondary containment is set up, safely stabilize the weight of trailer before any human accesses into trailer, remove obstacles (dividers, doors, ramps, cut trailer ties), and allow self-extrication. Cover "holes" in overturned trailer "floor" with a backboard or rubber mats. If trapped or recumbent, sedate and assess a plan for cutting or manipulation to extricate animal. Ensure egress openings (minimum 4-ft wide and as tall as possible) provide structural integrity. Pole syringe can induce IM sedation without a human entering the trailer. Triage, Treat, or Euthanize based on injuries. Plan egress path for leading the animal to a safe area off the roadway or directly to transport.

Manipulations to Consider: Sideways Slide/Drag, Forward Assist, Backwards Slide/Drag, Cast Horse Roll.

Note: *Most frequent injuries reported by practitioners are head, neck, and lower leg injuries – at impact horses fall forward into the chest bar or bulkhead area. The first area to absorb the blow is the face and neck, then lower legs are injured as the animal scrambles to stand up.*

Note: *A common scenario with high mortality rates are horse trailer floor failures – shock, severe injuries, and pain, and animals rarely have relevant muscle, bone, ligament, or tendon anatomy available to make a surgical attempt for recovery.*

### Horse and/or Rider Hit by Vehicle on the Roadway

If first on scene – ensure traffic is controlled, stabilize medical needs of injured person. If horse is lying on top of the person, consider immediate sedation/anesthesia/euthanasia to prevent further rider injury. Move the horse off the person (coordinated with EMS personnel). Triage, Treat, or Euthanize horse based on injuries. Coordinate transportation resources early.

Manipulations to consider: Sideways Slide/Drag, Forward Assist, Backwards Slide/Drag, Cast Horse Roll.

### Loose Horses in the Roadway

If first on scene – ensure traffic is controlled, limit bystanders chasing horses, use a judas horse to attempt to lure horses off roadway (also try using grain or hay) then attempt to halter at least one animal. Use of portable fence panels or construction fencing can be employed to guide animals to safer areas. Triage, Treat, or Euthanize animals based on injuries. Coordinate transportation resources early.

### Horse Trapped in Mud, Pond, Well, Pool, Septic Tank, or Lake Edge

Keep people out of the entrapment while making plans and marshalling resources. Handler supports animal's head and neck with any form of floatation and halter if safe access is possible, consider pumping the hole dry, may need Nicopolous Needle to emplace webbing under the equine through water or mud, may need to inject air or water through mud lances to break suction of mud. Treat for hypothermia and prevent accidental hypothermia (Morauw and Gimenez 2014) and sequela from crush syndrome. Remember sedation will cause horse to drop head potentially into water and may lead to drowning.

Manipulations to consider: Sideways Slide/Drag, Forward Assist, Vertical Lift using Sling.

### Horse Laterally or Sternally Recumbent on the Ground (May Be Entrapped or Entangled)

Keep people away from the legs, animal handler should use a halter and their position to keep the horse down until entrapment is cut away. Protect the head and downside eye with a head protector.

Manipulations to consider: Sideways Slide/Drag, Forward Assist, Backward Slide/Drag, Cast Horse Roll, Vertical Lift using Sling.

### Horse in Anterior or Dorsal Recumbency Position (Entrapped or Entangled)

Keep people away from the legs, animal handler should use a halter and their position to keep the horse controlled until entrapment is cut away. Protect head and eyes with head protector.

Manipulations to consider: Sideways Slide/Drag, Forward Assist, Backward Slide/Drag, Cast Horse Roll, Vertical Lift using Sling.

### Horse Fallen Through Surface Ice

Keep people off the ice while making plans from shore and marshalling resources. Fire/Rescue must be called, and surface ice rescue PPE utilized. Handler tries to support animal's head and neck with any form of floatation and halter only if easy to do; small ponds or holes may be pumped dry. Cutting ice blocks then pushing them under surrounding ice to make a clear path to shore is easiest method, use chainsaws or ice saws. Remove vegetation at the egress point. Use Rescue Glide or plywood to protect edges during sideways drag. Hypothermia and accidental hypothermia are common.

Manipulations to consider: Sideways Slide/Drag over Surface of Ice, Lead or Forward Assist through cleared path in water, Vertical Lift using Sling.

### Competition Emergency (Three-Day Event, Rodeo, Racing, Show Jumping, Endurance, etc.)

Designated Handler gets control of horses' head for triage. Injured people are first priority. Decide upon extrication method, if horse will be mobile or recumbent for transport, or euthanize on site. Consider use of tarps held up by people to block view for euthanasia, cover head and eyes with towel, then roll onto Glide and load in trailer. Do not drag dead horses with chains by a tractor.

Manipulations to consider: Sideways Slide/Drag, Rescue Glide, Vertical Lift using Sling.

### Horse Trapped in Smoking or Burning Structure (Barn, Trailer, Arena)

Veterinarian should be called immediately with the fire/rescue responders to be able to provide immediate triage and treatment. Rarely will practitioners arrive before the fire department – rescue of people and horses out of the barn (Gimenez et al. 2008b, Gimenez 2011; Morauw and Gimenez 2014) may be done from outside wall stall openings even if there is live smoke and fire, but no one is allowed inside the interior aisle of a burning structure until fire department gives permission (due to concerns for collapse, toxic gases, and direct injury from heat). Instead, be prepared to conduct primary triage of evacuated animals for burn injuries (external, but more commonly internal), evaluate efficiently for immediate treatment at farm or transport to referral, or conduct immediate euthanasia of severe burn cases. The most common problems associated with barn fire injuries in horses include immediate carbon monoxide inhalation and subsequent hypoxia, various degrees of cutaneous burn injury, burn shock associated with rapid percutaneous fluid loss, smoke injury to the respiratory system, including severe inflammation and edema and secondary pneumonia (see *Chapter 22: Triage and Management of Injuries Associated with Fire and Flood Exposure*). Emergency triage at the farm may include delivering intranasal oxygen, fluid therapy to manage shock, rinsing burned skin with cool water to slow skin injury, decrease inflammation with NSAIDs and begin systemic antibiotics to prevent secondary infection. Tracheostomy may also be required to provide oxygen and prevent upper respiratory obstruction, especially with severe edema and tissue sloughing. Burn injury debridement and skin grafting may also be required during the healing process. In addition, increased nutritional requirements are required in horses following burn injury because of the high energy demands of healing. Use a scribe to take notes as you conduct triage and provide initial treatment – especially at scenes involving large numbers of animals – this will help with later reports and keeping track of first aid, aggressive treatment/therapy, under emotional duress.

*Special mention*: Some fires are later deemed arson – treat every fire scene as a crime scene. To be able to prosecute arsonists for cruelty, law enforcement will want at the minimum the veterinarian's detailed reports and may wish to have a full necropsy by a pathologist.

Manipulations: None. Prevention and Mitigation strategies are strongly suggested.

## Conclusion

Local equine practitioners are the first responder of preference for incidents involving horses (Shearer and Ramirez 2021); emergency 911 services will call you. Prior coordination with local law enforcement, fire/rescue, and emergency management offices will lead to improved outcomes for victims, owners, and responders on scene (Thompson et al. 2015). Individual preparation and training, effective use of simple LAR equipment, personnel positioning and standardized extrication techniques give professional results. Immediate treatment in situ as well as after extrication improves the prognosis for many horses.

### Case Example 34.1 Emergent Down Horse

Patient: *three-year-old Percheron/Belgian cross mare, 1800 pounds, 17 hands*
History: *Draft Horse fell onto the surface of the ice at least 12 h ago – was dragged off the ice to land by regional large animal response team and firefighters with Ice Rescue PPE using webbing around the body (not the head and neck); veterinarian was called. Horse couldn't stand and was hypothermic* (Figure 34.6).

Step 1: immediate patient stabilization

1) *Initiate Treatment for Regular Hypothermia – Warm and Dry the horse without stimulating the skin/causing Accidental Hypothermia. Insulate from wind and cold, warming blankets, forced air heaters, rectally administer warmed fluids, etc.*
2) *Provide intranasal oxygen (2 L soda bottle cut in half fits over nose with taped line)*
3) *Record Temperature, Respiratory and Heart rate, and evaluate distress*
4) *Evaluate mucous membranes for perfusion status*
5) *Get horse Sternal and support in Recovery Position**
6) *Provide warmed fluids, pain control, anti-inflammatory and antibiotic medications*

*Perform a quick, yet focused patient assessment to evaluate the following*

1) *Wounds*
2) *Head Trauma*
3) *Prevent Accidental Hypothermia*
4) *Wounds, Hemorrhage, and Bruising*
5) *Inhalation of Water (depends on whether immersed or not)*
6) *Rib or Leg fracture (common if animal goes through ice)*
7) *Blood samples for laboratory assessment (kidney and muscle damage, etc.)*

* The RECOVERY POSITION for equines is sternal recumbency – as soon as the animal is capable of being rolled to sternal without hurting a handler, it can be supported at the shoulder (Figure 34.6). The sternal recovery position allows the animal more efficient respirations, returns normal mentation and thermoregulation faster, thus allowing it to attempt to stand sooner. *Encouraging an animal to stand when it is not mentally or physically capable of doing so can result in severe injury to the animal or bystanders as it falls again.*

*History Questions to Ask the Owner*

(Unwitnessed or Witnessed fall to recumbency or failure to rise) When was the last time the horse was seen standing or in normal positions? Is the animal trapped in an obstacle (i.e., inside a trailer, feeder, tree branches, or ditch)? Has the equine eaten anything? Did anyone give any drugs or treatment before the veterinarian arrived? Did horse fall over backward, or to the side? Can you get TPR safely? Did you get photo or short video of situation?

(Owner Consult – over phone on the way to location) Give Directives for First aid while waiting for Veterinarian: CALL 911 for fire rescue assistance. Do not go out onto surface of pond ice. IF ABLE FROM A SAFE POSITION: Get a towel, heavy shirt, riding pad or horse blanket under the horses' head to protect the downside eye. Use Blanket to Protect from further cooling. Put on a halter and lead for head control. Remove all obstacles from the immediate area that the horse could kick or roll into. Stay out of the way of the legs and hooves and let the animal rest while waiting for the arrival of veterinarian. Provide hay for insulation, and if horse is interested in eating.

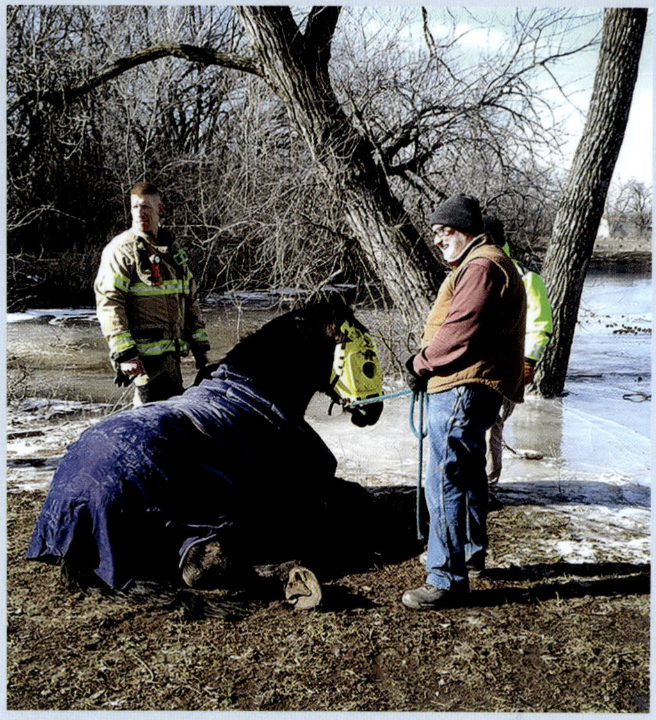

**Figure 34.6** A 3-year-old Percheron/Belgian cross immediately after being dragged by webbing and ropes off the surface of an icy pond (horse was down on the ice for 12 h). The horse had a low body temperature and was unable to stand. Immediate stabilization included treatment for hypothermia (drying and warming blankets), warmed fluids, and getting animal to recovery position (sternal) – here the firefighter is stabilizing the animal in sterna recumbency at the shoulder.

Step 2: formulating a plan

Once the horse is stable, further assess the animal to determine Manipulation, Lifting, and Transportation options with the goal of the horse being able to recover and stand on its own:

1) *Manipulation of the Horse to Sternal Recovery Position in situ*
2) *Encouragement of the Horse to Standing in situ*
3) *Manipulation and Transport of the Horse to Better Footing (Figure 34.7a, b) or Warm/Dry Location for long-term monitoring, evaluation, and treatment (i.e., Stall or Arena area)*
4) *Manipulation and Transport of the Horse on a Rescue Glide sked into a trailer for Delivery to Definitive Treatment (i.e., veterinary clinic)*
5) *Manipulation and Sling Vertical Lift for temporary support to allow animal to stand (Figure 34.8a, b).*

Step 3: manipulation and sling lifting guidelines

Working with the emergency response team and owner – choices can be made to provide ground transport to better rehabilitation conditions while in lateral recumbency and/or short-term sling lifting support (with the goal of allowing the animal to stand and support its own weight, not maintaining its full weight in the sling)

- Use of sked/glides and equine slings require prior training and team practice – there are numerous commercially available systems available – but safety of the handler and team members working around the horse while attaching webbing, hobbles, slings, and either pulling or lifting is paramount. Chemical restraint is normally utilized unless the horse is completely debilitated.
- Winches or Mechanical Advantage can be attached to the sked or Glide to pull the weight to another location – but not to any part of the horse's body or limbs. Head and neck is not an attachment point for pulling – only for a halter for guidance.
- Most types of slings feature support of the pelvic and pectoral girdles of the appendicular skeleton – but it is possible for a horse to fall or slide out if chest and butt straps are not properly placed. Appropriate heavy equipment must be selected for use that is tall enough and heavy enough to withstand lifting a potentially struggling horse.

(a) (b)

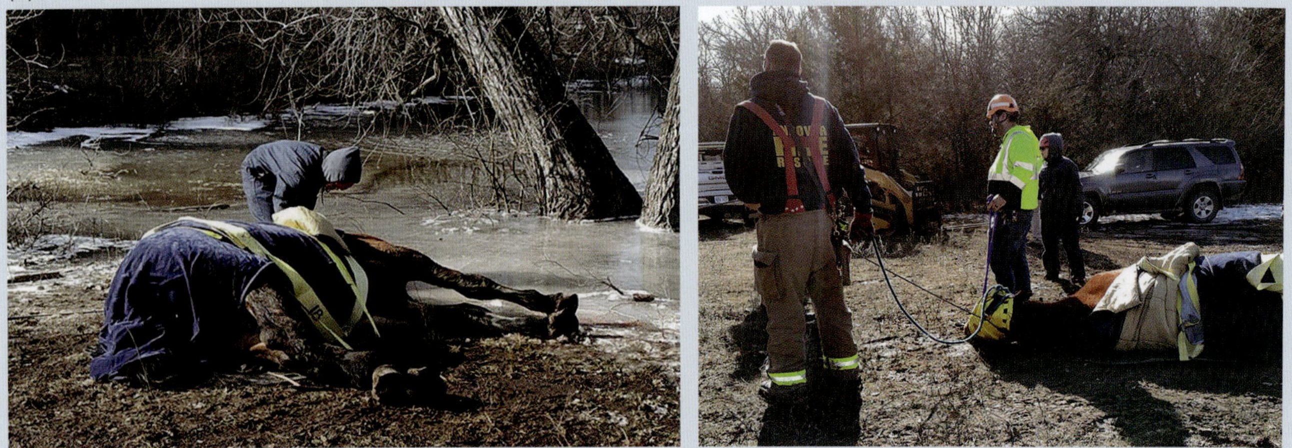

**Figure 34.7** (a, b) A decision was made by the owner, veterinarian, and emergency response team to move the animal to better footing to allow her to roll and attempt to stand. Sedation was given, straps were placed for sideways drag onto a sked, then animal was pulled up the hill to a better position using the winch on a truck attached to the Glide. Note the use of head protection to prevent injury to the facial nerves or eyes. Häst Becker Sling straps were then emplaced to allow a vertical sling lift to support the horse standing.

(a) (b)

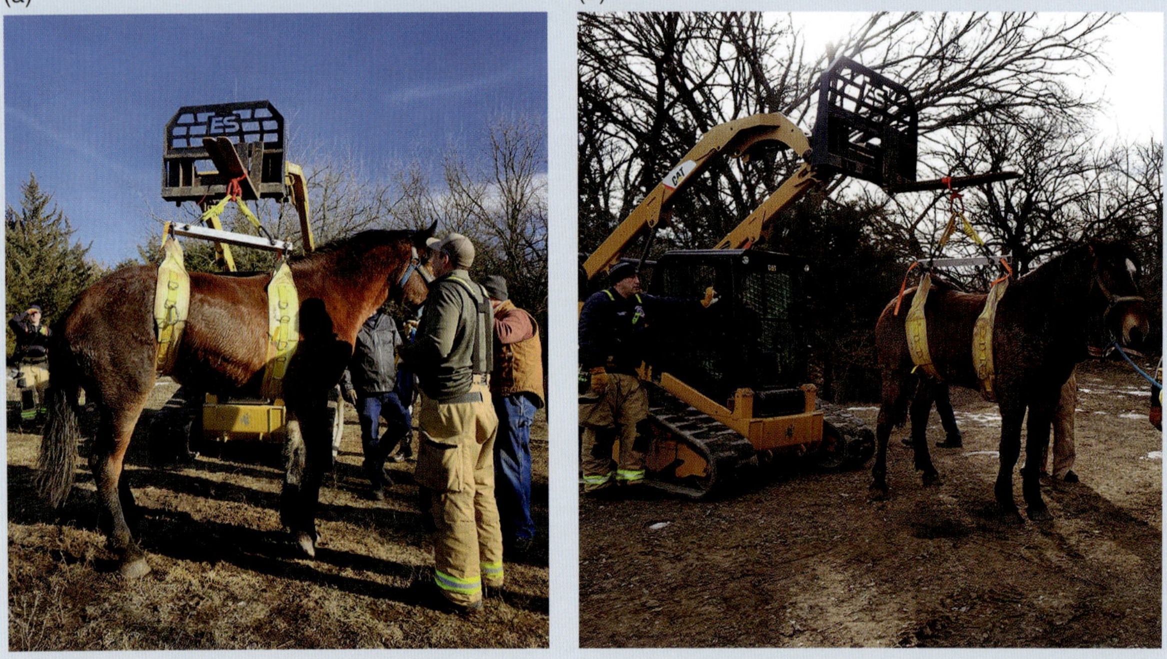

**Figure 34.8** (a, b) Horse is vertically lifted from recumbency using the Häst Becker Sling by appropriate mechanical equipment locally sourced. By providing vertical sling lift, the horse was able to put weight on the leg gradually and eventually support its own weight – as it woke up from sedation. *Use of a chest and butt strap is normally recommended – not used here.

Step 4: safety, assessment, and monitoring

Serial patient monitoring is essential during and after emergency response because horses may have muscle and nerve trauma or inability to thermoregulate normally and may develop serious complications even several days or longer following injury.

- Routine assessment should include a physical exam including monitoring of respiratory and heart rates, mentation, and quality of effort to rise.

- Selection of a method of physical or chemical restraint requires consideration of the situation, the behavior and size of the animal, personal protective equipment availability, and cooperation of the veterinary team responding.
- Laterally recumbent equines tend to go into a catatonic state for short periods interrupted by thrashing or flailing in attempts to get sternal or stand. Plugging the ears to reduce sounds, covering the eyes (downside to prevent injury and upside to prevent visual stimulation), and limiting touch to reduce struggling may reduce stimulation while being evaluated.
- Equids that endure long periods of recumbency often incur muscle, nerve and other soft-tissue and/or bone injury. These animals frequently require sling lift as well as significant nursing care, and generally have a poorer prognosis.
- Laterally recumbent equines cannot thermoregulate well, they may undergo myositis of their muscles on the down side, and their oxygen saturation will decrease over time in that position due to the lack of normal function of the downside lung (whether sedated, anesthetized, or not).

Step 5: decision making during triage

Difficult decisions face the emergency clinician working with ice-associated falls and long-time recumbent patients (Figure 34.9).

- Hypothermic patients may require long-term monitoring and support before recovering their ability to stand or to thermoregulate normally. If client does not have facilities or financial ability to prevent wind and weather affecting horse during recovery, consider euthanasia.
- Down horses may panic – failure in attempts to stand or serious fall again may cause head injury. These horses can injure a person and themselves – they should be held in lateral recumbency while evaluated by a veterinarian – possibly sedated immediately, or euthanasia considered.
- As a guideline, horses do not do well in long-term recumbency nor long-term sling lifting – their welfare, client financial considerations, and ability to provide sling lifting support versus recumbency should be measured when making decisions.

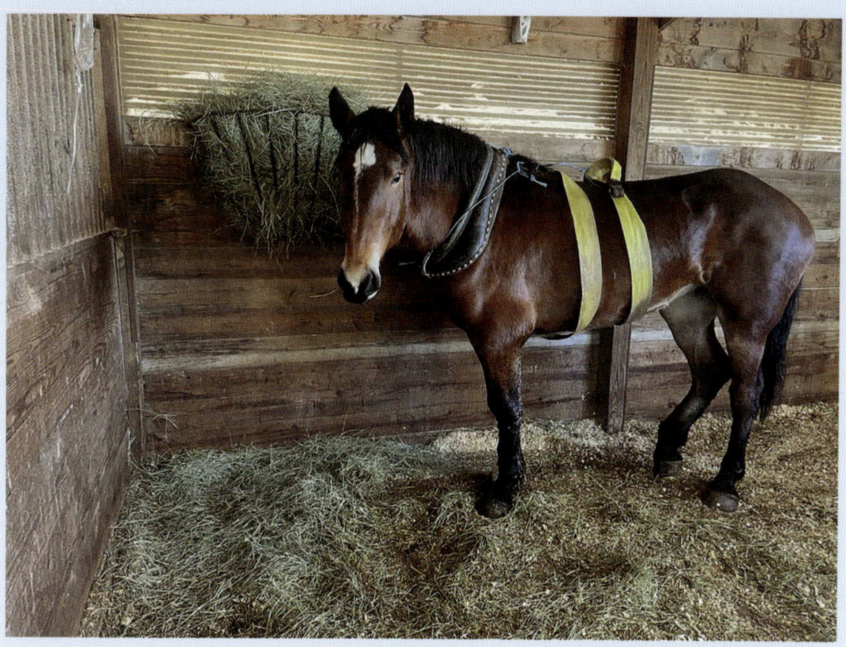

**Figure 34.9** Over the ensuing two weeks, the horse laid down normally but was unable to get up on her own if muddy or wet conditions – muscle injury and kidney function laboratory assays revealed minimal damage. The owner resorted to leaving lifting straps on the horse full time (in case of laying down) while in a stall. Horse was rehabilitated with exercise, and veterinarian provided regular monitoring to ensure thermoregulatory system return to normal and musculoskeletal healing.

## Photo Credits and Case Details

Andover, Kansas Fire-Rescue; Butler County, Kansas Animal Response Team, CERT Team, and Emergency Management; Brian Begley, owner; Jason Kiser, DVM.

## References


AVMA Policy on Euthanasia (2020). Edition. https://www.avma.org/KB/Policies/Documents/euthanasia.pdf (accessed 11 August 2021).

Emergency Management Institute (2021). Federal emergency management agency. ICS 100 training. https://training.fema.gov/is/courseoverview.aspx?code=IS-100.c (accessed 11 August 2021).

Gardner, R. (2012). Caring for the down horse. In: *Manual of Equine Emergencies*, 4e (ed. J.A. Orsini and T.J. Divers), 626–633. Philadelphia: Saunders.

Gimenez, T.G. (November 1, 2011). Tech Rescue: Accidental hypothermia calls in horses, Firehouse. https://www.firehouse.com/home/article/10445948/firefighter-technical-rescue-horse-hypothermia (accessed 26 August 2021).

Gimenez, T. (2012). The golden hours of equine emergency rescue. *Equine Vet.* 2: 26–29.

Gimenez, R. (2015). Trailer or vehicle crashes. In: *Equine Medicine*, 7e (ed. K.A. Sprayberry and N.E. Robinson), 1–5. St. Louis: Elsevier/Saunders.

Gimenez, R.M. and McConnico, R. (December 1–5, 2018). How to develop an equine veterinary facility all-hazards sheltering and evacuation plan. *Proceedings, Am Assoc Equine Pract,* San Francisco, CA 64: 74–86.

Gimenez, R.M. and Smith, S. (November 17–21, 2017). How to manipulate a recumbent horse (entrapment, clinical, or technical emergency rescue situations). *Proceedings, Am Assoc Equine Pract*, San Antonio, TX 63: 403–412.

Gimenez, T., Gimenez, R.M., Baker, J.L., and Johannessen, D.T. (December 4–8, 2002). How to effectively perform emergency rescue of equines. *Proceedings, Am Assoc Equine Pract,* Orlando, FL 48: 276–281.

Gimenez, R.M., Gimenez, T., Stafford, K. et al. (December 4–8, 2004). How to employ recumbent transport, perform a simple vertical lift, and perform proper helicopter slingload of horses. *Proceedings, Am Assoc Equine Pract*, Denver, CO 50: 433–446

Gimenez, R.M., Gimenez, T., and Stafford, K. (2004). Implementation of the equine rescue glide. *J. Vet. Emerg. Crit. Care* 14: S1–S17.

Gimenez, T., Gimenez, R., and May, K. (ed.) (2008a). *Technical Large Animal Emergency Rescue*. New York: John Wiley & Sons.

Gimenez, R.M., Dwyer, R., Woods, J. and Gimenez, T. (December 6–10, 2008b). A review of strategies to prevent and respond to fires affecting the horse industry. *Proceedings, Am Assoc Equine Pract*, San Diego, CA 54: 160–179.

Gimenez, T., Gimenez, R.M., and Mansmann, R.A. (2012). Disaster medicine and technical emergency rescue. In: *Manual of Equine Emergencies*, 4e (ed. J.A. Orsini and T.J. Divers), 634–645. Philadelphia: Saunders.

Husted, R., Egli, M., and Davenport, A. (December 5–9, 2020). How to safely restrain a laterally recumbent horse. *Proceedings, Am Assoc Equine Pract,* Las Vegas, NV 66: 466–472.

Madigan, J.E. (1993). Evaluation of a new sling support device for horses. *J. Equine Vet. Sci.* 13: 260–263.

Madigan, J., Costa, L., Nieves, S. et al. (2019a). Evaluation of a simplified loops system for emergency rescue lifting of the stranded or recumbent horse. *Animals* 9 (8): 511. https://doi.org/10.3390/ani9080511 (accessed 20 August 2021).

Madigan, J., Costa, L., Nieves, S. et al. (2019b). Description of placement procedures for common methods used in equine emergency rescue using a simplified loops system. *Animals* 9 (8): 529. https://doi.org/10.3390/ani9080529 (accessed 20 August 2021).

Morauw, C. and Gimenez, R.M. (December 6-10, 2014). How to configure an equine facility to prevent and better respond to barn fires. *Proceedings, Am Assoc Equine Pract*, Salt Lake City, UT 60: 440–450.

Riley, C.B., Noble, B.R., Bridges, J. et al. (2016). Horse injury during non-commercial transport: findings from researcher-assisted intercept surveys at southeastern Australian equestrian events. *Animals* 6 (11): 65. https://doi.org/10.3390/ani6110065.

Shearer, J.K. and Ramirez, A. (2021). *Procedures for Humane Euthanasia: Humane Euthanasia of Sick, Injured and/or Debilitated Livestock*. Iowa State University Humane Euthanasia Training, Iowa State University Extension. https://vetmed.iastate.edu/vdpam/about/focus-areas/dairy/dairy-extension/humane-euthanasia (accessed 11 August 2021).

Thompson, K., Leighton, M., and Riley, C. (2015). Helping hands, hurting hooves: towards a multidisciplinary paradigm of large animal rescue. *Aust. J. Emerg. Manag.* 30: 53–58. https://www.researchgate.net/publication/275963796_Helping_hands_hurting_hooves_Towards_a_multidisciplinary_paradigm_of_large_animal_rescue (accessed 20 August 2021).

# 35

# Emergency Welfare Response

*Rachel Gardner*

*BW Furlong and Associates, Oldwick, NJ, USA*

Veterinarians may be faced with equine welfare cases on an emergency basis. These cases can be challenging, in part because they require a distinct two-pronged approach that differs from management of most other situations encountered in equine emergency medicine. First, the individual patient(s) must be evaluated and treated. While there may be a single or few horses presented, situations may arise where large numbers of horses are affected which require triage to provide veterinary attention where it is needed most. Secondly, investigating, documenting, and reporting the situation may be required. Veterinarians play a vital role in working with both animal welfare investigators and law enforcement to provide for horses that have experienced abuse or neglect. It is important that veterinarians are familiar with how to manage situations of possible equine maltreatment as records and documentation may subsequently be used in a court of law.

## Patient Evaluation

It is critically important that as thorough a physical examination as possible be performed. In some cases, multiple and sometimes large numbers of horses may be involved. The number of horses and behavior of the horses may preclude thorough physical examination in some situations. Exam findings should be systematically recorded (Figure 35.1).

Horses should first be evaluated in their environment, if applicable and possible, to make an assessment of demeanor, mentation, vocalization, and behavior. If there are multiple horses, this initial assessment will likely help determine which horses should be prioritized for examination and treatment. Components of an initial assessment are summarized in Box 35.1.

### Physical Exam

- Whether presented with a group of horses or a single horse, it is important to identify each horse.
  - Age, breed, gender, and a description of the color or markings should be recorded. An estimate of age and breed should be made if not known.
  - Any identification such as a brand, tattoo, or microchip should be recorded.
- Body weight should be estimated using a weight tape and body condition score (BCS) should be determined using the Henneke Body Condition Scoring system (Table 35.1; Henneke et al. 1983).
  - Both visual exam and palpation should be used to determine BCS.
  - It is important to note that many factors can affect the BCS including feed availability, feeding practices, dental disease, reproductive status, environmental conditions, concurrent disease, energy demands, herd dynamics, and parasitic infections.
  - Not all under conditioned horses are neglected. Poor condition must be supported by other clinical signs in order to be considered starvation.

*Emergency Triage of the Horse*, First Edition. Edited by Rolfe M. Radcliffe and Jamie J. Kopper.
 Published 2026 by John Wiley & Sons, Inc.
Companion website: www.wiley.com/go/radcliffe/triage

EQUINE EXAM FORM

CASE #: ____________ DATE: ____________ TIME: _________ HORSE ID: ______________
EXAMINING VETERINARIAN: ______________ LOCATION: __________________________
GENDER: ________ COLOR: _____________ BRAND/TATTOO/MICROCHIP: _____________
MARKINGS: ______________________________ SCARS: ___________________________
AGE: ____________(note if estimated) BREED: ________________________ (note if estimated)
BODY CONDITION SCORE (1–9): _______ WEIGHT: _______ (weight tape estimate)
HEIGHT: _____h
BEHAVIOR (docile, aggressive, compulsive, manic): ______________________________

PHYSICAL EXAMINATION NOTES:

Subjective: bright alert responsive dull depressed
Objective: T: _______P: ______ R: ______ hydration status: ______________

Cardiovascular: MM: _______ CRT: ________ heart auscultation: ___________
Respiratory: nostrils: __________ lung auscultation: ____________ _________
Ophthalmic exam
Ears:
Lymph Nodes:
Integument: skin: __________ haircoat: ____________ wounds: ________________
Musculoskeletal: joints_____digital pulses: _____ lameness: __________hooves: _______
Neurologic: mentation: bright obtunded lethargic stuporous comatose
cranial nerves: __________ ataxia: ________________________
GI: Oral exam: ______________ abd. auscultation: __________ manure: _________
Genito urinary: external genitalia: ____________ urine: _______ if mare: ☐ suspect pregnant?

Collected: Coggins Chem CBC Fecal

Other diagnostics:

Additional notes:

Assessment:

Plan/Treatment:

ENVIRONMENT NOTES:

Shelter: Stabled Pasture/paddock w/ adequate shelter None
Shelter: Adequate size Inadequate
(Describe)_____________________________________________________

Fencing: Adequate Inadequate
(Describe type, condition, safety hazards)________________________________
Enclosure size: # of horses: ______ # of other animals: ______ (note species) __________

Manure accumulation: Minimal Moderate Heavy
Ammonia Odor: None Minimal Significant
Fly presence: Minimal fly burden Moderate fly burden Significant fly infestation

Water: Freely available Adequate Quality that does not discourage consumption
Not Freely available Inadequate Quality
Hay availability: Adequate quality + quantity Adequate quality, inadequate quantity
Inadequate quality, adequate quantity Inadequate quality + quantity
Other Feed (if available): Adequate quality + quantity Adequate quality, inadequate quantity
Inadequate quality, adequate quantity Inadequate quality + quantity

Additional notes:

**Figure 35.1** Equine exam form. *Source:* Adapted from AAEP Equine Exam Form.

**Box 35.1 Components of an initial assessment**

- Physical examination
  - Weight, BCS
  - Vital signs
  - Thorough examination
- Diagnostic testing
  - CBC
  - Serum biochemistry
  - Fecal floatation
  - Coggins test
  - +/– Vitamin E and selenium
  - +/– Others based on examination

**Table 35.1** Henneke body condition score chart.

| Score | Condition | Description |
|---|---|---|
| 1 | Poor | Horse is extremely emaciated. Spinous processes, ribs, tailhead, tuber coxae, and tuber ischii projecting prominently. Bone structure of withers, shoulders, and neck easily noticeable. No fatty tissue can be felt |
| 2 | Very thin | Horse is emaciated. Slight fat covering over base of spinous processes, transverse processes of lumbar vertebrae feel rounded. Spinous processes, ribs, tailhead, tuber coxae, and tuber ischii prominent. Withers, shoulders, and neck structures faintly discernible |
| 3 | Thin | Fat build up about halfway on spinous processes, transverse processes cannot be felt. Slight fat cover over ribs. Spinous processes and ribs easily discernible. Tailhead prominent, but individual vertebrae cannot be visually identified. Tuber coxae appear rounded, but easily discernible. Tuber ischii not distinguishable. Withers, shoulders, and neck accentuated |
| 4 | Moderately thin | There is a negative crease along back. Faint outline of ribs discernable. Tailhead prominence depends on conformation, fat can be felt around it. Tuber coxae not discernable. Withers, shoulders, and neck not obviously thin |
| 5 | Moderate | Back level. Ribs cannot be visually distinguished but can be easily felt. Fat around tailhead beginning to feel spongy. Withers appear rounded over spinous processes. Shoulders and neck blend smoothly into body |
| 6 | Moderately fleshy | May have slight crease down back. Fat over ribs feels spongy. Fat around tailhead feels soft. Fat beginning to be deposited along the side of the withers, behind the shoulders and along the sides of the neck |
| 7 | Fleshy | May have crease down back. Individual ribs can be felt, but noticeable filling between ribs with fat. Fat around tailhead is soft. Fat deposited along withers, behind shoulders, and along the neck |
| 8 | Fat | Crease down back. Difficult to feel ribs. Fat around tailhead very soft. Area along withers filled with fat. Area behind shoulder filled with fat. Noticeable thickening of neck. Fat deposited along inner thighs |
| 9 | Extremely fat | Obvious crease down back. Patchy fat appearing over ribs. Bulging fat around tailhead, along withers, behind shoulders and along neck. Fat along inner thighs may rub together. Flank filled with fat |

*Source:* Henneke et al. (1983)/The Bureau of Land Management.

- A thorough physical exam should be performed, starting with vital signs.
  - Thorough cardiothoracic auscultation should be performed taking note of heart rate, rhythm, and the presence of cardiac murmurs. Tachycardia or cardiac murmurs may suggest anemia or systemic response to disease beyond malnutrition. Mucous membranes should be assessed for hydration, color, and capillary refill time.
  - When possible, a basic oral exam should be performed to assess for the presence of severe dental disease.
  - The skin and coat should be evaluated for condition, and for the presence of parasites, or wounds.
  - The hooves should be evaluated for signs of disease such as thrush, laminitis or canker, and for overgrowth suggestive of neglect.
  - The eyes and ears should be evaluated.
  - If applicable, the horse should be walked to assess for lameness or ataxia.

### Diagnostic Testing

- Samples for diagnostic testing should be taken prior to initiation of any treatment.
- A complete blood count (CBC) should be performed to look for evidence of dehydration, anemia, and changes in the white blood cell count suggestive of underlying disease.
- A serum biochemistry panel should be performed to evaluate for hypoproteinemia that may be present with malnutrition or protein losing disorders and to evaluate for concurrent diseases such as renal or hepatic disease.
- Testing of serum electrolyte concentrations should be performed, recognizing that serum values may not accurately reflect total body stores.
- Testing of vitamin E and selenium concentrations may be indicated if white muscle disease is suspected.
- The combination of hypoproteinemia, hyperbilirubinemia, and hypertriglyceridemia may be present in malnourished horses.
- Fecal flotation and a Coggin's test should be performed.
- Further diagnostic testing such as radiographs should be performed as deemed necessary based on physical exam findings.
- Use of reference laboratories is superior to testing in-house in welfare cases due to possible concerns with legality.

## Next Steps

Following the initial exam, it must be decided how to proceed with the case(s). Options include:

- Treatment of the individual horse(s) on premises
- Referral to a veterinary center for more intensive care/monitoring
- Seizure of the horse by authorities to a welfare group
- Recommendations for euthanasia are outlined in Box 35.2

### Transport Considerations

- Weak or malnourished horses present unique challenges.
- Horses should ideally be shipped in open stock-type trailers or trailers with box stalls due to risk of falling.
- Horses should not be tied due to risk of injury if they fall.
- Bed the trailer deeply in the event of collapse.

## Refeeding

The reintroduction of feed to previously starved or malnourished horses must be done carefully. Refeeding syndrome is a well-documented sequela to reintroduction of feed in previously starved animals.

- In horses with refeeding syndrome, the introduction of carbohydrates, particularly glucose, causes insulin release. Insulin prevents the release of free fatty acids and results in intracellular influx of glucose and electrolytes. This process decreases serum concentrations of glucose and electrolytes. Hypokalemia, hypophosphatemia, and hypomagnesemia are the most common electrolyte deficiencies encountered, and hypophosphatemia is believed to be the most likely cause of progressive weakness. Vitamin and trace mineral deficiencies are also common.

**Box 35.2 Recommendations for Euthanasia**

- Euthanasia may be recommended if the prognosis is considered grave, or if the animal is suffering and transport to a facility for further treatment is either impossible or would also carry a grave prognosis.
- The opinion of a second veterinarian is recommended if possible.
- Owner consent should be obtained.
- If owner consent cannot be obtained, welfare authorities should be involved and authorized witnesses should be present.
- If euthanasia is required, antemortem samples should be obtained, and a complete post-mortem exam performed, ideally by a board certified pathologist.

**Box 35.3 Clinical signs of refeeding syndrome**

- Cardiac arrhythmias or insufficiency
- Peripheral edema
- Respiratory failure
- Neurological signs
- Rhabdomyolysis
- Seizures

- Clinical signs generally occur within three weeks of reintroduction of feed. Common clinical signs (Box 35.3) include cardiac arrhythmias or insufficiency, peripheral edema, respiratory failure, neurologic signs, rhabdomyolysis, and seizures. Death may occur in severe cases within 1–19 days of refeeding with a mean of 7.9 days (Whiting et al. 2005).
- The risk of refeeding syndrome may be higher with parenteral nutrition; therefore, enteral feeding is recommended when possible.
- Increased fecal water content may occur but does not change appetite or hydration status as seen with infectious colitis (Whitham and Stull 1998).
- Guidelines for feeding to help prevent refeeding syndrome include:
  - Provide calories at or below the daily requirement, starting with up to 50% of the daily energy requirement.
  - Utilize feeds low in carbohydrates to decrease the insulin response.
  - Small, frequent meals of forage with a low non-structural carbohydrate content are recommended. Bagged forages with known non-structured carbohydrate content are useful for this purpose.
  - Alfalfa may be preferable to grass hay due to higher phosphorus and magnesium content.
  - Administer parenteral thiamine.
  - Monitor plasma glucose and correct hypo- or hyperglycemia.
  - Treat hypophosphatemia with IV, oral, or rectal phosphorus-containing sterile enema solutions.
  - Monitor serum electrolyte concentrations prior to and during refeeding.
  - Monitor vital signs during refeeding.
- If signs of refeeding syndrome occur:
  - Decrease or discontinue feeding until electrolyte derangements are resolved.
  - Provide a balanced electrolyte solution with supplemental dextrose to avoid hypoglycemia.
- Other complications of feed deprivation include:
  - Delayed gastric emptying.
  - Decreased nutrient absorption.

## Recumbent Horses

Severely undernourished horses may be unable to stand or unable to rise.

- An attempt should be made to determine the cause of recumbency.
- Horses that are recumbent for 12–18 h may be unable to move into sternal recumbency and are unlikely to be able to stand unassisted. When down to 36–48 h, horses will become unaware of their surroundings and exhibit paddling and tetany. When down for over 48 h, horses will become anorectic and semi-comatose (Finnochio 1994).
- The prognosis is poor for horses that are recumbent, and grave for horses recumbent for over 24 h.
- Horses that are unable to rise on their own or with assistance should be turned every two to six hours for adequate musculoskeletal perfusion and ventilation of the down lung, and should be assisted to stay in sternal recumbency when possible (Nout and Reed 2005).

*Supplemental therapies*

- Severely weak or debilitated horses may require frequent nursing care.
- Intravenous fluids may be necessary in dehydrated and debilitated horses.
- Antibiotic therapy may be indicated for horses with wound infections, decubital ulcers, pneumonia, or other infections.

*Prognosis*

- Prognosis depends on severity and duration of the disease processes, and presence of comorbidities
- Fatality rates for cases of equine starvation are reported to be from 14 to 20% (Finnochio 1994; Witham and Stull 1998; Whiting et al. 2005).
- Time of death is reported to range from 1 to 19 days after refeeding with an average of 7.9 days (Whiting et al. 2005).
- Return to appropriate body condition takes approximately 3–10 months (Witham and Stull 1998; Whiting et al. 2005).

## Non-clinical Responsibilities

Veterinarians also play a critical role in animal abuse cases outside of patient evaluation, diagnosis, and treatment.

- If an owner or caretaker is available, a complete history, including diet, husbandry practices, and any recent veterinary care should be obtained and recorded.
- If animal abuse is suspected and authorities have not been alerted, it is the responsibility of the veterinarian to do so.
- It is essential that accurate and thorough documentation of all findings on the initial exam be taken at the time of the exam.
- Both descriptive notes and photographs with case identification should be taken.
- Full detailed descriptions and photographs of the conditions of the premises should be taken.
- A complete statement should be prepared which includes the following (adapted from Touroo and Eller 2016):
  - Names of investigators
  - Reason for exam
  - Date/time/location of exam
  - Signalment of all animals examined
  - Details on observations of the premises
  - Medical history of the horses if known
  - Details of the clinical exam findings
  - Diagnostic test results and interpretation
  - Differential diagnoses
  - Treatments provided and response to treatment
- Always seek a second opinion when unsure of a diagnosis or recommendation for treatment

**Case Example 35.1 Emergency Welfare Response**

You receive a call from your local animal control officer that they have been alerted about a possible neglected horse that is located within your veterinary practice range. They request you meet them at the farm that afternoon to evaluate the horse.

*What Is Your Initial Course of Action?*

You meet the animal control officer at the farm and discuss your plan with them. You carefully evaluate the premises, look for evidence of other animals, and document your findings. With the help of the animal control officer, you identify and photograph the horse for documentation purposes. You then perform a complete physical examination on the horse. The physical examination reveals generalized weakness, a thick, dull haircoat with numerous areas of alopecia and malodor from the oral cavity. You conclude that the alopecia is due to dermatitis, most likely dermatophilosis based on your clinical exam. Gentle oral exam reveals buccal and lingual erosions due to enamel points. You estimate body weight to be 785 lbs (357 kg) using a weight tape, and assign the horse a BCS of 2/9. You carefully document and photograph your findings.

You had not observed any other animals on the property, so you evaluate the area carefully. You observe a small tub with dirty water that appears to be the only water source. The pasture in which the horse is housed has minimal grass, and there is no hay in the pasture for the horse. You look in an adjacent small barn, the only other structure on the property, and find several bales of hay which are partially moldy. No other feed or forage is present.

You discuss your findings with the animal control officer who indicates he has been in contact with the owner. The owner reportedly was elderly and not in good physical condition, and had recently had financial difficulties. He could no longer afford to purchase adequate feed for the horse and was physically unable to attend to the horse more than every few days. The animal control officer states that he has a rescue group willing to take the horse and the owner is willing to surrender the horse.

The animal control officer arranges for the rescue group to come with a trailer to transport the horse to their facility and they arrive an hour later. The animal control officer handles all transactions and change of ownership. ***What do you recommend to the rescue group?***

You recommend taking samples from the horse to run a complete blood count, serum chemistry panel, electrolyte and mineral panel, fecal egg count, and Coggin's test. You assist them in loading the horse in the trailer, ensuring that he is loose in a well-bedded box stall. You give them recommendations for feeding which include small, frequent forage-based meals, starting with approximately 2 lbs/day of alfalfa hay and 2 lbs/day of a bagged chopped forage with low NSC content, divided into 8–12 evenly spaced feedings over 24 h. You recommend increasing the feed very slowly after 48 h if he is improving and eating well. You recommend waiting approximately two weeks before performing most routine procedures such as vaccination or deworming. However, due to the horse's oral ulcers, you recommend rechecking the horse in a few days and plan to consider dental evaluation and treatment at this time. You then go back to your office to ship all of the labwork to a reference laboratory and ensure all of your findings have been clearly documented.

## References


Finocchio, E.J. (1994). Equine starvation: recognition and rehabilitation of the recumbent, malnourished horse. *Large Anim. Vet.* 49: 6–10.

Henneke, D.R., Potter, G.D., Kreider, J.L., and Yeates, B.F. (1983). Relationship between condition score, physical measurements and body fat percentage in mares. *Equine Vet. J.* 15: 371–372.

Nout, Y.S. and Reed, S.M. (2005). Management and treatment of the recumbent horse. *Equine Vet. Educ.* 17: 324–336.

Touroo, R. and Eller, N. (2016). The equine veterinarian's role in potential cases of animal abuse. *Am. Assoc. Equine Pract.* 62: 199–207.

Whitham, C.L. and Stull, C.L. (1998). Metabolic responses of chronically starved horses to refeeding with three isoenergetic diets. *J. Am. Vet. Med. Assoc.* 212: 691–696.

Whiting, T.L., Salmon, R.H., and Wruck, G.C. (2005). Chronically starved horses: predicting survival, economic, and ethical considerations. *Can. Vet. J.* 46 (4): 320–324.

# Part 5

# Appendices

# Appendix 1

## Reference Values for Adult Horses, Foals and Adult Donkeys

*Jenifer R. Gold*

*Gold Equine Medicine Consulting, Florence, MT, USA*

## Reference Values for Adult Horses and Foals

**Table A1.1** Biochemistry panel reference intervals for adult horses.

| Measure | Unit | Reference range |
|---|---|---|
| Albumin | g/dL | 2.5–4.2 |
| Alkaline phosphatase (ALP) | U/L | 109–315 |
| Ammonia | μg/dL | 19–94 |
| Aspartate aminotransferase (AST) | U/L | 205–555 |
| Bile acids | μg/mL | 0.4–3.5 |
| Bilirubin (total) | mg/dL | 0.1–1.9 |
| Blood urea nitrogen (BUN) | mg/dL | 8–27 |
| Calcium | mg/dL | 10.7–13.4 |
| Carbon dioxide $TCO_2$ | mEq/L mmol/L | 24–31 |
| Chloride | mEq/L mmol/L | 94–102 |
| Cholesterol | mg/dL | 51–109 |
| Creatinine kinase (CK) | U/L | 90–270 |
| Creatinine | mg/dL | 0.6–1.8 |
| Fibrinogen | mg/dL | 150–375 |
| Gamma glutamyl transferase (GGT) | U/L | 12–45 |
| Globulins | g/dL | 2.6–4.0 |
| Glucose | mg/dL | 72–114 |
| L-lactate | mmol/L | <2.0 |
| Magnesium | mg/dL | 1.6–2.5 |
| Phosphorus | mg/dL | 1.9–5.4 |
| Potassium | mEq/L mmol/L | 2.7–4.9 |
| Sodium | mEq/L mmol/L | 132–141 |
| Sorbitol dehydrogenase (SDH) | U/L | 0.3–7.0 |
| Total plasma protein | g/dL | 4.6–6.9 |
| Triglycerides | mg/dL | 11–52 |

*Source:* Southwood (2013), Fielder (2022a).

*Emergency Triage of the Horse*, First Edition. Edited by Rolfe M. Radcliffe and Jamie J. Kopper.

Published 2026 by John Wiley & Sons, Inc.
Companion website: www.wiley.com/go/radcliffe/triage

**Table A1.2** Biochemistry panel reference intervals for foals 24 h and 1 month of age.

| Measure | Unit | 24 h old | 1 month |
|---|---|---|---|
| Albumin | g/dL | 2.0–5.0 | 0.9–3.5 |
| Alkaline phosphatase (ALP) | U/L | 861–2671 | 210–866 |
| Ammonia | µg/dL | Low | Low |
| Aspartate aminotransferase (AST) | U/L | 146–340 | 252–440 |
| Bile acids | µg/mL | 10-6-30.2 | 3.7–6.9 |
| Bilirubin (total) | mg/dL | 1.6–5.0 | 1.0–1.6 |
| Blood urea nitrogen (BUN) | mg/dL | 9–40 | 6–21 |
| Calcium | mg/dL | 9.5–13.4 | 10.7–13.1 |
| Carbon dioxide $TCO_2$ | mEq/L mmol/L | 21–34 | 22–32 |
| Chloride | mEq/L mmol/L | 90–114 | 97–109 |
| Cholesterol | mg/dL | 11.7–58.8 | 7.4–23.5 |
| Creatinine kinase (CK) | U/L | 40–909 | 81–585 |
| Creatinine | mg/dL | 1.2–4.3 | 1.1–1.8 |
| Fibrinogen | mg/dL | 201–301 | 150–375 |
| Gamma glutamyl transferase (GGT) | U/L | 18–43 | 17–99 |
| Globulins | g/dL | 1.8–3.6 | 1.8–3.6 |
| Glucose | mg/dL | 121–233 | 130–216 |
| L-lactate | mmol/L | 0.5–1.8 | 0.5–1.8 |
| Magnesium | mg/dL | 0.6–1.1 | 0.9–2.7 |
| Phosphorus | mg/dL | 3.7–7.4 | 5.0–9.3 |
| Potassium | mEq/L mmol/L | 3.6–5.6 | 3.8–5.4 |
| Sodium | mEq/ Lmmol/L | 123–159 | 136–154 |
| Sorbitol dehydrogenase (SDH) | U/L | 1.0–18 | 0.1–6.1 |
| Total plasma protein | g/dL | 5.2–8.0 | 5.1–7.1 |
| Triglycerides | mg/dL | 30–193 | 45–155 |

*Source:* Southwood (2013), Gold (2024).

**Table A1.3** Adult horse hematology reference intervals.

| Erythrocyte and leukocyte indices | Reference range |
|---|---|
| Red blood cells ($\times 10^6$ cells/µL) | 6.2–10.2 |
| HCT % | 34–46% |
| Hemoglobin (g/dL) | 11.8–15.9 |
| MCV (fL) | 43–55 |
| MCH (pg) | 15–20 |
| RDW (%) | 16.2–19.3 |
| White blood cells ($\times 10^3$ cells/µL) | 5.2–10.1 |
| Segmented neutrophils ($\times 10^3$ cells/µL) | 2.7–6.6 |
| Band neutrophils ($\times 10^3$ cells/µL) | 0 |
| Lymphocytes ($\times 10^3$ cells/µL) | 1.2–4.9 |
| Monocytes | 0–0.6 |
| Eosinophils ($\times 10^3$ cells/µL) | 0–1.2 |
| Basophils ($\times 10^3$ cells/µL) | 0–0.2 |
| Platelets ($\times 10^3$ cells/µL) | 94–232 |

*Source:* Southwood (2013), Cornell University, Animal Health Diagnostic Center (2025).

**Table A1.4** Horse foal hematology reference intervals.

| Erythrocyte and leukocyte indices | Neonatal < 24 h | Neonatal to 1 Month |
|---|---|---|
| Red blood cells ($\times 10^6$ cells/μL) | 8.2–11 | 7.9–11.1 |
| HCT % | 32–46 | 29–41 |
| Hemoglobin (g/dL) | 12–16.6 | 10.9–15.3 |
| MCV (fL) | 33–41 | |
| MCH (pg) | 13–15.5 | |
| RDW (%) | 18–20 | |
| White blood cells ($\times 10^3$ cells/μL) | 5.2–10.1 | 5.3–12.1 |
| Segmented neutrophils ($\times 10^3$ cells/μL) | 2.7–6.6 | 2.8–9.3 |
| Band neutrophils ($\times 10^3$ cells/μL) | 0 | 0 |
| Lymphocytes ($\times 10^3$ cells/μL) | 1.2–4.9 | 1.4–2.3 |
| Monocytes | 0–0.6 | 0.03–0.5 |
| Eosinophils ($\times 10^3$ cells/μL) | 0–1.2 | 0–0.1 |
| Basophils ($\times 10^3$ cells/μL) | 0–0.2 | 0–0.08 |
| Platelets ($\times 10^3$ cells/μL) | 129–409 | 136–468 |

*Source:* Southwood (2013), Cornell University, Animal Health Diagnostic Center 2025.

**Table A1.5** Blood gas reference intervals for adult horses.

| Measure | Unit | Reference range |
|---|---|---|
| pH | | 7.32–7.44 |
| $HCO_3$ | mEq/L | 24–30 |
| $PaCO_2$ | mmHg | 36–46 |
| $PvCO_2$ | mmHg | 38–48 |
| $PaO_2$ | mmHg | 80–112 |
| $PvO_2$ | mmHg | 37–56 |

*Source:* Fielder (2022b).

**Table A1.6** Blood gas reference intervals for neonatal foals.

| Measure | Unit | Reference range |
|---|---|---|
| pH | | 7.38–7.4 |
| $HCO_3$ | mEq/L | 25.1–27.3 |
| $PaCO_2$ | mmHg | 44–47 |
| $PvCO_2$ | mmHg | 45.4–63.1 |
| $PaO_2$ | mmHg | 55.2–58.8 |
| $PvO_2$ | mmHg | 16.6–52.7 |
| $SaO_2$ | % | 95–100 |
| $SvO_2$ | % | 39.9–84.88 |

*Source:* Gold (2024), Hodgson (1987).

## Reference Values for Adult Donkeys

**Table A1.7** Serum biochemistry reference intervals for adult donkeys.

| Measure | Unit | Reference range |
|---|---|---|
| Albumin | g/dL | 2.0–3.6 |
| Aspartate aminotransferase (AST) | U/L | 223–555 |
| Bilirubin (total) | mg/dL | 0–0.2 |
| Blood urea nitrogen (BUN) | mg/dL | 3.0–20 |
| Calcium | mg/dL | 10.9–12.7 |
| Chloride | mEq/L mmol/L | 94–106 |
| Cholesterol | mg/dL | 54–112 |
| Creatinine kinase (CK) | U/L | 95–500 |
| Creatinine | mg/dL | 0.6–1.5 |
| Gamma glutamyl transferase (GGT) | U/L | 10–55 |
| Globulins | g/dL | 2.9–4.8 |
| Glucose | mg/dL | 58–117 |
| Magnesium | mg/dL | 1.2–2.4 |
| Phosphorus | mg/dL | 2.2–5.0 |
| Potassium | mEq/L mmol/L | 3.4–5.7 |
| Sodium | mEq/L mmol/L | 127–140 |
| Sorbitol dehydrogenase (SDH) | U/L | 2.0–10 |
| Total protein | g/dL | 5.7–7.8 |
| Triglycerides | mg/dL | 30–190 |

**Table A1.8** Hematology reference intervals for adult donkeys.

| Erythrocyte and leukocyte indices | Reference range |
|---|---|
| Red blood cells ($\times 10^6$ cells/μL) | 4.4–8.8 |
| HCT % | 28–53 |
| Hemoglobin (g/dL) | 9.3–17.5 |
| MCV (fL) | 53–68 |
| MCH (pg) | 18–23 |
| RDW (%) | 16.1–19.4 |
| White blood cells ($\times 10^3$ cells/μL) | 5.8–16.0 |
| Segmented neutrophils ($\times 10^3$ cells/μL) | 2.2–8.5 |
| Band neutrophils ($\times 10^3$ cells/μL) | 0 |
| Lymphocytes ($\times 10^3$ cells/μL) | 1.5–9.9 |
| Monocytes ($\times 10^3$ cells/μL) | 0–1.0 |
| Eosinophils ($\times 10^3$ cells/μL) | 0–1.7 |
| Basophils ($\times 10^3$ cells/μL) | 0–0.1 |
| Platelets ($\times 10^3$ cells/μL) | 84–380 |

*Source:* Goodrich and Webb (2024).

## References

Cornell University, Animal Health Diagnostic Center, College of Veterinary Medicine. (2025). Routine hemogram testing intervals. https://www.vet.cornell.edu/animal-health-diagnostic-center/laboratories/clinical-pathology/reference-intervals/hematology-advia-2120 (accessed May 2025).

Fielder, S.E. (2022a). *Serum biochemical analysis reference ranges*. Merck Manual. https://www.merckvetmanual.com/special-subjects/reference-guides/serum-biochemical-analysis-reference-ranges.

Fielder, S.E. (2022b). *Blood-gas analysis reference ranges*. Merck Manual. https://www.merckvetmanual.com/special-subjects/reference-guides/blood-gas-analysis-reference-ranges.

Gold, J. (2024). Clinical chemistry in the foal. In: *Equine Neonatal Medicine* (ed. D.M. Wong and P.A. Wilkins). Wiley https://doi.org/10.1002/9781119617228.ch44.

Goodrich, E.L. and Webb, J.L. (2024). Complete blood count and biochemistry reference intervals for healthy adult donkeys in the United States. *Animals* 2018: 14. https://doi.org/10.3390/ani14142018.

Hodgson, D.R. (1987). Blood gas and acid-base changes in the neonatal foal. *Vet. Clin. North Am. Equine Pract.* 3 (3): 617–629.

Southwood, L.L. (ed.) (2013). *Practical Guide to Equine Colic*, 1ste edn. © 2013 John Wiley & Sons, Inc. Wiley.

# Appendix 2

## Equine Emergency Medications and Fluids

*Maia R. Aitken*[1] *and Eric L. Schroeder*[2]

[1] *Department of Clinical Studies - New Bolton Center, University of Pennsylvania School of Veterinary Medicine, Kennett Square, PA, USA*
[2] *Galbreath Equine Center, College of Veterinary Medicine, The Ohio State University, Columbus, OH, USA*

*Emergency Triage of the Horse*, First Edition. Edited by Rolfe M. Radcliffe and Jamie J. Kopper.

Companion website: www.wiley.com/go/radcliffe/triage

**Table A2.1** Common emergency medications and doses.

| Medication | Indications, mechanism of action/effect | Dose | Route | Concentration | Example: 500 kg adult (50 kg foal when specified) *for concentration listed only | Precautions |
|---|---|---|---|---|---|---|
| Acepromazine | Tranquilizer, sedation, peripheral vasodilator | 0.02–0.05 mg/kg q6–8 h | IV, IM | 10 mg/mL | 1 – 2.5 mL | May cause hypotension, paraphimosis |
| Acetaminophen | Analgesia, COX-3 inhibitor | 20–25 mg/kg q12 h | PO | 500 mg tablet | 20–25 tablets | |
| Acetazolamide | Prevention of HYPP attack, Diuretic, Carbonic anhydrase inhibitor | 2–4 mg/kg q6–12 | PO | 250 mg tablets | 4–8 tablets | |
| Acetylcysteine | Mucolytic, anticollagenase | 50–140 mg/kg<br>0.25–1 g q6–8 h | PO or slowly IV<br>Nebulization | 100–200 mg/mL | 100 mg/mL: 250–700 mL<br>200 mg/mL: 125 mL–350 mL<br>Nebulized: 100 mg/mL: 1–10 mL<br>200 mg/mL: 0.5–5 mL | |
| N-Acetyl-L-cysteine powder | Retention enema for meconium impaction | 8 g powder and 22.5 g sodium bicarbonate in 200 mL water | PR | | | Sedation necessary for foal, used Foley catheter |
| Acetylsalicylic acid (aspirin) | Antithrombotic, COX-1 inhibitor | 15–20 mg/kg q48 h | PO | 325 mg tablet | 23–31 tablets | |
| Albuterol | Bronchodilator, beta2 adrenergic agonist | 720 µg q4–6 h | Inhaler<br>Nebulization | 90 µg/actuation | 8 actuations | Do not use in hypokalemia |
| Allopurinol | Antioxidant | 5 mg/kg q4–6 | IV, PO | 16.67 mg/mL<br>(500 mg/30 mL) | 150 mL | |
| Altrenogest | Progestin<br>Pregnancy maintenance, estrus suppression | 0.044–0.088 mg/kg q24 | PO | 2.2 mg/mL | 10–20 mL | Wear gloves when handling |
| Amantadine | Antiviral | 10–20 mg/kg q8 h | PO | 100 mg capsule | 11–12 capsules | Can cause seizures and sudden death in high doses |
| Amikacin | Antibiotic, aminoglycoside | 15–25 mg/kg q24 h foal<br>10–15 mg/kg q24 h adult | IV, IM<br>IV<br>IVRLP-1/4–1/3 systemic dose | 250 mg/mL | 50 kg foal:<br>3–5 mL IV, IM<br>500 kg adult:<br>20–30 mL IV | Nephrotoxic |

| | | | | | | |
|---|---|---|---|---|---|---|
| Aminocaproic acid | Antifibrinolytic, lysine analog, | 40 mg/kg bolus<br>20 mg/kg q6 h | IV bolus<br>IV CRI | 250 mg/mL | IV Bolus: 80 mL IV, then 40 mL IV q6 h | |
| | | 52.5 mg/kg bolus over 15 minutes then 0.25 mg/kg/min | | | IV CRI: 105 mL over 15 minutes, then 30 mL/h | |
| Aminophylline | Bronchodilator, respiratory stimulant, diuretic | 4–10 mg/kg q8–12 h<br>2–5 mg/kg q8–12 h | PO<br>IV (diluted slowly) | 200 mg tablets<br>25 mg/mL | 10–25 tablets<br>40–100 mL IV (diluted, slowly) | |
| Amiodarone | Antiarrhythmic, class III antiarrhythmic | 5–7 mg/kg | IV | 50 mg/mL | 50–70 mL | Potassium channel blocker |
| Ammonium chloride | Urinary acidifier | 90–330 mg/kg q24 h | PO | 5, 25, 100 g per bottle | 45–165 g | Contraindicated in renal failure |
| Amoxicillin clavulanic acid | Antibiotic, potentiated beta lactam | 10–30 mg/kg q6–8 h | PO | 250 mg tablets | 50 kg foal: 2–6 tablets | Foals only |
| Amphotericin B | Antifungal | 0.3–1 mg/kg q24–48 h | IV slowly | 5 mg/mL | 30–100 mL | Dilute in 1 L D5W |
| Ampicillin sodium | Antibiotic, beta lactam | 15–50 mg/kg q8–12 h | IV, IM | 40 mg/mL | 188–625 mL | |
| Ampicillin trihydrate | | 11–22 mg/kg q8–12 h | IM | | 138–275 mL | |
| Antivenin | Viperid antidote | 1–5 vials | IV slowly | 10 mL vial | 1–5 vials | |
| Atipamezole | Alpha-2 reversal, Alpha-2 antagonist | 0.05–0.2 mg/kg | IV slowly<br>IM | 5 mg/mL | 5–20 mL | May cause excitement or adverse cardiac effects when IV |
| Atracurium | Neuromuscular blocker | 0.1–0.2 mg/kg | IV | 10 mg/mL | 5–100 mL | Causes paralysis |
| Atropine | Bradycardia, bronchodilation, organophosphate toxicity, parasympatholytic | 0.005–0.01 mg/kg for bradycardia<br>0.014–0.02 mg/kg for bronchodilation<br>0.15 mg/kg for organophosphate toxicity | IV | 15 mg/mL | 0.2–0.3 mL<br>1.4–2 mL<br>15 mL | May cause tachycardia, ileus, mydriasis |
| Azathioprine | Immunosuppressant, purine analog | 2–3 mg/kg q12–24 | PO | 50 mg tab | 20–30 tablets | |
| Azithromycin | Antibiotic, macrolide | 10 mg/kg q24 h | PO | 100 mg tablet<br>250 mg tablet | 50 tablets<br>20 tablets | May cause hyperthermia, risk of fatal colitis in adults |
| Beclomethasone | Airway anti-inflammatory, corticosteroid | 3–8 mcg/kg q12–24 h | Inhaler | 40 mcg/puff, 80 mcg/puff | 38–100 puffs (40 mcg inhaler)<br>19–50 puffs (80 mcg inhaler) | |

(*Continued*)

**Table A2.1** (Continued)

| Medication | Indications, mechanism of action/effect | Dose | Route | Concentration | Example: 500 kg adult (50 kg foal when specified) *for concentration listed only | Precautions |
|---|---|---|---|---|---|---|
| Benazepril | Diuresis, angiotensin-converting enzyme inhibitor | 0.5 mg/kg q24 | PO | 40 mg tab | 6.25 tablets | |
| Benztropine mesylate | Fluphenazine toxicity, priapism, Anticholinergic | 0.02–0.04 mg/kg | IV | 1 mg/mL | 10–20 mL | |
| | | 0.04 mg/kg | PO | 1 mg tab | 20 tablets | |
| Bethanecol | Urinary retention, ileus, Parasympathomimetic | 0.03–0.04 mg/kg q6–8 | SQ, IV | 5 mg/mL | 3–4 mL | |
| | | 0.22–0.45 mg/kg q6–8 | PO | | 22–45 mL | |
| Bismuth subsalicylate | Antidiarrheal | 1–4.5 mL/kg q4–12 | PO | 262/15 mL | 0.5–2.25 L | |
| Boldenone undecylenate | Anabolic steroid | 1.1 mg/kg | IM | Variable concentrations | Variable | |
| Bretylium | Ventricular fibrillation, class III antiarrhythmic | 5–10 mg/kg every 10 minutes | IV | 50 mg/mL | 50–100 mL | Do not exceed 10 mg/kg in adults |
| Bumetanide | Diuresis, loop diuretic | 15 µg/kg | IV, IM | 0.25 mg/mL | 30 mL | |
| Buprenorphine | Analgesia, opioid partial agonist | 0.001–0.01 mg/kg | IV | 0.3 mg/mL | 1.7–17 mL | May cause ileus, excitement |
| | | 0.004–0.006 mg/kg | IM | | 6.7–10 mL | Controlled III |
| Butorphanol tartrate | Analgesia, opioid partial agonist | 200.5–3.1 mg/kg | IV, IM | 10 mg/mL | 0.5–5 mL | Controlled IV |
| | | 13–22 µg/kg/h | CRI | | 0.65–1.1 mL/h | |
| Butylscopolammonium bromide | Antispasmodic, Anticholinergic | 0.3 mg/kg | IV, IM, SQ | 20 mg/mL | 7.5 mL | Contraindicated in glaucoma, causes tachycardia |
| Ca-EDTA | Lead Chelation, Chelator | 37.5 mg/kg q12 | IV slowly | 50 mg/mL | 375 mL | |
| Caffeine | Hypoventilation, Respiratory stimulant | 10 mg/kg loading | PO, PR | 200 mg tab | 500 kg adult: 25 tablets, then 6.25–7.5 tablets | Hyperexcitability with doses >40 mg/kg |
| | | 2.5–3 mg/kg q12–24 | | | 50 kg foal: 2.5 tablets, then 0.6–0.75 tablets | |
| Calcium gluconate | Treatment for hypocalcemia, hyperkalemia | 150–200 mg/kg | IV slowly | 230 mg/mL | 326–434 mL | |
| Canigliflozin | Insulin dysregulation, sodium-glucose cotransporter 2 inhibitors (SGLT2i) | 0.6 mg/kg q24 h | PO | 100 mg tablets | 3 tablets | |

| | | | | | | |
|---|---|---|---|---|---|---|
| Carbamazepine | Seizures, anticonvulsant, sodium channel blocker | 2–8 mg/kg q6–8 h | PO | 200 mg tablets | 5–20 tablets | |
| Carprofen | NSAID, COX-2 preferential inhibitor | 1.4 mg/kg q24 h | IV<br>PO | 50 mg/mL<br>100 mg tablets | 14 mL<br>7 tablets | |
| Cefazolin | Antibiotic, first-generation cephalosporin | 11–22 mg/kg q6–8 h 200 mg | IV | 1 g, 2 g vials | Variable depending on dilution used | |
| Cefepime | Antibiotic, fourth-generation cephalosporin | 2.2 mg/kg q8 h adults<br>11 mg/kg q8 h foals | IV, IM | 500 mg, 1 g, 2 g vials | Variable depending on dilution used | |
| Cefoperazone | Antibiotic, third-generation cephalosporin | 30 mg/kg q8 h | IV | 40 mg/mL | 500 kg adult: 375 mL<br>50 kg foal: 37.5 mL | |
| Cefotaxime | Antibiotic, third-generation cephalosporin | 40–50 mg/kg q6–8 h | IV | 20 mg/mL | 50 kg foal: 100–125 mL | |
| Cefoxitin | Antibiotic, second-generation cephalosporin | 20 mg/kg q6 h | IV, IM | 1 g vial | Variable depending on dilution used | |
| Cefpodoxime proxetil | Antibiotic, third-generation cephalosporin | 10 mg/kg q6–12 h | PO | 200 mg tablets | 50 kg foal: 2.5 tablets | |
| Cefquinome | Antibiotic, fourth-generation cephalosporin | 1–2.5 mg/kg q6–12 h | IV, IM | 25 mg/mL | 500 kg adult: 20–50 mL<br>50 kg foal: 2–5 mL | |
| Ceftazidime | Antibiotic, third-generation cephalosporin | 20–50 mg/kg q6–12 h | IV, IM | 40 mg/mL | 50 kg foal: 25–62.5 mL | |
| Ceftiofur sodium (*Naxcel*®) | Antibiotic, third-generation cephalosporin | 2.2–5 mg/kg q6–24 h | IV, IM | 50 mg/mL | 500 kg adult: 22–50 mL<br>50 kg foal: 2.2–5 mL | |
| Ceftiofur crystalline free acid<br>(*Excede*®) | Antibiotic, third-generation cephalosporin | 6.6 mg/kg<br>q4 days | IM | 200 mg/mL | 16.5 mL | DO NOT GIVE IV<br>Maximum 7 mL per injection site |
| Ceftriaxone | Antibiotic, third-generation cephalosporin | 20–25 mg/kg q12 h | IV, IM | 100 mg/mL | 50 kg foal: 10–12.5 mL | |
| Cephalexin | Antibiotic, first-generation cephalosporin | 25 mg/kg q6 h | PO | 500 mg tab | 2.5 tablets | |

(*Continued*)

**Table A2.1** (Continued)

| Medication | Indications, mechanism of action/effect | Dose | Route | Concentration | Example: 500 kg adult (50 kg foal when specified) *for concentration listed only | Precautions |
|---|---|---|---|---|---|---|
| Cephalothin | Antibiotic, first-generation cephalosporin | 20 mg/kg q6 h | IV, IM | 1 or 2 g vials | Variable depending on dilution | |
| Cephapirin | Antibiotic, first-generation cephalosporin | 20–30 mg/kg | IV, IM | 500 mg vials | Variable depending on dilution | May cause diarrhea, anaphylaxis reported, available as intramammary preparation |
| Cetirizine | Antihistamine, metabolite of hydroxyzine | 0.2–0.4 mg/kg q12 h | PO | 10 mg tabs | 10–20 tablets | |
| Charcoal | Adsorbent | 0.5–1 g/kg | PO | 200 mg/mL | 1.25–2.5 L | |
| Chloramphenicol | Antibiotic, protein synthesis inhibitor | 50 mg/kg q6 h | PO | 500 mg tabs<br>Compounded paste<br>Ophthalmic ointment | 50 tablets | Wear gloves when handling |
| Ciclisonide (*Aservo Equihaler®*) | Equine asthma, Glucocorticoid | 8 actuations q12 h | Inhaler | 343 mcg/actuation | 8 actuations | No evaluation for use in pregnant mares |
| Cimetidine | Gastric ulcers/Gastroprotectant | 6.6 mg/kg q6–8 | IV | 150 mg/mL | 22 mL | |
| | H2 antagonist | 16–25 mg/kg q6–8 | PO | 800 mg tab | 10–16 tablets | |
| Cisapride | Ileus, Promotility agent, 5 HT4 agonist | 0.1–1 mg/kg q4–8 | PO | 10 mg tab | 5–50 tablets | May cause arrhythmias |
| Clarithromycin | Antibiotic, macrolide | 7.5 mg/kg q12 h | PO | 500 mg tab | 50 kg foal: 0.75 tablets | Risk of severe colitis in adults |
| Clavulanic acid-ticarcillin | Antibiotic, potentiated beta lactam | 100 mg/kg loading then 50 mg/kg q6 h | IV | 3.1 and 31 g vials | Variable depending on dilution | |
| Clenbuterol | Equine asthma, bronchodilator | 0.8–3.2 μg/kg q12<br>0.5 μg/kg q8 h | IV,PO<br>Nebulizer | 72.5 μg/mL | 5.5–22 mL<br>3.4 mL | May cause tachycardia, anxiety at high doses. DO NOT combine nebulizer with systemic administration |
| Clopidogrel | Hypercoagulation, platelet activator inhibitor | 4 mg/kg loading<br>2 mg/kg q24 | PO | 75 mg tab | 27 tablets, then 13 tablets | |

| | | | | | | |
|---|---|---|---|---|---|---|
| Dalteparin | Hypercoagulation, low-molecular-weight heparin | 50–100 U/kg q24 h | SQ | 25,000 U/mL | 1–2 mL | |
| Dantrolene | Rhabdomyolysis, malignant hyperthermia, Muscle relaxant | 10 mg/kg loading | PO | 100 mg capsules | 50 capsules, then 12.5–25 capsules | Sedation at high doses |
| | | 2.5–5 mg/kg q8–24 | | | | |
| | | 2–4 mg/kg q1–2 | IV | 20 mg vial | Variable depending on dilution | |
| Desferrioxamine | Iron toxicity, iron chelator | 10 mg/kg | IM, IV slowly | 500 mg vials | Variable depending on dilution | |
| Detomidine hydrochloride | Sedative | 5–40 μg/kg | IV, IM | 10 mg/mL | 0.25–2 mL | |
| | Alpha-2 agonist | 30–40 μg/kg | Epidural | | 1.5–2 mL | |
| | | 8.4 μg/kg loading then 0.5 μg/kg/min | CRI | | 0.42 mL, then 1.5 mL/h | |
| Dexamethasone | Glucocorticoid | 0.02–0.2 mg/kg | IV, IM | 2 mg/mL | 5–50 mL | Use with caution in equine metabolic syndrome (EMS), prolonged high dose may cause abortion, if given PO 30–60% bioavailable |
| | Anti-inflammatory to immunosuppressive | | | | | |
| Dexmedetomidine | Sedative | 2.5–10 μg/kg | IV, IM | 0.5 mg/mL | 2.5–10 mL | |
| | Alpha-2 agonist | | | | | |
| Dextrose | Hypoglycemia, partial parenteral nutrition | 0.5 mL/kg bolus or 4–8 mg/kg per min as a 5–10% solution | IV | 500 mg/mL | 250 mL | For immediate treatment of severe hypoglycemia |
| Diazepam | Anticonvulsant | 0.05–0.44 mg/kg adult | IV | 5 mg/mL | 500 kg adult: | Schedule IV controlled substance |
| | Sedative | 0.01–0.2 mg/kg foal | | | 5–44 mL | |
| | Preanesthetic | | | | 50 kg foal: 0.1–2 mL | |
| Digoxin | Positive inotrope, cardiac glycoside | 0.0022–0.0075 mg/kg q12 | IV | 0.1 mg/mL | 11–37.5 mL | May cause colic signs |
| | | 0.011–0.0175 mg/kg q12 | PO | | 55–87.5 mL | |
| Di-tri-octahedral smectite (Biosponge®) | Diarrhea, intoxication, intestinal adsorbent | 0.5–3 pounds per adult | PO or NGT | Paste or powder | 500 kg adult: 0.5–3 lbs | |
| | | q6–q24 h | | | 50 kg foal: 2.5–5 mL | |
| | | 0.5–1 mL/10 kg foal | | | | |
| Diltiazem | Rate control during atrial fibrillation conversion, calcium channel blocker | 0.125 mg/kg | IV over 2 minutes | 5 mg/mL | 12.5 mL | Not to exceed 1 mg/kg |

*(Continued)*

**Table A2.1** (Continued)

| Medication | Indications, mechanism of action/effect | Dose | Route | Concentration | Example: 500 kg adult (50 kg foal when specified) *for concentration listed only | Precautions |
|---|---|---|---|---|---|---|
| Dimercaprol | Heavy metal intoxication, chelating agent | 5 mg/kg then 3 mg/kg q6 h for 24 h | IM | 100 mg/mL | 25 mL, then 15 mL | Must be used acutely |
| Dinoprost tromethamine | Abortifacient, prostaglandin F2a | 0.011–0.022 mg/kg | IM | 5 mg/mL | 1.1 mL–2.2 mL | |
| Diphenhydramine hydrochloride | Allergic reaction, antihistamine | 0.5–2 mg/kg | IV (slowly) IM | 50 mg/mL | 5–20 mL | |
| Dipyrone | Anti-inflammatory, antipyretic, COX 3 inhibition | 10–22 mg/kg | IV, IM | 500 mg/mL | 10–22 mL | |
| Dobutamine | Hypotension, positive inotrope | 0.5–15 μg/kg/min | IV CRI | 12.5 mg/mL | 1.2–36 mL/h | Do not exceed 10 μg/kg/min in adults |
| Domperidone | Hypogalactia/agalactia, dopamine agonist, | 1.1 mg/kg q12 h | PO | 110 mg/mL | 5 mL | |
| Dopamine | Hypoperfusion, catecholamine | 1–20 μg/kg/min | IV CRI | 40 mg/mL | 0.75–15 mL/h | |
| | Low dose increased renal perfusion | | | | | |
| | High dose beta 1 agonist | | | | | |
| Doxapram | Hypoventilation, CNS/respiratory stimulant | 0.2–0.5 mg/kg | IV | 20 mg/mL | 5–12.5 mL | |
| Doxycycline | Antibiotic, tetracycline | 10 mg/kg q12 h | PO | 100 mg tab | 50 tablets | |
| Doxylamine succinate | Allergic Reaction Antihistamine | 0.5 mg/kg q6–12 h | IV slowly, IM, SQ | 11.36 mg/mL | 22 mL | |
| Edrophonium | Avermectin, atropine toxicity, anticholinesterase | 0.5–1 mg/kg | IV | 10 mg/mL | 25–50 mL | |
| Enalapril | Diuresis, angiotensin-converting enzyme inhibitor | 1 mg/kg q12–24 h | PO | 20 mg tab | 25 tablets | |
| Enoxaparin | Hypercoagulation, low-molecular-weight heparin | 40–80 U/kg or 0.4–0.8 mg/kg q24 h | SQ | 100 mg/mL | 2–4 mL | |
| Enrofloxacin | Antibiotic, fluoroquinolone | 5–7.5 mg/kg q24 h | IV, PO | 100 mg/mL | 25–37.5 mL | May cause oral ulceration; may cause arthropathy in foals |

| | | | | | | |
|---|---|---|---|---|---|---|
| Ephedrine | Hypotension, sympathomimetic | 0.02–0.1 mg/kg | IV | 50 mg/mL | 0.2–1 mL | May cause CNS stimulation, tachycardia, hypertension |
| Epinephrine | Hypotension, alpha and beta adrenergic agonist | 0.01–0.05 mg/kg | IV, IM | 1:1,000 (1 mg/mL) | 500 kg adult: 5–25 mL<br>50 kg foal: 0.5–2.5 mL | |
| Epoetin alfa | Anemia, synthetic erythropoietin | 50 U/kg q7 days | SQ | 4000 U/mL | 6.25 mL | May cause aplastic anemia |
| Ertugliflozin | Reduce hyperinsulinemia, manage metabolic associated laminitis, sodium-glucose cotransporter 2 inhibitors (SGLT2i) | 0.025–0.05 mg/kg q24 h | PO | 5 mg tab<br>15 mg tab | 2.5–5 tablets<br>0.8–1.7 tablets | May cause inappetence, elevated GGT |
| Erythromycin | Ileus, antibiotic Macrolide | 25–30 mg/kg q6–12 h foals | IV | 100 mg/mL | 50 kg foal: 12.5–15 mL | May cause severe colitis in adults |
| | Prokinetic | 0.5–2.2 mg/kg q6 h | IV | | 500 kg adult: 2.5–11 mL | |
| Etodolac | Analgesia, COX-2 selective | 20 mg/kg q12–24 h | PO | 500 mg tab | 20 tablets | |
| **Euthanasia solution, see Pentobarbital** | | | | | | |
| Famotidine | Gastric ulcers, $H_2$ receptor antagonist | 0.23–0.5 mg/kg q8–12 h | IV | 10 mg/mL | 11.5–25 mL | |
| | | 2.8–4 mg/kg q8–12 h | PO | 20 mg tab | 70–100 tablets | |
| Fentanyl | Analgesia, mu opioid agonist | 3–6 μg/kg/h | IV CRI | 0.05 mg/mL | 500 kg adult: 30–60 mL/h<br>50 kg foal: 3–6 mL/h | May cause ileus, schedule II controlled substance |
| Firocoxib | Analgesia, COX-2 selective | 0.1 mg/kg q24 h<br>(0.3 mg/kg loading) | PO | 57 mg tablets<br>Or oral paste | 2.5 tablets, then 1 tablet | |
| Florfenicol | Antibiotic, phenol antibiotic | 20 mg/kg q24–48 h | IM | 300 mg/mL | 33 mL | |
| Fluconazole | Antifungal | 8–14 mg/kg loading<br>4–5 mg/kg q12–24 h | PO | 200 mg tab | 20–35 tablets, then 10–12.5 tablets | |
| Flumazenil | Midazolam reversal, benzodiazepine antagonist | 0.011–0.022 mg/kg | IV slowly | 0.1 mg/mL | 55–110 mL | |

(*Continued*)

**Table A2.1** (Continued)

| Medication | Indications, mechanism of action/effect | Dose | Route | Concentration | Example: 500 kg adult (50 kg foal when specified) *for concentration listed only | Precautions |
|---|---|---|---|---|---|---|
| Flunixin meglumine | Analgesia, COX 1&2 inhibitor | 0.25–1.1 mg/kg q8–12 h | IV, PO | 50 mg/mL<br>Or oral paste | 2.5–11 mL | IM injections may be associated with clostridial myositis. Do not exceed 2.2 mg/kg dose in 24 h |
| Fluprostenol sodium | Luteolytic, abortifacient, prostaglandin F analog | 2.2 μg/kg | IM | 50 μg/mL | 22 mL | |
| Fluticasone (*Flovent*) | Equine asthma, glucocorticoid | 10 puffs q12 h | Inhaler | 220 mcg/puff | 10 puffs | |
| Fomepizole 4-methylpyrazole (*4MP, Antizol-vet*) | For ethylene glycol toxicity, synthetic alcohol dehydrogenase inhibitor | 20 mg/kg initial<br>15 mg/kg after 17 h<br>5 mg/kg after 25 h<br>5 mg/kg after 36 h | IV | 50 mg/mL | 200 mL, then 150 mL, then 50 mL | May cause phlebitis (dilution recommended) |
| Furosemide | Diuresis, loop diuretic | 1–2 mg/kg<br>0.12 mg/kg/h | IV, SQ, IM<br>CRI | 50 mg/mL | 10–20 mL<br>1.2 mL/h | |
| Gabapentin | Analgesia, GABA (gamma-iminobutyric acid) analog | 5–60 mg/kg q8–24 h | PO | 300 mg tablets | 8.3–33.3 tablets | |
| Gamithromycin | Antibiotic, macrolide | 6 mg/kg q6 d | IM | 150 mg/mL | 50 kg foal: 2 mL | Risk of severe colitis in adults |
| Ganciclovir | EHV-1 infection, prophylaxis, antiviral | 2.5 mg/kg q8 h (1st day) then q12 h | IV | 50 mg/mL | 25 mL | |
| Gentamicin sulfate | Antibiotic, aminoglycoside | 6.6–10 mg/kg q24 h | IV, IM | 100 mg/mL | 33–50 mL | Nephrotoxic |
| Glycopyrrolate | Bronchoconstriction, bradycardia, antimuscarinic agent, | 0.002–0.01 mg/kg | IV | 0.2 mg/mL | 5–25 mL | May cause ileus |
| Griseofulvin | Antibiotic, fungistatic antibiotic | 10 mg/kg q24 h | PO | 2.5 g packets | 5.0 g (2 packets) | |
| Guaifenesin | Anesthesia, central-acting muscle relaxant, expectorant | 60–90 mg/kg | IV | 50 mg/mL | 600–900 mL | Administer as a 5% solution |
| Heparin, unfractionated | Hypercoagulation, anticoagulant | 40–100 U/kg q6 h | IV, SQ | 1000 U/mL | 20–50 mL | |

| | | | | | | |
|---|---|---|---|---|---|---|
| Hydralazine | Hypertension, phthalazine derivative vasodilator | 0.5–1.5 mg/kg q12 h | PO | 50 mg tablets | 5–15 tablets | |
| | | 0.5 mg/kg | IV | 10 mg/mL | | |
| Hydrochlorothiazide | Diuresis, thiazide diuretic | 0.56 mg/kg q24 h | PO | 25 mg/mL | 11.2 mL | |
| Hydrocortisone | Inflammation, glucocorticoid | 0.2–0.4 mg/kg q4 h | IV | 50 mg/mL | 500 kg adult: 2–4 mL | |
| | | | | | 50 kg foal: 0.2–0.4 mL | |
| Hydromorphone | Analgesia, opiate | 0.01–0.04 mg/kg | Epidurally | 2 mg/mL | 2.5–10 mL | |
| Hydroxyzine hydrochloride | Allergic reaction, antihistamine | 1–1.5 mg/kg q8–12 h | PO | 100 mg tablets | 5–7.5 tablets | |
| | | 0.5–1 mg/kg q12 h | IM | 25 mg/mL | 10–20 mL | |
| Imidocarb | Babesia and theileria treatment Antiprotozoal | 2.2–4 mg/kg q24 h for 3 days | IM, SQ | 120 mg/mL | 9.2 mL–16.7 mL | |
| Imipenem | Antibiotic, carbapenem | 10–15 mg/kg q6–8 h | IV | 10 mg/mL | 500–750 mL | Dilute with saline or fluids, may cause phlebitis |
| Imipramine | Headshaking, tricyclic antidepressant | 1–2 mg/kg q8–12 h | PO | 50 mg tablets | 10–20 tablets | |
| Insulin (Regular) | Hyperglycemia, hyperkalemia, Pancreatic hormone | 0.1–0.2 U/kg | IV,SQ, IM | 100 U/mL | 500 kg adult: 0.5–1 mL | Use with concurrent dextrose administration for hyperkalemia |
| | | 0.1–1 U/kg/h | CRI | | 0.5–5 mL/h | |
| | | | | | 50 kg foal: 0.05–0.5 mL | |
| Iodide potassium | Fungal infection, antifungal | 22–67 mg/kg q24 h | PO, IV | | Variable depending on dilution | 1 g is soluble in 0.7 mL water |
| Ipratropium bromide | Bronchospasm, equine asthma, anticholinergic | 0.2–0.5 μg/kg (5–8 actuations) q8 h | Inhaler | 18 μg/actuation | 5–14 actuations | |
| Isoflupredone acetate | Inflammation, corticosteroid | 0.02 mg/kg q24 h | IM | 2 mg/mL | 5 mL | |
| Isoproterenol | Bradycardia, beta-adrenergic agonist | 0.05–0.2 μcg/kg/min | CRI | 0.2 mg/mL | 7.5–30 mL/h | |
| Isoxsuprine | Vasoconstriction, peripheral vasodilator | 0.6–1.32 mg/kg q12 h | PO | 20 mg tablets | 15–33 tablets | Oral bioavailability poor |
| | | 0.4–1.2 mg/kg q24 h | IM | 5 mg/mL | 40–120 mL | |
| Itraconazole | Fungal infection, triazole antifungal | 5 mg/kg q24 h | PO | 100 mg tablets, compounded solution | 25 tablets | Oral bioavailability improved with solution |
| Ivermectin | Parasite infection, avermectin anthelmintic | 200 μg/kg | PO | 10 mg/mL | 10 mL | |
| Kaolin/pectin | Diarrhea, aluminum silicate adsorbent, antidiarrheal | 4–8 mL/kg q12 h | PO | 8% kaolin, 0.8% pectin solution | 2–4 L | |

(*Continued*)

**Table A2.1** (Continued)

| Medication | Indications, mechanism of action/effect | Dose | Route | Concentration | Example: 500 kg adult (50 kg foal when specified) *for concentration listed only | Precautions |
|---|---|---|---|---|---|---|
| Ketamine | Dissociative anesthetic, NMDA antagonist | 1–2 mg/kg | IV | 100 mg/mL | 5–10 mL | Schedule III Controlled substance |
| | | 0.2 mg/kg q2 h | IM | | 0 mL | |
| | | 0.01–0.04 mg/kg/min | CRI | | 3–12 mL | |
| Ketoprofen | Analgesia, COX 1&2 inhibitor | 1.1–2.2 mg/kg q12–24 h | IV | 100 mg/mL | 5.5–11 mL | |
| Lactulose | Hyperammonemia, disaccharide laxative, ammonia reducer | 0.2 mL/kg q6–12 h | PO | 666 mg/mL (10 g/15 mL) | 100 mL | May cause diarrhea |
| Levamisole | Antinematodal parasiticide, immune stimulant | 2–10 mg/kg q24 h | PO | 50 mg tablets | 20–100 tablets | |
| Levetiracetam | Seizures, pyrrolidone-derivative antiepileptic | 32 mg/kg q12 h | PO, IV | 250-, 750-, 1000 mg tablets, 100 mg/mL solution | 500 kg adult: 64 tablets (250 mg), 21 tablets (750 mg), 16 tablets (1000 mg) | |
| | | | | | 16 mL | |
| | | | | | 50 kg foal: 6.4 tablets (250 mg), 2 tablets (750 mg), 1.6 tablets (1,000 mg) | |
| | | | | | 1.6 mL | |
| Levothyroxine | Hypothyroidism, weight loss, thyroid hormone | 0.01–0.1 mg/kg q24 h | PO | 12 mg per teaspoon powder | 0.4–4.1 teaspoons | |
| Lidocaine | Sodium channel blocker local anesthetic, antiarrhythmic | 0.25–1 mg/kg bolus | IV slowly | 20 mg/mL | 6.25–25 mL | Excitement, seizures, ataxia may occur if administered quickly IV |
| | | 1.3 mg/kg loading dose, then 0.05 mg/kg/min | CRI | | 32.5 mL, then 75 mL/h | |
| | | 0.2–0.25 mg/kg | Epidural | | 5–6.25 mL | |
| Magnesium sulfate, enteral (*Epsom salts*) | Constipation, osmotic laxative | 0.2–1 g/kg q24hr | PO | | 100–500 g | Dilute in water |
| Magnesium sulfate, parenteral | Electrolyte for treatment of ventricular tachyarrhythmia, hypomagnesemia | 2.2–5.6 mg/kg/min for 10 min | CRI | 0.5 g/mL | 132–336 mL/h | Do not exceed 25 g IV total dose |
| | | 50–100 mg/kg q24 h | IV slowly | | 50–100 mL | |
| Mannitol | Osmotic diuretic | 0.25–2 g/kg q6–24 h | IV slowly | 200 mg/mL | 500 kg adult: 625–5000 mL | Examine product for crystal sedimentation, contraindicated in intracrainal hemorrhage, pulmonary edema, anuria |
| | | | | | 50 kg foal: 62.5–500 mL | |

| | | | | | | |
|---|---|---|---|---|---|---|
| Marbofloxacin | Antibiotic, fluoroquinolone | 2–3 mg/kg | PO | 100 mg tablets | 10–15 tablets | |
| Medetomidine | Sedation, alpha-2 adrenergic agonist | 5–7 µg/kg q2–4 h | IV | 1 mg/mL | 2.5–3.5 mL | |
| | | 3.5 µg/kg/h | CRI | | 1.75 mL/h | |
| Meloxicam | Analgesia, COX-2 selective | 0.6 mg/kg q12 h | IV | 5 mg/mL solution | 60 mL | |
| | | 0.6 mg/kg q12–24 h | PO | 15 mg tablets | 20 tablets | |
| Meperidine hydrochloride | Analgesia, opiate | 0.55–2.2 mg/kg q4–8 h | IV, IM | 50 mg/mL | 5.5–22 mL | May cause excitement and hypotension given IV |
| Meropenem | Antibiotic, carbapenem | 10–15 mg/kg q8 h | IV | 1 g vials | 5–7.5 g (vials) | |
| Metformin | Hyperglycemia, reduces gluconeogenesis | 15–30 mg/kg q8 h | PO | 1,000 mg tablets | 7.5–15 tablets | |
| Methadone | Analgesia, opioid | 0.1–0.22 mg/kg | IV, IM | 10 mg/mL | 5–11 mL | Schedule II controlled substance |
| Methocarbamol | Muscle relaxant | 40–60 mg/kg q12–24 h | PO | 500 mg tablets | 40–60 tablets | |
| | | 10–25 mg/kg q6 h | IV | 100 mg/mL | 50–125 mL | |
| Methylene blue | Thiazine dye for methemoglobinemia | 5–8.8 mg/kg | IV slowly | 10 mg/mL | 250–440 mL | Contraindicated in renal insufficiency |
| Methylprednisolone sodium succinate | Inflammation, glucocorticoid | 10–30 mg/kg | IV slowly | 125 mg/mL | 40–120 mL | |
| Metoclopramide | Ileus, prokinetic agent, D2 receptor antagonist | 0.1–0.5 mg/kg q4–8 h | SQ | 5 mg/mL | 10–50 mL | May cause extrapyramidal CNS signs |
| | | 0.04 mg/kg/h | CRI | | 4 mL/h | |
| Metronidazole | Antibiotic/ antiprotozoal, nitroimidazole | 15–25 mg/kg q6–8 h | PO, PR | 500 mg tablets | 500 kg adult: 15–25 tablets | May result in anorexia, per rectum administration is 50% bioavailability of PO |
| | | 10–15 mg/kg q8–12 h | PO foals | 5 mg/mL | 50 kg foal: 1–1.5 tablets | |
| | | 15–20 mg/kg q8–12 h | IV | | 150–200 mL | |
| Midazolam | Seizures, benzodiazepine | 0.1–0.2 mg/kg | IV | 5 mg/mL | 500 kg adult: 10–20 mL | Schedule IV controlled substance |
| | | 0.04–0.12 mg/kg/h | CRI | | 4–12 mL/h | |
| | | | | | 50 kg foal: 1–2 mL | |
| | | | | | 0.4–1.2 mL/h | |
| Milk Thistle | Hepatic dysfunction, antifibrotic, immunomodulatory agent | 20 mg/kg q12 h | PO | Various formulations | Variable depending on formulation | |
| Milrinone | Pulmonary hypertension, heart failure, phosphodiesterase-III inhibitor | 10 µg/kg/min | CRI (short-term) | 1 mg/mL | 300 mL/h | May cause ventricular arrhythmias |
| | | 0.5–1 mg/kg q12 h | IV | | 250–500 mL | |

(*Continued*)

**Table A2.1** (Continued)

| Medication | Indications, mechanism of action/effect | Dose | Route | Concentration | Example: 500 kg adult (50 kg foal when specified) *for concentration listed only | Precautions |
|---|---|---|---|---|---|---|
| Mineral oil | Enteric lubricant, marker of GI transit | 5–9 mL/kg | NGT | n/a | 2.5–4.5 L | |
| Misoprostol | Right dorsal colitis, glandular gastric ulcers, abortigenic, prostaglandin E1 analog | 2.5–5 μg/kg q12–24 h | PO | 200 μg tablets | 12.5 tablets | Do not use in pregnant horses<br>May cause colic |
| Morphine sulfate | Analgesia, opioid | 0.05–0.1 mg/kg<br>0.01 mg/kg | IV,IM<br>Epidural (must be preservative free) | Various concentrations | Variable depending on concentration | May cause CNS excitement |
| Moxidectin | Parasite infestation, avermectin anthelmintic | 0.4–0.5 mg/kg | PO | 20 mg/mL | 10–12.5 mL | |
| Naloxone | Analgesia, opioid antagonist | 0.01–0.03 mg/kg | IV | 0.4 mg/mL | 12.5–37.5 mL | |
| Naproxen | Analgesia, COX 1 &2 inhibitor | 5 mg/kg<br>10 mg/kg q12–24 h | IV<br>PO | 100 mg/mL, 500 mg tablets | 25 mL<br>10 tablets | |
| Neomycin | Antibiotic, aminoglycoside | 8–20 mg/kg q8–24 h | PO | 50 mg/mL | 80–200 mL | May cause diarrhea |
| Neostigmine | Ileus, prokinetic, parasympathomimetic | 0.005–0.02 mg/kg q4–6 h | SQ, IM | 2 mg/mL | 1.25–5 mL | May cause cramping |
| Nitazoxanide | antiprotozoal | 25–50 mg/kg | PO | 500 mg tablets | 25–50 tablets | |
| Norepinephrine | Hypotension, alpha-1 and 2 adrenergic agonist | 0.05–1 μg/kg/min | CRI | 1 mg/mL | 25–50 mL | Dose not to exceed 10 mcg/kg/min |
| Octreotide acetate | Insulin dysregulation, synthetic somatostatin analog | 0.5–5 μg/kg q6 h | SQ | 200 μg/mL | 1.25–12.5 mL | |
| Omeprazole | Gastric ulcers, proton pump inhibitor | 1–4 mg/kg q24 h | PO | Oral paste | See syringe | |
| Oxfendazole | Parasite infestation, benzimidazole anthelmintic | 10 mg/kg | PO | 90.6 mg/mL | 55 mL | |
| Oxibendazole | Parasite infestation, benzimidazole anthelmintic | 10–15 mg/kg | PO | 100 mg/mL | 50–75 mL | |

| | | | | | | |
|---|---|---|---|---|---|---|
| Oxymorphone | Analgesia, opioid | 0.02–0.03 mg/kg | IV, SQ, IM | 1 mg/mL | 10–15 mL | Schedule II controlled substance |
| Oxytetracycline | Antibiotic, tetracycline | 6.6 mg/kg q12 h<br>30–60 mg/kg for contracted foals | IV slowly<br>IV slowly | 100 mg/mL, 200 mg/mL | 500 kg adult: 33 mL (100 mg/mL), 16.5 mL (200 mg/mL)50 kg foal: (contracture)<br>15–30 mL (100 mg/mL)<br>7.5–15 mL (200 mg/mL) | Nephrotoxic |
| Oxytocin | Uterine involution, induction of parturition, esophageal relaxation, hypothalamic hormone | 2.5–20 U q4–6 h for uterine involution<br>75 U for induction of parturition<br>0.11–0.22 U/kg for esophageal relaxation | IV, IM, SQ<br>IV over 1 h<br>IV | 20 U/mL | 0.125–1 mL<br>3.9 mL<br>2.75–5.5 mL | May see signs of cramping or colic |
| Penicillamine D | Copper toxicity, monothiol chelating agent | 3 mg/kg q6 h | PO | 250 mg capsules | 6 capsules | |
| Penicillin ($K^+$ or $Na^+$) | Antibiotic, beta lactam | 22 000–44,000 U/kg q6 h<br>4–11 U/kg/h | IV<br>CRI | Concentration depends on dilution | Variable depending on concentration | |
| Penicillin procaine G | Antibiotic, beta lactam | 22 000–44,000 U/kg q12 h | IM | 300,000 U/mL | 37–73 mL | *Do not administer IV,* procaine reactions may cause collapse |
| Pentazocine | Analgesia, partial opiate agonist | 0.3–0.6 mg/kg | PO, IV | 30 mg/mL | 5–10 mL | |
| Pentobarbital | Euthanasia, barbiturate | 85 mg/kg | IV | 390 mg/mL | 109 mL | Schedule III controlled substance |
| Pentoxifylline | Fibrosis, increased ed. blood cell deformity, synthetic xanthine | 7.5–10 mg/kg q8–12 h | PO | 400 mg tablets | 9.5–12.5 tablets | Do not mix with water |
| Pergolide | Pars pituitary intermedia dysfunction (PPID) dopamine receptor agonist | 0.0017–0.01 mg/kg q24 h | PO | 1 mg tablets | 0.85–5 tablets | |
| Perphenazine | Fescue toxicity, domain receptor inhibitor | 0.3–0.5 mg/kg q8 h | PO | 16 mg tablets | 9–15.5 tablets | |
| Phenazopyridine | Pollakiuria, straining to urinate urinary tract mucosal anesthetic | 4–10 mg/kg q8–12 h | PO | 100, 200 mg tablets | 20–50 tablets (100 mg)<br>10–25 tablets (200 mg) | Will cause yellow urine staining |

(*Continued*)

Table A2.1 (Continued)

| Medication | Indications, mechanism of action/effect | Dose | Route | Concentration | Example: 500 kg adult (50 kg foal when specified) *for concentration listed only | Precautions |
|---|---|---|---|---|---|---|
| Phenobarbital | Seizures, barbiturate | 2–10 mg/kg q8–12 h | PO | 100 mg tablets | 500 kg adult: 10–50 tablets | Schedule IV controlled substance |
| | | 5–12 mg/kg | IV slowly | 130 mg/mL | 19–46 mL | |
| | | Foals: 2–3 mg/kg | IV slowly | | 50 kg foal: 0.77–1.15 mL | |
| Phenoxybenzamine | Hypertension, alpha adrenergic antagonist | 0.4 mg/kg q6 h | PO | 10 mg capsules | 20 capsules | |
| Phenylbutazone | Analgesia, COX 1&2 inhibitor | 2.2–4.4 mg/kg q12 h | PO, IV | 1 g tablets, 200 mg/mL | 1–2 tablets<br>5.5–11 mL | Perivascular injections may cause severe inflammation or necrosis |
| Phenylephrine | Hypotension, nephrosplenic ligament entrapment, alpha-1 agonist | 0.2–1 µg/kg/min | CRI | 10 mg/mL | 0.6–3 mL/h | Secondary bradycardia |
| | | 0.04 mg/kg for nephrosplenic ligament entrapment | IV | | 2 mL qs to 60–1,000 mL, administered slowly while monitoring heart rate | |
| Phenylpropanolamine | Urinary incontinence sympathomimetic amine | 0.5–2 mg/kg q8–12 h | PO | 25, 50, 75 mg tablets | 10 tablets (25 mg), 5 tablets (50 mg), 3.5 tablets (75 mg) | |
| Phenytoin | Seizures, voltage-gated sodium channel blocker | 5–20 mg/kg | IV | 50 mg/mL | 50 mL | |
| | | 20 mg/kg q12 h, then 10–15 mg/kg | PO | 100 mg capsules | 250 capsules, then 50–75 capsules | |
| | | 2–7.5 mg/kg q12 h | PO | | 10–37.5 capsules | |
| Physostigmine | Anti-cholinergic toxicity, cholinesterase inhibitor | 0.6 mg/kg | IV | 1 mg/mL | 300 mL | |
| Pimobendan | Heart failure, phosphodiesterase III inhibitor, inodilator | 0.25 mg/kg q24 h | IV, PO | 0.75 mg/mL | 167 mL | |
| Pioglitazone | Insulin dysregulation, thiazolidinediones | 2 mg/kg q24 h | PO | 15, 30, 45 mg tablets | 66.5 tablets (15 mg), 33.5 tablets (30 mg), 22 tablets (45 mg) | |
| Piperazine | Parasite infestation, GABA agonist | 110 mg/kg | PO | paste | See supplied dosing syringe | |
| Piroxicam | Analgesia, COX 1&2 inhibitor | 80–100 mg q24 h per 500 kg horse | PO | 10 mg capsules | 8–10 capsules | |
| Polymyxin B | Antibiotic, polypeptide bactericidal, LPS binding | 1,000–6,000 U/kg q8 h | IV slowly, diluted | 500,000 U vials | 1–6 vials | Nephrotoxic |

| | | | | | | |
|---|---|---|---|---|---|---|
| Ponazuril | EPM treatment, triazine antiprotozoal | 5–10 mg/kg q24 h (15 mg/kg loading) | PO | paste | See supplied dosing syringe | |
| Potassium bromide | Seizures, anticonvulsant | 25–90 mg/kg q24 h | PO, IV | 250 mg/mL | 50 mL | |
| Pralidoxime (2-PAM) | Organophosphate toxicity, quaternary ammonium oxime cholinesterase reactivator | 20 mg/kg q4–6 h | IV | 300 mg/mL | 3.3 mL | Not effective in carbamate toxicity |
| Praziquantel | Tapeworm treatment, pyrazinoisoquinoline anthelmintic | 1.5 mg/kg | PO | Paste, 34 mg tablets | 22 tablets | |
| Prednisolone | Anti-inflammatory or immunosuppressive, glucocorticoid | 0.4–1.6 mg/kg q24 h | PO | 20 mg tablets | 10–40 tablets | |
| Prednisolone sodium succinate | Anti-inflammatory or immunosuppressive, glucocorticoid | 2–5 mg/kg | IV | 10 mg/mL, 50 mg/mL | 100–250 mL (10 mg/mL), 20–50 mL | |
| | | 10 mg/kg q6 h | IV | | 50 mL (10 mg/mL), 100 mL (50 mg/mL) | |
| Pregabalin | Seizures, voltage-gated calcium channel blocker | 2–4 mg/kg q8 h | PO | 300 mg capsules | 3–7 capsules | |
| Procainamide | Ventricular tachycardia, class-1 antiarrhythmic | 1 mg/kg/min | CRI | 100 mg/mL | 300 mL/h | May see hypotension, neurological, colic signs |
| Progesterone (in oil) | Hormone, maintenance of pregnancy | 0.8 mg/kg q24 h | IM | 50 mg/mL | 8 mL | |
| Propafenone | Tachyarrhythmias, antiarrhythmic | 0.5–1 mg/kg in 5% dextrose | IV slowly | 300 mg capsules | 3–4 capsules | May see colic or neurological signs |
| | | 2 mg/kg q8 h | PO | | | |
| Propantheline bromide | Antispasmodic, antimuscarinic | 0.067 mg/kg | IV | | Variable depending on concentration | |
| Propofol | Anesthetic, short-acting hypnotic | 2–4 mg/kg | IV | 10 mg/mL | 500 kg adult: 100–200 mL<br>50 kg foal: 10–20 mL | May cause respiratory depression |
| Propranolol | Hypertension, dysrhythmias, beta-adrenergic blocker | 0.03–0.05 mg/kg | IV | 1 mg/mL | 15–25 mL | |
| | | 0.38–0.78 mg/kg q8 h | PO | 160 mg tablets | 1–2.5 tablets | |
| Psyllium | Constipation, bulk laxative | 0.25–1 g/kg q6–24 h | PO, NGT | | 125–500 g | Mix with cold water |
| Pyrantel pamoate | Parasite infestation, pyrimidine = derivative anthelmintic | 6.6–13.2 mg/kg | PO | 50 mg/mL | 66–132 mL | |

(*Continued*)

**Table A2.1** (Continued)

| Medication | Indications, mechanism of action/effect | Dose | Route | Concentration | Example: 500 kg adult (50 kg foal when specified) *for concentration listed only | Precautions |
|---|---|---|---|---|---|---|
| Pyrilamine maleate | Allergic reaction, injectable antihistamine | 1 mg/kg q12 h<br>0.44 mg/kg foal | IV slowly, IM, SQ | 50 mg/mL | 500 kg adult: 10 mL<br>50 kg foal: 4.4 mL | |
| Pyrimethamine | Antibiotic, anti-protozoal, aminopyrimidine agent, folic acid inhibitor | 1–2 mg/kg q24 h | PO | 25 mg tablets | 20–40 tablets | |
| Quinapril | Diuresis, angiotensin-converting enzyme (ACE) inhibitor | 0.25–0.5 mg/kg q24 h | PO | 40 mg tablets | 3–6.25 tablets | Low oral bioavailability |
| Quinidine gluconate | Atrial fibrillation, class I antiarrhythmic | 0.5–2.2 mg/kg q10 min to effect | IV | 80 mg/mL | 3–13.75 mL | Do not exceed 12 mg/kg total dose |
| Quinidine sulfate | Atrial fibrillation, class I antiarrhythmic | 20–22 mg/kg q2 h to effect | NGT | 300 mg tablets | 33–37 tablets | Do not exceed six doses, may cause neurological, colic signs, paraphimosis, urticaria, laminitis |
| Ranitidine | Gastric ulcers, H2 receptor antagonist | 6.6 mg/kg q6–8 h<br>0.9–1.5 mg/kg q6–8 h | PO<br>IV, IM | 300 mg tablets, 25 mg/mL | 11 tablets<br>18–30 mL | Off market in US |
| Rifampin | Antibiotic, rifamycin | 5–10 mg/kg q12 h | PO | 300 mg capsules | 8–17 capsules | |
| Rimantadine | Viral infection, antiviral | 30 mg/kg q12 h | PO | 100 mg tablets | 160 tablets | |
| Romifidine | Sedation, alpha-2 agonist | 0.04–0.12 mg/kg q2-4 h | IV, IM | 10 mg/mL | 2–6 mL | |
| S-adenosylmethionine (SAM-e) | Hepatitis, anti-inflammatory, monoamine producer | 10–20 mg/kg q24 h | PO | 425 mg tablets | 12–23.5 tablets | |
| Salbutamol | Equine asthma, bronchoconstriction, beta 2 agonist, short-acting bronchodilator | 1–2 mcg/kg q8–12 h | Inhaler | 100 mcg actuations | 5–10 actuations | |
| Salmeterol | Equine asthma, bronchoconstriction, beta 2 agonist, long-acting bronchodilator | 0.5 mcg/kg q12 h | Inhaler | 50 mcg actuations | 5 actuations | |

| | | | | | | |
|---|---|---|---|---|---|---|
| Sarmazenil | Partial benzodiazepine inverse agonist<br>Moxidectin intoxication | 0.04 mg/kg | IV | Not currently available in the US | | |
| Selenium-vitamin E | For deficiency | 1 mL/100 lb | IM | 2.5 mg Se and 68 U vitamin E per mL | 500 kg adult: 10 mL<br>50 kg foal: 1 mL | |
| Sildenafil citrate | Pulmonary hypertension, phosphodiesterase V inhibitor | 0.2–0.6 mg/kg q4–8 h | PO | 25, 100 mg tablets | 4–12 tablets (25 mg)<br>1–3 tablets (100 mg) | Contraindicated in hypotensive patients |
| Sodium bicarbonate | Alkalinizing agent, for quinidine toxicity | 0.5–1 mEq/kg | IV | 1 mEq/mL, 8.4% | 250–500 mL | See Chapter 28 for information regarding use in patients with a metabolic acidosis |
| Sodium iodide | For actinobacillosis | 100 mg/kg q24 h<br>20–40 mg/kg q24hr | IV<br>PO | 200 mg/mL | 250 mL (IV)<br>50–100 mL (PO) | |
| Sodium nitrate | For cyanide toxicity | 16 mg/kg | IV | 10 mg/mL | 800 mL | |
| Sodium thiosulfate | For cyanide or arsenic poisoning | 30–50 mg/kg | IV slowly | 300 mg/mL | 50–83 mL | |
| Sotalol | Tachyarrhythmia, non-selective beta blocker, class III antiarrhythmic | 2.5–4 mg/kg q24 h | PO | 160 mg tablets | 8–12.5 tablets | |
| Stanozolol | Anabolic steroid | 0.55 mg/kg | IM | 50 mg/mL | 5.5 mL | May give once weekly up to four weeks |
| Sucralfate | Gastroprotectant | 20–40 mg/kg q6–8 h | PO | 1 g tablets | 500 kg adult: 10–20 tablets<br>50 kg foal: 1–2 tablets | Give two hours apart from other medications as it can decrease their bioavailability |
| Terbutaline | Bronchoconstriction, beta agonist, bronchodilator | 0.04–0.13 mg/kg q8–12 h | PO | 5 mg tablets | 4–13 tablets | |
| Thiabendazole | Parasite infestation, benzimidazole anthelmintic, antifungal | 50–100 mg/kg | PO | 500 mg tablets | 50–100 tablets | |
| Thiamine, vitamin B1 | For deficiency, CNS injury, lead poisoning | 1–10 mg/kg q12–24 h | IV, SQ, IM | 200 mg/mL | 500 kg adult:<br>2.5–25 mL<br>50 kg foal: 0.25–2.5 mL | |

(*Continued*)

**Table A2.1** (Continued)

| Medication | Indications, mechanism of action/effect | Dose | Route | Concentration | Example: 500 kg adult (50 kg foal when specified) *for concentration listed only | Precautions |
|---|---|---|---|---|---|---|
| Ticarcillin | Antibiotic, beta lactam | 50 mg/kg q6 h | IV, IM | | Variable depending on concentration | |
| Ticarcillin-clavulanate | Antibiotic, beta lactam with potentiator | 50 mg/kg q6hr | IV | 3.1 and 31 g vials | Variable depending on concentration | |
| Tiletamine and zolazepam (Telazol) | Anesthesia, dissociative anesthetic/tranquilizer | 1.1–2.2 mg/kg | IV | 100 mg/mL | 5.5–11 mL | Schedule III controlled substance |
| Tissue plasminogen activator (tPA) | Thrombosis dissolution, Thrombolytic | 4–16 mg diluted in 1 L isotonic fluid | Intrapleural | 250 µg/mL (0.25 mL syringes) | 16–64 mL | |
| Tolazoline | Sedation, alpha 2 antagonist | 0.5–2 mg/kg | IV slowly | 100 mg/mL | 2.5–10 mL | Rapid administration may cause hypotension, arrhythmias |
| Tramadol | Analgesia, opioid | 4 mg/kg | IV | 50 mg/mL | 40 mL | |
| | | 10 mg/kg | PO | 50 mg tablets | 100 tablets | |
| Tranexamic acid | Bleeding, lysine analog, antifibrinolytic | 10 mg/kg q8–12 h | IV slowly | 100 mg/mL | 50 mL | |
| | | 20 mg/kg q6 h | PO | 650 mg tablets | 15.5 tablets | |
| Trimethoprim-sulfa (diazine methoxazole) | Antibiotic, folic acid inhibitors/sulfonamide | 20–30 mg/kg q12 h | PO, IV | 960 mg tablets, 480 mg/mL | 10.5–16 tablets | |
| Tripelennamine HCl | Allergic reaction, antihistamine | 1 mg/kg q6–12 h | IM | 20 mg/mL | 26 mL | Do not give IV |
| Ursodiol | Cholestasis, bile acid | 15 mg/kg q24 h | PO | 500 mg tablets | 15 tablets | |
| Valacyclovir | Antiviral | 27–30 mg/kg q8 h for 2 days, then 18 mg/kg q12 h | PO | 500 mg tablets | 27–30 tablets, then 18 tablets | |
| Vancomycin | Antibiotic, glycopeptide | 7.5 mg/kg q8 h | IV | 50 mg/mL (requires further dilution) | 75 mL | |
| | | 300 mg in saline | IVRLP | | 6 mL | |
| Vasopressin (ADH) | Hypothalamic–pituitary gland axis dysfunction, Hormone, vasopressor | 0.05–0.8 U/kg | IV | 20 U/mL | 1.25–20 mL | |
| | | 0.0005–0.001 U/kg/min | CRI | | 0.75–1.5 mL/h | |
| Verapamil | Anti-arrhythmic, calcium channel blocker | 0.025–0.05 mg/kg q30 min | IV | 2.5 mg/mL | 5–10 mL | Do not exceed 0.2 mg/kg total dose |

| | | | | | | |
|---|---|---|---|---|---|---|
| Vitamin C | Antioxidant | 0.2–1 g/kg q24 h | PO | 1 g tablets, | 100–1000 tablets | |
| | | 30 mg/kg q12–24 h | IV slowly | 250 mg/mL | 60 mL | |
| Vitamin E | Neuroprotectant | 6.6 U/kg | IM | Variable | Variable depending on concentration | Not all forms are bioavailable to the horse |
| | | 10–20 U/kg q24 h | PO | | | |
| Vitamin $K_1$ | Rodenticide toxicity | 0.5–2 mg/kg | SQ, IM | 10 mg/mL | 25–100 mL | Do not administer IV |
| Voriconazole | Triazole antifungal | 3–4 mg/kg q12–24 h | PO | 200 mg capsules | 8–10 capsules | |
| Xylazine | Sedation, alpha-2 adrenergic agonist | 0.2–1 mg/kg q8–12 h | IV, IM | 100 mg/mL | 1–5 mL | May cause tachypnea in febrile patients, may cause aggression |
| | | 0.17 mg/kg | Epidural | | 0.85 mL | |
| Yohimbine | Alpha-2 agonist (sedation) reversal, alpha-2 adrenergic antagonist | 0.075–0.12 mg/kg | IV slowly | 2 mg/mL | 18.75–30 mL | May cause tachycardia |
| Yunnan baiyao | Bleeding, traditional Chinese herb | 10 mg/kg q8 h | PO | 250 mg capsules | 20 capsules | Can be applied topically to source of hemorrhage, no evidence of *in vivo* hemostatic changes |

IV - intravenous; IM - intramuscular; PO - by mouth; NGT - by nasogastric tube; CRI - continuous rate infusion; IVRLP - intravenous regional limb perfusion.

Table A2.2 Crystalloid fluids.

| Fluid type | Osmolarity (mOsm/L) | pH | SID | Components (mEq/L) |
|---|---|---|---|---|
| Plasmalyte-A | 295 | 7.4 | 50 | Na 140<br>K 5<br>Cl 98<br>Mg 3<br>Acetate 27<br>Gluconate 23 |
| Normosol-R | 295 | 7.4 | 50 | Na 140<br>K 5<br>Cl 98<br>Mg 3<br>Acetate 27<br>Gluconate 23 |
| Lactated Ringer's solution | 273 | 6.5 | 28 | Na 130<br>K 4<br>Cl 109<br>Ca 3<br>Lactate 28 |
| Hartmann's solution | 278 | 6.5 | 29 | Na 131<br>K 5<br>Cl 111<br>Ca 4<br>Lactate 29 |
| D5W | 254 (0) | 4.3 | 0 | 5% Dextrose |
| 0.45% NaCl | 154 | 5.6 | 0 | Na 77<br>Cl 77 |
| 0.9% NaCl | 308 | 5.6 | 0 | Na 154<br>Cl 154 |
| 7.2% NaCl hypertonic saline | 2464 | 5.6 | 0 | Na 1232<br>Cl 1232 |

Table A2.3 Colloids.

| Type | Type | Concentration/components | Molecular weight (Da) | Dose |
|---|---|---|---|---|
| Albumin (human) | Natural | 250 mg/mL | 69,000 | 250–750 mg/kg/h |
| Equine plasma (fresh frozen) | Natural | Total solid protein concentration varies | 69,000 (albumin) | 5–20 mL/kg |
| Hextend | Synthetic | 6% hetastarch<br>670/0.75 in 0.9% NaCl<br>4:1 (C2:C6) | 670,000 | 5–10 mL/kg<br>Max 20 mL/kg/d |
| Vetstarch/Voluven | Synthetic | 6% tetrastarch<br>130/0.4 in 0.9% NaCl<br>9:1 (C2–C6) | 130 000 | 5–10 mL/kg<br>Max 50 mL/kg/d |
| Dextran 70 | Synthetic | Alpha-1,6-glucans | 70,000 | 5–10 mL/kg |
| 23.4% Hypertonic saline + 6% hydroxyethylstarch (HES) (1:2.5 ratio) | Synthetic | Combination of hypertonic saline and HES solution to prolong effects of increases in intravascular volume | Depends on which HES product is used | 3–5 mL/kg |

# Appendix 3

## Emergency Treatment Protocols

*Jamie J. Kopper*

*Department of Veterinary Clinical Sciences, College of Veterinary Medicine, Iowa State University, Ames, IA, USA*

## Electrolyte Disturbances

### Hyperkalemia

Management of hyperkalemia is a medical emergency that requires prompt reduction of potassium levels to prevent fatal cardiac arrythmias. Horses with serum potassium levels >5.5 mEq/L require immediate attention.

Step 1: Re-evaluate the sample, particularly if the result is unexpected. Blood samples that are not analyzed promptly may be hyperkalemic secondary to red blood cell lysis.

Step 2: If hyperkalemia is confirmed or suspected based on clinical picture, perform an ECG to monitor for associated cardiac changes including tall narrow T waves, prolonged QRS complex and PR interval, depressed ST segments, depressed p waves, atrial standstill and ventricular arrythmias.

Step 3: Begin treatment to lower blood potassium levels and increase cardiac threshold voltage as described in the table below (Table A3.1, also present in Chapter 13, Table 13.1). Ideally intravenous fluids will not contain potassium (i.e., 0.9% NaCl or 0.45% NaCl). However, if potassium-free fluids are not available, the use of isotonic replacement formulas (i.e., Lactated Ringer's solution or Normosol-R) contains a relatively small amount of potassium and should be acceptable.

Step 4: Assess the patient for causes of hyperkalemia to address the underlying disease. Common causes include uroperitoneum (Chapter 13), rhabdomyolysis (Chapter 8) or intravascular hemolysis, and renal failure (Chapter 13).

### Hyponatremia

Serum sodium concentrations less than 115–120 mEq/L in adult horses need to be corrected with care, particularly if they are chronic (i.e., >48 hours duration) due to the risk of osmotic demyelination with too rapid of a correction. Careful correction requires frequent monitoring of serum electrolytes and continuous intravenous fluid therapy which is most easily accomplished in a hospital with 24-hour care.

Step 1: Determine if patient has chronic (>48 hours) or acute (<48 hours) hyponatremia. This is best determined with pre-existing serum electrolyte values. When in doubt it is best to assume chronicity, as osmotic demyelination due to over-correction may not be reversible and can be fatal.

Step 1a: If the hyponatremia is acute the sodium can be rapidly corrected. This can be accomplished by addressing the underlying condition resulting in sodium loss and provision of isotonic replacement fluids (enteral or intravenously) or 7.2% NaCl.

Step 2: For patients with unknown or chronic hyponatremia slow correction should be pursued to prevent the development of osmotic demyelination. Unless the patient is displaying seizure-like activity, the goal is to increase serum sodium levels by 0.5–1 mEq/L per hour and by no more than 12 mEq/day. Patients should have serum electrolytes rechecked regularly to ensure that overcorrection is not occurring.

*Emergency Triage of the Horse*, First Edition. Edited by Rolfe M. Radcliffe and Jamie J. Kopper.

Companion website: www.wiley.com/go/radcliffe/triage

**Table A3.1** Emergency drugs for patients with hyperkalemia.

| Drug | Dosage | Mechanism of action | Per 1 L for 50 kg foal | Per 5 L for 500 kg adult |
|---|---|---|---|---|
| 23% calcium gluconate | 0.25–0.5 mL/kg IV over 5–10 minutes | Does not lower serum potassium<br>Increases cardiac threshold voltage | ~12–25 mL | ~125–250 mL |
| 50% dextrose | 0.35–0.5 g/kg IV over 3–5 minutes | Promotes translocation of potassium intracellularly | 35–50 mL | 350–500 mL |
| 8.4% sodium bicarbonate | 1–2 mEq/kg over 15 minutes | Promotes translocation of potassium intracellularly | 50–100 mL | 500–1,000 mL |

Step 2a: *For patients with neurologic sequela* due to hyponatremia (i.e., seizures) an initial correction can be made more rapidly (i.e., initially increase in the patient's serum sodium concentration by 4–6 mEq/L).

Step 3: Depending on the starting serum sodium concentration and the desired serum sodium concentration intravenous fluids of the desired sodium concentration can be created. The Adrogué–Madias formula (Anrogué and Madias, 2000) is used to estimate the effect of infusate on change in serum sodium concentration, although it frequently under-estimates the effect; thus, frequent assessment of that patient's serum electrolytes is imperative.

Adrogué–Madias formula: Change in serum Na+ = (infusate Na+-serum Na+)/(total body water +1)

Step 3a: To make infusates that are less sodium rich, a replacement formula can be combined with 0.45% NaCl or sterile water in varying proportions.

Step 4: Determine and treat the cause of the hyponatremia so that ongoing losses can be minimized. Common causes in horses include gastrointestinal loss (i.e., diarrhea) combined with consumption of free water, severe renal disease, uroperitoneum, sweat losses combined with consumption of free water and salivary loss (i.e., dysphagia, etc.). Access to free water may need to be removed during correction period.

### Hypernatremia

Serum sodium concentrations greater than 160 mEq/L in adult horses need to be corrected with care, particularly if they are chronic (i.e., >48 hours durations) due to the risk of cerebral edema with too rapid correction. Careful correction requires frequent monitoring of serum electrolytes and continuous intravenous fluid therapy which is most easily accomplished in a hospital with 24-hour care.

Step 1: Determine if patient has chronic (>48 hours) or acute (<48 hours) hypernatremia. This is best determined with pre-existing serum electrolyte values; however, in veterinary patients this information is often not available. When in doubt it is best to assume chronicity, as damage due to cerebral edema from over-correction often is not reversible and may be fatal.

Step 1a: If the hypernatremia is known to be acute the sodium can be rapidly corrected. This can be accomplished by addressing the underlying condition resulting in sodium loss and provision of isotonic replacement solutions for maintenance fluids (enteral or intravenously).

Step 2: For patients with unknown or chronic hypernatremia slow correction should be pursued to prevent the development of cerebral edema. Unless the patient is displaying seizure-like activity, the goal is to decrease serum sodium levels by 0.5–1 mEq/L/h and by no more than 12 mEq/day. Patients should have serum electrolytes rechecked regularly to ensure that overcorrection is not occurring.

Step 2a: *For patients with neurologic sequela* due to hypernatremia (i.e., seizures) an initial correction can be made more rapidly (i.e., decrease in the patient's serum sodium concentration 4–6 mEq/L).

Step 3: Depending on the starting serum sodium concentration and the desired serum sodium concentration intravenous fluids can be custom created. The Adrogué–Madias formula is used to estimate the effect of infusate on change in serum sodium concentration, although it frequently under-estimates the effect; thus, frequent assessment of that patient's serum electrolytes is imperative.

Adrogué–Madias formula: Change in serum Na+ = (infusate Na+-serum Na+)/(total body water +1)

Step 3a: To make infusates that are more sodium rich, hypertonic saline (i.e., 7.2% NaCl) can be added to traditional replacement or maintenance formulas.

Step 4: Determine the cause of the hypernatremia. The most frequent cause of hypernatremia in horses is lack of access to free water which may be combined with the administration of replacement intravenous fluids or hypertonic saline. Horses that are unable to drink and are receiving intravenous fluids (i.e., replacement formulas or hypertonic saline) should be carefully monitored to prevent the development of hypernatremia.

## Airway Emergencies

Please see Chapter 11 for additional details regarding respiratory emergencies.

### Acute Asthma Exacerbation

Step 1: After performing a thorough physical examination to rule out other causes of tachypnea (i.e., bronchopneumonia, pleuropneumonia, etc.) remove/modify environmental triggers if possible.
Examples: Wet the hay, provide all pelleted diet, remove round bale, house outside.

Step 2: Unless contra-indicated due to other co-morbidities administer systemic corticosteroids (dexamethasone IV or IM 0.05 mg/kg) and begin a slow taper (i.e., decrease by 25–50% every ~7 days unless clinical signs return) for anti-inflammatory effects.

Step 3: Provide bronchodilation and anti-inflammatory support. A list of medications for emergent aerosol and systemic treatment is provided in Table A3.2. Please refer to the ACVIM Consensus statement on Inflammatory Airway disease (Couetil et al. 2016) for longer-term management plans.

### Broncho and Pleural Pneumonia

Step 1: Obtain transtracheal aspirate (TTA) sample for cytology to confirm septic inflammation and culture. Steps to performing a TTA are described in Chapter 4.

Step 2: If moderate-to-significant volumes of pleural effusion are present a thoracocentesis can be performed for therapeutic and diagnostic purposes as described in Chapter 4. Submission of pleural fluid for culture should not replace a TTW sample, but submitting both samples may increase the number of organisms identified (Arroyo et al. 2017). Depending on the degree of severity, the thoracic trocar catheter may be left in place for continued drainage, occluded for intermittent drainage or removed.

Step 3: If septic inflammation is confirmed and empirical antimicrobials need to be initiated before receiving culture and sensitivity results the ideal antimicrobial choice is broad spectrum, including anaerobic coverage if there is a high index

**Table A3.2** Bronchodilator and anti-inflammatory medications for horses with equine asthma.

| Drug | Dose | Route | Notes |
|---|---|---|---|
| Albuterol | 1–2 μg/kg q1–3 hours (Couetil et al. 2016) | Aerosolized | Bronchodilator |
| Budesonide | 1800 μg/500 kg horse q12 hours (Lavoie et al. 2019) | Aerosolized | Corticosteroid |
| Ciclesonide (Aservo EquiHaler(R)) | 2744 μg/horse q12 hours for 5 days, then 4116 μg/horse q24 hours for 5 days | Aerosolized | Corticosteroid<br>Ciclesonide is a prodrug, activated in the airway epithelium. |
| Clenbuterol | 0.8–3.2 μg/kg PO q12 hours | PO | Bronchodilator |
| Dexamethasone | 0.05 mg/kg q24 hours (Couetil et al. 2016; Leguillette et al. 2017) | IV, IM | Corticosteroid<br>Can be given PO, but lower bioavailability |
| Fluticasone | 1–6 μg/kg q12 hours (Couetil et al. 2016) | Aerosolized | Corticosteroid |
| Ipatropium | 0.2–0.4 μg/kg q8–12 hours (Couetil et al. 2016)<br>2–3 μg/kg in 0.02% solution for q8–12 hours (Couetil et al. 2016) | Aerosolized<br>Ultrasonic nebulization | Bronchodilator |

**Table A3.3** Common antimicrobial choices for broncho and pleural pneumonia.

| Medications | Dose | Comments |
|---|---|---|
| Penicillin | Penicillin procaine G: 22,000 IU/kg IM q12 hours<br>Potassium penicillin: 22,000 IU/kg IV q6 hours | |
| Gentamicin | Gentamicin: 6.6 mg/kg IV q24 hours*<br>Gentamicin: 2 mg/kg nebulized q24 hours (McKenzie and Murray, 2020) | *Several studies have questioned the need for higher doses of gentamicin for systemic administration (7.7–10 mg/kg) (Bauquier et al. 2015; Schoster et al. 2021). |
| Penicillin | Penicillin procaine G: 22,000 IU/kg IM q12 hours<br>Potassium penicillin: 22,000 IU/kg IV q6 hours | |
| Enrofloxacin | Enrofloxacin: 5.5 mg/kg IV q24 hours (Giguere et al. 1996)<br>Enrofloxacin: 7.5 mg/kg PO q24 hours (Giguere et al. 1996) | |
| Ceftiofur | Ceftiofur sodium: 2.2 mg/kg IV or IM q12 hours<br>Ceftiofur crystalline-free acid: 6.6 mg/g day 0, 4, then every 7 days (Fultz et al. 2014) | |
| Trimethoprim sulfamethoxazole | Trimethoprim sulfamethoxazole: 30 mg/kg PO q12 hours | Each component (trimethoprim, sulfamethoxazole) is bacteriostatic, but may have bactericidal activity when combined at appropriate concentrations. |
| +/− metronidazole | Metronidazole: 15–25 mg/kg PO q6 hours (Sweeney et al. 1986) | Addition of metronidazole can increase the spectrum of activity against anaerobic organisms if indicated.<br>Metronidazole can be given per rectum, but has low bioavailability (~30%) (Steinman et al. 2000) |

of suspicion for anaerobic components, with bactericidal activity. Table A3.3 provides several commonly used antimicrobial combinations in adult horses that fulfill these requirements. The ideal choice depends on many factors including severity of disease, suspected etiology (i.e., severe pleural pneumonia after aspiration secondary to esophageal obstruction vs mild bronchopneumonia post viral infection), patient factors (i.e., compliance), and owner factors (i.e., skill giving IM injections, ability to maintain an intravenous catheter, etc.).

Step 4: Depending on results of the culture and sensitivity an initial response to treatment antimicrobial selection may be modified.

**Pulmonary Edema** – See **Chapter 11**

## Abdominal Emergencies

**Colic – Adult – See Chapter 10**
**Colic – Neonate – See Chapter 20**

### Colitis – Adult

Step 1: Determine if the patient is dehydrated and develop a fluid plan. An example is provided in Table A3.4.

Step 2: Determine if colloid therapy is necessary. Indications for needing colloid (natural or synthetic) include severe hypoproteinemia with tachycardia and hemoconcentration that does not respond to resuscitation with crystalloid fluids.

**Table A3.4** Example intravenous fluid plan for an adult horse.

| Fluid requirement | Example 500 kg patient |
|---|---|
| Maintenance: 1–2 mL/kg/h | 0.5–1 L/h |
| % dehydrated (estimate) | 6% dehydrated = 30 L (0.06 × Bwt) |
| Ongoing losses (estimate) | 2 L/h |
| Total estimated fluid requirement for 24 hours | 90–102 L |
| Fluid plan | 20 L bolus, then 3 L/h |

Step 3: Determine if empirical antimicrobial therapy is necessary.

Step 3a: If Potomac Horse Fever (i.e., enteric disease due to *Neorickettsia risticii*) or *Lawsonia intracellularis* are high on the differential list empirical treatment with oxytetracycline (6.6 mg/kg IV q12 hours) may be indicated.

Step 3b: If diarrhea is suspected to be due to *Clostridioides difficile* or *Clostridium perfringens* treatment with metronidazole (15–25 mg/kg PO q12 hours) may be indicated.

Step 3c: If the patient is profoundly leukopenic, treatment with broad-spectrum antimicrobials may be indicated as prophylaxis for bacterial translocation. Examples of broad-spectrum antimicrobial combinations can be found in Table A3.3.

Step 3d: In many instances, treatment with antimicrobials is not necessary and may even be contraindicated (i.e., suspected antimicrobial associated diarrhea, equine coronavirus, *Salmonella* spp.) due to risks of exacerbating intestinal dysbiosis.

Step 4: Determine if anti-inflammatory or analgesic medication such as a non-steroidal anti-inflammatory drug (NSAID) is indicated. Dosages for these medications can be found in Chapter 31.

Step 4a: Use of an NSAID may be indicated in horses showing signs of colic (for analgesic properties) and/or meeting systemic inflammatory response syndrome (SIRS) criteria (for anti-inflammatory properties).

Step 4b: Due to the potential adverse effects of NSAIDs (i.e., acute kidney injury, colonic epithelial injury, decreased intestinal epithelial healing) NSAIDs should be used judiciously with efforts taken to mitigate the risk of adverse effects such as ensuring appropriate hydration.

Step 4c: If additional analgesia is needed adjunctive agents such as a continuous rate infusion of lidocaine and/or butorphanol can provide analgesia with fewer adverse effects.

## Colitis – Neonatal

Step 1: Address electrolyte derangements, evidence of acute kidney injury and/or other organ dysfunction as described elsewhere in this appendix.

Step 2: For neonates, with an IgG of less than 800 mg/dL, consider including a plasma transfusion as part of your fluid therapy. Plasma can be transfused as 20 mL/kg doses (i.e., 1 L/50 kg foal) to effect, with up to 60 mL/kg in a 24-hour period.

Step 3: Determine if the patient is dehydrated and develop a fluid plan. An example is provided in Table A3.5.

Step 4: In neonates with diarrhea, broad-spectrum antimicrobials are usually indicated as prophylaxis for sepsis and secondary localized sites of infection. The ideal antimicrobial(s) is/are broad-spectrum, bactericidal and administered parenterally, as gastrointestinal motility and absorption may be altered. Also see Chapters 20 and 31. Table A3.6 also provides commonly used antimicrobials in neonatal foals.

Step 5: Determine if anti-inflammatory medication such as a non-steroidal anti-inflammatory drug (NSAID) is indicated. Chapter 31 includes commonly used anti-inflammatory and analgesic medications in horses and foals.

Step 5a: Judicious use of an NSAID may be indicated in foals showing signs of colic (for analgesic properties) and/or meeting systemic inflammatory response syndrome (SIRS) criteria (for anti-inflammatory properties).

Step 5b: Due to the potential adverse effects of NSAIDs (i.e., acute kidney injury, colonic injury, decreasing intestinal mucosal healing) they should be used judiciously with efforts taken to mitigate the risk of adverse effects such as ensuring appropriate hydration.

Step 5c: If additional analgesia is needed adjunctive agents such as a continuous rate infusion of lidocaine and/or butorphanol can provide analgesia with fewer adverse effects.

**Table A3.5** Example of intravenous fluid plan for a neonatal foal.

| Fluid requirement | Example 50 kg patient |
|---|---|
| Maintenance: 3–5 mL/kg/h[a] | 150–250 mL/h |
| % dehydrated (estimate) | 6% dehydrated = 3 L (0.06 × Bwt) |
| Ongoing losses (estimate) | 0.25 L/h |
| Total estimated fluid requirement for 24 hours | ~12.6–15 L |
| Option A | 2 L bolus, then 0.5 L/h |
| Option B | 2 L bolus q4 hours |

[a] There are numerous "maintenance" fluid rates used for neonatal foals. This is an example of one; however, you can use the formula of your choice. Reassessment and adjustment of the fluid plan is imperative.

**Table A3.6** Commonly used antimicrobials in neonatal foals.

| Antimicrobial(s) and dosage(s) | Class | Comments |
|---|---|---|
| Amikacin: 25 mg/kg IV q24 hours | Aminoglycoside | May be used in combination with a beta-lactam antimicrobial to increase spectrum of activity against. Use with caution in foals with azotemia or in foals at risk for acute kidney injury due to nephrotoxicity. Ideally, use with therapeutic drug monitoring. |
| Ceftiofur sodium: 5 mg/kg IV, IM q12 hours (Meyer et al. 2009) | Beta-lactam | |
| Ceftiofur crystalline-free acid: 13.2 mg/kg SQ q48 hours (Pusterla et al. 2017) | Beta-lactam | |
| Gentamicin: 8–16 mg/kg IV q24 hours | Aminoglycoside | May be used in combination with a beta-lactam antimicrobial to increase spectrum of activity against. Use with caution in foals with azotemia or in foals at risk for acute kidney injury due to nephrotoxicity. Ideally, use with therapeutic drug monitoring. |
| Potassium penicillin: 22,000 IU/kg IV q6 hours | Beta-lactam | Infuse slowly over five minutes |

Step 6: Foals that continue to show signs of colic despite analgesia warrant further evaluation for potential lesions requiring surgical exploration and correction and/or may need to be held off nursing to allow for gastrointestinal rest. Foals that are not allowed to nurse typically need partial or total parenteral nutrition.

**Esophageal obstruction** – See **Chapter 10**
**Grain overload** – See **Chapter 10**

## Hepatitis

Hepatitis is discussed in Chapter 21. In lieu of a definitive diagnosis, the following are general supportive care measurements that can be considered for treatment of undifferentiated hepatitis. Depending on the case, options are provided below:

Anti-inflammatory medications: Anti-inflammatory medications can be used for analgesia and to decrease inflammation associated with hepatitis. Reducing inflammation may help decrease the risk of fibrosis. Commonly used anti-inflammatories medications for horses with hepatitis are summarized in Table A3.7.

**Table A3.7** Anti-inflammatory medications used in horses with hepatitis.

| Drug | Dose | Comments |
|---|---|---|
| Dimethyl sulfoxide (DMSO) | 0.5–1 g/kg diluted to a 10% solution IV q24 hours × 3–5 days | May solubilize calcium bilirubinate, which is a common component of equine choleliths. |
| NSAIDs | 1.1 mg/kg IV, PO q12 hours | |
| Flunixin meglumine | 0.9 mg/kg IV, PO once, then | |
| Firocoxib | 0.3 mg/kg IV, PO q24 thereafter | |
| Pentoxyifylline | 8.5 mg/kg IV q12 hours (Liska et al. 2006)<br>10 mg/kg PO q12 hours (Liska et al. 2006) | Anti-inflammatory and immune-modulating effects.<br>Increases red blood cell flexibility and reduces hepatic fibrosis in humans. |
| Prednisolone | 1 mg/kg PO q24 hours | May be helpful for chronic-active lymphocytic plasmacytic hepatitis. Should not be used unless infectious causes have been ruled out. |

**Table A3.8** Hepatoprotectants.

| Compound | Dose | Comments |
|---|---|---|
| N-acetylcysteine | 70 mg/kg IV q6 hours for 8 treatments | No pharmacokinetic or dynamic studies in horses. |
| S-adenosylmethionine (SAMe) | 20 mg/kg PO q24 hours | No pharmacokinetic or dynamic studies performed in horses. |
| Silibinin (milk thistle extract) | 6.5–26 mg/kg PO (Hackett et al. 2013)<br>Due to the low oral bioavailability dosing frequency was not extrapolated | <1% oral bioavailability in horses (Hackett et al. 2013). |
| Vitamin E | 20 IU/kg PO q24 hours | Anti-oxidant and anti-inflammatory effects. |

Hepatoprotectants: Hepatoprotectants may be employed for their potential anti-oxidant, hepatocellular membrane-stabilizing, and anti-fibrotic activities (Table A3.8). Unfortunately, little work has been done with most of these medications in horses, and doses are often extrapolated from other species.

Antimicrobials: If a bacterial cause is suspected and culture and sensitivity data is not available antimicrobial therapy can be instituted. In general, antimicrobials should be broad spectrum, include activity against those commonly found in the intestinal tract, amenable to long-term administration, provide adequate concentrations in the bile, and should not require P450 metabolism. Some examples of commonly used antimicrobials are provided in Table A3.9.

Step 7: Ensure that the patient is consuming adequate nutrition. This is important to prevent mobilization of lipids which increase the risk of secondary hepatic complications such as hepatic lipidosis. If the patient is unwilling to consume an adequate amount of feed, nutrition should be provided enterally or via partial parenteral nutrition.

## Hepatic Encephalopathy

Step 1: If sedation is necessary, it should be used with caution due to altered drug metabolism associated with hepatic insufficiency. Low doses of alpha-2 agonists (i.e., xylazine, detomidine hydrochloride) are ideal. Benzodiazepines should be avoided.

Step 2: Begin intravenous fluid therapy to provide maintenance fluid requirements and correct existing deficits. Table A3.4 provides a template for establishing a fluid plan for adult horses.

Step 3: Consider treatments outlined in Table A3.10, which are designed to reduce absorption of ammonia from the gastrointestinal tract.

Step 4: Treatments aimed to decrease cerebral edema can be considered as described in Table A3.11.

**Table A3.9** Common antimicrobials for treatment of bacterial hepatitis.

| Antimicrobial(s) | Dose(s) | Comments |
|---|---|---|
| Ceftiofur | Ceftiofur sodium: 2.2 mg/kg IV or IM q12 hours | |
| Penicillin | Penicillin procaine G: 22,000 IU/kg IM q12 hours<br>Potassium penicillin: 22,000 IU/kg IV q6 hours | |
| Gentamicin | Gentamicin: 6.6 mg/kg IV q24 hours* | *Several studies have questioned the need for higher doses of gentamicin (7.7–10 mg/kg) (Bauquier et al. 2015; Schoster et al. 2021). |
| Penicillin | Penicillin procaine G: 22,000 IU/kg IM q12 hours<br>Potassium penicillin: 22,000 IU/kg IV q6 hours | Enrofloxacin can also be considered as a monotherapy, if the degree of suspicion for anaerobic bacteria is low. |
| Enrofloxacin | Enrofloxacin: 5.5 mg/kg IV q24 hours (Giguere et al. 2014)<br>Enrofloxacin: 7.5 mg/kg PO q24 hours (Giguere et al. 2014) | |
| Trimethoprim sulfamethoxazole | 30 mg/kg PO q12 hours | |
| +/− Metronidazole | Metronidazole: 15–25 mg/kg PO q6 hours (Sweeney et al. 1986) | The addition of metronidazole can increase the spectrum of activity against anaerobic organisms if indicated.<br>Metronidazole can be given per rectum, but has low bioavailability (~30%) (Steinman et al. 2000). |

**Table A3.10** Medications to decrease intestinal absorption of ammonia.

| Drug | Dose | Comments |
|---|---|---|
| Lactulose | 0.2–0.5 mL/kg PO q6–8 hours | Poorly absorbed by the small intestine and acidifies the intestinal contents leading to decreased absorption of ammonia. |
| Mineral oil | 2 mL/kg via nasogastric intubation | May decrease absorption of ammonia from the gastrointestinal tract. |
| Neomycin | 10–30 mg/kg PO q6 hours | Suppresses enteric ammonia-producing bacteria.<br>More nephrotoxic than gentamicin – do not use for more than a couple days. |

**Table A3.11** Treatments to decrease cerebral edema.

| Drug | Dose | Comments |
|---|---|---|
| Furosemide | 1 mg/kg IV, IM q8–12 hours | |
| Mannitol | 0.25–2 g/kg as a 20% solution IV over 20–30 minutes | Must be warmed to prevent crystallization at room or colder temperatures.<br>Administer with filter to prevent administration of precipitant. |
| 7.2% NaCl | 4–6 mL/kg IV | |

### Acute Kidney Injury

Acute Kidney Injury (AKI) can occur for several reasons such as conditions resulting in decreased renal blood flow and exposure to nephrotoxins.

Step 1: Determine if a nephrotoxin is contributing to the current AKI. If so, eliminate the source if possible.
Step 2: If there are any significant electrolyte derangements address and/or take them into consideration as described elsewhere in this appendix.
Step 3: Estimate any current fluid deficits, ongoing losses, and maintenance requirements to establish a fluid therapy plan. An example of this is provided in Table A3.12.
 Step 3a. If the patient has not urinated after three 20 mL/kg IV fluid boluses, the patient should be closely re-evaluated to ensure that the patient is not anuric and in renal failure or that the patient does not have a urinary obstruction or uroperitoneum. If any of the above are identified, the patient should be referred to a tertiary hospital for further management.
 Step 3b: Fluid therapy can also be accomplished using enteral or rectal fluids. Initial fluid deficits are best corrected using intravenous fluids as volume deficits resulting in poor perfusion may decrease the absorption of enterally or rectally administered fluids. However, long term, many of these patients would benefit from fluids that are less sodium and chloride rich than commercially available intravenous replacement formulas used in horses.
Step 4: Continue to monitor serum biochemistry and urine-specific gravity values approximately every 24 hours. Ideally, elevations in creatinine will improve by 50% every 24 hours. Patients with isosthenuria require especially close monitoring when discontinuing fluid support as they are unable to concentrate their urine.

**Reproductive Emergencies** – See **Chapter 14**

**Castration Complications**
**Dystocia**
**Paraphimosis**
**Periparturient Hemorrhage**
**Uterine prolapse**

## Neurological Emergencies

Approaches to neurological emergencies are also covered in Chapter 15.

### Ataxia

Step 1: Perform a thorough history, physical exam, and neurological examination including assessment of mentation, cranial nerve function, and gait assessment.
Step 2: For horses that are at risk for falling, consider early referral. Transportation, diagnostics, and institution of care is better for standing horses versus recumbent horses.

**Table A3.12** Fluid therapy template for an adult horse with AKI.

| Fluid requirement | Example 500 kg patient |
|---|---|
| Maintenance: 1–2 mL/kg/h | 0.5–1 L/h |
| % dehydrated (estimate) | 5% dehydrated = 25 L (0.05 × Bwt) |
| Ongoing losses (estimate) | 0 |
| Total estimated fluid requirement for 24 hours | 37–49 L |
| Fluid plan | 10 L IV fluid bolus, repeated up to two times until patient urinates, then 2 L/h |

Step 3: Institute biosecurity protocols and contact your state veterinarian if contagious disease (i.e., Equine Herpes Myeloencephalopathy, EHM) is on your differential list.

Step 4: Ultimately, the treatment plan will be dependent on your diagnosis and differential list. However, Table A3.13 provides general supportive care and considerations:

## Head Trauma

Step 1: If the horse is recumbent, elevate the horse's head 30° to decrease cerebral swelling.

Step 2: The use of anti-inflammatory medications, anti-oxidants, and hyperosmolar agents may be needed or used in horses with head trauma depending on the injury and clinical signs. Table A3.14 summarizes these therapies.

**The recumbent horse – Chapter 15**
**Seizures – Chapter 15**

**Table A3.13** General treatments for horses with ataxia.

| Medication | Purpose | Dose | Comments |
|---|---|---|---|
| NSAIDs | Anti-inflammatory, analgesia | Firocoxib – 0.9 mg/kg IV, PO then 0.3 mg/kg q24 hours<br>Flunixin meglumine – 1.1 mg/kg IV, PO q12 hours<br>Phenylbutazone – 4.4 mg/kg IV,PO | |
| Steroids | Anti-inflammatory | Dexamethasone – 0.05–0.1 mg/kg IV, IM, PO q24 hours<br>Prednisolone – 1 mg/kg PO q24 hours | |
| Dimethyl sulfoxide (DMSO) | Anti-inflammatory, anti-oxidant | 0.5–1 g/kg diluted to a 10% solution IV q24 hours × 3–5 days | There is little experimental evidence to support beneficial effects of DMSO in horses, but it is commonly used.<br>Administration of solutions greater than 10% can result in red blood cell lysis. |
| Vitamin E | Anti-inflammatory, anti-oxidant | 20 IU/kg PO | Low vitamin E levels are implicated for Equine Degenerative Myeloencephalopathy (EDM).<br>Water-soluble forms of vitamin E are the most bioavailable to horses. |
| Anti-protozoal | Treatment for EPM | Marquis® (Ponazuril): 5 mg/kg PO q24 hours<br>Protazil® (Diclazuril): 1 mg/kg PO q24 hours<br>Rebalance® (Sulfadiazine and pyrimethamine): 20 mg/kg sulfadiazine, 1 mg/kg pyrimethamine | In some instances, treatment for EPM may be instituted while waiting for confirmatory diagnostic testing. |
| Anti-viral | Treatment for EHM | Gancyclovir: 2.5 mg/kg IV q8 hours for 24 hours, then 2.5 mg/kg IV q12 hours (Carmicheal et al. 2013)<br>Valacyclovir: 27 mg/kg PO q8 hours for 2 days, then 18 mg/kg PO q12 hours (Maxwell et al. 2017) | Valacyclovir is most effective when administered prophylactically (Maxwell et al. 2017) |

**Table A3.14** Medications for use in horses with head trauma.

| Group, medication | Dose | Comments |
|---|---|---|
| Anti-inflammatory medication, NSAIDs | Firocoxib – 0.9 mg/kg IV, PO then 0.3 mg/kg q24 hours<br>Flunixin meglumine – 1.1 mg/kg IV, PO q12 hours<br>Phenylbutazone – 4.4 mg/kg IV,PO | |
| Anti-inflammatory medication, steroids | Dexamethasone – 0.05–0.1 mg/kg IV, IM, PO q24 hours<br>Prednisolone – 1 mg/kg PO q24 hours | In humans, routine use of steroids in patients with traumatic brain injury, is no longer recommended due to increased association with mortality. |
| Hyperosmolar, mannitol | Mannitol: 0.25–2 g/kg as a 20% solution IV over 20–30 minutes | Must be warmed to prevent crystallization at room or colder temperatures.<br>Administer with filter to prevent administering precipitant. |
| Hyperosmolar, 7.2% NaCl | 4–6 mL/kg IV over 15 minutes | |
| Anti-inflammatory and anti-oxidant, DMSO | 0.5–1 g/kg diluted to a 10% solution IV q24 hours × 3–5 days | Solutions greater than 10% can result in red blood cell lysis. |
| Anti-inflammatory, anti-oxidant, Vitamin E | 20 IU/kg PO q24 hours | |
| Anti-epileptic, Diazepam | 0.05–0.1 mg/kg IV (to effect) | |
| Anti-epileptic, Phenobarbital | Loading dose: 6–12 mg/kg IV, then 6–12 mg/kg PO q12 hours | Therapeutic serum concentrations range from 15 to 40 µg/mL. |

## Cardiovascular Emergencies

Cardiovascular emergencies are covered in detail in Chapter 12

**Dysrhythmia**
**Congestive heart failure**
**Cardiopulmonary resuscitation**

## Neonatal Emergencies

Neonatal emergencies are also covered in Chapter 20.

### Neonatal Maladjustment Syndrome, Neonatal Encephalopathy

Also referred to as hypoxic ischemic syndrome, barker foal syndrome, dummy foal syndrome, and others.

Neonates with abnormal behavior and/or mentation are also at high risk for sepsis, and many times should be treated as such unless proven otherwise. Given the wide variety in severity of neonatal maladjustment, below are some general guidelines. If the foal is unable to stand or nurse appropriately referral to a 24-hour care facility is indicated.

Step 1: If the foal is less than 12 hours of age, has not consumed colostrum, is not showing signs of colic, and has intestinal motility, pass a nasogastric tube and administer colostrum.

Step 2: If the foal has not received colostrum, has failure of passive transfer, or has shown additional clinical signs consistent with sepsis begin prophylactic broad-spectrum antimicrobial therapy as outlined under sepsis (Table A3.6).

Step 3: In foals that do not have rib fractures or other co-morbidities the Madigan squeeze technique can be used.

Step 4: Although there are few clinical trials to examine the benefits of anti-oxidants and hyperosmolar therapy a number of them are commonly used. Table A3.15 provides commonly used therapies in foals with suspected neonatal maladjustment syndrome

Step 5: If the foal is having seizures the medications listed in Table A3.16 can be used for seizure control. Foals having seizures should be referred to a hospital with 24-7 care.

## Sepsis

Recumbent neonates or those requiring intravenous fluid therapy, enteral feedings, or other frequent treatments are best managed in a referral hospital. Early referral for aggressive intervention significantly improves survival and decreases the risk of secondary complications.

Step 1: Collect baseline diagnostic information including complete blood count, serum biochemistry, IgG, blood gas (arterial or venous), and blood cultures. If significant electrolyte or blood glucose derangements are identified treat as indicated.

**Table A3.15** Anti-oxidant and hyperosmolar therapy for neonatal foals.

| Medication | Dose | Rationale | Comments |
|---|---|---|---|
| DMSO | 0.5–1 g/kg diluted to a 10% solution IV q24 hours × 3–5 days | Anti-inflammatory, Anti-oxidant | Concentrations greater than 20% can result in hemolysis. |
| Mannitol | 0.25–1 g/kg IV as a 20% solution over 20 minutes | Decreases cerebral edema. | Mannitol needs to be kept warm to prevent precipitation and should be administered using a filter. |
| $MgSO_4$ | 0.05 mg/kg/h × 1 hour, then 0.025 mg/kg/h | Blocks the release of glutamate and antagonizes influx of calcium at NMDA channels. | |
| Thiamin | 10–20 mg/kg IV diluted in intravenous fluids every 12 hours | May have a role in preventing glutamate-induced cell death | Give diluted to decrease to risk of anaphylactic reaction. |
| Vitamin C | 0.5–1 g/kg PO or IV q24 hours | Anti-oxidant and neuroprotective effects | |
| Vitamin E | 20 IU/kg PO q24 hours | Anti-inflammatory | Water-soluble vitamin E is most bioavailable to horses. |

**Table A3.16** Anti-epileptic medications for neonatal foals.

| Medication | Dose | Comments |
|---|---|---|
| Diazepam | 0.1–0.4 mg/kg IV or PR | |
| Levetiracetam | 32 mg/kg IV, PO q12 hours (Macdonald et al. 2018) | This dose was established using the immediate-release formula for PO administration |
| Midazolam | 0.04–0.1 mg/kg IV, IM bolus<br>0.02–0.06 mg/kg/h | |
| Pentobarbital | 2–10 mg/kg IV once | |
| Phenobarbital | 20 mg/kg IV loading dose, then 8 mg/kg IV q8 hours (Spehar et al. 1984) | Can cause respiratory depression. |
| Phenytoin | 2–10 mg/kg IV or PO q4 hours for six doses, then q12 hours | |
| Potassium bromide | 10 mg/kg PO q8 hours<br>60 mg/kg PO q24 hours | |

Step 2: Institute broad-spectrum antimicrobial therapy. Ideally, the antimicrobial therapy will be broad spectrum and bactericidal. Table A3.6 provides several frequently used options in neonates.

Step 3: Assess the foal's perfusion parameters (physical exam, blood lactate, blood pressure) to determine if volume resuscitation is necessary. Begin with a 20 mL/kg bolus with intravenous isotonic replacement fluids, followed by reassessment. This may be repeated up to three times. If hypoglycemia was identified on initial evaluation the 20 mL/kg fluid bolus should include 1–5% dextrose and be administered to effect.

Step 4: If indicated based on IgG levels or albumin levels, administer 20 mL/kg of plasma intravenously. This may be repeated up to 3 times in a 24-hour period to achieve adequate IgG levels and should be considered as part of the overall fluid therapy plan.

Step 5: If perfusion parameters do not improve with intravenous fluid and plasma administration more aggressive treatment with inotropic medications is needed – referral is indicated.

### Ruptured Bladder

Step 1: Address electrolyte derangements as described earlier in this section under "electrolyte derangements." The most common concerns are hyperkalemia and hyponatremia.

Step 2: Aseptically, place a urinary catheter to divert urine.

Step 3: Depending on the degree of peritoneal effusion, you may consider aseptically placing an abdominal drain with a closed drainage system to limit the development of peritonitis.

Step 4: If placing urinary and/or abdominal drains place on broad-spectrum prophylactic antimicrobials.

Step 5: Refer to a hospital for surgical repair of the bladder.

### Uroperitoneum

See **Chapters 13 and 20**.

## Orthopedic Emergencies

Orthopedic emergencies are also covered in Chapters 8 and 23.

### Cellulitis

Step 1: If exudate is readily available or if there are fluid pockets amenable to aspiration on ultrasonographic evaluation of the limb, obtain a sample for culture and sensitivity testing.

Step 2: Begin broad-spectrum antimicrobial treatment. Commonly used antimicrobial agents are provided in Table A3.17.

Step 3. Depending on the location of the cellulitis a regional limb perfusion may also be considered. Chapter 5 describes performing regional limb perfusions in horses. Table A3.18 provides commonly used first-line antimicrobials and doses for regional limb perfusions in horses. Dose ranges are those reported for use in 500 kg horses.

Step 4: Apply a pressure bandage to reduce edema and swelling.

Step 5: Institute anti-inflammatory and analgesia therapy as described in Chapter 31

Step 6: Depending on the degree of lameness decide if cushion support is indicated for the contra-lateral limb as prophylaxis for contra-lateral limb laminitis.

**Fracture**
See **Chapters 8 and 23**
**Myopathies (Acute)**
See **Chapter 8**

**Table A3.17** Broad-spectrum antimicrobials commonly used in adults with cellulitis.

| Medication(s) | Dose(s) |
|---|---|
| Penicillin | Potassium penicillin: 22,000 IU/kg IV q6 hours;<br>Penicillin procaine G: 22,000 IU/kg IM q12 hours |
| Gentamicin | 6.6 mg/kg IV q24 hours |
| Penicillin | Potassium penicillin: 22,000 IU/kg IV q6 hours;<br>Penicillin procaine G: 22,000 IU/kg IM q12 hours |
| Enrofloxacin | Enrofloxacin: 5.5 mg/kg IV q24 hours (Giguere et al. 1996)<br>Enrofloxacin: 7.5 mg/kg PO q24 hours (Giguere et al. 1996) |
| Ceftiofur | 2.2 mg/kg IV, IM q12 hours |
| Trimethoprim sulfamethoxazole | 30 mg/kg PO q12 hours |
| Doxycycline | 10 mg/kg PO q12 hours |

**Table A3.18** First-line antimicrobials for regional limb perfusions in horses.

| Medication | Dose |
|---|---|
| Ceftiofur | 2 g in 100 mL of 0.9% NaCl |
| Amikacin | 125 mg–2 g in 100 mL of 0.9% NaCl |
| Gentamicin | 100 mg–1 g in 100 mL of 0.9% NaCl |

## Septic Synovitis

Septic synovial structures often warrant referral for aggressive treatment. The steps below are initial steps that may be taken prior to referral.

Step 1: After confirmation of a suspected synovial structure, while the needle is still in place consider lavaging the joint with 1 L of isotonic crystalloid fluids by placing a second needle to serve an egress canula.

Step 2: Prior to removing the last needle, if samples have already been obtained for culture and sensitivity, consider administering intra-articular antimicrobials. Table A3.19 provides commonly used intra-articular antimicrobials in horses. Doses are provided per 500 kg horse.

Step 3: Provide the patient with anti-inflammatory and analgesia medication as needed for pain.

Step 4: Further treatment may include repeated lavage, intra-articular or regional limb perfusion administration of antimicrobials, and/or systemic administration of anti-microbials.

**Table A3.19** Antimicrobials for intra-articular injection.

| Medication | Dose |
|---|---|
| Amikacin | 31.25 mg–500 mg |
| Ceftiofur | 150 mg |
| Gentamicin | 150 mg–1 g |

## References


Anrogué, H.J. and Madias, N. (2000). Hyponatremia. *N. Engl. J. Med.* 342: 1581–1589.

Arroyo, M.G., Slovis, N.M., Moore, G.E., and Taylor, S.D. (2017). Factors associated with survival in 97 horses with septic pleuropneumonia. *J. Vet. Intern. Med.* 31 (3): 894–900.

Bauquier, J.R., Boston, R.C., Sweeney, R.W. et al. (2015). Plasma peek and trough gentamicin concentrations in hospitalized horses receiving intravenously administered gentamicin. *J. Vet. Intern. Med.* 29 (6): 1660–1666.

Carmichael, R.J., Whitfield, C., and Maxwell, L.K. (2013). Pharmacokinetics of ganciclovir and valganciclovir in the adult horse. *J. Vet. Pharmacol. Ther.* 36 (5): 441–449.

Couetil, L.L., Cardwell, J.M., Gerber, V. et al. (2016). Inflammatory airway disease of horses – revised consensus statement. *J. Vet. Intern. Med.* 30 (2): 503–515.

Fultz, L., Giguere, S., Berghaus, L.J., and Davis, J.L. (2014). Plasma and pulmonary pharmacokinetics of desfuroylceftiofur acetamide after weekly administration of ceftiofur crystalline free acid to adult horses. *Equine Vet. J.* 46 (2): 252–255.

Giguere, S., Sweeney, R.W., and Belanger, M. (1996). Pharmacokinetics of enrofloxacin in adult horses and concentration of the drug in serum, body fluids and endometrial tissues after repeated intragastrically administered doses. *Am. J. Vet. Res.* 57 (7): 1025–1030.

Hackett, E.S., Mama, K.R., Twedt, D.C., and Gustafson, D.L. (2013). Pharmacokinetics and safety of silibinin in horses. *Am. J. Vet. Res.* 74 (10): 1372–1332.

Lavoie, J.P., Leclere, M., Rodrigues, N. et al. (2019). Efficacy of inhaled budesonide for the treatment of severe equine asthma. *Equine Vet. J.* 51 (3): 401–407.

Leguillette, R., Tohver, T., Bond, S.L. et al. (2017). Effect of dexamethasone and fluticasone on airway hyperresponsiveness in horses with Inflammatory Airway Disease. *J. Vet. Intern. Med.* 31 (4): 1193–1201.

Liska, D.A., Akucewich, L.H., Marsella, R. et al. (2006). Pharmacokinetics of pentoxyifylline and its 5-hydroxyhexyl metabolite after oral and intravenous administration of pentoxifylline to healthy adult horses. *Am. J. Vet. Res.* 67 (9): 1621–1627.

Macdonald, K.D., Hart, K.A., Davis, J.L. et al. (2018). Pharmacokinetics of the anticonvulsant levetiracetam in neonatal foals. *Equine Vet. J.* 50 (4): 532–536.

Maxwell, L.K., Bentz, B.G., Gililam, L.L. et al. (2017). Efficacy of the early administration of valacyclovir hydrochloride for the treatment of neuropathogenic equine herpesvirus type-1 infection in horses. *Am. J. Vet. Res.* 78 (10): 1126–1139.

McKenzie, H. and Murray, M.J. (2020). Concentrations of gentamicin in serum and bronchial lavage fluid after intravenous and aerosol administration of gentamicin to horses. *J. Vet. Intern. Med.* 61 (10): 1185–1190.

Meyer, S., Giguere, S., Rodriguez, R. et al. (2009). Pharmacokinetics of intravenous ceftiofur sodium and concentration in body fluids of foals. *J. Vet. Pharmacol. Ther.* 32 (4): 309–316.

Pusterla, N., Hall, T.L., Wetzlich, S.E. et al. (2017). Pharmacokinetic parameters for single- and multi-dose regiments for subcutaneous administration of a high-dose ceftiofur crystallin-free acid to neonatal foals. *J. Vet. Pharmacol. Ther.* 40 (1): 88–91.

Schoster, A., Amsler, M., Kirchgaessner, C. et al. (2021). Gentamicin plasma concentrations in hospitalized horses and retrospective minimal inhibitory concentrations of gram-negative equine pathogens. *J. Vet. Emerg. Crit. Care* 31 (3): 323–330.

Spehar, A.M., Hill, M.R., Mayhew, I.G., and Hendeles, L. (1984). Preliminary study on the pharmacokinetics of phenobarbital in the neonatal foal. *Equine Vet. J.* 16 (4): 368–371.

Steinman, A., Gips, M., Lavy, E. et al. (2000). Pharmacokinetics of metronidazole in horses after intravenous, rectal and oral administration. *J. Vet. Pharmacol. Ther.* 23 (6): 353–357.

Sweeney, R.W., Sweeney, C.R., Soma, L.R. et al. (1986). Pharmacokinetics of metronidazole given to horses by intravenous and oral routes. *Am. J. Vet. Res.* 47 (8): 1726–1729.

# Index



*Emergency Triage of the Horse*, First Edition. Edited by Rolfe M. Radcliffe and Jamie J. Kopper.

Companion website: www.wiley.com/go/radcliffe/triage

## l

## m



## n

## t